MOSBY'S
FAMILY PRACTICE SOURCEBOOK
EVIDENCE-BASED EMPHASIS

Visit our website at **www.mosby.com**

MOSBY'S
FAMILY PRACTICE SOURCEBOOK
EVIDENCE-BASED EMPHASIS

KENNETH G. MARSHALL, M.D.

Department of Family Medicine
University of Western Ontario
London, Ontario, Canada

Mosby

A Harcourt Health Sciences Company
St. Louis   London   Philadelphia   Sydney   Toronto

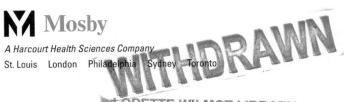

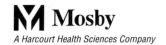

Mosby
A Harcourt Health Sciences Company

Acquisitions Editor: Elizabeth M. Fathman
Project Manager: Patricia Tannian
Book Design Manager: Gail Morey Hudson
Cover Designer: Teresa Breckwoldt

Mosby, Inc.
A Harcourt Health Sciences Company
11830 Westline Industrial Drive
St. Louis, Missouri 63146

Printed in United States of America

International Standard Book Number 1-55664-469-8

00 01 02 03 04 CL/MV 9 8 7 6 5 4 3 2 1

To

front-line family physicians

whose domain embraces all aspects of clinical medicine

Preface

As in the two previous editions of *Mosby's Family Practice Sourcebook,* I have collected from the literature a vast amount of pertinent up-to-date information and have presented it in an easy-to-read integrated fashion. I have taken this approach because I think most of us absorb new information better when it is presented in context.

The third edition of the *Family Practice Sourcebook* has been extensively revised with new material culled from over 750 articles published in 1999 in 96 different medical journals. All told, the book contains more than 4000 references, the vast majority from articles published within the last 5 years. Although I have been responsible for most of this work, Dr. Michael Evans from the University of Toronto has used his expertise in critical appraisal to thoroughly revise the section on mood disorders.

Extensively updated topics include gastroesophageal reflux disease, Barrett's esophagus, and esophageal carcinoma; *Helicobacter pylori* and nonulcer dyspepsia; beta-blockers and spironolactone for heart failure; homocysteine and coronary artery disease; chronic fatigue syndrome and fibromyalgia; hormone replacement therapy; surgical correction of refractive errors; male infertility; concussion in the athlete; screening for colon cancer, diabetes, and prostate cancer; causes of chronic cough; the circumcision controversy; new drugs for dementia, Parkinson's disease, diabetes, and obesity; shaken baby syndrome; urine testing for sexually transmitted diseases; chronic prostatitis; and screening of relatives of patients with subarachnoid hemorrhages for aneurysms.

The medical literature is full of "pearls," often embedded in pages and pages of turgid text. I pride myself in having become a fairly expert miner. I hope you enjoy the material I have extracted and compiled for you.

Kenneth G. Marshall, M.D.

Preface to the First Edition

No family physician, no matter how competent and dedicated, can acquire or keep in his or her head the vast and changing body of medical data that is needed for adequate care of patients. My goal in writing this annual book is to supplement the already extensive knowledge and skills of practicing family physicians with an up-to-date database that can be accessed quickly and easily.

This book deals primarily with conditions seen and treated by family physicians in an outpatient setting. Some material on inpatient treatment is included, primarily so that office-based family physicians have information with which to counsel patients or their families. Community health issues are also part of the text because prevention of disease is an important part of our mandate.

The *Family Practice Sourcebook* is not a textbook, and only rarely is an attempt made to cover all aspects of any medical condition. Rather, this is an up-to-date, annual reference manual dealing with selected aspects of a wide variety of subjects chosen because of their usefulness or interest for family physicians. Many of the entries are practical therapeutic programs for disorders such as acne, Parkinson's disease, or sexually transmitted diseases, while others cover the background data required by family physicians for making rational decisions about controversial issues such as cholesterol or prostate-specific antigen screening. I hope this text will facilitate the practice of "evidence-based," or if that is not possible, at least "reference-based" office medicine. To help achieve this, almost all of the data in this text has been extracted from recent articles in the medical literature and in most cases the full citations appear at the end of each topic.

HOW TO USE THIS BOOK
Finding Your Way Around the Text

There are six ways of finding your way around the text:
1. Index. Using the index is the most efficient way of finding what you want quickly. Drugs are listed by both generic and trade names.
2. Table of contents. The table of contents lists the major subject areas covered.
3. Inside front and back covers. A more detailed table of contents is given that corresponds to the outlines described below.
4. Outlines. At the beginning of each subject area listed in the table of contents is an outline of topics covered in that section.
5. Cross references. Related subjects are listed beneath the section and topic headings ("See also . . . ").
6. Random perusal. This is the most fun. It requires a bit of time and if possible a winter evening in front of a crackling fire.

Organization of the Text

The overall organization is alphabetical as in a glossary. First-level headings as listed in the table of contents are based on anatomical systems (Cardiovascular System," "Gastrointestinal System") or specialties ("Gynecology," "Ophthalmology"), although a few important medical problems such as "Alcohol" and "Smoking" are also included at this level. Subheadings also tend to be in alphabetical order, but exceptions are made when the natural flow of content makes this inappropriate.

Topics that do not easily fit into one of the first-level headings are listed alphabetically under the major heading "Miscellaneous." Examples are "Bed Rest Complications," "Bites," "Informed Consent," "Leg Cramps," and "Multiple Chemical Sensitivities."

Where drugs are available in Canada but not the United States, or where the trade names in Canada differ from those in the United States, the proprietary names are underlined.

Errors

I have tried to minimize errors in this volume, but I cannot guarantee that none are present. Therefore anyone using this book should verify the accuracy of the contents, particularly in terms of drugs and dosages, before basing patient treatment on them.

Kenneth G. Marshall, M.D.

In the second edition of *Mosby's Family Practice Sourcebook* I have modified much of the text by integrating into it information and perspectives obtained from reviewing hundreds of articles from the recent medical literature. The result is an up-to-date, succinct, and readable review of data that are relevant to office-based family practice.

An accessible overview such as this is particularly important in the era of proliferating clinical guidelines. Family physicians are overwhelmed by them, and all too often they provide little help: Have recent guidelines been published on this topic? If so, where? Did I receive them? If I did, where are they? Are there several guidelines on the same topic? If there are, which should I use? Which ones are evidence based? If I find the appropriate guideline, can I easily extract from it the information I need?

Hibble and associates collected all the guidelines that were available in 22 general practices in Great Britain. They ended up with 855, which formed a pile 68 cm (27 inches) high and weighing 28 kg (61 lb). Some of the guidelines were so detailed that they were presented in small book format. As Gray put it, "The present position is intolerable [and a major effort has to be directed into managing] knowledge and know how." Slawson and Shaughnessy's objective of "Patient Oriented Evidence that Matters (POEM)" seems to be the ideal one for busy primary care practitioners. My goal has been to make this book a "POEM."

Kenneth G. Marshall, M.D.

Acknowledgments

As was the case with previous editions of this book, I have received unstinting support from the administration, colleagues, and residents in the Department of Family Medicine at the University of Western Ontario. I am very grateful.

Dr. Michael Evans from the University of Toronto played a major part in reviewing and revising the section on mood disorders. I very much appreciate his wisdom and his skills in critical appraisal.

Lynn Dunikowski, Christine Ingram, Lorraine Schoel, and Trixie Usselman from the Canadian Library of Family Medicine have done a superb job in finding and supplying me with the hundreds of articles I have requested over the past year. They have been a key factor in turning a concept into a book.

If you haven't had the fortune (sometimes I think it is a misfortune) of publishing a book, you are unlikely to appreciate the importance of good editors. Liz Fathman, my acquisitions editor, has done a first-class job of supporting me in the production of the manuscript for this text. As always, project manager Trish Tannian exemplifies high-quality professionalism—under her guidance a rough manuscript becomes a polished text.

The comments of readers are particularly valuable. I thank all of you who have taken the time to give me feedback on the first or second edition of this book.

Contents

MOSBY'S
FAMILY PRACTICE SOURCEBOOK
EVIDENCE-BASED EMPHASIS

ALCOHOL

(See also alcoholic hepatitis)

Topics covered in this section

EPIDEMIOLOGY AND NATURAL HISTORY OF EXCESSIVE ALCOHOL INTAKE

The estimated 1-year prevalence of alcohol use disorder in the United States is 7.4% and among patients in family practices is greater than 15%.[1] A U.S. survey of college students found that 84% drank and that 44% met the criteria for binge drinking (five or more drinks in a row at least once in the past 2 weeks). Nineteen percent of the students were frequent binge drinkers, and half of these reported alcohol-related problems such as injuries and participation in unplanned sex.[2]

A long-term follow-up of two cohorts of white men in Boston sheds light on the natural history of alcoholism. Members of one group were from working class and welfare families in inner-city Boston, and the other group was Harvard sophomores. By age 60, 33% of the core city men and 21% of the Harvard graduates had at some point during their lives met the criteria of alcohol abuse given in the *Diagnostic and Statistical Manual of Mental Disorders,* ed. 3 *(DSM-III).* Prognosis for permanent abstinence was excellent after 5 to 6 years of teetotalism, but the relapse rate after 2 years of abstinence was 41%. The odds of returning to controlled drinking were poor. Although the incidence of alcohol abuse was greater in working class men than in university graduates, the rate of abstinence by the age of 60 was twice as great in the working class men as in the Harvard alumni. The natural history of alcohol abuse was not one of relentless progression, but rather of persistence with fluctuations.[3]

Heredity is an important risk factor for alcohol abuse. In one study, one third of first-degree relatives of alcoholic subjects were also alcoholics. The same study found that with the exception of cannabis, drug abuse was not a risk factor for alcohol abuse in first-degree relatives.[4] Alcoholics frequently have anxiety disorders, especially social phobias. Although common sense suggests that alcohol ameliorates social anxiety, the bulk of evidence fails to support this view. Alcohol is not a social lubricant.[5]

◣ REFERENCES ◪

1. Burge SK, Schneider FD: Alcohol-related problems: recognition and intervention, *Am Fam Physician* 59:361-370, 1999.
2. Wechsler H, Davenport A, Dowdall G, et al: Health and behavioral consequences of binge drinking in college—a national survey of students at 140 campuses, *JAMA* 272:1672-1677, 1994.
3. Vaillant GE: A long-term follow-up of male alcohol abuse, *Arch Gen Psychiatry* 53:243-249, 1996.
4. Merikangas KR, Stolar M, Stevens DE, et al: Familial transmission of substance use disorders, *Arch Gen Psychiatry* 55:973-979, 1998.
5. Himle JA, Abelson JL, Haghightgou H, et al: Effect of alcohol on social phobic anxiety, *Am J Psychiatry* 156:1237-1243, 1999.

DEFINITION OF HIGH-RISK DRINKING

A number of alcohol use disorders have been described, ranging from mildly excessive (heavy) drinking to full-blown dependence with withdrawal symptoms and major disruption of social and occupational activities. The following is one classification[1]:

1. Heavy drinking
2. Hazardous drinking
3. Harmful drinking
4. Abuse
5. Dependence

There is no consensus in the literature as to how many drinks per week constitute heavy or hazardous drinking. The U.S. National Institute on Alcohol Abuse and Alcoholism defines heavy drinking as more than 14 drinks a week or more than four drinks during an occasion for men, more than seven drinks a week or more than three drinks during an occasion for women, and more than seven drinks a week for anyone over the age of 65.[2] A British working group put the upper limit of sensible drinking at three to four drinks per day for men and two to three per day for women.[3]

One definition of hazardous drinking is more than 21 drinks a week or more than seven drinks per occasion at least three times a week for men or more than 14 drinks per week or more than five drinks during an occasion at least three times a week for women.[1]

Drinking is defined as harmful if the patient is suffering physical or psychological harm as a result of alcohol use but does not meet the criteria for abuse or dependency.[1]

Heavy, hazardous, and harmful drinking can be treated more successfully than abuse and dependency. For this reason identification of the level of the patient's alcohol use by the primary care practitioner is important (see discussion of alcohol screening questionnaires).[1]

◣ REFERENCES ◪

1. Reid MC, Fiellin DA, O'Connor PG: Hazardous and harmful alcohol consumption in primary care, *Arch Intern Med* 159:1681-1689, 1999.

2. National Institute on Alcohol Abuse and Alcoholism: *The physicians' guide to helping patients with alcohol problems,* NIH pub no 95-3769, Washington, DC, 1995, US Government Printing Office.
3. Interdepartmental Working Group: *Sensible drinking,* London, 1995, Department of Health.

DEFINITIONS OF STANDARD DRINKS

A standard drink contains approximately 13.6 grams of alcohol and is the equivalent of:

12 ounces (360 ml) of regular strength beer	5% alcohol
5 ounces (150 ml) of table wine	12% alcohol
1.5 ounces (45 ml) of spirits	40% alcohol

ALCOHOL SCREENING QUESTIONNAIRES

Numerous alcohol screening questionnaires have been developed, some of which are short and simple and some long and complex. For example, the CAGE questionnaire has four questions, TWEAK five, AUDIT (Alcohol Use Disorders Identification Test) and BMAST (Brief Michigan Alcoholism Screening Test) 10, and MAST (Michigan Alcoholism Screening Test) 25. Each answer is scored, and if positive answers surpass a predetermined point, the test is said to be positive. A review of the literature suggests that the cutoffs should be lower for women than for men.

The CAGE questionnaire is as follows[1]:

C	Have you ever felt the need to CUT down on your drinking?
A	Has anyone ever ANGERED you by criticizing your drinking?
G	Have you ever felt GUILTY over consequences of drinking?
E	Have you ever had an EYE OPENER (morning drink)?

Scoring: Each positive response gets 1 point.

This is the TWEAK questionnaire[1]:

T	Tolerance. How many drinks can you hold ("hold" version: more than six drinks indicates tolerance), or how many drinks does it take before you begin to feel the first effects of the alcohol? ("high" version: more than three drinks indicates tolerance)
W	Worried. Have close friends or relatives worried or complained about your drinking in the past year?
E	Eye openers. Do you sometimes take a drink in the morning when you first get up?
A	Amnesia. Has a friend or family member ever told you about things you said or did while you were drinking that you could not remember?
K	Kut down. Do you sometimes feel the need to cut down on your drinking?

Scoring: Score 2 points for a yes answer to Tolerance and Worried and 1 point for the remainder. The usual cutoff point is 3.

Below is the AUDIT questionnaire[2]:

1. How often do you have a drink containing alcohol?
   (1) Monthly or less often
   (2) Two to four times a month
   (3) Two or three times a week
   (4) Four or more times a week
2. How many drinks do you have on a typical day when you are drinking?
   (1) One or two
   (2) Three or four
   (3) Five or six
   (4) Seven to nine
3. How often do you have six or more drinks on one occasion?
   (1) Monthly or less often
   (2) Monthly
   (3) Weekly
   (4) Daily or almost daily
4. How often during the last year have you found that you were not able to stop drinking once you had started?
   (1) Monthly or less often
   (2) Monthly
   (3) Weekly
   (4) Daily or almost daily
5. How often during the last year have you failed to do what was normally expected from you because of drinking?
   (1) Monthly or less often
   (2) Monthly
   (3) Weekly
   (4) Daily or almost daily
6. How often during the last year have you needed a first drink in the morning to get yourself going after a heavy drinking session?
   (1) Monthly or less often
   (2) Monthly
   (3) Weekly
   (4) Daily or almost daily
7. How often during the last year have you had a feeling of guilt or remorse after drinking?
   (1) Monthly or less often
   (2) Monthly
   (3) Weekly
   (4) Daily or almost daily
8. How often during the last year have you been unable to remember what happened the night before because you had been drinking?
   (1) Monthly or less often
   (2) Monthly
   (3) Weekly
   (4) Daily or almost daily
9. Have you or someone else been injured as a result of your drinking?
   (2) Yes, but not in the last year
   (4) Yes, during the last year
10. Has a relative, a friend, or a doctor or other health worker been concerned about your drinking or suggested you cut down?
    (2) Yes, but not in the last year
    (4) Yes, during the last year

Scoring: Each of the ten questions in the AUDIT questionnaire is scored from 0 to 4; a "never" answer receives a score of 0. A total score of 8 is suggestive of an alcohol use disorder.

For the detection of heavy, hazardous, and harmful drinking the AUDIT questionnaire seems more appropriate than the MAST, CAGE, or TWEAK questionnaires, which do not ask the quantity of alcohol consumed or distinguish between past and present drinking. Several trials have found that the AUDIT questionnaire has not only high sensitivity and specificity, but equally important, a high positive predictive value (most people with a positive test have an alcohol use disorder).[2]

The Alcohol Risk Assessment and Intervention program of the College of Family Physicians of Canada suggests that an initial screening question be, "Has alcohol ever caused a problem for you or your family?" If the response is positive, the CAGE questionnaire should be administered, followed by specific questions to elicit the quantity of alcohol taken[3]:

1. Number of drinks taken on the days when the patient drinks
2. Number of days per week the patient drinks
3. Total weekly number of drinks
4. Maximum number of drinks taken in any 24-hour period in the previous month

Both the Canadian Task Force on Preventive Health Care[4] and the U.S. Preventive Services Task Force[5] give a "B" recommendation for screening adolescents and adults for alcohol intake.

───────────── ◈ **REFERENCES** ◈ ─────────────

1. Bradley KA, Boyd-Wickizer J, Powell SH, et al: Alcohol screening questionnaires in women: a critical review, *JAMA* 280:166-171, 1998.
2. Reid MC, Fiellin DA, O'Connor PG: Hazardous and harmful alcohol consumption in primary care, *Arch Intern Med* 159:1681-1689, 1999.
3. Alcohol Risk Assessment and Intervention (ARAI): *Resource manual for family physicians,* Toronto, 1994, College of Family Physicians.
4. Canadian Task Force on the Periodic Health Examination: *Canadian guide to clinical preventive health care,* Ottawa, 1994, Canada Communication Group—Publishing, pp 488-498.
5. US Preventive Services Task Force: *Guide to clinical preventive services,* ed 2, Baltimore, 1996, Williams & Wilkins, pp 567-582.

DETRIMENTAL EFFECTS OF ALCOHOL

(See also abuse; alcoholic hepatitis; fetal alcohol syndrome; hypertension; motor vehicle accidents; poverty)

Several studies of drinking and mortality have reported a J-curve with a shallow dip in total mortality at lower amounts of drinking and increases in total mortality at higher levels of alcohol intake.[1,2] The reduction is due to a decrease in cardiovascular disease (see discussion of beneficial effects of alcohol below), while the increase is due to accidents, violence (including homicide and suicide), certain cancers, cirrhosis, and hemorrhagic strokes. Alcohol-induced morbidity includes social disruption,[3] hallucinations, delirium tremens, personality changes, violence, accidents, cirrhosis of the liver, pancreatitis, gastritis, hypertension,[4] cardiomyopathy, dysrhythmias, strokes,[5] subarachnoid hemorrhages, degenerative diseases of the nervous system, seizures, community-acquired pneumonias,[6] adult respiratory distress syndrome,[7] fetal abnormalities, and cancers of the mouth, pharynx, larynx, esophagus, and liver. The incidence of breast cancer is believed to be increased in those who drink alcohol,[8] and even having five drinks or fewer per week can decrease fertility.[9] Most of these conditions are discussed elsewhere in the text.

Binge drinking of six or more bottles of beer in one session has been reported to be associated with increased mortality from accidents, violence, and myocardial infarction.[10]

Women who drink alcohol are particularly prone to liver disease. An increased risk of cirrhosis is found with an alcohol intake only half that which increases the risk of cirrhosis in men.[11]

Between 80% and 95% of persons with a substance abuse problem are smokers. Evidence suggests that smoking cessation does not endanger sobriety and may even facilitate it.[12]

Hangovers are probably not directly related to ethanol but rather to other constituents of alcoholic beverages, such as methanol. Between 25% and 50% of drinkers who have become intoxicated do not get hangovers.[13] The incidence of hangovers varies with the beverage drunk. In one study from the 1970s volunteers drank equal concentrations of alcohol but in different types of drinks. The severity of hangovers was related in decreasing order to brandy, red wine, rum, whisky, white wine, gin, vodka, and pure ethanol.[14] Hangovers can be ameliorated by rehydration and by nonsteroidal antiinflammatory drugs, particularly if they are taken before retiring at night.[13]

───────────── ◈ **REFERENCES** ◈ ─────────────

1. Ashley MF, Ferrence R, Room R, et al: Moderate drinking and health: report of an international symposium, *Can Med Assoc J* 151:809-828, 1994.
2. Friedman GK, Klatsky AL: Is alcohol good for your health? (editorial), *N Engl J Med* 329:1882-1883, 1993.
3. Room R: Alcohol consumption and social harm, *Contemp Drug Probl* 23:373-388, 1996.
4. Marmot MG, Elliott P, Shipley MJ, et al: Alcohol and blood pressure: the INTERSALT study, *BMJ* 308:1263-1267, 1994.
5. Gill JS, Zezulka AV, Shipley MJ, et al: Stroke and alcohol consumption, *N Engl J Med* 315:1041-1046, 1986.
6. Fernandez-Sola J, Junque A, Estruch R, et al: High alcohol intake as a risk and prognostic factor for community-acquired pneumonia, *Arch Intern Med* 155:1649-1654, 1995.
7. Moss M, Bucher B, Moore FA, et al: The role of chronic alcohol abuse in the development of acute respiratory distress syndrome in adults, *JAMA* 275:50-54, 1996.

8. Smith-Warner SA, Spiegelman D, Yaun S-S, et al: Alcohol and breast cancer in women: a pooled analysis of cohort studies, *JAMA* 279:535-540, 1998.

9. Jensen TK, Hjollund NH, Henriksen TB, et al: Does moderate alcohol consumption affect fertility? Follow up study among couples planning first pregnancy, *BMJ* 317:505-510, 1998.

10. Kauhanen J, Kaplan GA, Goldberg DE: Beer binging and mortality: results from the Kuopio ischaemic heart disease risk factor study, a prospective population based study, *BMJ* 315:846-851, 1997.

11. Lieber CS: Medical disorders of alcoholism, *N Engl J Med* 333:1058-1065, 1995.

12. McIlvain HE, Bobo JK, Leed-Kelly A, et al: Practical steps to smoking cessation for recovering alcoholics, *Am J Physician* 57:1869-1876, 1998.

13. Calder I: Hangovers: not the ethanol—perhaps the methanol (editorial), *BMJ* 314:2-3, 1997.

14. Pawan GL: Alcoholic drinks and hangover effects, *Proc Nutr Soc* 32:15A, 1973.

BENEFICIAL EFFECTS OF ALCOHOL

Most epidemiological studies suggest that moderate drinking is associated with a 40% to 60% relative reduction of coronary artery disease risk.[1-9] This effect is present in both women[3,4,8] and men[4-9] and is also found in persons with type 2 diabetes.[8] Benefit is seen primarily in older adults because the risk of coronary artery disease is greater in that population. Protection against coronary artery disease has been reported with as little as one drink every second day and is associated with alcohol in any form: red wine, white wine, beer, or spirits.[1,4,5,10] A study of male British physicians found that those who had eight to 14 drinks per week had a relative mortality rate 30% lower than that of nondrinkers, while the heaviest drinkers had about the same mortality as the nondrinkers.[5] In a Danish trial of men without overt ischemic heart disease the risk of an initial cardiac event was greatest in abstainers, intermediate for those taking one to 21 drinks per week, and lowest among those imbibing more than 22 drinks per week.[9] A prospective French study found that men who drank one to three glasses of wine each day had a decreased total mortality rate, which was related to decreases in cardiovacular disease and cancer. Heavy drinkers had an increased mortality rate.[7] In contrast, a study of Scottish workingmen failed to find any beneficial effect from drinking.[11]

A 1999 analysis of the U.S. Physicians' Health Study concluded that the risk of sudden cardiac death was decreased in men who imbibed two to six drinks a week compared with abstainers and those taking two or more drinks a day.[6]

Postulated mechanisms by which moderate alcohol intake leads to a decreased risk of cardiovascular disease include an antithrombotic effect, an increase in high-density lipoprotein, inhibition of the oxidation of low-density lipoprotein, and enhanced insulin sensitivity.[12]

Because of the potential for abuse, few workers in the field recommend that abstainers be advised to drink moderately or that very occasional drinkers be advised to increase their alcohol consumption in order to decrease their risk of coronary artery disease.[13] This view is supported by the finding that on a population basis a higher average mean consumption of alcohol is associated with higher rates of problem drinking.[14] A critical factor in this debate is an individual's age. Cardiovascular benefits are achieved only in the middle aged and elderly, and very few drinks per week are required for this purpose. Younger individuals receive no cardiovascular benefit, whereas risks are linear with no known lower limits.[15]

Moderate alcohol consumption appears to help protect against peripheral vascular disease,[16] type 2 diabetes,[17] and ischemic stroke.[18,19] Alcoholic beverages have in vitro antimicrobial properties against enteric pathogens, and in a few outbreaks of food poisoning those consuming alcohol were found to have lower attack rates than abstainers.[20] An epidemiological study from Germany found an inverse dose-response relationship between reported alcohol consumption and *Helicobacter pylori* infection.[21]

―――――――――― ⚕ REFERENCES ⚕ ――――――――――

1. Ashley MF, Ferrence R, Room R, et al: Moderate drinking and health: report of an international symposium, *Can Med Assoc J* 151:809-828, 1994.

2. Thun MJ, Lopez AD, Monaco JH, et al: Alcohol consumption and mortality among middle-aged and elderly U.S. adults, *N Engl J Med* 337:1705-1714, 1997.

3. Fuchs CS, Stampfer MJ, Colditz GA, et al: Alcohol consumption and mortality among women, *N Engl J Med* 332:1245-1250, 1995.

4. McElduff P, Dobson AJ: How much alcohol and how often? Population based case-control study of alcohol consumption and risk of a major coronary event, *BMJ* 314:1159-1164, 1997.

5. Doll R, Peto R, Hall E, et al: Mortality in relation to consumption of alcohol: 13 years' observation on male British doctors, *BMJ* 309:911-918, 1994.

6. Albert CM, Manson JE, Cook NR, et al: Moderate alcohol consumption and the risk of sudden cardiac death among US male physicians, *Circulation* 100:944-950, 1999.

7. Renaud SC, Guéguen R, Schenker J, et al: Alcohol and mortality in middle-aged men from eastern France, *Epidemiology* 9:184-188, 1998.

8. Valmadrid CT, Klein R, Moss SE, et al: Alcohol intake and the risk of coronary heart disease mortality in persons with older-onset diabetes mellitus, *JAMA* 282:239-246, 1999.

9. Hein HO, Suadicani P, Gyntelberg F: Alcohol consumption, serum low density lipoprotein cholesterol concentration, and risk of ischaemic heart disease: six year follow up in the Copenhagen male study, *BMJ* 312:736-741, 1996.

10. Gaziano JM, Hennekens CH, Godfried SL, et al: Type of alcoholic beverage and risk of myocardial infarction, *Am J Cardiol* 83:52-57, 1999.

11. Hart CL, Davey Smith G, Hole DJ, et al: Alcohol consumption and mortality from all causes, coronary heart disease, and stroke: results from a prospective cohort study of Scottish men with 21 years of follow up, *BMJ* 318:1725-1729, 1999.

12. Kiechl S, Willeit J, Rungger G, et al: Alcohol consumption and atherosclerosis: what is the relation? Prospective results from the Bruneck Study, *Stroke* 29:900-907, 1998.

13. Criqui MH, Golomb BA: Should patients with diabetes drink to their health? (editorial), *JAMA* 282:279-280, 1999.

14. Colhoun H, Ben-Shlomo Y, Dong W, et al: Ecological analysis of collectivity of alcohol consumption in England: importance of average drinker, *BMJ* 324:1164-1168, 1997.

15. Doll R: One for the heart, *BMJ* 315:1664-1668, 1997.

16. Camargo CA Jr, Stampfer MJ, Glynn RJ, et al: Prospective study of moderate alcohol consumption and risk of peripheral arterial disease in US male physicians, *Circulation* 95:577-580, 1997.

17. Perry IF, Wannamethee SG, Walker MK, et al: Prospective study of risk factors for development of non-insulin dependent diabetes in middle aged British men, *BMJ* 310:560-564, 1995.

18. Sacco RL, Elkind M, Boden-Albala B, et al: The protective effect of moderate alcohol consumption on ischemic stroke, *JAMA* 281:53-60, 1999.

19. Berger K, Ajani U, Kase CS, et al: Light-to-moderate alcohol consumption and the risk of stroke among U.S. male physicians, *N Engl J Med* 341:1557-1564, 1999.

20. Klontz KC: Does imbibing alcohol protect against enteric pathogens? (editorial), *Epidemiology* 10:207-208, 1999.

21. Brenner H, Berg G, Lappus N, et al: Alcohol consumption and *Helicobacter pylori* infection: results from the German National Health and Nutrition Survey, *Epidemiology* 10:214-218, 1999.

EFFECTS OF ALCOHOL ON LABORATORY TESTS
(See also alcoholic hepatitis)

Gamma-glutamyl transferase (γ-GT) levels are often increased when two to five or more drinks per day are taken regularly over 7 or more days. However, the sensitivity of this test is poor, especially concerning young alcohol-dependent adults and non-alcohol-dependent heavy drinkers.[1] With abstinence or diminution of drinking, the γ-GT concentration usually reverts to normal after 2 to 6 weeks.[2] γ-GT levels are not reliable indicators of the quantity of alcohol imbibed by those who continue to drink.[2]

The mean corpuscular volume has been variously reported to be raised in between one fourth and three fourths of alcohol-dependent drinkers.[1] The serum aspartate aminotransferase (AST) and serum alanine aminotransferase (ALT) levels are increased in about the same proportion of alcohol-dependent drinkers.[1] If some degree of alcoholic hepatitis is present, both the AST and ALT levels are elevated but rarely more than five times normal. Usually the elevation of AST is greater than that of ALT.

⚑ REFERENCES ⚑

1. Alcohol Risk Assessment and Intervention (ARAI): *Resource manual for family physicians,* Toronto, 1994, College of Family Physicians.

2. Kahan M: Identifying and managing problem drinkers, *Can Fam Physician* 42:661-667, 1996.

TREATMENT OF ALCOHOLISM
(See also seizures)

Brief Interventions by Family Physicians

For most problem drinkers, brief interventions by family physicians are the first line of management.[1] Even asking patients about their drinking habits has been reported to change behavior in 5% of patients at risk.[2] A 10- to 15-minute counseling session by a physician or nurse has significantly reduced the alcohol consumption of both male and female high-risk drinkers.[3]

Family physicians may also play an important role in helping patients avoid relapse after they have stopped drinking. The risk of relapse is 50% to 80% during the first year. Preventive measures include establishing a strong, positive relationship with the patient; scheduling frequent follow-up visits, which may be as brief as 5 minutes; mobilizing family and other social supports; encouraging participation in 12-step programs; identifying precipitants to craving and relapse and forcefully recommending that patients avoid such situations; facilitating changes to a healthier life-style; treating comorbid psychiatric illnesses; and, where possible, collaborating with specialists in addiction. When relapse does occur, physicians can help patients see this as a learning experience rather than proof of utter failure.[4]

Opiate Antagonists, Acamprosate, and Disulfiram

Several but not all controlled trials have shown that the opiate receptor antagonist naltrexone (ReVia) helps prevent relapses in alcoholic patients who have become abstinent. It decreases craving for alcohol but does not induce a disulfiram reaction. Nalmefene (Revex), which is also an opiate antagonist, proved effective in a well-performed pilot study. Acamprosate is not available in North America, but European studies have shown it to increase abstinence rates. The role of disulfiram (Antabuse) is controversial. It has been used for a number of years and many clinicians swear by it, but controlled clinical trials have not shown it to be of value.[5,6] The usual dose is 250 to 500 mg each morning.

Antidepressants

Depression has long been known to be associated with alcoholism, but whether the alcoholism causes the depression or vice-versa is uncertain. In one study of depressed alcoholics who had been abstinent for a median of 8 days, desipramine (Norpramin, Pertofrane) was compared with placebo.[7] The desipramine-treated group had a significantly greater amelioration of depression than the control subjects; whether this decreased the recidivism rate for drinking could not be determined. A specific problem encountered in this study was that some patients were encouraged to discontinue desipramine by their Alcoholics Anonymous groups.[7] Imipramine (Tofranil) safely and effectively relieves symptoms of depression in actively drinking alcoholics.[8] Lithium has not proved to be of value.[5]

Acute Withdrawal Syndromes

Acute alcohol withdrawal syndromes require specific management. These syndromes can be classified as follows[9]:

1. Minor withdrawal symptoms. Symptoms often develop within 3 to 6 hours of the beginning of abstinence and include anxiety, tremulousness, insomnia, and in some patients tachycardia, sweating, gastrointestinal distress, and headaches. Symptoms usually abate within 24 to 36 hours.

2. Delirium tremens. Delirium tremens affects only 4% to 5% of alcoholics who abstain from drinking. The syndrome consists of disorientation, agitation, hallucinations (usually visual), diaphoresis, hypertension, and mild fever. The illness begins 2 to 4 days after the last episode of drinking and usually lasts 2 to 5 days. It is rare before the age of 30 and is seen mainly in those who have had more than five or six drinks per day over a prolonged period. The death rate is about 5%.

3. Alcohol hallucinations. Some alcoholics experience hallucinations (usually visual) without having delirium tremens. The onset is usually during the first day of abstinence, and the hallucinations resolve within 48 hours. Patients remain oriented.

4. Alcoholic withdrawal seizures. About 3% of abstaining alcoholics have withdrawal seizures. These are usually generalized and come on 12 to 24 hours after withdrawal.

The mainstay of management of all the withdrawal syndromes is an adequate dose of a long-acting benzodiazepine. This prevents some of the more serious syndromes if given early. The most commonly used drugs are diazepam (Valium) and chlordiazepoxide (Librium). Oral doses vary according to the clinical situation but traditionally range from 20 to 100 mg q6h for chlordiazepoxide and from 5 to 20 mg q6h for diazepam.[9] Since many alcoholics are subject to cross-addiction to other drugs, including benzodiazepines, only the limited number of doses required for withdrawal should be prescribed.

Although a 1999 metaanalysis did not show that one benzodiazepine was superior to another for the treatment of acute alcohol withdrawal,[10] some workers prefer diazepam because it is more rapidly absorbed than is chlordiazepoxide.[11] A technique useful for supervised outpatients is "front loading." Suitable candidates are those who manifest minor withdrawal symptoms and may or may not have hallucinations with insight. Patients with elevated temperatures or hallucinations without insight need inpatient treatment.[12] Before withdrawal, thiamin 100 mg should be given intramuscularly (since alcoholics have poor gastric absorption).[11]

A protocol for front loading with diazepam is 20 mg po every hour for three doses if patients weigh less than 76.5 kg (168 pounds), 20 mg every hour for four doses if they weigh 76.5 to 90 kg (168 to 198 pounds), and 20 mg every hour for five doses if they weigh more than 90 kg (198 pounds). If a patient has had major withdrawal symptoms in the past, these doses may be doubled. Usually no further diazepam is needed, although a few patients require a repeat of the procedure the next day.[11] If chlordiazepoxide is used, a suggested regimen is 100 to 200 mg po q2-4h until sedation is achieved followed by 50 to 100 mg q4-6h as needed for 24 hours. A few patients need 50 to 100 mg q4-6h on day 2 or even day 3.[12]

12-Step Programs

Do 12-step programs such as Alcoholics Anonymous work? There have been no large, randomized controlled studies: participation in the programs is voluntary, and anonymity is sacrosanct. Furthermore, each group is autonomous, so practices differ somewhat. The outcomes for inpatient programs, which have been more intensively studied, may not apply to outpatient programs.[13,14] Cross-sectional evidence suggests that those who join and stay with the programs have higher rates of abstinence.[13-15] A comparison of cognitive behavioral therapy and 12-step programs among U.S. veterans found equal improvement in both groups, as well as equally high rates of recidivism; as in so many studies there were no untreated control subjects.[15] An additional merit of 12-step programs is the friendship network that develops among participants.[16]

According to Khantzian and Mark,[13,17] 12-step programs are effective because they deal with the basic character deficits that lead to substance abuse. A character trait predisposing to substance abuse appears to be a defect in the functioning or regulation of feelings. Some individuals experience excessive emotions, such as unbearable rage, dread, despair, or even elation. Others have a deficit of emotions; they cannot access any feelings, are unable to define their feelings (alexithymia), or have no subjective feelings but express these suppressed emotions through somatization. Inability to modulate emotions often leads to the devaluation of self or others.[13] For example, a minor slight may make a person feel worthless and despicable and at the same time perceive the individual responsible for the affront as hateful, ignorant, or scornful. Most alcoholics have a strikingly deficient sense of self-worth, and they drink to try to overcome the shame resulting from their low self-esteem. They feel that others would not like or respect them and therefore have difficulty initiating and maintaining any sort of intimate relationship. They often mobilize defense mechanisms that enable them to deny the need for others through pseudo–self-sufficiency: a sense of invincibility, pride, arrogance, and bravado and a life-style oriented toward action. Many addicted individuals also demonstrate behavior inimical to self-care beyond that induced by the substance abuse itself. Such behavior often precedes the onset of addiction. Examples include lack of appropriate prevention or treatment of disease, financial irresponsibility, and physical risk taking.[13,17]

Alcoholics Anonymous and other 12-step programs function as support groups with the goal of helping addicts not only stop drinking, but also resolve underlying difficulties in their physical, emotional, and spiritual lives. The leadership of a group rotates among all members on a regular basis so that a cult is unlikely to develop. Through the group process individuals realize they cannot control substance abuse on their own. They come to admit their own vulnerability and the value of caring for themselves, being cared for by others in the group, and caring for others. The group process breaks through denial and deals with dysfunctional character traits.[13,17]

Spirituality is an important part of 12-step programs, which is a godsend for many and an initial stumbling block for others. Spirituality is difficult to define but involves a sense that the universe has a deeper structure of being or purpose than is evident in the apparently meaningless hustle of daily life. The therapeutic value of spirituality is that it leads many people to perceive their inner values, purpose, direction, and responsibilities, and this helps them to value and cherish themselves and others. Some believe that spirituality has a divine origin, while for others it is a purely personal or humanistic experience.[13]

◈ REFERENCES ◈

1. O'Connor PG, Schottenfeld RS: Patients with alcohol problems, *N Engl J Med* 338:592-602, 1998.
2. Anderson P, Scott E: The effect of general practitioners' advice to heavy drinking men, *Br J Addict* 87:891-900, 1992.
3. Ockene JK, Adams A, Hurley TG, et al: Brief physician- and nurse practitioner–delivered counseling for high-risk drinkers, *Arch Intern Med* 159:2198-2205, 1999.
4. Friedmann PD, Saitz R, Samet JH: Management of adults recovering from alcohol or other drug problems: relapse prevention in primary care, *JAMA* 279:1227-1231, 1998.
5. Garbutt JC, West SL, Carey TS, et al: Pharmacological treatment of alcohol dependence: a review of the evidence, *JAMA* 281:1318-1325, 1999.
6. Swift RM: Drug therapy for alcohol dependence, *N Engl J Med* 340:1482-1490, 1999.
7. Mason BJ, Kocsis JH, Ritvo EC, et al: A double-blind, placebo-controlled trial of desipramine for primary alcohol dependence stratified on the presence or absence of major depression, *JAMA* 275:761-767, 1996.
8. McGrath PJ, Nunes EV, Stewart JW, et al: Imipramine treatment of alcoholics with primary depression: a placebo-controlled clinical trial, *Arch Gen Psychiatry* 53:232-240, 1996.
9. Yost DA: Alcohol withdrawal syndrome, *Am Fam Physician* 54:657-664, 1996.
10. Holbrook AM, Crowther R, Lotter A, et al: Meta-analysis of benzodiazepine use in the treatment of acute alcohol withdrawal, *Can Med Assoc J* 160:649-655, 1999.
11. Mezciems PE: Withdrawal strategies for outpatients: alcohol, benzodiazepine, barbiturate, and opiate addictions, *Can Fam Physician* 42:1745-1752, 1996.
12. Prater CD, Miller KE, Zylstra RG: Outpatient detoxification of the addicted or alcoholic patient, *Am Fam Physician* 60:1175-1182, 1999.
13. Khantzian EJ, Mack JE: How AA works and why it's important for clinicians to understand, *J Substance Abuse Treatment* 11:77-92, 1994.
14. Tonigan JS, Toscova R, Miller WR: Meta-analysis of the literature on Alcoholics Anonymous: sample and study characteristics moderate findings, *J Studies Alcohol* 57:65-72, 1995.
15. Ouimette PC, Finney JW, Moos RH: Twelve-step and cognitive-behavioral treatment for substance abuse—a comparison of treatment effectiveness, *J Consult Clin Psychol* 65:230-240, 1997.
16. Humphreys K, Noke JM: The influence of posttreatment mutual help group participation on the friendship networks of substance abuse patients, *Am J Community Psychol* 25:1-16, 1997.
17. Khantzian EJ: The 1994 Distinguished Lecturer's Address: Alcoholics Anonymous—cult or corrective: a case study, *J Substance Abuse Treatment* 12:157-165, 1995.

ANTIBACTERIALS

Topics covered in this section

Antimicrobial Resistance
Pediatric Doses
Antibacterials, Specific Drugs

ANTIMICROBIAL RESISTANCE

It is well known that antimicrobial use in hospitals facilitates the emergence of resistant strains of microorganisms. A study from Iceland suggests that the same phenomenon occurs outside of the hospital. Nasopharyngeal swabs from children in five different communities were cultured for pneumococcal carriage. Organisms resistant to penicillin were far more likely to be found in communities where total antibiotic sales for children as recorded in pharmacies were high than in those where they were low.[1] A concerted effort was made in Finland to decrease the use of macrolides because of emerging resistance of group A streptococci to these antibiotics. The effort was successful, and the frequency of resistant strains decreased.[2]

Inappropriate antibiotic prescription for upper respiratory tract infections and bronchitis is rampant in the United States, on the order of 50% for both adults[3] and children.[4] In the case of children, family physicians are worse offenders than pediatricians.[4] Parental demands may be a powerful factor leading to inappropriate antibiotic prescriptions; a survey of U.S. pediatricians found that one third of them occasionally or frequently complied with such parental requests.[5] Another study found that inappropriate prescription of antibiotics by pediatricians was determined not by actual parental expectations that they be prescribed, but

Table 1   Cephalosporins

Name	Usual adult dose	Usual child dose
First Generation		
Cephalexin (Keflex)	250-500 mg qid	20-50 mg/kg/day in 4 divided doses
Second Generation		
Cefaclor (Ceclor)	250-500 mg tid	20-40 mg/kg/day in 2-3 divided doses
Cefuroxime axetil (Ceftin)	250-500 mg bid	20-30 mg/kg/day in 2 divided doses
Cefprozil (Cefzil)	250-500 mg bid	15-30 mg/kg/day in 2 divided doses
Third Generation		
Cefdinir (Omnicef)	300-600 mg once daily	14 mg/kg/day as a single dose
Cefixime (Suprax)	400 mg once daily	8 mg/kg/day as a single dose
Cefpodoxime (Vantin)	100-200 mg bid	10 mg/kg/day in 2 divided doses
Ceftibuten (Cedax)	400 mg once daily	9 mg/kg/day as a single dose

rather by physicians' perceptions of such expectations. In this study the degree of parental satisfaction correlated with the quality of physician-parent communication, not with whether antibiotics were prescribed.[6] If you talk to your patients, you can throw away the prescriptions.

◣ REFERENCES ◢

1. Arason VA, Kristinsson KG, Sigurdsson JA, et al: Do antimicrobials increase the carriage rate of penicillin resistant pneumococci in children? Cross sectional prevalence study, *BMJ* 313:387-391, 1996.
2. Seppälä H, Klaukka T, Vuopio-Varkila J, et al: The effect of changes in the consumption of macrolide antibiotics on erythromycin resistance in group A streptococci in Finland, *N Engl J Med* 337:441-446, 1997.
3. Gonzales R, Steiner JF, Sande MA: Antibiotic prescribing for adults with colds, upper respiratory tract infections, and bronchitis by ambulatory care physicians, *JAMA* 278:901-904, 1997.
4. Nyquist A-C, Gonsales R, Steiner JF, et al: Antibiotic prescribing for children with colds, upper respiratory tract infections, and bronchitis, *JAMA* 279:875-877, 1998.
5. Bauchner H, Pelton SI, Klein JO: Parents, physicians, and antibiotic use, *Pediatrics* 103:395-398, 1999.
6. Mangione-Smith R, McGlynn EA, Elliott MN, et al: The relationship between perceived parental expectations and pediatrician antimicrobial prescribing behavior, *Pediatrics* 103:711-718, 1999.

PEDIATRIC DOSES

The usual method of calculating pediatric doses is as follows: If weight is given in pounds, divide by 2.2 to obtain weight in kilograms. Multiply weight in kilograms by recommended daily dose. Divide daily dose by frequency of dosage (e.g., by 3 if dosage is tid).

A shortcut for determining an antibiotic dose when the recommended dosage is 40 mg/kg/day is the rule of 6. For example, if you want to give 40 mg/kg/day in three divided doses (e.g., of amoxicillin, amoxicillin-clavulanate [Augmentin, Clavulin], erythromycin-sulfisoxazole [Pediazole], penicillin V, or cefaclor [Ceclor]), multiply the child's

Table 2   Fluoroquinolones

Name	Usual adult dose	Usual child dose
Ciprofloxacin (Cipro)	250-500 mg (occasionally 750 mg) bid; 100 mg bid for 3 days for uncomplicated urinary tract infections	Not indicated
Levofloxacin (Levaquin)	500 mg once daily	Not indicated
Norfloxacin (Noroxin)	400 mg bid	Not indicated
Ofloxacin (Floxin)	200-400 mg bid	Not indicated
Sparfloxacin (Zagam)	200 mg once daily	Not indicated
Trovafloxacin (Trovan)	200 mg once daily	Not indicated

weight in pounds by 6, and the result is the number of milligrams required for each of the three daily doses.[1]

◣ REFERENCES ◢

1. Reynolds RD: Shortcuts for calculating the dose of pediatric medications, *Am Fam Physician* 54:878, 1996.

ANTIBACTERIALS, SPECIFIC DRUGS

Tables 1 to 6 list the generic names, some of the trade names, and usual doses of selected antibiotics used in the care of ambulatory patients. Optimal doses vary with different clinical conditions, and these are not always indicated in the tables. A reputable drug reference should be consulted before prescribing.

Cephalosporins

Selected cephalosporins are listed in Table 1.

Fluoroquinolones (Table 2)

Quinolones are contraindicated in pediatric patients because studies in immature experimental animals have shown dam-

Table 3   Macrolides

Name	Usual adult dose	Usual child dose
Azithromycin (Zithromax)	500 mg as single dose on day 1 followed by 250 mg daily on days 2-5; 1 g as single dose for *Chlamydia*	10 mg/kg/day on day 1 as single dose followed by 5 mg/kg/day on days 2-5 for otitis media; 12 mg/kg/day as single dose for 5 days for pharyngitis or tonsillitis
Clarithromycin (Biaxin)	250-500 mg bid	15 mg/kg/day in 2 divided doses
Dirithromycin (Dynabac)	500 mg once daily	Age 12 years and older only
Erythromycin base	250-500 mg qid or 333 mg tid	30-50 mg/kg/day in 3-4 divided doses
Erythromycin ethylsuccinate-sulfisoxazole (Pediazole)		30-50 mg/kg/day of erythromycin in 3-4 divided doses

Table 4   Penicillins

Name	Usual adult dose	Usual child dose
Benzathine penicillin G	2.4 million units IM as a single dose for primary or secondary syphilis	
Penicillin G (benzylpenicillin)	For IM and IV use only	
Penicillin V potassium, phenoxymethylpenicillin (Pen-Vee)	300 mg (500,000 units) tid-qid	25-50 mg/kg/day (40,000-90,000 units/kg/day) given in 3 or 4 divided doses
Penicillinase Resistant		
Cloxacillin (Tegopen, Orbenin)	250-500 mg qid	25-50 mg/kg/day in 4 divided doses
Dicloxacillin (Dycill, Dynapen, Pathocil)	125-250 mg qid	12.5-25 mg/kg/day in 4 divided doses
Aminopenicillins		
Amoxicillin (Amoxil)	250-500 mg q8h	25-50 mg/kg/day in 3 divided doses
Amoxicillin plus clavulanate potassium (Augmentin, Clavulin)	250-500 mg of amoxicillin q8h or 875 mg q12h	25-50 mg/kg/day of amoxicillin in 3 divided doses

age to the cartilage of weight-bearing joints. Tendon ruptures (shoulder, hand, and Achilles) have been reported as complications of treatment with quinolones.[1] Acute liver failure and death have been reported with the use of trovafloxacin (Trovan). The U.S. Food and Drug Administration advises restricting the drug to patients with very serious or life-threatening infections that are unlikely to respond to other drugs.[2]

Fosfomycin

Fosfomycin (Monurol) is a broad-spectrum antibiotic that is generally used as a single 3-g dose treatment for uncomplicated urinary tract infections. The product comes in a single 3-g dose sachet containing the granules, which are dissolved in one-half cup of water before the medication is taken.

Lincosamides

The most frequently used lincosamide is clindamycin (Cleocin, Dalacin). It is particularly effective against aerobic gram-positive organisms, such as streptococci and staphylococci, and anaerobes. The usual oral dosage is 150 to 300 mg q6h.

Macrolides (Table 3)

Erythromycin can raise to toxic levels the serum concentrations of a variety of drugs metabolized by the cytochrome P450 system. These include theophylline (Theo-Dur, Uniphyl), the antihistamines astemizole (Hismanal) and terfenadine (Seldane), digoxin, carbamazepine (Tegretol), warfarin (Coumadin), and cisapride (Propulsid).

The reputed advantages of azithromycin are once a day doses, fewer gastrointestinal side effects than with erythromycin, and better coverage of gram-negative organisms, particularly *Haemophilus influenzae* and *Moraxella catarrhalis,* including beta-lactamase-producing strains. It is effective against gram-positive organisms but is slightly less potent than other macrolides.

Penicillins

Penicillins are listed in Table 4.

Sulfonamides (Table 5)

A frequently prescribed sulfonamide is trimethoprim-sulfamethoxazole (Septra, Bactrim). The usual pediatric dose is 6 mg/kg/day of trimethoprim and 30 mg/kg/day of sulfamethoxazole in 2 divided doses. This translates roughly as follows:

Under 2 years	2.5 ml of pediatric suspension bid
2-5 years	2.5-5 ml of pediatric suspension bid
6-12 years	5-10 ml of pediatric suspension or 2-4 pediatric tablets bid

Table 5   Sulfonamides

Name	Usual adult dose	Usual child dose
Trimethoprim-sulfamethoxazole (TMP-SMX) (Septra, Bactrim)	1 DS tablet bid	6 mg/kg/day of trimethoprim and 30 mg/kg/day of sulfamethoxazole in 2 divided doses
Erythromycin ethylsuccinate–sulfisoxazole (Pediazole)		30-50 mg/kg/day of erythromycin in 3-4 divided doses

Table 6   Tetracyclines

Name	Usual adult dose	Usual child dose
Tetracycline hydrochloride (Achromycin V)	250-500 mg qid	25-50 mg/kg/day in 4 divided doses (over 8-12 years of age)
Doxycycline (Vibramycin)	100 mg bid on day 1 followed by 100 mg/day	4.4 mg/kg/day on day 1 in 2 divided doses followed by 2.2 mg/kg/day as a single daily dose (over 8-12 years of age)
Minocycline (Minocin)	200 mg on day 1 followed by 100 mg/day	4 mg/kg/day on day 1 followed by 2 mg/kg/day (over 8-12 years of age)

Tetracyclines (Table 6)

Tetracyclines may be partly inactivated by iron preparations and by bismuth subsalicylate. Because they are deposited in growing bones and teeth, they are contraindicated in pregnancy and during lactation and in general should not be given to children under the age of 13 (Canadian recommendations) or under the age of 8 (American recommendations).

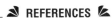

REFERENCES

1. Nightingale SL: New fluoroquinolone warning label, *JAMA* 276:774, 1996.
2. Nightingale SL: Trovafloxacin public health advisory, *JAMA* 282:19, 1999.

BREAST DISEASES

Topics covered in this section

Breast, Benign
Breast Cancer

BREAST, BENIGN
Breast Cysts

If the fluid aspirated from a breast cyst is not bloody, and if on palpation the breast lump has completely disappeared, the specimen does not have to be sent for cytological analysis. If the fluid is bloody, or if the lump does not completely disappear or recurs, surgical consultation is indicated.[1]

REFERENCES

1. Mahoney L, Heisey R, Watson B: Breast cyst aspiration (practice tips), *Can Fam Physician* 44:2093, 1998.

Breast Implants

(See also breast feeding; functional somatic syndromes; multiple chemical sensitivities)

Both a 1995 follow-up report of the Nurses' Health Study[1] and a 1998 retrospective population-based study in Sweden[2] were unable to find any association between breast implants and connective tissue diseases. A number of other studies have failed to show a correlation between breast implants and specific connective tissue diseases such as rheumatoid arthritis,[3] scleroderma,[4] and systemic lupus erythematosus.[5] The only study to date showing a correlation between implants and connective tissue diseases was a retrospective cohort study of women self-reporting both implants and the diagnosis of connective tissue disease; the relative risk was 1.24.[6] In this study the diagnoses were not verified, which is particularly important because the assessment was made after the widely publicized U.S. Food and Drug Administration ban on breast implants.[7] Despite the lack of scientific evidence, courts have awarded huge settlements to plaintiffs. Such court decisions have widespread implications for the future of health care in the United States, both because they foster an antiscientific approach to medical issues and because companies are increasingly unwilling to produce medical devices under the current product liability system.[7]

Silicone breast implants have a limited life span. By 15 years 50% will have leaked or ruptured. According to some authorities, all women who have had implants for 10 or more years should be carefully assessed, usually by magnetic resonance imaging, for leakage or rupture of the prostheses. They also recommend the removal of all prostheses that have been in place for 15 years.[8]

── ◆ **REFERENCES** ◆ ──

1. Sánchez-Guerrero J, Colditz GA, Karlson EW, et al: Silicone breast implants and the risk of connective-tissue diseases and symptoms, *N Engl J Med* 332:1666-1670, 1995.
2. Nyrén O, Yin L, Josefsson S, et al: Risk of connective tissue disease and related disorders among women with breast implants: a nation-wide retrospective cohort study in Sweden, *BMJ* 316:417-422, 1998.
3. Dugowson CE, Daling J, Koepsell T, et al: Silicone breast implants and risk for rheumatoid arthritis (abstract), *Arthritis Rheum* 35(suppl):S66, 1992.
4. Hochberg MC, Miller R, Wigley FM: Frequency of augmentation mammoplasty in patients with systemic sclerosis: data from the Johns Hopkins–University of Maryland Scleroderma Center, *J Clin Epidemiol* 48:565-569, 1995.
5. Strom BL, Reidenberg MM, Freundlich B, et al: Breast silicone implants and risk of systemic lupus erythematosus, *J Clin Epidemiol* 47:1211-1214, 1994.
6. Hennekens CH, Lee I-M, Cook NR, et al: Self-reported breast implants and connective-tissue diseases in female health professionals: a retrospective cohort study, *JAMA* 275:616-621, 1996.
7. Angell M: Shattuck Lecture—evaluating the health risks of breast implants: the interplay of medical science, the law, and public opinion, *N Engl J Med* 334:1513-1518, 1996.
8. Beekman WH, Feitz R, Hage JJ, et al: Life span of silicone gel–filled mammary prostheses, *Plast Reconstr Surg* 100:1723-1726, 1997.

Breast Pain

(See also alternative medicine)

Mastalgia can be divided into the two broad categories of cyclical premenstrual breast pain and noncyclical breast pain. Two thirds of women with mastalgia have cyclical pain. Many women with breast pain worry that this is a symptom of cancer. Reassurance after a careful examination is often the only therapy required. Three drugs that have been used for cyclical breast pain are gamma linolenic acid (Evening Primrose Oil), bromocriptine (Parlodel), and danazol (Cyclomen).[1]

Evening Primrose Oil is extracted from the seeds of the evening primrose (a flower that opens its blooms in the evening) and contains gamma linolenic acid, linoleic acid, and vitamin E. It is available without prescription. The usual dosage is 6 to 8 capsules daily in divided doses. Three small randomized trials of this compound for patients with mastalgia have shown favorable results with few reported adverse effects.[2] However, a certain amount of skepticism is in order because Evening Primrose Oil has been promoted as beneficial for a wide variety of ailments aside from mastalgia, including atopic dermatitis, rheumatoid arthritis, diabetic neuropathy, multiple sclerosis, various cancers, Raynaud's phenomenon, ulcerative colitis, preeclampsia, premenstrual syndrome, hot flashes, Sjögren's syndrome, schizophrenia, and hyperactivity.[3]

Bromocriptine is usually started as a single daily dose of 1.25 mg and is increased by 2.5 mg every 2 to 4 weeks as necessary. The usual dosage for mastalgia is 2.5 mg bid. The initial dosage of danazol is 100 to 150 mg bid with reduction to about 100 mg/day once symptoms are controlled. Therapy with danazol is usually continued for 6 to 9 months. Both bromocriptine and danazol have significant side effects. The major one for bromocriptine is nausea, while for danazol the adverse effects are related to the medication's androgenic effects and include weight gain, fluid retention, fatigue, decrease in breast size, hirsutism, atrophic vaginitis, hot flashes, acne, greasy skin, depression, and hoarse voice. All except hoarseness are said to be reversible when the medication is discontinued.

── ◆ **REFERENCES** ◆ ──

1. Mansel RE: Breast pain, *BMJ* 309:866-868, 1994.
2. Mansel RE, Pye JK, Hughes LE: Effects of essential fatty acids on cyclical mastalgia and non-cyclical breast disorders. In Horrobin DF, ed: *Omega-6 essential fatty acids: pathophysiology and roles in clinical medicine,* New York, 1990, Wiley-Liss, pp 557-566.
3. Kleijnen J: Evening primrose oil: currently used in many conditions with little justification (editorial), *BMJ* 309:824-825, 1994.

BREAST CANCER

This section is primarily a discussion of techniques for preventing breast cancer in the general population. What should be done for high-risk women is unknown. Some authors recommend early surveillance of this group with breast self-examination, clinical breast examinations, and mammography.[1]

── ◆ **REFERENCES** ◆ ──

1. Chart PL, Franssen E: Management of women at increased risk for breast cancer: preliminary results from a new program, *Can Med Assoc J* 157:1235-1242, 1997.

Risk Factors and Primary Prevention

(See also hormone replacement therapy; oral contraceptives)

Table 7 lists some of the established and probable risk factors for breast cancer.[1-17]

The incidence of breast cancer increases progressively with age.[1,2,6] However, the rate of increase slows at the time of the menopause, presumably because of estrogen withdrawal (see below).[6]

After increasing age the next most significant risk factor for breast cancer is a family history of the disease. A small proportion of women with a strong family history have identifiable genetic mutations in the BRCA1 or BRCA2 gene.[2] Hereditary breast cancer is discussed in the next section.

The breast cancer rate in the West is five to seven times that in Asia. However, women of Japanese origin whose

Table 7 Breast Cancer Risk Factors

Well-Documented Risk Factors

Increasing age[1,2]
Family history of breast cancer or genetic mutations[1,2]
Geographical location (West versus Asia)[1]
History of proliferative breast dysplasia[1-3]
History of fibroadenoma[3]
Radiation[2,4]
Menarche before age 12[1,2]
First pregnancy over age 30[1,2]
Failure to breast feed[4,5*]
Delayed menopause[2,6]
Hormone replacement therapy for ≥5 years[2,6-8]
Oral contraceptives[9]
Elevated bone density[10]
Postmenopausal body mass index >35[1,2,6,11]

Possible Risk Factors

Alcohol[12]
Diet[2,13-15]
Smoking[2,16]
Sedentary life-style[2,17,18]

*Elevated risk reported only for breast cancer developing in premenopausal women.

families moved to Hawaii acquired Western rates within two generations.[1]

Women with a history of benign breast disease with proliferative epithelial patterns[1-3] or fibroadenomas[3] have a slightly increased risk of breast cancer. In both instances the risk varies according to the degree of histological atypia.[1,3]

A rare but important risk factor for breast cancer is previous radiation exposure such as that used in the treatment of childhood Hodgkin's disease.[2,4]

Changes in the hormonal milieu appear to affect breast cancer risk. Early menarche and late first pregnancies increase the risk slightly,[1,2] as does failure to breast feed.[5] The menopause is protective, and thus the incidence of breast cancer in premenopausal women is higher than that of postmenopausal women of equivalent age. The earlier the menopause, whether natural or surgically induced, the greater the protective effect.[6] Hormone replacement therapy is associated with clinically important increases in incidence[6] and mortality rate[7,8] from breast cancer (see discussion of hormone replacement therapy—adverse effects). Use of birth control pills is associated with a slightly increased risk of breast cancer, a risk that dissipates completely within 10 years of discontinuing the medication.[9] Women with high bone densities[10] and obese postmenopausal women[1,2,6,11] have increased rates of breast cancer; in both cases higher estrogen levels probably account for the findings. Paradoxically, obesity is associate with a decreased risk of premenopausal breast cancer, probably because obese women have higher rates of anovulation.[11]

Alcohol is probably a risk factor for breast cancer, although this has not been conclusively proved.[12] High-fat di-

ets have been suggested as a risk factor, but this has not been substantiated in a pooled analysis of seven cohort studies[13] or in a 1999 report from the Nurses' Health Study.[14] Further data from the Nurses' Health Study indicated that premenopausal women who ate five or more servings of fruit or vegetables each day had a decreased risk of breast cancer.[15]

Both active and passive smoking have been reported to be associated with an increased risk of breast cancer. This is particularly evident for women exposed to passive cigarette smoke before the age of 12 years.[16]

An epidemiological study of over 25,000 Norwegian women reported that regular exercise was associated with a decreased risk of breast cancer.[17] An evaluation of the Nurses' Health Study concluded that moderate exercise was associated with a modest reduction in the risk of breast cancer.[18]

Some studies have indicated that induced abortion is associated with an increased risk of breast cancer. The unlikeliness of such a connection is suggested by a 1997 report on the entire at-risk female population of Denmark, in which population registries were used to determine the rates of both induced abortion and breast cancer; no increased risk from induced abortion was detected.[19]

≥ REFERENCES ≤

1. McPherson K, Steel CM, Dixon JM: Breast cancer—epidemiology, risk factors and genetics, *BMJ* 309:1003-1006, 1994.
2. Warner E, Heisey RE, Goel V, et al: Hereditary breast cancer: risk assessment of patients with a family history of breast cancer, *Can Fam Physician* 45:104-112, 1999.
3. Fitzgibbons PL, Henson DE, Hutter RV: Benign breast changes and the risk for subsequent breast cancer—an update of the 1985 consensus statement, *Arch Pathol Lab Med* 122:1053-1055, 1998.
4. Bhatia S, Robison LL, Oberlin O, et al: Breast cancer and other second neoplasms after childhood Hodgkin's disease, *N Engl J Med* 334:745-751, 1996.
5. Furberg H, Newman B, Moorman P, et al: Lactation and breast cancer risk, *Int J Epidemiol* 28:396-402, 1999.
6. Beral V, Bull D, Doll R, et al (Collaborative Group on Hormonal Factors in Breast Cancer): Breast cancer and hormone replacement therapy: collaborative reanalysis of data from 51 epidemiological studies of 52,704 women with breast cancer and 108,411 women without breast cancer, *Lancet* 350:1047-1059, 1997.
7. Colditz GA, Hankinson SE, Hunter DJ, et al: The use of estrogens and progestins and the risk of breast cancer in postmenopausal women, *N Engl J Med* 332:1589-1593, 1995.
8. Grodstein F, Stampfer MJ, Colditz A, et al: Postmenopausal hormone therapy and mortality, *N Engl J Med* 336:1769-1775, 1997.
9. Collaborative Group on Hormonal Factors in Breast Cancer: Breast cancer and hormonal contraceptives: collaborative reanalysis of individual data on 53,297 women with and 100,239 women without breast cancer from 54 epidemiological studies, *Lancet* 347:1713-1727, 1996.

10. Zhang Y, Kiel DP, Kreger BE, et al: Bone mass and the risk of breast cancer among postmenopausal women, *N Engl J Med* 336:611-617, 1997.

11. Huang Z, Hankinson SE, Colditz GA, et al: Dual effects of weight and weight gain on breast cancer risk, *JAMA* 278:1407-1411, 1997.

12. Smith-Warner SA, Spiegelman D, Yaun S-S, et al: Alcohol and breast cancer in women: a pooled analysis of cohort studies, *JAMA* 279:535-540, 1998.

13. Hunter DJ, Spiegelman D, Adami H-O, et al: Cohort studies of fat intake and the risk of breast cancer—a pooled analysis, *N Engl J Med* 334:356-361, 1996.

14. Holmes MD, Hunter DJ, Colditz GA, et al: Association of dietary intake of fat and fatty acids with risk of breast cancer, *JAMA* 281:914-920, 1999.

15. Zhang S, Hunter DJ, Forman MR, et al: Dietary carotenoids and vitamins A, C, and E and risk of breast cancer, *J Natl Cancer Inst* 91:547-556, 1999.

16. Lash TL, Aschengrau A: Active and passive cigarette smoking and the occurrence of breast cancer, *Am J Epidemiol* 149:5-12, 1999.

17. Thune I, Brenn T, Lund E, et al: Physical activity and the risk of breast cancer, *N Engl J Med* 336:1269-1275, 1997.

18. Rockhill B, Willett WC, Hunter DJ, et al: A prospective study of recreational physical activity and breast cancer risk, *Arch Intern Med* 159:2290-2296, 1999.

19. Melbye M, Wohlfahrt J, Olsen J, et al: Induced abortion and the risk of breast cancer, *N Engl J Med* 336:81-85, 1997.

Family History of Breast Cancer
(See also informed consent; prevention; screening)

BRCA1 and BRCA2 mutations

Two genetic mutations, BRCA1 and BRCA2, account for approximately half of all hereditary breast cancers; the genetic causes of the other half have not yet been determined. Although women with the BRCA1 mutation were originally believed to be at an 80% to 90% risk for breast cancer and a 40% to 65% risk for ovarian cancer by the age of 70, more recent data suggest that the risks for these women, as well as those with BRCA2 mutations, are high but considerably lower than these figures.[1] In a Canadian study the calculated risk of BRCA1 mutations leading to breast cancer was 60% and for BRCA2 28%.[2] Aside from having a markedly increased risk of breast and ovarian cancer, carriers of the BRCA1 mutation are at a somewhat increased risk of colon cancer (and if they are male, prostate cancer), while carriers of the BRCA2 mutation appear to have an increased risk of pancreatic cancer (and if they are male, prostate cancer).[3] Breast cancer is more likely to develop by age 40 in carriers of BRCA1 and BRCA2 mutations who have had children than in nulliparous carriers.[4]

The most important clue that a woman has hereditary breast cancer is a strong family history of breast cancer, but even among women with such histories BRCA mutations are rare.[5,6] A 1997 study from Philadelphia found that only 16% of women with documented breast cancer and a strong family history of breast cancer (average four cases) had BRCA1 linkages, and the figure dropped to 7% if the women did not also have a family history of ovarian cancer. Higher rates of BRCA1 were found in women who were of Ashkenazi Jewish ancestry or whose family members had had breast cancer diagnosed before the age of 55, ovarian cancer, or both breast and ovarian cancer.[6]

Almost all the breast cancers in Ashkenazi Jewish women who carry BRCA1 or BRCA2 mutations develop before the age of 50 or occur in women with a first-, second-, or third-degree relative who has had ovarian cancer.[2]

The benefits and harm of screening women for BRCA genetic defects remain uncertain.[1,2,7,8] If screening is undertaken, the optimal approach is first to test a family member with breast or ovarian cancer who is considered to be at increased risk of carrying the mutations. If a specific mutation is detected in the family member with cancer but not in the screened relative, the relative can be reassured that her risk for breast cancer is that of the general population. On the other hand, if no specific mutation is detected in the family member with cancer or in the relative being screened, the result is uncertain; the screened relative cannot be reassured that her risk is low, since half of familial breast cancers are unrelated to BRCA mutations.[1]

If a specific genetic defect is detected in a screened woman, optimal management is uncertain. Bilateral mastectomies and oophorectomies reduce but do not eliminate the risk of breast and ovarian cancers, and the effectiveness of surveillance for breast or ovarian cancer in these high-risk women is uncertain. Prophylactic tamoxifen (Nolvadex) is an option (see later discussion), but data on its efficacy for this population of patients are unavailable.[1]

Which women should be considered for genetic screening? Although about 20% of women in the general population have a family history of breast cancer, less than 5% are at high risk for hereditary breast cancer and only a small proportion of these actually have detectable genetic defects. An algorithm developed by Warner and associates[5] suggests referral for genetic counseling in the following circumstances:

1. Three or more relatives on one side of the family have had breast or ovarian cancer.

2. Two or more first- or second-degree relatives on one side of the family have had breast or ovarian cancer.

3. One or more first- or second-degree relatives have had breast cancer before the age of 50, bilateral breast cancer, breast and ovarian cancer, breast cancer in association with Jewish ancestry, or male breast cancer.

Selective estrogen receptor modulators for high-risk women

An approach that has generated a great deal of controversy is the use of tamoxifen, a selective estrogen receptor modulator (SERM), for the primary prevention of breast cancer in women at increased risk of breast cancer. The National Surgical Adjuvant Breast and Bowel Project

(NSABP) in the United States enrolled women over age 60, as well as younger women who had a strong family history of breast cancer or who had had lobular carcinoma in situ. Their BRCA status was not determined. The women were treated with either tamoxifen 20 mg/day or a placebo. The study was stopped prematurely after about 4 years because the group taking tamoxifen had a 49% relative reduction in invasive breast cancer (268 women had to be treated for 1 year to prevent one invasive cancer) and a 50% relative reduction in ductal carcinoma in situ. Whether this intervention can prevent breast cancer deaths and how long tamoxifen can be given safely are unknown. In the NSABP study a significant increase in early-stage endometrial carcinoma and thromboembolic disease (stroke, pulmonary embolism, and deep vein thrombosis) occurred in the tamoxifen-treated group. Three patients in the tamoxifen group died of pulmonary embolism, whereas none in the placebo group died from this cause.[9] Both an Italian[10] and a British[11] trial of tamoxifen for the prevention of breast cancer failed to show any benefit.

At present there is no evidence that tamoxifen has benefit for the primary prevention of breast cancer in the general population, and even for those at high risk, evidence of benefit is at best tenuous.[12]

A 3-year trial of another SERM, raloxifene (Evista), for osteoporosis in postmenopausal women reported a decreased incidence of breast cancer and no increase in endometrial cancer, but an increased incidence of thrombophlebitis and pulmonary embolism.[13] The long-term harm/benefit ratio of raloxifene in the prevention of breast cancer or breast cancer mortality has not been established, and the drug should probably be limited to clinical trial settings.[14]

To keep the preceding information in perspective, the reader should remember that more than 75% of women in whom breast cancer develops have no known risk factors.[5]

⚡ REFERENCES ⚡

1. Heissey RE, Carroll JC, Warner E, et al: Hereditary breast cancer: identifying and managing BRCA1 and BRCA2 carriers, *Can Fam Physician* 45:114-124, 1999.
2. Warner E, Foulkes W, Goodwin P, et al: Prevalence and penetrance of BRCA1 and BRCA2 gene mutations in unselected Ashkenazi Jewish women with breast cancer, *J Natl Cancer Inst* 91:1241-1247, 1999.
3. Easton D et al for the Breast Cancer Linkage Consortium: Cancer risks in BRCA2 mutation carriers, *J Natl Cancer Inst* 91:1310-1316, 1999.
4. Jernström H, Lerman C, Ghadirian P, et al: Pregnancy and risk of early breast cancer in carriers of BRCA1 and BRCA2, *Lancet* 354:1846-1850, 1999.
5. Warner E, Heisey RE, Goel V, et al: Hereditary breast cancer: risk assessment of patients with a family history of breast cancer, *Can Fam Physician* 45:104-112, 1999.
6. Couch FJ, De Shano ML, Blackwood MA, et al: BRCA1 mutations in women attending clinics that evaluate the risk of breast cancer, *N Engl J Med* 336:1409-1415, 1997.
7. Kodish E, Wiesner GL, Mehlman M, et al: Genetic testing for cancer risk: how to reconcile the conflicts, *JAMA* 279:179-181, 1998.
8. Carroll JC, Heisey RE, Warner E, et al: Hereditary breast cancer: psychosocial issues and family physicians' role, *Can Fam Physician* 45:126-132, 1999.
9. Fischer B, Costantino JP, Wickerham DL, et al: Tamoxifen for prevention of breast cancer: report of the National Surgical Adjuvant Breast and Bowel Project P-1 Study, *J Natl Cancer Inst* 90:1371-1388, 1998.
10. Veronesi U, Maisonneuve P, Costa A, et al: Prevention of breast cancer with tamoxifen: preliminary findings from the Italian randomised trial among hysterectomised women, *Lancet* 352:93-97, 1998.
11. Powles T, Eeeles R, Ashley S, et al: Interim analysis of the incidence of breast cancer in the Royal Marsden Hospital tamoxifen randomised chemoprevention trial, *Lancet* 352:98-101, 1998.
12. Goel V: Tamoxifen and breast cancer prevention: what should you tell your patients? (editorial), *Can Med Assoc J* 158:1615-1617, 1998.
13. Cummings SR, Eckert S, Krueger KA, et al: The effect of raloxifene on risk of breast cancer in postmenopausal women: results from the MORE randomized trial, *JAMA* 281:2189-2197, 1999.
14. Chlebowski RT, Collyar DE, Somerfield MR, et al (American Society of Clinical Oncology Working Group on Breast Cancer Risk Reduction Strategies): Tamoxifen and raloxifene, *J Clin Oncol* 17:1939-1955, 1999.

Lifetime Risk of Breast Cancer
(See also ductal carcinoma in situ)

Widely published figures from Great Britain state that a woman's lifetime risk for breast cancer is 1 in 12. In the United States the equivalent figure is 1 in 8.[1] Such figures are deceptive for three main reasons[1,2]:

1. Lifetime risk figures apply only to the relatively few women who live to a ripe old age. When life table analyses are performed, a different picture emerges. For example, the lifetime risk of breast cancer for a woman between 30 and 34 years of age is 1 in 625, for a 50-year-old is 1 in 18, and for a 75-year-old is 1 in 13.[1] Another useful way of evaluating breast cancer risk is to determine the probability that the disease will develop within the next decade. This risk is higher in older than in younger women, but no matter what the age, it is never greater than 1 in 34.[2]
2. Mortality from breast cancer is much lower than incidence, in part because of improved treatment and in part because many of the cases diagnosed with mammography such as ductal carcinoma in situ are relatively innocuous (see below). The probability of a woman's dying of breast cancer by age 34 is 1:2873, by age 54 is 1:136, and by age 75 is 1:39. Overall, 70% of women treated for breast cancer are still alive 10 years later.[1]

3. Many people interpret lifetime risk figures to mean that breast cancer is a greater health risk than other potentially preventable diseases such as coronary artery disease and lung cancer, which kill many more women than does breast cancer.[1,2] For example, if a cohort of 1000 women is followed for 85 years from the time of birth, 33 will have died of breast cancer and 203 will have died of cardiovascular disease. No matter what age bracket is considered, breast cancer never accounts for more than 20% of deaths.[2]

◁ REFERENCES ▷

1. Bunker JP, Houghton J, Baum M: Putting the risk of breast cancer in perspective, *BMJ* 317:1307-1309, 1998.
2. Phillips K-A, Glendon G, Knight JA: Putting the risk of breast cancer in perspective, *N Engl J Med* 340:141-144, 1999.

Breast Self-Examination

(See also breast examination by health professionals; mammography; prevention; screening)

The evidence that breast self-examination is beneficial is inconclusive,[1-6] and such examination may even be detrimental[1]:

1. The overall positive predictive value of breast self-examination has been reported to be 12% (88% false-positive rate). Breast self-examination reveals many benign lesions, leading to anxiety, anesthesia, and surgery.[1]
2. A Finnish cohort study reported a benefit from breast self-examination.[2] Two case-control trials of this procedure (one from Canada and one from the United States) found a slight decrease in death or advanced disease among the relatively few women in the programs who practiced proficient self-examination, but not among those who were not proficient.[3,4] Proficiency in the Canadian study was defined as a combination of visual inspection, use of the fingerpads for palpation, and palpation with the three middle fingers. In this study each woman was seen annually and counseled on performing breast self-examination by specially trained nurses.[3] One year after the first visit about a third of the women were deemed proficient at breast self-examination, and after 4 years (and four training sessions) about two thirds were proficient.[5] The preliminary results of the only satisfactory randomized prospective trial of breast self-examination published to date showed no benefit after 5 years. Definitive results will not be available until the trial has run for several more years.[6]

Both the Canadian Task Force on Preventive Health Care[7] and the U.S. Preventive Services Task Force[8] give breast self-examination a "C" recommendation. The American Academy of Family Physicians[9] recommends the procedure.

◁ REFERENCES ▷

1. Frank JW, Mai V: Breast self-examination in young women: more harm than good? *Lancet* 2:654-657, 1985.
2. Gastrin G, Miller AB, To T, et al: Incidence and mortality from breast cancer in the Mama Program for breast screening in Finland 1973-86, *Cancer* 73:2168-2174, 1994.
3. Harvey BJ, Miller AB, Baines CJ, et al: Effect of breast self-examination techniques on the risk of death from breast cancer, *Can Med Assoc J* 157:1205-1212, 1997.
4. Newcomb PA, Weiss NS, Storer BA, et al: Breast self-examination in relation to the occurrence of advanced breast cancer, *J Natl Cancer Inst* 83:260-265, 1991.
5. Harvey BJ, Miller AB, Baines CJ, et al: Breast self-examination techniques (response to letter), *Can Med Assoc J* 158:870, 1998.
6. Thomas DB, Gao DL, Self SG, et al: Randomized trial of breast self-examination in Shanghai: methodology and preliminary results, *J Natl Cancer Inst* 89:355-365, 1997.
7. Canadian Task Force on the Periodic Health Examination: *Canadian guide to clinical preventive health care,* Ottawa, 1994, Canada Communication Group—Publishing, pp 788-795.
8. US Preventive Services Task Force: *Guide to clinical preventive services,* ed 2, Baltimore, 1996, Williams & Wilkins, pp 73-87.
9. American Academy of Family Physicians: *Age charts for periodic health examination,* Kansas City, Mo, 1994, The Academy (reprint no 510).

Breast Examinations by Health Professionals

(See also breast self-examination; mammography)

Only one series of investigations, the Canadian National Breast Screening Studies (NBSS), has compared physical examination alone with mammography plus physical examination (in almost all cases, physical examination was performed by trained nurses). All other mammographic studies have compared mammography plus physical examination against no systematic examination. After 7 years of follow-up in the NBSS, no decrease in death rates was found in the mammography plus physical examination cohorts compared with the physical examination only cohorts.[1,2] The results of these studies suggest that much of the benefit attributed to mammography is actually a result of clinical examination of the breasts.

Elmore and associates[3] have reported that by the time women have had 10 breast examinations by health professionals, 6.2% of those who did not have cancer will have had breast biopsies.

Guidelines vary as to when physicians should perform breast examinations for cancer detection. The Canadian Task Force on Preventive Health Care gives a "D" recommendation to physician breast examination (and mammography) of women 40 to 49 years of age but an "A" recommendation to performing both these examinations annually on women 50 to 69 years of age.[4]

The U.S. Preventive Services Task Force gives a "C" recommendation for clinical breast examinations alone in women 40 to 69 years of age.[5] However, it gives an "A" recommendation to screening mammography every 1 to 2 years with or without annual clinical breast examinations for women 50 to 69 years of age.[5]

Annual physician breast examinations beginning at 40 years of age are recommended by many other U.S. organizations, including the American Cancer Society,[6] American College of Radiology,[7] American Medical Association,[8] and American College of Obstetricians and Gynecologists.[9] The American Academy of Family Physicians goes even further, recommending examination by a physician every 1 to 3 years beginning at age 30.[10]

In a study of U.S. women over 50 years of age, one third of those seen by male physicians underwent mammography but no clinical breast examination, whereas only 5% of those seen by female physicians had mammography and no clinical breast examination.[11] Since examination of the breasts by physicians may account for some or all of the apparent positive benefits of mammographic screening (see preceding discussion), the findings of this study are worrisome.

--- **REFERENCES** ---

1. Miller AB, Baines C, To T, et al: Canadian National Breast Screening Study. 1. Breast cancer detection and death rates among women aged 40-49 years, *Can Med Assoc J* 147:1459-1476, 1992.
2. Miller AB, Baines CJ, To T, et al: Canadian National Breast Screening Study. 2. Breast cancer detection and death rates among women aged 50 to 59 years, *Can Med Assoc J* 147:1477-1488, 1992.
3. Elmore JG, Barton MB, Moceri VM, et al: Ten-year risk of false positive screening mammograms and clinical breast examinations, *N Engl J Med* 338:1089-1096, 1998.
4. Canadian Task Force on the Periodic Health Examination: *Canadian guide to clinical preventive health care*, Ottawa, 1994, Canada Communication Group—Publishing, pp 788-795.
5. US Preventive Services Task Force: *Guide to clinical preventive services*, ed 2, Baltimore, 1996, Williams & Wilkins, pp 73-87.
6. American Cancer Society: *Guidelines for the cancer-related checkup: an update*, Atlanta, 1993, The Society.
7. Dodd GD: Screening for breast cancer, *Cancer* 72:1038-1042, 1993.
8. Council on Scientific Affairs, American Medical Association: Mammographic screening in asymptomatic women aged 40 years and older, *JAMA* 261:2535-2542, 1989.
9. American College of Obstetricians and Gynecologists: *The obstetrician-gynecologist and primary-preventive health care*, Washington, DC, 1993, The College.
10. American Academy of Family Physicians: *Age charts for periodic health examination*, Kansas City, Mo, 1994, The Academy (reprint no 510).
11. Burns RB, Freund KM, Ash AS, et al: As mammography use increases, are some providers omitting clinical breast examination? *Arch Intern Med* 156:741-744, 1996.

Mammography

(See also breast examinations by health professionals; breast self-examination; informed consent; prevention; screening)

Intervals between mammographic screenings

(See also controversies and uncertainties about mammographic screening; efficacy of mammography)

The intervals between mammographic screenings usually vary between 1 and 3 years. Cancers that are diagnosed in the intervals between screenings are called "interval cancers." One British report found that the number of interval cancers expressed as a percentage of the underlying incidence was 31% during the first year after screening, 52% in the second year, and 82% in the third year. On this basis the authors suggest that a 3-year interval is too long.[1] However, a 1995 metaanalysis of all the major studies found no difference in mortality between women screened annually and those screened every 2 to 2½ years.[2]

Mammography performed on women under 50 years of age is less sensitive than for women over 50. In one study the sensitivity of breast cancer detection by mammography in women over 50 years of age determined after 25 months of follow-up was 85.7% whereas that for women under 50 with the same length of follow-up was 71.4%.[3] The increased breast density of younger women, which makes the detection of cancers more difficult, has been offered as an explanation for this phenomenon, but a more likely reason is that tumors often grow more quickly in this younger population.[4] The particularly low screening sensitivity in women under 40 years of age who have a strong family history of breast cancer lends indirect support to this hypothesis. Whether screening women under 50 years of age has benefit is controversial (see later discussion of controversies and uncertainties about mammographic screening), but if such a program were undertaken in this age group, annual screening would seem indicated.[4]

--- **REFERENCES** ---

1. Woodman CBJ, Threlfall AG, Boggis CR, et al: Is the three year breast screening interval too long—occurrence of interval cancers in NHS breast screening programmes North Western Region, *BMJ* 310(6974):224-226, 1995.
2. Kerlikowske K, Grady D, Rubin SM, et al: Efficacy of screening mammography: a meta-analysis, *JAMA* 273:149-154, 1995.
3. Kerlikowske K, Grady D, Barclay J, et al: Effect of age, breast density, and family history on the sensitivity of first screening mammography, *JAMA* 276:33-38, 1996.
4. Tabar L, Fagerberg G, Chen H, et al: Efficacy of breast cancer screening by age: new results from the Swedish Two-County trial, *Cancer* 75:2507-2517, 1995.

Major mammographic screening programs

Ten of the major randomized controlled trials of mammographic screening with references are listed below (Two-County is actually two trials). The reason for recording them here is that the benefits and adverse consequences of mammographic screening are not fully established. Family physicians have to keep up to date with the literature on the subject, and almost every article refers to one or more of these studies.

Health Insurance Plan of Greater New York (HIP)[1]	United States
Two-County (Kopparberg and Ostergotland)[2]	Sweden
Malmö[3]	Sweden
Stockholm[4]	Sweden
Gothenburg[5]	Sweden
Edinburgh[6,7]	United Kingdom
National Breast Screening Study—1 (NBSS-1)[8]	Canada
National Breast Screening Study—2 (NBSS-2)[9]	Canada
Finland[10]	Finland

❧ REFERENCES ❧

1. Shapiro S: *Periodic screening for breast cancer: the Health Insurance Plan Project and its sequelae, 1963-1986,* Baltimore, Md, 1988, Johns Hopkins University Press.
2. Tabar L, Fagerberg G, Chen H, et al: Efficacy of breast cancer screening by age: new results from the Swedish Two-County trial, *Cancer* 75:2507-2517, 1995.
3. Andersson I, Aspegren K, Janzon L, et al: Mammographic screening and mortality from breast cancer: the Malmö Mammographic Screening trial, *BMJ* 297:943-948, 1988.
4. Frisell J, Lidbrink E, Hellstrom L, et al: Follow-up after 11 years: update of mortality results in the Stockholm mammographic screening trial, *Breast Cancer Res Treat* 45:263-270, 1997.
5. Bjurstam N, Bjorneld L, Duffy SW, et al: The Gothenburg Breast Screening Trial: first results on mortality, incidence, and mode of detection for women ages 39-49 years at randomization, *Cancer* 80:2091-2099, 1997.
6. Roberts MM, Alexander FE, Anderson TJ, et al: Edinburgh trial of screening for breast cancer: mortality at seven years, *Lancet* 335:241-246, 1990.
7. Alexander FE, Anderson TJ, Brown HK, et al: 14 Years of follow-up from the Edinburgh randomised trial of breast-cancer screening, *Lancet* 353:1903-1908, 1999.
8. Miller AB, Baines CJ, To T, et al: Canadian National Breast Screening Study. 1. Breast cancer detection and death rates among women aged 40 to 49 years, *Can Med Assoc J* 147:1459-1476, 1992.
9. Miller AB, Baines CJ, To T, et al: Canadian National Breast Screening Study. 2. Breast cancer detection and death rates among women aged 50 to 59 years, *Can Med Assoc J* 147:1477-1488, 1992.
10. Hakama M, Pukkala E, Heikkilä M, et al: Effectiveness of the public health policy for breast cancer screening in Finland: population based cohort study, *BMJ* 314:864-867, 1997.

Efficacy of mammographic trials

(See also controversies and uncertainties about mammographic screening; evidence-based medicine; surrogate outcomes)

Women aged 40 to 49 years. Whether screening mammography for women under 50 years of age is beneficial is controversial, mainly because only two trials have demonstrated statistically significant decreases in mortality for women in this age group and the validity of these findings is questionable (see later discussion). An overview of five combined Swedish trials (including the Gothenburg trial) published in 1993 found a 13% mortality reduction in the 40- to 49-year age group, but this was not statistically significant.[1] A 1993 metaanalysis of eight randomized trials involving the same age group by Fletcher and associates[2] also failed to show any statistically significant decrease in mortality. In 1995 three metaanalyses of randomized trials of mammography in women under 50 years of age were published. The first reviewed seven randomized trials involving 160,000 women and found no benefit from the intervention.[3] The second concluded that there was a trend toward decreased mortality after 10 to 12 years of follow-up, but in the opinion of the authors, even if this trend were to be verified with time and further studies, screening beginning at 50 years of age would probably achieve the same benefit.[4] In contrast, the third 1995 metaanalysis, that of Smart and associates,[5] concluded that the previous reports were erroneous and that mammographic screening indeed produced a statistically significant decrease in mortality in this age group, provided the Canadian National Breast Screening Study—1 (NBSS-1) was excluded.

The NBSS-1 program that Smart and co-workers chose to exclude from their metaanalysis showed an increase in breast cancer mortality in the screened group compared with the control group.[6] A number of workers have criticized the randomization process of this study,[5,7] but a careful review by two eminent outside epidemiologists failed to find fault with the randomization.[8]

One of the most controversial studies of mammography for women in their forties is the Gothenburg study, published in 1997. It reported a 45% relative reduction of mortality (the absolute reduction is on the order of 0.13%) in this age group.[9] Some epidemiologists question the effectiveness of the randomization process and therefore treat the results with skepticism (see controversies and uncertainties about mammographic screening).[10]

Long-term follow-up results of the Edinburgh breast screening project were reported in a 1999 *Lancet* article. Women who entered the program between ages 45 and 49 and continued in it after age 50 showed slight benefit; the number of women who were screened only between ages 45 and 49 was small, and the results were "equivocal."[11]

A comprehensive analysis of the controversies surrounding mammographic screening of women in their forties was published by Antman and Shea[12] in *JAMA* in April 1999. The issue is discussed further in the later section on controversies and uncertainties about mammographic screening.

Women 50 to 69 years of age. Mortality for women aged 50 to 64 on entry to the Health Insurance Plan of Greater New York (HIP) study,[13] and for women aged 50 to 69 on entry to all the Swedish trials,[1] was significantly reduced. The relative mortality rates of women who had mammography in the combined Swedish studies were 0.72 for women 50 to

59 years of age and 0.69 for women 60 to 69.[2] The absolute mortality reduction rates were much smaller (see below). There was no decrease in mortality in the NBSS-2 study of Canadian women aged 50 to 59 at entry[14] or in the Malmö trial in Sweden.[15] A statistically insignificant decrease occurred in the Finnish trial,[16] and an equivocally significant benefit was shown in the Edinburgh trial.[11] A metaanalysis of all the major studies reported in 1995 concluded that mammography resulted in a decreased cancer death rate in women between the ages of 50 and 74 after a follow-up period of 7 to 9 years.[4]

Until the publication of an article by Gøtzsche and Olsen[17] in the *Lancet* in January 2000, it was generally accepted that mammography leads to a decrease in breast cancer mortality in women aged 50 to 69. Gøtzsche and Olsen claim that the evidence supporting this view is flawed and that "screening for breast cancer with mammography is unjustified."[17] They base this stand on their assessment of the randomization processes of the various major trials; according to their calculations the randomization process was flawed in all trials but the two that showed no benefit (Malmö[15] and Canadian[14]). This article is stirring up a great deal of controversy—an accompanying editorial by de Koning[18] has already challenged many of the authors' assumptions.

Women over 70 years of age. Whether mammography decreases breast cancer mortality in women aged 70 or over is unknown because randomized trials have not included enough women in this age group to draw any meaningful conclusions. For women with comorbid medical conditions such as coronary artery disease or diabetes, the chances of dying from breast cancer are remote. Even without comorbid conditions life expectancy in the elderly is limited, and diagnosing and treating slowly progressive lesions such as ductal carcinoma in situ would be unlikely to offer any benefit.[19]

◣ REFERENCES ◢

1. Nyström L, Rutqvist LE, Wall S, et al: Breast cancer screening with mammography: overview of Swedish randomised trials, *Lancet* 34:973-978, 1993.
2. Fletcher SW, Black W, Harris R, et al: Report of the International Workshop on Screening for Breast Cancer, *J Natl Cancer Inst* 85:1644-1656, 1993.
3. Glasziou PP, Woodward AJ, Mahon CM: Mammographic screening trials for women aged under 50: a quality assessment and meta-analysis, *Med J Aust* 162:625-629, 1995.
4. Kerlikowske K, Grady D, Rubin SM, et al: Efficacy of screening mammography: a meta-analysis, *JAMA* 273:149-154, 1995.
5. Smart CR, Hendrix RE, Rutledge JH, et al: Benefit of mammography screening in women ages 40-49, *Cancer* 75:1619-1626, 1995.
6. Miller AB, Baines CJ, To T, et al: Canadian National Breast Screening Study. 1. Breast cancer detection and death rates among women aged 40 to 49 years, *Can Med Assoc J* 147:1459-1476, 1992.
7. Leitch AM: Controversies in breast cancer screening, *Cancer* 76(suppl 10):2064-2069, 1995.
8. Bailar JC III, MacMahon B: Randomization in the Canadian National Breast Screening Study: a review for evidence of subversion, *Can Med Assoc J* 156:193-199, 1997.
9. Bjurstam N, Bjorneld L, Duffy SW, et al: The Gothenburg Breast Screening Trial: first results on mortality, incidence, and mode of detection for women ages 39-49 years at randomization, *Cancer* 80:2091-2099, 1997.
10. Nelson NJ: The mammography consensus jury speaks out, *J Natl Cancer Inst* 89:344-47, 1997.
11. Alexander FE, Anderson TJ, Brown HK, et al: 14 Years of follow-up from the Edinburgh randomised trial of breast-cancer screening, *Lancet* 353:1903-1908, 1999.
12. Antman K, Shea S: Screening mammography under age 50, *JAMA* 281:1470-1472, 1999.
13. Shapiro S, Venet W, Strax P, et al: *Periodic screening for breast cancer: the Health Insurance Plan project and its sequelae, 1963-1986,* Baltimore, 1988, Johns Hopkins University Press.
14. Miller AB, Baines CJ, To T, et al: Canadian National Breast Screening Study. 2. Breast cancer detection and death rates among women aged 50 to 59 years, *Can Med Assoc J* 147:1477-1488, 1992.
15. Andersson I, Aspegren K, Janzon L, et al: Mammographic screening and mortality from breast cancer: the Malmö Mammographic Screening Trial, *BMJ* 297:943-948, 1988.
16. Hakama M, Pukkala E, Heikkilä M, et al: Effectiveness of the public health policy for breast cancer screening in Finland: population based cohort study, *BMJ* 314:864-867, 1997.
17. Gøtzsche PC, Olsen L: Is screening for breast cancer with mammography justifiable? *Lancet* 355:129-134, 2000.
18. de Koning HJ: Assessment of nationwide cancer-screening programmes (editorial), *Lancet* 355:80-81, 2000.
19. Smith-Bindman R, Kerlikowske K: Is there a downside to elderly women undergoing screening mammography? (editorial), *J Natl Cancer Inst* 90:1322-1323, 1998.

Effect of reporting methods on perception of benefits of mammography

(See also absolute risk reduction; numbers of patients who need to be screened or treated; relative risk reduction)

Although the reported relative reduction of death from breast cancer in women over 50 years of age who have had mammography looks impressive for many of these trials (14% to 40%), the absolute risk reduction is much smaller. For example, a relative mortality reduction of 35% in the Health Insurance Plan of New York (HIP) trial translates into an absolute reduction in breast cancer deaths of 0.02% (2 per 10,000). Put another way, in the HIP trial 5061 women would have had to be screened to prevent one breast cancer death.[1,2] In the five combined Swedish studies the overall relative decrease in breast cancer mortality for women 40 to 74 years of age was 24%. The absolute figures were 0.3:1000 at 6 years, 0.7:1000 at 9 years, and 1.2:1000 at 12 years.[3]

In a 1995 evaluation of several randomized controlled studies of mammography, two Canadian surgeons calculated the number of women who would have to be screened in each trial to save one life annually. Their figures are[4]:

Health Insurance Plan of New York	7,086
Swedish National Board of Health (Two-County)	13,665
Stockholm	15,703
Edinburgh	20,322
Malmö	63,264
Canadian National Breast Screening Study	No evidence of any lives saved

The results of the Finnish breast screening program published in 1997 reported that 10,000 women had to be screened to save one life.[5] Gøtzsche and Olsen[6] calculated that if the Swedish trials are unbiased and therefore valid (a hypothesis they question; see preceding discussion), 1000 women would have to be screened every 2 years for 12 years to prevent one breast cancer death.

Whether mammographic screening of women in their forties saves lives at all is controversial, as discussed elsewhere in the text. However, if some of the published figures are accepted at face value, six times more women in their forties would have to be screened to save a life than would be required for women in their sixties.[7]

❧ REFERENCES ❧

1. Dixon T: Breast screening: time for translation? (editorial), *Can Fam Physician* 37:2544-2548, 1991.
2. Scrabanek P: Mass mammography: the time for reappraisal, *Int J Technol Assess Health Care* 5:423-430, 1989.
3. Nyström L, Rutqvist LE, Wall S, et al: Breast cancer screening with mammography: overview of Swedish randomised trials, *Lancet* 341:973-978, 1993.
4. Wright CJ, Mueller CB: Screening mammography and public health policy: the need for perspective, *Lancet* 346:29-32, 1995.
5. Hakama M, Pukkala E, Heikkilä M, et al: Effectiveness of the public health policy for breast cancer screening in Finland: population based cohort study, *BMJ* 314:864-867, 1997.
6. Gøtzsche PC, Olsen L: Is screening for breast cancer with mammography justifiable? *Lancet* 355:129-134, 2000.
7. Antman K, Shea S: Screening mammography under age 50, *JAMA* 281:1470-1472, 1999.

Adverse effects of mammography

(See also attitudes, physician; prevention; screening)

Psychological distress is common in women who are recalled for further investigations after a routine mammogram.[1-4] Lerman and associates[1] studied women 3 months after they who had undergone thorough workup for "highly suspicious" mammograms and had been found not to have cancer; 41% were worried that they had breast cancer, and 17% reported decreased ability to participate fully in activities of daily life. A prospective Australian study of women undergoing mammography found that those recalled for repeat mammograms experienced increased psychological, social, and physical distress compared with women who were not recalled.[2] However, these symptoms did not persist beyond 1 month (none of the women studied were found to have breast cancer); what did persist was anxiety about breast cancer.[2] A British study evaluated women who had been recalled for further evaluation after screening mammography and had been found not to have cancer. Five months after they were told they did not have cancer, adverse psychological consequences (such as trouble sleeping, change in appetite, depression or unhappiness as a result of thoughts of breast cancer) were still being experienced by 59% of women who were followed up with an early repeat mammogram (usually in 6 months), 61% of those who had had a surgical biopsy, and 44% of those who had had fine needle aspiration cytology. The prevalence of psychological distress in the control group who had had normal screening mammograms was 10%.[3]

Concern has been raised that women who have had false-positive mammograms may be reluctant to participate in further mammographic screening programs. According to one retrospective[5] and one prospective[6] study, this did not occur; if anything the experience reinforced the need for further screening.

How many women undergoing mammography receive false-positive reports? If only women who have biopsies are analyzed, the ratio is about 3:1.[4] From the psychological viewpoint a more realistic evaluation is the malignancy rate among all women who are recalled for further evaluation as a result of a mammogram report. Shades of gray and risk spectrum are not part of most people's conception of illness; to many, any recall means cancer.[8] In most studies 5% to 14% of women having mammograms are recalled.[7,9,10] As a specific example, in a 1991-1992 Scottish program, in which the recall rate of 7.3% was on the low end of the spectrum, 8.6% of those recalled had cancer and 91.4% did not.[7] Elmore and associates[10] found that over a 10-year screening period during which the median number of mammograms performed was four, 24% of women had false-positive results (defined as recall for any reason). The authors calculated that the cumulative false-positive rate after 10 mammograms (one mammogram every 2 years from age 50 to 70) would be 49% and that 18.6% of women without cancer would be subjected to biopsies.

Open surgical breast biopsies are not innocuous. One study found that 92% of women had "a lot of pain," felt sick for 3 days, or missed 3 days of work; 94% reported decreased arm movement on the affected side for over a week; and most had diminished sexual feelings in the breast for over 2 weeks.[5]

Since abnormal mammograms requiring follow-up testing often generate anxiety, it is important to know how rapidly follow-up examinations are performed. According to one study of American women over the age of 65, only 15% of those requiring diagnostic (as opposed to an initial screening) mammography had it on the same day, 40% had it within a month, and another 40% waited 4 to 8 months, probably because the radiologists' recommendations were to repeat the testing in that time interval. When biopsies were required, almost half the women had to wait more than 3 weeks.[9]

As pointed out in the section on the efficacy of mammographic screening, inadequate numbers of women over the age of 70 have been studied to determine whether the procedure is beneficial. Despite this, over one fourth of American women older than 80 years of age are sent for mammographic screening. Since octogenarians have limited life expectancy, and since a high percentage of the breast cancers detected by mammography are either ductal carcinomas in situ (see below) or small invasive tumors, the chance that the lesions would impair the quality of life of these women is remote.[11]

The usual false-negative rate for mammograms is 10% for women 50 to 69 years of age. For women aged 40 to 49 it is as high as 25%.[12] The danger of a false-negative result is unwarranted reassurance of a patient who actually has cancer.

Failure to obtain fully informed consent for mammographic screening may also cause harm. Women under the age of 50 have been shown to overestimate their risk of dying of breast cancer in the next 10 years 20 fold and to overestimate the benefit of screening 6 fold.[13] If women are not informed of the actual figures and the pros and cons of screening, they may choose to participate in a program on the basis of false assumptions and suffer adverse effects as a result.[14] Most articles on mammography downplay or avoid any discussion of the adverse effects; as Dixon[15] points out, it is the family physician, not the mammographer, who has to deal with the emotional havoc that this can induce.

The major adverse physical effect of mammography is pain. In one study about 90% of women experienced some pain, about 30% had moderately severe pain, and 5% to 15% reported severe pain[16]; in another study 60% complained of some pain and 5% of severe pain.[17]

❧ REFERENCES ❧

1. Lerman C, Trock B, Rimer BK, et al: Psychological and behavioral implications of abnormal mammograms, *Ann Intern Med* 114:657-661, 1991.
2. Lowe JB, Balanda KP, Del Mar C, et al: Psychologic distress in women with abnormal findings in mass mammography screening, *Cancer* 85:1114-1118, 1999.
3. Brett J, Austoker J, Ong G: Do women who undergo further investigation for breast screening suffer adverse psychological consequences? A multi-centre follow-up study comparing different breast screening result groups five months after their last breast screening appointment, *J Public Health Med* 20:396-403, 1998.
4. Lindfors KK, O'Connor J, Acredolo CR, et al: Short-interval follow-up mammography versus immediate core biopsy of benign breast lesions: assessment of patient stress, *AJR* 171:55-58, 1998.
5. Pisano ED, Earp J, Schell M, et al: Screening behavior of women after a false-positive mammogram, *Radiology* 208:245-249, 1998.
6. Burman ML, Taplin SH, Herta DF, et al: Effect of false-positive mammograms on interval breast cancer screening in a health maintenance organization, *Ann Intern Med* 131:1-6, 1999.
7. Balmy WR, Wilson ARM, Pantoic J, et al: Screening for breast cancer, *BMJ* 309:1076-1079, 1994.
8. Wardle J, Pope R: The psychological costs of screening for cancer, *J Psychosom Res* 36:609-624, 1992.
9. Welch HG, Fisher ES: Diagnostic testing following screening mammography in the elderly, *J Natl Cancer Inst* 90:1389-1392, 1998.
10. Elmore JG, Barton MB, Moceri VM, et al: Ten-year risk of false positive screening mammograms and clinical breast examinations, *N Engl J Med* 338:1089-1096, 1998.
11. Smith-Bindman R, Kerlikowske K: Is there a downside to elderly women undergoing screening mammography? (editorial), *J Natl Cancer Inst* 90:1322-1323, 1998.
12. National Institutes of Health Consensus Development Panel: National Institutes of Health Consensus Development Conference Statement: Breast cancer screening for women ages 40-49, Jan 21-23, 1997, *J Natl Cancer Inst* 89:1015-1026, 1997.
13. Black WC, Nease RF, Tosteson AN: Perceptions of breast cancer risk and screening effectiveness in women younger than 50 years of age, *J Natl Cancer Inst* 87:720-731, 1995.
14. Harris R, Leininger L: Clinical strategies for breast cancer screening: weighing and using the evidence, *Ann Intern Med* 122:539-547, 1995.
15. Dixon T: Breast screening: time for translation? (editorial), *Can Fam Physician* 37:2544-2548, 1991.
16. Kornguth PJ, Keefe FJ, Conaway MR: Pain during mammography: characteristics and relationship to demographic and medical variables, *Pain* 66:187-194, 1996.
17. Aro AR, Absetz-Ylöstalo P, Eerola T, et al: Pain and discomfort during mammography, *Eur J Cancer* 32A:1674-1679, 1996.

Controversies and uncertainties about mammographic screening

(See also ductal carcinoma in situ; efficacy of mammographic trials; guidelines for mammographic screening; informed consent; length bias; prevention; screening)

One problem in assessing the efficacy of mammography is trying to determine whether a decrease of breast cancer deaths is due to early detection or to more effective treatment for all stages of the disease. For example, a study of breast cancer deaths from England and Wales found that the incidence of breast cancers in screened women increased sharply after the introduction of screening (an expected effect of this intervention) while the mortality from breast cancer had begun to level off before the introduction of screening and dropped sharply within 3 years of its institution. In the opinion of the authors the decline in death rates occurred too soon to be explained by screening and might be the result of an increasing use of tamoxifen.[1]

Most of the major mammographic studies used a combination of mammography and physical examination of the breasts in the study group and no breast examinations in the control group. It is therefore uncertain how much of the decline in mortality rates in women over the age of 50 is attributable to physical examination of the breasts and how much to mammography.[2] In the Canadian National Breast Screening Studies (NBSS), which showed no decrease in mortality after 7 years of follow-up, physical examination and mammography were used in the study group and physical examination in the control group.[2,3] If physical examination alone is an important modality for decreasing breast cancer mortality, this may account for the failure of the NBSS to demonstrate a decreased mortality in women over the age of 50 who had mammography.

Another controversial issue about mammography is the clinical importance of diagnosing ductal carcinoma in situ. Carcinoma in situ accounts for nearly half of all mammographically diagnosed breast cancers, but whether the detection and treatment of this lesion decrease mortality is unknown (see later discussion of ductal carcinoma in situ). One hypothesis is that length bias accounts for much of the observed benefit of mammography: mammography may preferentially detect tumors, such as ductal carcinoma in situ, that have very slow growth rates and little or no propensity to spread even if untreated. A report from Yale gives some support to this. The recurrence and mortality rates were lower among women with breast cancers detected by mammography than among those with cancers detected by other means even when tumors of identical TNM stages were compared.[4]

A current controversial issue is whether mammography in women between 40 and 49 years of age decreases mortality. The conclusions of some relevant studies are summarized in the earlier discussion of the efficacy of mammographic trials. The Malmö and Gothenburg trials have shown statistically significant decreases in mortality in this age group, and the methodology of the latter is suspect.[5] Relatively few women in the Edinburgh trial were screened only between the ages of 45 and 49, and the results for this group were equivocal.[6] The only metaanalysis to show a decrease in mortality excluded the NBSS-1. A further problem is that in most trials the majority of women in their forties have been in the late forties, giving little data for analysis of screening women early in this age group. Finally, an estimated one third to more than two thirds[5] of the benefit noted is the result of "age creep"; that is, women began a screening program in their forties, but their cancer was not diagnosed until they were over 50.[5,6] Clearly these women would have done as well if screening had started at 50.

In January 1997 the majority report of a National Institutes of Health expert consensus conference concluded that current evidence (including results of the Gothenburg trial) did not warrant a universal recommendation for mammographic screening of women aged 40 to 49. Instead, it proposed that with help from her physician, each women should decide for herself. This recommendation caused such an outcry among breast cancer screening advocates, including politicians, that a few months later the National Cancer Institute bowed to political pressure and recommended that women between 40 and 49 who have an average risk of breast cancer undergo mammographic screening every 1 to 2 years.[8,9]

My view of the controversy over mammography for women between the ages of 40 and 49 is that since benefits are uncertain, mammography is not innocuous (see discussion of the adverse effect of mammographic screening procedures), and the Canadian Task Force on Preventive Health Care gives the procedure a "D" recommendation and the U.S. Preventive Services Task Force gives it a "C," the odds are that the intervention will do more harm than good. Obviously, individual patients have the right to make up their own minds. To do so, they need to be informed of the pros and cons of this preventive modality. This is essentially the perspective of Pauker and Kassirer,[10] who consider the choice a tossup.

❧ REFERENCES ❧

1. Quinn M, Allen E (United Kingdom Association of Cancer Registries): Changes in incidence of and mortality from breast cancer in England and Wales since introduction of screening, *BMJ* 311:1391-1395, 1995.
2. Miller AB, Baines CJ, To T, et al: Canadian National Breast Screening Study. 2. Breast cancer detection and death rates among women aged 50 to 59 years, *Can Med Assoc J* 147:1477-1488, 1992.
3. Miller AB, Baines C, To T, et al: Canadian National Breast Screening Study. 1. Breast cancer detection and death rates among women aged 40-49 years, *Can Med Assoc J* 147:1459-1476, 1992.
4. Moody-Ayers SY, Wells CK, Feinstein AR: *Does the reduced breast cancer mortality after mammography screening represent cure, early detection or discovery of relatively "benign" tumors?* (abstract), Robert Wood Johnson-Clinical Scholars Program, 1996 National Meeting, Key Largo, Fla, November 1996.
5. Nelson NJ: The mammography consensus jury speaks out, *J Natl Cancer Inst* 89:344-347, 1997.
6. Alexander FE, Anderson TJ, Brown HK, et al: 14 Years of follow-up from the Edinburgh randomised trial of breast-cancer screening, *Lancet* 353:1903-1908, 1999.
7. National Institutes of Health Consensus Development Panel: National Institutes of Health Consensus Development Conference Statement: Breast cancer screening for women ages 40-49, Jan 21-23, 1997, *J Natl Cancer Inst* 89:1015-1026, 1997.
8. Baines CF: Breast-cancer screening: will the controversy never end? *Can J Diagn* 15:65-71, 1998.
9. Ernster VL: Mammographic screening for women aged 40 through 49: a guidelines saga and a clarion call for informed decision making, *Am J Publ Health* 87:1103-1106, 1997.
10. Pauker SG, Kassirer JP: Contentious screening decisions: does the choice matter? (editorial), *N Engl J Med* 336:1243-1244, 1997.

Guidelines for mammographic screening
(See also breast examination by health professionals; breast self-examination; clinical practice guidelines; prevention; screening)

The recommendations of the Canadian Task Force on Preventive Health Care are that women aged 50 to 69 years have annual physical examinations of the breast and annual mammography ("A" recommendation).[1] Screening by physical examination of the breasts and mammography is not recommended for women under 50 ("D" recommendation).[1] The recommendations of the U.S. Preventive Services Task Force are that women aged 50 to 69 have screening mammography every 1 to 2 years with or without annual clinical breast examinations.[2] The Task Force gives a "C" recommendation for both mammography and clinical breast examination for women aged 40 to 49 and for those over 70.[2]

Most Canadian, British, and European organizations concur with the policy of not screening women under 50.[1] However, many U.S. organizations, such as the American Cancer Society,[3] American College of Radiology,[4] American Medical Association,[5] and American College of Obstetricians and Gynecologists,[6] have endorsed mammographic screening of women aged 40 to 59. In 1997 the U.S. National Cancer Institute recommended that women aged 40 to 49 and at average risk of breast cancer have mammographic screening every 1 to 2 years.[7] At about the same time the American Cancer Society changed its recommendation for this age group from screening mammography every 1 to 2 years to annual screening mammography.[3]

REFERENCES

1. Canadian Task Force on the Periodic Health Examination: *Canadian guide to clinical preventive health care,* Ottawa, 1994, Communication Group—Publishing, pp 788-795.
2. US Preventive Services Task Force: *Guide to clinical preventive services,* ed 2, Baltimore, 1996, Williams & Wilkins, pp 73-87.
3. Leitch AM, Dodd GD, Costanza M, et al: American Cancer Society guidelines for the early detection of breast cancer: update 1997, *CA Cancer J Clin* 47:150-153, 1997.
4. Dodd GD: Screening for breast cancer, *Cancer* 72:1038-1042, 1993.
5. Council on Scientific Affairs, American Medical Association: Mammographic screening in asymptomatic women aged 40 years and older, *JAMA* 261:2535-2542, 1989.
6. American College of Obstetricians and Gynecologists: *The obstetrician-gynecologist and primary-preventive health care,* Washington, DC, 1993, American College of Obstetricians and Gynecologists.
7. Marwick C: Final mammography recommendation? *JAMA* 277:1181, 1997.

Prognosis and Staging

The most important factor determining the prognosis of breast cancer is the presence of positive axillary nodes. The more positive nodes present, the worse the prognosis.[1,2]

However, even the presence of multiple positive nodes is not necessarily an immediate death sentence; in one study the actuarial 10-year survival of women with more than 10 positive nodes was 29%.[3] If nodes are negative, tumor size is the dominant factor in determining prognosis.[1] Other factors of prognostic importance include estrogen-receptor concentration and histological grade.[2]

Survival of women with metastatic breast cancer varies with the site of metastases. For those with bone or skin metastases it may be years, whereas for those with hepatic metastases or lymphangitic spread in the lungs it is months.[2]

REFERENCES

1. Berkowitz LD, Love N: Adjuvant systemic therapy for breast cancer: issues for primary care physicians, *Postgrad Med* 98:85-94, 1995.
2. Phillips DM, Balducci L: Current management of breast cancer, *Am Fam Physician* 53:657-665, 1996.
3. Walker MJ, Osborne MD, Young DC, et al: The natural history of breast cancer with more than 10 positive nodes, *Am J Surg* 169:575-579, 1995.

Ductal Carcinoma in Situ
(See also mammography; surrogate outcomes)

Ductal carcinoma in situ (DCIS) is an important disease because it is detectable by mammography and as a result the incidence of the disorder has skyrocketed in the past decade.[1,2] In the United States in 1992 DCIS accounted for about 12% of all breast cancers that were diagnosed but between 30% and 40% of those diagnosed by mammography.[1] Between 1985 and 1995, 43% of breast cancers diagnosed in women aged 40 to 49 were ductal carcinomas in situ, while for women aged 30 to 39 the percentage was 92%.[1]

DCIS is found in 6% to 18% of autopsies of women dying of other diseases.[1] Although it seems likely that some cases of DCIS will become invasive over a 15- to 25-year period, it is unknown which will and which will not and, by extension, whether detecting these lesions by mammography saves lives (see discussion of controversies and uncertainties about mammographic screening).[4]

A decade ago it was thought that all cases of DCIS were multicentric and therefore the usual treatment was mastectomy. It is now clear that the vast majority of cases are localized and are amenable to local resection.[5] An 8-year prospective follow-up study published in 1998 compared lumpectomy to lumpectomy plus radiation. The cumulative risk of invasive and noninvasive breast cancers in the ipsilateral breast was 27% in those treated by lumpectomy alone and 12% in those treated by lumpectomy plus radiation therapy; 1% of women treated by lumpectomy and 2.5% of those treated by lumpectomy plus radiation died of breast cancer. On the basis of these data, lumpectomy plus radiation therapy is the current treatment of choice for DCIS.[6] That this approach might not always be best is suggested by a subsequent study that carefully assessed surgical margins of the resected lesions in three dimensions; if the margins were 1 mm or more, radiation therapy did not produce an additional benefit.[7]

In addition to local resection and radiation therapy, tamoxifen may be beneficial for some patients with DCIS. In one study patients with DCIS who had been taking this drug for 5 years had a decreased incidence of invasive and non-invasive cancer in both the ipsilateral and contralateral breasts, but they also had increased rates of endometrial cancer and thrombophlebitis.[8]

That axillary lymph node dissection is not indicated for patients with ductal carcinoma in situ is well established.[2,5] Nevertheless, data from the United States indicate that half of patients with DCIS undergo axillary dissection.[5]

Lobular carcinoma in situ is a different entity from ductal carcinoma in situ. It cannot be detected by mammography and is an incidental finding in breast biopsies performed for other reasons. It is not an anatomical precursor of breast cancer but is a risk factor for breast cancer in either breast.

✎ REFERENCES ✎

1. Ernster VL, Barclay J, Kerlikowske K, et al: Incidence of and treatment for ductal carcinoma in situ of the breast, *JAMA* 275:913-918, 1996.
2. Silverstein MJ: Ductal carcinoma in situ of the breast, *BMJ* 317:734-739, 1998.
3. Page DL, Dupont WD, Rogers LW, et al: Continued local recurrence of carcinoma 15-25 years after a diagnosis of low grade ductal carcinoma in situ of the breast treated only by biopsy, *Cancer* 76:1197-1200, 1995.
4. National Institutes of Health Consensus Development Panel: National Institutes of Health Consensus Development Conference Statement: Breast cancer screening for women ages 40-49, Jan 21-23, 1997, *J Natl Cancer Inst* 89:1015-1026, 1997.
5. Page DL, Simpson JF: Ductal carcinoma in situ—the focus for prevention, screening, and breast conservation in breast cancer (editorial), *N Engl J Med* 340:1499-1500, 1999.
6. Fisher B, Dignam J, Wolmark N, et al: Lumpectomy and radiation therapy for the treatment of intraductal breast cancer: findings from National Surgical Adjuvant Breast and Bowel Project B-17, *J Clin Oncol* 16:441-452, 1998.
7. Silverstein MJ, Lagios MD, Groshen S, et al: The influence of margin width on local control of ductal carcinoma in situ of the breast, *N Engl J Med* 340:1455-1461, 1999.
8. Fisher B, Dignam J, Wolmark N, et al: Tamoxifen in treatment of intraductal breast cancer: National Surgical Adjuvant Breast and Bowel Project B-24 randomised controlled trial, *Lancet* 353:1993-2000, 1999.
9. Winchester DJ, Menck HR, Winchester DP: National treatment trends for ductal carcinoma in situ of the breast, *Arch Surg* 132:660-665, 1997.

Management of Breast Cancer
(See also alternative medicine; follow-up of cancer patients who have had curative treatments; hormone replacement therapy)

Investigations in patients with early stage breast cancer
The basic workup for patients with early stage breast cancer is chest x-ray examination, complete blood cell counts, and liver function tests. Bone or liver scans or liver ultrasound evaluation is of little or no additional value. More intensive workup may be indicated for patients with stage T3-4 or N2 tumors. Most patients with metastatic disease have symptoms or signs suggesting tumor spread.[1]

Extensive follow-up investigations of patients who have been treated for early-stage breast cancer are contraindicated (see discussion of follow-up of cancer patients who have had curative treatments).

✎ REFERENCES ✎

1. Samant R, Ganguly P: Staging investigations in patients with breast cancer: the role of bone scans and liver imaging, *Arch Surg* 134:551-553, 1999.

Delay in diagnosis and treatment of breast cancer
Delay in the diagnosis and treatment of breast cancer may occur at the level of the patient or her medical providers; provider delay may be due to delay in surgical consultation or to a delay in diagnostic and therapeutic interventions by the surgeons.[1] Although some studies have reported a small increase in mortality when combined patient and provider delay was 3 to 6 months,[2] a recent British study failed to find any evidence that provider delays of over 3 months increased mortality.[3]

✎ REFERENCES ✎

1. Coates AS: Breast cancer: delays, dilemmas, and delusions (editorial), *Lancet* 353:1112-1113, 1999.
2. Richards MA, Westcombe AM, Love SB, et al: Influence of delay on survival in patients with breast cancer: a systematic review, *Lancet* 353:1119-1126, 1999.
3. Sainsbury R, Johnston C, Haward B: Effect on survival of delays in referral of patients with breast-cancer symptoms: a retrospective analysis, *Lancet* 353:1132-1135, 1999.

Timing of surgery according to menstrual phase
A number of studies have reported that survival of breast cancer patients is greater if surgery takes place in the second half of the menstrual cycle. In some studies this effect was limited to node-positive patients, and in others it was related to the estrogen or progesterone receptor status or the size of the tumor.[1] Other studies have found no such correlation.[2] A recent report from the Memorial Sloan-Kettering Cancer Center in New York found that mortality was lowest when surgery was performed at the time of ovulation and highest when it was performed at or near the time of menstruation in women treated in the late 1970s and early 1980s but that no such correlation was evident in women treated in the late 1980s.[1]

During the menstrual cycle changes occur not only in estrogen and progesterone levels, but also in immune function, hepatic function, hemostasis, adhesion molecules, angiogenesis, and DNA repair. Theoretically any of these could contribute to tumor spread.[1]

At present there is no consensus on whether limiting breast cancer surgery to certain periods of the menstrual cycle decreases mortality.[1]

➤ REFERENCES ➤

1. Harlap S, Zauber AG, Pollack DM, et al: Survival of premenopausal women with breast carcinoma: effects of menstrual timing of surgery, *Cancer* 83:76-88, 1998.
2. Wobbes T, Thomas CM, Segers MF, et al: The phase of the menstrual cycle has no influence on the disease-free survival of patients with mammary carcinoma, *Br J Cancer* 69:599-600, 1994.

Lumpectomy and axillary node dissection
(See also adjuvant systemic therapy; practice patterns)

Numerous well-designed, randomized prospective trials of early-stage breast cancer have shown no differences in mortality rates between local tumor resection plus radiation therapy and modified radical mastectomy.[1] Thus with few exceptions, breast-conserving surgery followed by local radiation is the treatment of choice for women with stage I or II breast cancer whether or not the tumor is centrally located and whether or not axillary lymph nodes are involved. The presence of an implant is not a contraindication to local resection.[2] Radiation therapy is usually given 5 days a week (Monday through Friday) for 5 consecutive weeks. If both radiation therapy and chemotherapy (see later discussion) are to be given, chemotherapy is generally administered first.[1]

In patients with invasive breast cancer, axillary dissection has traditionally been considered essential for staging and for assessing the need for adjuvant hormonal or chemotherapy (see later discussion of adjuvant systemic therapy).[3] However, axillary dissection causes considerable morbidity, including lymphedema, numbness, pain, limitation of arm movement, and increased risk of infection.[4] In one study close to three fourths of women subjected to axillary node dissection experienced one or more of these symptoms even many years after the procedure.[5]

Since axillary dissection is associated with considerable morbidity and contributes little or nothing to decreasing mortality rates, alternatives are being sought. Women with infiltrating breast carcinomas smaller than 0.5 cm probably do not require axillary node dissection because they almost never have axillary metastases.[6] A novel surgical approach is to attempt to identify the node or nodes that receive the initial lymph drainage from the tumor (sentinel nodes). A colored dye or a radioactive material is injected in the region of the tumor, and at surgery one or a very few nodes that are colored or radioactive are selectively resected. If no tumor is found in the sentinel nodes, the chance that other nodes are involved is very small and axillary dissection can be avoided. The procedure is technically difficult and remains experimental.[7]

A more radical view is that axillary dissection is rarely indicated for patients with breast cancer because with the exception of women who have purely intraductal carcinomas or very small invasive cancers, all patients with breast cancer are given chemotherapy, hormonal therapy, or a combination of the two regardless of nodal status (see adjuvant systemic therapy below).[8,9]

Rates of local resection and of mastectomy for early stage breast cancer vary considerably among geographical regions (see discussion of practice patterns).

➤ REFERENCES ➤

1. Kotwall CA: Breast cancer treatment and chemoprevention, *Can Fam Physician* 45:1917-1924, 1999.
2. Margolese RG (Steering Committee on Clinical Practice Guidelines for the Care and Treatment of Breast Cancer): 3. Mastectomy or lumpectomy? The choice of operation for clinical stages I and II breast cancer, *Can Med Assoc J* 158(suppl 3):S15-S21, 1998.
3. McCready DR, Cantin J (Steering Committee on Clinical Practice Guidelines for the Care and Treatment of Breast Cancer): 4. Axillary dissection, *Can Med Assoc J* 158(suppl 3):S22-S26, 1998.
4. Warmuth MA, Bowen, Prosnitz LR, et al: Complications of axillary lymph node dissection for carcinoma of the breast: a report based on a patient survey, *Cancer* 83:1362-1368, 1998.
5. Hack TF, Katz J, Robson LS, et al: Physical and psychological morbidity after axillary lymph node dissection for breast cancer, *J Clin Oncol* 17:143-149, 1999.
6. Saiz E, Toonkel R, Poppiti RJ Jr, et al: Infiltrating breast carcinoma smaller than 0.5 centimeters: is lymph node dissection necessary? *Cancer* 85:2206-2211, 1999.
7. McMasters KM, Giuliano A, Ross MI, et al: Sentinel-lymph-node biopsy for breast cancer—not yet the standard of care, *N Engl J Med* 339:990-995, 1998.
8. Parmigiani G, Berry DA, Winer EP, et al: Is axillary lymph node dissection indicated for early-stage breast cancer? A decision analysis, *J Clin Oncol* 17:1465-1473, 1999.
9. Ganz PA: The quality of life after breast cancer—solving the problem of lymphedema (editorial), *N Engl J Med* 340:383-385, 1999.

Adjuvant systemic therapy
(See also lumpectomy and axillary node dissection)

Decisions about whether women with invasive breast cancer would benefit from adjuvant hormonal treatment or chemotherapy are based on numerous factors such as menopausal status, the presence or absence of axillary node metastases, tumor size, histological type, degree of anaplasia, and estrogen receptor status. Most patients with breast cancer benefit from one or a combination of these therapeutic modalities, with combination therapy generally giving superior results.[1,2] Polychemotherapy over a 3- to 6-month period has been shown to decrease both recurrence and mortality rates in premenopausal and postmenopausal women regardless of nodal status and whether they were taking tamoxifen. The absolute 10-year survival benefit for women over age 50 was 2% to 3%; it was considerably higher in premenopausal women.[2] Women who may not require adjuvant systemic therapy are those with purely intraductal cancers and those with negative axillary nodes who have only microinvasion or small tumors with favorable histological characteristics.[1]

Tamoxifen (Nolvadex) acts on breast tissue as an antiestrogenic agent and is the usual drug of choice when hormonal therapy is indicated. It has proved effective in premenopausal and postmenopausal women up to the age of 69 whose tumors are estrogen receptor positive; it is probably not indicated for estrogen receptor–negative tumors. The optimal duration of treatment is 5 years, and no further benefit is obtained by more prolonged administration.[1] The usual dose of tamoxifen is 20 mg/day. Side effects include hot flashes and irregular periods. The incidence of endometrial cancer is slightly increased, and the risk of thromboembolism is elevated to about that of women taking oral contraceptive pills.

Combination chemotherapy is generally given as four to six courses at intervals of 3 to 4 weeks. Standard protocols include fluorouracil, doxorubicin (Adriamycin), and cyclophosphamide (FAC); fluorouracil, epirubicin, and cyclophosphamide (FEC); doxorubicin and cyclophosphamide (AC); and cyclophosphamide, methotrexate, and fluorouracil (CMF). In one study the addition of four cycles of paclitaxel to the AC regimen improved survival.[1] A Dutch study found that 28% of women with breast cancer who had undergone six courses of CMF treatment had detectable cognitive impairments, compared with 12% in a control group of women with breast cancer who did not have postoperative chemotherapy.[3] Cognitive deficits were even more common in women with high-risk cancers who received high-dose adjuvant chemotherapy with hematopoietic rescue (see later discussion).

Patients with inflammatory breast cancer or with locally advanced tumors that have invaded the skin or chest wall should receive preoperative chemotherapy. This usually shrinks the tumors enough to make previously inoperable lesions resectable. The 10-year survival rate for these cancers is approximately 30%.[1]

Some centers are providing high-dose chemotherapy with hematopoietic rescue using autologous stored marrow or peripheral blood stem cells. This strategy allows much higher doses of chemotherapy than would otherwise be possible. It is used for high-risk patients with breast cancer, that is, those with multiple nodes involved or with inflammatory breast cancer. Whether such therapy is effective has not been determined.[5] One well-known complication of chemotherapy is cognitive deficits, which may have particular importance when very high doses are used.[4] Preliminary results of five trials released in 1999 reported benefits in one and no benefit in four.[6]

──────── ◣ REFERENCES ◢ ────────

1. Hortobagyi GN: Treatment of breast cancer, *N Engl J Med* 339:974-984, 1998.
2. Early Breast Cancer Trialists' Collaborative Group: Polychemotherapy for early breast cancer: an overview of the randomised trials, *Lancet* 352:930-942, 1998.
3. Schagen SB, van Dam FS, Muller MJ, et al: Cognitive deficits after postoperative adjuvant chemotherapy for breast carcinoma, *Cancer* 85:640-650, 1999.
4. van Dam FS, Schagen SB, Muller MJ, et al: Impairment of cognitive function in women receiving adjuvant treatment for high-risk breast cancer: high-dose versus standard-dose chemotherapy, *J Natl Cancer Inst* 90:210-218, 1998.
5. Ragaz J, Jackson SM, Le N, et al: Adjuvant radiotherapy and chemotherapy in node-positive premenopausal women with breast cancer, *N Engl J Med* 337:956-962, 1997.
6. Gottlieb S: Bone marrow transplants do not help in breast cancer, *BMJ* 318:1093, 1999.

Metastatic breast cancer
(See also osteoporosis; pain)

Initial systemic therapy for metastatic breast cancer is usually hormonal. First-line drugs in this class are the antiestrogens such as raloxifene (Evista) or toremifene (Fareston), second-line agents are aromatase inhibitors such as anastrozole (Arimidex), third-line are progestins such as megestrol (Megace), and fourth-line are androgens. When patients become refractory to hormonal treatment, chemotherapy is given. Standard protocols are cyclophosphamide, methotrexate, and fluorouracil (CMF) or doxorubicin (Adriamycin) and cyclophosphamide (AC). Second-line therapy often consists of paclitaxel (Taxol) or docetaxol (Taxotere); vinorelbine (Navelbine) may be used as third-line therapy.[1] One randomized prospective study of patients with metastatic breast cancer that compared low-dose single-agent therapy with standard drug combinations found no difference in survival between the two groups but an improved quality of life among those receiving the single agent.[2]

High-dose chemotherapy with hematopoietic rescue for patients with metastatic breast cancer has been evaluated in a few small studies; so far no survival benefit has been documented.[3]

Monthly 2-hour IV infusions of the bisphosphonate drug pamidronate (Aredia) in patients with breast cancer and bone metastases who were receiving chemotherapy resulted in later onset of skeletal complications, less bone pain, and better quality of life than in control subjects. Few adverse effects were reported.[4] Daily ingestion of another bisphosphonate, clodronate (Ostac), over a 2-year period by patients with breast cancer at high risk of metastases reduced the incidence of both bony and visceral metastases.[5]

──────── ◣ REFERENCES ◢ ────────

1. Hortobagyi GN: Treatment of breast cancer, *N Engl J Med* 339:974-984, 1998.
2. Joensuu H, Heikkinen M, Suonio E, et al: Combination chemotherapy versus single-agent therapy as first- and second-line treatment in metastatic breast cancer: a prospective randomized trial, *J Clin Oncol* 16:3720-3730, 1998.
3. Antman KH, Heitjan DF, Hortobagyi GN: High-dose chemotherapy for breast cancer, *JAMA* 282:1701-1703, 1999.

4. Theriault RL, Lipton A, Hortobagyi GN, et al: Pamidronate reduces skeletal morbidity in women with advanced breast cancer and lytic bone lesions: a randomized, placebo-controlled trial, *J Clin Oncol* 17:846-854, 1999.

5. Diel IJ, Solomayer E-F, Costa SD, et al: Reduction in new metastases in breast cancer with adjuvant clodronate treatment, *N Engl J Med* 339:357-363, 1998.

Hormone replacement therapy in patients with breast cancer

Hot flashes are often a greater problem for women with breast cancer than for other women because they can be precipitated or aggravated by chemotherapy that inhibits ovarian function or by the antiestrogenic effect of tamoxifen. Most authorities consider estrogen replacement therapy to be contraindicated in women who have had breast cancer, although this remains controversial.[1] A 1994 review of the literature on the subject did not find studies documenting adverse effects of giving estrogen replacement therapy to postmenopausal women who had had breast cancer.[2] Since then a number of other studies have not shown that estrogen replacement therapy increased breast cancer risk, but all have been small and many were retrospective evaluations. No large prospective randomized controlled trials dealing with this issue have been reported.[3]

One alternative to estrogens for controlling hot flashes in women who have had breast cancer is the use of a progestogen. In 1994 a short-term study of low-dose (20 mg bid) megestrol acetate (Megace) in women who had had breast cancer (and in men who had had orchiectomies) found that the control of hot flashes was equal to that reported for estrogen use. As with estrogens, the beneficial effect was often delayed until a few weeks after the beginning of treatment and commonly persisted for weeks after the drug was withdrawn. No significant side effects were found in this study except for a paradoxical increase in the amount of flushing in the first few days of treatment. Long-term adverse effects have not been determined. At the doses used, appetite was not stimulated.[4]

Another method of attempting to control hot flashes is the use of clonidine (Catapres, Dixarit) 0.025 mg, 2 tablets bid. Overall, this drug has not been very effective.[5]

◣ REFERENCES ◤

1. Carpenter JS, Andrykowski, Cordova M, et al: Hot flashes in postmenopausal women treated for breast carcinoma: prevalence, severity, correlates, management, and relation to quality of life, *Cancer* 82:1682-1691, 1998.

2. Cobleigh MA, Berris RF, Bush T, et al: Estrogen replacement therapy in breast cancer survivors: a time for change, *JAMA* 272:540-545, 1994.

3. Vassilopoulou-Sellin R, Asmar L, Hortobagyi GN, et al: Estrogen replacement therapy after localized breast cancer: clinical outcome of 319 women followed prospectively, *J Clin Oncol* 17:1482-1487, 1999.

4. Loprinzi CL, Michalak JC, Quella SK, et al: Megestrol acetate for the prevention of hot flashes, *N Engl J Med* 33:347-352, 1994.

5. Goldberg RM, Loprinzi CL, O'Fallon JR, et al: Transdermal clonidine for ameliorating tamoxifen-induced hot flashes, *J Clin Oncol* 12:155-158, 1994.

Pregnancy and invasive breast cancer

No evidence has shown that women who have invasive breast cancer diagnosed during pregnancy have a worse prognosis than do nonpregnant women.[1]

Numerous studies of patients with breast cancer who subsequently became pregnant have failed to demonstrate any adverse effect of pregnancy on prognosis. At present it seems advisable for women with stage I disease (tumor 2 cm or smaller and negative nodes) or stage II disease (tumor 2 cm or greater with or without movable axillary nodes, or movable axillary nodes but no palpable tumor) to delay pregnancy for 2 years simply because most tumor recurrences occur within that time period. Women with stage III disease (any local extension of tumor, or inflammatory breast cancer, or matted or fixed axillary nodes) should probably delay pregnancy for 5 years. Those with stage IV disease (distant metastases) should avoid pregnancy.[1]

Among women who have had breast cancer the fertility rate is decreased because of chemotherapy-induced ovarian dysfunction.[1]

◣ REFERENCES ◤

1. Averette HE, Mirhashemi R, Moffat FL: Pregnancy after breast carcinoma: the ultimate medical challenge, *Cancer* 85:2301-2304, 1999.

CARDIOVASCULAR SYSTEM

(See also congenital anomalies—congenital heart disease)

Topics covered in this section

Abdominal Aortic Aneurysm
Arrhythmias
Cardiac Arrest
Cardiomyopathy
Coronary Artery Disease
Electrocardiograms
Heart Failure
Hypertension
Valvular Heart Disease
Vascular Disease

ABDOMINAL AORTIC ANEURYSM
(See also attitudes, physician; informed consent; prevention; screening)

Smoking is a major risk factor for the development of abdominal aortic aneurysms.[1]

The rate of rupture increases significantly for aneurysms greater than 5 cm in diameter. In a Mayo Clinic population study of the yearly rate of rupture based on the size of aneurysm as determined by the last ultrasound, no ruptures occurred in those less than 4 cm and the rates were 1% for those 4 to 4.99 cm and 11% for those 5 to 5.99 cm. Rates of growth varied widely among individuals and from one period of time to another in the same individual. The authors recommended serial ultrasound examinations at annual intervals for aneurysms less than 4 cm in diameter and every 6 months for those between 4 and 5 cm. They also advised elective surgery once the aneurysm reached a diameter of 5 cm.[2] Although this is reasonable advice, Mason and associates[3] estimated that 72% of patients with untreated abdominal aortic aneurysms die of other causes and that operating on three individuals electively would be necessary to prevent one rupture.

The overall mortality rate for ruptured aortic aneurysms is about 80%. Two thirds of patients die before reaching the hospital, and of those who are operated on, more than one third die within 30 days.[4] In contrast, the operative mortality for elective resection of aneurysms is 5% to 6%.[5] A randomized controlled trial in the United Kingdom, in which open surgery was compared with ultrasonographic surveillance for aneurysms 4 to 5.5 cm in diameter, found no long-term benefit from surgery but a short-term survival disadvantage in that the 30-day mortality rate for the surgical patients was 5.8%.[5]

Endovascular grafting is a new method of controlling abdominal aortic aneurysms that is being developed in a number of specialized centers. In this procedure a graft is inserted via the femoral artery and is held in place by expandable stents. Only about half the patients with abdominal aortic aneurysms are suitable candidates for this procedure. Short- and medium-term results are comparable to those of open surgical repairs, but long-term results have not yet been reported.[6]

Although a number of vascular surgeons have advocated abdominal ultrasound screening, evidence supporting this is controversial. Mason and associates[3] recommend against it, not only because of the physical morbidity and mortality of surgery, but also because of the possible psychological harm to patients who are told they have an aneurysm, even if it is too small to warrant surgery at the time of diagnosis. The Canadian Task Force on Preventive Health Care[7] and the U.S. Preventive Services Task Force[8] give screening abdominal physical examination and screening abdominal ultrasound a "C" recommendation.

REFERENCES

1. Lederle FA, Johnson GR, Wilson SE, et al: Prevalence and associations of abdominal aortic aneurysm detected through screening, *Ann Intern Med* 126:441-449, 1997.
2. Reed WW, Hallett JW Jr, Damiano MA, et al: Learning from the last ultrasound: a population-based study of patients with abdominal aortic aneurysm, *Arch Intern Med* 157:2064-2068, 1997.
3. Mason JM, Wakeman AP, Drummond MF, et al: Population screening for abdominal aortic aneurysm: do the benefits outweigh the costs? *J Public Health Med* 15:154-160, 1993.
4. Norman PE, Semmens JB, Lawrence-Brown MM, et al: Long term relative survival after surgery for abdominal aortic aneurysm in Western Australia: population based study, *BMJ* 317:852-856, 1998.
5. UK Small Aneurysm Trial Participants: Mortality results for randomised controlled trial of early elective surgery or ultrasonographic surveillance for small abdominal aortic aneurysms, *Lancet* 352:1649-1655, 1998.
6. D'Ayala M, Hollier LH, Marin ML: Endovascular grafting for abdominal aortic aneurysms, *Surg Clin North Am* 78:845-862, 1998.
7. Canadian Task Force on the Periodic Health Examination: *Canadian guide to clinical preventive health care,* Ottawa, 1994, Canada Communication Group—Publishing, pp 672-678.
8. US Preventive Services Task Force: *Guide to clinical preventive services,* ed 2, Baltimore, 1996, Williams & Wilkins, pp 67-72.

ARRHYTHMIAS
Atrial Fibrillation
(See also anticoagulation; cerebrovascular accidents; subclinical hyperthyroidism; transient ischemic attacks)

Epidemiology and complications
The prevalence of atrial fibrillation in developed countries increases with age. Between 60 and 69 years of age the prevalence is 3% to 4%, whereas for those over 70 it is estimated to be 9%.[1] Most patients have underlying heart disease, such as coronary artery disease, valvular disease, or cardiomyopathy, or systemic disorders, such as alcohol excess or alcohol withdrawal, hyperthyroidism, cocaine or amphetamine intoxication, electrolyte imbalance, or the postoperative state.

The major complication of atrial fibrillation is stroke. In the pooled data of five randomized trials of patients with atrial fibrillation, the annual risk of stroke in patients younger than 65 with no risk factors was 1%, whereas it was 8.1% in patients older than 75 with one or more risk factors. The risk was the same whether atrial fibrillation was constant or paroxysmal. Risk factors include prosthetic valves, previous strokes or transient ischemic attacks, diabetes, hypertension, and coronary artery disease.[2] The risk of stroke in patients with lone atrial fibrillation is very low (see later discussion on lone atrial fibrillation).

A small pilot case-control study of patients who had non-valvular atrial fibrillation and were not taking anticoagulants found that those with fibrillation performed less well on a battery of neuropsychological tests than did control subjects with no fibrillation. The authors postulated that this may have been due to small subclinical cerebral infarcts in the group experiencing fibrillation.[3]

◣ REFERENCES ◢

1. Ezekowitz MD, Levine JA: Preventing stroke in patients with atrial fibrillation, *JAMA* 281:1830-1835, 1999.
2. Atrial Fibrillation Investigators: Risk factors for stroke and efficacy of antithrombotic therapy in atrial fibrillation: analysis of pooled data from five randomized controlled trials, *Arch Intern Med* 154:1449-1457, 1994.
3. O'Connell JE, Gray CS, French JM, et al: Atrial fibrillation and cognitive function: case-control study, *J Neurol Neurosurg Psychiatry* 65:386-389, 1998.

Rate control and cardioversion

The rapid rate that often occurs with atrial fibrillation can be controlled with pharmacological or electrical conversion to sinus rhythm, often with maintenance pharmacotherapy, or by rate control alone without attempting to convert to sinus rhythm. Although conversion to sinus rhythm might seem the optimal approach, this has not been proved to decrease morbidity or mortality. Furthermore, any antiarrhythmic drug may be toxic. Three randomized trials to resolve this issue are in progress.[1]

If cardioversion is planned for new-onset atrial fibrillation, it is important to realize that up to half the patients will revert to sinus rhythm spontaneously. The success of cardioversion by whatever means is better if the arrhythmia is treated within 24 to 48 hours of onset.[2,3] A variety of pharmacological agents are effective for restoring sinus rhythm; all are potentially toxic. Examples are class IA agents such as quinidine or procainamide (Pronestyl), class IC agents such as flecainide (Tambocor) or propafenone (Rythmol), and the class III agent ibutilide (Corvert). Amiodarone (Cordarone) and sotalol (Betapace, Sotacor), which are also class III agents, do not appear to be effective in converting recent-onset atrial fibrillation. Digoxin (Lanoxin) is also ineffective for this purpose.[1] An alternative to pharmacological cardioversion is electrical rhythm reversion, which is effective in up to 90% of patients.[2]

Since one of the major complications of cardioversion by any method is systemic embolization, current guidelines advise anticoagulation before and after the procedure, even though scant evidence supports or refutes this approach.[3] The American College of Chest Physicians recommends that patients who have had fibrillation for more than 24 to 48 hours and who do not require emergency cardioversion be given anticoagulants for 3 weeks before cardioversion is undertaken and for 4 weeks after it has been accomplished.[4]

The value of attempting to maintain sinus rhythm with pharmacological agents is controversial. Without treatment, only about one fourth of patients who have successfully un-

dergone cardioversion will remain in sinus rhythm after 1 year, whereas with maintenance antiarrhythmic drugs about half will still be in sinus rhythm after 1 year.[2] Quinidine has been associated with an increased death rate and is no longer used for maintenance purposes. Unfortunately, all the other drugs also have adverse effects, and whether it is better to use maintenance pharmacotherapy or simply to control the rate and give anticoagulants is unknown.[2,3]

If anticoagulation and rate control are the goals of therapy, the drug of choice is a beta-blocker or either of the calcium channel blockers verapamil (Isoptin, Calan) or diltiazem (Cardizem). Amiodarone also controls the atrial fibrillation rate in maintenance doses of about 200 mg/day, but it is not widely used because of potential adverse effects, especially pulmonary toxicity.[5] Digoxin is not a good drug for rate control; although it controls resting rate, it does not control the rate when sympathetic tone is increased as during acute illness, thyrotoxicosis, or exercise. For patients whose rate cannot be adequately controlled with medications, radiofrequency energy applied to the atrioventricular node via an intracardiac catheter may modify the node sufficiently to control the ventricular rate in 75% of cases; in the remainder, complete atrioventricular block results and a permanent pacemaker is required.[6]

◣ REFERENCES ◢

1. Dell'Orfano JT, Luck JC, Wolbrette DL, et al: Drugs for conversion of atrial fibrillation, *Am Fam Physician* 58:471-480, 1998.
2. Masoudi FA, Goldschlager N: The medical management of atrial fibrillation, *Cardiol Clin* 15:689-719, 1997.
3. Jung F, DiMarco JP: Antiarrhythmic drug therapy in the treatment of atrial fibrillation, *Cardiol Clin* 14:507-520, 1996.
4. Laupacis A, Albers G, Dalen J, et al: Antithrombotic therapy in atrial fibrillation, *Chest* 108(suppl 4):352S-359S, 1995.
5. Antman EM: Maintaining sinus rhythm with antifibrillatory drugs in atrial fibrillation, *Am J Cardiol* 78(suppl 4):67-72, 1996.
6. Morady F: Radio-frequency ablation as treatment for cardiac arrhythmias, *N Engl J Med* 340:534-544, 1999.

Anticoagulation and aspirin
(See also anticoagulants; cerebrovascular accidents)

Numerous clinical trials have conclusively shown that warfarin (Coumadin) in doses adjusted to maintain the international normalized ratio (INR) between 2 and 3 helps to prevent strokes in patients with atrial fibrillation. Fixed low-dose warfarin that maintains INR levels below 2 is not effective, nor are combinations of fixed low-dose warfarin and aspirin.[1]

The greatest risk with warfarin therapy is major hemorrhage, and this increases with age and INR levels above 3. In the Stroke Prevention in Atrial Fibrillation (SPAF) II trial the incidence of intracerebral hemorrhage was high enough nearly to offset the benefits, particularly in those over the age of 75, but in almost all cases where this occurred the INR was above 3.[2] A Danish study found that among patients receiving adjusted-dose warfarin aimed at maintaining the INR between 2 and 3, the annual rate of major bleeding was 1.1%, which was not significantly different from the rate in patients treated only with aspirin. In this study age was not a risk factor for major bleeding in patients taking warfarin.[3] Aside from INR above 3, recognized risk factors for hemorrhage are a past history of serious gastrointestinal bleeding, alcoholism, use of NSAIDs, and poor compliance with medications. Risk of falling has often been seen as a contraindication to anticoagulation. According to one decision analysis, if possible falling is the only contraindication, the benefits of warfarin far outweigh the risks, even in those over 75 years of age.[4]

In general, an INR of 2 is equivalent to a prothrombin time (PT) of 1.3, an INR of 3 to a PT of 1.5, and an INR of 4 to a PT of 2.

An overview of studies that evaluated the role of aspirin in preventing stroke in patients with atrial fibrillation concluded that although less effective than warfarin, aspirin reduced the risk of stroke by about 21%, with no clear relationship to dose.[5] A 1999 metaanalysis of the Cochrane database came to similar conclusions about aspirin but noted that it primarily prevented nondisabling strokes; benefits from warfarin were much greater than those achieved with aspirin and were particularly marked in patients who had had a previous stroke or transient ischemic attack.[6]

The risk of stroke in patients with atrial fibrillation increases greatly if the patient is older than 75 years or has comorbid conditions such as a previous stroke or transient ischemic attack, coronary artery disease, heart failure, previous hypertension, diabetes, mitral stenosis, prosthetic heart valves, or thyrotoxicosis. The risk is particularly high if the patient has several of these comorbid conditions. Unless warfarin is strictly contraindicated, it should be given to patients with comorbid conditions.[1]

Patients with lone atrial fibrillation (no associated hypertension, cardiac disease, or pulmonary disease) who are under 60 years of age do not require antithrombotic treatment; those over 60 should probably receive aspirin or warfarin, with the choice determined by the number of other risk factors for stroke the patient may have.[7] The value of aspirin for such patients is supported by a randomized controlled trial of elderly low-risk patients with atrial fibrillation recruited from Dutch general practices; aspirin was as effective as standard-dose warfarin in preventing strokes and vascular deaths.[8]

Warfarin's role in treating atrial fibrillation in the very elderly has not been established. According to Ackermann,[9] no study has shown that warfarin is more beneficial than aspirin for persons over the age of 80. He suggests that in this age group anticoagulation may cause more harm than good. In contrast English and Channer[10] and Gulløv and coworkers[3] believe that all patients with fibrillation should receive anticoagulants regardless of age, unless they have absolute contraindications.

❧ REFERENCES ❧

1. Albers GW: Choice of antithrombotic therapy for stroke prevention in atrial fibrillation: warfarin, aspirin, or both? *Arch Intern Med* 158:1487-1491, 1998.
2. Stroke Prevention in Atrial Fibrillation Investigators: Warfarin versus aspirin for prevention of thromboembolism in atrial fibrillation: Stroke Prevention in Atrial Fibrillation II Study, *Lancet* 343:687-691, 1994.
3. Gulløv AL, Koefoed BG, Petersen P: Bleeding during warfarin and aspirin therapy in patients with atrial fibrillation: the AFASAK 2 study, *Arch Intern Med* 159:1322-1328, 1999.
4. Man-Son-Hing M, Nichol G, Lau A, et al: Choosing antithrombotic therapy for elderly patients with atrial fibrillation who are at risk for falls, *Arch Intern Med* 159:677-685, 1999.
5. Atrial Fibrillation Investigators: The efficacy of aspirin in patients with atrial fibrillation, *Arch Intern Med* 157:1237-1240, 1997.
6. Hart RG, Benavente O, McBride R, et al: Antithrombotic therapy to prevent stroke in patients with atrial fibrillation: a meta-analysis, *Ann Intern Med* 131:492-501, 1999.
7. Kopecky SL, Gersh BJ, McGoon MD, et al: Lone atrial fibrillation in elderly persons: a marker for cardiovascular risk, *Arch Intern Med* 159:1118-1122, 1999.
8. Hellemons BS, Langenberg M, Lodder J, et al: Primary prevention of arterial thromboembolism in non-rheumatic atrial fibrillation in primary care: randomised controlled trial comparing two intensities of coumarin with aspirin, *BMJ* 319:958-964, 1999.
9. Ackermann RJ: Anticoagulant therapy in patients aged 80 years or more with atrial fibrillation: more caution is needed (editorial), *Arch Fam Med* 6:105-110, 1997.
10. English KM, Channer KS: Managing atrial fibrillation in elderly people (editorial), *BMJ* 318:1088-1089, 1999.

Paroxysmal Atrial Fibrillation

Paroxysmal atrial fibrillation makes up over 40% of cases of fibrillation, but it has not been as well studied as persistent atrial fibrillation. From the evidence available it seems prudent to treat paroxysmal atrial fibrillation in a manner identical to persistent atrial fibrillation.[1] Sotalol has generally been considered the drug of choice for paroxysmal atrial fibrillation, but a comparative crossover study of sotalol 80 mg bid and atenolol 50 mg once daily found that they were equally effective in diminishing the number and frequency of episodes of fibrillation.[2] Digoxin should not be used for patients with paroxysmal atrial fibrillation, since it does not reduce the frequency of episodes or control the heart rate during attacks. Digoxin is contraindicated in patients with Wolff-Parkinson-White syndrome.[3]

❧ REFERENCES ❧

1. Aboaf AP, Wolf PS: Paroxysmal atrial fibrillation: a common but neglected entity, *Arch Intern Med* 156:362-367, 1996.

2. Steeds RP, Birchall AS, Smith M, et al: An open label, random-ised, crossover study comparing sotalol and atenolol in the treatment of symptomatic paroxysmal atrial fibrillation, *Heart* 82:170-175, 1999.

3. Masoudi FA, Goldschlager N: The medical management of atrial fibrillation, *Cardiol Clin* 15:689-719, 1997.

Supraventricular Arrhythmias
(See also palpitations)

Two thirds of cases of paroxysmal supraventricular tachy-cardia are atrioventricular nodal reentrant tachycardias, and most of the remainder are due to an accessory atrioventric-ular pathway. Radiofrequency ablation under fluoroscopic control is effective and has few adverse effects in the vast majority of cases.[1,2] Radiofrequency ablation is also effec-tive in patients with Wolff-Parkinson-White syndrome and in many cases of atrial flutter.[1]

◼ REFERENCES ◼

1. Morady F: Radio-frequency ablation as treatment for cardiac arrhythmias, *N Engl J Med* 340:534-544, 1999.

2. Calkins H, Yong P, Miller JM, et al: Catheter ablation of acces-sory pathways, atrioventricular nodal reentrant tachycardia, and the atrioventricular junction: final results of a prospective, mul-ticenter clinical trial, *Circulation* 99:262-270, 1999.

Pacemakers and Implantable Defibrillators
(See also cardiac arrest)

Rapid advances in technology have led to the develop-ment of single-lead cardioverter-defibrillators. The genera-tor for these devices is usually implanted in the left pectoral area, and access to the heart is obtained via the left subcla-vian vein. Cardioverter-defibrillators are used primarily for patients with life-threatening ventricular arrhythmias. The apparatus can sense heart rates and institute a variety of re-medial maneuvers. It can provide demand ventricular pac-ing in cases of bradycardia; when tachycardia is detected, it can institute competitive rapid pacing to interrupt the reen-try circuit, or if that fails, it can defibrillate the heart.[1] Com-parative studies have shown that cardioverter-defibrillators are more effective than antiarrhythmic drugs.[1,2]

Patients with cardioverter-defibrillators are usually exam-ined every 3 to 4 months in a cardiac electrophysiology laboratory where the device is "interrogated" by means of a wand placed over the generator.

Patients may detect shocks from the device. In general an isolated shock can be assessed electively in the cardiac labo-ratory, but repetitive shocks require emergency assessment.[1]

Most household electromagnetic devices such as mi-crowave ovens do not adversely affect cardioverter-defibrillators, but large industrial motors and arc welding equipment may do so.[1] Cellular telephones can interfere with implanted pacemaker functions when held over the pacemaker, but holding the phone over the ear does not cause problems.[3]

Patients with implantable defibrillators have reportedly suffered syncope and shocks as a result of standing for a while close to electronic surveillance equipment in stores. Simply walking by the equipment seems to be safe.[4]

◼ REFERENCES ◼

1. Groh WJ, Foreman LD, Zipes D: Advances in the treatment of arrhythmias: implantable cardioverter-defibrillators, *Am Fam Physician* 57:297-307, 1998.

2. Antiarrhythmics Versus Implantable Defibrillators (AVID) In-vestigators: A comparison of antiarrhythmic drug therapy with implantable defibrillators in patients resuscitated from near-fatal ventricular arrhythmias, *N Engl J Med* 337:1576-1583, 1997.

3. Hayes DL, Wang PJ, Reynolds DW, et al: Interference with car-diac pacemakers by cellular telephones, *N Engl J Med* 336:1473-1479, 1997.

4. Santucci PA, Haw J, Trohman RG, et al: Interference with an implantable defibrillator by an electronic antitheft-surveillance device, *N Engl J Med* 339:1371-1374, 1998.

Palpitations

Palpitations are common presenting complaints in primary care; in one general medical outpatient clinic they were noted in 16% of patients.[1] In a Harvard study of 130 patients who were referred for Holter monitoring because of palpita-tions, the group had a 28% lifetime prevalence of panic dis-order, which was six times the rate in control subjects.[2]

Although anxiety disorders may cause palpitations, par-oxysmal supraventricular tachycardia may mimic the symp-toms of panic disorder.[3] In one study of patients with con-firmed supraventricular tachycardia, two thirds of the patients met the criteria for panic disorder given in the *Di-agnostic and Statistical Manual of Mental Disorders,* edi-tion 4 *(DSM-IV).* Frequent symptoms included dizziness, shortness of breath, sweating, chest pain, fear of dying, flushing, tremulousness, and numbness. After definitive therapy, usually radiofrequency ablation, only 11% of pa-tients whose symptoms had originally fulfilled the diagnos-tic criteria of panic disorder continued to experience such symptoms.[3]

The diagnosis of paroxysmal supraventricular tachycar-dia is usually easy if an electrocardiogram (ECG) can be obtained during an episode; otherwise it is difficult. The resting ECG of some patients may exhibit the delta-wave typical of Wolff-Parkinson-White syndrome, but this is rela-tively uncommon. Holter monitoring, which records and saves all data over a 24-hour period, detects only a few cases because most patients do not have episodes of tachy-cardia during the monitoring period.[3] An alternative is the continuous-loop recorder, which the patient wears for up to 2 weeks. Data are monitored continuously but are saved for later analysis only if the patient manually activates the sys-tem when symptoms occur.[4]

Most ambulatory patients investigated for palpitations are found to have either normal sinus rhythm or benign atrial or ventricular ectopy. The treatment of choice for these conditions is reassurance; in a few instances beta-blockers are needed. Most cases of supraventricular tachycardia and several variants of ventricular tachycardia are curable with radiofrequency ablation.[4]

REFERENCES

1. Kroenke K, Arrington ME, Mangelsdorff AD: The prevalence of symptoms in medical outpatients and the adequacy of therapy, *Arch Intern Med* 150:1685-1689, 1990.
2. Barsky AJ, Cleary PD, Coeytaux RR, et al: The clinical course of palpitations in medical outpatients, *Arch Intern Med* 155:1782-1788, 1995.
3. Lessmeier TJ, Gamperling D, Johnson V, et al: Unrecognized paroxysmal supraventricular tachycardia: potential for misdiagnosis as panic disorder, *Arch Intern Med* 157:537-543, 1997.
4. Zimetbaum P, Josephson ME: Evaluation of patients with palpitations, *N Engl J Med* 338:1369-1373, 1998.

CARDIAC ARREST

(See also aviation medicine; exercise; heart failure; informed consent; pacemakers and implantable defibrillators; sports medicine; sudden infant death syndrome)

Ventricular arrhythmia resulting from coronary artery disease causes 80% of sudden cardiac deaths. Beta-blockers have a significant protective effect against this event in both hypertensive and post–myocardial infarction patients.[1] Beta-blockers are also protective against sudden cardiac death in patients with congestive heart failure.[2] For patients with previous documented ventricular tachycardia or ventricular fibrillation, an implantable cardioverter defibrillator is generally the treatment of choice.[2]

Numerous cohort studies have examined the relationship of fish consumption and sudden cardiac death. Most have shown a decrease in sudden cardiac deaths among those who ate fish as infrequently as once a week or even once a month, but no decrease in nonfatal cardiac events. A plausible explanation is that n-3 polyunsaturated fatty acids or some other component of fish is antiarrhythmic. On the basis of this evidence it seems reasonable to recommend that everyone eat fish once a week and that patients with cardiac disease have two helpings of fish a week.[3] Moderate leisure activity such as walking or gardening has also been shown to decrease the risk of primary cardiac arrest.[4]

Hospitalized elderly patients with acute medical problems have a 10% to 17% chance of surviving to discharge after a cardiopulmonary resuscitation (CPR), although if they have chronic illnesses associated with a life expectancy of less than 1 year their chance is less than 5%.[5] Some studies have found that even after a successful resuscitation, close to half the survivors have significant residual functional deficits,[6] whereas others report that 75% of survivors are able to live independently.[7]

Patients grossly overestimate their chances of recovery; in requesting advance directives, physicians and hospitals must give them accurate data so that they can give reasonable informed consent.[5] A factor contributing to their overly optimistic expectations of CPR may be the messages received from U.S. television programs such as *ER, Chicago Hope,* and *Rescue 911,* which portray an inordinately high success rate for resuscitation.[8] The major British medical television dramas *Casualty, Cardiac Arrest,* and *Medics* seem to give a more realistic perspective on the outcomes of this intervention.[9]

The results of resuscitation in nursing homes are abysmal, with virtually no long-term survivors. For the very few who survive to discharge, quality of life is awful.[10]

Reported overall survival rates after cardiac arrests outside of hospitals vary from 1.4% to 18%.[11] Results are slightly better if a bystander has initiated CPR[11,12] but markedly better if the arrest was witnessed by paramedics equipped with defibrillators.[12] A Scottish study found that about 40% of patients who had been successfully resuscitated away from a hospital were discharged without significant neurological sequelae.[13] Current evidence suggests that although both ventilation and external chest compression should be given in cases of arrest outside the hospital, chest compression alone can give good results.[11]

The automatic external defibrillator is a recent advance in CPR. This device, which is applied to a patient with no clinically detected pulse, senses cardiac rhythm and, if it detects a rapid ventricular tachycardia or ventricular fibrillation, automatically delivers a countershock.[11]

A study from the Hospital for Sick Children in Toronto found that only 15% of children with out-of-hospital cardiac or respiratory arrests who were resuscitated in the emergency room survived to discharge and that all of the survivors were left with neurological deficits. The authors concluded that except for cases of severe hypothermia or episodes of recurrent (as opposed to persistent) arrest, continuation of resuscitation for out-of-hospital cardiac arrests is futile after 20 minutes or after the two doses of epinephrine have been administered.[14]

Most advance directives made by ambulatory patients are inaccessible to the health care team when a patient is transferred to a hospital and are therefore not used.[15]

REFERENCES

1. Kendall MJ, Lynch KP, Hjalmarson A, et al: Beta-blockers and sudden cardiac death, *Ann Intern Med* 123:358-367, 1995.
2. Goldberger JJ: Treatment and prevention of sudden cardiac death: effect of recent clinical trials, *Arch Intern Med* 159:1281-1287, 1999.
3. Kromhout D: Fish consumption and sudden cardiac death (editorial), *JAMA* 279:65-66, 1998.
4. Lemaitre RN, Siscovick DS, Raghunathan TE, et al: Leisure-time physical activity and the risk of primary cardiac arrest, *Arch Intern Med* 159:686-690, 1999.
5. Murphy DJ, Burrows D, Santilli S, et al: The influence of the probability of survival on patients' preferences regarding cardiopulmonary resuscitation, *N Engl J Med* 330:545-549, 1994.

6. FitzGerald JD, Wenger NS, Califf RM, et al: Functional status among survivors of in-hospital cardiopulmonary resuscitation, *Arch Intern Med* 156:72-76, 1996.

7. de Vos R, de Haes HC, Koster RW, et al: Quality of survival after cardiopulmonary resuscitation, *Arch Intern Med* 159:249-254, 1999.

8. Diem SJ, Lantos JD, Tulsky JA: Cardiopulmonary resuscitation on television: miracles and misinformation, *N Engl J Med* 334:1578-1582, 1996.

9. Gordon PN, Williamson S, Lawler PG: As seen on TV: observational study of cardiopulmonary resuscitation in British television medical dramas, *BMJ* 317:780-783, 1998.

10. Awoke S, Mouton CP, Parrott M: Outcomes of skilled cardiopulmonary resuscitation in a long-term-care facility: futile therapy? *J Am Geriatr Soc* 40:593-595, 1992.

11. Ballew KA: Cardiopulmonary resuscitation, *BMJ* 324:1462-1465, 1997.

12. Norris RM (United Kingdom Heart Attack Study Collaborative Group): Fatality outside hospital from acute coronary events in three British health districts, 1994-5, *BMJ* 316:1065-1070, 1998.

13. Cobbe SM, Dalziel K, Ford I, et al: Survival of 1476 patients initially resuscitated from out of hospital cardiac arrest, *BMJ* 312:1633-1637, 1996.

14. Schindler MB, Bohn D, Cox PN, et al: Outcome of out-of-hospital cardiac or respiratory arrest in children, *N Engl J Med* 335:1473-1479, 1996.

15. Morrison RS, Olson E, Mertz KR, et al: The inaccessibility of advance directives on transfer from ambulatory to acute care settings, *JAMA* 274:478-482, 1995.

CARDIOMYOPATHY
Hypertrophic Cardiomyopathy

In recent years the diagnosis of asymptomatic hypertrophic cardiomyopathy through molecular genetic assays has become possible. As a result of such studies, it has become clear that the disorder is more common (1:500) than was previously thought and that most patients have no or only mild symptoms. When annual mortality rates are calculated for unselected patients (in contrast to those from tertiary referral centers), they are about 1% or less[1]; this is about the expected mortality of the general population.[2]

Hypertrophic cardiomyopathy is not always a progressive disease, and in some patients the symptoms abate over time. Prognostic indicators of a more severe course are advanced symptoms at the time of diagnosis, atrial fibrillation, basal outflow obstruction, severe ventricular hypertrophy, nonsustained ventricular tachycardia on Holter monitoring, family history of premature deaths from this disorder, and prior cardiac arrest.[2]

The drugs of choice for patients with hypertrophic cardiomyopathy who are in heart failure are beta-blockers or verapamil (Calan, Covera-HS, Isoptin). Both slow the heart, and the prolonged diastole allows increased filling of the ventricles. However, these drugs do not protect patients against sudden death.[1] Prophylactic drugs have not shown value in asymptomatic or mildly symptomatic patients.

These patients should be encouraged to lead normal lives, but intense physical training or competitive athletics should probably be discouraged.[1] A few patients appear to benefit from antiarrhythmic agents such as amiodarone (Cordarone), implantable cardioverter-defibrillators, or heart transplants.[2]

Dilated Cardiomyopathy

Idiopathic dilated cardiomyopathy is the major indication for heart transplantation in both adults and children. The condition is 2.5 times as common in males as in females, and 2.5 times as common in blacks as in whites. The disorder may develop in children or the elderly, but most patients are between 20 and 50 years of age. At the time of clinical presentation, heart failure is usually advanced.[3] Dilated cardiomyopathy develops in about 8% of HIV-positive patients; this appears to result from a virus-induced myocarditis in most cases.[4]

The prognosis of dilated cardiomyopathy is variable. Some patients remain stable for years, and others have a progressive downhill course. The average 5-year mortality is about 20%.[3] An observational cohort study found that adding metoprolol (Lopressor) to the usual treatment with angiotensin-converting enzyme (ACE) inhibitors and diuretics reduced mortality and the need for cardiac transplantation.[5]

━━━━━━━━━━ ◤ REFERENCES ◢ ━━━━━━━━━━

1. Spirito P, Seidman CE, McKenna WJ, et al: The management of hypertrophic cardiomyopathy, *N Engl J Med* 336:775-785, 1997.

2. Maron BJ, Casey SA, Poliac LC, et al: Clinical course of hypertrophic cardiomyopathy in a regional United States cohort, *JAMA* 281:650-655, 1999.

3. Dec GW, Fuster V: Idiopathic dilated cardiomyopathy, *N Engl J Med* 331:1564-1575, 1994.

4. Barbaro G, Di Lorenzo G, Grisorio B, et al: Incidence of dilated cardiomyopathy and detection of HIV in myocardial cells of HIV-positive patients, *N Engl J Med* 339:1093-1099, 1998.

5. Di Lenarda A, Gavazzi MA, Gregori D, et al: Long term survival effect of metoprolol in dilated cardiomyopathy, *Heart* 79:337-344, 1998.

CORONARY ARTERY DISEASE
(See also cardiac arrest; gastroesophageal reflux)

Over the last three decades the mortality rate from coronary artery disease has decreased by 2% to 4% per year in the United States. About one fourth of the decline can be attributed to primary prevention and three fourths to secondary prevention and improved treatment.[1]

━━━━━━━━━━ ◤ REFERENCES ◢ ━━━━━━━━━━

1. Hunink MG, Goldman L, Tosteson AN, et al: The recent decline in mortality from coronary heart disease, 1980-1990: the effect of secular trends in risk factors and treatment, *JAMA* 277:535-542, 1997.

Risk Factors for Coronary Artery Disease

(See also cardiac arrest; exercise; gastroesophageal reflux; hypertension; lipids; menopause; myocardial infarction; obesity; polycystic ovarian syndrome; poverty; smoking; vitamins)

The major established risk factors for coronary artery disease are age, male sex, family history, smoking, obesity, hypertension, physical inactivity, diabetes mellitus, elevated cholesterol, elevated low-density lipoprotein-cholesterol (LDL-C), and reduced high-density lipoprotein-cholesterol (HDL-C).[1] Other proven or putative risk factors are poverty; diet; elevated triglyceride levels; polycystic ovarian syndrome; elevated serum homocysteine levels; low serum levels of certain B vitamins; *Chlamydia pneumoniae, Helicobacter pylori,* and cytomegalovirus infections; peripheral vascular disease; sexual intercourse; cocaine use; oral contraceptives in smokers; and depression. Many of these are discussed elsewhere in the text; some are considered below.

The single biggest risk for coronary artery disease is being human. As Rose[2] pointed out, the most common cause of death in men with no apparent risk factors for coronary artery disease is coronary artery disease, and coronary artery disease is also the leading cause of death among U.S. women.[3] Women tend to acquire coronary artery disease 10 years later than men, but once women have had a myocardial infarction, their overall prognosis is worse than that of men. Female diabetics are more prone to coronary artery disease than are male diabetics, and women smokers have a higher risk of coronary artery disease than do men smokers.[4]

Another important risk factor is poverty.[5] Epidemiological evidence also suggests that diets low in fish[6] or fiber (fruits, vegetables, and particularly cereals)[7] and the presence of peripheral vascular disease[8] are risk factors.

Children with homocystinuria have marked elevations of plasma homocysteine and suffer from premature vascular disease.[9] A number of epidemiological studies have documented an association between elevated plasma homocysteine levels (normal fasting levels are 5 to 15 μmol/L) and coronary artery disease, cerebrovascular accidents, and peripheral vascular disease.[9] It has been postulated that homocysteine might lead to atherosclerosis through its ability to damage endothelium (see discussion of lipids).[10] Although vitamin supplements, particularly of folic acid, reduce plasma homocysteine levels, whether elevated homocysteine levels promote atherogenesis or whether lowering homocysteine levels decreases cardiovascular morbidity or mortality is unknown.[9]

In the Nurses' Health Study, women taking more than 400 μg of folate and more than 3 mg of vitamin B$_6$ per day had the lowest rates of coronary artery disease.[11] In view of the proven benefits of a daily supplement of 400 μg of folate in preventing congenital anomalies in pregnant women, as well as the possibility that such supplements might decrease the risk of vascular disease, one editorial writer recommends that all adults take a daily multivitamin containing 400 μg of folic acid.[12] As might be expected with such a controversial issue, another writer voices skepticism about such an approach.[13] (The mandatory fortification of cereals with folate in the United States may not replace the need for a vitamin supplement because cereal often contains as little as 100 μg of folate per serving.[12])

The American Heart Association opposes screening the general population for elevated plasma levels of homocysteine but acknowledges that some researchers test "high-risk patients." If elevated homocysteine levels are to be treated, the initial recommendation is a diet rich in folic acid and vitamins B$_6$ and B$_{12}$. If that is ineffective, multivitamins containing 400 μg of folic acid, 2 mg of vitamin B$_6$, and 6 μg of vitamin B$_{12}$ are prescribed.[9]

Increasing evidence indicates that inflammation plays an important role in the development of atherosclerosis, and some studies have suggested that infection with *Chlamydia pneumoniae,* cytomegalovirus, or *Helicobacter pylori* may be the etiological factor responsible for such inflammation.[14] Antibodies to *C. pneumoniae*[15] and *H. pylori*[16] have been reported to be more common in patients who have had myocardial infarctions than in control subjects, monocytes containing *C. pneumoniae* have been identified in atherosclerotic plaques,[17] and a case-control study of patients after a first-time acute myocardial infarction found that they were less likely to have taken tetracyclines or quinolones in the previous 3 years than were control subjects.[18] On the other hand, a prospective nested case-control study of women found no association between imunoglobulin G antibody titers to *C. pneumoniae, H. pylori,* herpes simplex virus, or cytomegalovirus and the risk of cardiovascular disease.[19] At present the evidence supporting chronic infection as a cause of coronary artery disease is provocative but unproved,[14-19] and evidence is insufficient to recommend antibiotics as a means of preventing coronary artery disease.[14,18,19]

The absolute risk that sexual intercourse will trigger myocardial infarction in a healthy individual is about 1 in 1 million, while for someone who has had a previous infarct it is about 20 per million. Regular exercise reduces these minimal risks even further for both healthy persons and post–myocardial infarction patients.[20]

Cocaine use may lead to myocardial infarction within an hour by causing vasospasm, platelet aggregation, and increased myocardial oxygen demand. Questions about use of cocaine should be asked of all patients seeking treatment for chest pain thought to be of cardiogenic origin.[21]

Psychosocial factors may alter risk factors for coronary artery disease by affecting health-related behaviors such as smoking and exercise (in most studies considered to be confounding variables), through direct pathophysiological changes, or by altering access to and quality of medical care. A systematic review of prospective cohort studies suggests that type A personality, hostility, depression, anxiety, work stress, and poor social supports are associated with increased risk of coronary artery disease. Among patients with known coronary artery disease all these factors except type A personality are associated with a worse prognosis.[22]

Risk assessment protocols for cholesterol screening and the treatment of dyslipidemias are discussed in the section on lipids.

≥ REFERENCES ≤

1. Hoeg JM: Evaluating coronary heart disease risk: tiles in the mosaic, *JAMA* 277:1387-1390, 1997.
2. Rose G: High-risk and population strategies of prevention: ethical considerations, *Ann Med* 21:409-413, 1989.
3. Mosca L, Grundy SM, Judelson D, et al: Guide to preventive cardiology for women, *Circulation* 99:2480-2484, 1999.
4. Thomas JL, Braus PA: Coronary artery disease in women: a historical perspective, *Arch Intern Med* 158:333-337, 1998.
5. Morrison C, Woodward M, Leslie W, et al: Effect of socioeconomic group on incidence of, management of, and survival after myocardial infarction and coronary death: analysis of community coronary event register, *BMJ* 314:541-546, 1997.
6. Daviglus ML, Stamler J, Orencia A, et al: Fish consumption and the 30-year risk of fatal myocardial infarction, *N Engl J Med* 336:1046-1053, 1997.
7. Rimm EB, Ascherio A, Giovannucci E, et al: Vegetable, fruit, and cereal fiber intake and risk of coronary heart disease among men, *JAMA* 275:447-451, 1996.
8. McKenna M, Wolfson S, Kuller L: The ratio of ankle and arm arterial pressure as an independent predictor of mortality, *Atherosclerosis* 87:119-128, 1991.
9. Malinow MR, Bostom AG, Krauss RM: Homocyst(e)ine, diet, and cardiovascular diseases: a statement for healthcare professionals from the Nutrition Committee, American Heart Association, *Circulation* 99:178-182, 1999.
10. Nappo F, De Rosa N, Marfella R, et al: Impairment of endothelial functions by acute hyperhomocysteinemia and reversal by antioxidant vitamins, *JAMA* 281:2113-2118, 1999.
11. Rimm EB, Willett WC, Hu FB, et al: Folate and vitamin B_6 from diet and supplements in relation to risk of coronary heart disease among women, *JAMA* 279:359-364, 1998.
12. Oakley GP Jr: Eat right and take a multivitamin (editorial), *N Engl J Med* 338:1060-1061, 1998.
13. Kuller LH, Evans RW: Homocysteine, vitamins, and cardiovascular disease (editorial), *Circulation* 98:196-199, 1998.
14. Folsom AR: Antibiotics for prevention of myocardial infarction? Not yet! *JAMA* 281:461-462, 1999.
15. Strachan DP, Carrington D, Mendall MA, et al: Relation of *Chlamydia pneumoniae* serology to mortality and incidence of ischaemic heart disease over 13 years in the Caerphilly prospective heart disease study, *BMJ* 318:1035-1040, 1999.
16. Danesh J, Peto R: Risk factors for coronary heart disease and infection with *Helicobacter pylori:* meta-analysis of 18 studies, *BMJ* 316:1130-1132, 1998.
17. West RR: *Chlamydia pneumoniae* infection and ischaemic heart disease: the story so far (editorial), *BMJ* 1039-1040, 1999.
18. Meier CR, Derby LE, Jick SS, et al: Antibiotics and risk of subsequent first-time acute myocardial infarction, *JAMA* 281:427-431, 1999.
19. Ridker PM: Inflammation, infection, and cardiovascular risk: how good is the clinical evidence? (editorial), *Circulation* 97:1671-1674, 1998.
20. Muller JE, Mittleman MA, Maclure M, et al (Determinants of Myocardial Infarction Onset Study Investigators): Triggering myocardial infarction by sexual activity: low absolute risk and prevention by regular physical exertion, *JAMA* 275:1405-1409, 1996.
21. Mittleman MA, Mintzer D, Maclure M, et al: Triggering of myocardial infarction by cocaine, *Circulation* 99:2737-2741, 1999.
22. Hemingway H, Marmot M: Psychosocial factors in the aetiology and prognosis of coronary heart disease: systematic review of prospective cohort studies, *BMJ* 318:1460-1467, 1999.

Primary Prevention of Coronary Artery Disease

(See also alcohol; aspirin; cardiac arrest; exercise; hormone replacement therapy; hypertension; lipids; obesity; relative risk reduction; risk factors for coronary artery disease; smoking; vitamin E)

Standard recommendations for the primary prevention of coronary artery disease include exercise, low-fat diet, avoidance of smoking, control of hypertension, avoidance of obesity, lipid-lowering strategies, and hormone replacement therapy.[1] The regular ingestion of aspirin, ACE inhibitors, warfarin, vitamin E, folate and vitamin B_6 (to lower homocysteine levels), cereal fiber, fish, garlic, and a Mediterranean diet has also been suggested. Most of these modalities are discussed elsewhere in the text; the roles of aspirin, ACE inhibitors, warfarin, fish, and garlic are reviewed in the ensuing paragraphs.

Aspirin

Two well-publicized studies of the preventive effects of aspirin on healthy physicians (primary prevention) have been published. The British Doctors' Trial compared male physicians between the ages of 50 and 78 taking 500 mg of aspirin daily over a 6-year period against a similar group who avoided aspirin-containing products.[2] No significant differences were found in the endpoints of myocardial infarction, strokes (except for slightly more disabling strokes in the acetylsalicylic acid [ASA]-treated group), and total cardiovascular mortality. In the Physicians' Health Study of U.S. male physicians ranging in age from 40 to 84 years, the treated group was given 325 mg of ASA every second day and the control group a placebo. At the end of 5 years there were no differences in cardiovascular mortality. The aspirin-treated group had a slight increase in hemorrhagic stroke and a 44% reduction in myocardial infarctions.[3] The latter figure, although statistically significant, represents a relative, not an absolute, risk reduction rate (see discussion of relative risk reduction). Because the overall incidence of cardiovascular disease was low in the studied population, the relative risk reduction for myocardial infarction of 44% translates into an absolute reduction rate of 0.4%.[4,5] In other words, four nonfatal myocardial infarctions were prevented by treating 1000 men with aspirin for 5 years.[5]

A more recent study that enrolled high-risk men without known coronary artery disease was the British Thrombosis

Prevention Trial, which had a median follow-up period of close to 7 years. Those in the aspirin arm of the study received one 75-mg slow-release tablet daily. No decrease in mortality was recorded, and a slight increase in hemorrhagic strokes occurred. The relative reduction of nonfatal myocardial infarctions was 32%, for an absolute reduction rate of 0.27%. In other words, treating 1000 men for 1 year prevented three nonfatal myocardial infarctions.[6]

The Hypertension Optimal Treatment (HOT) trial, which recruited approximated equal numbers of men and women, included a comparison of placebo and 75 mg of aspirin per day. The abstract in *Lancet* reported that those taking aspirin had a 15% reduction in major cardiovascular events and a 36% reduction in myocardial infarctions. Translating these relative reduction figures into numbers of persons who needed to be treated gives the following results: 1000 individuals had to take aspirin for 1 year to prevent 1.6 major cardiovascular events and 1.5 myocardial infarctions (in the case of diabetics, 2.5 myocardial infarctions). There was no decrease in mortality in the aspirin group. There was also no increase in strokes, but there was a significant increase in major bleeding, mainly from the nose and gastrointestinal tract.[7]

Because prophylactic aspirin benefits only a small number of men without known coronary artery disease and can have serious adverse effects (see discussion of aspirin), its widespread use for coronary artery disease prophylaxis is probably not indicated. High-risk diabetic patients may be an exception. On the basis of expert opinion the American Diabetes Association recommends the prophylactic use of low-dose aspirin for patients with type 1 or type 2 diabetes who are obese, smoke, or have hypertension, dyslipidemia, microalbuminuria or macroalbuminuria, or a family history of coronary artery disease.[8]

If medications are considered necessary for the primary prevention of coronary artery disease, aspirin appears to be as effective as the far more expensive statins.[9]

Angiotensin-converting enzyme inhibitors

The Heart Outcomes Prevention Evaluation (HOPE) study, published in January 2000, reported that ramipril (Altace) 10 mg/day resulted in a marked decrease in cardiovascular events and cardiovascular deaths not only in patients with known coronary artery disease, but also in high-risk patients (e.g., with peripheral vascular disease, previous stroke, and diabetes plus at least one other risk factor) without known coronary artery disease.[10] (See also discussion of secondary prevention of coronary artery disease.)

Warfarin

Low-intensity warfarin (Coumadin) has been shown to decrease the incidence and mortality rate of myocardial infarctions in men at high risk of coronary artery disease. However, it is associated with an increased incidence of fatal and nonfatal hemorrhagic strokes.[6,9]

Fiber

Results of the Nurses' Health Study suggest that high-fiber diets, particularly from cereal sources, are protective against coronary artery disease. Although high-fiber diets lead to a slight lowering of total and LDL cholesterol, this does not completely explain their beneficial effect.[11] (Lipid-lowering diets and the Mediterranean diet are discussed in the section on treatment of elevated lipids.)

Fish

Although a number of studies have shown an inverse correlation between fish consumption and coronary artery disease or total mortality, numerous others have not.[12] If eating fish has a cardiac benefit, it probably stems from the n-3 polyunsaturated fatty acids found in marine vertebrates. This is discussed further in the sections on cardiac arrest and secondary prevention of coronary artery disease.

Garlic

Garlic has been touted as an agent for preventing vascular disease because it is reputed to lower blood pressure and lipids. However, two randomized controlled trials did not show a reduction of lipid levels as a result of the regular ingestion of garlic.[13,14]

≈ REFERENCES ≈

1. Grundy SM, Balady GJ, Criqui MH, et al: Guide to primary prevention of cardiovascular disease: a statement for health-care professionals from the Task Force on Risk Reduction, *Circulation* 95:2329-2331, 1997.
2. Peto R, Gray R, Collins R, et al: Randomised trial of prophylactic daily aspirin in British male doctors, *Br Med J Clin Res Ed* 296:313-316, 1988.
3. Steering Committee of the Physicians' Health Study Research Group: Final report on the aspirin component of the ongoing Physicians' Health Study, *N Engl J Med* 321:129-135, 1989.
4. Rees MK: Use of low-dose aspirin as a preventive measure (letter), *Am Fam Physician* 52:766, 768, 1995.
5. Marshall KG: Use of low-dose aspirin as a preventive measure (letter), *Am Fam Physician* 52:761, 766, 1995.
6. Medical Research Council's General Practice Research Framework: Thrombosis Prevention Trial: randomised trial of low-intensity oral anticoagulation with warfarin and low-dose aspirin in the primary prevention of ischaemic heart disease in men at increased risk, *Lancet* 351:233-241, 1998.
7. Hansson L, Zanchetti A, Carruthers SG, et al: Effects of intensive blood-pressure lowering and low-dose aspirin in patients with hypertension: principal results of the Hypertension Optimal Treatment (HOT) randomised trial; HOT study group, *Lancet* 351:155-1762. 1998
8. American Diabetes Association: Aspirin therapy in diabetes, *Diabetes Care* 21(suppl 1):S45-S46, 1998.
9. Verheugt FW: Aspirin, the poor man's statin? (editorial), *Lancet* 351:227-228, 1998.
10. Heart Outcomes Prevention Evaluation Study Investigators: Effects of an angiotensin-converting-enzyme inhibitor, ramipril, on cardiovascular events in high-risk patients, *N Engl J Med* 342:145-153, 2000.

11. Wolk A, Manson JE, Stampfer MJ, et al: Long-term intake of dietary fiber and decreased risk of coronary heart disease among women, *JAMA* 281:1998-2004, 1999.

12. Ascherio A, Rimm EB, Stampfer MJ, et al: Dietary intake of marine n-3 fatty acids, fish intake, and the risk of coronary disease among men, *N Engl J Med* 332:977-982, 1995.

13. Berthold HK, Sudhop T, von Bergmann K: Effect of a garlic oil preparation on serum lipoproteins and cholesterol metabolism: a randomized controlled trial, *JAMA* 279:1900-1902, 1998.

14. Isaacsohn JL, Moser M, Stein EA, et al: Garlic powder and plasma lipids and lipoproteins: a multicenter, randomized, placebo-controlled trial, *Arch Intern Med* 158:1189-1194, 1998.

Secondary Prevention of Coronary Artery Disease

(See also cerebrovascular accidents; exercise; hypertension; hormone replacement therapy; lipids; Mediterranean diet; myocardial infarction; peripheral vascular disease; primary prevention of coronary artery disease; smoking; vitamin E)

Secondary prevention strategies for coronary artery disease are numerous. Guidelines include such items as smoking cessation, diet, exercise, lipid-lowering agents, aspirin, clopidogrel (Plavix), beta-blockers, ACE inhibitors, postmenopausal hormone replacement therapy, blood pressure control, n-3 polyunsaturated fatty acids,[1] and vitamin E.[2] Most of these are discussed elsewhere in the text. Aspirin, clopidogrel, warfarin, beta-blockers, ACE inhibitors, and n-3 polyunsaturated fatty acids are discussed in the ensuing paragraphs.

Aspirin

In the Swedish Angina Pectoris Aspirin Trial, patients with stable angina who had not had a myocardial infarction were treated with 75 mg of ASA or a placebo. Over a 4-year period there was a relative reduction of 34% in myocardial infarctions and sudden deaths in the aspirin-treated group. The absolute rate reduction of cardiovascular events was 51:1000 over 4 years or 5.1%. This reduction is more than 10 times greater than that reported for asymptomatic men in the Physicians' Health Study mentioned previously.[3] Similar results have been reported from the Multicenter Myocardial Ischemia Research Group. Patients were enrolled in this study within 6 months of the development of myocardial infarction or unstable angina. Cardiac events, including cardiac deaths, were markedly reduced in patients taking aspirin (250 to 325 mg/day), and this protective effect was particularly pronounced among patients who had had thrombolysis. Cardiac mortality at 2 years was 1.6% for patients taking aspirin and 5.4% for nonusers. Total cohort mortality was also reduced in the aspirin users.[4] One set of evidence-based guidelines recommends long-term use of 75 mg of aspirin daily for patients with stable or unstable angina or who had a myocardial infarction more than 1 month previously. For acute myocardial infarction the recommended dose is 150 mg/day continued for 1 month.[5]

The bottom line is that all patients with coronary artery disease should be taking aspirin unless the drug is strictly contraindicated.

Clopidogrel

Clopidogrel (Plavix) is an antithrombogenic agent related to ticlopidine (Ticlid) but with far fewer adverse effects. In a study of patients with known vascular disease (ischemic stroke, myocardial infarction, or peripheral vascular disease), 325 mg of aspirin daily was compared with 75 mg of clopidogrel. Patients taking clopidogrel had fewer myocardial infarctions, ischemic strokes, or vascular deaths than patients taking aspirin. The relative risk reduction of clopidogrel over aspirin was 8.7%. In other terms, 24 major events occurred in 1000 patients treated for 1 year with aspirin versus 19 in 1000 patients treated for 1 year with clopidogrel.[6] However, most of the increased benefit of clopidogrel over aspirin occurred in patients with peripheral vascular disease. At present, aspirin appears to be the drug of first choice for post–myocardial infarction patients. Clopidogrel is reserved for those who do not respond to aspirin or who cannot take it.[7]

Warfarin

Patients with coronary artery disease who are given warfarin in doses that maintain the INR above 2 have fewer cardiac events and more hemorrhages than patients taking placebos; warfarin is no more effective in preventing cardiac events than is aspirin.[8]

Beta-blockers

Beta-blockers without intrinsic sympathomimetic activity are cardioprotective; they reduce mortality after infarction, limit infarct size, and decrease arrhythmias and sudden death.[9] Unless strictly contraindicated, beta-blockers should be prescribed for all patients with coronary artery disease.

Angiotensin-converting enzyme inhibitors

A large multicenter international study (HOPE study) of the ACE inhibitor ramipril (Altace) selected men and women over the age of 55 who were known to have or were at high risk for coronary artery disease (e.g., history of stroke, peripheral vascular disease, or diabetes plus at least one other risk factor such as smoking or hypertension). Excluded were patients with heart failure, known low ejection fractions, or uncontrolled hypertension and those already taking ACE inhibitors. All patients received standard medical therapy, which often included aspirin and beta-blockers. Patients were assigned at random to receive 10 mg of ramipril once daily or a placebo. The study was stopped prematurely after 4.5 years because a clear benefit from ramipril therapy had been established. Those taking the active drug had a significant decrease in total mortality, cardiovascular mortality, cardiac arrests, myocardial infarctions, strokes, revascularization procedures, heart failure, and complications of diabetes. Benefits could not be explained by the very small decrease in blood pressure noted in the treated group[10] but were probably related to inhibition of the renin-angiotensin-aldosterone system at the tissue level.[11] Whether other ACE inhibitors have equal cardioprotective effects has not been established.

n-3 Polyunsaturated fatty acids

A prospective study of myocardial infarction survivors found that a daily supplement of n-3 polyunsaturated fatty acids (eicosapentaenoic acid plus docosahexanoic acid) in the form of a gelatin capsule was associated with a significant decrease in mortality, nonfatal myocardial infarction, and stroke. The quantity of n-3 polyunsaturated fatty acids in each capsule was the equivalent to that found in 100 g of fatty fish.[12]

⚓ REFERENCES ⚓

1. Smith SC Jr, Blair SN, Criqui MH, et al: Preventing heart attack and death in patients with coronary disease: Consensus Panel statement of the American Heart Association, *Circulation* 92:2-4, 1995.
2. Stephens NG, Parsons A, Schofield PM, et al: Randomised controlled trial of vitamin E in patients with coronary disease: Cambridge Heart Antioxidant Study (CHAOS), *Lancet* 347:781-786, 1996.
3. Juul-Möller S, Edvardsson N, Jahnmatz B, et al: Double-blind trial of aspirin in primary prevention of myocardial infarction in patients with stable chronic angina pectoris, *Lancet* 340:1421-1425, 1992.
4. Goldstein RE, Andrews M, Hall WJ, et al (Multicenter Myocardial Ischemia Research Group): Marked reduction in long-term cardiac deaths with aspirin after a coronary event, *J Am Coll Cardiol* 28:326-330, 1996.
5. Eccles M, Freemantle N, Mason J (North of England Aspirin Guideline Development Group): North of England evidence based guideline development project: guideline on the use of aspirin as secondary prophylaxis for vascular disease in primary care, *BMJ* 316:1303-1309, 1998.
6. CAPRIE Steering Committee: A randomised, blinded, trial of clopidogrel versus aspirin in patients at risk of ischaemic events (CAPRIE), *Lancet* 348:1329-1339, 1996.
7. Gorelick PB, Born GV, D'Agostino RB, et al: Therapeutic benefit: aspirin revisited in light of the introduction of clopidogrel, *Stroke* 30:1716-1721, 1999.
8. Anand SS, Yusuf S: Oral anticoagulant therapy in patients with coronary artery disease: a meta-analysis, *JAMA* 282:2058-2067, 1999.
9. Kendall MJ, Lynch KP, Hjalmarson A, et al: Beta-blockers and sudden cardiac death, *Ann Intern Med* 123:358-367, 1995.
10. Heart Outcomes Prevention Evaluation Study Investigators: Effects of an angiotensin-converting-enzyme inhibitor, ramipril, on cardiovascular events in high-risk patients, *N Engl J Med* 342:145-153, 2000.
11. Francis GS: ACE inhibition in cardiovascular disease (editorial), *N Engl J Med* 342:201-202, 2000.
12. Marchioli R et al (GISSI Prevenzione Investigators): Dietary supplementation with n-3 polyunsaturated fatty acids and vitamin E after myocardial infarction: results of the GISSI-Prevenzione trial, *Lancet* 354:447-455, 1999.

Angina

(See also coronary artery bypass grafting, angioplasty, and stenting)

Stable angina

All patients with angina should be taking aspirin and beta-blockers (unless strictly contraindicated) because these two drugs are cardioprotective (see earlier discussion of secondary prevention of coronary artery disease). If aspirin cannot be used, clopidogrel (Plavix) should be prescribed. Associated risk factors such as smoking, elevated lipid levels, diabetes, obesity, and a sedentary life-style should be aggressively treated.[1]

In patients with stable angina, proper use of nitroglycerin improves quality of life through symptom control. Short-acting nitroglycerin products may be given as sublingual tablets (Nitrostat) or sprays (Nitrolingual) to treat individual anginal attacks or can be taken prophylactically before an activity known to induce angina. Isosorbide dinitrate (Isordil) comes in both oral and sublingual formulations; its rate of onset of action is slower than nitroglycerin, but its duration of action is up to 1 hour, so it is particularly useful as a prophylactic agent before activity. Long-acting nitrates include transdermal patches (Transderm-Nitro, Minitran), sustained-release isosorbide dinitrate (Isordil Tembids), standard-formulation isosorbide mononitrate (ISMO, Monoket), and sustained-release isosorbide mononitrate (Imdur). Because of nitrate tolerance, daily drug-free periods are required. Sustained-release isosorbide mononitrate is given once a day. Standard-formulation isosorbide mononitrate or sustained-release isosorbide dinitrate may be given twice a day provided that no more than 7 hours elapses between doses. Patches should be removed after 12 to 14 hours.[2] Patients taking nitrates must not use sildenafil (Viagra).

Beta-blockers are excellent drugs for controlling angina, but if they are contraindicated, calcium channel blockers might be considered because they increase coronary blood flow and are effective in the symptomatic management of angina. However, because some of the shorter acting formulations have been associated with an increased incidence of myocardial infarction, calcium channel blockers are no longer considered first-line agents for the treatment of either angina or hypertension (see discussion of calcium channel blockers in the section on hypertension). If calcium channel antagonists are needed, a long-acting nondihydropyridine drug should be chosen and short-acting dihydropyridine derivatives should be avoided.[1]

The role of bypass surgery or angioplasty in the management of angina is discussed in the section on coronary artery bypass grafting, angioplasty, and stenting.

Unstable angina

Braunwald[3] classifies unstable angina as follows:

Class I. New-onset severe or accelerated angina developing within the past 2 months. Frequency of anginal episodes three or more per day. For patients who had stable angina, the episodes have become more frequent, last longer, are more severe, or are brought on by lesser degrees of exercise. No rest pain.

Class II. Angina at rest within the last month but not the past 48 hours (angina at rest subacute).

Class III. Angina at rest within the last 48 hours (angina at rest acute).

A number of studies have shown that the administration of aspirin to patients with unstable angina decreases fatal and nonfatal myocardial infarctions by 51% to 72%. Usual practice in the United States is to administer an initial dose of at least 160 mg/day followed by daily doses of between 80 and 325 mg indefinitely.[4] A set of guidelines for the United Kingdom recommends a daily dose of 75 mg over an indefinite period.[5] Ticlopidine (Ticlid) or clopidogrel (Plavix) should be used for patients who cannot take aspirin.[4]

The addition of unfractionated heparin (regular IV heparin)[6] or low-molecular-weight heparin[7] to aspirin for patients with unstable angina decreases both myocardial infarction and death rates. Current data suggest that low-molecular-weight heparin is superior to unfractionated heparin for this purpose[7] and that it should be given for at least 1 month to patients who have not had invasive therapy (angioplasty or coronary artery bypass surgery).[8] Beta-blockers should be given to all patients with unstable angina, and nitrates are probably beneficial.[4] Thrombolytic therapy is contraindicated for patients with unstable angina.[4]

The role of invasive therapy for unstable angina is controversial and is discussed in more detail in the section on coronary artery bypass grafting, angioplasty, and stenting. A 1999 randomized trial comparing conservative (aspirin and low-molecular-weight heparin) with invasive therapy for patients with unstable angina found that invasive therapy led to three fewer cardiac events per hundred patients after 6 months but no statistically significant reduction in mortality. The benefits of invasive interventions accrued between 3 and 6 months after the presenting event, not during the first 3 months, and therefore initial treatment of all patients with aspirin and low-molecular-weight heparin seems safe even if invasive therapy is to be the ultimate choice.[9]

In one study about half of patients with unstable angina required revascularization procedures in the first year, with the rate highest for those with Braunwald class III angina. The mortality rate for all unstable angina patients was 6% in the first year and 2% to 3% in subsequent years. The Braunwald classification was not useful as a predictor of 7-year mortality.[10]

◣ REFERENCES ◢

1. Gibbons RJ, Chatterjee K, Daley J: ACC/AHA/ACP-ASIM guidelines for the management of patients with chronic stable angina: executive summary and recommendations: a report of the American College of Cardiology/American Heart Association Task Force on Practice Guidelines (Committee on Management of Patients With Chronic Stable Angina), *Circulation* 99:2829-2848, 1999.
2. Parker JD, Parker JO: Nitrate therapy for stable angina pectoris, *N Engl J Med* 338:520-531, 1998.
3. Braunwald E: Unstable angina: a classification, *Circulation* 80:410-414, 1989.
4. Yeghiazarians Y, Braunstein JB, Askari A, et al: Unstable angina pectoris, *N Engl J Med* 342:101-114, 2000.
5. Eccles M, Freemantle N, Mason J (North of England Aspirin Guideline Development Group): North of England evidence based guideline development project: guideline on the use of aspirin as secondary prophylaxis for vascular disease in primary care, *BMJ* 316:1303-1309, 1998.
6. Oler A, Whooley MA, Oler J, et al: Adding heparin to aspirin reduces the incidence of myocardial infarction and death in patients with unstable angina: a meta-analysis, *JAMA* 276:811-815, 1996.
7. Zed PJ, Tisdale JE, Borzak S: Low-molecular-weight heparins in the management of acute coronary syndromes, *Arch Intern Med* 159:1849-1857, 1999.
8. Wallentin L, Swahn E, Kontny F, et al: Long-term low-molecular-mass heparin in unstable coronary-artery disease: FRISC II prospective randomised multicentre study, *Lancet* 354:701-707, 1999.
9. Wallentin L, Swahn E, Kontny F, et al: Invasive compared with non-invasive treatment in unstable coronary-artery disease: FRISC II prospective randomised multicentre study, *Lancet* 354:708-715, 1999.
10. van Domburg RT, van Miltenburg-van Zijl AD, Veerhoek RJ, et al: Unstable angina: good long-term outcome after a complicated early course, *J Am Coll Cardiol* 31:1534-1539, 1998.

Coronary Artery Bypass Grafting, Angioplasty, and Stenting

(See also anesthesia; informed consent; investigations; myocardial infarction; performance reports; practice patterns)

The number of invasive cardiac procedures performed varies widely among geographical regions. This is discussed under variations in medical care in the section on practice patterns.

Coronary artery bypass grafting (CABG) has been clearly shown to decrease mortality in patients with the following[1]:

1. Left mainstem coronary artery disease
2. Multivessel disease involving the proximal left anterior descending artery
3. Two-vessel disease with proximal left anterior descending artery narrowing and either impaired left ventricular function or demonstrable ischemia on noninvasive testing.

At present, data are insufficient to determine whether percutaneous transluminal coronary angioplasty (PTCA) is as effective as CABG in reducing mortality in patients who meet the above criteria.[1]

For patients with angina who have single-vessel disease or multiple-vessel disease not involving the proximal left anterior descending coronary artery and whose left ventricular systolic function is normal, medical therapy, angioplasty, and bypass surgery have been shown to be equally effective, and therefore the choice for a particular patient can be individualized.[2,3] In this group of patients bypass is associated with greater initial morbidity but results in better control of angina and less need for repeat interventions. Angioplasty has a lower immediate morbidity, but there is a greater risk of recurrent angina requiring medical therapy or further interventions. In one study of patients with multivessel disease, 31% of patients who initially had PTCA had a subsequent CABG within 5 years.[4]

Objective measurements of the degree of angina such as the threshold of activity that will precipitate an attack are not sufficient in themselves to determine the best therapeutic modality. Patients differ considerably in how they tolerate symptoms, so their preferences are an important factor to be considered in reaching a decision.[5,6] Since the perioperative mortality of CABG is as high as 4%,[5] even some patients with left mainstem coronary artery disease may refuse the operation on this basis alone.[6]

In the United States either PTCA or CABG is often routinely performed on patients with acute coronary syndromes, including unstable angina and Q-wave and non-Q-wave infarction. This is done even though several large prospective studies have shown no benefit from such aggressive therapy compared with medical management. According to a *New England Journal of Medicine* editorial in 1998, the only patients with acute coronary syndromes who should undergo angiography or revascularization are those who remain symptomatic despite medical treatment or who have evidence of systolic dysfunction.[7] An editorial in *JAMA* went so far as to claim that the ever-increasing number of angiography procedures in the United States is caused largely by a proliferation of interventional cardiologists eager to perform these procedures, using the rationalization that such interventions improve "quality of life."[8]

Skepticism about interventional strategies for acute coronary syndromes has to be reevaluated in the light of two 1999 publications. The FRISC II study showed that patients with unstable angina treated with invasive therapy had a decreased event rate (but not a decreased mortality rate) compared with those receiving medical therapy,[9] and Zijlstra and colleagues[10] from the Netherlands found that after 5 years patients with acute myocardial infarction who were randomly assigned to undergo immediate angioplasty had less mortality and morbidity than those randomly selected to receive streptokinase. The practical significance of these studies is uncertain: few hospitals have the facilities or expertise to offer 24-hour angioplasty services; new drugs such as platelet glycoprotein IIb/IIIa receptor inhibitors are now available to be used in conjunction with thrombolytic therapy; and stenting is becoming a standard adjunct to angioplasty. Future studies may demonstrate that immediate medical therapy followed at a later date by "elective" angioplasty is the treatment of choice for acute coronary syndromes.[11]

An important factor in deciding whether a patient should undergo angioplasty is the volume of procedures performed in the institution where the procedure will take place. The rate of major complications and death appears to be much lower in centers performing 400 to 600 or more procedures per year compared with those performing fewer than 400. Furthermore, both patient mortality and the need for same-day CABG surgery are greater for individual cardiologists performing fewer than 75 PTCA procedures per year.[12] Updated guidelines of the American College of Cardiology and American Heart Association suggest that angioplasty rather than thrombolysis should be used only if it can be performed within 90 minutes of admission; is performed by a physician who does more than 75 such procedures a year; and takes place in a center that has a well-staffed catheter laboratory that carries out more than 200 angioplasty procedures a year and that has backup cardiac surgery facilities.[13]

Cerebral complications from coronary artery bypass are common. In one multicenter study such adverse events occurred in 6.1% of patients. Half of them had either fatal cerebral injury or nonfatal strokes, and the other half had a new deterioration of intellectual function or a new onset of seizures.[14]

The optimal revascularization procedure for diabetic patients is uncertain.[4,15] Diabetic patients subject to PTCA have higher in-hospital mortality and nonfatal myocardial infarction rates than do nondiabetic patients having the same procedure. They also have twice the mortality rate after 9 years of follow-up.[12] The adverse effects are probably related to the greater degree of vascular disease in these patients. Preliminary evidence indicates that diabetic patients taking insulin or oral hypoglycemic agents do better after CABG than after PTCA.[4] In one study the mortality rate of this category of patients 5 years after CABG was 20% whereas it was 45% 5 years after PTCA.[4]

The technical aspects of percutaneous coronary revascularization are in a constant state of change. Atherectomy and laser angioplasty came into vogue in the late 1980s and are now declining in frequency, whereas the placement of intracoronary stents is increasing.[16] By 1999 between 60% and 70% of angioplasties were associated with placement of stents. Stents decrease the frequency of restenosis but so far have not led to decreased rates of myocardial infarction or death.[17] Until recently patients receiving stents were placed on the dual-antiplatelet therapy of aspirin plus ticlopidine (Ticlid) for a few weeks after the procedure.[18] Since ticlopidine can cause fatal hematological reactions (see discussion of transient ischemic attacks), whether the benefits outweigh the harm is uncertain. The current solution to this problem is to use clopidogrel (Plavix) instead of ticlopidine.[19,20]

❧ REFERENCES ❧

1. Gibbons RJ, Chatterjee K, Daley J: ACC/AHA/ACP-ASIM Guidelines for the management of patients with chronic stable angina: executive summary and recommendations; a report of the American College of Cardiology/American Heart Association Task Force on Practice Guidelines (Committee on Management of Patients With Chronic Stable Angina), *Circulation* 99:2829-2848, 1999.
2. Hamm CW, Reimers J, Ischinger T, et al: A randomized study of coronary angioplasty compared with bypass surgery in patients with symptomatic multivessel coronary disease, *N Engl J Med* 331:1037-1043, 1994.
3. King SB III, Lembo NJ, Weintraub WS, et al: A randomized trial comparing coronary angioplasty with coronary bypass surgery, *N Engl J Med* 331:1044-1050, 1994.
4. Bypass Angioplasty Revascularization Investigation (BARI) Investigators: Comparison of coronary bypass surgery with angioplasty in patients with multivessel disease, *N Engl J Med* 335:217-225, 1996.
5. Nease RF Jr, Kneeland T, O'Connor GT, et al: Variation in patient utilities for outcomes of the management of chronic stable angina: implications for clinical practice guidelines, *JAMA* 273:1185-1190, 1995.
6. Hlatky MA: Patient preferences and clinical guidelines (editorial), *JAMA* 273:1219-1220, 1995.
7. Lange RA, Hillis LD: Use and overuse of angiography and revascularization for acute coronary syndromes (editorial), *N Engl J Med* 338:1838-1839, 1998.
8. Graboys TB: Coronary angiography (editorial), *JAMA* 282: 184-185, 1999.
9. Wallentin L, Swahn E, Kontny F, et al: Invasive compared with non-invasive treatment in unstable coronary-artery disease: FRISC II prospective randomised multicentre study, *Lancet* 354:708-715, 1999.
10. Zijlstra F, Hoorntje JC, de Boer M-J, et al: Long-term benefit of primary angioplasty as compared with thrombolytic therapy for acute myocardial infarction, *N Engl J Med* 341:1413-1419, 1999.
11. Faxon DP, Heger JW: Primary angioplasty—enduring the test of time (editorial), *N Engl J Med* 341:1464-1465, 1999.
12. Hannan EL, Racz M, Ryan T, et al: Coronary angioplasty volume-outcome relationships for hospitals and cardiologists, *JAMA* 279:892-898, 1997.
13. Ryan TJ, Antman EM, Brooks NH, et al: 1999 update: ACC/AHA guidelines for the management of patients with acute myocardial infarction, *J Am Coll Cardiol* 34:890-911, 1999.
14. Roach GW, Kanchuger M, Mangano M, et al: Adverse cerebral outcomes after coronary bypass surgery, *N Engl J Med* 335:1857-1863, 1996.
15. Kip KE, Faxon DP, Detre KM, et al: Coronary angioplasty in diabetic patients—the National Heart, Lung, and Blood Institute Percutaneous Transluminal Corollary Angioplasty Registry, *Circulation* 94:1818-1825, 1996.
16. Hasdai D, Berger PB, Bell MR, et al: The changing face of coronary interventional practice: the Mayo Clinic experience, *Arch Intern Med* 157:677-682, 1997.
17. Jacobs AK: Coronary stents—have they fulfilled their promise? (editorial), *N Engl J Med* 341:2005-2006, 1999.
18. Topol EJ: Coronary-artery stents—gauging, gorging, and gouging (editorial), *N Engl J Med* 339:1702-1704, 1998.
19. Wang X, Oetgen M, Maida R, et al: The effectiveness of the combination of Plavix and aspirin versus Ticlid and aspirin after coronary stent implantation (abstract), *J Am Coll Cardiol* 33(2 suppl A):13A, 1999.
20. Klein LW, Calvin JE: Use of clopidogrel in coronary stenting: what was the question? (editorial), *J Am Coll Cardiol* 34:1895-1898, 1999.

Myocardial Infarction

(See also cardiac arrest; coronary artery bypass grafting and angioplasty; practice patterns; risks of exercise; smoking)

Panic disorder presenting as possible myocardial infarction

A series of 441 consecutive consenting patients with chest pain seen in the emergency room of a major Montreal teaching hospital specializing in heart disease was evaluated as to etiology and underlying psychiatric disorders. One fourth of these patients met the criteria for panic attacks in the *Diagnostic and Statistical Manual of Mental Disorders,* edition 3 revised *(DSM-III-R),* and of this group one fourth had suicidal thoughts in the week before being seen in the emergency room. In addition, close to 60% of patients with panic disorder had other Axis I psychiatric diagnoses, mainly generalized anxiety disorder, agoraphobia, major depression, and dysthymia. In only 2% of cases was the panic disorder recognized by the attending staff cardiologists in the emergency room. Seventy-five percent of the patients with panic disorder were discharged from the emergency room with the diagnosis "noncardiac chest pain."[1]

❧ REFERENCES ❧

1. Fleet RP, Dupuis G, Marchand A, et al: Panic disorder in emergency department chest pain patients—prevalence, comorbidity, suicidal ideation, and physician recognition, *Am J Med* 101:371-380, 1996.

Office or home management of suspected acute myocardial infarction

In cases of suspected myocardial infarction, rapid transfer to an emergency facility for consideration of thrombolytic therapy is paramount (in general, thrombolytic therapy is not given if symptoms have persisted for more than 12 hours). If time permits, an immediate ECG should be obtained and sent with the patient along with previous ECGs if available. This is because changing electrocardiographic patterns, especially ST segment changes or new-onset left bundle-branch block, support the diagnosis of myocardial infarction and determine whether thrombolytic therapy is indicated (enzyme changes are often not seen for at least 3 to 4 hours).[1]

Aspirin has been shown to reduce mortality, so a half to one aspirin should be given stat.[2] Chewing and swallowing aspirin results in a more rapid antiplatelet effect than occurs from swallowing intact tablets.[2] Aspirin should not be omitted because of a vague history of allergy or a remote history of gastrointestinal bleeding. The administration of aspirin does not interfere with subsequent thrombolytic therapy.[1]

A randomized double-blind study from Scotland showed a significant decrease in death rate measured at 30 months among patients with suspected acute myocardial infarctions who received intravenous thrombolytic therapy with 30 units of anistreplase (Eminase) at home from their general practitioners compared with patients who received similar therapy only after arrival at the hospital.[3]

─────────── ☙ **REFERENCES** ❧ ───────────

1. Collins R, Peto R, Baigent C, et al: Aspirin, heparin, and fibrinolytic therapy in suspected acute myocardial infarction, *N Engl J Med* 336:847-860, 1997.
2. Feldman M, Cryer B: Aspirin absorption rates and platelet inhibition times with 325-mg buffered aspirin tablets (chewed or swallowed intact) and with buffered aspirin solution, *Am J Cardiol* 84:404-409, 1999.
3. Rawles J: Magnitude of benefit from earlier thrombolytic treatment in acute myocardial infarction: new evidence from Grampian Region Early Anistreplase Trial (GREAT), *BMJ* 312:212-215, 1996.

Secondary prevention of myocardial infarction
(See also exercise; hypertension; lipids; practice patterns; smoking)

Risk stratification. For optimal provision of secondary prevention measures, patients who have had a myocardial infarction should be stratified according to their degree of risk for further coronary events. This is best performed by testing left ventricular function with echocardiography and assessing ischemia with exercise testing.[1]

The first-year mortality rate after a myocardial infarction is zero to 2% if the post–myocardial infarction exercise stress test is negative, but if it is positive, the total cardiac event rate is about 25%.[1] In recent years the interval between myocardial infarction and exercise testing has been decreasing, and in some centers symptom-limited testing is being done as early as 4 to 7 days after the cardiac event. Usually one of two protocols is recommended: submaximal testing at 4 to 7 days followed by symptom-limited testing

at 3 to 6 weeks, or symptom-limited testing at 2 to 3 weeks. Patients who have contraindications to exercise stress testing have a much higher mortality rate than those who are able to undergo the test.[2]

Left ventricular function as determined by echocardiography is the single most important determinant of risk after myocardial infarction. The 1-year mortality rate varies from 3% when the ejection fraction is greater than 50% to more than 40% when the ejection fraction is less than 30%.[1]

Management guidelines
Recent guidelines for management of patients after myocardial infarction include the following recommendations[1]:

1. Evaluate left ventricular function by echocardiography.
2. Evaluate residual ischemia by exercise testing if possible.
3. Start low-dose aspirin immediately if it is not contraindicated, and continue it indefinitely.
4. Start beta-blockers immediately if they are not contraindicated, and continue them indefinitely.
5. Start ACE inhibitors before discharge for all patients with a left ventricular ejection fraction less than 40%. (See below for updated recommendations.)
6. Give anticoagulants for at least 3 months if the patient has extensive abnormalities of left ventricular wall motion or demonstrable left ventricular thrombus.
7. Modify coronary risk factors through smoking cessation, exercise, control of hypertension, and control of dyslipidemia. The goals for the last mentioned are a low-density lipoprotein-C concentration less than 2.6 mmol/L (100 mg/dl), a high-density lipoprotein-C concentration greater than 0.9 mmol/L (35 mg/dl), and a triglyceride level less than 1.58 mmol/L (140 mg/dl).

Post–myocardial infarction exercise, beta-blockers, aspirin, anticoagulants, and ACE inhibitors are discussed in the ensuing paragraphs. The remaining recommendations are dealt with elsewhere in the text. An important and controversial aspect of post–myocardial infarction management is the role of invasive cardiac procedures such as CABG and angioplasty, which varies greatly among geographical areas. This is discussed under variations in medical care in the section on practice patterns.

Exercise. Metaanalysis of randomized controlled studies of rehabilitation exercise in post–myocardial infarction patients has shown a 25% relative reduction in mortality during the first 3 years of follow-up.[3] Regular exercise also decreases the slightly raised relative risk of triggering myocardial infarction during sexual intercourse.[4] Symptom-limited exercise testing is considered essential before a cardiac rehabilitation program.[2]

Beta-blockers. If not strictly contraindicated, beta-blockers should be prescribed for all post–myocardial infarction patients because they decrease mortality rates.[1,5-8] Any beta-blocker without intrinsic sympathomimetic activity (ISA) may be used. In clinical trials large doses have been administered, and these are listed below. However, one recent study has found that patients treated with half or less of the doses listed had even better outcomes than those who received the maximum doses shown here[5]:

Metoprolol (Lopressor)	100 mg bid
Propranolol (Inderal)	60-80 mg tid
Atenolol (Tenormin)	100 mg/day

Beta-blocker therapy should probably be continued indefinitely.[1] In most instances patients with relative or presumed contraindications to beta-blockers should not be deprived of these drugs. Gottleib and associates[6] found that these drugs decreased mortality rates among post–myocardial infarction patients who were very old or had other illnesses, including diabetes mellitus, chronic obstructive pulmonary disease, and heart failure. They were also effective in patients with non-Q-wave infarctions.[6]

In practice, beta-blockers are underused after myocardial infarctions. In one U.S. study of patients discharged from hospital after a myocardial infarction, only about one third of "good candidates" and one half of "ideal candidates" received these drugs, regardless of whether they were treated by cardiologists, internists, or family practitioners.[7] In an evaluation of patients with recurrent myocardial infarctions, 44% of patients were taking beta-blockers but the rate was lower for the elderly.[8]

Aspirin. Aspirin in doses of 75 to 325 mg/day has been well documented to decrease morbidity and mortality in old and young men and women who have had myocardial infarctions. Benefit has been noted even when aspirin was started weeks or years after the initial infarction (see discussion of secondary prevention of coronary artery disease).[9] Clinical practice guidelines from the United Kingdom recommend a dosage of 150 mg/day for the first month following infarction and then 75 mg/day indefinitely.[10] Unfortunately, not all eligible patients take aspirin. One U.S. study of patients with recurrent myocardial infarctions found that overall 53% were taking the drug but the rate was significantly lower among women and the elderly,[8] and another reported that only three fourths of "ideal candidates" were prescribed aspirin.[7]

Clopidogrel. Clopidogrel (Plavix), like ticlopidine (Ticlid), inhibits platelet aggregation, but so far it does not appear to have the serious adverse effects of ticlopidine. Clopidogrel is the drug of choice for the secondary prevention of myocardial infarctions in patients who cannot take aspirin.[11]

Anticoagulants. Anticoagulation has been shown to decrease morbidity and mortality in post–myocardial infarction patients.[12] Oral anticoagulants are widely used in Europe, whereas aspirin is the drug of choice in North America. There are no good recent comparisons of the two modalities.[13] Three months of anticoagulation is recommended for post–myocardial infarction patients who have

significant abnormalities of left ventricular wall motion or who are shown to have a left ventricular thrombus.[1]

ACE inhibitors. A systematic review of post–myocardial infarction patients given a 4- to 6-week course of oral ACE inhibitors started within 36 hours of infarction found a small but significant decrease in 30-day mortality compared with those not given the drug. This benefit was greatest for subgroups of patients at increased risk of mortality. Two alternative recommendations emerged from this review. Barring contraindications, a 4- to 6-week course of an ACE inhibitor should be given either to all post–myocardial infarction patients or only to post–myocardial infarction patients at increased risk of mortality, such as those with anterior infarction, tachycardia, heart failure, or diabetes.[14] A 1999 meta-analysis of randomized controlled trials confirmed the value of ACE inhibitors in decreasing total mortality in post–myocardial infarction patients.[15]

≈ REFERENCES ≈

1. Deedwania PC, Amsterdam EA, Vagelos RH (California Cardiology Working Group on Post-MI Management): Evidence-based, cost-effective risk stratification and management after myocardial infarction, *Arch Intern Med* 157:273-280, 1997.
2. Gibbons RJ, Balady GJ, Beasley JW, et al: ACC/AHA guidelines for exercise testing: a report of the American College of Cardiology/American Heart Association Task Force on Practice Guidelines (Committee on Exercise Testing), *J Am Coll Cardiol* 30:260-311, 1997.
3. US Department of Health and Human Services, Public Health Service, Agency for Health Care Policy and Research: *Cardiac rehabilitation,* Clinical Practice Guideline No 17, 1995.
4. Muller JE, Mittleman MA, Maclure M, et al (Determinants of Myocardial Infarction Onset Study Investigators): Triggering myocardial infarction by sexual activity: low absolute risk and prevention by regular physical exertion, *JAMA* 275:1405-1409, 1996.
5. Barron HV, Viskin S, Lundstrom RJ, et al: ß-Blocker dosages and mortality after myocardial infarction: data from a large health maintenance organization, *Arch Intern Med* 158:449-453, 1998.
6. Gottleib SS, McCarter RJ, Vogel RA: Effect of beta-blockade on mortality among high-risk and low-risk patients after myocardial infarction, *N Engl J Med* 339:489-497, 1998.
7. Frances CD, Go AS, Dauterman DW, et al: Outcome following acute myocardial infarction, *Arch Intern Med* 159:1429-1436, 1999.
8. McCormick D, Gurwitz JH, Lessard D, et al: Use of aspirin, ß-blockers, and lipid-lowering medications before recurrent acute myocardial infarction: missed opportunities for prevention? *Arch Intern Med* 159:561-567, 1999.
9. Antiplatelet Trialists' Collaboration: Collaborative overview of randomised trials of antiplatelet therapy. I. Prevention of death, myocardial infarction, and stroke by prolonged antiplatelet therapy in various categories of patients, *BMJ* 308:81-106, 1994.

10. Eccles M, Freemantle N, Mason J (North of England Aspirin Guideline Development Group): North of England evidence based guideline development project: guideline on the use of aspirin as secondary prophylaxis for vascular disease in primary care, *BMJ* 316:1303-1309, 1998.

11. Gorelick PB, Born GV, D'Agostino RB, et al: Therapeutic benefit: aspirin revisited in light of the introduction of clopidogrel, *Stroke* 30:1716-1721, 1999.

12. ASPECT Research Group: Effect of long-term oral anticoagulant treatment on mortality and cardiovascular morbidity after myocardial infarction, *Lancet* 343:499-503, 1994.

13. Cairns JA, Markham BA: Economics and efficacy in choosing oral anticoagulants or aspirin after myocardial infarction (editorial), *JAMA* 273:965-967, 1995.

14. Franzosi MG, Santoro E, Zuanetti G, et al (ACE Inhibitor Myocardial Infarction Collaborative Group): Indications for ACE inhibitors in the early treatment of acute myocardial infarction: systematic overview of individual data from 100,000 patients in randomized trials, *Circulation* 97:2202-2212, 1998.

15. Domanski MJ, Exner DV, Borkowf CB, et al: Effect of angiotensin converting enzyme inhibition on sudden cardiac death in patients following acute myocardial infarction, *J Am Coll Cardiol* 33:598-604, 1999.

ELECTROCARDIOGRAMS

A long tradition in primary care holds that routine ECGs are a valuable part of the periodic health examination of middle-aged or elderly patients. This is a myth.[1] The cardiogram has poor sensitivity and specificity for Q-wave myocardial infarction in asymptomatic individuals, and the positive predictive value for this entity for 60-year-old men is calculated to be only 3%.[1] T-wave and ST segment changes are so common and so nonspecific that they do not help identify patients at risk of coronary artery disease. The U.S. Preventive Services Task Force gives screening ECGs for middle-aged and elderly men and women a "C" recommendation. They give a "D" recommendation for routine periodic health visits or routine pre–sports participation examinations in adolescents or young adults.[2]

A common argument for performing electrocardiography is to have ECGs available as a baseline in case cardiac symptoms develop in the future. The assumption is that the ECG will be relatively recent and rapidly accessible at whatever emergency room the patient goes to when symptoms of coronary artery disease develop. If the ECG is available, it will probably be helpful, but if cardiograms are going to be taken for this reason, the possible benefits for the very few must be weighed against the significant number of false-positive findings that would inevitably cause distress for both patients and physicians.

◣ REFERENCES ◤

1. Health Services Utilization and Research Commission: Anatomy of a practice guideline: tradition, science, and consensus on using electrocardiograms in Saskatchewan, *Can Fam Physician* 41:37-48, 1995.

2. US Preventive Services Task Force: *Guide to clinical preventive services,* ed 2, Baltimore, 1996, Williams & Wilkins, pp 3-14.

HEART FAILURE

The following is the New York Heart Association classification of congestive heart failure:

Class I	Symptoms with unusual activity (manual labor)
Class II	Symptoms with usual activity (light yard work, sexual intercourse)
Class III	Symptoms with self-care activity (dressing, making bed)
Class IV	Symptoms at rest and worse with activity

Prognosis

The overall 5-year survival rate of patients with congestive heart failure is poor. Among U.S. Medicare patients in heart failure who were 67 years or older, 19% of back men, 16% of white men, 25% of black women, and 23% of white women survived 6 years from diagnosis.[1] The annual death rates for various degrees of heart failure based on the New York Heart Association classifications are estimated as follows[2]:

Class II	5% to 10% per year
Class III	10% to 20% per year
Class IV	20% to 50% per year

About half of the deaths from cardiac causes are sudden, and one fourth of these occur without prior worsening of the heart failure.[2]

◣ REFERENCES ◤

1. Croft JB, Giles WH, Pollard RA, et al: Heart failure survival among older adults in the United States: a poor prognosis for an emerging epidemic in the Medicare population, *Arch Intern Med* 159:505-510, 1999.

2. Dracup K, Baker DW, Dubar SB, et al: Management of heart failure. II. Counseling, education, and lifestyle modifications, *JAMA* 272:1442-1446, 1994.

Systolic and Diastolic Heart Failure

Systolic heart failure is caused by a decreased contractility of the heart and is associated with dilation, which is often seen as an enlarged heart on chest roentgenogram. It is the type of heart failure with which most people are familiar and is much more common than diastolic failure. In systolic failure the left ventricular ejection fraction is usually less than 40%.[1]

Diastolic heart failure is the inability of the heart to relax properly. Decreased cardiac compliance leads to inadequate filling of the ventricles during diastole. The chest roentgenogram may show no increase in heart size, and the left ventricular ejection fraction is often greater than 40%. In fact, pure diastolic dysfunction may be defined as an elevated end-diastolic pressure without chamber enlargement.[1] Some of the causes of diastolic failure are hypertrophic cardiomyopathy, aortic stenosis, hypertension, and conditions such as cardiac amyloidosis and extensive scarring from coronary artery disease in which cardiac interstitial tissue is increased. An element of diastolic failure is particularly common in elderly or hypertensive patients.[1] Diastolic failure is sometimes detected by noting the changes in the indices of ventricular filling during an echocardiogram, but its sensitivity and specificity are poor.[2] If a patient has evidence of systemic or pulmonary venous congestion in the absence of left ventricular enlargement, the odds are high that diastolic failure is a major component of the failure.[1]

A number of patients have a combination of systolic and diastolic failure. Physicians should not rule out heart failure in a patient with dyspnea on effort, orthopnea, and decreased energy just because the heart size is normal.[1] According to one set of clinical guidelines, any patient with symptoms suggestive of heart failure should undergo echocardiography or, as a second choice, radionuclide ventriculography.[2] The history, physical examination, and chest roentgenogram may not allow differentiation among systolic or diastolic dysfunction, valvular disease, or even noncardiac causes of the patient's symptoms.[1]

REFERENCES

1. Cohn JN: The management of chronic heart failure, *N Engl J Med* 335:490-498, 1996.
2. Heart Failure Guideline Panel: Heart failure: management of patients with left ventricular systolic dysfunction, *Am Fam Physician* 50:603-616, 1994.

Diet and Exercise
(See also exercise; nutrition)

Except in severe failure the maximum daily salt intake should be 3 g, which can be achieved by avoiding salty food and by not adding salt to food after it has been cooked. Patients with severe failure (e.g., those requiring at least 80 mg of furosemide per day) should limit their salt intake to 2 g per day. This involves avoiding milk products, prepared foods, and canned foods and is unpalatable for most patients.[1]

Data on alcohol in congestive heart failure are inconclusive. Alcohol is obviously contraindicated in alcoholic cardiomyopathy. In other cases expert opinion is that patients should not have more than one drink per day.[1]

Patients with stable heart failure should be encouraged to exercise regularly by walking or bicycling on flat terrain.[1,2] A 1999 randomized controlled trial of patients with stable heart failure found that in addition to improving quality of life, exercise decreased mortality rates.[3]

REFERENCES

1. Dracup K, Baker DW, Dubar SB, et al: Management of heart failure. II. Counseling, education, and lifestyle modifications, *JAMA* 272:1442-1446, 1994.

2. Willenheimer R, Erhardt L, Cline C, et al: Exercise training in heart failure improves quality of life and exercise capacity, *Eur Heart J* 19:774-781, 1998.
3. Belardinelli R, Georgiou D, Cianci G, et al: Randomized, controlled trial of long-term moderate exercise training in chronic heart failure, *Circulation* 99:1173-1182, 1999.

Pharmacotherapy

Mild cases of congestive heart failure can be managed by an ACE inhibitor alone or an ACE inhibitor combined with a diuretic. Moderately severe failure is managed by an ACE inhibitor combined with a diuretic and digoxin. Severe failure is managed as above with the addition of a second diuretic (metolazone) and usually a second vasodilator (long-acting nitrates or hydralazine).[1] Most patients also benefit from the careful addition of a beta-blocker,[2,3] and spironolactone (Aldactone) has proved beneficial in patients with severe failure.[4]

REFERENCES

1. Heart Failure Guideline Panel, Rockville, Maryland: Heart failure: management of patients with left ventricular systolic dysfunction, *Am Fam Physician* 50:603-616, 1994.
2. Pepper GS, Lee RW: Sympathetic activation in heart failure and its treatment with β-blockade, *Arch Intern Med* 159:225-234, 1999.
3. Cleland JG, McGowan J, Clark A: The evidence for β blockers in heart failure: equals or surpasses that for angiotensin converting enzyme inhibitors (editorial), *BMJ* 318:824-825, 1999.
4. Pitt B, Zannad F, Remme WJ, et al: The effect of spironolactone on morbidity and mortality in patients with severe heart failure, *N Engl J Med* 341:709-717, 1999.

ACE inhibitors
(See also cough; urticaria and angioedema)

A metaanalysis of a large number of studies using different ACE inhibitors in congestive heart failure showed them to reduce symptoms, total mortality, and hospitalization rates in a broad range of patients. Those with the lowest ejection fractions benefited the most.[1] According to a number of studies,[2-4] high doses are more effective than low doses (e.g., lisinopril 32.5 to 35 mg/day compared with 2.5 to 5 mg/day[4]). Despite clear-cut evidence that ACE inhibitors are the drugs of choice for congestive failure, a recent survey found that only 46% of U.S. patients with the condition received drugs in this class when treated by cardiologists, and only 22% when treated by other physicians.[5]

ACE inhibitors should be used with caution in patients who have diminished renal function. If the creatinine level is greater than 3 mg/dl (250 μmol/L), only half the usual dose of ACE inhibitor should be given and it should be titrated upward slowly. ACE inhibitors should not be given to patients whose potassium concentration is 5.5 mEq/L

(5.5 mmol/L) or greater.[6] In the absence of renal failure or heart failure, hyperkalemia is relatively uncommon. Minimal degrees of hyperkalemia after starting ACE inhibitors rarely progress to dangerous levels except in patients over the age of 70 or those who have a serum urea nitrogen level greater than 25 mg/dl (8.9 mmol/L); patients in these two categories should be monitored closely or changed to another class of drugs.[7]

Cough caused by ACE inhibitors is nonproductive. Although it may develop within hours of starting the medication, a latent period of weeks or even months is more common. Cough is not always a reason for stopping an ACE inhibitor because the benefits of the drug may outweigh the distress caused by the symptom.[6] Some patients obtain symptomatic relief with sulindac (Clinoril), indomethacin (Indocin, Indocid), nifedipine (Adalat, Procardia), or inhaled cromolyn (sodium cromoglycate, Intal), but a physician would rarely want to prescribe NSAIDs for a patient who is in heart failure. For patients who cannot tolerate ACE inhibitors, an angiotensin II inhibitor may be substituted (see below).

Other notable adverse reactions to ACE inhibitors are hypotension after the first dose, angioedema, and abnormalities of taste. Angioedema does not necessarily develop during the early days of therapy,[9] but if patients who have had an episode of this disorder continue taking the drug, they are at high risk for recurrent episodes.[10]

ACE inhibitors increase and aspirin inhibits prostaglandin production. The effect of these conflicting pharmacological effects in patients with heart failure who are taking both ACE inhibitors and aspirin has not been established. Whether clopidogrel (Plavix) or warfarin should be substituted for aspirin in such situations will be determined only by randomized controlled trials.[11]

Many of the available ACE inhibitors and their usual maintenance doses are listed in Table 8.

Table 8 ACE Inhibitors

Drug	Usual dose
Benazepril (Lotensin)	10-20 mg/day as a single dose
Captopril (Capoten)	25-50 mg bid or tid
Cilazapril (Inhibace)	2.5-5 mg/day as a single dose
Enalapril (Vasotec)	5-40 mg/day as a single dose or bid
Fosinopril (Monopril)	20 mg as a single daily dose
Lisinopril (Zestril, Prinivil)	10-40 mg/day as a single dose
Moexipril (Univasc)	7.5-30 mg/day in 1 or 2 divided doses
Perindopril (Coversyl)	4-8 mg/day as a single dose
Quinapril HCl (Accupril)	10-20 mg/day as a single dose
Ramipril (Altace)	2.5-10 mg/day as a single dose
Trandolapril (Mavik)	2-4 mg/day as a single dose

▧ REFERENCES ▨

1. Garg R, Yusuf S: Overview of randomized trials of angiotensin-converting enzyme inhibitors on mortality and morbidity in patients with heart failure, *JAMA* 273:1450-1456, 1995.
2. van Veldhuisen DJ, Genth-Zotz S, Brouwer J, et al: High-versus low-dose ACE inhibition in chronic heart failure: a double-blind, placebo-controlled study of Imidapril, *J Am Coll Cardiol* 32:1811-1818, 1998.
3. Luzier AB, Forrest A, Adelman M, et al: Impact of angiotensin-converting enzyme inhibitor underdosing on re-hospitalization rates in congestive heart failure, *Am J Cardiol* 82:465-469, 1998.
4. Packer M, Poole-Wilson PA, Armstrong PW, et al: Comparative effects of low and high doses of the angiotensin-converter enzyme inhibitor, lisinopril on morbidity and mortality in chronic heart failure, *Circulation* 100:2312-2318, 1999.
5. Stafford RS, Saglam D, Blumenthal D: National patterns of angiotensin-converting enzyme inhibitor use in congestive heart failure, *Arch Intern Med* 157:2460-2464, 1997.
6. Baker DW, Konstam MA, Bottoriff M, et al: Management of heart failure. I. Pharmacologic treatment, *JAMA* 272:1361-1366, 1994.
7. Reardon LC, Macpherson DS: Hyperkalemia in outpatients using angiotensin-converting enzyme inhibitors: how much should we worry? *Arch Intern Med* 158:26-32, 1998.
8. Irwin RS, Boulet LP, Cloutier MM, et al: Managing cough as a defense mechanism and as a symptom: a consensus panel report of the American College of Chest Physicians, *Chest* 114(suppl 2):133S-181S, 1998.
9. Forslund T, Tohmo H, Weckstrom G, et al: Angio-oedema induced by enalapril, *J Intern Med* 238:179-181, 1995.
10. Brown NJ, Snowden M, Griffin MR: Recurrent angiotensin-converting enzyme inhibitor–associated angioedema, *JAMA* 278:232-233, 1997.
11. Teerlink JR, Massie BM: The interaction of ACE inhibitors and aspirin in heart failure: torn between two lovers (editorial), *Am Heart J* 138:193-197, 1999.

Angiotensin II antagonists

Some of the available angiotensin II receptor antagonists and their usual doses are listed in Table 9. They do not cause cough but occasionally cause angioedema, which may manifest itself at varying time intervals after the drug is

Table 9 Angiotensin II Inhibitors

Drug	Usual dose
Candesartan Cilexetil (Atacand)	8-32 mg/day as a single daily dose
Eprosartan (Teveten)	400-800 mg/day as a single dose or bid
Irbesartan (Avapro)	150-300 mg/day as a single daily dose
Losartan (Cozaar)	25-100 mg/day as a single daily dose
Telmisartan (Micardis)	40-80 mg/day as a single daily dose
Valsartan (Diovan)	80-320 mg/day as a single daily dose

started.[1] Studies are in progress to determine whether these drugs are as effective as ACE inhibitors in prolonging life in patients with congestive heart failure or after a myocardial infarction and whether they prevent nephropathy in diabetic patients. One trial comparing captopril to losartan in patients with class II to IV heart failure reported equal benefit for controlling failure but a lower total mortality rate in the losartan-treated cohort, apparently because of a decrease in sudden cardiac death.[2]

◣ REFERENCES ◢

1. Van Rijnsoever EW, Kwee-Zuiderwijk WJ, Feenstra J: Angioneurotic edema attributed to the use of losartan, *Arch Intern Med* 158:2063-2065, 1998.
2. Pitt B, Segal R, Martinez FA, et al: Randomised trial of losartan versus captopril in patients over 65 with heart failure (Evaluation of Losartan in the Elderly Study, ELITE), *Lancet* 349:747-752, 1997.

Diuretics

(See also specific antihypertensive drugs)

The standard diuretic for the outpatient treatment of congestive heart failure is a loop diuretic such as furosemide (Lasix),[1] although in mild cases a thiazide can sometimes be used.[2] Few patients need more than 80 mg of furosemide per day if the drug is combined with an ACE inhibitor or metolazone (Zaroxolyn) or both.[1] If the response to a moderate morning dose of a loop diuretic is inadequate, larger morning doses are unlikely to be effective; more frequent moderate doses spread throughout the day often result in diuresis. In refractory cases the addition of a thiazide may result in diuresis, but care must be taken because the diuresis may be profound and cause cardiovascular collapse.[3] One retrospective study of patients with heart failure reported an increased rate of arrhythmic deaths in patients treated with non-potassium-sparing diuretics (with or without potassium supplementation) compared with those treated with potassium-sparing diuretics alone or a combination of potassium-sparing and non-potassium-sparing diuretics.[4]

Volume depletion should be avoided because it makes the dose of an ACE inhibitor difficult to titrate. Once the excess fluid volume is controlled, patients should weigh themselves every morning. If the weight changes by more than 1 to 2 kg, medication reassessment is indicated.[1]

Metolazone may be added to the furosemide–ACE inhibitor regimen when necessary. Dosage is 2.5 to 5 mg po daily or every 2 days for a few days at a time. Metolazone is usually given 1 hour before the furosemide, and careful monitoring of potassium is required.[2] Only exceptionally does metolazone have to be continued on a long-term basis.

If elderly patients with congestive heart failure who are taking thiazide diuretics are also given NSAIDs, they are at risk of worsening failure and the need for hospitalization.[5]

◣ REFERENCES ◢

1. Baker DW, Konstam MA, Bottoriff M, et al: Management of heart failure. I. Pharmacologic treatment, *JAMA* 272:1361-1366, 1994.
2. Cohn JN: The management of chronic heart failure, *N Engl J Med* 335:490-498, 1996.
3. Brater DC: Diuretic therapy, *N Engl J Med* 339:387-395, 1998.
4. Cooper HA, Dries DL, Davis CE, et al: Diuretics and risk of arrhythmic death in patients with left ventricular dysfunction, *Circulation* 100:1311-1315, 1999.
5. Heerdink ER, Leufkens HG, Herings RM, et al: NSAIDs associated with increased risk of congestive heart failure in elderly patients taking diuretics, *Arch Intern Med* 158:1108-1112, 1998.

Digoxin

Withdrawal of digoxin (Lanoxin) from patients with heart failure who are receiving diuretics alone (PROVED trial)[1] or with ACE inhibitors (RADIANCE trial)[2] worsens the left ventricular ejection fraction, functional status, and exercise capacity. A pooled analysis of these two studies concluded that optimal therapy for patients with severe systolic dysfunction was triple therapy with an ACE inhibitor, a diuretic, and digoxin.[3] This view is supported by the Digitalis Investigation Group (DIG) study, which reported that patients randomly assigned to receive digoxin in addition to diuretics and ACE inhibitors had the same mortality rate as those not receiving digoxin but had fewer hospitalizations.[4]

At present digoxin has the greatest value for patients with severe heart failure. A loading dose is not required. The usual adult dose is 0.125 to 0.25 mg/day, and in most cases 0.125 mg is adequate, especially in the elderly.

◣ REFERENCES ◢

1. Uretsky BF, Young JB, Shahidi FE, et al (PROVED Investigative Group): Randomized study assessing effect of digoxin withdrawal in patients with mild to moderate chronic congestive heart failure: results of the PROVED trial, *J Am Coll Cardiol* 22:955-962, 1993.
2. Packer M, Gheorghiade M, Young JB, et al: Withdrawal of digoxin from patients with chronic heart failure treated with angiotensin-converting enzyme inhibitors: RADIANCE Study, *N Engl J Med* 329:1-7, 1993.
3. Young JB, Gheorghiade M, Uretsky BF, et al: Superiority of "triple" drug therapy in heart failure: insights from the PROVED and RADIANCE trials, *J Am Coll Cardiol* 32:686-692, 1998.
4. Garg R, Gorlin R, Smith T, et al (Digitalis Investigation Group): The effect of digoxin on mortality and morbidity in patients with heart failure, *N Engl J Med* 336:525-533, 1997.

Vasodilators

In 1986 the combination of hydralazine (Apresoline) and isosorbide dinitrate (Isordil, Coradur) was found to reduce both morbidity and mortality in congestive heart failure.[1] This regimen has since been replaced by ACE inhibitors, which are more effective, but the combination is still used in patients who cannot tolerate ACE inhibitors.[2] If the combination is used, the maintenance doses are usually high. Hydralazine is given as 25 to 75 mg tid or qid with a maximum daily dose of 300 mg, and isosorbide dinitrate as 10 to 40 mg tid or qid with a maximum daily dose of 240 mg. At the higher doses of hydralazine, drug-induced lupus may be a complication. Clinical benefits of these regimens may not be apparent for the first few weeks of treatment.

❧ REFERENCES ❧

1. Cohn JN, Archibald DG, Ziesche S, et al: Effect of vasodilator therapy on mortality in chronic congestive heart failure: results of a Veterans Administration Cooperative Study, *N Engl J Med* 314:1547-1552, 1986.
2. Grauer K, Clark DS, Ruoff GE: *Cardiovascular disease: update on management of heart failure, acute myocardial infarction, and cardiac arrhythmias* (an *American Family Physician* monograph), St Louis, 1998, American Academy of Family Physicians.

Beta-blockers

Recent metaanalyses have shown that beta-blockers given to patients with moderately severe heart failure whose condition has been stabilized with ACE inhibitors, diuretics, and in many cases digoxin decrease mortality and hospital admissions and improve ejection fractions and functional status. In a number of studies carvedilol (Coreg), which has combined beta- and alpha$_1$-blocking functions as well as antioxidant effects, seemed to be more effective than other beta-blockers,[1,2] but a 1999 study comparing carvedilol and metoprolol (Betaloc, Lopresor) found no difference in efficacy between the two drugs.[3] According to Cleland and associates,[4] beta-blockers are at least as effective as ACE inhibitors in decreasing mortality from heart failure.

Heart failure activates the adrenergic system, and this may be detrimental through a variety of mechanisms. Catecholamines may lead to increased myocardial oxygen consumption,[5] have a direct toxic effect on the myocytes,[5] and activate the renin-angiotensin system, causing sodium retention and venous and arterial constriction, which increases preload and afterload.[6] Beta-blockers counter these effects. If they are used, initial doses should be very small and titrated upward at about weekly intervals. Full therapeutic benefit may take 1 to 3 months.[4,6] A direct antiarrhythmic effect of beta-blockers is suggested by a trial of bisoprolol (Zebeta), which led to a 42% decrease in sudden cardiac deaths among patients with heart failure in the treatment arm of the study.[7]

Carvedilol (and other beta-blockers) should generally not be started until the patient's condition has been stabilized with diuretics, ACE inhibitors, and perhaps digoxin and neither fluid overload nor hypotension is present. The initial dose of carvedilol is 3.125 mg bid, and one recommended protocol is to double the dose every 2 weeks to a maximum of 25 mg bid for patients weighing 85 kg (187 lb) or less and 50 mg bid for those over that weight.[8,9] Patients should monitor their weight daily and report to the physician if it increases by more than about 1 kg (2.2 lb).[8] The benefits of carvedilol may not be apparent for weeks or even months. Even if symptoms are not relieved, the drug should be continued because it may improve survival.[9]

Although carvedilol is generally considered to be contraindicated in patients with severe decompensated heart failure (class IV),[9] preliminary evidence indicates that many patients can benefit from careful administration of the drug provided they are not in cardiogenic shock, severely hypotensive or bradycardic, or in intractable pulmonary edema.[10]

❧ REFERENCES ❧

1. Lechat P, Packer M, Chalon S, et al: Clinical effects of ß-adrenergic blockade in chronic hear failure: a meta-analysis of double-blind, placebo-controlled, randomized trials, *Circulation* 98:1184-1191, 1998.
2. Heidenreich PA, Lee TT, Massie BM, et al: Effect of beta-blockade on mortality in patients with heart failure: a meta-analysis of randomized clinical trials, *J Am Coll Cardiol* 30:27-34, 1997.
3. Kukin ML, Kalman J, Charney RH, et al: Prospective randomized comparison of effect of long-term treatment with metoprolol or carvedilol on symptoms, exercise, ejection fraction, and oxidative stress in heart failure, *Circulation* 99:2645-2651, 1999.
4. Cleland JG, McGowan J, Clark A: The evidence for β blockers in heart failure: equals or surpasses that for angiotensin converting enzyme inhibitors (editorial), *BMJ* 318:824-825, 1999.
5. Haim M, Shotan A, Boyko V, et al: Effect of beta-blocker therapy in patients with coronary artery disease in New York Heart Association classes II and III, *Am J Cardiol* 81:1455-1460, 1998.
6. Drugs for chronic heart failure, *Med Lett* 38:92-94, 1996.
7. CIBIS-II Investigators and Committees: The Cardiac Insufficiency Bisoprolol Study II (CIBIS-II): a randomised trial, *Lancet* 353:9-13, 1999.
8. Vanderhoff BT, Ruppel HM, Amesterdam PB: Carvedilol: the new role of beta blockers in congestive heart failure, *Am Fam Physician* 58:1627-1634, 1998.
9. Frishman WH: Carvedilol, *N Engl J Med* 339:1759-1765, 1998.
10. Macdonald PS, Keogh AM, Aboyoun CL, et al: Tolerability and efficacy of carvedilol in patients with New York Heart Association class IV heart failure, *J Am Coll Cardiol* 33:924-931, 1999.

Spironolactone

Aldosterone levels are markedly increased in congestive heart failure and cause a variety of deleterious effects, including sodium retention, potassium loss, inhibition of myocardial uptake of norepinephrine, and myocardial fibrosis. Because ACE inhibitors only transiently suppress aldosterone production, a randomized placebo-controlled trial of the aldosterone blocking agent spironolactone (Aldactone) for patients with severe heart failure already being treated with ACE inhibitors, loop diuretics, and in most cases digoxin was instituted. The initial dose was 25 mg once daily, and after 8 weeks it was increased to 50 mg/day if the patient's condition did not improve. If hyperkalemia (≥ 6 mmol/L [≥ 6.0 mEq/L]) developed, the dose was reduced to 25 mg every other day. Patients receiving spironolactone had lower death and hospitalization rates and less progression of heart failure. Hyperkalemia was rarely a problem, and only a few men suffered from painful gynecomastia. Few patients were taking beta-blockers, so what the effect of combining beta-blockers and aldosterone would be in severe failure is unknown.[1]

REFERENCES

1. Pitt B, Zannad F, Remme WJ, et al: The effect of spironolactone on morbidity and mortality in patients with severe heart failure, *N Engl J Med* 341:709-717, 1999.

HYPERTENSION

(See also hypertensive disorders of pregnancy)

Definition and Epidemiology

The definitions of hypertension according to the *Sixth Report of the Joint National Committee on Detection, Evaluation, and Treatment of High Blood Pressure (JNC VI)* are recorded in Table 10. The blood pressure should be recorded with the patient in the sitting position with the arm at heart level, and the mean of two readings taken 2 minutes apart should be used. The patient should have been resting for at least 5 minutes and have abstained from caffeine or smoking for at least 30 minutes. Normal readings are <130/85 mm Hg. If the initial pressures are ≥ 180 mm Hg systolic or ≥ 110 mm Hg diastolic, further evaluation or institution of treatment should take place within a week. Elevated levels of lesser degrees should be reevaluated within 1 month for relatively high readings and within 2 months for lesser degrees of elevation.[1]

It has been estimated that 25% of the adult U.S. population has hypertension. The prevalence is higher in blacks than whites and increases with age. The mean increase in blood pressure from ages 30 to 65 is 20 mm Hg systolic and 10 mm diastolic.[2] Among untreated persons with hypertension 70% die of heart failure or coronary artery disease, 15% of cerebral hemorrhage, and 10% of uremia.[3]

Blood pressure has a circadian pattern. It plateaus at its highest level during the day, falls during the evening to reach its lowest level after midnight, and rises steeply again in the early morning before waking.[4]

REFERENCES

1. Joint National Committee on Detection, Evaluation, and Treatment of High Blood Pressure: Sixth report of the Joint National Committee on Detection, Evaluation, and Treatment of High Blood Pressure, *Arch Intern Med* 157:2413-2416, 1997.
2. Kannel WB: Blood pressure as a cardiovascular risk factor: prevention and treatment, *JAMA* 275:1571-1576, 1996.
3. Kligman EW: Hypertension. In Mengel MB, Schwiebert LP, eds: *Ambulatory medicine: the primary care of families,* Norwalk, Conn, 1993, Appleton & Lange, pp 415-425.
4. Wever MA: Hypertension as a risk factor syndrome: therapeutic implications, *Am J Med* 94(suppl 4 A):4A-24A, 1993.

Laboratory Investigations

The usual laboratory investigations for patients with hypertension are aimed at assessing target organ damage and other risk factors for coronary artery disease. These are urinalysis; complete blood cell count; measurement of electrolytes, creatinine, and fasting glucose; lipid profile; and 12-lead ECG. Other investigations are optional and directed by the clinical findings.[1,2]

REFERENCES

1. Joint National Committee on Detection, Evaluation, and Treatment of High Blood Pressure: Sixth report of the Joint National Committee on Detection, Evaluation, and Treatment of High Blood Pressure, *Arch Intern Med* 157:2413-2416, 1997.
2. Feldman RD, Campbell N, Larochelle P, et al: 1999 Canadian recommendations for the management of hypertension, *Can Med Assoc J* 161(suppl 12):S1-S22, 1999.

Secondary Hypertension

Except among persons who drink alcohol to excess, secondary hypertension is rare. Investigations for secondary hypertension are necessary only when it is clinically suspected. The following are important causes of the condition[1]:

1. Alcohol
2. Medications (e.g., oral contraceptives, NSAIDs, sympathomimetics such as appetite suppressants and decongestants)
3. Renal parenchymal disease
4. Renovascular disease
5. Coarctation of the aorta
6. Cushing's syndrome
7. Primary hyperaldosteronism

Table 10   Definition of Hypertension

Blood pressure	Systolic (mm Hg)	Diastolic (mm Hg)
Optimal	<120	<80
Normal	<130	<85
High normal	130-139	85-89
Hypertension	140+	90+
Stage 1 (mild)	140-159	90-99
Stage 2 (moderate)	160-179	100-109
Stage 3 (severe)	≥ 180	≥ 110

Modified from Joint National Committee on Prevention, Detection, Evaluation and Treatment of High Blood Pressure: Sixth report of the Joint National Committee on the Prevention, Detection, Evaluation and Treatment of High Blood Pressure, *Arch Intern Med* 157:2413-2446, 1997.

8. Pheochromocytoma
9. Thyroid dysfunction (hyperthyroidism or hypothyroidism)

Secondary hypertension may be suspected on the basis of the history, physical examination, or basic hypertensive investigations. It should be seriously considered in young patients or those with onset after the age of 55 years. Alcohol and drug use should be determined for all patients, as should the presence or absence of physical stigmata of Cushing's disease. The femoral artery pulsations and leg blood pressure should be checked as a screen for coarctation of the aorta in all young hypertensive patients. An abnormal urinalysis may point to renal disease, hypokalemia to primary hyperaldosteronism, and an abnormal thyroid-stimulating hormone level to thyroid disease.[1]

The following are other clues to secondary hypertension[1]:

1. Abrupt onset of hypertension
2. Severe hypertension (diastolic ≥110 mm Hg)
3. Rapid worsening of hypertension
4. Hypertension resistant to treatment

Although not formally recognized as a cause of secondary hypertension, hyperventilation (as is commonly seen in panic disorders) can raise blood pressure.[2,3] This diagnosis of hyperventilation is often missed.[3] Closely related to (and perhaps even synonymous with) hyperventilation-induced hypertension is a condition called "severe paroxysmal hypertension" or "pseudopheochromocytoma." Patients have recurring episodes of hypertension associated with symptoms typical of panic attacks, but they deny experiencing anxiety or stress before the onset of the episodes. Peak blood pressures can exceed 200/110 mm Hg.[4]

❧ REFERENCES ❧

1. Adcock BB, Ireland RB Jr: Secondary hypertension: a practical diagnostic approach, *Am Fam Physician* 55:1263-1270, 1997.
2. Todd GP, Chadwick IG, Yeo WW, et al: Pressor effect of hyperventilation in healthy subjects, *J Hum Hypertens* 9:119-122, 1995.
3. Kaplan NM: Anxiety-induced hyperventilation: a common cause of symptoms in patients with hypertension (editorial), *Arch Intern Med* 157:945-948, 1997.
4. Mann SJ: Severe paroxysmal hypertension (pseudopheochromocytoma), *Arch Intern Med* 159:670-674, 1999.

White Coat Hypertension

In patients with "white coat" or "office" hypertension, blood pressure readings are elevated when taken by physicians in their offices but normal when recorded at home or by ambulatory blood pressure monitoring. The incidence of white coat hypertension is about 20% in the population of patients with mild hypertension as recorded in physicians' offices. Although there is some controversy about this issue, most investigators have found that white coat hypertension diagnosed by ambulatory blood pressure monitoring is not associated with increased morbidity.[1]

White coat hypertension also occurs in treated hypertensive patients. In one study of hypertensive patients without end organ damage who failed to respond to medication, 54% of the women and 20% of the men demonstrated a white coat response as determined by 24-hour ambulatory monitoring.[2] (Normal daytime ambulatory monitoring was defined as 139/89 mm Hg or less, or systolic readings 20 mm Hg and diastolic readings 15 mm Hg lower than clinic readings.)

Certain precautions may reduce the frequency of white coat hypertension. Blood pressure should be measured with recently calibrated sphygmomanometers using correct cuff size, and measurements should be taken with the patient in a sitting position. Patients should have been resting for at least 5 minutes and should have abstained from coffee and cigarettes for at least 30 minutes.[3] Caffeine[3] and cocaine[4] can raise the blood pressure acutely and should be avoided by patients who are coming in for blood pressure checks. Le Pailleur and associates[5] found that if patients talked while the blood pressure was being taken, the measurements were a mean of 17 mm Hg systolic and 13 mm Hg diastolic higher than those taken when the patients were silent. Having patients read while the measurement was taken lowered the blood pressure even further.

Appel and Stason[6] reviewed the literature comparing office-based readings taken by physicians, office-based readings taken by nurses or technicians, ambulatory blood pressure monitoring, and patient self-monitoring. The most significant finding was that end organ damage correlated much better with ambulatory blood pressure readings than with office readings. Within the office, readings by physicians were higher than readings by nurses or technicians. Data were insufficient to make a definitive statement about the value of patient self-monitoring.

The role of ambulatory blood pressure in monitoring patients with hypertension was evaluated in a randomized controlled trial in Belgium. The initiation and monitoring of pharmacotherapy were based on either office readings or ambulatory readings, but the treating physician was blinded to which system was used. Left ventricular hypertrophy was used as a surrogate endpoint for morbidity. Twenty-six percent of patients in the ambulatory monitoring group required no pharmacotherapy versus 7% in the regular care group, and for those requiring drugs, dosage levels were significantly lower for those in the ambulatory monitoring group. Left ventricular mass was not increased in the ambulatory monitoring group compared with the regular care group.[7]

A number of studies have found that self-monitoring of blood pressure at home gives results similar to ambulatory blood pressure monitoring. What remains controversial is a definition of normal values for self-monitoring or ambulatory blood pressure results. Since home-recorded levels are always lower that office-measured levels, 135/85 mm Hg may be a realistic upper limit of normal for home readings.[8] The *JNC VI* set 135/85 mm Hg[3] and a Canadian task force 135/83 mm Hg[9] as the upper limits of normal blood pressure for mean daytime ambulatory readings.

What approach should family physicians take? Obviously they should make sure that their patients have abstained from caffeine or cocaine before the time the blood pressure is to be measured and have them refrain from talking during the procedure. Appel and Stason[5] suggest that if office readings by physicians are high, several more readings be taken by nurses or technicians (most of the trials showing beneficial effects of lowering blood pressure depended on nurse or technician readings). If blood pressure is still elevated when measured by nurses or technicians, the patients should be assessed for end-organ damage and other cardiovascular risk factors, and if either is present, they should be treated; if neither is present, home self-measurements or ambulatory monitoring should be undertaken and treatment decisions should be based on these readings.[6] Spence disagrees and recommends treating all patients with "office" hypertension until such time as randomized controlled trials show that it is safe not to do so.[10] I side with Appel and Stason.

─────────────── ◢ REFERENCES ◣ ───────────────

1. Pickering TG: White coat hypertension: to treat or not to treat? (editorial), *Am Fam Physician* 52:48, 58, 1995.
2. MacDonald MB, Laing GP, Wilson MP, et al: Prevalence and predictors of white-coat response in patients with treated hypertension, *Can Med Assoc J* 161:265-269, 1999.
3. Joint National Committee on Detection, Evaluation, and Treatment of High Blood Pressure: Sixth report of the Joint National Committee on Detection, Evaluation, and Treatment of High Blood Pressure, *Arch Intern Med* 157:2413-2416, 1997.
4. Brecklin CS, Gopaniuk-Folga A, Kravetz T, et al: Prevalence of hypertension in chronic cocaine users, *Hypertension* 11: 1279-1283, 1998.
5. Le Pailleur C, Helft G, Landais P, et al: The effects of talking, reading, and silence on the "white coat" phenomenon in hypertensive patients, *Am J Hypertens* 11:203-207, 1998.
6. Appel LJ, Stason WB: Ambulatory blood pressure monitoring and blood pressure self-measurement in the diagnosis and management of hypertension, *Ann Intern Med* 118:867-882, 1993.
7. Staessen JA, Byttebier G, Buntinx F, et al: Antihypertensive treatment based on conventional or ambulatory blood pressure measurement: a randomized controlled trial, *JAMA* 278:1065-1072, 1997.
8. Mengden T, Schwartzkopff B, Strauer BE: What is the value of home (self) blood pressure monitoring in patients with hypertensive heart disease? *Am J Hypertens* 11:813-819, 1998.
9. Feldman RD, Campbell N, Larochelle P, et al: 1999 Canadian recommendations for the management of hypertension, *Can Med Assoc J* 161(suppl 12):S1-S22, 1999.
10. Spence JD: Withholding treatment in white-coat hypertension: wishful thinking (editorial), *Can Med Assoc J* 161:275-276, 1999.

Pseudohypertension

Pseudohypertension is found in 2% to 5% of elderly patients and may raise both the systolic and diastolic readings by as much as 20 to 30 mm Hg.[1] The diagnosis may be suspected in patients with very high readings and no signs of end organ damage, in patients who do not respond to intensive pharmacological therapy, and in those who have postural hypotension after minimal therapy.[2] The traditional confirmatory test on physical examination is Osler's maneuver, which consists of inflating the blood pressure cuff above the systolic reading while palpating the radial or brachial artery. If the artery can still be felt as a nonpulsatile cord when the cuff is inflated above the systolic reading, Osler's maneuver is positive and the patient probably has pseudohypertension.[1] Not all workers agree that this is a sensitive or specific test; Belmin and associates[3] found it insensitive and also found that a significant number of normotensive patients were Osler test positive.

─────────────── ◢ REFERENCES ◣ ───────────────

1. Messerli FH, Ventura HO, Amodeo C: Osler's maneuver and pseudohypertension, *N Engl J Med* 312:1548-1551, 1985.
2. Fifth report of the Joint National Committee on Detection, Evaluation, and Treatment of High Blood Pressure (JNC V), *Arch Intern Med* 153:154-183, 1993.
3. Belmin J, Visintin J-M, Salvatore R, et al: Osler's maneuver: absence of usefulness for the detection of pseudohypertension in an elderly population, *Am J Med* 98:42-49, 1995.

Abdominal Bruits and Renovascular Hypertension

Between 7% and 31% of young individuals have abdominal bruits. Screening for such bruits in normotensive individuals is not indicated. However, about 80% of patients with angiographically documented renal artery stenosis have bruits; the specificity is particularly high if there is a systolic-diastolic bruit. The absence of a bruit does not rule out renovascular hypertension.[1]

─────────────── ◢ REFERENCES ◣ ───────────────

1. Turnbull JM: Is listening for abdominal bruits useful in the evaluation of hypertension? *JAMA* 274:1299-1301, 1995.

Efficacy of the Treatment of Hypertension

Lowering blood pressure has been documented to decrease the incidence of coronary artery disease, stroke, congestive heart failure, and all-cause mortality.[1] It also decreases the rate of progression of renal failure[1] and the risk for left ventricular hypertrophy.[2] In many randomized controlled trials, benefits have been obtained with only modest lowering of pressures, such as a 5 to 6 mm Hg reduction for diastolic readings.[3] Treatment of isolated systolic hypertension in the elderly reduces the incidence of stroke and coronary artery disease.[4-6]

Thus far the major studies proving decreased morbidity and mortality rates through the treatment of hypertension have involved diuretics and beta-blockers.[1] However, new trials are finding that other classes of drugs also decrease morbidity and mortality. A Scandinavian randomized prospective trial of hypertensive patients age 70 to 84 found equal benefit from diuretics, beta-blockers, calcium channel blockers, and ACE inhibitors.[7]

Antihypertensive therapy is effective in women, men, and the elderly.[1] Whether treating hypertension in the very elderly (those over 80 years of age) is beneficial is controversial (see later discussion of factors influencing the choice of drugs).

⚓ REFERENCES ⚓

1. Joint National Committee on Detection, Evaluation, and Treatment of High Blood Pressure: Sixth report of the Joint National Committee on Detection, Evaluation, and Treatment of High Blood Pressure, *Arch Intern Med* 157:2413-2416, 1997.
2. Moser M, Hebert PR: Prevention of disease progression, left ventricular hypertrophy and congestive heart failure in hypertension treatment trials, *J Am Coll Cardiol* 27:1214-1218, 1996.
3. Hebert PR, Moser M, Mayer J, et al: Recent evidence on drug therapy of mild to moderate hypertension and decreased risk of coronary heart disease, *Arch Intern Med* 153:578-581, 1993.
4. Systolic Hypertension in the Elderly Program Cooperative Research Group: Prevention of stroke by antihypertensive drug treatment in older persons with isolated systolic hypertension: final results of the Systolic Hypertension in the Elderly Program (SHEP), *JAMA* 265:3255-3264, 1991.
5. Staessen JA, Fagard R, Thijs L, et al (Systolic Hypertension in Europe [Syst-Eur] Trial Investigators): Randomised double-blind comparison of placebo and active treatment for older patients with isolated systolic hypertension, *Lancet* 350:757-764, 1997.
6. Liu L, Wang JG, Gong L, et al (Systolic Hypertension in China [Syst-China] Collaborative Group): Comparison of active treatment and placebo in older Chinese patients with isolated systolic hypertension, *J Hypertens* 16:1823-1829, 1998.
7. Hansson L, Lindholm LH, Ekbom T, et al: Randomised trial of old and new antihypertensive drugs in elderly patients: cardiovascular mortality and morbidity the Swedish Trial in Old Patients with Hypertension-2 study, *Lancet* 354:1751-1756, 1999.

Life-Style Modifications or Pharmacotherapy?

An important concept in the management of hypertension that is emphasized by the *JNC VI* is risk stratification of patients. Hypertensive patients at increased risk of complications are male, are over the age of 60, have a family history of cardiovascular disease, smoke, and have coronary artery disease, left ventricular hypertrophy, heart failure, peripheral vascular disease, nephropathy, retinopathy, diabetes, or dyslipidemia. The *JNC VI* recommends life-style modifications for all hypertensive patients. Those whose pressures are less than 160 mm Hg systolic or 100 mm Hg diastolic and who do not have target organ damage, clinical cardiovascular disease, or diabetes may be given an initial 6- to 12-month trial of life-style modifications without drugs. Pharmacotherapy should be instituted in those with pressures greater than or equal to 160 systolic or 100 diastolic and in those with lower readings who have target organ damage, clinical cardiovascular disease, or diabetes.[1]

⚓ REFERENCES ⚓

1. Joint National Committee on Detection, Evaluation, and Treatment of High Blood Pressure: Sixth report of the Joint National Committee on Detection, Evaluation, and Treatment of High Blood Pressure, *Arch Intern Med* 157:2413-2416, 1997.

Nonpharmacological Treatment of Hypertension
(See also alcohol; exercise; NSAIDs; obesity)

The following are some of the nonpharmacological treatment modalities for hypertension. Many of these are discussed more fully in the ensuing paragraphs.
1. Discontinue smoking.
2. Lose weight.
3. Exercise.
4. Discontinue or diminish alcohol consumption.
5. Discontinue NSAIDs if possible.
6. Change diet.

Smoking cessation
Smoking is not a risk factor for hypertension as such, but because it is a major cardiovascular risk factor, quitting is particularly important for hypertensive patients.[1]

Weight reduction
Significant lowering of blood pressure occurs in a large proportion of patients who lose 4.5 kg (10 lb).[1] Such moderate weight loss allowed older adults whose hypertension was well controlled with antihypertensive medications to discontinue the drugs and still maintain normal blood pressure levels. The benefit of weight loss was even more marked when combined with modest salt reduction.[2] Whether weight loss can be maintained for more than short periods of time is doubtful (see discussion of obesity).[3]

Exercise
Regular aerobic exercise such as 3 hours of brisk walking per week has been shown to reduce both the systolic and diastolic blood pressure in mild, moderate, and severe hypertension.[4] A study of Japanese men found that those who walked to work had a decreased risk of hypertension.[5]

Reduction in alcohol intake
A 1994 study found that individuals who have less than three drinks per day did not show any elevation of blood pressure. However, drinking more than that, even if in the form of binge drinking, caused a rise in blood pressure.[6] An evaluation of heavy drinkers in Spain found that 42% were hypertensive while drinking but only 12% were hypertensive after 1 month of abstinence.[7] The pressor effect of alcohol begins within a few days of starting to drink and recedes within a few days of discontinuing alcohol; weekend binge drinkers have their highest readings on Mondays, and these become progressively lower throughout the week.[8]

Nonsteroidal antiinflammatory drugs

A large number of elderly patients with hypertension may have the disorder simply because they are taking, or have recently taken, NSAIDs. In one study 41% of elderly patients with hypertension had used NSAIDs in the previous year as compared with 26% of younger control subjects. The higher the dosage of NSAIDs, the more likely that the patients were started on antihypertensive therapy.[9] In a metaanalysis of a number of studies an Australian group found that on average NSAIDs elevated supine mean blood pressure by 5 mm Hg. Furthermore, NSAIDs antagonized the blood pressure–lowering effect of antihypertensive drugs, particularly beta-blockers. Diuretics and vasodilators were less affected.[10]

Dietary changes

The blood pressure–lowering effect of decreased dietary sodium intake varies among individuals.[1] Although one metaanalysis concluded that only a minority of hypertensive patients have a significant drop in blood pressure through salt limitation,[11] a recent study of elderly patients whose hypertension was well controlled by medication found that modest salt restriction allowed many to discontinue their drugs and remain normotensive. This benefit was even greater if those who were obese also lost weight.[2] For patients taking antihypertensive drugs, lowering salt intake often enhances their effect. The *JNC VI* recommends that dietary sodium be restricted to no more than 100 mmol/day (6 g of sodium chloride or 2.4 g of sodium).[1] For hypertensive patients with renal failure greater degrees of salt restriction often result in significant lowering of blood pressure.[12] There is no good evidence that sodium restriction for the general population would decrease the incidence of hypertension.[13]

In the United States 75% of sodium comes from processed foods. Foods high in salt include canned soups, bouillon cubes, smoked meat, smoked fish, bacon, ham, marinades, commercial sauces (ketchup, Worcestershire sauce, mustard), salt-covered snacks (chips, nuts), and some mineral waters. Some medications high in salt are Alka-Seltzer, Bromo-Seltzer, and Rolaids.

In normotensive persons and patients with mild hypertension, a short-term diet that was high in fruits and vegetables (8 to 10 servings a day) and rich in potassium and magnesium lowered blood pressures. This effect was augmented when low-fat dairy products containing plenty of calcium were added to the high–fruit and vegetable diet.[14] A 1999 metaanalysis found that calcium supplementation or diets high in calcium resulted in statistically significant[15] but clinically insignificant[16] reduction of both systolic and diastolic pressures. Caffeine can raise the blood pressure acutely but is not a cause of persistently elevated levels.[1] Excessive licorice ingestion may induce a hyperaldosterone-like syndrome with hypertension and a hypokalemic metabolic alkalosis.[17]

❧ REFERENCES ❧

1. Joint National Committee on Detection, Evaluation, and Treatment of High Blood Pressure: Sixth report of the Joint National Committee on Detection, Evaluation, and Treatment of High Blood Pressure, *Arch Intern Med* 157:2413-2416, 1997.
2. Whelton PK, Appel LJ, Espeland MA, et al: Sodium reduction and weight loss in the treatment of hypertension in older persons: a randomized controlled trial of nonpharmacologic interventions in the elderly (TONE), *JAMA* 279:839-846, 1998.
3. Freis ED: Improving treatment effectiveness in hypertension, *Arch Intern Med* 159:2517-2521, 1999.
4. Cléroux J, Feldman RD, Petrella RJ: Lifestyle modifications to prevent and control hypertension. 4. Recommendations on physical exercise training, *Can Med Assoc J* 160(suppl 9): S21-S28, 1999.
5. Hayashi T, Tsumura K, Suematsu C, et al: Walking to work and the risk for hypertension in men: the Osaka Health Survey, *Ann Intern Med* 130:21-26, 1999.
6. Marmot MG, Elliott P, Shipley MJ, et al: Alcohol and blood pressure: the INTERSALT study, *BMJ* 308:1263-1267, 1994.
7. Aguilera MT, de la Sierra A, Coca A, et al: Effect of alcohol abstinence on blood pressure: assessment by 24-hour ambulatory blood pressure monitoring, *Hypertension* 33:653-657, 1999.
8. Wannamethee G, Shaper AG: Alcohol intake and variations in blood pressure by day of examination, *J Hum Hypertens* 5:59-67, 1991.
9. Gurwitz FH, Avorn J, Bohn RL, et al: Initiation of antihypertensive treatment during nonsteroidal anti-inflammatory drug therapy, *JAMA* 272:781-786, 1994.
10. Johnson AG, Nguyen TV, Day RO: Do nonsteroidal anti-inflammatory drugs affect blood pressure? A meta-analysis, *Ann Intern Med* 121:289-300, 1994.
11. Midgley JP, Matthew AG, Greenwood CM, et al: Effect of reduced dietary sodium on blood pressure: a meta-analysis of randomized controlled trials, *JAMA* 275:1590-1597, 1996.
12. Moore MA, Epstein M, Agodoa L, et al: Current strategies for management of hypertensive renal disease, *Arch Intern Med* 159:23-28, 1999.
13. Graudal NA, Galløe AM, Garred P: Effects of sodium restriction on blood pressure, renin, aldosterone, catecholamines, cholesterols, and triglyceride: a meta-analysis, *JAMA* 279:1383-1391, 1998.
14. Appel LF, Moore TJ, Obarzanek E, et al: A clinical trial of the effects of dietary patterns on blood pressure, *N Engl J Med* 336:1117-1124, 1997.
15. Griffith LE, Guyatt GH, Cook RJ, et al: The influence of dietary and nondietary calcium supplementation on blood pressure: an updated metaanalysis of randomized controlled trials, *Am J Hypertens* 12:84-92, 1999.
16. Cappuccio FP: The "calcium antihypertension theory" (editorial), *Am J Hypertens* 12:93-95, 1999.
17. Heikens J, Fliers E, Endert E, et al: Liquorice-induced hypertension—a new understanding of an old disease: case report and brief review, *Netherlands J Med* 47:230-234, 1995.

Pharmacological Treatment of Hypertension
Optimal blood pressure levels

When treating hypertension, what level of blood pressure readings should one aim for? Is there a J-curve—does morbidity or mortality increase if target blood pressures are maintained below a certain level? The Hypertension Optimal Treatment (HOT) randomized trial (which excluded patients with isolated systolic hypertension) found no evidence of a J-curve and concluded that if 1000 patients achieved a pressure of 140/90 mm Hg, five to 10 cardiovascular events would be prevented per year. Lower levels gave only slight additional benefit but were not harmful.[1] In contrast, the Systolic Hypertension in the Elderly Program (SHEP) found a slight increase in cardiovascular events in patients whose diastolic pressure was lowered below 70 mm Hg and a more marked increase in those whose diastolic level reached 60 mm Hg or less.[2]

According to the Joint National Committee on the Detection, Evaluation and Treatment of High Blood Pressure, current evidence favors lowering pressures to levels achieved in clinical trials (usually below 140 systolic and 90 diastolic) for most patients and to below 130/85 for diabetic patients.[3] Levels below 130/85 mm Hg might also be a reasonable goal for patients in renal failure, and some workers recommend target levels of 120/75 mm Hg for blacks patients or those with renal disease and protein excretion greater than 1 g/day.[4] The 1999 British Hypertension Society guidelines advise readings below 140/85 mm Hg in nondiabetic patients and below 140/80 mm Hg in those with diabetes.[5]

—————————— ◤ REFERENCES ◣ ——————————

1. Hansson L, Zanchetti A, Carruthers SG, et al: Effects of intensive blood-pressure lowering and low-dose aspirin in patients with hypertension: principal results of the Hypertension Optimal Treatment (HOT) randomised trial; HOT Study Group, *Lancet* 351:155-1762, 1998.
2. Somes GW, Pahor M, Shorr RI, et al: The role of diastolic blood pressure when treating isolated systolic hypertension, *Arch Intern Med* 159:2004-2009, 1999.
3. Joint National Committee on Prevention, Detection, Evaluation and Treatment of High Blood Pressure: Sixth report of the Joint National Committee on the Prevention, Detection, Evaluation and Treatment of High Blood Pressure, *Arch Intern Med* 157:2413-2446, 1997.
4. Moore MA, Epstein M, Agodoa L, et al: Current strategies for management of hypertensive renal disease, *Arch Intern Med* 159:23-28, 1999.
5. Ramsay LE, Williams B, Johnston GD, et al: British Hypertension Society guidelines for hypertension management 1999: summary, *BMJ* 319:630-635, 1999.

Single-drug versus multiple-drug treatment

The recommendations of the *JNC VI* are to start with a low dose of one drug (preferably a diuretic or beta-blocker) and increase the dose gradually over several weeks. If ad-

equate control has not been achieved after the full dose has been reached, and if there are no significant adverse effects, a drug from another class (preferably a diuretic if it has not already been used) should be added. If this results in good control, it would be reasonable to try decreasing the dose of the original drug or discontinue it completely. If the patient experiences significant side effects while receiving the original drug, that drug should be discontinued and an antihypertensive from another class substituted.[1] If the blood pressure is over 200 mm Hg systolic or 115 mm Hg diastolic, a single agent will rarely give adequate control.[2]

A good case can be made for using a combination of antihypertensive drugs from the onset of treatment: adequate control often cannot be achieved with a single drug, or if it is, a high dose is required; good control is often rapidly achieved with the initial doses of combination drugs; adverse effects are fewer with combination drugs because the dose of each is low; compliance is improved with combination drugs because of simplified dosing (often a single combination pill each day) and fewer adverse effects. Some of the more effective combination pills are diuretics plus beta-blockers or diuretics plus ACE inhibitors.[3]

Noncompliance probably accounts for nearly half of all failures in the treatment of hypertension.[4]

—————————— ◤ REFERENCES ◣ ——————————

1. Joint National Committee on Prevention, Detection, Evaluation and Treatment of High Blood Pressure: Sixth report of the Joint National Committee on the Prevention, Detection, Evaluation and Treatment of High Blood Pressure, *Arch Intern Med* 157:2413-2446, 1997.
2. Kaplan NM, Gifford RW Jr: Choice of initial therapy for hypertension, *JAMA* 275:1577-1580, 1996.
3. Freis ED: Improving treatment effectiveness in hypertension, *Arch Intern Med* 159:2517-2521, 1999.
4. Stephenson J: Noncompliance may cause half of antihypertensive drug "failures," *JAMA* 228:313-314, 1999.

Factors influencing the choice of drugs

Many factors influence the choice of antihypertensive drugs. Although all classes of antihypertensives have been shown equally effective in lowering blood pressure, the *JNC VI* recommendation is to use either a diuretic or a beta-blocker as initial treatment unless a specific clinical reason exists for choosing another class of drugs. The rationale is that these are the drugs that have most frequently been shown to decrease morbidity and mortality in randomized controlled trials.[1] A 1999 Canadian task force includes ACE inhibitors along with low-dose thiazides or beta-blockers as first-line monotherapy.[2]

Support for using thiazides as first-line drugs comes from a 1999 systematic review in which low-dose diuretics were found to reduce the risk of death, stroke, coronary artery disease, and cardiovascular events, whereas high-dose thiazide therapy, beta-blocker therapy, and calcium channel blocker therapy did not decrease the risk of death or coronary artery disease (ACE inhibitors were not assessed).[3]

The Captopril Prevention Project (CAPPP) published in 1999 compared conventional treatment (beta-blockers or diuretics) with captopril for the management of hypertension. Cardiovascular mortality was lower and the incidence of fatal and nonfatal strokes higher among those taking captopril, while rates of myocardial infarction were similar in the two groups.[4]

Table 11 is an outline summary of additional factors that influence the prescriber's choice of antihypertensives. This table should be considered a broad guide with many exceptions. Most of these determinants are discussed in more detail in the ensuing text.

Reduction of left ventricular hypertrophy. Reduction of left ventricular hypertrophy is important because it is associated with improved prognosis. No evidence has shown that any one class of antihypertensives is superior to another in reducing left ventricular hypertrophy.[2,5]

Quality of life. No one class of antihypertensive agent is clearly superior to another in terms of quality of life. A 4-year follow-up of patients with mild hypertension taking a placebo or low doses of one of five classes of drugs (beta-blockers [acebutolol], calcium channel blockers [amlodipine], diuretics [chlorthalidone], alpha$_1$-blockers [doxazosin], ACE inhibitors [enalapril]) found that quality of life improved in all groups, including those taking placebo.[6]

Cost. Antihypertensive drugs vary greatly in cost. The least expensive in most cases is a generic diuretic or beta-blocker.

Age of patient. Isolated systolic hypertension is primarily a disease of the elderly and is much more prevalent in women. Low-dose diuretics such as hydrochlorothiazide 12.5 to 25 mg/day[7] or calcium channel blockers[8] have been shown to decrease the morbidity and mortality caused by coronary artery disease in elderly hypertensive patients.

A subgroup analysis of randomized controlled trials of antihypertensive treatment concluded that treating 100 patients age 80 and over prevented one nonfatal stroke per year and that such treatment also decreased the incidence of major cardiovascular events and heart failure. It did not decrease mortality.[9] The benefits and harm of treating hypertension in the very elderly can be determined only through randomized controlled trials.

According to the *JNC VI*, the drug of first choice for elderly hypertensives is low-dose thiazide diuretics.[1] A Canadian task force considers both low dose-thiazides and long-acting dihydropyridine calcium channel blockers to be first-choice agents.[2] In elderly patients without known coronary artery disease, beta-blockers are less effective than diuretics in lowering blood pressure, and they do not decrease cardiovascular morbidity and mortality in this population. However, beta-blockers are effective in elderly patients with cardiovascular diseases (such as myocardial infarctions) for which this class of drug is indicated.[10]

Table 11   Choice of Drugs in the Treatment of Hypertension

Clinical factor	Preferred drugs	Drugs of less value/comments
Reduction of left ventricular hypertrophy	Any antihypertensive drug	
Quality of life	Low dose; few side effects	High dose; significant side effects
Cost	Thiazides, beta-blockers	New drugs
Elderly	Thiazides	Beta-blockers
Black race	Diuretics, calcium channel blockers, alpha$_1$-blockers	Beta-blockers, ACE inhibitors
Arthritis		Discontinue NSAIDs or use aspirin or sulindac (Clinoril)
Angina	Beta-blockers, calcium channel blockers	
History of myocardial infarction	Beta-blockers	
Heart failure	ACE inhibitors, thiazides, ?angiotensin II antagonists	Beta-blockers often beneficial
Diabetes	ACE inhibitors, beta-blockers, low-dose thiazides	Beta-blockers and thiazides not contraindicated
Chronic renal failure	ACE inhibitors, diuretics	
Hyperlipidemia	ACE inhibitors, calcium channel blockers, alpha$_1$-blockers	Thiazides and beta-blockers not contraindicated; may be drugs of first choice
Chronic obstructive pulmonary disease		Beta-blockers
Benign prostatic hypertrophy	Alpha$_1$-blockers	
Peripheral vascular disease	Beta-blockers	
Depression		?Calcium channel blockers, ?beta-blockers

?, The indications or contraindications to these drugs are controversial. Some of these are discussed in the text here or in the sections dealing with specific drugs.

Race. Blacks may not respond as well as whites to beta-adrenergic blockers or ACE inhibitors.[11]

Angina. Angina or a history of a myocardial infarction is a strong indication for beta-blockers, whereas chronic obstructive lung disease is almost always a contraindication for this class of drugs.[1,2]

Arthritis. Arthritis is often treated with NSAIDs, but they tend either to cause hypertension or to counter the therapeutic effect of many antihypertensive drugs.

Diabetes mellitus. Because of the very high risk of cardiovascular and renal disease in patients with both diabetes and hypertension, the U.S. National Heart, Lung and Blood Institute[12] and the American Diabetes Association[13] have recommended that the target blood pressure for such individuals be 130/85 mm Hg.[2] Support for tight control comes from a United Kingdom Prospective Diabetes Study Group (UKPDS) report of hypertensive patients with type 2 diabetes who were treated with either a beta-blocker or an ACE inhibitor as first-line therapy (other drug classes were added if necessary). Mean blood pressures obtained were 144/82 mm Hg, and the incidence of macrovascular events, diabetes-related mortality, and visual loss was significantly lower than in the control group, who had a mean pressure of 154/87 mm Hg.[14]

Antihypertensive medications may decrease glucose tolerance, and thiazide diuretics are commonly considered the worst offenders. They are not. All classes of antihypertensives decrease glucose tolerance over the short term, and multiple-drug regimens are more likely to do so than single-drug treatments.[15] However, the decreased glucose tolerance of thiazides seems to be self-limited and disappears with time.[16] Therefore low-dose thiazides are acceptable treatment for diabetic patients provided that glucose levels are carefully monitored.[17] For example, the Systolic Hypertension in the Elderly Program (SHEP) found that both diabetic and nondiabetic patients treated with low-dose thiazides (chlorthalidone) had decreased rates of cardiovascular events (fatal and nonfatal strokes and fatal and nonfatal myocardial infarctions) compared with a control group receiving placebo. The absolute reduction rates were actually higher in diabetic than in nondiabetic patients because of their underlying high risk levels (see discussion of disease prevalence and risk reduction).[18]

Use of ACE inhibitors to decrease the risk of diabetic nephropathy in hypertensive diabetic patients has been generally recommended. A 1998 UKPDS report of tight blood pressure control in hypertensive diabetics using either the ACE inhibitor captopril (Capoten) or the beta-blocker atenolol (Tenormin) found that both drugs were equally effective in preventing renal disease (both also decreased the incidence of visual loss and macrovascular disease). This suggests that the protective factor is the effective lowering of blood pressure, not a specific class of antihypertensives.[19]

Beta-blockers are the only class of antihypertensives that have been shown to be cardioprotective; since persons with diabetes are at high risk of coronary events, beta-blockers are probably one of the drugs of choice for these patients.[20] This view is strongly supported by a 1996 Israeli report of type 2 diabetic patients with coronary artery disease. The 3-year mortality rate among those treated with beta-blockers was 7.8% compared with a 14% rate for those not taking beta-blockers.[21] Although these drugs may mask the symptoms of hypoglycemia in patients who are taking hypoglycemic agents, this is only a relative contraindication.

Hyperlipidemias. There is no good evidence that specific classes of antihypertensive drugs increase the risk of cardiovascular complications. The choice of antihypertensive drugs for hypertensive patients with hyperlipidemia should be the same as for hypertensive patients with normal lipid profiles.[2]

Chronic renal failure. The most important goal in the treatment of hypertension in patients with renal failure is to achieve good control ($\leq$130/85 mm Hg) by whatever means are effective, and this often means using multiple drugs. Whenever possible ACE inhibitors should be used because they have documented renal protective effects beyond that brought about by blood pressure control. In most cases diuretics are needed because of the salt and water retention that is usually part of renal failure. In severe failure thiazides are ineffective and loop diuretics are required.[22]

If a patient has a creatinine level above 30 mg/dl (250 μmol/L), ACE inhibitors should be started at low doses and the creatinine level monitored closely. ACE inhibitors should not be used if the potassium is 5.5 mmol/L or greater.[23]

Heart failure. ACE inhibitors are the drugs of first choice in hypertensive patients with heart failure.[2]

Benign prostatic hyperplasia. The drug of first choice for hypertensive patients with symptomatic benign prostatic hyperplasia is an alpha$_1$-blocker such as terazosin (Hytrin).[24]

Peripheral vascular disease. Beta-blockers may be used safely in cases of mild or moderate peripheral vascular disease.[2] Since peripheral vascular disease is a marker for widespread atherosclerosis, beta-blockers (without intrinsic ISA) may be the drugs of choice for hypertensive patients with peripheral vascular disease because of their cardioprotective effects.

Depression. Beta-blockers are commonly believed to cause or aggravate depression; however, several studies have failed to show such a correlation.[25,26]

▲ REFERENCES ▲

1. Joint National Committee on Detection, Evaluation, and Treatment of High Blood Pressure: Sixth report of the Joint National Committee on Detection, Evaluation, and Treatment of High Blood Pressure, *Arch Intern Med* 157:2413-2416, 1997.
2. Feldman RD, Campbell N, Larochelle P, et al: 1999 Canadian recommendations for the management of hypertension, *Can Med Assoc J* 161(suppl 12):S1-S22, 1999.

3. Wright JM, Lee C-H, Chambers GK:. Systematic review of antihypertensive therapies: does the evidence assist in choosing a first-line drug? *Can Med Assoc J* 161:25-32, 1999.

4. Hansson L, Lindholm LH, Niskanen L, et al: Effect of angiotensin-converting-enzyme inhibition compared with conventional therapy on cardiovascular morbidity and mortality in hypertension: the Captopril Prevention Project (CAPPP) randomised trial, *Lancet* 353:611-616, 1999.

5. Dunn FG, Pfeffer MA: Left ventricular hypertrophy in hypertension (editorial), *N Engl J Med* 340:1279-1280, 1999.

6. Grimm RH Jr, Grandits GA, Cutler FA, et al: Relationships of quality-of-life measures to long-term lifestyle and drug treatment in the treatment of mild hypertension study, *Arch Intern Med* 157:638-648, 1997.

7. Pearce KA, Furberg CD, Rushing J: Does antihypertensive treatment of the elderly prevent cardiovascular events or prolong life? A meta-analysis of hypertension treatment trials, *Arch Fam Med* 4:943-950, 1995.

8. Staessen JA, Fagard R, Lutgarde T, et al (Systolic Hypertension in Europe Trial Investigators): Subgroup and per-protocol analysis of the randomized European Trial on Isolated Systolic Hypertension in the Elderly, *Arch Intern Med* 158:1681-1691, 1998.

9. Gueyffier F, Bulpitt C, Boissel J-P, et al: Antihypertensive drugs in very old people: a subgroup meta-analysis of randomised controlled trials, *Lancet* 353:793-796, 1999.

10. Messerli FH, Grossman E, Goldbourt U: Are ß-blockers efficacious as first-line therapy for hypertension in the elderly? A systematic review, *JAMA* 279:1903-1907, 1998.

11. Hall WD, Reed JW, Flack JM, et al: Comparison of the efficacy of dihydropyridine calcium channel blockers in African American patients with hypertension, *Arch Intern Med* 158:2029-2034, 1998.

12. National High Blood Pressure Education Program Working Group report on hypertension in diabetes, *Hypertension* 23:145-158, 1994.

13. American Diabetes Association: Clinical practice recommendations 1996: diagnosis and management of nephropathy in patients with diabetes mellitus, *Diabetes Care* 19(suppl 1):S103-S106, 1996.

14. UK Prospective Diabetes Study Group: Tight blood pressure control and risk of macrovascular and microvascular complications in type 2 diabetes: UKPDS 38, *BMJ* 317:703-713, 1998.

15. Gurwitz JH, Bohn RL, Glynn RJ, et al: Antihypertensive drug therapy and the initiation of treatment for diabetes mellitus, *Ann Intern Med* 118:273-278, 1993.

16. Freis ED: The efficacy and safety of diuretics in treating hypertension, *Ann Intern Med* 122:223-226, 1995.

17. Moser M: Management of hypertension, part I, *Am Fam Physician* 53:2295-2302, 1996.

18. Curb JD, Pressel SL, Cutler JA, et al: Effect of diuretic-based antihypertensive treatment on cardiovascular disease risk in older diabetic patients with isolated systolic hypertension, *JAMA* 276:1866-1892, 1996.

19. UK Prospective Diabetes Study Group: Efficacy of atenolol and captopril in reducing risk of macrovascular and microvascular complications in type 2 diabetes: UKPDS 39, *BMJ* 317:713-720, 1998.

20. Kendall MJ, Lynch KP, Hjalmarson A, et al: Beta-blockers and sudden cardiac death, *Ann Intern Med* 123:358-367, 1995.

21. Jonas M, Reicherreiss H, Boyko V, et al: Usefulness of beta-blocker therapy in patients with non-insulin-dependent diabetes mellitus and coronary artery disease, *Am J Cardiol* 77:1273-1277, 1996.

22. Moore MA, Epstein M, Agodoa L, et al: Current strategies for management of hypertensive renal disease, *Arch Intern Med* 159:23-28, 1999.

23. Baker DW, Konstam MA, Bottoriff M, et al: Management of heart failure. I. Pharmacologic treatment, *JAMA* 272:1361-1366, 1994.

24. Hill SJ, Lawrence SL, Lepor H: New use for alpha blockers: benign prostatic hyperplasia, *Am Fam Physician* 49:1885-1888, 1994.

25. Wurzelmann J, Frishman WH, Aronson M, et al: Neuropsychological effects of antihypertensive drugs, *Cardiol Clin* 4:689-701, 1987.

26. Prisant LM, Spruill WJ, Fincham JE, et al: Depression associated with antihypertensive drugs, *J Fam Practice* 33:481-485, 1991.

Step-down therapy

As many as one third of patients whose hypertension has been well controlled for at least a year may be able to decrease or even discontinue their medications.[1] No recent guidelines for this have been published. It is generally agreed that such an undertaking should be implemented gradually, that close follow-up is indicated after medications are stopped, and that success is most likely in patients who have made significant life-style improvements.[1,2] One suggested protocol from 1987 is that if patients taking more than one antihypertensive drug are normotensive for 6 to 12 months, all but one drug may be gradually withdrawn. Patients who remain normotensive for 6 to 12 months while taking one medication and whose pretreatment pressure was only mildly elevated may have all medications discontinued.[3]

❧ REFERENCES ❧

1. Froom J, Trilling JS, Yeh S-S, et al: Withdrawal of antihypertensive medications, *J Am Board Fam Pract* 10:249-258, 1997.

2. Joint National Committee on Prevention, Detection, Evaluation and Treatment of High Blood Pressure: Sixth report of the Joint National Committee on the Prevention, Detection, Evaluation and Treatment of High Blood Pressure, *Arch Intern Med* 157:2413-2446, 1997.

3. Dannenberg AL, Kannel WB: Remission of hypertension: the "natural" history of blood pressure treatment in the Framingham Study, *JAMA* 257:1477-1483, 1987.

Specific antihypertensive drugs

(See also benign prostatic hypertrophy; detrusor overactivity; heart failure; pharmaceuticals; stress incontinence; urticaria and angioedema)

Diuretics and diuretics combined with potassium-sparing agents. Hypokalemia secondary to thiazide drugs is dose dependent[1] and is not usually a problem with doses less than 25 mg/day. One reason for treating even mild hypokalemia is that low potassium levels are associated with elevations of blood pressure.[2] Although oral supplements of potassium chloride are traditionally given to counter hypokalemia, the use of a potassium-sparing agent such as amiloride, triamterene, or spironolactone in conjunction with a thiazide should be considered for hydrochlorothiazide doses of 25 mg/day or more (Table 12). There is evidence that this decreases the risk of primary cardiac arrest compared with control patients receiving equivalent doses of thiazides with or without potassium supplementation.[3] Some of the available combined products are Dyazide, Moduretic or Moduret, and Aldactazide.

Other reputed adverse effects of thiazides are elevated cholesterol and glucose levels. When low doses are used, both of these effects tend to be short lived and either to disappear with long-term therapy[4] or at least not to be progressive.[5] In the Systolic Hypertension in the Elderly Program (SHEP) program, in which chlorthalidone (Hygroton) in doses of 12.5 to 25 mg/day was the primary therapeutic agent, diabetic patients had as great a decrease in cerebrovascular accidents and strokes as did nondiabetic patients.[5]

Potassium supplementation. If hypokalemia is induced by diuretics, prescribing a combination of a thiazide and a potassium-sparing diuretic is often best (see earlier discussion of diuretics). Foods high in potassium include milk products, fruits, meat, and vegetables. A large number of commercial potassium supplements are available; the usual dose for oral replacement is about 20 mEq/day.

Calcium channel blockers. Traditional calcium channel blockers that block the L-channels are divided into three classes (Table 13). All calcium channel blockers increase coronary artery flow and are therefore antianginal agents. Verapamil has the most marked negative inotropic effect of all these agents. Verapamil and to a lesser extent diltiazem decrease atrioventricular node conduction and are therefore useful in patients with paroxysmal supraventricular tachycardia or atrial fibrillation with a rapid ventricular response.[6] Both verapamil and diltiazem may be used in patients with angina who are taking nitrates because these agents do not tend to cause reflex tachycardia.

It has been known for some time that calcium channel blockers have no cardioprotective effect after myocardial infarction.[6] Of more concern are reports of an association between both short-acting[7] and long-acting[8] calcium channel blockers and myocardial infarction, but the true significance of this is uncertain because other reports have not shown such a correlation.[9] There are also reports that these agents may lead to increased perioperative bleeding.[10] Some reports have claimed an association between calcium channel blockers and gastrointestinal hemorrhages,[11] but others have failed to confirm this finding.[12] Although some studies have found an increased risk of cancer in patients taking calcium channel blockers,[13] others report no such association.[14] An increased risk of suicide has been reported among patients taking these drugs.[15]

The current role of calcium channel blockers is controversial. Furberg[16] recommends considering any calcium channel blocker a third-line drug until controlled trials prove the safety of the newer formulations, whereas Stanton[17] advises no restriction of use pending the results of large randomized trials. I support a cautious approach to the use of calcium channel blockers.

Beta-blockers (Table 14). Beta-blockers decrease heart rate, systolic blood pressure, myocardial contractility, and myocardial oxygen demand. Beta-blockers without ISA are the only antihypertensive drugs shown to be cardioprotective;

Table 12 Diuretics and Diuretics Combined with Potassium-Sparing Agents

Drug	Usual dose
Diuretics	
Hydrochlorothiazide (Hydrodiuril, Esidrix, HCTZ)	12.5-25 mg qam
Chlorthalidone (Hygroton)	25 mg qam
Indapamide (Lozide)	1.25-2.5 mg qam
Spironolactone (Aldactone)	25-100 mg qam
Diuretics Plus K⁺ Sparing Agents	
Hydrochlorothiazide 50 mg plus amiloride 5 mg (Moduretic, Moduret)	½ tablet qam
Hydrochlorothiazide 25 mg plus triamterene 50 mg (Dyazide)	½ tablet qam
Spironolactone 25 mg plus hydrochlorothiazide 25 mg (Aldactazide)	1 tablet qam

Table 13 Calcium Channel Blockers

Drug	Usual dose
Benzothiazepine Derivatives	
Diltiazem (Cardizem, Tiazac)	30-60 mg tid-qid for short acting; 60-180 mg bid for SR; 180-360 mg as a single dose for controlled delivery
Papaverine-Like Compounds	
Verapamil (Isoptin, Calan, Covera-HS)	80 tid for short acting; 180-240 mg as single dose for extended-release tablets
Dihydropyridine Derivatives	
Amlodipine besylate (Norvasc)	5-10 mg/day as a single dose
Felodipine (Renedil, Plendil)	2.5-10 mg/day as a single dose
Isradipine (DynaCirc)	2.5-5 mg bid for short acting; 5-10 mg/day as single dose for extended release
Nicardipine (Cardene)	20-40 mg tid for short acting; 30-60 mg bid for extended release
Nifedipine (Adalat, Procardia)	10-20 mg bid for short acting; 30-90 mg/day as a single dose for extended release
Nisoldipine (Sular)	20-40 mg/day as a single dose

Table 14 Beta-blockers

Drug	Usual dose
Nonselective, Without ISA	
Nadolol (Corgard)	80-240 mg/day as a single dose
Propranolol (Inderal)	40-160 mg bid for short acting; 80-320 mg once a day for extended release
Timolol (Blocadren)	5-30 mg bid
Selective, Without ISA	
Atenolol (Tenormin)	50-100 mg/day as a single dose
Metoprolol (Lopresor, Toprol-XL)	50-100 mg bid for short acting; 100 mg/day as a single dose for extended release
Nonselective, with ISA	
Pindolol (Visken)	5-15 mg bid
Selective, with ISA	
Acebutolol (Sectral)	100-400 mg bid
Beta-Adrenergic and Alpha$_1$-Blocking Agents	
Labetalol (Trandate)	200-400 mg bid
Carvedilol (Coreg)	12.5 mg bid

ISA, Intrinsic sympathomimetic activity.

Table 15 ACE Inhibitors and Angiotensin II Antagonists

Drug	Usual dose
ACE Inhibitors	
Benazepril (Lotensin)	10-20 mg/day as a single dose
Captopril (Capoten)	25-50 mg bid or tid
Cilazapril (Inhibace)	2.5-5 mg/day as a single dose
Enalapril (Vasotec)	5-40 mg/day as a single dose or bid
Fosinopril (Monopril)	20 mg/day as a single daily dose
Lisinopril (Zestril, Prinivil)	10-40 mg/day as a single dose
Moexipril (Univasc)	7.5-30 mg/day as a single dose or bid
Perindopril (Coversyl)	4-8 mg/day as a single dose
Quinapril HCl (Accupril)	10-20 mg/day as a single dose
Ramipril (Altace)	2.5-10 mg/day as a single dose
Trandolapril (Mavik)	2-4 mg/day as a single dose
Angiotensin II Antagonists	
Candesartan cilexetil (Atacand)	8-32 mg/day as a single dose
Eprosartan (Teveten)	400-800 mg/day as a single dose or bid
Irbesartan (Avapro)	150-300 mg/day as a single dose
Losartan (Cozaar)	25-100 mg/day as a single dose
Telmisartan (Micardis)	40-80 mg/day as a single dose
Valsartan (Diovan)	80-320 mg/day as a single dose

Table 16 Alpha$_1$-Adrenergic Blocking Agents

Drug	Usual dose
Terazosin (Hytrin)	1-5 mg/day as a single dose
Prazosin (Minipress)	2-5 mg tid
Doxazosin (Cardura)	1-8 mg/day as a single dose

they reduce mortality after infarction, limit infarct size, and decrease arrhythmias and sudden death. Beta-blockers may mask some of the symptoms of hypoglycemia in diabetic patients taking hypoglycemic medications, but except for patients with recurrent hypoglycemic episodes this is not a contraindication to using these agents, since the cardioprotective benefits far outweigh this adverse effect. Although beta-blockers without intrinsic ISA may cause a slight lowering of HDL-cholesterol and some elevation of triglycerides, the clinical significance of these changes is unknown; there are no human or animal data showing that beta-blockers promote atherogenesis. Beta-blockers with intrinsic ISA activity do not adversely affect lipid profiles, but since they are not a good choice for cardioprotection, they have little role in the treatment of hypertension. Heart failure is only a relative contraindication for beta-blocker drugs,[18] while peripheral vascular disease is not a contraindication.[19]

Beta-blockers are commonly believed to cause or aggravate depression. However, not all studies show such a correlation.[20]

Beta-blockers may lead to or aggravate urinary incontinence because of detrusor overactivity. This is because beta-adrenergic stimulation normally inhibits the detrusor muscle.[21]

Sotalol is not indicated for the treatment of hypertension.

ACE inhibitors and angiotensin II–blocking agents (Table 15). ACE inhibitors may cause disorders of taste, cough in up to 25% of patients, and rarely angioedema. An alternative for patients unable to tolerate ACE inhibitors is to try an angiotensin II–blocking agent. A more complete discussion of ACE inhibitors may be found in the section on heart failure.

Angiotensin II receptor antagonists are as effective as ACE inhibitors in lowering blood pressure, but as yet few published studies have examined whether they prolong life in patients with congestive heart failure or after a myocardial infarction or whether they prevent nephropathy in diabetics. They do not cause cough, rarely cause angioedema, and occasionally cause hyperkalemia.[22-24]

Alpha$_1$-adrenergic blocking agents (Table 16). Reflex tachycardia often occurs in patients treated with alpha$_1$-blocking agents who are not also taking beta-blockers. Alpha$_1$-blockers inhibit the alpha-adrenergic receptors of the internal bladder sphincter and may lead to incontinence. On the other hand, they may relieve the symptoms of benign prostatic hyperplasia.

≥ REFERENCES ≤

1. Knauf H: The role of low-dose diuretics in essential hypertension, *J Cardiovasc Pharmacol* 22(suppl 6):S1-S7, 1993.
2. Whelton PK, He J, Cutler JA, et al: Effects of oral potassium on blood pressure: meta-analysis of randomized controlled clinical trials, *JAMA* 277:1624-1632, 1997.
3. Siscovick DS, Raghunathan TE, Psaty BM, et al: Diuretic therapy for hypertension and the risk of primary cardiac arrest, *N Engl J Med* 330:1852-1857, 1994.
4. Freis ED: The efficacy and safety of diuretics in treating hypertension, *Ann Intern Med* 122:223-226, 1995.

5. Savage PJ, Pressel SL, Curb JD, et al: Influence of long-term, low-dose, diuretic-based, antihypertensive therapy on glucose, lipid, uric acid, and potassium levels in older men and women with isolated systolic hypertension: the Systolic Hypertension in the Elderly Program, *Arch Intern Med* 158:741-751, 1998.

6. Raspa RF, Wilson CC: Calcium channel blockers in the treatment of hypertension, *Am Fam Physician* 48:461-470, 1993.

7. Furberg CD, Psaty BM, Meyer JV: Nifedipine: dose-related increase in mortality in patients with coronary heart disease, *Circulation* 92:1326-1331, 1995.

8. Estacio RO, Jeffers BW, Hiatt W, et al: The effect of nisoldipine as compared with enalapril on cardiovascular outcomes in patients with non-insulin-dependent diabetes and hypertension, *N Engl J Med* 338:645-652, 1998.

9. Abascal VM, Larson MG, Evans JC, et al: Calcium antagonists and mortality risk in men and women with hypertension in the Framingham Heart Study, *Arch Intern Med* 158:1882-1886, 1998.

10. Zuccalà G, Pahor M, Landi F, et al: Use of calcium antagonists and need for perioperative transfusion in older patients with hip fracture: observational study, *BMJ* 314:643-644, 1997.

11. Pahor M, Guralnik JM, Furberg CD, et al: Risk of gastrointestinal hemorrhage with calcium antagonists in hypertensive patients over 67, *Lancet* 347:1061-1066, 1996.

12. Suissa S, Bourgault C, Barkun A, et al: Antihypertensive drugs and the risk of gastrointestinal bleeding, *Am J Med* 105:230-235, 1998.

13. Pahor M, Guralnik JM, Salive ME, et al: Do calcium channel blockers increase the risk of cancer? *Am J Hypertens* 9:695-699, 1996.

14. Rosenberg L, Rao RS, Palmer JR, et al: Calcium channel blockers and the risk of cancer, *JAMA* 279:1000-1004, 1998.

15. Lindberg G, Bingefors K, Ranstam J, et al: Use of calcium channel blockers and risk of suicide: ecological findings confirmed in population based cohort study, *BMJ* 316:741-745, 1998.

16. Furberg CD: Should dihydropyridines be used as first-line drugs in the treatment of hypertension? The con side, *Arch Intern Med* 155:2157-2161, 1995.

17. Stanton AV: Calcium channel blockers: the jury is still out on whether they cause heart attacks and suicide (editorial), *BMJ* 316:1471-1473, 1998.

18. Kendall MJ, Lynch KP, Hjalmarson A, et al: Beta-blockers and sudden cardiac death, *Ann Intern Med* 123:358-367, 1995.

19. Radack K, Deck C: Beta-adrenergic blocker therapy does not worsen intermittent claudication in subjects with peripheral arterial disease: a meta-analysis of randomized controlled trials, *Arch Intern Med* 151:1705-1707, 1991.

20. Prisant LM, Spruill WJ, Fincham JE, et al: Depression associated with antihypertensive drugs, *J Fam Pract* 33:481-485, 1991.

21. Mold JW: Pharmacotherapy of urinary incontinence, *Am Fam Physician* 54:673-680, 1996.

22. Losartan for hypertension, *Med Lett* 37:57-58, 1995.

23. Gradman AH, Arcuri KE, Goldberg AI, et al: A randomized, placebo-controlled, double-blind, parallel study of various doses of losartan potassium compared with enalapril maleate in patients with essential hypertension, *Hypertension* 25:1345-1350, 1995.

24. Valsartan for hypertension, *Med Lett* 39:43-44, 1997.

VALVULAR HEART DISEASE

(See also anticoagulants; endocarditis prophylaxis; screening)

Heart Murmurs in Children

The ability of pediatric cardiologists to differentiate functional from organic murmurs in children by history and physical examination alone is excellent. Features suggesting organic disease include a pansystolic murmur, a murmur intensity of grade 3 or higher, and an abnormal second heart sound.[1]

Aortic Stenosis

A long latent period occurs during the presymptomatic phase of aortic stenosis. Once symptoms such as angina, syncope, or heart failure occur, the mortality rate is very high over the next 2 to 5 years. In general, stenotic aortic valves should be replaced as soon as the patient is symptomatic. Age is not a contraindication, and results are usually excellent.[2]

Aortic Insufficiency

In a 1994 study, nifedipine in doses of 20 mg bid was given to asymptomatic patients with aortic insufficiency who had normal left ventricular ejection fractions. This resulted in a significant delay in the need for valve replacement compared with the control group. The rationale for treatment with nifedipine is that arteriolar vasodilation increases forward flow and decreases the amount of aortic regurgitation.[3]

Mitral Stenosis

Percutaneous balloon mitral commissurotomy appears to be the procedure of choice for most patients with mitral stenosis.[4]

Mitral Valve Prolapse

Mitral valve prolapse has a community prevalence rate of 2.4%. Two variants can be distinguished with two-dimensional echocardiography. In the common benign form the valves are anatomically normal (normal variant mitral valve prolapse), and in a rare but serious variant, which is usually seen in older men or in patients with connective tissue diseases, they are deformed (primary mitral valve prolapse). Adverse sequelae such as cerebrovascular accidents, progressive severe mitral insufficiency, or endocarditis are generally limited to patients with primary mitral valve prolapse. Anxiety, atypical chest pain, and palpitations are not caused by mitral valve prolapse.[5]

Antibiotic prophylaxis against infective endocarditis is mandatory for patients with primary mitral valve prolapse, especially those with a systolic murmur. Prophylaxis for patients with normal variant mitral valve prolapse and no murmur is unnecessary.[5]

Prosthetic Valves

The two major types of prosthetic valves are mechanical valves and tissue valves. Mechanical valves may be caged-ball (Starr-Edwards), single-tilting-disk (e.g., Medtronic-Hall, Bjork-Shiley), or bileaflet-tilting-disk (e.g., St. Jude). The most common tissue valve is the porcine heterograft valve. Porcine heterograft valves usually last 10 to 15 years and do not require long-term anticoagulation; mechanical valves last longer but require anticoagulation. Failure of porcine valves is usually gradual, so the replacement surgery can be elective.[6,7]

The surgical mortality of valve replacement depends largely on the patient's individual risk factors. Isolated aortic valve replacement in an otherwise healthy person has a 30-day mortality rate of 1% to 5%, while that for isolated mitral valve replacement is 2% to 8%.[6]

The risk of thrombosis depends on the type of mechanical valve; it is greatest for the caged-ball valves, least for the bileaflet-tilting-disk, and intermediate for the single-tilting-disk. One set of recommendations is that the INR should be maintained between 4 and 4.9 for patients with caged-ball valves or multiple prosthetic valves, between 3 and 3.9 for those with single-tilting-disk valves, and between 2.5 and 2.9 for those with bileaflet-tilting-disk valves. Patients with porcine heterografts may be given anticoagulants to achieve an INR between 2 and 3 for the first 3 months. Modifications of these recommendations are required for patients at risk of bleeding such as the very elderly.[7] The authors of a French study concluded that INR levels of 2 to 3 are acceptable for patients with single St. Jude bileaflet-tilting-disk valves implanted in the aortic or mitral regions.[8] Hirsh and associates[9] recommend INR levels of 2.5 to 3.5 for all mechanical prosthetic valves.

⚕ REFERENCES ⚕

1. McCrindle BW, Shaffer KM, Kan JS, et al: Cardinal clinical signs in the differentiation of heart murmurs in children, *Arch Pediatr Adolesc Med* 150:169-174, 1996.
2. Carabello BA, Crawford FA Jr: Valvular heart disease, *N Engl J Med* 337:32-41, 1997.
3. Scognamiglio R, Rahimtoola SH, Fasoli G, et al: Nifedipine in asymptomatic patients with severe aortic regurgitation and normal left ventricular function, *N Engl J Med* 331:689-694, 1994.
4. Farhat MB, Ayari M, Maatouk F, et al: Percutaneous balloon versus surgical closed and open mitral commissurotomy: seven-year follow-up results of a randomized trial, *Circulation* 97:245-250, 1998.
5. Nishimura RA, McGoon MD: Perspectives on mitral-valve prolapse, *N Engl J Med* 341:48-50, 1999.
6. Katz NM: Current surgical treatment of valvular heart disease, *Am Fam Physician* 52:559-568, 1995.
7. Vongpatanasin W, Hillis D, Lange RA: Prosthetic heart valves, *N Engl J Med* 335:407-416, 1996.
8. Acar J, Iung B, Boissel JP, et al: AREVA: multicenter randomized comparison of low-dose versus standard-dose anticoagulation in patients with mechanical prosthetic heart valves, *Circulation* 94:2107-2112, 1996.
9. Hirsh J, Dalen JE, Deykin D, et al: Oral anticoagulants: mechanism of action, clinical effectiveness, and optimal therapeutic range, *Chest* 108(suppl 4):231S-246S, 1995.

VASCULAR DISEASE
(See also transient ischemic attacks)

Arterial Disease

Peripheral vascular disease
(See also coronary artery disease)

In patients with claudication the risk of death from all causes is four to seven times greater and the risk of dying of cardiovascular disease within 10 years is 15 times greater than the respective risks of patients who do not have claudication. The 5-year mortality rate for patients with claudication is 29%.[1] The mortality rate is particularly high in diabetic patients.[2] Claudication itself improves spontaneously in 40% of patients, and in only 7% does it progress to the point that amputation is required within the next 5 years.[3]

An objective measurement of peripheral vascular disease is the ankle-brachial index (ABI), which is determined by using Doppler probes to measure systolic pressures over the posterior tibial or dorsalis pedis arteries and comparing them with the branchial artery systolic pressure. Normally the ankle pressure is higher than the brachial pressure, so in normal individuals the index is greater than 1. Any value less than 1 is abnormal, and patients with rest pain usually have values less than 0.5. Some patients with peripheral vascular disease have a normal ABI at rest but an abnormal one after exercising or taking a vasodilator drug such as papaverine (augmented ABI).[4] Most cases of peripheral vascular disease seen in family medicine are easily diagnosed on the basis of history and physical examination. I am unaware of any evidence that obtaining an ABI improves the clinical outcome of these patients.

First-line treatment for intermittent claudication is smoking cessation and exercise.[3] In one study patients were instructed to walk for at least 30 minutes three times per week and continue walking to a point at which the claudication pain was near maximal. After 6 months the distance walked to onset and to maximal claudication pain increased by 120% to 180%.[5] Whether smoking cessation leads to improved walking distance is uncertain because of the poor quality of most studies,[3] but even if no improvement is achieved, smoking should be anathema to patients with claudication because of its adverse effect on coronary artery disease.

Pentoxifylline (Trental), usually given as 400 mg bid or tid, has been clearly shown to increase pain-free walking distances. Because the quantitative effect is small, however, the drug's clinical usefulness for many patients is uncertain. Pentoxifylline is believed to decrease blood viscosity by making red blood cells more pliable.[3] One study found that verapamil (Isoptin, Calan, Covera-HS) in doses of 120 to 480 mg/day gave some symptomatic improvement.[6] Cilostazol (Pletal) has been recently approved by the U.S. Food and Drug Administration for the treatment of claudication (with a usual dosage of 100 mg bid). According to the *Medical Letter*, cilostazol has been shown to be moderately effective and may be worth trying in patients who cannot participate in exercise programs. There are concerns that it may prove cardiotoxic.[7]

Prophylactic aspirin given over long periods to asymptomatic men is associated with a slight decrease in the need for vascular surgery.[8] Patients with peripheral vascular disease have a very high incidence of coronary artery disease, and prophylactic aspirin is a reasonable option for this reason alone. An alternative is clopidogrel (Plavix), which in doses of 75 mg/day has been shown to decrease the risk of myocardial infarction, stroke, and vascular death in patients with peripheral vascular disease.[9,10]

Another prophylactic drug that should probably be prescribed for all patients with peripheral vascular disease is the ACE inhibitor ramipril (Altace). In the HOPE study patients treated with ramipril 10 mg/day had a decreased risk of coronary events, strokes, and total mortality.[11] Chelation therapy has no role in the treatment of peripheral vascular disease.[12]

◤ REFERENCES ◢

1. Criqui MG, Langoer RD, Fronek A, et al: Mortality over a period of 10 years in patients with peripheral arterial disease, *N Engl J Med* 326:381-386, 1992.
2. Barzilay JI, Kronmal RA, Bittner V, et al: Coronary artery disease in diabetic and nondiabetic patients with lower extremity arterial disease: a report from the Coronary Artery Surgery Study Registry, *Am Heart J* 135:1055-1062, 1998.
3. Girolami B, Bernardi E, Prins MH, et al: Treatment of intermittent claudication with physical training, smoking cessation, pentoxifylline or nafronyl, *Arch Intern Med* 159:337-345. 1999.
4. Steinmetz OK, Cole CW: Noninvasive blood flow tests in vascular disease, *Can Fam Physician* 39:2405-2416, 1993.
5. Gardner AW, Poehlman ET: Exercise rehabilitation programs for the treatment of claudication pain: a meta-analysis, *JAMA* 274:975-980, 1995.
6. Bagger JP, Helligsoe P, Randsbaek F, et al: Effect of verapamil in intermittent claudication: a randomized double-blind, placebo-controlled, cross-over study after individual dose-response assessment, *Circulation* 95:411-414, 1997.
7. Cilostazol for intermittent claudication, *Med Lett* 41:44-46, 1999.
8. Goldhaber SZ, Manson JE, Stampfer MJ, et al: Low-dose aspirin and subsequent peripheral arterial surgery in the Physicians' Health Study, *Lancet* 340:143-145, 1992.
9. CAPRIE Steering Committee: A randomised, blinded, trial of clopidogrel versus aspirin in patients at risk of ischaemic events (CAPRIE), *Lancet* 348:1329-1339, 1996.
10. Gorelick PB, Born GV, D'Agostino RB, et al: Therapeutic benefit: aspirin revisited in light of the introduction of clopidogrel, *Stroke* 30:1716-1721, 1999.
11. Heart Outcomes Prevention Evaluation Study Investigators: Effects of an angiotensin-converting-enzyme inhibitor, ramipril, on cardiovascular events in high-risk patients, *N Engl J Med* 342:145-153, 2000.
12. van Rij AM, Solomon C, Packer SG, et al: Chelation therapy for intermittent claudication: a double-blind, randomized, controlled trial, *Circulation* 90:1194-1199, 1994.

Raynaud's phenomenon

Most cases of Raynaud's phenomenon are idiopathic and develop in women in their twenties and thirties. Underlying diseases to be ruled out include lupus, scleroderma and other types of vasculitis, myeloproliferative disorders, and cryoglobulinemia.[1] The risk that connective tissue disease will develop in patients with primary Raynaud's phenomenon is low, but the exact incidence is uncertain. In one metaanalysis, which included studies from rheumatology and immunology referral centers, the rate was a little more than 10%. This figure is certainly too high because of referral bias; many patients with Raynaud's phenomenon do not seek medical attention. Clinical predictors of progression included abnormalities of the nailfold capillaries, telangiectasia, puffy fingers, and sclerodactyly.[2] Symptomatic treatment involves keeping the patient warm, especially the extremities, and in some cases administering long-acting calcium channel blockers such as long-acting nifedipine (Adalat XL) or felodipine (Renedil, Plendil).[1]

◤ REFERENCES ◢

1. Keystone EC: Appropriate management of Raynaud's disease, *Patient Care Can* 7:14, 1996.
2. Spencer-Green G: Outcomes in primary Raynaud phenomenon: a meta-analysis of the frequency, rates, and predictors of transition to secondary diseases, *Arch Intern Med* 158:595-600, 1998.

Venous Disease
Thrombophlebitis

(See also anticoagulants; hormone replacement therapy; oral contraceptives; pulmonary embolism)

Difficulty making the clinical diagnosis. The clinical diagnosis of deep vein thrombosis is notoriously difficult, and most patients have no suggestive signs or symptoms.[1] Among patients who do have symptoms or signs suggestive of phlebitis, only about one fourth actually have the condition. The accuracy of diagnosis among patients with symptoms can be greatly improved by using a clinical prediction guide. One point is given for each of the following factors[2]:

1. Active cancer
2. Paralysis or plaster immobilization of a lower limb
3. Recent confinement to bed for more than 3 days or recent major surgery
4. Localized tenderness along the deep venous system
5. Swelling of the entire leg
6. Calf swelling greater than 3 cm compared with the unaffected leg, as measured 10 cm below the tibial tuberosity
7. Pitting edema (greater than in the unaffected limb)
8. Superficial collateral veins

Two points are subtracted if there is good reason to suspect an alternative diagnosis such as a Baker's cyst. The patient has a high probability of DVT with scores of 3 or higher, moderate probability if the score is 1 or 2, and low probability if it is zero or a negative number.[2]

From a clinical viewpoint, all symptomatic patients should still be investigated. If a patient with a high or moderate probability of DVT has negative findings on ultrasonography, a venogram or serial testing is indicated. These options are also indicated if someone with a low probability has a positive ultrasonography result. On the other hand, ultrasonography negative for DVT in a patient with low probability of the condition does not require further investigation, whereas positive ultrasonography in patients with high or moderate probabilities is an indication for immediate treatment.[2]

Two practical, noninvasive procedures for assessing the presence of DVT are impedance plethysmography and compression ultrasonography. Neither is reliable for detecting isolated calf thrombophlebitis.[2] In most centers compression ultrasonography is now the procedure of choice.[3]

Ultrasonography. Real-time ultrasonography processes the images rapidly enough to show the examiner what is going on at that instant. When it is used to diagnosis DVT, the probe is usually placed over the femoral vein in the groin and over the popliteal vein in the popliteal fossa. Each vein is compressed with the probe, and if the lumen is no longer visible, there is no contained thrombus.[3]

Proximal versus distal thrombosis. The distinction between proximal and distal (calf only) DVT is important because patients with thrombi limited to the calf rarely have pulmonary emboli, and if they do, the emboli are generally inconsequential. Neither impedance plethysmography nor ultrasound can rule out calf vein thrombosis, and since a certain percentage of calf vein thrombi propagate proximally, serial measurements are necessary to detect this eventuality. Various requirements for the number of repeat examinations have been published. One recent study evaluated patients with two ultrasound examinations 1 week apart; of all abnormal results, only 3% were found solely on the second visit. No treatment was given to patients with negative results on either the first or the second evaluation. After 6 months of follow-up only 0.7% of patients who had negative results on the two initial evaluations showed clinical evidence of thromboembolic disease.[3]

Risk factors. Risk factors may be divided into those that are reversible and those that are permanent.[4] Reversible risk factors include trauma, surgery, temporary immobilization, travel, estrogen treatment, infection, Baker's cyst, and pregnancy.[4] Even "minor" surgery may be associated with a high incidence of thrombophlebitis; in one series of arthroscopies calf or proximal deep vein thrombophlebitis developed in 18% of the patients as documented by venography.[5] One case-control study found that travel of 4 hours or more (mean 5.2) by plane, train, or car increased the odds ratio of thrombophlebitis fourfold.[6] Permanent risk factors include inherited disorders of coagulation, malignancy, permanent immobilization, and idiopathic recurrent thromboembolic episodes.[4] Probable permanent risk factors are smoking and central abdominal obesity.[7]

Inherited disorders of coagulation. Some of the inherited disorders of coagulation inhibitors that predispose to thrombophlebitis are the thrombophilias, which include antithrombin III, protein C, and protein S deficiencies[8]; activated protein C resistance (which is usually caused by inheriting a mutation in factor V—factor V Leiden)[8]; and G20210A prothrombin mutation.[9] Factor V Leiden is found in about 5% of individuals of European ancestry and between 11% and 21% of those with venous thromboembolism. Patients with factor V Leiden alone do not appear to be at major risk for recurrent thromboembolism, but if both G20210A prothrombin mutation and factor V Leiden are present, the risk is very high.[9] Whether women who want oral contraceptives should be screened for factor V Leiden is discussed in the section on oral contraceptives.

The antiphospholipid antibody syndrome consists of recurrent venous or arterial thrombosis; recurrent spontaneous abortions, usually in the second trimester; and the presence of antiphospholipid antibodies (anticardiolipin antibodies or lupus anticoagulant). Many cases are in patients with systemic lupus erythematosus.[10] Stroke is one of the most serious complications of the antiphospholipid antibody syndrome. Treatment is lifelong warfarin (Coumadin)[10] except during pregnancy, when aspirin, heparin, or a combination of the two is used.[11]

Cancer and thrombophlebitis. Although patients with cancer have long been known to have a higher risk of thromboembolic disease, extensive investigations looking for malignancy are not indicated for patients in whom thrombophlebitis develops.[12,13] A thorough history, a physical examination including a pelvic examination, a chest x-ray examination, and "routine" blood tests should suffice because when cancer is related to a thrombotic event, the diagnosis of malignancy is often suspected at the time of initial presentation on the basis of clinical findings.[12,13] In cases with no clinical suggestion of malignancy, approximately 88 patients would have to be investigated to find one cancer and many of the malignancies detected by this method would be incurable.[13]

Trauma and thrombophlebitis. A study from Sunnybrook Hospital in Toronto using serial impedance plethysmography and lower extremity contrast venography found that 58% of trauma patients had DVT and in 18% of cases proximal DVT was present. Of 201 patients, only three (1.5%) had clinical symptoms or signs suggesting the disorder. None of the patients had received prophylaxis against thromboembolism at the time of the study.[14]

Prevention of thrombophlebitis. A variety of methods have been used to prevent deep vein thrombosis in patients at risk. Physical measures include graduated compression stockings and intermittent external pneumatic compression of the lower extremities. Drugs that are commonly used include warfarin, IV heparin, and low-molecular-weight heparin. Aspirin is not as effective as other modalities of prevention.[1]

Treatment of thrombophlebitis. The traditional initial treatment of thrombophlebitis is 5 days of IV (unfractionated) heparin followed by oral anticoagulation (warfarin) therapy for at least 3 months. Such therapy reduces the incidence of recurrent thrombosis from 25% to less than 4%. A simpler, more cost-effective method of initiating therapy is to use subcutaneous low-molecular-weight heparin (LMWH) or heparinoids administered on an outpatient basis (Table 17). Metaanalyses comparing LMWH with unfractionated heparin suggest that not only is LMWH more effective than unfractionated heparin, but it results in fewer major bleeding episodes.[15] Warfarin is contraindicated in pregnancy.

LMWH does not normally alter the partial thromboplastin time, so this is not monitored during therapy; INR is monitored in the usual way to control the level of concomitantly given warfarin. Heparin can cause thrombocytopenia through the development of heparin-dependent IgG antibodies, usually after 5 days of treatment. This complication appears to be less common in patients treated with LMWH than in those treated with unfractionated heparin.[16]

The optimal duration of therapy with anticoagulants is an area of controversy. The risk of recurrent thromboembolism is low in patients who have thrombosis limited to the calf veins and also in patients who have had a reversible risk factor such as surgery compared with those who have permanent risk factors such as cancer or those with idiopathic DVT. In the opinion of Hirsh, patients with a single episode of DVT associated with reversible risk factors that are no longer present should receive anticoagulants for 4 to 6 weeks if the thrombus is limited to the calf and for 12 weeks if proximal vein thrombosis is present. The optimal duration of anticoagulation for patients without reversible risk factors who have had proximal venous thrombosis or pulmonary embolism is uncertain but probably should be at least 6 months.[8] This view is substantiated by a 1999 report that studied patients with no known risk factors who had had an initial episode of proximal venous thrombosis or pulmonary embolism. All patients were given anticoagulants for 3 months, and thereafter half were given placebo and half continued on warfarin. The study was terminated after only 10 months because the calculated annual recurrence rate in the placebo group was 27% compared with 1% in the anticoagulated group.[17]

If patients with a initial episode of thrombophlebitis are known to have a thrombophilia, longer periods of anticoagulation such as 1 to 3 years are probably indicated, but the optimal duration is unknown because the risk of hemorrhage may outweigh the benefits.[8] One decision analysis model of carriers of factor V Leiden who had had a single thromboembolic event concluded that anticoagulation for periods of over a year would result in more major hemorrhages than pulmonary emboli prevented.[18]

The management of recurrent thrombophlebitis is also uncertain. A Swedish study found that after a second episode of thromboembolism, anticoagulation for a prolonged period resulted in fewer recurrences than occurred in those receiving anticoagulants for 6 months.[19] On an empirical basis, Ginsberg[20] recommended treating patients with two episodes of thromboembolism for 1 year and those with three or more episodes for life. Bedridden cancer patients might require lifelong anticoagulation.[4]

Inferior vena cava filters can be placed through the transcutaneous route, which is being done more and more frequently.[21] Reputed indications are patients in whom anticoagulation is contraindicated and those with free-floating proximal vein thrombi. The latter is a tenuous indication, since the risk of pulmonary embolism in patients taking anticoagulants is no higher in those with free-floating thrombi than in those with obstructing thrombi.[22] The efficacy of inferior vena cava filters has not been well studied. One 2-year randomized trial comparing inferior vena cava filters to 3 months of anticoagulation found no difference in mortality but an increased incidence of subsequent thrombophlebitis in the cohort with inferior vena cava filters.[21]

Postthrombotic syndrome develops in an estimated 50% or more of patients with symptomatic DVT, usually within 2 years of the initial thrombotic episode. Wearing made-to-measure below-knee compression stockings during the day over a 2-year period (two new stockings every 6 months) decreases the risk by 50%.[23]

The management of excessively high INRs is discussed under anticoagulants in the hematology section.

Table 17   Low-Molecular-Weight Heparins and Heparinoids

Drug	Usual dose for postoperative prophylaxis against deep vein thrombosis
Low-Molecular-Weight Heparins	
Ardeparin (Normiflo)	50 anti-Xa U/kg q12h
Dalteparin (Fragmin)	200 anti-Xa U/kg subcutaneously once daily
Enoxaparin (Lovenox)	40 mg subcutaneously once daily
Tinzaparin (Innohep)	175 anti-Xa U/kg once daily
Heparinoids	
Danaparoid (Orgaran)	750 anti-Xa U bid

⟆ REFERENCES ⟆

1. Weinmann EE, Salzman EW: Deep-vein thrombosis, *N Engl J Med* 331:1630-1641, 1994.
2. Anand SS, Wells PS, Hunt D, et al: Does this patient have deep vein thrombosis? *JAMA* 279:1094-1099, 1998.
3. Cogo A, Lensing AW, Koopman MM, et al: Compression ultrasonography for diagnostic management of patients with clinically suspected deep vein thrombosis: prospective cohort study, *BMJ* 316:17-20, 1998.
4. Hirsh J: The optimal duration of anticoagulant therapy for venous thrombosis (editorial), *N Engl J Med* 332:1710-1711, 1995.
5. Demers C, Marcoux S, Ginsberg JS, et al: Incidence of venographically proved deep vein thrombosis after knee arthroscopy, *Arch Intern Med* 158:47-50, 1998.

6. Ferrari E, Chevallier T, Chapelier A, et al: Travel as a risk factor for venous thromboembolic disease: a case-control study, *Chest* 115:440-444, 1999.

7. Hansson P-O, Eriksson H, Wellin L, et al: Smoking and abdominal obesity: risk factors for venous thromboembolism among middle-aged men, *Arch Intern Med* 159:1886-1890, 1999.

8. Hirsh J: Duration of anticoagulant therapy after first episode of venous thrombosis in patients with inherited thrombophilia (editorial), *Arch Intern Med* 157:2174-2177, 1997.

9. De Stefano V, Martinelli I, Mannucci PM, et al: The risk of recurrent deep venous thrombosis among heterozygous carriers of both factor V Leiden and the G20210A prothrombin mutation, *N Engl J Med* 341:1801-1806, 1999.

10. Khamashta MA, Cuadrado MJ, Mujic F, et al: The management of thrombosis in the antiphospholipid-antibody syndrome, *N Engl J Med* 332:993-997, 1995.

11. Rai R, Cohen H, Dave M, et al: Randomised controlled trial of aspirin and aspirin plus heparin in pregnant women with recurrent miscarriage associated with phospholipid antibodies (or antiphospholipid antibodies), *BMJ* 314:253-257, 1997.

12. Hettiarachchi RJ, Lok J, Prins MH, et al: Undiagnosed malignancy in patients with deep vein thrombosis, *Cancer* 83:180-185, 1998.

13. Sørensen HT, Mellemkjaer L, Steffensen FH, et al: The risk of a diagnosis of cancer after primary deep venous thrombosis or pulmonary embolism, *N Engl J Med* 338:1169-1173, 1998.

14. Geerts WH, Code KI, Jay RM, et al: A prospective study of venous thromboembolism after major trauma, *N Engl J Med* 331:1601-1606, 1994.

15. Siragusa S, Cosmi B, Piovella F, et al: Low-molecular-weight heparins and unfractionated heparin in the treatment of patients with acute venous thromboembolism: results of a meta-analysis, *Am J Med* 100:269-277, 1996.

16. Warkentin TE, Levine MN, Hirsh J, et al: Heparin-induced thrombocytopenia in patients treated with low-molecular-weight heparin or unfractionated heparin, *N Engl J Med* 332:1330-1335, 1995.

17. Kearon C, Gent M, Hirsh J, et al: A comparison of three months of anticoagulation with extended anticoagulation for a first episode of idiopathic venous thromboembolism, *N Engl J Med* 340:901-907, 1999.

18. Sarasin FP, Bounameaux H: Decision analysis model of prolonged oral anticoagulant treatment in factor V Leiden carriers with first episode of deep vein thrombosis, *BMJ* 316:95-99, 1998.

19. Schulman S, Granqvist S, Holmström M, et al: The duration of oral anticoagulant therapy after a second episode of venous thromboembolism, *N Engl J Med* 336:393-398, 1997.

20. Ginsberg JS: Management of venous thromboembolism, *N Engl J Med* 335:1816-1828, 1996.

21. Decousus H, Leizorovicz, Parent F, et al: A clinical trial of vena caval filters in the prevention of pulmonary embolism in patients with proximal deep-vein thrombosis, *N Engl J Med* 338:409-415, 1998.

22. Pacouret G, Alison D, Pottier J-M, et al: Free-floating thrombus and embolic risk in patients with angiographically confirmed proximal deep venous thrombosis: a prospective study, *Arch Intern Med* 157:305-308, 1997.

23. Brandjes PM, Büller HR, Heijboer H, et al: Randomised trial of effect of compression stockings in patients with symptomatic proximal-vein thrombosis, *Lancet* 349:759-762, 1997.

Pulmonary embolism
(See also thrombophlebitis)

The risk factors for pulmonary embolism are similar to those for thrombophlebitis and include trauma, surgery, heart failure, immobilization, cancer, and inherited disorders of coagulation. Important additional risk factors are obesity, smoking, and hypertension.[1]

Symptoms of pulmonary embolism include tachypnea and tachycardia, which are quite nonspecific.[2] Blood gas concentrations are not sensitive enough to rule out pulmonary embolism. In one study 30% of patients with pulmonary emboli had a PaO_2 of more than 80 mm Hg,[3] while in another study between 8% and 23% had a normal A-a gradient.[4] In a third investigation 30% of patients with pulmonary embolism but no past history of cardiopulmonary disease had no diminution of the PaO_2 or the $PaCO_2$ and also had normal A-a gradients.[5] Among patients with pulmonary emboli and a prior history of cardiopulmonary disease, 14% had all three values in the normal range.[5]

The standard investigative technique for suspected pulmonary embolism is a ventilation/perfusion (V/Q) lung scan.[2] This is a two-step procedure in which the pulmonary distribution of inhaled radioactive material (ventilation scan) is compared with the pulmonary distribution of intravenously injected radioactive material (technetium-99m). In a classic case of pulmonary embolism the ventilation scan is normal and the perfusion scan shows multiple perfusion defects. A "mismatch" occurs between the ventilation and perfusion scans.[2]

V/Q scans are reported as "normal," "low probability," "intermediate probability," and "high probability." In one study a pulmonary embolus was found in none of the patients with a "normal" scan, only 5% of those with a "low-probability" scan, 30% of those with "intermediate" results, and 90% of those with a "high-probability" scan.[6] Among those with "intermediate" results, 30% had a pulmonary embolism. Unfortunately, 50% to 70% of reports are in the intermediate range.[2] A suggested algorithm for this type of report, or for a low-probability report when the clinical probability of pulmonary embolism is high, is to perform duplex scanning of the leg veins; if this is negative and the patient's condition is stable, it is often safe simply to follow with serial duplex scanning or plethysmography of the leg veins because recurrent pulmonary embolism is extremely rare in the absence of proximal deep vein thrombosis.[2,7] A new technology that may be used for patients with "intermediate" V/Q scan results is helical computed tomography of the thorax. It has a sensitivity of 67% to 87% and a specificity of over 95%.[8]

Subcutaneous low-molecular-weight heparin is reported to be as effective as IV unfractionated heparin in the treatment of pulmonary embolism.[9,10]

◥ REFERENCES ◤

1. Goldhaber SZ, Grodstein F, Stampfer MJ, et al: A prospective study of risk factors for pulmonary embolism in women, *JAMA* 277:642-645, 1997.
2. Bergus GU, Barloon TS, Kahn D: An approach to diagnostic imaging of suspected pulmonary embolism, *Am Fam Physician* 53:1259-1266, 1996.
3. Cvitanic O, Marino PL: Improved use of arterial blood gas analysis in suspected pulmonary embolism, *Chest* 95:48-51, 1989.
4. Stein PD, Goldhaber SZ, Henry JW: Alveolar-arterial oxygen gradient in the assessment of acute pulmonary embolism, *Chest* 107:139-143, 1995.
5. Stein PD, Goldhaber SZ, Henry JW, et al: Arterial blood gas analysis in the assessment of suspected acute pulmonary embolism, *Chest* 109:78-81, 1996.
6. Gottschalk A, Sostman HD, Coleman RE, et al: Ventilation-perfusion scintigraphy in the PIOPED study. II. Evaluation of the scintigraphic criteria and interpretations, *J Nucl Med* 34:1119-1126, 1993.
7. Hull RD, Raskob GE, Ginsberg JS, et al: A noninvasive strategy for the treatment of patients with suspected pulmonary embolism, *Arch Intern Med* 154:289-297, 1994.
8. Siegel MJ, Evens RG: Advances in the use of computed tomography, *JAMA* 281:1252-1254, 1999.
9. Büller HR, Gent M, Gallus AS, et al (Columbus Investigators): Low-molecular-weight heparin in the treatment of patients with venous thromboembolism, *N Engl J Med* 337:657-662, 1997.
10. Simmoneau G, Sors H, Charbonnier B, et al: A comparison of low-molecular-weight heparin with unfractionated heparin for acute pulmonary embolism, *N Engl J Med* 337:663-669, 1997.

Varicose veins

A variety of lower leg symptoms such as heaviness, aching, swelling, cramps, restless legs, itch, and tingling have been attributed to varicose veins. A population survey in Edinburgh found a high incidence of such symptoms in individuals with and without varicose veins; the authors concluded that in only a small minority of patients might surgery relieve these types of symptoms. Since previous studies have failed to show that early surgery prevents venous ulcers, improved cosmetic appearance remains one of the few specific indications for operative intervention.[1]

◥ REFERENCES ◤

1. Bradbury A, Evans C, Allan P, et al: What are the symptoms of varicose veins? Edinburgh vein study cross sectional population survey, *BMJ* 318:353-356, 1999.

Venous ulcers

(See also ulcer, dermal)

Chronic venous ulcers result from dysfunction of the venous valves, which allows reflux of blood, increasing the pressure in the venous system. In some cases this is secondary to thrombophlebitis. If the valves of the perforating veins are also incompetent, the pressure is transmitted to the dermal capillaries with dilation of the capillaries and leakage of plasma and both red and white blood cells. Activation of the extruded white blood cells leads to the release of various toxic products that cause tissue destruction and ulceration.[1]

Venous ulcers are almost always located in an edematous limb in the region of the malleoli; the surrounding skin shows the typical pigmentation and induration of chronic venous insufficiency. Conservative treatment consists primarily of compression,[1,2] which may be accomplished with graded elastic compression stockings (with a 30- to 40-Torr gradient), elastic bandages, inelastic compression bands attached with Velcro (CircAid), or Unna gel paste gauze boots. Surgical interventions that can be used in selected cases consist of the stripping of superficial veins and at times the interruption of perforating veins; the latter can be performed through an endoscope, decreasing the degree of skin scarring.[1]

◥ REFERENCES ◤

1. Angle N, Bergan JJ: Chronic venous ulcer, *BMJ* 314:1019-1022, 1997.
2. Fletcher A, Cullum N, Sheldon TA: A systematic review of compression treatment for venous leg ulcers, *BMJ* 315:576-580, 1997.

CENTRAL NERVOUS SYSTEM

Topics covered in this section

Amaurosis Fugax
Amyotrophic Lateral Sclerosis
Cerebral Palsy
Cerebrovascular Accidents
Concussion
Creutzfeldt-Jakob Disease and Bovine Spongiform Encephalopathy
Dementia
Headaches
Multiple Sclerosis
Myasthenia Gravis
Neoplasms
Neuropathy
Parkinson's Disease
Restless Legs Syndrome
Seizures
Spasticity
Subarachnoid Hemorrhage
Syncope
Tourette's Syndrome
Transient Global Amnesia
Tremors

AMAUROSIS FUGAX
(See also cerebrovascular accidents)

About half of all cases of amaurosis fugax are due to atherosclerosis, and in patients over 40 years of age it is the likely etiology. Spasm is a much more common cause in young individuals with no other evident disease or with a history of migraines; in these cases the course is usually benign. Lupus is a rare cause.[1,2] Effective symptomatic treatment of patients with amaurosis fugax caused by spasm is nifedipine 60 mg/day (20 mg of the regular formulations tid or Adalat XL 60 mg once daily).

▲ REFERENCES ▲

1. Winterkorn JMS, Kupersmith M, Wirtschafter JD, et al: Brief report: treatment of vasospastic amaurosis fugax with calcium-channel blockers, *N Engl J Med* 329:396-398, 1993.
2. Gautier J-C: Amaurosis fugax (editorial), *N Engl J Med* 329:426-427, 1993.

AMYOTROPHIC LATERAL SCLEROSIS

Amyotrophic lateral sclerosis (ALS, motor neuron disease, Lou Gehrig disease) usually affects the middle aged and has a slight male preponderance. It is characterized by upper and lower motor neuron lesions, so patients tend to have fasciculations and to demonstrate signs of spasticity. Most patients die within 5 years, but a few survive longer. The prognosis is worse for those with the bulbar form of the disease and for older patients. The cause of ALS is unknown, and no cure has been found. Riluzole (Rilutek) has been shown to slow the rate of progression of disease in a few patients but does not alter its natural history.[1]

▲ REFERENCES ▲

1. Walling AD: Amyotrophic lateral sclerosis: Lou Gehrig's disease, *Am Fam Physician* 59:1489-1496, 1999.

CEREBRAL PALSY

Probably only 10% of cases of cerebral palsy result from complications at the time of delivery.[1]

▲ REFERENCES ▲

1. Bakketeig LS: Only a minor part of cerbral palsy cases begin in labour (editorial), *BMJ* 319:1016-1017, 1999.

CEREBROVASCULAR ACCIDENTS
(See also amaurosis fugax; atrial fibrillation; subarachnoid hemorrhage; transient ischemic attacks; vertigo)

Risk Factors for Stroke
(See also lipids)

Six of the most important medical risk factors for stroke are hypertension, myocardial infarction, atrial fibrillation, diabetes mellitus, elevated blood lipid levels, and asymptomatic carotid artery stenosis. Major life-style risk factors are cigarette smoking, excessive alcohol use, lack of physical activity, and a diet deficient in fruits and vegetables.[1]

The risk of stroke is increased in patients with migraines, especially those who are smokers, have hypertension, or are taking oral contraceptives; however, the absolute number of women affected is small.[2] Women using low-dose contraceptives who are not hypertensive and do not smoke have very little increased risk of stroke even if they are over the age of 35.[3] Hormone replacement therapy appears to be associated with a decreased, not an increased, incidence of stroke.[4,5] Case-control studies have shown an increased risk of stroke in users of amphetamines and cocaine.[6] A prospective study of middle-aged men in Finland found that those who had the highest level of expressed anger were at elevated risk of stroke.[7]

McCormack and associates[8] have published an easily comprehensible nomogram integrating multiple risk factors so that the chance that a particular person will have a cerebrovascular accident within 10 years can be calculated.

Silent cerebral infarction (infarcts found on radiological examination in patients without corresponding clinical symptoms) occurs in 11% of the general population. Major risk factors are hypertension and smoking.[9]

▲ REFERENCES ▲

1. Gorelick PB, Sacco RL, Smith DB, et al: Prevention of a first stroke: a review of guidelines and a multidisciplinary consensus statement from the National Stroke Association, *JAMA* 281:1112-1120, 1999.
2. Chang CL, Donaghy M, Poulter N (World Health Organisation Collaborative Study of Cardiovascular Disease and Steroid Hormone Contraception): Migraine and stroke in young women: case-control study, *BMJ* 318:13-18, 1999.
3. Schwartz SM, Petitti DB, Siscovick DS, et al: Stroke and use of low-dose oral contraceptives in young women: a pooled analysis of two US studies, *Stroke* 29:2277-2284, 1998.
4. Finucane FF, Madans JH, Bush TL, et al: Decreased risk of stroke among postmenopausal hormone users, *Arch Intern Med* 153:73-79, 1993.
5. Faldeborn M, Persson I, Terent A, et al: Hormone replacement therapy and the risk of stroke: follow-up of a population-based cohort in Sweden, *Arch Intern Med* 153:1201-1209, 1993.
6. Petitti DB, Sidney S, Quesenberry C, et al: Stroke and cocaine or amphetamine use, *Epidemiology* 9:596-600,1998.
7. Everson SA, Kaplan GA, Goldberg DE, et al: Anger expression and incident stroke: prospective evidence from the Kuopio Ischemic Heart Disease Study, *Stroke* 30:523-528, 1999.
8. McCormack JP, Levine M, Rangno RE: Primary prevention of heart disease and stroke: a simplified approach to estimating risk of events and making drug treatment decisions, *Can Med Assoc J* 157:422-428, 1997.
9. Howard G, Wagenknecht LE, Cai J, et al: Cigarette smoking and other risk factors for silent cerebral infarction in the general population, *Stroke* 29:913-917, 1998.

Prevention of Strokes

(See also atrial fibrillation; exercise; lipids; performance reports; screening; smoking; transient ischemic attacks)

Life-style and medical interventions

A decreased incidence of strokes has been reported from the adequate treatment of hypertension,[1] leisure-time physical activity such as walking or swimming,[2] discontinuation of smoking,[3] adequate management of atrial fibrillation,[4] treatment of TIAs,[5] diet high in fruits and vegetables,[6] and according to one study of ischemic strokes, moderate alcohol intake.[7] Aspirin given to asymptomatic individuals is not effective for the primary prevention of strokes.[8] A metaanalysis of lipid-lowering interventions in hyperlipidemic individuals found a significant reduction in the risk of strokes among those treated with 3-hydroxy-3-methylglutaryl coenzyme A (HMG-CoA) reductase inhibitors, but no reduction among those receiving other classes of lipid-lowering drugs.[9] Pravastatin (Pravachol) reduced the incidence of both strokes and TIAs in post–myocardial infarction patients with average serum cholesterol levels.[10]

Endarterectomy

Endarterectomy for asymptomatic patients with carotid stenosis decreases the risk of ipsilateral stroke by a relative rate of about 30%. The absolute benefit is only 2%, and about 50 patients must be operated on to prevent one stroke over the next 3 years. Since many strokes are not disabling, the number of patients who would have to have surgery to prevent one disabling stroke is considerably higher.[11]

Two other important considerations when weighing the harm and benefits of carotid endarterectomy are coexisting illness in the patients and the morbidity and mortality rates of the procedure. In the randomized controlled trials that showed benefit from the procedure, most of the patients selected were otherwise well and the endarterectomies were performed in institutions and by surgeons with considerable experience and documented low morbidity and mortality rates. In the real world of practice these criteria are often not met. Far more patients have coexisting illness, and surgical outcomes tend to be poorer than in the clinical trials.[12,13] Even if surgical procedures are successful, they may not benefit the patients because far more individuals with asymptomatic carotid artery stenosis will suffer cardiac events than cerebrovascular events. In one Toronto study of patients with asymptomatic carotid stenosis, cardiac events outnumbered strokes by 4.5 to 1 and cardiac deaths outnumbered stroke deaths by 12 to 1.[14]

Whether screening for carotid bruits is effective is questionable. Carotid bruits are present in more than 5% of the population older than the age of 65,[15] but their sensitivity for the detection of carotid artery stenosis of greater than 70% is low.[16] In the Asymptomatic Carotid Atherosclerosis Study (ACAS) 25% of the patients had no bruit on the affected side,[16] and in another study the false-negative rate for severe disease was 43%.[17] The positive predictive value of a carotid bruit for significant stenosis is also low; one of the higher reported figures was 37%.[17]

Finding even a few cases of asymptomatic carotid stenosis might be considered worthwhile if a simple intervention such as aspirin prophylaxis for asymptomatic carotid stenosis were efficacious. In a double-blind placebo-controlled study to evaluate aspirin's effectiveness for prevention, patients with at least 50% stenosis in one or both carotid arteries were assigned to receive aspirin 325 mg/day or placebo. At the end of 2 years the two groups showed no difference in total mortality or ischemic events, including TIAs, strokes, myocardial infarctions, and unstable angina.[18]

The Canadian Task Force on Preventive Health Care gives a "D" recommendation both to screening for carotid artery bruits and to endarterectomy in asymptomatic patients. It gives a "C" recommendation to medical therapy for patients with asymptomatic carotid stenosis.[19] The U.S. Preventive Services Task Force gives a "C" recommendation to screening for carotid artery bruit but does not give a specific recommendation for carotid endarterectomy in asymptomatic individuals.[20] The 35 members of the Canadian Stroke Consortium published a report in early 1997 stating that evidence was insufficient to recommend either screening for carotid disease or carotid endarterectomy in asymptomatic patients.[21] The guidelines of both the American Heart Association[22] and the Canadian Neurosurgical Society[23] state that the upper limit for combined death and stroke after carotid endarterectomy in asymptomatic individuals should be 3%. Unfortunately, these data are not readily available to most referring physicians or their patients; this is a good reason for the publication of performance reports (see discussion of performance reports).[24]

The role of endarterectomies in the management of symptomatic carotid stenosis is discussed below under transient ischemic attacks.

--- **REFERENCES** ---

1. SHEP Cooperative Research Group: Prevention of stroke by antihypertensive drug treatment in older persons with isolated systolic hypertension: final results of the Systolic Hypertension in the Elderly Program (SHEP), *JAMA* 265:3255-3264, 1991.
2. Agnarsson U, Thorgeirsson G, Sigvaldason H, et al: Effects of leisure-time physical activity and ventilatory function on risk for stroke in men: the Reykjavík Study, *Ann Intern Med* 130:987-990, 1999.
3. Whisnant JP, Homer D, Ingall TJ, et al: Duration of smoking is the strongest predictor of severe extracranial carotid artery atherosclerosis, *Stroke* 21:707-714, 1990.
4. Atrial Fibrillation Investigators: Risk factors for stroke and efficacy of antithrombotic therapy in atrial fibrillation: analysis of pooled data from five randomized controlled trials, *Arch Intern Med* 154:1449-1457, 1994.

5. Antiplatelet Trialists' Collaboration: Collaborative overview of randomised trials of antiplatelet therapy. I. Prevention of death, myocardial infarction, and stroke by prolonged antiplatelet therapy in various categories of patients, *BMJ* 308:81-106, 1994.

6. Joshipura KJ, Ascherio A, Manson JE, et al: Fruit and vegetable intake in relation to risk of ischemic stroke, *JAMA* 282:1233-1239, 1999.

7. Sacco RL, Elkind M, Boden-Albala B, et al: The protective effect of moderate alcohol consumption on ischemic stroke, *JAMA* 281:53-60, 1999.

8. Manson JE, Stampfer MJ, Colditz GA, et al:. A prospective study of aspirin use and primary prevention of cardiovascular disease in women, *JAMA* 266:521-527, 1991.

9. Bucher HC, Griffith LE, Guyatt GH: Effect of HMGcoA reductase inhibitors on stroke: a meta-analysis of randomized, controlled trials, *Ann Intern Med* 128:89-95, 1998.

10. Plehn JF, Davis BR, Sacks FM, et al: Reduction of stroke incidence after myocardial infarction with pravastatin: the Cholesterol and Recurrent Events (CARE) study, *Circulation* 99:216-223, 1999.

11. Benavanete O, Moher D, Pham B: Carotid endarterectomy for asymptomatic carotid stenosis: a meta-analysis, *BMJ* 317:1477-1480, 1998.

12. Wennberg DE, Lucas FL, Birkmeyer JD, et al: Variation in carotid endarterectomy mortality in the Medicare population: trial hospitals, volume, and patient characteristics, *JAMA* 279:1278-1281, 1998.

13. Cebul RD, Snow RJ, Pine R, et al: Indications, outcomes, and provider volumes for carotid endarterectomy, *JAMA* 279:1282-1287, 1998.

14. Norris JW, Zhu CZ, Bornstein NM, et al: Vascular risks of asymptomatic carotid stenosis, *Stroke* 22:1485-1490, 1991.

15. Wiebers DO, Whisnant JP, Sandok BA, et al: Prospective comparison of a cohort with asymptomatic carotid bruit and a population-based cohort without carotid bruit, *Stroke* 21:984-988, 1990.

16. Executive Committee for the Asymptomatic Carotid Atherosclerosis Study: Endarterectomy for asymptomatic carotid artery stenosis, *JAMA* 273:1421-1428, 1995.

17. Davies KN, Humphrey PR: Do carotid bruits predict disease of the internal carotid arteries? *Postgrad Med J* 70:433-435, 1994.

18. Cote R, Battista RN, Abrahamowicz M, et al: Lack of effect of aspirin in asymptomatic patients with carotid bruits and substantial carotid narrowing, *Ann Intern Med* 123:649-655, 1995.

19. Canadian Task Force on the Periodic Health Examination: *Canadian guide to clinical preventive health care,* Ottawa, 1994, Canada Communication Group—Publishing, pp 691-704.

20. US Preventive Services Task Force: *Guide to clinical preventive services,* ed 2, Baltimore, 1996, Williams & Wilkins, pp 53-61.

21. Perry JR, Szalai JP, Norris JW (Canadian Stroke Consortium): Consensus against both endarterectomy and routine screening for asymptomatic carotid artery stenosis, *Arch Neurol* 54:25-28, 1997.

22. Moore WS, Barnett HJ, Beebe HG, et al: Guidelines for carotid endarterectomy: a multidisciplinary consensus statement from the Ad Hoc Committee, American Heart Association, *Circulation* 91:566-579, 1995.

23. Findlay JM, Tucker WS, Ferguson GG, et al: Guidelines for the use of carotid endarterectomy: current recommendations from the Canadian Neurosurgical Society, *Can Med Assoc J* 157:653-659, 1997.

24. Chassin MR: Appropriate use of carotid endarterectomy (editorial), *N Engl J Med* 339:1468-1471, 1998.

Management of Strokes

Both the American Heart Association and the American Academy of Neurology recommend the use of IV tissue plasminogen activator (t-PA) in selected patients when it can be administered within 3 hours of the onset of stroke symptoms. Selection criteria include absence of significant hypertension and use of computed tomography (CT) or magnetic resonance imaging (MRI) to rule out hemorrhage.[1,2] These recommendations were based on the National Institute of Neurological Disorders and Stroke (NINDS) trial, a randomized, placebo-controlled study that found a small but significant improvement in functional outcome at 3 months in patients receiving t-PA, but at the cost of an increase in intracerebral hemorrhage (6.4% versus <1%).[3] (When measured after 12 months, benefits in the NINDS trial were maintained; t-PA treatment of 100 patients prevented moderate to severe disability in 11 to 13 additional patients compared with those receiving placebo.[4]) A European trial of t-PA for stroke found no benefit and an intracerebral hemorrhage rate of 20%.[5] This discrepancy has been explained away on the grounds that the doses of t-PA were higher than those used in the NINDS study[6]; that the window of opportunity for administering the drug was up to 6 hours from the onset of symptoms, not 3 hours as in the NINDS trial[6]; and that numerous errors were made in the interpretation of the CT scans before treatment.[7] The last-mentioned phenomenon alone would appear to be a major obstacle to the widespread use of thrombolytic therapy; in one study of physician accuracy in interpreting CT scans in cases of suspected stroke, intracerebral hemorrhage was missed in 18% of cases.[8] Streptokinase trials to date have had an unacceptable rate of hemorrhage.[6]

How many patients suffering from strokes meet the inclusion criteria for t-PA therapy? In one Texas center that strongly advocates the intervention, the reported rate was 6% to 7% of patients,[6] while in a Copenhagen series it was 5%.[9] However, since stroke patients who die or make a full recovery do not benefit from t-PA, the percentage of patients in the Copenhagen series who might have benefited from t-PA was calculated as only 0.4%.[9] Although some workers are enthusiastic proponents of t-PA for strokes, others are skeptical, believing that more research is required before its widespread use is promoted.[9,10]

Two large multicenter studies have shown that daily aspirin in doses of 160 mg[11] or 300 mg[12] given as soon as possible after an ischemic stroke resulted in slightly fewer deaths or recurrent strokes in the first weeks and in fewer deaths or dependent patients after several months.[12] According to 1998 guidelines from the United Kingdom, anyone who has had a stroke should take 75 mg of aspirin daily for an indefinite period.[13]

The antithrombogenic agent clopidogrel (Plavix) given as a daily dose of 75 mg to patients with a history of stroke, myocardial infarction, or peripheral vascular disease decreased the risk of further strokes, myocardial infarctions, or vascular deaths (see discussion of coronary artery disease).[14]

Unfractionated heparin is frequently used for patients with ischemic strokes, but this is controversial because there is no conclusive proof that it is beneficial or safe.[12,15] A trial of IV heparinoid showed benefits at 7 days, but by 3 months none was detectable.[15]

❧ REFERENCES ❧

1. Adams HP Jr, Brott TG, Furlan AJ, et al: Guidelines for thrombolytic therapy for acute stroke: a supplement to the guidelines for the management of patients with acute ischemic stroke; a statement for healthcare professionals from a special writing group of the Stroke Council, American Heart Association, *Stroke* 27:1711-1718, 1996.
2. Practice advisory: thrombolytic therapy for acute ischemic stroke—summary statement; report of the Quality Standards Subcommittee of the American Academy of Neurology, *Neurology* 47:836-839, 1996.
3. National Institute of Neurological Disorders and Stroke rt-PA Stroke Study Group: Tissue plasminogen activator for acute ischemic stroke, *N Engl J Med* 333:1581-1587, 1995.
4. Kwiatkowski TG, Libman RB, Frankel M, et al: Effects of tissue plasminogen activator for acute ischemic stroke at one year, *N Engl J Med* 340:1781-1787, 1999.
5. European Cooperative Acute Stroke Study (ECASS): Intravenous thrombolysis with recombinant tissue plasminogen activator for acute hemispheric stroke, *JAMA* 274:1017-1025, 1995.
6. Grotta J: t-PA: should thrombolytic therapy be the first-line treatment for acute ischemic stroke? The best current option for most patients, *N Engl J Med* 337:1310-1313, 1997.
7. Fisher M, Bogousslavsky J: Further evolution toward effective therapy for acute ischemic stroke, *JAMA* 279:1298-1303, 1998.
8. Schriger DL, Kalafut M, Starkman S, et al: Cranial computed tomography interpretation in acute stroke: physician accuracy in determining eligibility for thrombolytic therapy, *JAMA* 279:1293-1297, 1998.
9. Jørgensen HS, Nakayama H, Kammersgaard LP, et al: Predicted impact of intravenous thrombolysis on prognosis of general population of stroke patients: simulation model, *BMJ* 319:288-289, 1999.
10. Caplan LR, Mohr JP, Kistler JP, et al: Should thrombolytic therapy be the first-line treatment for acute ischemic stroke? Thrombolysis—not a panacea for ischemic stroke, *N Engl J Med* 337:1309-1310, 1997.
11. CAST (Chinese Acute Stroke Trial) Collaborative Group: CAST: randomised placebo-controlled trial of early aspirin use in 20,000 patients with acute ischaemic stroke, *Lancet* 349:1641-1649, 1997.
12. International Stroke Trial Collaborative Group: The International Stroke Trial (IST): a randomised trial of aspirin, subcutaneous heparin, both, or neither among 19,435 patients with acute ischaemic stroke, *Lancet* 349:1569-1581, 1997.
13. Eccles M, Freemantle N, Mason J (North of England Aspirin Guideline Development Group): North of England evidence based guideline development project: guideline on the use of aspirin as secondary prophylaxis for vascular disease in primary care, *BMJ* 316:1303-1309, 1998.
14. CAPRIE Steering Committee: A randomised, blinded, trial of clopidogrel versus aspirin in patients at risk of ischaemic events (CAPRIE), *Lancet* 348:1329-1339, 1996.
15. Publications Committee for the Trial of ORG 10172 in Acute Stroke Treatment (TOAST) Investigators: Low molecular weight heparinoid, ORG 10172 (Danaparoid), and outcome after acute ischemic stroke, *JAMA* 279:1265-1272, 1998.

Transient Ischemic Attacks

(See also anticoagulants; aspirin; atrial fibrillation; informed consent; patient preferences and informed consent; performance reports; relative risk reduction; transient global amnesia; variations in medical practice)

Measures to reduce stroke risk factors in patients who have had TIAs or previous strokes include discontinuing smoking, rigorously controlling blood pressure, losing weight if obese, increasing physical activity, and taking statins if lipid levels are elevated. Specific drugs aimed at preventing future strokes are aspirin, ticlopidine (Ticlid), clopidogrel (Plavix), and anticoagulants (warfarin and heparin). Endarterectomy is beneficial for some patients.[1]

Aspirin

A collaborative overview of 145 randomized trials of antiplatelet therapy showed a relative reduction in strokes of 22% among patients with prior strokes or TIAs. This beneficial effect was noted among men, women, and the elderly with aspirin doses that averaged 75 to 325 mg/day.[2] A 1999 metaregression analysis of the dose-response effect of aspirin in patients who had suffered from TIAs found an overall reduction in strokes of 15%; doses of 50 mg/day were as effective as doses of 1500 mg/day.[3]

Ticlopidine and clopidogrel

Ticlopidine (Ticlid) has traditionally been prescribed for patients who cannot tolerate or do not respond to aspirin. Ticlopidine has many adverse side effects, some of which are fatal. There are few indications for its continued use, since the related drug clopidogrel (Plavix) is at least as effective as aspirin and so far appears to be devoid of serious sequelae.[4]

Anticoagulants

Warfarin is the drug of choice for all patients with atrial fibrillation.[1] The role of warfarin for noncardiac ischemic TIAs is uncertain; a number of clinicians use it for TIAs that have not responded to aspirin or for patients with progressive strokes who are already receiving aspirin.[5] A European randomized trial comparing aspirin and the anticoagulant drug phenprocoumon (Marcoumar) was prematurely discontinued because of an excess of major hemorrhagic events (primarily intracerebral hemorrhages) in the arm of the study receiving anticoagulants. However, in this study the target international normalized ratio (INR) was 3 to 4.5.[6] I am unaware of any recent published studies of the efficacy of anticoagulation when the INR is maintained between 2 and 3.

Endarterectomy

The risk of stroke in patients who have had a TIA is 12% to 13% in the first year and 30% to 35% after 5 years. The risk of a subsequent stroke in a patient who has already had a stroke is between 25% and 45% after 5 years.[7] Published prospective studies have reported an absolute decrease in ipsilateral strokes of about 15% to 17% over 2 years in selected patients undergoing carotid endarterectomy compared with a medically treated control group. These patients had a carotid stenosis of greater than 70%; had had previous TIAs, amaurosis fugax, or a nondisabling stroke in the appropriate carotid territory; and were less that 80 years old. Surgery was most beneficial for those with a very tight stenosis (90% to 99%) and was considerably less valuable for those with a stenosis less than 70% (80% as measured in the European trial).[8,9] Patients with a stenosis of 50% to 69% have only a moderate reduction in the risk of stroke, and this is eliminated if the combined risk of disabling stroke and death resulting from surgery exceeds 2%.[10] Surgery is riskier and less beneficial for women, who probably should not be treated operatively for stenosis less than 80% (90% as measured in the European trial).[11]

What is an acceptable morbidity and mortality rate for carotid endarterectomy in patients with TIAs? The consensus conference of the American Heart Association[7] and the guidelines of the Canadian Neurosurgical Society[12] put the upper limit for combined death and stroke from the operative procedure at 6% for patients who have had TIAs or mild strokes and at 3% for asymptomatic individuals. Since the overall death and stroke rate in the North American Symptomatic Carotid Endarterectomy Trial was 6.5%,[13] there must be few centers or surgeons meeting these standards. All candidates for carotid endarterectomy (and their family physicians) should become fully informed of the morbidity and mortality records of the surgeon and the center where the operation would be performed (see discussion of performance reports).[14] The role of endarterectomy in asymptomatic patients is discussed in the earlier section on prevention of strokes.

_____ ◣ **REFERENCES** ◤ _____

1. Wolf PA, Clagett P, Easton D, et al: Preventing ischemic stroke in patients with prior stroke and transient ischemic attack: a statement for healthcare professionals from the Stroke Council of the American Heart Association, *Stroke* 30:1991-1994, 1999.
2. Antiplatelet Trialists' Collaboration: Collaborative overview of randomised trials of antiplatelet therapy. I. Prevention of death, myocardial infarction, and stroke by prolonged antiplatelet therapy in various categories of patients, *BMJ* 308:81-106, 1994.
3. Johnson ES, Lanes SF, Wentworth CE III, et al: A metaregression analysis of the dose-response effect of aspirin on stroke, *Arch Intern Med* 159:1248-1253, 1999.
4. Gorelick PB, Born GV, D'Agostino RB, et al: Therapeutic benefit: aspirin revisited in light of the introduction of clopidogrel, *Stroke* 30:1716-1721, 1999.
5. Brown J, Bernstein M: Antithrombotic therapy for patients with stroke symptoms, *Can Fam Physician* 42:1724-1730, 1996.
6. Stroke Prevention In Reversible Ischemia Trial (SPIRIT) Study Group: A randomized trial of anticoagulants versus aspirin after cerebral ischemia of presumed arterial origin, *Ann Neurol* 42:857-865, 1997.
7. Moore WS, Barnett HJ, Beebe HG, et al: Guidelines for carotid endarterectomy: a multidisciplinary consensus statement from the Ad Hoc Committee, American Heart Association, *Circulation* 91:566-579, 1995.
8. North American Symptomatic Carotid Endarterectomy Trial Collaborators: Beneficial effects of carotid endarterectomy in symptomatic patients with high-grade stenosis (NIH), *N Engl J Med* 325:445-453, 1991.
9. European Carotid Surgery Trialists' Collaborative Group: MRC European Carotid Surgery Trial: interim results for symptomatic patients with severe (70-99%) or with mild (0-29%) carotid stenosis, *Lancet* 337:1235-1243, 1991.
10. Barnett HJ, Taylor W, Eliasziw M, et al (North American Symptomatic Carotid Endarterectomy Trial Collaborators): Benefit of carotid endarterectomy in patients with symptomatic moderate or severe stenosis, *N Engl J Med* 339:1415-1425, 1998.
11. European Carotid Surgery Trialists' Collaborative Group: Randomised trial of endarterectomy for recently symptomatic carotid stenosis: final results of the MRC European Carotid Surgery Trial (ECST), *Lancet* 351:1379-1387, 1998.
12. Findlay JM, Tucker WS, Ferguson GG, et al: Guidelines for the use of carotid endarterectomy: current recommendations from the Canadian Neurosurgical Society, *Can Med Assoc J* 157:653-659, 1997.
13. Ferguson GG, Eliasziw M, Barr HW, et al: The North American Symptomatic Carotid Endarterectomy Trial: surgical results in 1415 patients, *Stroke* 30:1751-1758, 1999.
14. Gorelick PB: Carotid endarterectomy: where do we draw the line? *Stroke* 30:1745-1750, 1999.

CONCUSSION

(See also seizures; sports medicine)

Concussion or mild traumatic brain injury may be associated with a loss of consciousness lasting less than 30 minutes or no loss of consciousness but a period of confusion that usually lasts less than an hour but may persist up to 24 hours. Amnesia is common but does not last more than 24 hours. Confusion may be apparent immediately after the injury or may develop gradually over a few minutes. Other early symptoms include headache, dizziness, imbalance, incoordination, and nausea and vomiting.[1] Any change in appearance or behavior (e.g., vacant facial appearance, inappropriate laughing or crying, forgetting plays if involved in athletic activity) may reflect neurological deficits.[2] Seizures that occur in the immediate posttraumatic period rarely presage the development of epilepsy; if they occur later, the prognosis for seizure disorder is guarded.[1]

A rare but serious consequence of concussion is the second-impact syndrome. If someone who suffered a mild concussion within the previous few hours or days has a second mild head injury, severe brain swelling and death may result.[3]

Among American high school sports, football is the leading cause of mild traumatic brain injury.[4] In a study of U.S. college football players, a single concussion did not appear to cause long-term neuropsychological deficits, but with two or more concussions the risk of permanent sequelae increased. This was particularly so among athletes who had underlying learning disabilities.[5] Multiple concussions were also found to result in an increased incidence of neuropsychological deficits among amateur soccer players in the Netherlands.[6]

Numerous guidelines for the management of athletes with concussion, based on expert opinion, have been developed.[2,3] If the symptoms of a first concussion last no longer than 15 minutes and if there has been no amnesia or loss of consciousness, the player can usually return to the game when asymptomatic or after a waiting period of 15 to 20 minutes. If symptoms of a first concussion last longer than 15 minutes, the athlete loses conciousness, or amnesia develops, he or she should be prohibited from playing for a week. The management of second and third concussions is controversial; all guidelines recommend removal from the sport for at least 2 weeks and some for 3 to 6 months.[3]

A study of 1382 patients from California who suffered head trauma with either loss of consciousness or amnesia for the event but who had a Glasgow Coma Scale score of 15 (no abnormalities) found that CT scans showed no significant clinical abnormalities in patients who did not have nausea or vomiting and who had no signs of depressed skull fracture such as lacerations, contusions, and swelling. Even among those with such symptoms and signs, abnormal CT scans leading to surgical intervention were rare. Only three patients (0.2%) in the entire study population required surgery.[7]

In many patients who have sustained mild traumatic brain injury the postconcussion syndrome develops. Somatic symptoms include headache, dizziness, tinnitus, and sometimes loss of hearing or olfaction. Sleep is often disturbed. Cognitive impairment may be manifested as difficulty with concentration, memory, word finding, executive functioning, and information processing but in some cases is detected only by neuropsychological testing.[1] (The term "executive functioning" refers to frontal lobe activities such as information processing, problem solving, organization, planning, judgment, abstract reasoning, and insight.[8]) Common emotional disturbances are irritability, anxiety, and depression. In the majority of cases symptoms resolve within 3 months. Young patients recover more rapidly than older ones. Patients who have not recovered completely by 3 months usually continue to improve over the ensuing 3 to 6 months. A few individuals who have had more severe inju-

ries (or multiple concussions[5,6]) never make a complete recovery.[1]

◪ REFERENCES ◪

---

1. Kushner D: Mild traumatic brain injury: toward understanding manifestations and treatment, *Arch Intern Med* 158:1617-1624, 1998.
2. Collins MW, Lovell MR, Mckeag DB: Current issues in managing sports-related concussion, *JAMA* 282:2283-2285, 1999.
3. Harmon KG: Assessment and management of concussion in sports, *Am Fam Physician* 60:887-892, 1999.
4. Powell JW, Barber-Foss KD: Traumatic brain injury in high school athletes, *JAMA* 282:958-963, 1999.
5. Collins MW, Grindel SH, Lovell MR, et al: Relationship between concussion and neuropsychological performance in college football players, *JAMA* 282:964-970, 1999.
6. Matser EJ, Kessels AG, Lezak MD, et al: Neuropsychological impairment in amateur soccer players, *JAMA* 282:971-973, 1999.
7. Miller EC, Derlet RW, Kinser D: Minor head trauma: is computed tomography always necessary? *Ann Emerg Med* 27:290-294, 1996.
8. NIH Consensus Development Panel on Rehabilitation of Persons with Traumatic Brain Injury: Rehabilitation of persons with traumatic brain injury, *JAMA* 282:974-983, 1999.

CREUTZFELDT-JAKOB DISEASE AND BOVINE SPONGIFORM ENCEPHALOPATHY

(See also dementia; insomnia; transfusions)

Creutzfeldt-Jakob disease (CJD) is one of the infectious diseases of the brain causing a spongiform encephalopathy. Like all of the transmissible spongiform encephalopathies it has a long incubation period. The disease usually affects individuals between 50 and 70 years of age and is manifested as a rapidly progressive dementia associated with myoclonus. The electroencephalogram commonly shows periodic sharp wave activity. The infectious agent has been labeled a "slow virus" or a "prion." About 10% of human cases of CJD have a familial autosomal dominant inheritance pattern, but even in this subgroup, tissue from the patient can transmit the disease to nonhuman primates. In the past the disease has been transmitted by corneal transplants, growth hormone harvested from cadaveric pituitary glands, dura mater grafts, and neurosurgical instruments. There have been no confirmed cases of person-to-person transmission or transmission through transfusions. Other human examples of this type of encephalopathy are kuru, described among cannibals in central New Guinea, the familial Gerstmann-Sträussler-Scheinker syndrome, and fatal familial insomnia. In animals similar disorders include bovine spongiform encephalopathy (BSE, "mad cow disease"), scrapie in sheep and goats, transmissible mink encephalopathy, and wasting disease of deer and elk.[1,2]

A major concern that surfaced in 1996 was the possibility that BSE could be transmitted to humans through eating contaminated beef. Not only was the disease unusual because of the age of the patients, but the initial manifestations were behavioral (psychiatric) rather than cognitive, and neuropathological findings were different from those seen in the usual form of CJD.[3] As of early 1999 there had been 38 confirmed cases of new variant CJD in the United Kingdom and one in France. Although the annual number of cases increased from 1995 through 1998, this is probably a result of increased surveillance, not a true increase in incidence.[4]

A WHO consensus conference held in April 1996 concluded that no definite link existed between BSE and this new form of CJD but that exposure to BSE was the most likely explanation. Subsequent analysis of the strains of prion found in the brains of patients with new variant CJD showed them to be similar to the strains found in cattle with BSE and different from the strains found in the usual forms of CJD, confirming that new variant CJD is the human equivalent of BSE.[5,6]

Expert opinion claims that new variant CJD is not transmitted through milk or milk products.[3] Whether the disease can be transmitted by blood transfusions is unknown.[4]

The incidence of BSE in cattle in the United Kingdom has diminished dramatically since a 1988 ban on feeding ruminant-derived proteins to ruminants. It is hoped that the incidence of human cases of new variant CJD will also decrease.[2]

--------------- ◢ **REFERENCES** ◣ ---------------

1. Haywood AM: Transmissible spongiform encephalopathies, *N Engl J Med* 337:1821-1828, 1997.
2. Johnson RT, Gibbs CJ: Creutzfeldt-Jakob disease and related transmissible spongiform encephalopathies, *N Engl J Med* 339:1994-2004, 1998.
3. Centers for Disease Control and Prevention: World Health Organization consultation on public health issues related to bovine spongiform encephalopathy and the emergence of a new variant of Creutzfeldt-Jakob disease, *JAMA* 275:1305-1306, 1996.
4. New variant CJD and the blood supply: Canadian Blood Services reacts (editor's preface), *Can Med Assoc J* 160:1681, 1999.
5. Bruce ME, Will RG, Ironside JW, et al: Transmissions to mice indicate that new variant CJD is caused by the BSE agent, *Nature* 389:498-501, 1997.
6. Hill AF, Desbruslais M, Joiner S, et al: The same prion strain causes VCJD and BSE, *Nature* 389:448-450, 1997.

DEMENTIA

(See also alternative medicine; anesthesia; coronary artery bypass grafting and angioplasty; Creutzfeldt-Jakob disease; hormone replacement therapy; smoking)

A retrospective study of 100 autopsy-confirmed cases of Alzheimer's disease found the typical natural history to be as follows. Diagnosis was made about 3 years after the onset of symptoms, institutionalization took place around 2 years later, and the patient died approximately 4 years after that. The mean total duration of disease in this series was 8.5 years. Subgroup analysis found that the course of Alzheimer's disease was longer when the disease was diag-

nosed before the age of 65, in those with a family history of the disease, and in women.[1]

In a Canadian study the estimated prevalence of dementia in people over the age of 65 was 8%. The age-standardized rate varied from 2.4% in those aged 65 to 74 to 34.5% for those over the age of 85. Alzheimer's disease accounted for the majority of cases. The male/female ratio of Alzheimer's disease is 3:1.[2] In a community study in Boston the estimated annual incidence of new-onset Alzheimer's disease was 0.6% for those 65 to 69, 3.3% for those 80 to 84, and 8.4% for those over 85.[3]

Persons with low educational achievement are at greater risk for Alzheimer's disease.[4] A study of nuns found an excellent correlation between "low idea density" and "low grammatical complexity" in autobiographies written when the women were in their early twenties and the development of Alzheimer's disease in old age.[5] The probable explanation for this phenomenon is that well-educated individuals have a "reserve" capacity that allows them to maintain good cognitive functioning in spite of age-related brain changes such as atrophy.[4] Evidence suggests that social isolation is a risk factor for dementia,[6] but it is also possible that dementing illnesses lead to social isolation.[7] Smoking is an independent risk factor for Alzheimer's disease.[8]

Behavioral or noncognitive symptoms are common in patients with Alzheimer's disease, and these often lead to extreme frustration on the part of caregivers. They include decreased initiative and increased stubbornness and suspiciousness. About half of patients have delusions, which are usually paranoid, and one fourth have hallucinations, which are often visual. Depression and anxiety are also common.[9]

Normal aging is associated with some deterioration in the speed of cognitive processing, memory, and executive functioning.[10] ("Executive functioning" or "executive control processes" refers to frontal lobe activities such as information processing, problem solving, organization, planning, judgment, abstract reasoning, and insight.) That a "sound body" contributes to a "sound mind" is supported by a trial in which sedentary elderly adults without dementia were assigned at random to either 6 months of regular aerobic exercise (walking) or 6 months of regular anaerobic exercise (stretching and toning). Aerobic exercise improved executive functioning; anaerobic exercise did not.[11]

Not every elderly person who complains of "memory problems" has early dementia; some have no abnormalities, and others may suffer from what is often labeled age-associated memory impairment (AAMI). Although generally a benign condition, AAMI is associated with a slightly increased risk of dementia.[10]

In one Canadian study of 196 patients with documented or suspected dementia, the prevalence of theoretically reversible lesions was 23%, but improvement of cognitive functioning with treatment was achieved in only seven cases (3.6%). No patients with severe cognitive impairments improved with treatment; of those with mild cognitive deficits who improved, two were treated for depression, two discontinued medications (benzodiazepine, benztropine), one was treated for hypothyroidism, one received a shunt for normal-pressure hydrocephalus, and one had a brain tumor resected.[12] Because treatable causes of dementia are so rare, only a limited number of routine investigations appear to be beneficial. Unfortunately, little agreement exists on the investigations to perform. Almost everyone obtains a complete blood cell count,[13,14] but there is little evidence that this is beneficial.[13] Tests to rule out metabolic abnormalities that may be reversible include thyroid function tests[7,13,14] and measurements of calcium,[7,13,14] electrolytes,[13,14] and glucose.[13,14] Whether vitamin B_{12} deficiency is associated with dementia is uncertain. Many apparently healthy elderly persons have low levels, and whether demented persons with low levels improve with treatment is unclear. A Canadian consensus conference on dementia recommends ordering the test only for patients with neurological signs or symptoms.[14] Serological tests for syphilis have low sensitivity and specificity, and neurosyphilis causing dementia is extremely rare. These syphilis tests should probably be limited to patients who are considered to be at risk on the basis of history or physical examination.[13]

Brain imaging to detect treatable causes of dementia such as brain tumors, subdural hematomas, or normal pressure hydrocephalus is rarely positive in patients who do not have suggestive findings on history or focal abnormalities on neurological examination.[13,14] Indications for CT scanning include age under 60, rapid (1 to 2 months) onset of symptoms, history of cancer, use of anticoagulants, and unexplained neurological symptoms, including disturbed gait.[14] A CT scan without contrast is adequate[7,14] unless the patient shows evidence of motor abnormalities on neurological examination, in which case MRI is the procedure of choice.[7]

Although some studies have suggested that estrogen is beneficial for cognitive functioning, this has not been confirmed by others (see discussion of hormone replacement therapy). Studies have also suggested that nonsteroidal antiinflammatory drugs (NSAIDs) decrease both the incidence of Alzheimer's disease[15] and its rate of progression once it is established.[16]

Two centrally acting cholinesterase inhibitors, tacrine (THA, Cognex), which is usually given as 10 to 40 mg qid, and donepezil (Aricept), which is usually given as 5 or 10 mg once daily, are available for the treatment of Alzheimer's disease. Only 25% of patients taking tacrine show improvement,[17] and approximately 30% have a threefold or greater elevation of liver enzyme levels, usually in weeks 6 to 8 of treatment.[18] In a trial of donepezil about a third of patients showed improvement as measured by clinician interview with input from caregivers, compared with 18% of those given placebo. Adverse effects of the drug were minimal.[19] Neither tacrine nor donepezil prevents progression of the disease, and patients' functional levels return to those of the control group when the drugs are discontinued.[20] Most

trials to date have evaluated patients with mild to moderate disease; there is no evidence that cholinesterase inhibitors are beneficial for severe or incipient disease.[21] Based on current evidence it appears that a small number of patients with mild or moderate Alzheimer's disease can obtain temporary benefits from these drugs.

Extracts of the plant *Ginkgo biloba* have been claimed to delay the progression of dementia. A 1998 systematic review of the literature uncovered only four acceptable randomized controlled trials. *Ginkgo biloba* appears to have a modest effect on cognitive functioning, but whether this has clinical significance in terms of altering behavior or improving daily functioning is unclear.[22]

Several double-blind randomized studies have compared selegiline, or L-deprenyl (Eldepryl), to placebo in the treatment of Alzheimer's disease. It has delayed progression of the disease over study periods ranging from 1 month to 2 years.[18,23] A multicenter placebo-controlled trial of vitamin E 1000 mg bid over a 2-year period found that the treated group had a significant delay in the progression of Alzheimer's disease.[23] Current data suggest that selegiline or alpha-tocopherol can delay the onset of the most advanced stages of dementia by 5 to 6 months; whether this is significant in a disease that usually spans a decade is uncertain.[24]

Agitation in patients with dementia may be due to a variety of causes, including medical conditions, constipation, pain, hunger, sleep deprivation, depression, or a change in the environment. Drugs are indicated if precipitating factors cannot be identified or rectified. The most frequently used agents are low-dose antipsychotics, usually given in the evening to help patients sleep and to counter evening agitation, or "sundowning."[18,20] One study of haloperidol found that daily doses of less than 1 mg were ineffective whereas daily doses of 2 to 3 mg controlled agitation. Extrapyramidal side effects developed in about 20% of patients receiving the higher doses. Atypical neuroleptic agents such as risperidone, olanzapine, or clozapine may have fewer neurological side effects, but hypotension may be a significant risk.[25] A European multicenter placebo-controlled trial found that although both low-dose risperidone (mean daily dose of 1.1 mg) and low-dose haloperidol (mean daily dose of 1.2 mg) were superior to placebo in controlling aggressiveness in patients with severely dementia, risperidone was more effective and had fewer adverse effects.[26]

Typical daily doses of neuroleptics in dementia are shown in Table 18.

Benzodiazepines may also be used for agitation. In comparative studies they have been better than placebos but less effective than antipsychotics. For patients who do not respond to antipsychotics or benzodiazepines, carbamazepine (Tegretol) or valproic acid (Depakene) may be tried.[20,25]

The literature on the management of inappropriate sexual behavior, such as groping, exhibitionism, and public masturbation, in demented persons is limited to case reports. Neuroleptics do not seem to be effective, but success has

Table 18   Neuroleptics for Agitation in Dementia

Drug	Starting dose (mg/day)	Maximum dose (mg/day)
Haloperidol (Haldol)	1	2-3
Thioridazine (Mellaril)	10-25	50-100
Risperidone (Risperdal)	0.5-1	4-6
Clozapine (Clozaril)	12.5	75-100

been reported with paroxetine (Paxil) 20 mg/day, clomipramine (Anafranil) built up to between 150 and 200 mg/day, and medroxyprogesterone acetate (Depo-Provera) 150 to 200 mg intramuscularly every 2 weeks.[27]

Patients with advanced dementia may have difficulty eating. No evidence has been presented that tube feeding is beneficial, and considerable evidence indicates that it is harmful.[28]

⚓ REFERENCES ⚓

1. Jost BC, Grossberg GT: The natural history of Alzheimer's disease: a brain bank study, *J Am Geriatr Soc* 43:1248-1255, 1995.
2. Canadian Study of Health and Aging Working Group: Canadian Study of Health and Aging: study methods and prevalence of dementia, *Can Med Assoc J* 150:899-912, 1994.
3. Hebert LE, Scherr PA, Beckett LA, et al: Age-specific incidence of Alzheimer's disease in a community population, *JAMA* 273:1354-1359, 1995.
4. Coffey CE, Saxton JA, Ratcliff G, et al: Relation of education to brain size in normal aging: implications for the reserve hypothesis, *Neurology* 53:189-196, 1999.
5. Snowdon DA, Kemper SJ, Mortimer JA, et al: Linguistic ability in early life and cognitive function and Alzheimer's disease in late life, *JAMA* 275:528-532, 1996.
6. Bassuk SS, Glass TA, Berkman LF: Social disengagement and incident cognitive decline in community-dwelling elderly persons, *Ann Intern Med* 131:165-173, 1999.
7. Haan MN: Can social engagement prevent cognitive decline in old age? (editorial), *Ann Intern Med* 131:220-221, 1999.
8. Ott A, Slooter AJ, Hofman A, et al: Smoking and risk of dementia and Alzheimer's disease in a population-based cohort study: the Rotterdam Study, *Lancet* 351:1840-1843, 1998.
9. Geldmacher DS, Whitehouse PJ: Evaluation of dementia, *N Engl J Med* 335:330-336, 1996.
10. Hänninen T, Hallikainen M, Koivisto K, et al: A follow-up study of age-associated memory impairment: neuropsychological predictors of dementia, *J Am Geriatr Soc* 43:1007-1015, 1995.
11. Kramer AF, Hahn S, Cohen NJ, et al: Ageing, fitness and neurocognitive function, *Nature* 400:418-419, 1999.
12. Freter S, Bergman H, Gold S, et al: Prevalence of potentially reversible dementias and actual reversibility in a memory clinic cohort, *Can Med Assoc J* 159:657-662, 1998.
13. Frank C: Dementia workup: deciding on laboratory testing for the elderly, *Can Fam Physician* 44:1489-1495, 1998.
14. Patterson CJ, Gauthier S, Bergman H, et al: The recognition, assessment and management of dementing disorders: conclusions from the Canadian Consensus Conference on Dementia, *Can Med Assoc J* 160(suppl 12):S1-S15, 1999.
15. Stewart WF, Kawas C, Corrada M, et al: Risk of Alzheimer's disease and duration of NSAID use, *Neurology* 48:626-632, 1997.
16. Rich JB, Rasmusson DX, Folstein MF, et al: Nonsteroidal anti-inflammatory drugs in Alzheimer's disease, *Neurology* 45:51-55, 1995.
17. Smucker WD: Maximizing function in Alzheimer's disease: what role for tacrine? *Am Fam Physician* 54:645-652, 1996.
18. Rabins P, Blacker D, Bland W, et al: Practice guideline for the treatment of patients with Alzheimer's disease and other dementias of late life, *Am J Psychiatry* 154(suppl):S1-S39, 1997.
19. Rogers SL, Doody RS, Mohs RC, et al: Donepezil improves cognition and global function in Alzheimer disease: a 15-week, double-blind, placebo-controlled study, *Arch Intern Med* 158:1021-1031, 1998.
20. Small GW, Rabins PV, Barry PP, et al: Diagnosis and treatment of Alzheimer disease and related disorder: consensus statement of the American Association for Geriatric Psychiatry, the Alzheimer's Association, and the American Geriatrics Society, *JAMA* 278:1363-1371, 1997.
21. Flicker L: Acetylcholinesterase inhibitors for Alzheimer's disease, *BMJ* 318:615-616, 1999.
22. Oken BS, Storzbach DM, Kaye JA: The efficacy of *Ginkgo biloba* on cognitive function in Alzheimer disease, *Arch Neurol* 55:1409-1415, 1998.
23. Sano M, Ernesto C, Thomas RG, et al: A controlled trial of selegiline, alpha-tocopherol, or both as treatment for Alzheimer's disease, *N Engl J Med* 336:1216-1222, 1997.
24. Mayeux R, Sano M: Treatment of Alzheimer's disease, *N Engl J Med* 341:1670-1679, 1999.
25. Devanand DP, Marder K, Michaels KS, et al: A randomized, placebo-controlled dose-comparison trial of haloperidol for psychosis and disruptive behaviors in Alzheimer's disease, *Am J Psychiatry* 155:1512-1520, 1998.
26. De Deyn PP, Rabheru K, Rasmussen A, et al: A randomized trial of risperidone, placebo, and haloperidol for behavioral symptoms of dementia, *Neurology* 53:946-955, 1999.
27. Levitsky AM, Owens NJ: Pharmacologic treatment of hypersexuality and paraphilias in nursing home residents, *J Am Geriatr Soc* 47:231-234, 1999.
28. Finucane TE, Christmas C, Travis K: Tube feeding in patients with advanced dementia: a review of the evidence, *JAMA* 282:1365-1370, 1999.

HEADACHES

Investigations of Patients with Chronic Headaches

Should patients with the clinical diagnosis of migraines or other types of benign chronic headaches have a CT or MRI scan? An evaluation of CT scans of 373 patients referred to a chronic headache clinic in a tertiary care center in London, Ontario, found two osteomas, one low-grade glioma, and one aneurysm. The only lesion treated was the aneurysm. The authors state that this detection rate is the same as might be expected in the general population without headaches.[1] A study of imaging and headaches in children concluded that imaging was indicated only if neurological abnormalities were found on examination, a good history could not be obtained, or the child was very young.[2] If imaging is considered necessary, CT is usually the procedure of choice.[3]

❧ REFERENCES ❧

1. Dumas MD, Pexman JHW, Kreeft JH: Computed tomography evaluation of patients with chronic headache, *Can Med Assoc J* 151:1447-1452, 1994.
2. Maytal J, Bienkowski RS, Patel M, et al: The value of brain imaging in children with headaches, *Pediatrics* 96:413-416, 1995.
3. Goh RH, Somers S, Jurriaans E, et al: Magnetic resonance imaging: application to family practice, *Can Fam Physician* 45:2118-2132, 1999.

Psychiatric Disorders and Headaches

The overall prevalence of headaches in children 9 to 15 years of age is 10%. Children with psychiatric disorders have twice as high a prevalence rate of headaches as those without psychiatric disorders. The most frequently associated psychiatric disorders are depression and anxiety disorders among girls and conduct disorder among boys.[1]

❧ REFERENCES ❧

1. Egger HL, Angold A, Costello EJ: Headaches and psychopathology in children and adolescents, *J Am Acad Child Adolesc Psychiatry* 37:951-958, 1998.

Chronic Daily Headaches
(See also migraines)

Many patients with migraines or other headaches are frequent users of analgesic drugs. This in itself can lead to withdrawal headaches, and a vicious circle of headaches–drugs–more headaches is established. Terms used to describe this type of headache include analgesic overuse headache, chronic daily headache, and transformed migraine (transformed from intermittent headaches to daily or almost daily headaches). Chronic tension headaches account for only a small proportion of chronic daily headaches. Patients with chronic daily headaches also frequently have anxiety or mood disorders.[1]

Almost any antimigraine drug, including aspirin, NSAIDs, acetaminophen, codeine, ergotamine, and sumatriptan, may be responsible for analgesic overuse headache,[1] and this may lead to abuse of any of these drugs. For example, a Danish study of sumatriptan use found that 5% of patients accounted for 40% of its total consumption.[2]

Although analgesic overuse is not the only cause of chronic daily headaches, it is thought to account for 50% to 75% of cases.[1] Such figures may be an artifact of specialty headache clinics; in a population survey of patients with chronic daily headache, analgesic abuse was reported in only 17% of cases.[3]

The clinical features are variable. Patients have daily or almost daily headaches that have variable locations and may be throbbing or steady. Patients often wake up with a headache. The headaches are often precipitated by physical exertion or intellectual effort, and the patient may have nausea, irritability, and difficulty concentrating.[1]

Prophylactic medications have little value in the management of chronic daily headaches as long as the patient continues to take analgesics on a regular basis. Treatment of the disorder consists of withdrawal of the analgesics. This may be done rapidly or slowly, but if a barbiturate (e.g., Fiorinal) is involved, the withdrawal should be slow. Although many patients improve within 1 week, it may take up to 3 months for the maximal effect of analgesic withdrawal to be noted.[1]

❧ REFERENCES ❧

1. Mathew NT: Transformed migraine, analgesic rebound, and other chronic daily headaches, *Neurol Clin* 15:167-186, 1997.
2. Gaist D, Tsiropoulos I, Sindrup SH, et al: Inappropriate use of sumatriptan: population based register and interview study, *BMJ* 316:1352-1353, 1998.
3. Castillo J, Munoz P, Guitera V, et al: Epidemiology of chronic daily headache in the general population, *Headache* 39:190-196, 1999.

Caffeine Withdrawal Headaches

The caffeine content of various beverages is as follows[1]:

6 ounces of brewed coffee	85-100 mg
6 ounces of instant coffee	65 mg
6 ounces of tea	40 mg
12 ounces of caffeinated soft drink	45 mg

Caffeine withdrawal symptoms usually begin within 12 to 24 hours of the last caffeine intake, reach their maximum in 20 to 48 hours, and last for about a week.[2] In a Dutch study, individuals withdrawing from four to six cups of coffee per day had a high incidence of headaches beginning on day 1 and persisting as long as 6 days (mean 2.3 days).[3] A U.S. study found that even individuals taking an average of two and a half cups of coffee per day had withdrawal symptoms; 52% had moderate or severe headaches, and 8% to 11% had significant symptoms of anxiety or depression.[4]

❧ REFERENCES ❧

1. Hughes JR: Clinical importance of caffeine withdrawal, *N Engl J Med* 327:1160-1161, 1992.
2. Griffiths RR, Woodson PP: Caffeine physical dependence: a review of human and laboratory animal studies, *Psychopharmacology (Berl)* 94:437-451, 1988.
3. Van Dusseldorp M, Katan MB: Headache caused by caffeine withdrawal among moderate coffee drinkers switched from ordinary to decaffeinated coffee: a 12 week double blind trial, *BMJ* 300:1558-1559, 1990.
4. Silverman K, Evans SM, Strain EC, et al: Withdrawal syndrome after the double-blind cessation of caffeine consumption, *N Engl J Med* 327:1109-1114, 1992.

Cluster Headaches

Men are affected by cluster headache six times as frequently as women. Alcohol is a frequent triggering factor. The pain is unilateral and severe, is usually centered around the eye, comes on suddenly, and frequently awakens the patient from sleep. The usual attack lasts about 45 minutes.[1] In one study the most common behavior observed during attacks of cluster headaches was walking with the trunk bent slightly forward while clutching the head, or sitting and rocking back and forth with the hands pressed over the painful area. Some patients banged their heads against a hard object, and others pressed a finger or thumb into the affected eye.[2]

Drugs used for treatment of the acute attack include sumatriptan (Imitrex), dihydroergotamine (DHE, Migranal), ergotamine tartrate (Medihaler-ergotamine), ergotamine tablets or suppositories (Cafergot, Wigraine), inhaled oxygen at 8 L/min for 10 minutes, and 2% to 4% lidocaine (Xylocaine) by nasal instillation.[1] If lidocaine is used, it is administered by having the patient lie on the bed with the head hanging over the edge so the neck is extended 45 degrees and the head is rotated 30 to 40 degrees toward the side of the headache. The lidocaine is slowly dropped into the nostril ipsilateral to the pain. If the nostril is plugged, a topical decongestant is given.[1,3] More information on the usual dosages of these drugs may be found in Tables 19 and 20.

Lithium carbonate in doses of 300 mg bid to qid is often effective for the prophylaxis of cluster headaches. Serum lithium levels need be only between 0.4 and 0.8 mEq/L (0.4 to 0.8 mmol/L). Prednisone and methysergide (Sansert) are also effective prophylactic drugs. Prednisone is given in doses of 40 to 80 mg/day for 1 to 2 weeks and then tapered and discontinued over the following week, and methysergide is usually taken as 2 to 4 mg tid with meals. During cluster periods ergotamine may be given hs or on a regular basis bid to abort the headaches. For some patients indomethacin (Indocin, Indocid) 25 to 50 mg tid prevents attacks.[1]

◤ REFERENCES ◣

1. Walling AD: Cluster headache, *Am Fam Physician* 47:1457-1463, 1993.
2. Blau JN: Behaviour during a cluster headache, *Lancet* 342:723-725, 1993.
3. Kittrelle J, Grouse D, Seybold M: Cluster headache: local anesthetic abortive agents, *Arch Neurol* 42:496-498, 1985.

Migraines

(See also caffeine withdrawal headaches; chronic daily headaches; cluster headaches; investigations of patients with chronic headaches; risk factors for stroke)

In North America 18% of women and 6% of men are estimated to suffer from migraines.[1] The association between migraines and stroke is equivocal (see discussion of risk factors for stroke). Many patients with migraines have superimposed withdrawal-type headaches from excessive use of medications to control the migraines (analgesic overuse headaches). Three fourths of women with migraines obtain relief with the onset of the menopause.[2]

The concept that the pain of migraine is directly caused by vascular hyperreactivity with initial vasoconstriction followed by vasodilation is no longer tenable. It is now thought that dysfunction of the serotonergic system in the brainstem activates trigeminal nerve fibers that supply blood vessels of the pia and dura mater. This results in the release of vasoactive substances, causing inflammation and pain around the vessels. Vasoconstriction and vasodilation are secondary phenomena. Serotonin is central to this process, which may explain the efficacy of dihydroergotamine and sumatriptan, agents that act on serotonin receptors.[3]

Migraines are divided into two main classes. Between 10% and 20% of patients have migraine with aura (classic migraine), and most of the remainder have migraine without aura (common migraine). A few patients have complicated migraines defined as neurological symptoms lasting for the duration of the headache and occasionally causing permanent sequelae. Well-known variants of this type are basilar, hemiplegic, and ophthalmoplegic migraines, the last usually occurring in children. Although migraines are classically unilateral and pulsatile, they are bilateral in 40% of cases and may be nonpulsatile. The criteria of the International Headache Society for making a diagnosis of migraine without aura state that there should be nothing in the history or physical examination to suggest that the headaches are caused by another disease, that the patient must have had at least five attacks of headache lasting 4 to 72 hours, and that these must have had at least two of the following characteristics[2-4]:

1. Unilateral
2. Pulsatile
3. Moderate to severe intensity
4. Aggravated by physical activity such as walking upstairs

In addition, the patient should experience at least one of the following associated symptoms[3,4]:

1. Nausea or vomiting
2. Photophobia, phonophobia

One of the most important principles of the pharmacological treatment of acute migraine attacks is to initiate therapy early in the attack using an effective dose of whatever drugs are chosen.[3] For anything but the mildest attack the chosen antimigraine drug should be combined with an antiemetic such as metoclopramide (Maxeran) or domperidone (Motilium). Not only will metoclopramide or domperidone decrease the symptom of nausea, but also they will facilitate the absorption of antimigraine drugs. Metoclopramide has the added advantage of providing some specific antimigraine effect.[5]

The initial choice of an antimigraine drug should be acetaminophen,[2] aspirin,[2] or a combination of these two agents plus caffeine.[6,7] Next on the list are NSAIDs, and if these fail, 5-HT$_1$ receptor agonists such as ergot derivatives or sumatriptan (Imitrex). Intense migraines persisting for many days may respond to a short course of oral steroids.[2] Very severe migraines usually respond to intravenous neuroleptics, dexamethasone, or metoclopramide.[3,4]

Acetaminophen or aspirin should be given as soon as possible after the onset of the migraine with initial doses of 650 to 1000 mg[3] or 650 to 1300 mg.[4] Enteric-coated aspirin should not be used because this formulation delays absorption.[3] The combination of acetaminophen 500 mg, aspirin 500 mg, and caffeine 130 mg as a single dose has been shown to control pain, nausea, photophobia, and phonophobia in adults with mild,[6] moderately severe,[6] and severe[7] migraines. A single oral dose of acetaminophen (15 mg/kg) is often effective in controlling migraines in children, but a single oral dose of ibuprofen (10 mg/kg) is said to be better.[8]

A variety of NSAIDs have proved beneficial (Table 19).[3,4] Capobianco and associates[3] favor naproxen if oral medications are tolerated or indomethacin suppositories if nausea and vomiting occur.

Several 5-HT$_1$ receptor agonists, or "triptans," of which sumatriptan is the best known, are now available (Table 19). The recurrence rate within 24 hours of successful treatment is 30% to 40%. A triptan should not be taken within 24 hours of using another triptan or an ergot derivative. A combination of triptans and selective serotonin reuptake inhibitors may induce the serotonin syndrome.[9] Triptans are often effective even if given after the headache has been present for some time and has become well established.

Ergot is an agonist of 5-HT$_1$ receptors but is less selective than sumatriptan. Ergotamine derivatives should be given as soon as possible after the onset of the migraine. Oral absorption is relatively poor, so for some patients rectal suppositories may be more effective. Because ergotamine derivatives may cause nausea and vomiting, the dose must be adjusted (cutting refrigerated suppositories in half or even quarters) to prevent this reaction.[3] Ergotamine is available as tablets or suppositories combined with caffeine (Cafergot, Wigraine), as sublingual tablets (Ergomar), and as a metered dose inhaler (Medihaler-ergotamine). The usual initial dose of tablets or suppositories is 1 to 2 mg, and these may be repeated every half hour to a maximum dosage of 6 mg. Dihydroergotamine is available for intramuscular injection (DHE) and has recently been formulated as a nasal spray (Migranal). The usual initial dose is 1 to 3 mg intramuscularly or 1 spray of 0.5 mg in each nostril.

Drug combinations for migraines include acetaminophen or aspirin with codeine and often caffeine; aspirin, caffeine, and the barbiturate butalbital with or without codeine (Fiorinal) or acetaminophen; and caffeine and butalbital (Esgic and Esgic Plus). Evidence supporting the efficacy of these drug combinations is poor, they may lead to addiction, and they are thought to be a major cause of rebound headaches that lead to chronic daily headaches.[4] Because of the risk of severe dependence, their use should be discouraged.[10]

Butorphanol (Stadol) is a mixed narcotic agonist-antagonist, administered by nasal insufflation, that is marketed for migraine treatment. Each spray contains about 1 mg of butorphanol, which has the analgesic equivalency of 5 mg of parenterally administered morphine. The median duration of pain relief in migraine is said to be 6 hours. A placebo-controlled study of 157 patients with migraines documented marked pain relief in 33% within 30 minutes, 47% within 1 hour, and 71% within 6 hours. Side effects, mainly dizziness, nausea, vomiting, and drowsiness, were prominent. Some patients also experienced confusion.[11] Butorphanol may be addictive and in some cases is sought by drug abusers.[12]

In a 1-month randomized placebo-controlled trial of ambulatory patients in a family medicine practice a 4% solution of intranasal lidocaine relieved a little over one third of migraines within 15 minutes with a relapse rate of 20% within 24 hours. In a 6-month follow-up open label trial, intranasal lidocaine relieved over 50% of migraines within 30 minutes, but as in the initial trial the relapse rate was 20%. Severe headaches responded less well than moderate ones, and lidocaine retained its effectiveness over the 6-month period.[13]

Intranasal lidocaine is administered by having the patient lie on a bed with the shoulders overhanging the edge and the head hyperextended as far as possible and rotated 30 degrees toward the side of the headache. With a 1-ml syringe, 0.5 ml of a 4% solution of lidocaine is dripped over a 30-second period into the nostril on the side of the headache. When this is completed, the head is maintained in the same position for another 30 seconds. If the migraine is bilateral, the procedure is repeated with the head turned to the opposite side. The patient then moves back up the bed and lies supine (no pillow) for 2 to 3 minutes. If the patient responds to the initial dose but relapses, the lidocaine treatment may be repeated.[13]

When other medications fail and the patient has had headaches for several days, a short course of oral prednisone often breaks a migraine cycle.[3]

A variety of drugs given IV or intramuscularly in the emergency room have aborted migraines. These include chlorpromazine (Thorazine, Largactil) 12.5 mg IV as an initial dose repeated every 30 minutes to a maximum of 37.5 mg,[3] prochlorperazine (Compazine, Stemetil) 7 to 10 mg IV stat,[14] metoclopramide (Maxeran) 7 to 10 mg IV stat,[15] dexamethasone 20 mg IV with or without 3.5 mg of prochlorperazine,[16] and ketorolac (Toradol) 60 mg intramuscularly.[17] Akathisia is a common sequela of a single IV dose of prochlorperazine.[18]

Table 19 lists some drugs and usual doses used in the treatment of acute migraine attacks.

Few randomized trials of the nonpharmacological treatment of migraines have been published, and the magnitude of the placebo effect in most reports is uncertain. Almost all patients find some relief from retiring to a dark room and attempting to sleep. Cold compresses applied to the head are reported to be useful.[19]

Table 19   Treatment of Acute Migraine Attacks

Drug	Usual dose
Simple Analgesics	
Acetaminophen	650-1300 mg stat
Aspirin	650-1300 mg stat
Acetaminophen 500 mg + aspirin 500 mg + caffeine 130 mg	A single dose stat
NSAIDs	
Diclofenac (Voltaren)	50-100 mg stat
Flurbiprofen (Ansaid, Froben)	100 mg stat
Ibuprofen (Motrin, Advil)	400-800 mg stat (10 mg/kg for children)
Indomethacin (Indocin, Indocid)	100 mg po or pr stat
Ketorolac (Toradol)	60 mg IM stat
Mefenamic acid (Ponstan)	500 mg stat
Naproxen (Anaprox)	550-825 mg stat
Serotonin Agonists ("Triptans")	
Naratriptan (Amerge)	1-2.5 mg po
Rizatriptan (Maxalt)	5-10 mg po (tablet or wafer)
Sumatriptan (Imitrex)	25-100 mg po; 6 mg sc; 1 nasal insufflation
Zolmitriptan (Zomig)	2.5-5 mg po
Ergot Derivatives	
Dihydroergotamine (Migranal)	1 spray (0.5 mg) each nostril; repeat once in 15 min prn
Dihydroergotamine (DHE)	1 mg IM stat; repeat q 1 hour × 2 prn
Ergotamine tartrate (Ergomar)	2 mg sl stat; repeat q 30 min × 2 prn
Ergotamine tartrate (Medihaler-ergotamine)	1 inhalation of 360 μg stat; repeat q 5 min × 5 prn
Ergotamine-caffeine (Cafergot)	2 tablets or 1 suppository stat; repeat with 1 tablet or ½ suppository q 30 min to maximum 6 tablets or 2 suppositories
Ergotamine–caffeine–belladonna alkaloids (Wigraine)	1-2 tablets or 1 suppository stat; repeat q 30 min to maximum 6 tablets or 2 suppositories
Drug Combinations	
Butalbital-ASA-caffeine with or without codeine (Fiorinal)	Addictive; not recommended
Butalbital-acetaminophen-caffeine (Esgic Plus)	Addictive; not recommended
Narcotics—Agonist-Antagonist	
Butorphanol tartrate (Stadol)	1 spray in 1 nostril stat; repeat × 1 in 30-60 min prn
Topical Nasal Anesthetics	
Lidocaine (Xylocaine)	Nasal instillation of 0.5 ml of 4% solution
Antiemetics	
Metoclopramide (Maxeran)	10 mg po stat
Domperidone (Motilium)	10-20 mg po stat
Steroids	
Prednisone	Variable, e.g., 60 mg/day × 4 days with tapering over 10-14 days
Parenteral Drugs in Emergency Room	
Chlorpromazine (Thorazine, Largactil)	12.5 mg IV as an initial dose repeated every 30 minutes to a maximum of 37.5 mg
Prochlorperazine (Compazine, Stemetil)	7-10 mg IV stat
Metoclopramide (Maxeran)	7-10 mg IV stat
Dexamethasone	20 mg IV with or without 3.5 mg of prochlorperazine
Ketorolac (Toradol)	60 mg IM

NSAIDs, Nonsteroidal antiinflammatory drugs.

Measures to prevent migraines focus on life-style modifications and, if necessary, pharmacotherapy (Table 20). The evidence that life-style factors contribute to migraines is largely anecdotal. Some of the more commonly accepted migraine triggers are bright or flickering lights, loud noises, strong odors, irregular sleeping patterns (sleeping in on weekends), missing meals, and specific dietary products, especially those containing nitrites, aspartame, or monosodium glutamate. Some of the foods that have been incriminated are alcohol, especially red wine; aged and processed cheese; aged, cured, or processed meats (hot dogs, bacon, smoked meat, many lunch meats); Chinese food (monosodium glutamate); chocolate; and caffeine-containing beverages. Biofeedback, relaxation therapy, and cognitive-

Table 20 Prophylaxis of Migraines

Drug	Usual dose
Beta-Blockers	
Atenolol (Tenormin)	50-200 mg/day
Metoprolol (Lopressor)	100-200 mg/day
Nadolol (Corgard)	40-240 mg/day
Propranolol (Inderal)	40-320 mg/day
Calcium Channel Blockers	
Flunarizine (Sibelium)	5-10 mg qhs
Verapamil (Calan, Isoptin)	240-480 mg/day
Tricyclic Antidepressants	
Amitriptyline (Elavil)	10-175 mg/day
Nortriptyline (Aventyl, Pamelor)	10-125 mg/day
Anticonvulsants	
Divalproex (Depakote)	250-1500 mg/day
Valproic acid (Depakene)	250-1500 mg/day
Nonsteroidal Antiinflammatory Drugs	
Naproxen sodium (Anaprox)	550 mg bid for 7 premenstrual days
Ergot Derivatives	
Methysergide (Sansert)	2-6 mg/day (drug holiday q 6 months)

behavioral therapy have reportedly decreased the frequency of migraines in some patients. Physiotherapy, osteopathy, chiropractic, transcutaneous electrical stimulation, acupuncture, naturopathy, and homeopathy are of doubtful value.[19]

Indications for pharmacological prophylaxis of migraines include more than two or three migraines a month, attacks lasting longer than 48 hours, severe attacks, and nonresponse to therapy. Between 55% and 65% of patients respond to prophylactic therapy, but amelioration of symptoms may be delayed for 1 to 2 months. In general it is wise to start with relatively low doses of prophylactic agents and raise them weekly if the response is inadequate.[3]

Beta-blockers are the agents of first choice (Table 20).[3] Beta-blockers with intrinsic sympathomimetic activity such as pindolol (Visken) and acebutolol (Sectral) are not effective.[4]

Most calcium channel blockers are of questionable value in the prophylaxis of migraines. Verapamil (Calan, Isoptin) seems to be marginally beneficial, the data for nifedipine are inconclusive, and diltiazem has not been adequately studied. If verapamil is used, the daily maintenance dose is 240 to 480 mg.[3] Flunarizine (Sibelium) has been effective at a usual maintenance dose of 5 to 10 mg qhs.[4]

Some patients respond well to tricyclic antidepressants such as amitriptyline (Elavil) with a usual daily maintenance dose of 10 to 175 mg or nortriptyline (Aventyl, Pamelor) in a daily maintenance dose of 10 to 125 mg.[3,4] An advantage of nortriptyline is that it has fewer anticholinergic side effects than amitriptyline.[4] Valproic acid (Depakene) and divalproex (Depakote) have been shown to be effective prophylactic agents for migraines with a daily maintenance

dose of 250 to 1500 mg.[3,4] For some patients daily use of NSAIDs is an effective prophylactic regimen.[3] Naproxen sodium (Anaprox) 550 mg bid may be used for 1 week a month before the menstrual period as prophylaxis against premenstrual migraines.[4]

The semisynthetic ergot preparation methysergide (Sansert) is a serotonin antagonist and an effective prophylactic agent against migraines. The daily maintenance dose is 2 to 6 mg. The major problem with the drug is that it can induce retroperitoneal or pleuropulmonary fibrosis with continuous use in about 1 in 1500 patients. Because of this it should be reserved for patients in whom other prophylactic endeavors have failed. Patients must taper the drug and take a 3- to 4-week drug holiday every 6 months.[3]

Other drugs that have been used for migraine prophylaxis but that have not been adequately studied are parthenolide (Tanacet 125 or "feverfew"), pizotyline (Sandomigran), and cyproheptadine (Periactin).[3]

❧ REFERENCES ❧

1. Stewart WF, Lipton RB, Celentano DD, et al: Prevalence of migraine headaches in the United States: relation to age, income, race, and other sociodemographic factors, *JAMA* 267:64-69, 1992.
2. Kumar KL, Cooney TG: Headaches, *Med Clin North Am* 79:261-286, 1995.
3. Capobianco DJ, Cheshire WP, Campbell JK: An overview of the diagnosis and pharmacologic treatment of migraine, *Mayo Clin Proc* 71:1055-1066, 1996.
4. Pryse-Phillips WE, Dodick DW, Edmeads JG, et al: Guidelines for the diagnosis and management of migraine in clinical practice, *Can Med Assoc J* 156:1273-1287, 1997.
5. Dahlöf CG, Hargreaves RJ: Pathophysiology and pharmacology of migraine: is there a place for antiemetics in future treatment strategies? *Cephalalgia* 18:593-604, 1998.
6. Lipton RB, Stewart WF, Ryan RE Jr, et al: Efficacy and safety of acetaminophen, aspirin, and caffeine in alleviating headache pain: three double-blind, randomized, placebo-controlled trials, *Arch Neurol* 55:210-217, 1998.
7. Goldstein J, Hoffman HD, Armellino JJ, et al: Treatment of severe, disabling migraine attacks in an over-the-counter population of migraine sufferers: results from three randomized, placebo-controlled studies of the combination of acetaminophen, aspirin, and caffeine, *Cephalalgia* 19:684-691, 1999.
8. Hamalainen ML, Hoppu K, Valkeila E, et al: Ibuprofen or acetaminophen for the acute treatment of migraine in children—a double-blind, randomized, placebo-controlled, crossover study, *Neurology* 48:103-107, 1997.
9. New "triptans" and other drugs for migraine, *Med Lett* 40:97-100, 1998.
10. Raja M, Altavista MC, Azzoni A, et al: Severe barbiturate withdrawal syndrome in migrainous patients, *Headache* 36:119-121, 1996.
11. Hoffert MJ, Couch JR, Diamond S, et al: Transnasal butorphanol in the treatment of acute migraine, *Headache* 35:65-69, 1995.

12. Canadian Adverse Drug Reaction Newsletter: Potential abuse of butorphanol nasal spray, *Can Med Assoc J* 156:1054-1056, 1997.

13. Maizels M, Scott B, Cohen W, et al: Intranasal lidocaine for treatment of migraine: a randomized, double-blind, controlled trial, *N Engl J Med* 276:319-321, 1996.

14. Coppola M, Yealy DM, Leibold RA: Randomized, placebo-controlled evaluation of prochlorperazine versus metoclopramide for emergency department treatment of migraine headache, *Ann Emerg Med* 26:541-546, 1995.

15. Ellis GL, Delaney J, DeHart DA, et al: The efficacy of metoclopramide in the treatment of migraine headache, *Ann Emerg Med* 22:191-195, 1993.

16. Saadah HA: Abortive migraine therapy in the office with dexamethasone and prochlorperazine, *Headache* 34:366-370, 1994.

17. Shrestha M, Singh R, Moreden J, et al: Ketorolac vs chlorpromazine in the treatment of acute migraine without aura: a prospective, randomized, double-blind trial, *Arch Intern Med* 156:1725-1728, 1996.

18. Drotts DL, Vinson DR: Prochlorperazine induces akathisia in emergency patients, *Ann Emerg Med* 34:469-475, 1999.

19. Pryse-Phillips WE, Dodick DW, Edmeads JG, et al: Guidelines for the nonpharmacologic management of migraine in clinical practice, *Can Med Assoc J* 59:47-54, 1998.

MULTIPLE SCLEROSIS

(See also investigations; labeling; pets; spasticity)

Multiple sclerosis (MS) is primarily a disease of young white adults. About 60% of cases occur in women. The disease is more common in northern than in tropical regions, and the incidence seems to be increasing.[1] The lifetime risk for a child whose mother has MS is 3% to 5%; the risk appears to be somewhat lower if the father has the disease.[2]

In 90% of cases MS begins between the ages of 20 and 50. The four most common initial symptoms, which occur with about equal frequency, are optic neuritis, numbness, weakness, and gait imbalance.[2] The disorder usually has a relapsing or remitting course, but in 10% to 15% of cases the course is progressive from the onset. Primary progressive MS tends to involve only one part of the nervous system, usually the spinal cord, and has a poor prognosis.[2,3] In more than half of patients with relapsing or remitting MS, secondary progressive disease eventually develops. Ten years after the onset of the disease 50% of patients cannot work, after 15 years 50% cannot walk unassisted, and after 25 years 50% cannot walk at all. In 10% of patients the disease is benign with little evidence of progression.[2]

MRI is the investigation of choice for confirming the diagnosis of MS when it is suspected clinically. However, MRI is negative in up to 10% of cases, and it is not 100% specific. In patients with MS, MRI almost always detects many more lesions than would be expected on the basis of clinical examination.[1] The presence of abnormal evoked potentials alone is not pathognomonic of MS. However, in the context of other clinical and laboratory findings, they may help confirm such a diagnosis. Visual evoked potentials and somatosensory evoked potentials are abnormal in more than three fourths of patients with MS, and brainstem auditory evoked responses are abnormal in more than half of such patients.[1]

A number of factors influence the prognosis of relapsing or remitting MS. The prognosis is better in younger patients, females, and those who have only a limited number of neuroanatomical areas affected, have primarily sensory symptoms, experience a complete first remission, and have limited deficits after 5 years. However, even after many years the course may become progressive and in that case the prognosis for permanent disability is grave.[4]

Acute relapses of MS are usually treated with corticosteroids. This shortens the duration of the relapse, but whether such therapy affects the ultimate course of the disease is unknown.[2,3]

Disease-modifying agents for relapsing-remitting MS include interferon and glatiramer. Both interferon beta-1a (Avonex) and interferon beta-1b (Betaseron, Rebif) injections have been shown to decrease the number of relapses and the number of plaques found on MRI scanning in patients with relapsing-remitting MS,[3] and beta-1a interferon has also been shown to delay the time to the onset of sustained progression.[5] Glatiramer (Copaxone) injections look promising for relapsing-remitting MS and may be considered as an alternative to interferon beta.[3]

The progressive forms of MS have usually been treated with drugs such as methotrexate, cyclophosphamide, or cyclosporine; benefits have been slight.[3] A 1998 study found that beta-1b interferon given to patients with secondary progressive MS significantly delayed neurological deterioration and the number of lesions detected with MRI.[6]

─────────────── ◥ **REFERENCES** ◤ ───────────────

1. Brod SA, Lindsey JW, Wolinsky JS: Multiple sclerosis: clinical presentation, diagnosis and treatment, *Am Fam Physician* 54: 1301-1311, 1996.

2. Rudick RA: A 29-year-old man with multiple sclerosis, *JAMA* 280:1432-1439, 1998.

3. Rudick RA, Cohen JA, Weinstock-Guttman B, et al: Management of multiple sclerosis, *N Engl J Med* 337:1604-1611, 1997.

4. Runmarker B, Andersen O: Prognostic factors in a multiple sclerosis incidence cohort with twenty-five years of follow-up, *Brain* 116:117-134, 1993.

5. PRISMS (Prevention of Relapses and Disability by Interferon β-1a Subcutaneously in Multiple Sclerosis) Study Group: Randomised double-blind placebo-controlled study of interferon β-1a in relapsing/remitting multiple sclerosis, *Lancet* 352: 1498-1504, 1998.

6. European Study Group on Interferon β-1b in Secondary Progressive MS: Placebo-controlled multicentre randomised trial of interferon β-1b in treatment of secondary progressive multiple sclerosis, *Lancet* 352:1491-1497, 1998.

MYASTHENIA GRAVIS
(See also paraneoplastic syndromes)

The incidence of myasthenia gravis occurs in two peaks. The first is in the second and third decades and involves mostly women; the second is in the sixth and seventh decades and involves mostly men. The pathogenesis of myasthenia gravis is an autoantibody destruction of acetylcholine receptors at the neuromuscular junctions.[1]

The traditional diagnostic test for myasthenia gravis is to give the patient an IV dose of 2 mg of edrophonium (Tensilon) and see whether muscle strength improves. A positive result is usually seen within 30 to 60 seconds, and the effect lasts about 5 minutes. Edrophonium inhibits the enzyme acetylcholinesterase, which normally inactivates acetylcholine. This allows the acetylcholine released into the neuromuscular junctions to act repeatedly with the acetylcholine receptors that still remain at the neuromuscular junctions. Another diagnostic test is the repetitive nerve stimulation test in which action potentials are recorded from the innervated muscle. The most specific test is an assay for acetylcholine-receptor antibodies. However, antibodies are found in only 85% of patients and in only 50% of those whose symptoms are limited to ocular muscle weakness.[1]

Treatment of myasthenia is effective, and the vast majority of patients are able to live normal lives. Thymectomy is indicated for any patient found to have a thymic tumor and for anyone with generalized myasthenia who is between the ages of puberty and 60. It has also been reported to be helpful for some patients with purely ocular myasthenia. Whether it is useful in those over the age of 60 who do not have a thymic tumor is uncertain. The standard medical treatment of myasthenia is pyridostigmine bromide (Mestinon). A few patients require long-term therapy with immunosuppressive drugs such as corticosteroids, azathioprine, or cyclosporine. IV immune globulin and plasma exchange are used to stabilize the condition of patients in myasthenic crisis or as perioperative therapy for patients undergoing thymectomy.[1]

REFERENCES

1. Drachman DB: Myasthenia gravis, *N Engl J Med* 330:1797-1810, 1994.

NEOPLASMS

Meningiomas are common intracranial neoplasms. Most are asymptomatic, and they either do not grow or grow very slowly. Optimal management of asymptomatic meningiomas is watchful waiting.[1]

An analysis of 19,000 patients with primary central nervous system neoplasms found that the overall 2- and 5-year survival rates were 36% and 28%, but prognosis varied greatly according to histological type and age (better for younger patients). For patients who survived 2 years, prognosis for survival was greatly improved, with an overall rate of 76%.[2]

The survival and quality of life of patients with single brain metastases were no better after surgery plus radiation therapy than after radiation therapy alone.[3]

REFERENCES

1. Go RS, Taylor BV, Kimmel DW: The natural history of asymptomatic meningiomas in Olmsted Country, Minnesota, *Neurology* 51:1718-1720, 1998.
2. Davis FG, McCarthy BJ, Freels S, et al: The conditional probability of survival of patients with primary malignant brain tumors: Surveillance, Epidemiology, and End Results (SEER) data, *Cancer* 85:485-491, 1999.
3. Mintz AH, Kestle J, Rathbone MP, et al: A randomized trial to assess the efficacy of surgery in addition to radiotherapy in patients with a single cerebral metastasis, *Cancer* 78:1470-1476, 1996.

NEUROPATHY

(See also diabetic neuropathy; herpes zoster)

Bell's Palsy

Bell's palsy may be incomplete or complete; the prognosis is better for patients with the incomplete form and for those under 40 years of age. Recovery usually commences in 6 weeks, and the median time to complete resolution of paresis is 6 weeks.[1]

Whether steroids (prednisone) improve the recovery rates in patients with Bell's palsy is a matter of controversy. Recent studies suggest that they do if started within 48 or perhaps 72 hours.[1-4] Pryse-Phillips[4] recommends 1 mg/kg up to a maximum dose of 70 mg given as a single morning dose for 4 days; no tapering is necessary. From their review of the literature Williamson and Whelan[1] recommend treating only patients with complete paralysis. They suggest 1 mg/kg of prednisolone (maximum of 80 mg) given for a maximum of 10 days.

REFERENCES

1. Williamson IG, Whelan TR: The clinical problem of Bell's palsy: is treatment with steroids effective? *Br J Gen Pract* 46:743-747, 1996.
2. Shafshak TS, Essa AY, Bakey FA: The possible contributing factors for the success of steroid therapy in Bell's palsy: a clinical and electrophysiological study, *J Laryngol Otol* 108:940-943, 1994.
3. Austin JR, Peskind SP, Austin SG, Rice DH: Idiopathic facial nerve paralysis: a randomized double blind controlled study of placebo versus prednisone, *Laryngoscope* 103:1326-1333, 1993.
4. Pryse-Phillips W: Oral steroid use in Bell's palsy, *Patient Care Can* 6:12, 1995.

Carpal Tunnel Syndrome

The normal pressure within a limb compartment is 7 to 8 mm Hg. In carpal tunnel syndrome the pressure is often 30 mm Hg. With wrist flexion or extension it may be as high as 90 mm Hg.[1]

Risk factors for carpal tunnel syndrome include female sex, increasing age, and obesity.[2] The most common medical cause of the condition is nonspecific flexor tenosynovitis in the wrist, and probably the next most common is an old Colles' fracture. Other medical conditions found in association with the disorder are diabetes, pregnancy, rheumatoid arthritis, hypothyroidism, amyloidosis, and acromegaly.[1] Whether some cases of carpal tunnel syndrome are occupationally related is controversial; often when this is thought to be the case, associated medical conditions are a more likely explanation.[2]

The diagnosis of carpal tunnel syndrome is often difficult. Many patients with typical symptoms of numbness, tingling, and weakness have normal electrophysiological tests, and conversely many individuals with electrophysiological evidence of median nerve mononeuropathy have no symptoms. To depress frustrated family physicians even more, trusted physical signs such as the Phalen and Tinel tests have poor sensitivity and specificity. Some clinicians base the diagnosis on history and physical findings alone, whereas others put considerable weight on nerve conduction velocity assessments.[3]

First-line medical treatment of carpal tunnel syndrome consists of avoiding activities and wrist positions that aggravate the condition, wearing wrist splints, and, in the opinion of many authorities, taking NSAIDs. The pressure in the carpal tunnel is lowest with the wrist in the neutral position (not the position of function), and pressure is increased not only by flexion and extension of the wrist, but also by holding objects, making a fist, and flexing the fingers against resistance. One minute of hand and wrist exercises (alternate flexion and extension of wrist and fingers 30 times in 1 minute) lowers the pressure and should be done every hour.[4] Splints that hold the wrist in the neutral position are particularly effective if worn at night.[1,5] Up to one fourth of patients treated with simple measures such as this have complete resolution of symptoms. In only one third of patients does serious weakness or thenar atrophy develop.[6]

The role of steroid injections into the carpal tunnel is controversial. The two main reasons for this are the risk of damaging the median nerve[7] and the fact that although short-term improvement is common, long-term remissions are less frequent.[1,8,9] For example, in one British study of such injections, short-term clinical improvement was recorded in half the patients but long-term improvement in only one fourth.[8] In contrast, a Dutch randomized controlled trial found that a single corticosteroid injection 4 cm proximal to the wrist creases resulted in improvement that was sustained for at least 1 year in half the patients. (Injection proximal to the carpal tunnel was considered safer than injection into the carpal tunnel and was also thought to be more beneficial, since swelling of the forearm proximal to the tunnel may

account for symptoms in some patients.[10]) Surgery is more likely to be required if the patient is over 50 years of age, has had the disease longer than 10 months, and has constant paresthesias.[1]

A prospective randomized double-blind comparison of a 4-week course of diuretics, NSAIDs, or oral corticosteroids for patients with mild to moderate carpal tunnel syndrome showed symptom improvement at 4 weeks in the corticosteroid groups and no improvement in the other groups. The corticosteroid group was treated with prednisolone 20 mg/day for the first 2 weeks and 10 mg/day for the second 2 weeks. How long the improvement persisted after discontinuation of the steroids is unknown.[9]

⊿ REFERENCES ⊾

1. Dawson DM: Entrapment neuropathies of the upper extremities, *N Engl J Med* 329:2013-2018, 1993.
2. Atcheson SG, Ward JR, Lowe W: Concurrent medical disease in work-related carpal tunnel syndrome, *Arch Intern Med* 158:1506-1512, 1998.
3. Franzblau A, Werner RA: What is carpal tunnel syndrome? (editorial), *JAMA* 282:186-187, 1999.
4. Seradge H, Jia YC, Owens W: In vivo measurement of carpal tunnel pressure in the functioning hand, *J Hand Surg* 20:855-859, 1995.
5. Weiss ND, Gordon L, Bloom T, et al: Position of the wrist associated with the lowest carpal-tunnel pressure—implications for splint design, *J Bone Joint Surg* 77A:1695-1699, 1995.
6. Yocum D: The many faces of carpal tunnel syndrome (editorial), *Arch Intern Med* 158:1496, 1998.
7. Kasten SJ, Louis DS: Carpal tunnel syndrome: a case of median nerve injection injury and a safe and effective method for injecting the carpal tunnel, *J Fam Pract* 43:79-82, 1996.
8. Irwin LR, Beckett R, Suman RK: Steroid injection for carpal tunnel syndrome, *J Hand Surg (Br)* 21:355-357, 1996.
9. Chang M-H, Chiang H-T, Lee SS, et al: Oral drug of choice in carpal tunnel syndrome, *Neurology* 51:390-393, 1998.
10. Dammers JW, Veering MM, Vermeulen M: Injection with methylprednisolone proximal to the carpal tunnel: randomised double blind trial, *BMJ* 319:884-886, 1999.

Guillain-Barré Syndrome

Guillain-Barré syndrome has traditionally been considered an immune-related inflammatory demyelinating polyneuropathy. However, many patients also have axonal degeneration. Symptoms of motor weakness (and often paresthesias) come on rapidly, and about one third of patients require treatment in an intensive care unit. The mortality rate is about 3%, maximum neurological deficits occur at 2 to 4 weeks, and 50% to 75% of patients recover completely within 6 to 12 months.[1,2]

In two thirds of cases a respiratory or gastrointestinal infection precedes the disease by 1 or 2 weeks.[1,2] A common precipitant of the syndrome is *Campylobacter jejuni* infection. In these situations patients often have axonal degeneration and recovery is slow, leaving residual deficits.[3]

Aside from supportive and rehabilitation care, therapeutic modalities that have been reported useful are plasma exchange and IV immune globulins with or without IV steroids.[2]

◥ REFERENCES ◤

1. Bolton CF: The changing concepts of Guillain-Barré syndrome (editorial), *N Engl J Med* 333:1415-1417, 1995.
2. Dematteis JA: Guillain-Barré syndrome: a team approach to diagnosis and treatment, *Am Fam Physician* 54:197-200, 1996.
3. Rees JH, Soudain SE, Gregson NA, et al: *Campylobacter jejuni* infection and Guillain-Barré syndrome, *N Engl J Med* 333:1374-1379, 1995.

Trigeminal Neuralgia

Trigeminal neuralgia usually affects otherwise healthy middle-aged adults, although in a few cases it is associated with MS or a tumor near the nerve root. The maxillary division of the trigeminal nerve is most often affected, and trigger sites are found on the face or in the mouth. Long-term spontaneous remissions are common, especially shortly after the onset of the disorder. Initial treatment is with carbamazepine (Tegretol), starting with a low dose and increasing as necessary until pain is relieved. This regimen is successful in 75% of cases. If control is not achieved, phenytoin (Dilantin) should be tried alone or along with carbamazepine. If control is still not achieved, baclofen (Lioresal) should be added.[1]

Surgery is indicated later in the course of the disease if symptoms remain. Various procedures are used, including neurectomy of trigeminal nerve branches and injury to the trigeminal ganglion by heat (radiofrequency thermal rhizotomy), mechanical pressure (trigeminal ganglion balloon microcompression), or chemicals (retrogasserian glycerol rhizotomy).[2] A surgical procedure that appears to have an excellent outcome is microvascular decompression of the trigeminal nerve through a retromastoid craniectomy. In a high percentage of affected patients the nerve root is compressed by a vessel, and pain is often relieved immediately by the decompression surgery.[1,2]

◥ REFERENCES ◤

1. Fields HL: Treatment of trigeminal neuralgia (editorial), *N Engl J Med* 334:1125-1126, 1996.
2. Barker FG II, Jannetta PJ, Bissonette DJ, et al: The long-term outcome of microvascular decompression for trigeminal neuralgia, *N Engl J Med* 334:1077-1083, 1996.

PARKINSON'S DISEASE

(See also neuroleptics; serotonin syndrome; tremors)

In a study of 467 Boston residents over the age of 65 the prevalence of parkinsonian signs (bradykinesia, gait disturbance, rigidity, and tremor) was about 15% for ages 65 to 74, 30% for ages 75 to 84, and 52% for those over 85. The death rate in study subjects with parkinsonian signs was twice the rate of those without them.[1] Smoking appears to have a protective effect against the development of Parkinson's disease.[2] No genetic predisposition to the disease has been found for those who acquire it after 50 years of age, but when it develops at or before 50, those affected have a strong familial predisposition.[3]

The differential diagnosis of Parkinson's disease includes essential tremor, progressive supranuclear palsy (Steele-Richardson-Olszewski syndrome), neuroleptic drugs, certain antiemetics such as metoclopramide,[4] and Wilson's disease.[5] Wilson's disease should be ruled out in any young individual with parkinsonian-like symptoms (or for that matter other neurological symptoms or psychiatric symptoms associated with neurological symptoms). Investigations of such individuals include a slit-lamp examination for Kayser-Fleischer rings, liver function tests, and an assessment of plasma ceruloplasmin levels, which are usually less than 200 mg/L (20 mg/dl) in patients who have the disease.[5]

The major pathophysiological defect in Parkinson's disease is a deficit of dopamine in the substantia nigra and other basal ganglia. Levodopa is used in therapy because dopamine does not cross the blood-brain barrier whereas levodopa does. In the body, levodopa is converted to dopamine by the enzyme aromatic-L-amino-acid decarboxylase. Dopamine is desirable in the central nervous system, but because of its side effects, it is undesirable elsewhere in the body. For this reason, levodopa is combined with inhibitors of aromatic-L-amino-acid decarboxylase that do not cross the blood-brain barrier (carbidopa in Sinemet and benserazide in Prolopa). The maximum required daily dose of carbidopa is 200 to 300 mg. Thus if a patient requires large doses of Sinemet, the 100/10 formulation should be given instead of the usual 100/25 form. The same principle applies for benserazide if Prolopa is used.

In North America a levodopa formulation (Sinemet, Prolopa) is usually the initial agent chosen for early Parkinson's disease, although accumulating evidence favors initiating therapy with dopamine agonists (see later discussion). Doses of levodopa should be small initially and increased gradually as required for symptom control. Nausea can be mitigated by giving the drug with meals or in some cases by giving domperidone (Motilium) 10 to 20 mg 30 to 60 minutes before each dose. This may be necessary only when the patient begins taking the drug.[6]

Levodopa/carbidopa (Sinemet) comes in both regular and controlled release formulations. As the disease progresses, the duration of symptom relief from each dose of the regular formulation wanes ("wearing off" effect). One therapeutic approach is to give more frequent doses of standard levodopa. Another is to add an agent that promotes gastric motility, such as cisapride (Propulsid). Alternatives are to switch to controlled release formulations of levodopa, to add a small dose of a dopaminergic agonist such as bromocriptine (Parlodel) or pergolide (Permax), or to add drugs that inhibit the metabolism of dopamine such as tolcapone (Tasmar)[7] or entacapone (Comtan).

Once a patient is taking 600 mg of levodopa a day, adding a dopamine agonist such as bromocriptine is generally recommended rather than just continuing to increase the dose of levodopa.[8] Some neurologists advocate adding dopamine agonists even earlier in the disease to reduce the levels of levodopa required and therefore produce more steady benefits and a lower incidence of levodopa-induced dyskinesias.[6] Initiating the treatment with drugs other than levodopa might lead to even better long-term control and fewer adverse effects such as levodopa-induced dyskinesias.[9] This approach may be facilitated by the Food and Drug Administration's approval in 1997 of two dopamine agonists, ropinirole (ReQuip) and pramipexole (Mirapex), for use as initial therapy for Parkinson's disease or as add-on therapy to levodopa. Early trials indicate that they are effective in both roles.[10] A 3-year randomized double-blind trial comparing bromocriptine to ropinirole as initial treatment in patients with early Parkinson's disease reported good control with both agents but better functional status in the group taking ropinirole.[11]

Patients who are on a stable regimen of carbidopa/levodopa and who are also taking a dopamine agonist may benefit from a switch to a different agonist if their condition begins to deteriorate. Such as change should be made by rapid titration, which is done by discontinuing the agonist the patient was taking on one day and giving the equivalent therapeutic dose of the new agonist the next day. Slow titration leads to clinical deterioration and the risk of serious injuries from falls.[12]

Apomorphine, which is a dopaminergic drug, may benefit selected patients with advanced Parkinson's disease who have fluctuating responses to levodopa with marked on-off oscillations or who have dyskinesias. The drug must be given by frequent subcutaneous injections or by continuous subcutaneous infusions, and its use must be preceded by domperidone administration for 3 days to prevent nausea, vomiting, and hypotension.[13]

Although selegiline (Deprenyl) was originally thought to be neuroprotective, this does not appear to be the case; the drug's benefit arises solely from its ability to control symptoms in mild cases. Like selegiline, amantadine (Symmetrel) may control symptoms in mild cases.[7]

Dyskinesias are a common complication of prolonged levodopa therapy. They are usually choreiform but may be dystonic or myoclonic; some amelioration comes about with lowering the dose of levodopa, but this may aggravate the parkinsonian symptoms.[14] A small double-blind placebo-controlled study of patients with advanced Parkinson's disease who were taking levodopa found that amantadine significantly decreased the frequency of dyskinesias as well the degree of motor fluctuations.[15] In some patients with dyskinesias, apomorphine may be helpful.[13]

Pallidotomy, a stereotactic neurosurgical operation that destroys a portion of the globus pallidus, usually controls dyskinesias on the contralateral side and to a lesser extent on the ipsilateral side, but surgical morbidity is high.[16] In a small number of patients with advanced Parkinson's disease, electrical stimulation of the subthalamic nuclei through electrodes implanted under stereoscopic guidance decreased the "off" periods and dyskinesias and permitted a lower dosage of levodopa.[17]

Anticholinergics such as trihexyphenidyl (Artane) or benztropine mesylate (Cogentin) may decrease tremor but are seldom useful for rigidity or bradykinesia. These drugs may cause confusion and should be avoided or used with caution.

Drugs used for the treatment of Parkinson's disease are listed in Table 21. The usual regimen is a low beginning dose followed by a gradual buildup of whatever drug or drugs are chosen. Before treatment begins, the practitioner should ensure that drugs such as metoclopramide (Maxeran) or a neuroleptic are not the cause of the clinical syndrome.

Table 21   Drugs for Parkinson's Disease

Drug	Usual dose
Dopamine Precursors	
Levodopa/carbidopa (Sinemet)	100/25 tid-qid; maximum 1000 mg of levodopa per day; controlled-release formulations have about 70% the bioavailability of regular tablets
Levodopa/benserazide (Prolopa)	100/25 tid-qid; maximum 1000 mg levodopa per day
Catechol-*O*-Methyltransferase Inhibitors	
Entacapone (Comtan)	200 mg with each dose of levodopa/carbidopa
Tolcapone (Tasmar)	100-200 mg tid
Dopamine Agonists	
Apomorphine	Variable—subcutaneous injections
Bromocriptine (Parlodel)	1.25-40 mg/day in 2-3 divided doses
Pergolide mesylate (Permax)	0.05-3 mg/day in 3 divided doses
Pramipexole (Mirapex)	0.125-1.5 mg tid
Ropinirole (Requip)	0.25-3 mg tid; maximum 8 mg/day
Dopaminergic Agents	
Amantadine (Symmetrel)	100 mg bid-tid
Selective Monoamine Oxidase Inhibitor Drugs (Type B)	
Selegiline or L-deprenyl (Eldepryl)	5 mg bid with breakfast and lunch
Anticholinergic Agents	
Trihexyphenidyl (Artane)	1-3 mg tid
Benztropine mesylate (Cogentin)	1-4 mg/day as a single or 2 divided doses
Antiemetics	
Domperidone (Motilium)	10-20 mg 30-60 min before medications causing nausea

The ability to drive a motor vehicle is often seriously impaired even in patients with mild Parkinson's disease. Accurate assessment of this problem is impossible in the usual office setting; formal psychological and psychomotor testing or driving tests are necessary to detect significant driving deficits.[18]

―――――― ◣ **REFERENCES** ◢ ――――――

1. Bennett DA, Beckett LA, Murray AM, et al: Prevalence of Parkinsonian signs and associated mortality in a community population of older people, *N Engl J Med* 334:71-76, 1996.
2. Gorell JM, Rybicki BA, Cole C, et al: Smoking and Parkinson's disease: a dose-response relationship, *Neurology* 52:115-119, 1999.
3. Tanner CM, Ottman R, Goldman SM, et al: Parkinson disease in twins: an etiologic study, *JAMA* 281:341-346, 1999.
4. Avorn J, Gurwitz JH, Bohn RL, et al: Increased incidence of levodopa therapy following metoclopramide use, *JAMA* 274:1780-1782, 1995.
5. Walshe JM, Yealland M: Wilson's disease: the problem of delayed diagnosis, *J Neurol Neurosurg Psychiatry* 55:692-696, 1992.
6. Kishore A, Snow BJ: Drug management of Parkinson's disease, *Can Fam Physician* 42:946-952, 1996.
7. Lang AE, Lozano AM: Parkinson's disease (second of two parts), *N Engl J Med* 339:1130-1143, 1998.
8. Calne DB: Treatment of Parkinson's disease, *N Engl J Med* 329:1021-1028, 1993.
9. Barone P, Bravi D, Bermejo-Pareja F, et al (Pergolide Monotherapy Study Group): Pergolide monotherapy in the treatment of early PD: a randomized controlled study, *Neurology* 53:573-579, 1999.
10. Pramipexole and ropinirole for Parkinson's disease, *Med Lett* 39:109-110, 1997.
11. Korcyn AD, Brunt ER, Larsen JP, et al: A 3-year randomized trial of ropinirole and bromocriptine in early Parkinson's disease, *Neurology* 53:364-370, 1999.
12. Goetz CG, Blasucci L, Stebbins GT: Switching dopamine agonists in advanced Parkinson's disease: is rapid titration preferable to slow? *Neurology* 52:1227-1229, 1999.
13. Chaudhuri KR, Clough C: Subcutaneous apomorphine in Parkinson's disease: effective yet under used (editorial), *BMJ* 316:641, 1998.
14. Olanow CW: A 61-year-old man with Parkinson's disease, *JAMA* 275:716-722, 1996.
15. Metman LV, Del Dotto P, van den Munckhof P, et al: Amantadine as treatment for dyskinesias and motor fluctuations in Parkinson's disease, *Neurology* 50:1323-1326, 1998.
16. Schrag A, Samuel M, Caputo E, et al: Unilateral pallidotomy for Parkinson's disease: results after more than 1 year, *J Neurol Neurosurg Psychiatry* 67:511-517, 1999.
17. Limousin P, Krack P, Pollak P, et al: Electrical stimulation of the subthalamic nucleus in advanced Parkinson's disease, *N Engl J Med* 339:1105-1111, 1998.
18. Heikkila V-M, Turkka J, Korpelainen J, et al: Decreased driving ability in people with Parkinson's disease, *J Neurol Neurosurg Psychiatry* 64:325-330, 1998.

RESTLESS LEGS SYNDROME
(See also insomnia)

Patients with the restless legs syndrome complain of a sensation of formications or other paresthesias often described as an aching, cramping, or crawling sensation deep in the legs, usually the calves. These occur at rest, usually at night, and are relieved by moving or walking. Associated symptoms include periodic movements during sleep (bed partners may complain of being kicked) and myoclonic jerks when awake. Insomnia is a common symptom and often the initial one, and in many cases the underlying restless legs syndrome is not diagnosed. The disorder is intermittent and may have prolonged remissions. An estimated 5% of the general population is affected, and there is sometimes a family history. The incidence of the disorder is higher in patients with iron deficiency anemia (25%) or receiving dialysis (30% to 40%). Other reported associated conditions are pregnancy, diabetes mellitus, polyneuropathy, and rheumatoid arthritis.[1,2]

The pathogenesis of the restless legs syndrome is uncertain, but alterations in dopamine functioning appear to be important. For this reason the first line of treatment has often been levodopa/carbidopa (Sinemet) or dopamine agonists such as bromocriptine (Parlodel), pergolide (Permax),[3] or more recently pramipexole (Mirapex).[4] The development of tolerance is a major problem with levodopa and bromocriptine, and sometimes a rebound daytime augmentation of symptoms occurs, which may be related to the short half-life of these drugs. Switching to longer acting drugs such as pergolide and pramipexole may resolve the problem.[4] Preliminary reports indicate that the antiepileptic drug gabapentin (Neurontin) is effective.[5] Benzodiazepines such as clonazepam (Rivotril) and opioids have long been known to suppress symptoms,[1,2,4] but because they are addictive, they should rarely if ever be used.

When prescribing medications for this condition, practitioners should start with low doses and increase them gradually. The usual dose of Sinemet 100/25 is ½ to 2 tablets hs, repeated during the night prn; that of bromocriptine is 1.25 to 7.5 mg hs; and that of pramipexole is 0.125 to 0.5 mg 2 hours before bedtime.

―――――― ◣ **REFERENCES** ◢ ――――――

1. Feigen A: Restless leg syndrome, *JAMA* 274:1191-1192, 1995.
2. O'Keeffe ST: Restless legs syndrome: a review, *Arch Intern Med* 156:243-248, 1996.
3. Wetter TC, Stiasny K, Winkelmann J, et al: A randomized controlled study of pergolide in patients with restless legs syndrome, *Neurology* 52:944-950, 1999.
4. Montplaisir J, Nicolas A, Devesle R, et al: Restless legs syndrome improved by pramipexole: a double-blind randomized trial, *Neurology* 52:938-943, 1999.
5. Adler CH: Treatment of restless legs syndrome with gabapentin, *Clin Neuropharmacol* 20:148-151, 1997.

SEIZURES

(See also alcoholism; anticonvulsants in pregnancy; bipolar disorder; concussion; febrile seizures; motor vehicle accidents; syncope; transient global anemia)

Seizures are classified as follows[1]:

1. Partial seizures (focal seizures). Partial seizures begin in one part of a cerebral hemisphere and may or may not become generalized. In simple partial seizures, consciousness is preserved and manifestations may include motor, somatosensory or special sensory, autonomic, or psychic symptoms. Complex partial seizures (temporal lobe seizures, psychomotor seizures) may start as a simple partial seizure that is followed by impaired consciousness, or consciousness may be impaired from the onset.
2. Generalized-onset seizures. Generalized-onset seizures have involvement of both cerebral hemispheres from the beginning. They are subcategorized as tonic-clonic (grand mal), absence (petit mal), atypical absence, myoclonic, tonic, and atonic.

The type of seizure may be determined if a reliable observer provides an accurate description of its course, but in other cases the diagnosis depends on video monitoring combined with electroencephalographic recordings (often repeated and sometimes recorded while the patient is hyperventilating or subject to photic stimulation).[1]

Recognized precipitating factors for seizures include alcohol and drug abuse, medications (e.g., neuroleptics, tricyclics), neoplasms, neurocysticercosis, previous head injury, and previous cerebrovascular accident.

The major causes of spontaneous loss of consciousness are seizures, pseudoseizures (conversion reactions), and syncope. Multifocal and generalized myoclonic jerks are commonly seen in syncope.[2] One study found that tongue biting (lacerations observed by a physician) had a sensitivity of 24% and a specificity of 99% for epilepsy. Lateral tongue biting was 100% specific for tonic-clonic seizures.[3]

Brief convulsive episodes immediately following head injury with rapid recovery are usually called posttraumatic seizures. However, the prognosis is excellent and they are probably not true epileptic reactions.[2]

About one third of patients with a single unprovoked seizure have recurrences, whereas three fourths of those with two or three unprovoked seizures have recurrences.[4] Recurrence is more likely if the patient had a previous serious central nervous system injury or has a family history of seizures, if the seizure was of the complex partial type, or if the EEG is abnormal.[5-7] In a study of 407 New York children with unprovoked seizures followed for a mean of 6.3 years, the overall recurrence rate by 8 years was 44%. Of the recurrences, 53% occurred within 6 months and 88% within 2 years. The best prognosis was among children who had seizures while they were awake and who had normal EEGs. Status epilepticus at the time of the initial seizure, having more than one seizure within 24 hours of the initial seizure,

or a past history of febrile seizures did not increase the risk of recurrences.[7]

A long-term prospective Finnish study found that two thirds of individuals who had had epilepsy (two or more seizures) in childhood were seizure free as adults, and of these, three fourths were not taking medication. However, many had diminished social functioning in interpersonal relations and at work. The mortality rate was increased in those whose seizures did not remit.[8]

Whether all patients who have had an unprovoked seizure require therapy is controversial. Treatment is known to decrease the frequency of recurrent seizures.[9-11] For example, in an Israeli study of adults between the ages of 18 and 50 with the new onset of a single unprovoked generalized tonic-clonic seizure, 45 patients were treated with carbamazepine (Tegretol) and 42 were given no antiseizure medications. At the end of 3 years 71% of the untreated patients had recurrent seizures compared with 22% of the treated patients.[11] However, treatment does not alter the long-term prognosis,[12,13] and therefore, if the risk of recurrence is low, the adverse effects of treatment may outweigh the benefits.[9] For low-risk children, withholding treatment may be acceptable in many cases because a single recurrent seizure may not have major adverse social or vocational implications. However, for many adults such an event may be perceived as catastrophic, and such patients may well choose therapy even if they are also at low risk.[14]

The usual recommendation for treatment of seizures with medications is to begin with a single drug, since 70% to 80% of patients treated with medications respond to such a regimen. If adequate control is not achieved with full therapeutic doses of a single drug in a compliant patient, a second drug is added. Doses are initially low and are increased gradually as necessary.[5,6] Marks and Garcia[14] suggest some important modifications to such a regimen. They advise increasing the level of the initial drug until complete seizure control is attained or until persistent unacceptable side effects occur, regardless of serum drug levels. They point out that many patients require so-called toxic levels for control and that in general the term "toxic levels" refers to an increased risk of dose-related adverse effects and not life-threatening situations. If a patient has further seizures once the maximum tolerated dose of a drug is achieved, a second drug should be added. As the dose of the second drug is increased to the maximum tolerated level, the dose of the initial drug is decreased and eventually discontinued so that the patient is once again receiving monotherapy.

Carbamazepine (Tegretol), phenytoin (Dilantin), and valproate (Depakene, Depakote, Epival) are considered by many to be the first-line drugs for both partial seizures and generalized tonic-clonic seizures.[5] Sustained release variants of carbamazepine (Tegretol-XR, Carbatrol) increase seizure control and decrease adverse effects.[15] Valproate is the preferred drug for myoclonic and atonic-type seizures, whereas absence seizures should be treated with ethosuximide (Zarontin) or valproate.[5,6] Since long-term use of phenytoin is associated with facial coarsening, gingival hyperplasia, and hirsutism, it may not appeal to everyone.[14]

A number of new antiepileptic drugs have been approved by the FDA as add-on treatments for patients with treatment-resistant partial or secondary generalized seizures (Table 22).[14,15] Many of these drugs have been shown in clinical trials to be effective as monotherapy for refractory partial seizures.[15] Felbamate (Felbatol) has been associated with hepatic failure and aplastic anemia, and its use is restricted to patients unresponsive to other therapies.[14,15]

A novel nonpharmacological treatment of refractory partial epilepsy is an implanted vagus nerve stimulator that is attached to the vagus nerve in the carotid sheath. The patient activates the device at the beginning of an aura or seizure. Its mechanism of action is unknown.[15]

When serum levels of antiepileptic drugs are drawn to determine whether therapeutic levels have been achieved, they should be obtained only after steady-state conditions have been reached. For phenytoin this is 6 days after starting or changing the dose, for carbamazepine and valproic acid it is 3 days, and for phenobarbital it is 20 days. Except for phenobarbital, which has an extremely long half-life, trough levels should be obtained. Immediate serum levels are indicated within 6 hours of a seizure or when toxicity or noncompliance is suspected.[16] In some patients seizures are controlled with subtherapeutic levels,[6] whereas others require "toxic" levels (see earlier discussion).[14]

After a period of good control, patients with epilepsy may be able to stop their medications. A variety of studies suggest that after 2 years of treatment without seizures, a little over two thirds of patients remain seizure free after stopping medications. This does not necessarily mean that 2 years of treatment improves the natural history of the disease; rather,

it may be a method of selecting patients who are most likely to remain seizure free with or without medications. Some factors that predict a higher risk of relapse in children who discontinue medications include partial epilepsy, older age at onset, and an epileptiform EEG while receiving medications. Since relapses in children are not harmful, discontinuing medications after 6 to 12 months may be safe for many, especially those at low risk of recurrence. Medications can be restarted if seizures recur.[17]

⚓ REFERENCES ⚓

1. Veilleux M: The keys to seizure management, *Can J CME* 11:113-123, 1999.
2. Sander JW, O'Donoghue MF: Epilepsy: getting the diagnosis right; all that convulses is not epilepsy (editorial), *BMJ* 314:158-159, 1997.
3. Benbadis SR, Wolgamuth BR, Goren H, et al: Value of tongue biting in the diagnosis of seizures, *Arch Intern Med* 155:2346-2349, 1995.
4. Hauser WA, Rich SS, Lee JR-J, et al: Risk of recurrent seizures after two unprovoked seizures, *N Engl J Med* 338:429-434, 1998.
5. Drugs for epilepsy, *Med Lett* 37:37-40, 1995.
6. Brodie MJ, Dichter MA: Antiepileptic drugs, *N Engl J Med* 334:168-175, 1996.
7. Shinnar S, Berg AT, Moshe SL, et al: The risk of seizure recurrence after a first unprovoked afebrile seizure in childhood—an extended follow-up, *Pediatrics* 98:216-225, 1996.
8. Sillanpää M, Jalava M, Kaleva O, et al: Long-term prognosis of seizures with onset in childhood, *N Engl J Med* 338:1715-1722, 1998.
9. Camfield P, Camfield C, Dooley J, et al: A randomized study of carbamazepine versus no medication following a first unprovoked seizure in childhood, *Neurology* 39:851-852, 1989.
10. First Seizure Trial Group: Randomized clinical trial on the efficacy of antiepileptic drugs in reducing the risk of relapse after a first unprovoked tonic-clonic seizure, *Neurology* 43:478-483, 1993.
11. Gilad R, Lampl Y, Gabbay U, et al: Early treatment of a single generalized tonic-clonic seizure to prevent recurrence, *Arch Neurol* 53:1149-1152, 1996.
12. Musicco M, Beghi E, Solari A (First Seizure Trial Group): Effect of antiepileptic treatment initiated after the first unprovoked seizure on the long-term prognosis of epilepsy, *Neurology* 44(suppl 2):A337-A338, 1994.
13. Shinnar S, Berg AT: Does antiepileptic drug therapy alter the prognosis of childhood seizures and prevent the development of chronic epilepsy? *Semin Pediatr Neurol* 1:111-117, 1994.
14. Marks WJ, Garcia PA: Management of seizures and epilepsy, *Am Fam Physician* 57:1589-1600, 1998.
15. Herman ST, Pedley TA: New options for the treatment of epilepsy, *JAMA* 280:693-694, 1998.
16. Schoenenberger RA, Tanasijevic MJ, Jha A, et al: Appropriateness of antiepileptic drug level monitoring, *JAMA* 274:1622-1626, 1995.
17. Peters AC, Brouwer OF, Geerts AT, et al: Randomized prospective study of early discontinuation of antiepileptic drugs in children with epilepsy, *Neurology* 50:724-730, 1998.

Table 22   Antiepileptic Drugs

Generic name	Trade name
Standard Drugs	
Carbamazepine	Tegretol
Ethosuximide	Zarontin
Phenobarbital	
Phenytoin	Dilantin
Primidone	Mysoline
Valproate (valproic acid, divalproex)	Depakene (valproic acid); Depakote, Epival (divalproex)
New Add-on Drugs	
Clobazam	Frisium
Felbamate	Felbatol
Gabapentin	Neurontin
Lamotrigine	Lamictal
Tiagabine	Gabitril
Topiramate	Topamax
Vigabatrin	Sabril

SPASTICITY

Three of the drugs used to decrease spasticity in patients with upper motor neuron disease, especially those with spinal cord transections and multiple sclerosis, are baclofen (Lioresal), dantrolene (Dantrium), and tizanidine (Zanaflex). The dosage should be low initially and increased gradually to the usual maintenance dosage, which for baclofen is 40 to 80 mg/day in 3 or 4 divided doses, for dantrolene 25 to 100 mg qid, and for tizanidine 12 to 36 mg tid. Dantrolene is less effective than baclofen or tizanidine.[1]

REFERENCES

1. Tizanidine for spasticity, *Med Lett* 39:62-63, 1997.

SUBARACHNOID HEMORRHAGE
(See also cerebrovascular accidents; prevention; screening)

Subarachnoid hemorrhage is a relatively common neurological condition with a greater prevalence rate than that of primary brain tumors or multiple sclerosis. Risk factors are personal history of a previous intracerebral aneurysm; family history of aneurysm; smoking; hypertension; excessive alcohol intake, particularly binge drinking; and certain heritable connective tissue disorders such as autosomal dominant polycystic kidney disease, Ehlers-Danlos syndrome, and Marfan's syndrome.[1]

The characteristic symptom of a subarachnoid hemorrhage is the sudden onset of severe headache. In some patients severe lower back pain with bilateral radicular pain develops as a result of the irritating properties of blood that has descended into the subarachnoid space surrounding the lower spinal cord. Between one third and one half of patients in whom a significant subarachnoid hemorrhage is found have had an unusual headache in the preceding days or weeks that was caused by a "warning leak"; physicians usually miss the significance of these. Classic physical findings are meningismus and subhyaloid fundal hemorrhages, with the latter found in about a quarter of the patients. CT scans without contrast medium identify 90% to 95% of patients with subarachnoid hemorrhages if obtained within 24 hours, but because blood is rapidly absorbed, the sensitivity of CT detection drops to 80% at 3 days and 70% at 5 days. MRI is not a sensitive way of diagnosing an acute subarachnoid hemorrhage but is a good technique for detecting intracranial aneurysms.[1] The mortality rate associated with subarachnoid hemorrhage is 50%.[2]

Magnetic resonance angiography screening for aneurysms in first-degree relatives of patients who have had a subarachnoid hemorrhage probably does more harm than good.[1,2] The lifetime risk of hemorrhage for someone with only one first-degree relative who has had a subarachnoid hemorrhage is 1% by the age of 50 and 2% by the age of 70.[1] A study from the Netherlands screened 626 first-degree relatives of 160 patients who had had a subarachnoid hemorrhage. Twenty-five relatives (4%) were found to have an-

eurysms, but in only 18 were the lesions suitable for surgical intervention. More than half of those who underwent surgery suffered some degree of permanent neurological deficit. The authors calculated that 149 relatives would have to be screened to prevent one lifetime subarachnoid hemorrhage and 298 would have to be screened to prevent one fatal subarachnoid hemorrhage.[2]

When more than one first-degree relative has had a subarachnoid hemorrhage (familial intracranial aneurysms), about 8% of the remaining first-degree relatives will have aneurysms; whether screening this high-risk population is beneficial is unknown[2] but seems unlikely.[3]

Morbidity and mortality from surgical clipping of aneurysms are considerable, ranging from about 6.5% in those under age 45 to 32% in those 65 or over.[4] An alternative management protocol is endovascular coil embolization (coiling) in which a neurointerventional radiologist inserts a number of detachable platinum coils into the aneurysm via a femoral artery catheter. Long-term outcomes of this technique have not been determined, but short-term benefits and complication rates are as good as or better than those with surgical clipping.[5]

REFERENCES

1. Schievink WI: Intracranial aneurysms, *N Engl J Med* 336:28-40, 1997.
2. Magnetic Resonance Angiography in Relatives of Patients with Subarachnoid Hemorrhage Study Group: Risks and benefits of screening for intracranial aneurysms in first-degree relatives of patients with sporadic subarachnoid hemorrhage, *N Engl J Med* 341:1344-1350, 1999.
3. Kirkpatrick PJ, McConnell RS: Screening for familial intracranial aneurysms: no justification exists for routine screening (editorial), *BMJ* 319:1512-1513, 1999.
4. International Study of Unruptured Intracranial Aneurysms Investigators: Unruptured intracranial aneurysms—risk of rupture and risks of surgical intervention, *N Engl J Med* 339:1725-1733, 1998.
5. Johnston SC, Dudley A, Gress DR, et al: Surgical and endovascular treatment of unruptured cerebral aneurysms at university hospitals, *Neurology* 52:1799-1805, 1999.

SYNCOPE
(See also seizures)

A number of elderly patients have a significant drop in blood pressure within 45 to 60 minutes after a meal. In one study of nursing home residents with a mean age of 80, 24% had a systolic pressure reduction of more than 20 mm Hg during the postprandial period. Those with a history of falls or syncope in the previous 6 months had a greater mean blood pressure loss than did patients without such a history.[1]

Mass fainting at rock concerts is common, especially in girls between 11 and 17 years of age. The cause seems to be a combination of fatigue, a long period of fasting (from standing in line for hours), compression by crowds, and hyperventilation as part of a panic attack.[2]

REFERENCES

1. Aronow WS, Ahn C: Postprandial hypotension in 499 elderly persons in a long-term health care facility, *J Am Geriatr Soc* 42:930-932, 1994.
2. Lempert T, Bauer M: Mass fainting at rock concerts (letter), *N Engl J Med* 332:1721, 1995.

TOURETTE'S SYNDROME
(See also attention deficit disorder; obsessive-compulsive disorder; sleepwalking)

Tics are repetitive stereotypical motor movements. Simple tics include shoulder jerking, eye blinking, picking movements of hands, sniffing, grunting, and animal sounds such as barking. Complex tics include flapping of arms, facial grimaces, kissing self or others, repeating words, and obscene language.[1]

Tics may be primary or secondary to some other disorder such as Huntington's chorea, Wilson's disease, Creutzfeldt-Jakob disease, or autism. Primary tics are classified as transient (lasting less than 1 year) or chronic. Tourette's syndrome is the most common form of chronic tic disorder.[1]

Tourette's syndrome usually begins as simple motor tics in young school-aged children. Boys are affected nine times as often as girls. Symptoms wax and wane but tend to peak between 9 and 11 years of age. One type of tic is commonly replaced by another. Patients with Tourette's syndrome can often voluntarily suppress tics for hours at a time when at work or school, but the tics tend to return in a rush once the affected person gets home. By adulthood 85% of patients are in remission or have markedly improved.[1] No correlation has been found between the severity of tics at the time of diagnosis and the ultimate outcome.[2] Coprolalia (the utterance of scatological terms) is rare.[1]

About half the patients with Tourette's syndrome also meet the diagnostic criteria for attention deficit/hyperactivity disorder (ADHD). One fourth to one third have obsessive-compulsive disorder or learning disabilities.[1]

Careful education of parents and teachers about the nature and natural history of Tourette's syndrome is essential and often allows the condition to be managed without pharmacological agents. Behavioral treatment that focuses on improving academic and social skills is recommended for all patients. An experienced physician may attempt to deal directly with Tourette symptoms, although this sometimes leads to a paradoxical exacerbation. Drugs that can be used to control symptoms are clonidine 0.05 mg bid to 1 mg qid; guanfacine (Tenex) 0.5 to 1.5 mg bid for children over age 12; haloperidol (Haldol); pimozide (Orap); and risperidone (Risperdal). For many patients the agents of first choice are clonidine or guanfacine. These medications have moderate efficacy in controlling tics and are often beneficial for comorbid conditions such as ADHD.[1]

REFERENCES

1. Bagheri M, Kerbeshian J, Burd L: Recognition and management of Tourette's syndrome and tic disorders, *Am Fam Physician* 59:2263-2272, 1999.
2. Leckman JF, Zhang H, Vitale A, et al: Course of tic severity in Tourette syndrome: the first two decades, *Pediatrics* 102:14-19, 1998.

TRANSIENT GLOBAL AMNESIA
(See also seizures; transient ischemic attacks)

Transient global amnesia is a strange syndrome in which patients, who are usually over the age of 50, experience a period of anterograde amnesia (inability to form new memories) lasting 1 to 8 hours. Patients tend to ask repetitive questions during the attack. They may be disoriented in terms of place and time, but otherwise cognition is unimpaired. No other neurological symptoms or signs are present. Patients may have some retrograde amnesia, but within a short time this decreases so that only amnesia for the attack itself persists. The cause of transient global amnesia is unknown. It is not a seizure or a TIA, and the prognosis is excellent. Within 5 years 3% to 20% of patients have a recurrence, and those with repetitive attacks are at a slightly increased risk for a seizure disorder. There is no increased risk of cerebrovascular accidents.[1]

If patients have no history of head trauma or previous neurological disorders, if a reliable witness is present who can describe the attack, and if a thorough history and physical examination fail to show evidence of other disorders, no investigation is required.[1]

REFERENCES

1. Brown J: Evaluation of transient global amnesia, *Ann Emerg Med* 30:522-526, 1997.

TREMORS
(See also Parkinson's disease)

Drugs that have proved effective for the treatment of essential tremor are beta-blockers such as propranolol (Inderal), metoprolol (Lopressor), and nadolol (Corgard) and the anticonvulsant primidone (Mysoline). The dosage range for propranolol is 80 to 320 mg/day and that for primidone 25 to 750 mg/day. Beta-blockers and primidone are equally effective; if one does not work, the other should be tried.[1] A preliminary placebo-controlled trial found that gabapentin (Neurontin) 400 mg tid was as effective as propranolol 40 mg tid.[2] Pharmacotherapy is more effective for hand and finger tremors than for head and voice tremors.[1]

REFERENCES

1. Charles PD, Esper GJ, Davis TL, et al: Classification of tremor and update on treatment, *Am Fam Physician* 59:1565-1572, 1999.
2. Gironell A, Kulisevsky J, Barbanoj M, et al: A randomized placebo-controlled comparative trial of gabapentin and propranolol in essential tremor, *Arch Neurol* 56:475-480, 1999.

COMMUNITY HEALTH

Topics covered in this section

PERIODIC HEALTH EXAMINATION

(See also attitudes, physician; evidence-based medicine; prevention; screening)

Three organizations in the forefront of making recommendations about the periodic health examination are the Canadian Task Force on Preventive Health Care,[1] the U.S. Preventive Services Task Force,[2] and the American College of Physicians.[3]

Evidence for the inclusion or exclusion of interventions from the periodic health examination as determined by the Canadian Task Force on Preventive Health Care and the U.S. Preventive Services Task Force is classified as follows:

A. There is good evidence to include.
B. There is fair evidence to include.
C. There is poor evidence to include.
D. There is fair evidence to exclude.
E. There is good evidence to exclude.

Examples of "A" and "B" recommendations for the general population from both the Canadian Task Force on Preventive Health Care and the U.S. Preventive Services Task Force are counseling on smoking cessation, prescribing folic acid for women at risk of pregnancy, fluoridation to prevent dental caries, mammography for women 50 to 69 years of age, and age-appropriate routine immunizations. Examples of "D" and "E" recommendations are periodic chest x-ray examinations to detect lung cancer, prostate specific antigen (PSA) screening of men over 50 to detect prostate cancer, pelvic examination to detect ovarian cancer, and urine dipstick examination to detect bladder cancer. The largest category is "C," which includes such items as mammography for women 40 to 49 years of age, screening of blood or urine for type 2 diabetes, and tonometry or funduscopy to detect glaucoma.[1,2]

❧ REFERENCES ❧

1. Canadian Task Force on the Periodic Health Examination: *Clinical preventive health care*, Ottawa, 1994, Canadian Communication Group—Publishing.
2. US Preventive Services Task Force: *Guide to clinical preventive services*, ed 2, Baltimore, 1996, Williams & Wilkins.
3. Eddy DM, editor: *Common screening tests*, Philadelphia, 1991, American College of Physicians.

PRACTICE PATTERNS

(See also acromegaly; attitudes, physician; cholecystectomy; consultations; coronary artery bypass grafting; investigations; lumpectomy; myocardial infarction; prescribing habits and the elderly; prevention; prevention of strokes; radical prostatectomy)

Variations in Medical Practice

Medical practice patterns vary among geographical locations and medical specialties.

Variations in local resection for breast cancer

Local resection (breast-conserving surgery) plus radiation therapy is as effective as mastectomy for stage I and II breast cancer.[1-3] The main exceptions are multiple tumors or a tumor of such a nature, usually because of its size, that local removal would have unacceptable cosmetic results.[1] Despite this, mastectomy continues to be a widely practiced procedure. The frequency with which it is performed varies considerably from one geographical region to another,[1-3] as well as from one surgeon to another in the same region.[4] A review of nine population-based cancer registries in the United States found that by 1995, 60% of women with stage I but only 39% of women with stage II breast cancer had had local resections.[3] The rates of local resection are higher in Canada than in the United States, but they vary among provinces; one review found that in British Columbia the rate was 44%, while in Ontario it was 68%.[2] Numerous factors have been cited to explain different treatment modalities in different locations, including accessibility of radiation therapy facilities, patients' preferences, and preferences of the attending surgeons.[2,3] In general, university-affiliated surgeons perform more breast-conserving operations.[2]

Variations in invasive cardiac procedures following myocardial infarctions

An international study involving two Canadian and three U.S. centers concluded that 1 year after a myocardial infarction (MI), Canadian patients had more cardiac symptoms and worse functional status than did those in the United States. This correlated with more visits to specialists and more invasive procedures in the U.S. cohort than in the Canadian.[5] On the other hand, a 1997 report on nearly 250,000 elderly Americans and nearly 10,000 elderly Ontario residents, all of whom had suffered an initial MI, found a slightly lower 30-day mortality rate in the U.S. cohort but no differences in mortality between the two groups at 1 year. In this study the rates of interventions for the United States versus Canada were 35% versus 7% for angiography, 12% versus 2% for percutaneous transluminal coronary angioplasty, and 11% versus 1% for coronary artery bypass surgery.[6] Other studies have also failed to find a correlation between the numbers of invasive cardiac procedures performed in the management of MI and mortality rates.[7,8] Within the United States itself the rates of invasive interventions after MI vary widely.[7] An enthusiasm for diagnostic testing may be an important reason for invasive cardiac procedures; positive stress tests lead to more angiograms, which in turn lead to more revascularization procedures.[8]

Variations in medical care after myocardial infarctions

Beta-blockers are prescribed for only half of elderly U.S. patients who have had an MI and who have no contraindications to this class of drugs. The rates of prescription vary from 30% to 77%, depending on geographical region.[9] A comparison of the outcomes of post-MI patients treated by cardiologists and primary care physicians in Pennsylvania found a decreased mortality rate among those treated by cardiologists. The difference may be due to experience, since the patients of primary care physicians who treated high numbers of patients with MIs also had improved mortality rates.[10] When direct comparisons are made of outcomes for patients treated by primary care physicians versus subspecialists, patient profiles and the role of consultations are usually omitted from consideration. A study of Minnesota hospitals found that patients with acute MIs cared for by primary care physicians were generally older and frailer than those looked after by cardiologists. The study also found that quality of care was often improved when generalists consulted with cardiologists.[11]

Variations in interventions to prevent stroke

A comparison of interventions prescribed by Western European and North American neurologists for the prevention of stroke in high-risk patients found that North Americans tended to prescribe high-dose and Europeans low-dose aspirin, that North Americans were more likely than Europeans to choose ticlopidine (Ticlid) as their second-choice drug, that Europeans were much more likely to prescribe warfarin than were North Americans, and that North Americans were more likely to recommend carotid endarterectomy for asymptomatic patients than were Europeans.[12]

Variations in rates of radical prostatectomy

It has been estimated that in 1989 a white male from Seattle had a 6.4% chance of undergoing radical prostatectomy by the time he was 75, whereas the odds in Connecticut were only 1.3%.[13] This is a fivefold difference.

Causes of variability in practice patterns

A probable reason for the marked variability in practice patterns from one region to another is that the norms of the local medical milieu have a more powerful influence on the behavior of individual physicians than does the national and international medical literature or national and international meetings. According to Greer,[14] a sequence of events has to take place within a particular milieu if a controversial innovation is to be introduced. The process begins when a "local innovator" enthusiastically adopts a new technology, but this in itself is insufficient to change the institutional practice. A local "opinion leader" usually has to endorse and support the change, experts in the technology have to be available in the local community to teach its application, and finally a "consensus" that it is desirable has to develop among the local physicians. There have been few randomized controlled trials documenting the influence of local leaders in changing medical opinion. One such study found a significant increase in prescribing aspirin and beta-blockers for post-MI patients treated in hospitals where designated local opinion leaders were promoting this form of therapy.[15]

Performance Reports

Outcomes for a variety of procedures vary from center to center or physician to physician. Better results have been shown to be associated with higher annual volumes in the management of myocardial infarction[16]; in cardiac surgery[17]; in the removal of pituitary adenomas for acromegaly[18]; in cases of complex cancer surgery such as pancreatectomy,[19] liver resection,[19] pelvic exenteration,[19] esophagectomy,[19] or radical prostatectomy[20]; and in liver transplantation.[21] One consequence of this variation in results has been a movement to publish consumer guides or report cards of performance data. A comparative guide to the outcomes of coronary bypass surgery in Pennsylvania (*Consumer Guide to Coronary Artery Bypass Graft Surgery*) has been widely distributed and is available without charge to anyone who requests a copy.[22,23] A survey of cardiologists and cardiac surgeons elicited considerable concern about such guides. The most important criticism was of the guide's failure to adjust adequately for risk (high-risk patients have poorer outcomes); the survey respondents feared that this type of publication might cause surgeons to refuse to operate on high-risk patients.[22] This concern appears to be unfounded because a study from New York State, where a similar program was established, found no increase in out-of-state coronary artery bypass procedures and an increase, not a decrease, in the number of high-risk patients undergoing surgery.[24] All of this may be academic, since only 12% of patients undergoing cardiac surgery in Pennsylvania were aware that consumer guides were available and less than 1% knew the rating of their hospital or surgeons.[23]

──────────── ◄ REFERENCES ► ────────────

1. Starreveld A: A surgical subculture: the use of mastectomy to treat breast cancer (editorial), *Can Med Assoc J* 156:43-45, 1997.
2. Goel V, Olivotto I, Hislop TG, et al: Patterns of initial management of node-negative breast cancer in two Canadian provinces, *Can Med Assoc J* 156:25-35, 1997.
3. Lazovich D, Solomon CC, Thomas DB, et al: Breast conservation therapy in the United States following the 1990 National Institutes of Health Consensus Development Conference on the treatment of patients with early stage invasive breast carcinoma, *Cancer* 86:628-637, 1999.

4. Moritz S, Bates T, Henderson SM, et al: Variation in management of small invasive breast cancers detected on screening in the former South East Thames regions: observational study, *BMJ* 315:1266-1272, 1997.

5. Mark DB, Naylor CD, Phil D, et al: Use of medical resources and quality of life after acute myocardial infarction in Canada and the United States, *N Engl J Med* 331:1130-1135, 1994.

6. Tu JV, Pashos CL, Naylor D, et al: Use of cardiac procedures and outcomes in elderly patients with myocardial infarction in the United States and Canada, *N Engl J Med* 336:1500-1505, 1997.

7. Guadagnoli E, Hauptman PJ, Ayanian JZ, et al: Variation in the use of cardiac procedures after acute myocardial infarction, *N Engl J Med* 333:573-578, 1995.

8. Wennberg DE, Kellett MA, Dickens JD Jr, et al: The association between local diagnostic testing intensity and invasive cardiac procedures, *JAMA* 275:1161-1164, 1996.

9. Krumholz HM, Radford MJ, Wang Y, et al: National use and effectiveness of ß-blockers for the treatment of elderly patients after acute myocardial infarction: National Cooperative Cardiovascular Project, *JAMA* 280:623-629, 1998.

10. Casale PN, Jones JL, Wolf FE, et al: Patients treated by cardiologists have a lower in-hospital mortality for acute myocardial infarction, *J Am Coll Cardiol* 32:885-889, 1998.

11. Willison DJ, Soumerai SB, McLaughlin TJ, et al: Consultation between cardiologists and generalists in the management of acute myocardial infarction, *Arch Intern Med* 158:1778-1783, 1998.

12. Masuhr F, Busch M, Einhäupl KM: Differences in medical and surgical therapy for stroke prevention between leading experts in North America and Western Europe, *Stroke* 29:339-345, 1998.

13. Lu-Yao GL, McLerran D, Wasson J, et al (Patient Outcomes Research Team): An assessment of radical prostatectomy: time trends, geographic variation, and outcomes, *JAMA* 269:2633-2636, 1993.

14. Greer AL: The state of the art versus the state of the science: the diffusion of new medical technologies into practice, *Int J Technol Assessment Health Care* 4:5-26, 1988.

15. Soumerai SB, McLaughlin TJ, Gurwitz JH: Effect of local medical opinion leaders on quality of care for acute myocardial infarction: a randomized controlled trial, *JAMA* 279:1358-1363, 1998.

16. Thiemann DR, Coresh J, Oetgen WJ, et al: The association between hospital volume and survival after acute myocardial infarction in elderly patients, *JAMA* 340:1640-1648, 1999.

17. Hannan EL, Racz M, Kavey R-E, et al: Pediatric cardiac surgery: the effect of hospital and surgeon volume on in-hospital mortality, *Pediatrics* 101:963-969, 1998.

18. Clayton RN, Stewart PM, Shalet SM, et al: Pituitary surgery for acromegaly: should be done by specialists (editorial), *BMJ* 319:588-589, 1999.

19. Begg CB, Cramer LD, Hoskins WJ, et al: Impact of hospital volume on operative mortality for major cancer surgery, *JAMA* 280:1747-1751, 1998.

20. Yao S-L, Lu-Yao G: Population-based study of relationships between hospital volume of prostatectomies, patient outcomes, and length of hospital stay, *J Natl Cancer Inst* 91:1950-1956, 1999.

21. Edwards EB, Roberts JP, McBride MA, et al: The effect of the volume of procedures at transplantation centers on mortality after liver transplantation, *N Engl J Med* 341:2049-2053, 1999.

22. Schneider EC, Epstein AM: Influence of cardiac-surgery performance reports on referral practices and access to care: a survey of cardiovascular specialists, *N Engl J Med* 335:251-256, 1996.

23. Schneider EC, Epstein AM: Use of public performance reports: a survey of patients undergoing cardiac surgery, *JAMA* 279:1638-1642, 1998.

24. Peterson ED, DeLong ER, Jollis JG, et al: The effects of New York's bypass surgery provider profiling on access to care and patient outcomes in the elderly, *J Am Coll Cardiol* 32:993-999, 1998.

PREVENTION

(See also informed consent; investigations; patient education; screening; statistics; wellness; as well as prevention entries in index)

Before participating in a preventive program, patients and their physicians should be able to answer the following questions[1]:

1. Are there any proven benefits?
2. If so, how great are they?
3. Are there potential adverse effects?
4. If so, what are they, how serious are they, and how frequently do they occur?

Some preventive programs such as accident prevention, avoidance of high-risk behavior, and selection of healthy life-style choices have virtually no adverse consequences. Even if the benefits have not been proved, there seems little harm in participating in such endeavors. On the other hand, preventive programs that involve screening for disease, classification of individuals into high- or low-risk categories for certain diseases, dietary interventions, or prophylactic drug regimens often have uncertain benefits and may have significant adverse consequences.[1]

Methods for reporting the benefits of preventive programs may have a profound influence on whether the programs appear useful.[1] The standard reporting methods are as follows[1]:

1. Relative reduction of morbidity or mortality rates
2. Absolute reduction of morbidity or mortality rates
3. Number of patients who need to be treated to prevent one adverse event
4. Total cohort mortality rates

Reporting methods for benefits are discussed in more detail under "Methods of Reporting Benefits of Clinical Trials" in the section on statistics. The essential clinical point is that although few participants in any screening program benefit, the use of relative reduction greatly exaggerates the apparent benefits. Relative reduction rates should never be used to make decisions about the clinical usefulness of a program.[1]

The clinical significance of the benefits of preventive programs may be misconstrued in many other ways, including these:

1. Surrogate rather than clinically significant outcomes are used (e.g., finding more "small" cancers is a surrogate outcome for decreased mortality rates).[2]
2. The risk level or disease prevalence of the population involved is not considered (e.g., lipid-lowering drugs are more effective for patients with proven coronary disease than for asymptomatic persons).[2]
3. The interval between the intervention and the benefit is not considered (e.g., if a decrease in prostate cancer death rates is ever proved to result from PSA screening, this benefit will not be evident until 10 years after radical prostatectomy).[2]
4. The duration of the intervention required to achieve the benefit is not considered (e.g., hormone replacement therapy must be given for several decades to prevent hip fractures).[2]
5. One benefit may be overshadowed by another (e.g., the value of exercise in the prevention of coronary artery disease and fractures may be deemphasized by the promotion of hormone replacement therapy for the same purpose).[2]
6. The observed benefit may be due to a "healthy user" effect rather than the intervention (e.g., women choosing hormone replacement therapy have a healthier life-style than those who choose not to take hormones).[3-5]
7. Benefits documented in clinical trials are assumed to occur in clinical practice (this is often not the case because the populations are different or compliance is less stringent).
8. There is publication bias (positive results of preventive interventions are more often published than are negative results).[2]
9. Studies showing positive results are preferentially cited (authors may cite positive studies more often than negative ones).[2]
10. False-negative results are present (if a study has inadequate power, a true beneficial result may not be shown—type II error).[2]

All preventive screening or case-finding programs have the potential for causing harm. In general, the degree of harm increases with each level of the "screening cascade." Harm is least at the initial level, which is the screening process itself, intermediate at the second level, which is the investigation of abnormal screening results, and greatest at the third level, which is the treatment of identified disorders. Examples of physical harm are breast pain from compression during mammography or syncope from a venipuncture at level 1 of the screening cascade, urinary tract infection from prostate biopsy or perforated colon from colonoscopy at level 2, and impotence or death as a result of radical prostatectomy or the precipitation of an eating disorder as a result of dietary therapy at level 3.[6]

The psychological and social harm of preventive programs may be categorized as follows[6]:

1. Anticipated discomfort or perception of adverse effects resulting from preventive interventions
2. Unpleasant interactions with health care workers
3. Time required for preventive programs
4. Excessive overall awareness of health
5. Anxiety while anticipating the results of a screening test
6. Anxiety induced by a positive screening test result
7. Distress from being labeled as "sick" or at "high risk"
8. Psychopathological effects directly induced by a therapeutic program (such as strict dieting)
9. False assurance of disease-free status as a result of a negative screening test

Screening-induced psychological distress is discussed in more detail in the section on screening below, and harm to society as a whole is dealt with in the section on wellness.

Since few persons participating in preventive screening programs benefit and many are harmed, failure to obtain informed consent before participation is unethical.[7-9] Unfortunately, obtaining informed consent is difficult because of biased promotional literature,[10,11] physicians' lack of knowledge, patients' problems assimilating data, and lack of time for the process to unfold.[7] Suggested ways to facilitate informed consent are for physicians to base their recommendations, whenever possible, on evidence-based guidelines, such as those put forward by the Canadian Task Force on Preventive Health Care and the U.S. Preventive Services Task Force, and for physicians to refrain from promoting a preventive program on the basis of relative reduction of morbidity rates. Patient information material (decision aids) should be used whenever it is available in a balanced form[7]; many brochures present a biased view that exaggerates benefits and glosses over adverse effects.[10,11]

The logistics of implementing systematic preventive programs in a physician's office is closely related to the organizational efficiency of the medical practice. McVea and associates[12] from the University of Nebraska surveyed eight midwestern practices that were interested enough in prevention to have requested "Put Prevention into Practice" (PPIP) kits from the American Academy of Family Practice. They found that even though all the clinicians were enthusiastic about prevention and reasonably knowledgeable about its benefits, none used the kits. Those offices that did not already have an organized system could not integrate the material into their routines, while well-organized offices had already made preventive interventions a part of their programs and had no need for the kits.

Specific aspects of prevention are covered in many sections of the text. Immediately following are the sections on screening, behavioral changes for prevention, and wellness.

➤ REFERENCES ➤

1. Marshall KG: Prevention. How much harm? How much benefit? 1. Influence of reporting methods on perception of benefits, *Can Med Assoc J* 154:1493-1499, 1996.
2. Marshall KG: Prevention. How much harm? How much benefit? 2. Ten potential pitfalls in determining the clinical significance of benefits, *Can Med Assoc J* 154:1837-1843, 1996.
3. Posthuma WF, Westendorp RG, Vandenbroucke JP: Cardioprotective effect of hormone replacement therapy in postmenopausal women: is the evidence biased? *BMJ* 308:1268-1269, 1994.
4. Rossouw JE: Estrogens for prevention of coronary heart disease: putting the brakes on the bandwagon, *Circulation* 94:2982-2985, 1996.
5. Grover SA: Estrogen replacement for women with cardiovascular disease: why don't physicians and patients follow the guidelines? (editorial), *Can Med Assoc J* 161:42-43, 1999.
6. Marshall KG: Prevention. How much harm? How much benefit? 3. Physical, psychological and social harm, *Can Med Assoc J* 155:169-176, 1996.
7. Marshall KG: Prevention. How much harm? How much benefit? 4. The ethics of informed consent for preventive screening programs, *Can Med Assoc J* 155:377-383, 1996.
8. Foster P, Anderson CM: Reaching targets in the national cervical screening programme: are current practices unethical? *J Med Ethics* 24:151-157, 1998.
9. Austoker J: Gaining informed consent for screening: is difficult—but many misconception need to be undone (editorial), *BMJ* 319:722-723, 1999.
10. Welch HG: Finding and redefining disease (editorial), *Effect Clin Pract* 2:96-99, 1999.
11. Coulter A: Evidence based patient information is important, so there needs to be a national strategy to ensure it (editorial), *BMJ* 317:225-226, 1998.
12. McVea K, Crabtree BF, Medder JD, et al: An ounce of prevention? Evaluation of the "Put Prevention into Practice" program, *J Family Pract* 43:361-369, 1996.

Screening

(See also abdominal aortic aneurysm; alcohol abuse; attitudes, physician; breast cancer; cervical cancer; clinical practice guidelines; colon cancer; congenital anomalies; consensus conferences; glaucoma; group B streptococci; hemochromatosis; hypothyroidism; informed consent; investigations; lipids; maternal serum screening; obesity; ovarian cancer; patient preferences; periodic health examination; pituitary incidentalomas; prevention; prostate cancer; testicular cancer; thyroid nodules; type 2 diabetes; urinalysis; wellness)

Screening is a public health program organized in such a way that an entire population is screened for a specified condition. Case finding is a program in which individual health care workers in practices and clinics screen their patients for one or more diseases.

Criteria justifying a screening program

Criteria that should be met to justify a screening program include the following[1]:

1. The disease in question should be a serious health problem.

2. There should be a presymptomatic phase during which treatment can change the course of the disease more successfully than in the symptomatic phase.
3. The screening procedure and the ensuing treatment should be acceptable to the public.
4. The screening procedure should have acceptable sensitivity and specificity.
5. The screening procedure and ensuing treatment should be cost effective.

Effect of screening on apparent prevalence rates

Increased imaging resolution or other techniques that detect small lesions lead to an apparent increase in prevalence rates. For example, ultrasound increases the detection of abdominal aneurysms threefold, but most are small. Computed tomography or magnetic resonance imaging detects many prolapsed disks in asymptomatic persons.[2] The incidence of prostate cancer has been increasing rapidly over the past two decades, probably because of an increase in diagnoses resulting from increased numbers of transurethral prostatic resections for benign disease in the period 1973-1986[3] and the increased use of PSA testing thereafter.[4] Ultrasound screening of the thyroid gland in asymptomatic patients resulted in a "nodule" detection rate of 67%.[5]

A closely related issue is disease definition. If the threshold for diagnosing a condition is lowered, the prevalence of the disease will increase. The 1997 decision of the American Diabetes Association to lower the fasting glucose threshold for diabetes from 7.8 mmol/L (140 mg/dl) to 7.0 mmol/L (126 mg/dl) created 1.7 million new diabetics in the United States. If proposed new diagnostic thresholds for diabetes, hypertension, hypercholesterolemia, and obesity are all implemented, 75% of the adult U.S. population will be labeled as diseased.[6]

Clinical significance of detecting small lesions in a screening program

Autopsy studies have shown an extremely high prevalence rate of some cancers. In a 1985 autopsy study from Finland, 2.5-mm slices of thyroid were examined. At least one papillary carcinoma was found in 36% of cases. By extrapolation, if even thinner slices had been obtained, almost 100% of autopsy subjects would have had papillary carcinoma.[7] Ductal carcinoma in situ is found in 6% to 18% of autopsies of women dying of other diseases. How many of these would have progressed to clinical cancer is unknown. This is an important issue because 30% to 40% of cancers diagnosed by mammography are ductal carcinomas in situ.[8]

Evidence that lowering diagnostic thresholds for diseases such as diabetes and hypercholesterolemia will decrease morbidity or mortality is absent or tenuous; in most instances guidelines are based on extrapolations from populations with more advanced disease. The certain result of lowering diagnostic thresholds will be an artifactual improvement in the outcomes of the identified diseases, since individuals with minimally elevated cholesterol, fasting glucose, or blood pressure will do better than those with more marked variations from the norm.[6] The harm of lowering thresholds is discussed below.

Lead time bias

Lead time bias is a failure to take into account the time of diagnosis of a disease.[2,9] As an example, assume that a hypothetical cancer kills everyone affected by it 10 years after its onset, regardless of what treatment is offered. If one cohort of patients with this disease goes through a screening process that detects the lesions and leads to tumor resection 3 or 4 years before they become symptomatic, the 5-year survival rate will be much higher than in a control cohort in which resection takes place only when the tumor becomes symptomatic (i.e., 3 or 4 years later in the natural history of the disease). If the follow-up is longer, however, survival rates would equalize for the two groups; in this example, everyone would be dead by 10 years.

Length bias

Length bias refers to the fact that cancers having a slow rate of progression are more likely to be detected by screening techniques than are rapidly growing cancers. These are the tumors with the best prognosis, and therefore they would be expected to have a better prognosis whether or not early treatment is instituted.[2,9]

Overdiagnosis bias

Overdiagnosis bias is the detection of pseudodisease, that is, subclinical disease that would not cause symptoms during the patient's life.[9] Detecting and treating such nonpathogenic conditions clearly results in excellent outcomes.

Efficacy of screening

Although some screening or case-finding programs have led to decreased morbidity or mortality (screening for phenylketonuria and thyroid-stimulating hormone in newborns, screening for bacteriuria in pregnant women, routine assessment of blood pressure, cervical cytology smears, and mammography in women between 50 and 69), others have not shown a benefit. For example, routine ultrasound screening of pregnant women at 15 to 22 weeks and 31 to 35 weeks has not improved perinatal outcome compared with control subjects who had ultrasound only if clinically indicated.[10] Other examples of screening or case-finding programs of no value, or unproved value, are digital rectal examination for the detection of prostate cancer, breast self-examination for the detection of breast cancer, examination of the skin for the detection of malignancy, examination of the testes for the detection of malignancy, periodic pelvic examinations for the detection of ovarian cancer, chest x-ray examination for the detection of lung cancer in smokers, sputum cytology for the detection of lung cancer in smokers, PSA screening for the detection of prostate cancer, measurement of blood cholesterol levels in asymptomatic average-risk children with the goal of decreasing cardiovascular mortal-

ity, assessment of blood glucose levels for the detection of diabetes mellitus in average-risk adults, and urine dipstick analysis for blood with the goal of detecting kidney, bladder, or ureteral malignancies. Most of the programs listed above are discussed and referenced elsewhere in the text, as well as in the reports of the U.S. Preventive Services Task Force[11] and the Canadian Task Force on Preventive Health Care.[12]

Adverse effects of screening

The adverse effects of screening are multiple, and many of these are discussed in the sections on prevention and wellness. The effect of screening programs on physicians and on patients' psychological states is dealt with here.

Effects of screening programs on physicians' practice patterns. Physicians are barraged with increasing numbers of guidelines recommending preventive screening interventions, and many are subject to audits assessing whether they comply adequately with these guidelines. There is concern that the increasing emphasis on prevention will take so much time and effort that physicians will be distracted from optimally diagnosing and treating the sick.[6,9]

Screening and psychological distress. Meador[13] points out that the search for disease may lead to the elimination of wellness, and Marteau[14] and Wardle and Pope[15] emphasize the degree of anxiety that screening procedures may invoke. Psychological distress may be manifested at several levels of screening programs. Some studies have found that publicity about screening programs in itself may arouse concern about having serious disease,[16] whereas others have found no such association.[17] Recalls for further tests, or the diagnosis of precancerous lesions such as cervical dysplasia or carcinoma in situ, are often seen by patients as a diagnosis of cancer.[15] False-positive results of cancer screening may lead to devastating psychological effects that sometimes persist for prolonged periods even after thorough investigations have ruled out malignancy.[15,18,19] True-positive results not only engender distress because of the diagnosis (particularly if incurable cancer is detected[15]), but also may lead to disruption of family relationships, difficulty obtaining insurance, and job discrimination.[20]

A factor that may increase patient anxiety about test results is a delay in receiving them or a failure to receive them. Many physicians do not have reliable methods of determining whether the tests they have ordered are reported, and even if they get them, many do not pass this information on to their patients.[21]

Not all studies have found adverse psychological effects from screening. For example, a coronary risk factor and lifestyle intervention study led by nurses in a number of general practices in Great Britain found that if anything the intervention group experienced less anxiety than the control group.[22]

Informed consent for screening

Informed consent is an important issue that is discussed in the earlier section "Prevention."

Clinical practice guidelines for screening

A confusing aspect of clinical guidelines for screening is that different organizations often produce contradictory recommendations. This occurs even though the evidence on which the recommendations are based is the same for all the organizations involved. The probable explanation is differing attitudes among the individuals who make up the issuing bodies (see discussion of physician attitudes).

Czaja and associates[23] point out that the recommendations of the Canadian Task Force on Preventive Health Care and the U.S. Preventive Services Task Force are more conservative than those of the National Cancer Institute and the American Cancer Society. The two task forces base their recommendations whenever possible on evidence from randomized controlled trials, whereas subspecialty groups such as the American Cancer Society more often accept "expert opinion."[24] Specialty societies are also more likely to emphasize the value of positive outcomes (such as finding "early" cancers) and to deemphasize any detrimental effects that may result from false-positive results in persons without disease.[24]

A survey of American physicians found that the majority followed more interventionist guidelines, which were also the most heavily publicized ones. In terms of specialties, surgeons tended to favor more aggressive screening than did family physicians or internists, and gynecologists favored aggressive screening for cancers in women. Older physicians and those in solo practice were more conservative than younger physicians but were also more likely to favor outmoded screening procedures such as annual chest x-ray examinations.[23] Remarks by focus groups of family physicians and patients in the province of Quebec revealed that most patients and many physicians value early diagnosis regardless of whether this would improve the outcome and that suspicion of "science" is common.[25] Goldbloom[26] suggests that part of the difficulty of giving up time-honored practices even when evidence shows them to be useless is that such practices are comforting rituals that act as anxiolytics for both patients and doctors.

Sometimes physicians follow only selected recommendations of a guideline while ignoring others, a practice that may vitiate any possible benefit of the intervention. PSA screening for prostate cancer is an example. Although both the U.S. Preventive Services Task Force[11] and the Canadian Task Force on Preventive Health Care[12] give PSA screening a "D" recommendation (good evidence not to perform the test), other organizations such as the American Urological Association disagree. In 1992 the American Urological Association specifically recommended PSA screening for men between the ages of 50 and 70.[27] (This has subsequently been modified to recommend screening for men over the age of 50 who have at least a 10-year life expectancy.) The reason for the cutoff at 70 was that the life expectancy of most men over that age was considered too short for benefit to accrue from radical prostatectomy. In practice, primary care physicians avidly screened men for PSA but paid little or no attention to the upper age limit.[28] Almost certainly because of this, a third of all radical prostatectomies in the United States are performed on men over the age of 70.[29]

◥ REFERENCES ◤

1. Feldman W: How serious are the adverse effects of screening? *J Gen Intern Med* (Sept/Oct suppl 5):S50-S53, 1990.
2. Black WC, Welch HG: Advances in diagnostic imaging and overestimations of disease prevalence and the benefits of therapy, *N Engl J Med* 328:1237-1248, 1993.
3. Potosky AL, Kessler L, Gridley G, et al: Rise in prostatic cancer incidence associated with increased use of transurethral resection, *J Natl Cancer Inst* 82:1624-1628, 1990.
4. Potosky AL, Miller BA, Albertsen PC, et al: The role of increasing detection in the rising incidence of prostate cancer, *JAMA* 273:548-552, 1995.
5. Ezzat S, Sarti DA, Cain DR, et al: Thyroid incidentalomas: prevalence by palpation and ultrasonography, *Arch Intern Med* 154:1838-1840, 1994.
6. Schwartz LM, Woloshin S: Changing disease definitions: implications for disease prevalence: analysis of the Third National Health and Nutrition Examination Survey, 1988-1994, *Eff Clin Pract* 2:76-85, 1999.
7. Harach HR, Franssila KO, Wasenius VM: Occult papillary carcinoma of the thyroid: a "normal" finding in Finland; a systematic autopsy study, *Cancer* 56:531-538, 1985.
8. Ernster VL, Barclay J, Kerlikowske K, et al: Incidence of and treatment for ductal carcinoma in situ of the breast, *JAMA* 275:913-918, 1996.
9. Welch HG: Finding and redefining disease (editorial), *Eff Clin Pract* 2:96-99, 1999.
10. Ewigman BG, Crane JP, Frigoletto FD, et al: Effect of prenatal ultrasound screening on perinatal outcome: RADIUS Study Group, *N Engl J Med* 329:821-827, 1993.
11. US Preventive Services Task Force: *Guide to clinical preventive services,* ed 2, Baltimore, 1996, Williams & Wilkins.
12. Canadian Task Force on the Periodic Health Examination: *Canadian guide to clinical preventive health care,* Ottawa, 1994, Canada Communication Group—Publishing.
13. Meador CK: The last well person, *N Engl J Med* 330:440-441, 1994.
14. Marteau TM: Psychological costs of screening: may sometimes be bad enough to undermine the benefits of screening, *BMJ* 299:527, 1989.
15. Wardle J, Pope R: The psychological costs of screening for cancer, *J Psychosom Res* 36:609-624, 1992.
16. Kottke TE, Trapp MA, Fores MM, et al: Cancer screening behaviors and attitudes of women in Southeastern Minnesota, *JAMA* 273:1099-1105, 1995.
17. Wardle J, Taylor T, Sutton S, et al: Does publicity about cancer screening raise fear of cancer? Randomised trial of the psychological effect of information about cancer screening, *BMJ* 319:1037-1038, 1999.
18. Lerman C, Trock B, Rimer BK, et al: Psychological and behavioral implications of abnormal mammograms, *Ann Intern Med* 114:657-661, 1991.

19. Brett J, Austoker J, Ong G: Do women who undergo further investigation for breast screening suffer adverse psychological consequences? A multi-centre follow-up study comparing different breast screening result groups five months after their last breast screening appointment, *J Pub Health Med* 20:396-403, 1998.

20. Macdonald KG, Doan B, Kelner M, et al: A sociobehavioural perspective on genetic testing and counselling for heritable breast, ovarian and colon cancer, *Can Med Assoc J* 154:457-464, 1996.

21. Boohaker EA, Ward RE, Uman JE, et al: Patient notification and follow-up of abnormal test results: a physician survey, *Arch Intern Med* 156:327-331, 1996.

22. Marteau TM, Kinmonth AL, Thompson S, et al: The psychological impact of cardiovascular screening and intervention in primary care: a problem of false reassurance? *Br J Gen Pract* 46:577-582, 1996.

23. Czaja R, McFall SL, Warnecke RB, et al: Preferences of community physicians for cancer screening guidelines, *Ann Intern Med* 120:602-608, 1994.

24. Hayward RSA, Steinberg EP, Ford DE, et al: Preventive care guidelines: 1991, *Ann Intern Med* 114:L758-L783, 1991.

25. Beaulieu M-D, Hudon E, Roberge D, et al: Practice guidelines for clinical prevention: do patients, physicians and experts share common ground? *Can Med Assoc J* 161:519-523, 1999.

26. Goldbloom RB: Prisoners of ritual (editorial), *Can Med Assoc J* 161:528-529, 1999.

27. American Urological Association: Early detection of prostate cancer and use of transrectal ultrasound. In American Urological Association: *1992 Policy statement book,* vol 4, Baltimore, 1992, The Association, p 20.

28. Fowler FJ, Bin L, Collins MM, et al: Prostate cancer screening and beliefs about treatment efficacy: a national survey of primary care physicians and urologists, *Am J Med* 104:526-532, 1998.

29. Murphy GP, Mettlin C, Menck H, et al: National patterns of prostate cancer treatment by radical prostatectomy: results of a survey by the American College of Surgeons Commission on Cancer, *J Urol* 152:1817-1819, 1994.

Behavioral Changes for Prevention

Behavioral or life-style change is an essential aspect of many preventive programs, but as everyone knows, this is an extraordinarily difficult undertaking for patients and physicians. Understanding why we behave as we do facilitates approaches to change. Six stages of change have been defined by Dr. James Prochaska.[1] By identifying and understanding them, physicians can direct interventions toward patients' current stages with the goal of helping the patients move to the next stage. This process takes time, and a reasonable goal is to advance from one stage to another at monthly intervals. The stages are as follows:

1. Precontemplation. Patients are not prepared to change, often feel that they are unable to do so, and may rationalize their reluctance by concluding that the cons outweigh the pros. Interventions that can be used at this stage include:
   a. Fully informing patients of the risks of their current behavior (e.g., smoking, sedentary life-style)
   b. Using life events, such as the death of a friend from an illness related to the same high-risk behavior, or the unhappiness of spouses or children with the behavior, as a reason for contemplating change
   c. Pointing out the benefits of change not only to themselves, but to their social environment (e.g., less risk that their children will smoke if they quit)

2. Contemplation. Patients in this stage are seriously considering changing their behavior within the next 2 to 6 months but not within the next month. Interventions in this stage may involve suggesting short-term, limited trials of change. Giving two or three choices, such as delaying the first cigarette of the morning by 30 minutes, cutting the daily consumption by five cigarettes, or refraining from smoking for 24 hours, often gives patients a feeling of empowerment and confidence so that they can move on to a more permanent program.

3. Preparation. Patients in this stage generally have a plan that they expect to implement within 1 month. Their major fear is that they may fail. Interventions include helping them formalize the details of the plan and supporting their self-confidence.

4. Action. Most of the published literature on life-style changes deals with this stage. This is the point at which nicotine patches are given or serious dieting or regular exercise begins. This phase usually takes 6 months, and relapses are frequent if patients let down their guard after just 2 or 3 months. One of the more important therapeutic interventions in this stage is frequent positive reinforcement for a job well done. As many social supports as possible should be mobilized; this means patients should tell a lot of people what they are trying to accomplish.

5. Maintenance. For most programs such as smoking cessation it takes at least 5 years before the risk of relapse becomes relatively low. Vigilance is required throughout the maintenance period. Continuing social supports should be mobilized.

6. Termination. Termination is a theoretical stage in which there is no risk of relapse. Some achieve it, but for most, prolonged maintenance is a more realistic goal.

◣ REFERENCES ◢

1. Prochaska JO: Why do we behave the way we do? *Can J Cardiol* 11(suppl A):20A-25A, 1995.

Wellness

"Wellness" or "health" is an evasive concept. In recent years, especially in North America, public concern about body functions and health has become an obsession.[1-8] A variety of phrases have been used to describe these attitudes, such as death-denying culture,[4] an unhealthy obsession with health,[5] tyranny of health,[6] coercive healthism,[7] war on death,[8] and cultural imperialism.[9]

Meador[2] suggests that the search for disease may lead to

the elimination of wellness. Barsky[1] points out that the health of Americans has increased immeasurably over the past few decades but the subjective conception of being well has diminished.

Several reasons have been proposed for our concerns about health. A straightforward one is that increase in life expectancy has allowed more people to live long enough to acquire chronic diseases. More important is an epidemic of health awareness publicity. Diet programs, exercise programs, health spas, and publications on health proliferate without limit,[1] and almost a quarter of the Internet is devoted to health.[10] Health has become a huge commercial market that is exploited and expanded by advertising. If you have a cold and watch television, you will see how medications bring about instant health. When this fails to work for you, you feel not only cheated, but unhealthy. Because not everyone has a specific illness, the health promotion (and advertising) organizations delve into potential hidden disasters such as elevated cholesterol levels, prostate cancer, or skin cancer. Even normal anatomical or physiological traits such as baldness, wrinkles, and a touch of plumpness are targeted, since they become profitable if considered as treatable diseases.[1]

Førde suggests that the ever increasing number of epidemiological reports on "risk" factors in daily life is promoting a life-style whose main focus is risk evasion. Since in his view acceptance of risk and uncertainty is necessary for self-realization and social functioning, a person obsessed with risk aversion is socially impaired. According to Førde, health promotion has become a form of "cultural imperialism"—a moral crusade to change basic cultural norms with no assurance that the overall effect will not be deleterious.[9]

Another reason for our decreased sense of wellness is that greater availability of medical care and the growth of medical technology have paradoxically harmed us. In many parts of the Western world people receive more medical care than ever before from an increasing variety of doctors who order escalating numbers of investigations. Investigations lead to more diagnoses and more treatments, but many of the detected "disorders"—impaired glucose tolerance, mildly elevated lipid levels, ductal carcinoma in situ of the breast, small prostate cancers, or angiographically demonstrable coronary artery narrowing—may never cause clinically significant adverse effects and are best classified as "pseudodiseases." Unfortunately, once pseudodiseases are discovered, healthy persons are labeled as "sick" and subjected to medical or surgical interventions that offer questionable benefit and in many cases have serious adverse effects. Furthermore, current medical practice patterns have increased both the volume and the complexity of physicians' workloads. Physicians become distracted, which may be why many patients who have had myocardial infarctions are not discharged on a regimen of aspirin or beta-blockers, or why patients often feel their doctors no longer listen to them.[11] A wonderful article illustrating the absurdities of excessive concern about health is "The Last Well Person" by Meador,[2] which appeared in the *New England Journal of Medicine* in 1994.

The perception of health as a precarious state besieged by a host of ailments destroys the concept of health as "physical, mental and social well-being,"[12] "something positive, a joyful attitude toward life,"[13] or "a buoyant life, full of zest."[14]

◈ REFERENCES ◈

1. Barsky AJ: The paradox of health, *N Engl J Med* 318:414-418, 1988.
2. Meador CK: The last well person, *N Engl J Med* 330:440-441, 1994.
3. Goodwin JS: Geriatrics and the limits of modern medicine, *N Engl J Med* 340:1283-1285, 1999.
4. Annas GJ: Reframing the debate on health care reform by replacing our metaphors, *N Engl J Med* 332:744-747, 1995.
5. Thomas L: Notes of a biology-watcher: the health-care system, *N Engl J Med* 293:1245-1246, 1975.
6. Fitzgerald FT: The tyranny of health, *N Engl J Med* 331:196-198, 1994.
7. Scrabanek P: *The death of humane medicine and the rise of coercive healthism,* Bury Saint Edmunds, Eng, 1994, Crowley Esmonde, pp 37-41.
8. Herman J: The ethics of prevention: old twists and new, *Br J Gen Pract* 46:547-549, 1996.
9. Førde OH: Is imposing risk awareness cultural imperialism? *Soc Sci Med* 47:1155-1159, 1998.
10. Holmer AF: Direct-to-consumer prescription drug advertising builds bridges between patients and physicians, *JAMA* 281: 380-382, 1999.
11. Fisher ES, Welch HG: Avoiding the unintended consequences of growth in medical care: how might more be worse? *JAMA* 281:446-453, 1999.
12. *Basic documents,* ed 35, Geneva, 1985, World Health Organization.
13. Sigerist HE: *The university at the crossroads: addresses and essays,* New York, 1946, Henry Schuman.
14. Breslow L: From disease prevention to health promotion, *JAMA* 281:1030-1033, 1999.

Bicycle Helmets
(See also motor vehicle accidents)

Head injuries cause 75% of bicycle-related deaths.[1,2] Three case-control studies reported that bicycle helmets reduced the risk of head injury by 85%,[3] 69%,[4] and 63%.[5] In a Canadian study of deaths from bicycle-related injuries in Ontario between 1986 and 1991, 75% of the deaths were due to head injuries but only 4% of those killed were wearing bicycle helmets.[2] In this study 91% of deaths were the result of collisions with motor vehicles, males outnumbered females 3.5:1, and the risk of being killed was four times greater at night than during the day.[2] In Victoria, Australia, mandatory bicycle helmet use was associated with a 51% decrease in the number of cyclists killed or hospitalized with head injuries.[6] A case-control study has also shown that helmets protect against upper face and midface injuries.[7]

All types of helmets (soft shelled and hard shelled) are protective for all age groups.[5] Children under 6 years of age do not require a different type of helmet.[5]

An argument given against mandatory use of bicycle helmets is that fewer people might bicycle and therefore fewer people would gain the health benefits of that activity.[8] Several letters to the editor published in the *British Medical Journal*[9-11] and *JAMA*[12,13] suggest that this has happened in Australian states where such laws have been enacted. In fact, the decrease in bicycle usage reported there was mainly in teenagers, while adult bicycling actually increased.[6,14] The peer-reviewed literature firmly supports the use of bicycle helmets as a protection against serious injury, and no solid evidence has been presented that mandatory helmet use decreases bicycle use.

◣ REFERENCES ◢

1. Friede AM, Azzara CV, Gallagher SS, et al: The epidemiology of injuries to bicycle riders, *Pediatr Clin North Am* 32:141-151, 1985.
2. Rowe BH, Rowe AM, Bota GW: Bicyclist and environmental factors associated with fatal bicycle-related trauma in Ontario, *Can Med Assoc J* 152:45-53, 1995.
3. Thompson RS, Rivara FP, Thompson DC: A case-control study of the effectiveness of bicycle safety helmets, *N Engl J Med* 320:1361-1367, 1989.
4. Thompson DC, Rivara FP, Thompson RS: Effectiveness of bicycle safety helmets in preventing head injuries: a case-control study, *JAMA* 276:1968-1973, 1996.
5. Thomas S, Acton C, Nixon J, et al: Effectiveness of bicycle helmets in preventing head injury in children: case-control study, *BMJ* 308:173-176, 1994.
6. Centers for Disease Control and Prevention: Mandatory bicycle helmet use—Victoria, Australia, *JAMA* 269(23):2967, 1993.
7. Thompson DC, Nunn ME, Thompson RS, et al: Effectiveness of bicycle safety helmets in preventing serious facial injury, *JAMA* 276:1974-1975, 1996.
8. DeMarco T: Helmet legislation could decrease cycling (letter), *Can Family Physician* 40:1703-1704, 1994.
9. Davis A: Cyclists should wear helmets: increasing the number of cyclists is more important (letter), *BMJ* 314:69, 1997.
10. Robinson DL: Cyclists should wear helmets: Australian laws making helmets compulsory deterred people from cycling (letter), *BMJ* 314:69-70, 1997.
11. Hillman M: Cyclists should wear helmets: health benefits of cycling greatly outweigh loss of life years from deaths (letter), *BMJ* 314:70, 1997.
12. Bayliss J: Do bicycle helmets protect, and should they be mandatory? (letter), *JAMA* 277:883, 1997.
13. Goldman D: Do bicycle helmets protect, and should they be mandatory? (letter), *JAMA* 277:883-884, 1997.
14. Thompson DC, Thompson RS: Do bicycle helmets protect, and should they be mandatory? (in reply to letters), *JAMA* 277:884, 1997.

Causes of Preventable Deaths in the United States

Any public health policy must be based in part on the frequency of occurrence of the disorders the policy aims to prevent. One estimate is that 19% of U.S. deaths could be prevented or delayed by cessation of smoking, 14% by exercise and diet, and 5% by abstention from excessive alcohol intake.[1]

◣ REFERENCES ◢

1. McGinnis JM, Foege WH: Actual causes of death in the United States, *JAMA* 270:2207-2212, 1993.

Guns
(See also suicide)

In 1994 guns were owned by 33% of urban, 39% of suburban, and 60% of rural U.S. households, and pistols made up more than 50% of the weapons in each category. Gun ownership is highest in southern and Rocky Mountain states. More guns are owned by men than women, whites than blacks, Republicans than Democrats, and persons whose parents owned a gun than those whose parents did not.[1]

An analysis of the type of gun used in firearm-related homicides and suicides in Milwaukee, Wisconsin, between 1991 and 1994 found that handguns accounted for 89% of the homicides and 71% of the suicides.[2]

According to 1989 U.S. data, firearms accounted for 11% of childhood deaths, 17% of deaths among adolescents aged 15 to 19, and 41% of deaths of black males aged 15 to 19.[3] Many high school students take guns to school. A Seattle survey found that 6% of the students had brought a handgun to school at least once,[4] and in Illinois a third of students had done so.[5] A survey of predominantly Hispanic adolescents in three New York City schools found that 21% carried a weapon to school and 42% reported having had a relative or close friend who was shot.[6] More recent data suggest some improvement. A survey of violence-related behavior in U.S. high school students found that between 1991 and 1997 both fighting and the carrying of weapons, including guns, decreased.[7]

Adequate storage of guns in the home requires that they be unloaded and locked. A survey of parents of children in 29 urban, suburban, and rural pediatric practices from across the United States found that a third of families reported owning at least one gun. Of gun-owning families, 61% had at least one unlocked gun and 15% had at least one loaded gun. Only 30% kept all guns unloaded and locked.[8]

In 1998 an 11-year-old and a 13-year-old boy in Jonesboro, Arkansas, stole an arsenal of high-powered assault rifles from the grandfather of one of them and ambushed a public school, killing four children and one teacher and wounding many others. The editor of the *New England Journal of Medicine*, Dr. Jerome Kassirer, pointed out that almost all commentaries on this incident focused on the psychological or social circumstances that might have led these boys to commit such atrocities, while very few dealt with the fact that had the children been unable to obtain weapons easily (i.e., if effective gun control laws had been in place), these deaths would not have occurred.[9]

In 1999 two adolescent boys killed a teacher, 13 fellow students, and themselves at Columbine High School in Littleton, Colorado. As in previous school shootings much of the commentary focused on psychosocial issues, but one proposal that seemed to be gaining support was personalized guns that could be fired only by the owners. Operating such guns would require either button codes or fingerprints, technologies that are already extant.[10]

Accidental shootings, which are usually self-inflicted by young males, are reported to be a common sequel of gun ownership.[11] Six published case-control studies have reported that the relative risk of suicide among persons with access to guns in their homes varies from 1.4 to 4.8,[12] and a California population-based cohort study found that the risk of suicide in the first week after the purchase of a handgun was 57 times that of the general population.[13] Only two case-control trials have dealt with homicides and access to guns in the home; the relative risk for those with access to guns was 2.2 and 2.7.[12] In Washington State 75% of the weapons used by children who shot themselves or others were stored in the home of the victim, a relative, or a friend.[14]

Statistics showing benefit from access to or use of guns usually come from questionnaires in which individuals are asked if they have successfully used guns to save lives or property.[12,15] Such case series carry little scientific weight.[12] Proponents of gun control interpret the literature as indicating that owning a gun increases a person's risk of death, whereas opponents claim that the medical literature on the topic is rife with publication and citation biases and that this is not a valid conclusion.[15]

◄ REFERENCES ►

1. Blendon RJ, Young JT, Hemenway D: The American public and the gun control debate, *JAMA* 275:1719-1722, 1996.
2. Hargarten SW, Karison TA, O'Brien M, et al: Characteristics of firearms involved in fatalities, *JAMA* 275:42-45, 1996.
3. Fingerhut LA, Kleinman FC: *Firearm mortality among children and youth: advance data from Vital and Health Statistics No 178*, Hyattsville, Md, 1989, National Center for Health Statistics, US Dept of Health and Human Services, Pub No PHS 90-1250.
4. Callahan CM, Rivara FP: Urban high school youth and handguns: a school-based survey, *JAMA* 267:3038-3042, 1992.
5. Koop CE, Lundberg GB: Violence in America: a public health emergency; time to bite the bullet back (editorial), *JAMA* 267:3075-3076, 1992. [Published errata appear in *JAMA* 268:3074, 1992, and 271:1404, 1994.]
6. Vaughan RD, McCarthy JF, Armstrong B, et al: Carrying and using weapons—a survey of minority junior high school students in New York City, *Am J Public Health* 86:568-572, 1996.
7. Brener ND, Simon TR, Krug EG, et al: Recent trends in violence-related behaviors among high school students in the United States, *JAMA* 282:440-446, 1999.
8. Senturia YD, Christoffel KK, Donovan M (Pediatric Practice Research Group): Gun storage patterns in US homes with children, *Arch Pediatr Adolesc Med* 150:265-269, 1996.
9. Kassirer JP: Private arsenals and public peril (editorial), *N Engl J Med* 338:1375-1376, 1998.
10. Teret SP, Webster DW: Reducing gun deaths in the United States: personalised guns would help—and would be achievable (editorial), *BMJ* 318:1160-1161, 1999.
11. Sinauer N, Annest JL, Mercy JA: Unintentional, nonfatal firearm-related injuries, *JAMA* 275:1740-1743, 1996.
12. Cummings P, Koepsell TD: Does owning a firearm increase or decrease the risk of death? *JAMA* 280:471-473, 1998.
13. Wintemute GJ, Parham CA, Beaumont JJ, et al: Mortality among recent purchasers of handguns, *N Engl J Med* 341:1583-1589, 1999.
14. Grossman DC, Reay DT, Baker SA: Self-inflicted and unintentional firearm injuries among children and adolescents: the source of the firearm, *Arch Pediatr Adolesc Med* 153:875-878, 1999.
15. Kleck G: What are the risks and benefits of keeping a gun in the home? *JAMA* 280:473-475, 1998.

In-Line Skating

Elbow and wrist guards have been shown to decrease injuries to the elbows and wrists of in-line skaters. Data documenting the efficacy of helmets in this sport are not yet available.[1]

◄ REFERENCES ►

1. Schieber RA, Branche-Dorsey CM, Ryan GW, et al: Risk factors for injuries from in-line skating and the effectiveness of safety gear, *N Engl J Med* 335:1630-1635, 1996.

Motor Vehicle Accidents

(See also alcohol; bicycle helmets; cocaine; exercise; posttraumatic stress disorder; prescriptions for elderly; sleep apnea; whiplash injury)

The last 75 years have seen a progressive decline in motor vehicle–related deaths per million vehicle miles traveled in the United States. In spite of this, motor vehicle accidents account for one third of injury-related deaths in the United States and are the leading cause of death among persons 1 to 24 years of age.[1]

Safety belts

Safety belts are the single most effective method of reducing injuries and deaths in motor vehicle accidents. Seat belt use is higher in jurisdictions with safety belt laws. Young men are among those least likely to use safety belts.[2]

Air bags

The safety and efficacy of air bags have been well documented. However, a number of childhood fatalities have been reported to result from air bag deployment when the child was sitting in the front passenger seat, particularly if he or she was unrestrained or in a rear-facing child safety seat. Although deployment of the passenger side air bag has reduced the overall risk of fatality for right front seat passengers by 18% in frontal crashes, the risk of death for children under 10 in the right front passenger seat has increased by 34%.[3]

Protective measures for children in cars

The American Academy of Pediatrics and the Centers for Disease Control and Prevention have made a number of recommendations about infant and child car seats, booster seats, use of seat belts, and positioning of children in vehicles, including the following:

1. No matter what the age, rear seats are safer than front seats.[4-6]

2. All infants should be in a backward-facing seat strapped into the back seat until they are 1 year of age and weigh 20 lb (9 kg). Such seats should never be placed in the front passenger seat.[4,6] The shoulder straps in rear-facing seats should be in the lowest slots until the child's growth places the shoulders above that slot. If the tilt of the car seat causes the infant's head to flop forward, a rolled towel or newspaper should be placed under the depressed edge of the seat, raising it enough to keep the infant's head resting against the back of the seat.[4]

3. Children between 20 lb (9 kg) and 40 lb (18 kg) should be placed in a forward-facing child seat that is fastened into the back seat.[4,6]

4. Once the child surpasses 40 lb (18 kg), a belt-positioning booster with lap and shoulder belts may be used.[4,6]

5. Booster seats should be used until the child is 58 inches (147 cm) tall, has a sitting height of 29 inches (74 cm), and weighs 80 lb (36 kg). Without a booster seat the lap and seat belts are inadequately positioned and not only may not be protective but may be harmful. Most children outgrow booster seats by about age 10.[5]

6. Ideally a child who has outgrown a booster seat should be in the back seat, but if he or she is in the front passenger seat, the seat should be pushed as far back as possible to avoid injury if the air bag deploys.[4,6]

Nonuse or misuse of restraint systems is responsible for numerous deaths and injuries. Children are twice as likely to be unrestrained if the driver is not using the seatbelt system. Misuse of child safety seats is common; the most frequent errors are failure to attach the seat tightly to the vehicle and failure to adjust the harness so that the child is held snugly in place.[6]

Alcohol

In the United States, motor vehicle accidents are the leading cause of death of all ages from 1 to 34 years, and slightly less than half of these fatal accidents are alcohol related. The cutoff point for blood alcohol levels in determining the above statistics is 0.1 g/dl (100 mg/dl). In the general population the risk of a motor vehicle accident has been shown to be much greater when this level is reached than at lower blood alcohol levels. However, lower levels are far from risk free. The risk begins to increase at levels of 0.02 g/dl (20 mg/dl), increases significantly at 0.05 g/dl (50 mg/dl), and increases rapidly at levels over 0.1 g/dl (100 mg/dl).[7] The risk of a fatal crash among drivers with blood alcohol levels of 0.05 to 0.09 g/dl is nine times greater than among those with no alcohol in the blood.[8]

Alcohol-impaired drivers are less likely to use seat belts than other drivers,[9] and children who are passengers in cars driven by drivers who have been drinking are less likely to be restrained.[10]

Evidence indicates that zero tolerance laws with respect to blood alcohol levels of drivers can dramatically decrease fatal motor vehicle accidents. This has been the case for drivers under the age of 21 in many U.S. states and for the entire population in Japan. In Maine a law that reduced the maximal allowable blood alcohol level to 0.05% for individuals with a previous conviction for driving while impaired cut the fatal accident rate for this population by 25%.[8]

Drivers 16 to 24 years of age are five times more likely to be involved in alcohol-related driving fatalities than drivers aged 35 to 64, and in many instances this increased risk occurs with very low levels of blood alcohol. The reasons are uncertain, but the risk-taking behavior of adolescents coupled with inexperience is thought to be the major factor. It is also probable that less alcohol is required to impair adolescents than older drivers.[11] Although the frequency of driving after drinking has declined among U.S. high school seniors over the past 15 years, it is still a common occurrence. A 1997 national survey of high school seniors reported that in the 2 weeks preceding the survey 18% had driven after drinking, 26% had ridden with someone who had been drinking, and 31% had either driven after drinking or ridden with someone who had been drinking.[12]

One of the medicolegal problems with the use of breathalyzers is that they require the person to blow into the device for a brief period. This has led to a number of court challenges in which individuals who had such conditions as asthma, chronic obstructive pulmonary disease, tracheostomy, or ankylosing spondylitis or who were experiencing severe emotional or physical distress were in some jurisdictions considered to have a reasonable excuse for not complying with police requests for breathalyzer tests.[13]

Seizures

The overall accident rate of drivers with controlled seizures is slightly increased and is comparable to the rates of patients with other significant medical disorders such as heart disease and diabetes. A short seizure-free period is the major risk factor for accidents in patients with seizure disorders; the risk is significantly reduced in those who have been seizure free for more than 6 to 12 months. The risk is also reduced in those who consistently have an aura before the onset of seizures.[14]

In the United States the seizure-free interval required to obtain a driver's license varies from 3 to 18 months depending on the state of residence. In practice this may have relatively little significance, since a high percentage of persons who have seizures never report their condition to the licensing authorities.[14]

Diabetes mellitus

No evidence has shown that the rate of motor vehicle accidents is higher in persons with type 1 diabetes than in the general population. However, in driving simulation tests, driving skills deteriorated significantly in type 1 diabetic patients with mild hypoglycemia (blood glucose levels of 2.6 to 3.6 mmol/L [47 to 65 mg/dl]). Half of the patients tested were unaware of these deficits and stated they would drive again under similar conditions. Patients with type 1 diabetes should be warned about this problem, encouraged to measure blood sugar before driving, and advised not to delay or miss meals on long trips.[15]

Speed

Increasing the speed limit is associated with an increased mortality rate.[16] It has been estimated that an increase in impact speed of 10% results in approximately a 40% increase in mortality for both restrained and unrestrained occupants of a vehicle.[17]

Fog

Fog distorts drivers' perceptions of speed—they think they are going more slowly than they actually are and so tend to accelerate.[18] In foggy conditions the driver should check the speedometer frequently.

Sleep deprivation

Serious sleep deprivation is common among long-distance truck drivers, especially those who drive at night, and is responsible for numerous accidents.[19] Sleep apnea is also a risk factor for motor vehicle accidents.[20]

Geriatric drivers

Elderly people drive relatively few miles and tend to be law abiding. Therefore they account for a small proportion of total road accidents. On the other hand, on a per mile traveled basis the accident rate is higher than for younger individuals; by age 85 and over it is three times that of other drivers and is exceeded only by that of teenage drivers. Older drivers involved in accidents are more likely to be killed than are younger persons; those over 85 have the highest death rate per accident of any group.[21] Use of long-acting benzodiazepines is associated with an increased rate of motor vehicle accidents in the elderly.[22]

Motorcycles

The death rate for motorcyclists is 35 times that of car occupants. Major injuries in motorcycle accidents are to the head and lower extremities. Helmets decrease fatal head injuries by 25%.[23]

Posttraumatic stress disorder

Posttraumatic stress disorder is a common sequel to motor vehicle accidents in both adults[24] and children.[25] In one study of children posttraumatic stress disorder was identified in one third of those who were involved in vehicle accidents but in only 3% of those who sustained a sports injury. In spite of this high incidence the condition is rarely identified in daily clinical practice.[25]

❧ REFERENCES ❧

1. Centers for Disease Control and Prevention: Motor-vehicle safety: a 20th century public health achievement, *JAMA* 281: 2080-2082, 1999.
2. Nelson DE, Bolen J, Kresnow M-J: Trends in safety belt use by demographics and by type of state safety belt law, 1987 through 1993, *Am J Public Health* 88:245-249, 1998.
3. Braver ER, Ferguson SA, Greene MA, et al: Reductions in deaths in frontal crashes among right front passengers in vehicles equipped with passenger air bags, *JAMA* 278:1437-1439, 1997.
4. Committee on Injury and Poison Prevention of the American Academy of Pediatrics: Selecting and using the most appropriate car safety seats for growing children: guidelines for counseling parents, *Pediatrics* 97:761-763, 1996.
5. Centers for Disease Control and Prevention: National Child Passenger Safety Week—February 14-20, 1999, *MMWR* 48: 83-84, 1999.
6. Winston FK, Durbin DR: Buckle up! is not enough: enhancing protection of the restrained child, *JAMA* 281:2070-2072, 1999.
7. Madden C, Cole TB: Emergency intervention to break the cycle of drunken driving and recurrent injury, *Ann Emerg Med* 26:177-179, 1995.
8. Hingson R, Heeren T, Winter M: Effects of Maine's 0.05% legal blood alcohol level for drivers with DWI convictions, *Public Health Rep* 113:440-446, 1998.
9. Foss RD, Beirness DJ, Sprattler K: Seat belt use among drinking drivers in Minnesota, *Am J Public Health* 84:1732-1737, 1994.
10. Centers for Disease Control and Prevention: Alcohol-related traffic fatalities involving children—United States, 1985-96, *JAMA* 279:104-105, 1998.
11. Augustyn M, Simons-Morton BG: Adolescent drinking and driving: etiology and interpretation, *J Drug Educ* 25:41-59, 1995.
12. O'Malley PM, Johnston LD: Drinking and driving among US high school seniors, 1984-1997, *Am J Public Health* 89:678-684, 1999.
13. Marks P: Drunk driving legislation: medicine and the law, *Medico-Legal J* 63:119-127, 1995.
14. Krauss GL, Krumholz A, Carter BA, et al: Risk factors for seizure-related motor vehicle crashes in patients with epilepsy, *Neurology* 52:1324-1329, 1999.
15. Clarke WL, Cox DJ, Gonder-Frederick LA, et al: Hypoglycemia and the decision to drive a motor vehicle by persons with diabetes, *JAMA* 282:750-754, 1999.
16. Rock SM: Impact of the 65 mph speed limit on accidents, deaths and injuries in Illinois, *Accid Anal Prevent* 27:207-214, 1995.

17. Joksch HC: Velocity change and fatality risk in a crash—a rule of thumb, *Accid Anal Prevent* 25:103-104, 1993.

18. Snowden RJ, Stimpson N, Ruddle RA: Speed perception fogs up as visibility drops (letter), *Nature* 392:450, 1998.

19. Mitler MM, Miller JC, Lipsitz JJ, et al: The sleep of long-haul truck drivers, *N Engl J Med* 337:755-761, 1997.

20. Terán-Santos J, Jiménez-Gómez A, Cordero-Guevara J (Co-operative Group Burgos-Santander): The association between sleep apnea and the risk of traffic accidents, *JAMA* 340:847-851, 1999.

21. Martinez R: Older drivers and physicians (editorial), *JAMA* 274:1060, 1995.

22. Hemmelgarn B, Suissa S, Huang A, et al: Benzodiazepine use and the risk of motor vehicle crash in the elderly, *JAMA* 278:27-31, 1997.

23. Rivara FP, Grossman DC, Cummins P: Injury prevention (first of two parts), *N Engl J Med* 337:543-548, 1997.

24. Blanchard EB, Hickling EJ, Vollmer AJ, et al: Short term follow up of post traumatic stress symptoms in motor accident vehicles, *Behav Res Ther* 33:369-377, 1995.

25. Stallard P, Velleman R, Baldwin S: Prospective study of post-traumatic stress disorder in children involved in road traffic accidents, *BMJ* 317:1619-1623, 1998.

Poverty

Within developed nations, poverty correlates with increased morbidity and mortality.[1-6] For example, the chance that an adolescent male in Harlem will live to be 65 has been shown to be 37%.[1] Causes of excess mortality among the poor vary from one region to another. The poor have an excess death rate from cardiovascular disease in all regions and from cancer in most. In certain urban areas HIV infection and homicides are the leading causes of death, while in others accidents top the list.[1]

Repeated studies have shown that in developed countries increases in mortality and morbidity correlate far more with relative poverty than with absolute poverty. The United States has one of the greatest income disparities in the world.[2] Societies with less income disparity tend to have more social cohesion and lower variances in mortality and morbidity rates among income groups.[3] Loss of social cohesiveness is in part a result of a decrease in the number of neighborhoods shared by rich and poor as the wealthy escape to more affluent districts. The poor are left to deal not only with their own economic and social problems, but also with the problems inherent in living in low-income neighborhoods. Municipal services are minimal, social supports borderline, schools second rate, and school dropout rates high. In such a milieu crime flourishes and economic productivity drops because of the lack of educated workers.[4]

It is frequently stated that much of the excess mortality among the poor is due to high-risk behaviors. In one nationwide U.S. study, smoking, alcohol excess, sedentary lifestyle, and obesity accounted for less than 15% of the excess mortality. Psychosocial stresses such as a lack of social supports or relationships, low self-esteem, loss of personal con-trol, racism, and classism may in themselves lead to higher mortality rates.[5]

The more affluent commonly assume that by moving to the suburbs they can escape the problems endemic to the decaying inner cities such as AIDS, tuberculosis, and violent crime. This is only partly true. Studies have documented that while rates of disease and violence in suburban communities are lower, they rise in direct proportion to the rise in the inner cities.[5] Rodrick and Deborah Wallace[6] conclude that poor neighborhoods in central cities have a great detrimental effect on the safety and health of a large proportion of the American population, including the wealthy.

A problem related to, but not necessarily synonymous with, poverty is unemployment. Unemployment is associated with an overall increase in mortality, greater use of health care services, and increased physical and psychological morbidity. Whether it causes these ills is uncertain.[7]

⚓ REFERENCES ⚓

1. Geronimus AT, Bound J, Waidmann TA, et al: Excess mortality among blacks and whites in the United States, *N Engl J Med* 335:1552-1558, 1996.

2. Lynch JW, Kaplan GA, Pamuk ER, et al: Income inequality and mortality in metropolitan areas of the United States, *Am J Public Health* 88:1074-1080, 1998.

3. Wilkinson RG: Socioeconomic determinants of health: health inequalities: relative or absolute material standards? *BMJ* 314:591-594, 1997.

4. Kawachi I, Kennedy BP: Health and social cohesion: why care about income inequality? *BMJ* 314:1037-1040, 1997.

5. Lantz PM, House JS, Lepkowski JM, et al: Socioeconomic factors, health behaviors, and mortality: results from a nationally representative prospective study of US adults, *JAMA* 279:1703-1708, 1998.

6. Wallace R, Wallace D: Socioeconomic determinants of health: community marginalisation and the diffusion of disease and disorder in the United States, *BMJ* 314:1341-1345, 1997.

7. Jin RL, Shah CP, Svoboda TJ: The impact of unemployment on health: a review of the evidence, *Can Med Assoc J* 153:529-540, 1995.

Tap Water Scalds

The risk of scalding from hot water depends on the water temperature and the duration of exposure. The usual home hot water heater is set at 60° C (140° F), and scalding at this temperature takes place in 5 to 6 seconds. Lowering the heater temperature to 49° C (120° F) will prevent many scalds in those most at risk (children under 5, the disabled, and the elderly) because at this temperature scalding occurs only after 9 minutes of exposure.[1]

⚓ REFERENCES ⚓

1. Huyer DW, Corkum SH: Reducing the incidence of tap-water scalds: strategies for physicians, *Can Med Assoc J* 156:841-844, 1997.

STATISTICS

(See also angina; ankylosing spondylitis; cholesterol; colon cancer; electrocardiograms; gestational diabetes; investigations; mammography; nonsteroidal antiinflammatory drug gastropathy; ovarian cancer; prevention; risk analysis; screening)

If you are like me, your eyes glaze over when you run across a term like statistical techniques. When we read the medical literature, we keep seeing such terms as p value, confidence intervals, type I error, type II error, and inadequate power, so to make sense of it we have to learn what they mean. Fortunately for the statistically illiterate, Guyatt and associates[1-4] from McMaster University have published a series of simple, clear articles on this topic in the *Canadian Medical Association Journal.*

Null Hypothesis

Many studies involve comparing the efficacy of one treatment with another treatment or a placebo. One way of determining if a statistically significant difference exists between treatments is for the study authors to start with the assumption that there will be no difference. This is called the null hypothesis. If the results clearly show that one treatment is superior to the other (see below), the null hypothesis is disproved.[1]

p Value

The p value is a way of recording probability. A p value of .01 is another way of saying that chance alone would account for the observed results in 1% of cases, while a p value of .05 means that chance alone would account for the results in 5% of cases.[1]

Statistical Significance

A study result is said to be statistically significant if the odds are that chance alone is unlikely to account for the results. By convention the boundary between statistically significant and statistically insignificant is a p value of .05. Any p value of .05 or less is statistically significant.[1]

Type I Error

A type I error is falsely concluding that an observed difference is due to the intervention being studied and not to chance alone. The lower the p value, the less likely that a type I error is present. However, with a p value of .05, any observed differences in results could be explained by chance alone in 5% of cases.[1]

Type II Error

A type II error is falsely concluding that no difference exists between two treatment plans (or a treatment and a placebo) when actually there is a difference. This error may occur because the study had inadequate power (see below).[1]

Power

If a study fails to disprove the null hypothesis, one reason may be that too few subjects were in the study to allow a true difference to become apparent. If this is the case, the study is said to have inadequate power and a type II error has occurred. The larger the sample, the less likelihood of inadequate power and a resulting type II error.[1]

Multiple Tests

When multiple independent tests or variables are assessed at the same time in any study, the odds that one of them will show a difference with a p value $\leq$.05 by chance alone increases with the number of variables assessed. If a single variable is assessed, the odds are 5%. If six variables are assessed, the odds are 26% (or 1 in 4), and for 10 variables the odds are 40%.[1]

In family medicine this problem is seen most frequently when a physician makes the mistake of ordering a batch of laboratory tests for a healthy person "just to make sure everything is all right." Ordering 10 tests is very easy, and if the physician does so, close to half the patients will have falsely abnormal results.

Point Estimate

If a study comparing a drug with a placebo shows that 35% of patients taking the placebo died at 1 year whereas only 30% of those taking the drug died, the difference of 5% is called the point estimate. One way of determining whether this point estimate is statistically significant is to calculate confidence intervals (see below).[2]

Confidence Intervals

The likelihood that the 5% difference in mortality rate described above under "Point Estimate" is due to chance rather than the drug being tested depends largely on the number of subjects assessed. If only 10 were in each group, the result might well be due to chance; if there were 1000, it might be due to the beneficial effects of the drug. This type of probability calculation can be quantified to produce confidence intervals around the point estimation. The wider the confidence intervals, the greater the chance that the observed point estimate is a result of chance, and the narrower they are, the greater the chance that the point estimate is due to the intervention applied.[2]

Methods of Reporting the Benefits of Clinical Trials

The benefits of clinical studies are usually reported in one of four ways.[3,5] These are relative risk reduction of morbidity or mortality (RRR), absolute risk reduction of morbidity or mortality (ARR), numbers of patients who need treatment to prevent adverse events (NNT), and total cohort morbidity or mortality. Mathematical formulas for calculating most of these figures have been given in a paper by Miller.[6] The meaning of these terms and their clinical significance are discussed in a simplified form in the ensuing paragraphs.

Relative reduction of risk

Relative reduction of risk or mortality is the percentage reduction of morbidity or mortality in a population that is subject to an intervention compared with a control population that is not subject to that intervention.[3] Thus a mammographic trial may report a 35% reduction in death rate from breast cancer in the mammographically screened population, or a cholesterol-lowering drug trial may report a 45% decrease in myocardial infarction rate in the treated compared with the control population.

The calculation of relative risk is demonstrated by the following example. A mammographic study enrolled 10,000 women in the screened group and 10,000 women in the control group. If after 10 years six women in the control group had died of breast cancer and only four in the screened group had died of this disease, these figures could be presented as percentages. In the screened group 0.04% of women died of breast cancer, while in the control group 0.06% died. The relative risk of dying of breast cancer in this study is 0.04/0.06 × 100 or 66%. Put another way, the relative risk of dying of breast cancer for a woman who had mammography is two thirds that of a woman who did not have mammography.

Once the relative risk is established, it is easy to determine the relative risk reduction. This is simply the reciprocal of the relative risk.[3] The relative risk in the screened population is 66%, so the relative reduction of risk has to be 34%. The latter figure is the one most often quoted in studies such as the one in the example. Although the study described here is hypothetical, a 34% relative reduction of risk is fairly representative of figures reported from actual mammographic screening programs (see discussion of mammography).

A 34% relative reduction of risk of dying of breast cancer looks impressive. However, the clinical significance of such relative risk or mortality reductions may be deceiving because they are often quite unrelated to the magnitude of the actual numbers, a trap into which many of us have fallen on more than one occasion. It is the absolute risk reduction and the numbers of patients who must be screened or treated for one beneficial event to accrue that are most important (see below).[5,6]

A term that needs mention but can be quickly forgotten by most of us is odds ratios. Odds ratios may be useful for statisticians, and the numbers are often close to relative reduction figures, but as far as I can determine, their main effect on family physicians is to induce confusion.

Absolute risk reduction

Absolute risk reduction or absolute mortality reduction is the actual morbidity rate or death rate of the screened population subtracted from the actual morbidity rate or death rate of the control population. As an example from the hypothetical mammographic screening program described in the previous section, we have already determined that after 10 years, four of 10,000 women in the screened group died of breast cancer, compared with six of 10,000 women in the unscreened control group. Expressed as percentages, these number are 0.04% and 0.06%. The absolute risk reduction (or mortality reduction) that can be attributed to screening is

0.06 to 0.04, or 0.02%. The most important point for patients and physicians to remember is that the small absolute risk reduction figure is far more important clinically than the larger relative risk reduction figure.

Numbers of patients who need to be screened

If a screening procedure or a therapeutic intervention is undertaken with the object of preventing adverse effects, many of the individuals screened or treated will not benefit from the intervention.[5] This is well illustrated in the mammography screening example discussed previously. The relative mortality reduction rate was 34%, and the absolute mortality reduction 0.02%. The latter figure means that two lives were saved by screening 10,000 women over a 10-year period or, putting it another way, 5000 women would have to be screened by mammography to save one life over a 5-year period. In comparing one study with another, it is often useful to standardize the results in terms of benefits observed after 1 year.[6] In this example, 50,000 women would have to be screened to save one life annually. As stated previously, the example given here is theoretical, but the figures used are close to those that have actually been reported (see discussion of mammography).

The usefulness of determining numbers of individuals who need to be screened is illustrated by a study from Rembold[7] at the University of Virginia. He compared the numbers of persons who would have to be screened for serum lipids, blood pressure, mammography, or occult blood in stool in order to save one life 5 years after initiation of treatment for detected abnormalities. His results were 418 for lipids, 274 for blood pressure when the diastolic pressure is lowered by 10 mm Hg, 1307 for blood pressure when the diastolic pressure is lowered by 5.7 mm Hg, 2451 for mammography, and 1274 for stool for occult blood. The results for lipids and blood pressure were expressed in terms of reduction in all-cause mortality, while for mammography and occult blood they were expressed as reduction in cancer-specific mortality.

Total cohort mortality rates

An important piece of information about any study is how the total mortality rates compare in the intervention group and the control group. If a therapeutic intervention, such as a cholesterol-lowering drug, decreases cardiovascular mortality in the treated cohort, but the total death rate of that cohort is unchanged or increased because of deaths from other causes such as cancer or suicide, clinicians would be hesitant about using such a drug on their patients.[5]

Disease prevalence or severity and risk reduction

An important association exists between the severity or prevalence of a disease and the absolute risk reduction, or the number of patients who need to be screened or treated to prevent one adverse effect. The greater the severity or prevalence of the disease, the higher the absolute risk reduction and the fewer patients who must be treated to prevent one adverse outcome.[8] Clinicians must be aware of this because the relative risk reduction does not necessarily vary with prevalence rates.

The following is an illustration: 1000 high-risk patients have a disease of such lethality that 500 of them will die within 1 year without treatment. If a treatment is available that reduces the risk of death by 50% (relative risk reduction of 50%), only 250 will die, an absolute mortality reduction of 25%. In comparison, 1000 low-risk patients have a disease that will kill two of them within 1 year without treatment. If the treatment reduces the risk of death by 50% (relative risk reduction of 50%), only one will die, an absolute reduction of 0.1%. The relative reduction rate is the same in both groups, but the clinical indications for treatment probably exist only in the former. These same figures can be presented as numbers of patients who must be treated to prevent one adverse event. In the high-risk group the number is 4, while in the low-risk group it is 1000.

Effect of Benefit Reporting Methods on Decision Making of Physicians and Patients

The discrepancies between relative reduction figures and absolute reduction figures or between relative reduction figures and number of patients who must be treated to prevent one adverse event are constantly influencing clinical decisions. For example, patients frequently ask their physicians if they should take an aspirin a day to prevent heart attacks. As Smith and Egger[9] point out, in virtually all the aspirin trials for the reduction of myocardial infarction, the relative reduction rate is about 40%. Using that figure alone, physicians might be tempted to put everyone on aspirin whether or not they have evidence of vascular disease or risks for vascular disease. However, the actual numbers of patients who need to be treated for 1 year to prevent one nonfatal myocardial infarction vary tremendously. For high-risk patients, such as those who have had a previous MI, the number is 100, whereas for low-risk patients, such as healthy British physicians, it is 1000.[9] If physicians base decisions on actual numbers of patients who need to be treated, they might be less likely to prescribe aspirin for healthy low-risk individuals.

Several studies have examined the way physicians respond to the various methods of reporting clinical benefits for preventive programs. All of them show that interventions (such as prescribing lipid-lowering agents) are more likely to ensue when benefits are presented as relative reduction figures than when they are given as absolute reduction figures or as the number of patients who must be treated to prevent one adverse event.[10,11] Methods of reporting benefits also have a major influence on patient decisions to participate or not participate in certain preventive interventions.[12]

Physicians who are advising their patients must try to be judicious. They should always remember that the methods of reporting benefits lead to cognitive biases on the part of both physicians and patients. They should not forget the principle stated by Rose[13] that in mass screening programs any one individual has only a very small chance of achieving any benefit and therefore this can easily be counterbalanced by a small risk.

Sensitivity of a test

Sensitivity is the percentage of test results that are positive among patients who have the disease for which one is testing.

Specificity of a test

Specificity is the percentage of test results that are negative in patients who do not have the disease for which one is testing.

Positive predictive value

The positive predictive value is the percentage of positive test results that are true positives. The positive predictive value varies directly with the prevalence of the disorder in the population being tested. If the disorder is uncommon, most test results will be false positives even if the specificity is high. For example, Westhoff and Randall[14] have calculated that if a test were developed for the detection of ovarian cancer that had a 98% specificity (only 2% of all positive tests were false positives), the most optimistic positive predictive value of the test for women 45 to 74 years of age would be 2%. This is based on the premise that approximately 2500 women would have to be screened to find one case of ovarian cancer. Such a screening test would involve considerable morbidity for many women, even if it saved a few lives. Further examples of the relationship of disease prevalence to the positive predictive value of a test can be found under "Investigations."

Surrogate outcomes

A surrogate or intermediate outcome is one that is used in a study instead of the truly desired clinical outcome. For example, if a study on the efficacy of a lipid-lowering drug uses as an endpoint the degree by which cholesterol is lowered in the treated cohort, this is a surrogate outcome for the true endpoints, which are cardiovascular events, cardiovascular deaths, or total mortality rates. The finding of small breast cancers by mammography is a surrogate outcome for a decreased death rate from breast cancer. In a study of the diagnosis and control of gestational diabetes, the incidence of large babies is a surrogate for neonatal or maternal morbidity and mortality. No guarantee can be provided that surrogate outcomes will eventually translate into the ultimately desired clinical outcomes.[8,15]

◣ REFERENCES ◤

1. Guyatt G, Jaeschke R, Heddle N, et al: Basic statistics for clinicians. 1. Hypothesis testing, *Can Med Assoc J* 152:27-32, 1995.

2. Guyatt G, Jaeschke R, Heddle N, et al: Basic statistics for clinicians. 2. Interpreting study results: confidence intervals, *Can Med Assoc J* 152:169-173, 1995.

3. Jaeschke R, Guyatt G, Shannon H, et al: Basic statistics for clinicians. 3. Assessing the effects of treatment: measures of association, *Can Med Assoc J* 152:351-357, 1995.

4. Guyatt G, Walter S, Shannon H, et al: Basic statistics for clinicians. 4. Correlation and regression, *Can Med Assoc J* 152:497-504, 1995.

5. Marshall KG: Prevention. How much harm? How much benefit? 1. Influence of reporting methods on perception of benefits, *Can Med Assoc J* 154:1493-1499, 1996.

6. Miller DB: Secondary prevention for ischemic heart disease: relative numbers needed to treat with different therapies, *Arch Intern Med* 157:2045-2052, 1997.

7. Rembold CM: Number needed to screen: development of a statistic for disease screening, *BMJ* 317:307-312, 1998.

8. Marshall KG: Prevention. How much harm? How much benefit? 2. Ten potential pitfalls in determining the clinical significance of benefits, *Can Med Assoc J* 154:1837-1843, 1996.

9. Smith GD, Egger M: Who benefits from medical interventions? (editorial), *BMJ* 308:72-74, 1994.

10. Bobbio M, Demichelis B, Giustetto G: Completeness of reporting trial results: effect on physicians' willingness to prescribe, *Lancet* 343:1209-1211, 1994.

11. Bucher HC, Weinbacher M, Gyr K: Influence of method of reporting study results on decision of physicians to prescribe drugs to lower cholesterol concentration, *BMJ* 309:761-764, 1994.

12. Hux JE, Naylor CD: Communicating the benefits of chronic preventive therapy: does the format of efficacy data determine patients' acceptance of treatment? *Med Decision Making* 15:152-157, 1995.

13. Rose G: Sick individuals and sick populations, *Int J Epidemiol* 14:32-38, 1985.

14. Westhoff C, Randall MC: Ovarian cancer screening: potential effect on mortality, *Am J Obstet Gynecol* 165:502-505, 1991.

15. Skrabanek P, McCormick J: *Follies and fallacies in medicine,* Glasgow, 1989, Tarragon Press.

DENTISTRY

(See also hormone replacement therapy)

Topics covered in this section

NOMENCLATURE

Dentists have different ways of identifying specific teeth. A common approach in the United States is to use a numerical system for naming the 32 adult teeth and an alphabetical system for the 20 primary teeth. For adult teeth number 1 is the upper right third molar (wisdom tooth) and from there the numbers move across the upper teeth so that the upper left third molar is 16. Number 17 is the lower left third molar, and the counting then moves across the lower teeth toward the right so that the right lower third molar is 32. For the primary teeth "A" is the upper right second molar, "J" the upper left second molar, "K" the lower left second molar, and "T" the lower right second molar.[1]

An international system that is used in many parts of Canada and the rest of the world divides the adult mouth into four equal quadrants, each containing eight teeth. Each quadrant has a number:

Right upper	1
Left upper	2
Left lower	3
Right lower	4

Within each quadrant, each tooth is also given a number, so that the medial incisor is 1 and the third molar 8. By use of a double number, the first to name the quadrant and the second the tooth, each tooth can be precisely identified. Thus 2-3 is the left upper canine and 4-8 is the right lower third molar or wisdom tooth.

In the international system the quadrants of a child's mouth are labeled 5 to 8:

Right upper	5
Left upper	6
Left lower	7
Right lower	8

As in the adult, each baby tooth within a quadrant is specifically identified, but with a letter rather than a number. The medial incisor is A, the lateral incisor B, the canine C, the first molar D, and the second molar E. Thus 6-C is the left upper canine and 8-E is the right lower second molar.

◥ REFERENCES ◤

1. Clark MM, Album MM, Lloyd RW: Preventive dentistry and the family physician, *Am Fam Physician* 53:619-626, 1996.

ANTIBIOTIC PROPHYLAXIS
Endocarditis Prophylaxis

(See also prosthetic joint infection; valvular heart disease)

In 1990 the American Heart Association (AHA) drew up guidelines for the prevention of bacterial endocarditis. The AHA advised using prophylactic antibiotics for all dental interventions that cause bleeding except for the bleeding produced by injection of a local anesthetic.[1] This covered a wide variety of procedures, many of which, such as fillings, crowns, and root canals, are not associated with significant bacteremia.[2] Antibiotics were to be given both 1 hour before the procedure and 6 hours afterward. Standard protocols for adults were[1]:

Amoxicillin	3 g po 1 hour before the procedure; 1.5 g 6 hours later *or*
Erythromycin	1 g po 2 hours before the procedure; 500 mg 6 hours later *or*
Clindamycin	300 mg po 1 hour before the procedure; 150 mg 6 hours later

In 1997 the AHA revised its guidelines for the prevention of endocarditis.[3] The new guidelines state that the only persons requiring prophylaxis are those at high or moderate risk of endocarditis—patients with prosthetic heart valves, a past history of endocarditis, congenital heart disease (except for isolated secundum atrial septal defect), acquired valvular disease, and hypertrophic cardiomyopathy. Patients with mitral valve prolapse usually need antibiotics only if they have a regurgitant murmur. The specific dental procedures for which prophylaxis is recommended include extractions, dental implant placement, periodontal surgery, and scaling or cleaning associated with bleeding. Antibiotic prophylaxis is not recommended for most local anesthetics, fillings, crowns, or root canals provided the latter do not extend beyond the apex of the tooth. However, if unexpected bleeding is encountered during one of these procedures, antibiotic prophylaxis may be given if the medication is taken no later than 4 hours after the intervention.[3]

Two major antibiotic regimens are recommended by the new guidelines[3]:

| Amoxicillin | 2 g po 1 hour before the procedure (children 50 mg/kg) *or* |
| Clindamycin | 600 mg po 1 hour before the procedure (children 20 mg/kg) |

The dose of amoxicillin has been decreased from 3 to 2 g, and postprocedure antibiotics are no longer considered necessary because of their long duration of action and the short period of bacteremia. Clindamycin has replaced erythromycin as the drug of choice for patients unable to take amoxicillin, but other alternatives are cephalexin 2 g (children 50 mg/kg) or azithromycin or clarithromycin 500 mg (children 15 mg/kg), all taken po 1 hour before the procedure.[3]

When prescribing prophylactic antibiotics, practitioners should inform patients that in the vast majority of cases bacterial endocarditis of oral origin is caused by poor oral hygiene, not dental procedures.[2,3] Therefore receiving regular dental care is particularly important, and patients should not avoid going to the dentist because they do not want to take antibiotics.

All guidelines for endocarditis prophylaxis are based on expert opinion because no prospective randomized controlled trials have shown that antibacterial prophylaxis for dental procedures is effective.[3-6] Indirect evidence suggests that it is, but even if this is so, only a small proportion of cases (4% to 19%) are related to procedures for which prophylaxis is recommended.[4] A study in the Netherlands has estimated that only 6% of cases of endocarditis could be prevented if 100% of patients requiring prophylactic antibiotics received them,[5] while a U.S. case-control study concluded that antibiotic prophylaxis for dental work failed to prevent any infections and that current guidelines should be reconsidered.[6]

◣ REFERENCES ◢

1. Dajani AS, Bisno AL, Chung KF, et al: Prevention of bacterial endocarditis: recommendations by the American Heart Association, *JAMA* 264:2919-2922, 1990.
2. Wahl MJ: Myths of dental-induced endocarditis, *Arch Intern Med* 154:137-144, 1994.
3. Dajani AS, Taubert KA, Wilson W, et al: Prevention of bacterial endocarditis: recommendations by the American Heart Association, *JAMA* 277:1794-1801, 1997.
4. Durack DT: Prevention of infective endocarditis, *N Engl J Med* 332:38-44, 1995.
5. Van der Meer JTM, van Wijk W, Thompson J, et al: Efficacy of antibiotic prophylaxis for prevention of native-valve endocarditis, *Lancet* 339:135-139, 1992.
6. Strom BL, Abrutyn E, Berlin JA, et al: Dental and cardiac risk factors for infective endocarditis: a population-based, case-control study, *Ann Intern Med* 129:761-769, 1998.

Prosthetic Joint Infection Prophylaxis
(See also endocarditis prophylaxis)

Whether patients with prosthetic joints should receive prophylactic antibiotics for dental treatments is controversial. No randomized trials dealing with this issue have been published, so recommendations are based on expert opinion.[1] Rather convincing case reports indicate that prosthetic joint infection may follow invasive dental procedures, particularly in patients at elevated risk of infection because of underlying conditions such as inflammatory arthritis, diabetes, or immunosuppression. However, the numbers involved are small, and how many cases of infection are prevented by antibiotic prophylaxis is unknown. Furthermore, morbidity from reactions to antibiotics might outweigh possible benefits.[2] In 1997 the American Academy of Orthopaedic Surgeons and the American Dental Association recommended against routine antibiotic prophylaxis for patients with joint arthroplasties but advised that prophylaxis might be considered for all patients during the first 2 years after arthroplasty placement and indefinitely for patients at elevated risk of infection. Such prophylaxis should be given only for dental procedures that are associated with an elevated risk of bacteremia (see previous discussion of endocarditis prophylaxis).[3]

◣ REFERENCES ◢

1. Uyemura MC: Antibiotic prophylaxis for medical and dental procedures: a look at AHA guidelines and controversial issues, *Postgrad Med* 98:137-140, 147, 151-152, 1995.

2. LaPorte DM, Waldman BJ, Mont MA, et al: Infections associated with dental procedures in total hip arthroplasty, *J Bone Joint Surg [Br]* 81-B:56-59, 1999.
3. American Dental Association: American Academy of Orthopaedic Surgeons: advisory statement: antibiotic prophylaxis for dental patients with total joint replacements, *J Am Dent Assoc* 128:1004-1007, 1997.

ANTICOAGULANTS

(See also anticoagulants in hematology section)

Because of an increased risk of thromboembolism, discontinuing anticoagulants before dental procedures such as extractions or gingival and alveolar surgery may be dangerous. The international normalized ratio (INR) should be maintained in the therapeutic range; any bleeding that occurs can be controlled by local measures.[1]

⚡ REFERENCES ⚡

1. Wahl MJ: Dental surgery in anticoagulated patients, *Arch Intern Med* 158:1610-1616, 1998.

AVULSED TOOTH

An avulsed tooth that is reimplanted within 30 minutes will survive in 90% of cases. After 30 minutes the success rate decreases by about 1% per minute. The avulsed tooth should be held by the crown, rinsed off in water (with a plug in the sink so that it is not lost down the drain), and reimplanted. The patient can hold it in place by biting gently on it through an overlying piece of gauze until he or she is seen by a dentist. If the physician or patient is unable to replace the tooth in the socket, it should rinsed and transported to the dentist in milk or water. Primary teeth need not be reimplanted.[1]

⚡ REFERENCES ⚡

1. Clark MM, Album MM, Lloyd RW: Medical care of the dental patient, *Am Fam Physician* 52:1126-1132, 1995.

DENTAL ABSCESS

A dental abscess can often be diagnosed by percussing the suspected tooth to see if this elicits pain. The emergency treatment of dental abscesses is penicillin plus analgesics.[1]

⚡ REFERENCES ⚡

1. Clark MM, Album MM, Lloyd RW: Medical care of the dental patient, *Am Fam Physician* 52:1126-1132, 1995.

DRUGS AND ORAL HEALTH

Any drug that inhibits salivation is likely to increase the incidence of dental caries, periodontal disease, and oral infections. Antidepressants, particularly tricyclics, are an important cause of this phenomenon. Patients taking such drugs should participate in a regimen of optimal oral hygiene, including use of fluorides. Salivary flow between meals may be stimulated by taking vitamin C tablets or chewing sugar-free gum. If the problem is serious, attempts should be made to change medications.[1]

⚡ REFERENCES ⚡

1. Peeters FP, deVries MW, Vissink A: Risk for oral health with the use of antidepressants, *Gen Hosp Psychiatry* 20:150-154, 1998.

FLUORIDES

The amount of fluoride children should receive and the ages at which it should be administered are controversial issues. Because a significant amount of fluoride is present in toothpaste, mouthwash, and even soft drinks and juices reconstituted with fluoridated water, many young children receive their daily fluoride requirements in this fashion even if their drinking water is not fluoridated. There is fear that excessive supplementation could lead to fluorosis.[1] Degrees of fluorosis vary; most cases in North America are so mild that the alterations in the enamel are visible only to experts.[2,3]

The optimal fluoridation levels of the water supply should be 0.6 or 0.7 to 1.2 ppm.[2-5] If the levels are below that, supplementation is indicated. The recommended doses and age at onset of supplementation vary according to both the fluoride level of the water supply and the viewpoints of the issuing organizations.[1-4] The trend has been to initiate fluoride supplementation later in life (2 to 3 years) and to give lower doses than were previously the case. This is done not only to prevent fluorosis, but also because the traditional view that fluorides had to be incorporated into the tooth enamel before tooth eruption is false and therefore administration of the agent can be delayed until after tooth eruption.[2,3] The American Academy of Pediatrics advises no supplementation before the age of 6 months regardless of the concentration of fluorides in the water; they recommend that from 6 months to 3 years children receive 0.25 mg/day only if the water supply fluorides are less than 0.3 ppm.[5] The Canadian Dental Association goes further and recommends no supplementation before the age of 3 years regardless of the fluoride concentration of the water.[2,3]

Whether or not fluoride supplements are given, young children should brush their teeth twice daily under adult supervision using only a pea-sized amount of (fluoridated) toothpaste, and they should be taught to spit it out, not swallow it.[1-3]

The Canadian Task Force on Preventive Health Care updated its evaluation of dental caries in 1995.[6] It gave "A" recommendations for fluoridation of the water supply, the use of fluoride dentifrices, daily fluoride supplementation when the water is not fluoridated, and annual or biannual professional application of topical fluorides. The latter is effective but costly and is therefore not recommended for the general populace. The U.S. Preventive Services Task Force also gives an "A" recommendation to fluoride supplementation if the fluoride concentration in the water supply is inadequate.[7]

❧ REFERENCES ❧

1. Raves J: MDS call for more study before endorsing dentists' new recommendations on fluoride, *Can Med Assoc J* 149:1820-1822, 1993.
2. Clark DC: Appropriate uses of fluorides for children: guidelines from the Canadian Workshop on the Evaluation of Current Recommendations Concerning Fluorides, *Can Med Assoc J* 149: 1787-1793, 1993.
3. Clark DC: Appropriate use of fluorides in the 1990s, *J Can Dent Assoc* 59:272-279, 1993.
4. Jakush J: New fluoride schedule adopted, *ADA News* 25:12, 14, 1994.
5. American Academy of Pediatrics Committee on Nutrition: Fluoride supplementation for children: interim policy recommendations, *Pediatrics* 95:777, 1995.
6. Lewis DW, Ismail AI (Canadian Task Force on the Periodic Health Examination): Periodic health examination, 1995 update. 2. Prevention of dental caries, *Can Med Assoc J* 152:836-846, 1995.
7. US Preventive Services Task Force: *Guide to clinical preventive services,* ed 2, Baltimore, 1996, Williams & Wilkins, pp 711-721.

PAIN

Nonsteroidal antiinflammatory drugs are, in general, the analgesics of choice for dental pain.[1]

❧ REFERENCES ❧

1. Seymour RA, Walton JG: Analgesic efficacy in dental pain, *Br Dent J* 153:291-298, 1982.

PERIODONTITIS

Gingivitis is inflammation that is limited to the gums. Periodontitis is inflammation of the gums that has extended into the periodontal area, causing destruction of periodontal ligaments and eventual loosening (loss of attachment) of affected teeth. As periodontitis advances, the gums recede and retract from around the roots of affected teeth, forming pockets. The process can be localized or generalized. In its most common form, periodontitis is a disease of older individuals. Smoking and diabetes are additional risk factors. Bacterial organisms play a significant role in the disease, although which of the many hundreds of species that inhabit the gums are primarily responsible is unknown. The goal of treatment is good oral hygiene in the form of brushing, flossing, and professional removal of calculus to reduce the bacteria that may populate periodontal pockets. Adjuvant measures are smoking cessation, 2-minute mouthwashes twice a day with agents such as 0.2% chlorhexidine, in some cases antibiotic treatment with one of the tetracyclines, and in more advanced cases surgery.[1]

❧ REFERENCES ❧

1. Watts TL: Periodontitis for medical practitioners, *BMJ* 316: 993-996, 1998.

DERMATOLOGY

(See also pruritus ani)

Topics covered in this section

Acne Vulgaris
Actinic Keratoses
Alopecia
Contact Dermatitis
Folliculitis
Hand-Foot-and-Mouth Disease
Hidradenitis Suppurativa
Hirsutism
Hyperhidrosis Palmaris
Melanoma
Pediculosis Pubis and Pediculosis Capitis
Phytophotodermatitis
Port-Wine Stains
Psoriasis
Rosacea
Scabies
Scalp Lotions, Steroid
Scalp Shampoos, Medicated
Seabather's Eruption
Sun Damage
Swimmer's Itch
Tattoos
Tinea
Topical Steroids
Ulcers, Dermal
Urticaria and Angioedema
Warts
Wrinkles and Skin Aging

ACNE VULGARIS

(See also oral contraceptives; polycystic ovarian syndrome)

About 80% of the population suffers from some degree of acne between the ages of 11 and 30. Acne develops earlier in girls than boys but affects boys more frequently and more severely.[1,2]

Pathogenesis

The basic pathogenetic factors in acne are an increased desquamation of epithelial cells, which block the follicular orifices, and an increased production of sebum. Sebum accumulating behind the obstruction favors the growth of *Propionibacterium acnes,* which is a normal commensal within the pilosebaceous units. *P. acnes* secretes lipolytic enzymes, leading to the release of free fatty acids, as well as secreting chemotactic factors that attract neutrophils. The hydrolytic enzymes of the neutrophils damage the follicular wall, and these, as well as the free fatty acids, are released into the tissues, causing inflammation.[1-3]

Clinical Manifestations

A whitehead or closed comedone is caused by accumulation of sebum behind a plugged pilosebaceous follicle. Continued distention leads to a partial protrusion from the follicular opening, which has the clinical appearance of an opened comedone or blackhead. The black color of a blackhead is due to melanin and oxidized lipids, not dirt. Once the sebaceous contents rupture into the dermis, the pattern becomes one of inflammatory acne with papule, and in more severe cases nodule or "cyst," formation. Acne usually develops at puberty when androgens stimulate the sebaceous follicles.[1-3] Premenstrual flares of acne are common because the follicular orifices become more obstructed at that time of the cycle.[1,2]

Specific Etiological Factors

Endocrine disorders with excess androgen production such as polycystic ovarian syndrome and Cushing's syndrome can cause acne. Medications known to be associated with acne include corticosteroids, androgens, certain oral contraceptives containing antiestrogenic progestins, phenytoin, barbiturates, lithium, isoniazid, cyclosporine, iodides, and bromides. Oil-based cosmetics and occupational exposure to oils are other known precipitants.[1]

Principles of Acne Vulgaris Therapy

Diet has no influence on acne. Vigorous scrubbing of the affected areas may aggravate rather than ameliorate the situation.[2] Gentle washing (20 minutes before the application of topical medications) is all that is required.[1,2]

Oil-based cosmetics and moisturizers should be avoided. If the patient insists on using cosmetics, they should be water based.[1]

Gels are more potent than creams. Gels are better for oily skin or for hot, humid climates, while creams are better for sensitive skins and cold, dry climates.[1,2]

Topical therapy should be started at low doses for short periods. Some drying, erythema, and scaling are to be expected. If they are not excessive, the duration of application is increased to 8 to 12 hours. The concentrations of topical medications may be increased, if necessary, at 4- to 8-week intervals.[1,2] A therapeutic response to any treatment modality may take 2 months.[1,2]

Blackheads may be removed with a comedone extractor, and whiteheads with a no. 25 needle. Comedone extraction hastens the resolution of the disorder.[1]

Most of the pharmacological agents target one or more of three pathogenetic mechanisms of acne production—excessive sebum production (estrogens, isotretinoin, spironolactone); abnormal desquamation of epithelial cells (isotretinoin, tretinoin, adapalene, azelaic acid, benzoyl peroxide); or *P. acnes* (antibiotics, benzoyl peroxide, azelaic acid).[2]

Sequence of Therapeutic Regimens in the Treatment of Acne Vulgaris

For noninflammatory acne the initial regimen of choice is tretinoin (Retin-A) or adapalene (Differin). These drugs decrease the adhesiveness of follicular epithelial cells and increase cell turnover. By doing this they inhibit the formation of comedones and hasten the expulsion of those already formed. Treatment should start with once-daily low doses and increase gradually.[3,4] The maximum benefit from tretinoin may not be evident for 3 to 4 months.[3] Adapalene is as effective as tretinoin but causes less irritation.[4] For patients with both comedonal and papulopustular acne a combination of tretinoin and a topical antibiotic such as erythromycin (Stievamycin) or tretinoin and a systemic antibiotic should be given.[2]

For mild papulopustular acne, benzoyl peroxide (Panoxyl, Desquam-X, Dermoxyl, Loroxide), a topical antibiotic such as erythromycin (Staticin), clindamycin (Cleocin T, Dalacin T), or a combination of erythromycin and benzoyl peroxide (Benzamycin) is the agent of first choice.[2,3] Benzoyl peroxide not only is a potent antibacterial agent that inhibits *P. acnes*, but also has mild comedolytic and exfoliant properties. If both tretinoin and benzoyl peroxide are used, one should be applied in the morning and the other in the evening. If a combination of tretinoin and 10% benzoyl peroxide is not effective or not tolerated, a topical antibiotic may be substituted for benzoyl peroxide. The topical antibiotic should not be applied at the same time as the tretinoin unless it is in a commercial formulation such as Stievamycin that combines tretinoin and erythromycin. A new topical antibacterial agent with some effect on comedogenesis is azelaic acid (Azelex).[2,3]

If tretinoin plus a topical antibiotic is ineffective, the patient requires oral antibiotics.[1] The oral antibiotics of choice are doxycycline (Vibra-Tabs) or minocycline (Minocin) in daily doses of 50 to 200 mg, or trimethoprim-sulfamethoxazole (Septra, Bactrim) as one regular tablet daily or bid or one double-strength tablet daily. Alternatives, which are probably less effective, are tetracycline and erythromycin. In general, the dose should not be reduced for 2 to 4 months.[2] Although concomitant use of antibiotics and oral contraceptives has been commonly believed to decrease the efficacy of the contraceptives, there is no good evidence supporting this claim in terms of the usual antibiotics for treating acne.[5] In cases of moderate or severe inflammatory acne the initial treatment should include oral antibiotics.[1,2] A 1999 case-control study has reported that a lupuslike syndrome is a rare complication of minocycline.[6]

Isotretinoin (Accutane) is an oral retinoid that is effective for widespread, severe, nodular cystic lesions. It is teratogenic, so proof that the patient is not pregnant and is using effective measures to prevent conception is essential before starting it.[3,7] Specifically, all women of childbearing age should be given verbal and written instructions about the teratogenic effect of the drug, have a negative pregnancy test before the drug is prescribed, start therapy after the second or third day of the next normal menstrual period, and preferably use two forms of contraception.[7] The usual treatment regimen is 4 to 5 months at a dosage of 0.1 to 1 mg/kg/day. Continued improvement may be noted for 4 to 5 months after the completion of therapy. Only 15% of patients require a second course of the drug.[3]

For women, spironolactone (Aldactone) 25 to 200 mg/day or oral contraceptives may help control acne. Third-generation oral contraceptives containing "selective" progestins such as desogestrel (Marvelon, Ortho-Cept) or norgestimate (Cyclen, Tri-Cyclen) are often recommended for acne treatment because they are thought to have few androgenic side effects. Beneficial effects may take 2 to 4 months to appear, and relapses commonly occur after the agents are discontinued.[2,3]

❧ REFERENCES ❧

1. Nguyen QH, Kim YA, Schwartz RA: Management of acne vulgaris, *Am Fam Physician* 50:89-96, 1994.
2. Leyden JJ: Therapy for acne vulgaris, *N Engl J Med* 336:1156-1162, 1997.
3. Brown SK, Shalita AR: Acne vulgaris, *Lancet* 351:1871-1876, 1998.
4. Adapalene for acne, *Med Lett* 39:19-20, 1997.
5. Rasmussen JE: The effect of antibiotics on the efficacy of oral contraceptives, *Arch Dermatol* 125:1562-1564, 1989.
6. Sturkenboom MC, Meier CR, Jick H, et al: Minocycline and lupuslike syndrome in acne patients, *Arch Intern Med* 159:493-497, 1999.
7. Atanackovic G, Koren G: Motherisk update: young women taking isotretinoin still conceive; role of physicians in preventing disaster, *Can Fam Physician* 45:289-292, 1999.

ACTINIC KERATOSES

Over a 10-year period about 10% of actinic keratoses develop into low-grade squamous cell carcinomas.[1] Such carcinomas rarely metastasize.[2] Not all actinic keratoses progress; some remain unchanged, and others undergo spontaneous regression.[2]

The treatment of choice for isolated lesions is destruction, usually with liquid nitrogen. Multiple lesions may be treated with topical 5-fluorouracil (5-FU, Efudex, Fluoroplex) or topical tretinoin (Retin-A).[1,2]

5-FU is applied twice daily (with gloves or a wooden spatula[1]) in concentrations of 1% to 2% for the face and lips and 5% for the scalp, neck, arms, hands, chest, and back.[2] The usual duration of therapy is 3 weeks for the face and lips and 4 to 8 weeks for other areas of the body.[2] Erythematous and necrotic reactions beginning 5 to 15 days after the onset of therapy are the norm. The degree of inflammation is aggravated by sun exposure and can be somewhat ameliorated by applying a moderate-potency topical steroid. One way of decreasing the degree of inflammation is to use lower concentrations of 5-FU (0.1% to 0.9%), but if this is done, treatment must continue until the last lesion resolves, which may take 2 to 3 months. Residual lesions may be treated with higher concentrations of 5-FU or by cryosurgery.[1] Another way of decreasing inflammation is to use a "pulsing" schedule in which 5% 5-FU is applied once or twice a week for 6 to 8 weeks.[2]

A once daily application of 0.1% tretinoin cream may be used to treat actinic keratoses, but applications have to continue for 12 to 15 months or even longer.[2]

❧ REFERENCES ❧

1. Schwartz RA: Therapeutic perspectives in actinic and other keratoses, *Int J Dermatol* 35:533-538, 1996.
2. Odom R: Managing actinic keratoses with retinoids, *J Am Acad Dermatol* 39:S74-S78, 1998.

ALOPECIA
Telogen Effluvium

A common cause of diffuse hair loss is telogen effluvium. This is hair loss resulting from psychological, physiological, or pathological stress. The disorder usually declares itself 2 to 4 months after the precipitating event, and up to 50% of hair may be lost. Specific causes include childbirth; surgery and anesthesia; crash dieting; infections; hypothyroidism; a variety of drugs, including antidepressants, lithium, beta-blockers, angiotensin-converting enzyme (ACE) inhibitors, and anticoagulants; and discontinuation of oral contraceptives. Hair regrows in 2 to 3 months if the precipitating condition is no longer present.[1]

Trichotillomania and Alopecia Areata

In trichotillomania broken-off hairs may be seen in the region of the alopecia. Patients with alopecia areata have "exclamation point" hairs around the periphery of the bald spots.[1] A variety of treatments may be used for alopecia areata: intralesional glucocorticoid injections, topical glucocorticoids, 5% topical minoxidil (Rogaine), topical anthralin, and topical immunotherapy (an experimental procedure available in only a few centers).[2]

Male Pattern Androgenic Alopecia

Male pattern alopecia is common; 30% of white men are affected by age 30 and 50% by age 50. Whites are affected four times as often as blacks.[3] The inheritance pattern is thought to be polygenic.[2]

The standard topical medication for male pattern baldness is minoxidil (Rogaine) applied to the scalp twice a day. If benefits ensue, they persist only as long as the drug continues to be applied.[2,3] About 15% of treated men have a medium regrowth of hair, 50% note a delay of further hair loss, and 35% have continuing hair loss. Dense hair growth is rare. In view of the data the main benefit of minoxidil appears to be a delay in further hair loss.[3] A 5% solution of minoxidil (Rogaine Extra Strength for Men) has recently been marketed; hair counts have shown the 5% solution to be more effective than the 2% solution,[2] but whether this translates into a clinically important improvement is uncertain.[4]

Another pharmacological approach to male pattern baldness is the use of finasteride (Propecia) 1 mg/day po (the trade name for finasteride 5 mg, used to treat benign prostatic hyperplasia, is Proscar). This drug decreases the level of circulating dihydrotestosterone by inhibiting the enzyme 5-alpha-reductase, which is necessary for the conversion of testosterone to the more potent dihydrotestosterone. After 2 years of treatment with finasteride two thirds of men have hair regrowth and almost all of the remaining have no further hair loss.[2,3] Some benefit may be noted within 4 months of initiating treatment, but a full 24-month trial should be undertaken before a final decision is made about the efficacy of the drug. Treatment must be continued indefinitely to maintain benefits, and for some individuals continuing treatment beyond 2 years may lead to even further scalp coverage.[2] Decreased libido is a rare but significant side effect that is reversible when the drug is discontinued.[3]

The most frequently used surgical treatment of male pattern baldness is hair transplantation from the occiput to the frontal and vertex areas. The transplanted follicles maintain their resistance to androgenic alopecia. Other surgical techniques involve excision of bald areas and the use of scalp flaps.[3]

Female Androgenetic Alopecia

Female androgenetic alopecia is common in women and is manifested as diffuse hair loss in the temporoparietal region and a more than usually apparent central part. The frontal hairline is usually maintained. Treatment of this condition with 2% minoxidil has resulted in minimal hair growth in about half of patients and moderate hair growth in 13%[5]; 5% minoxidil is no more effective than the 2% solution.[2] Women with androgenic alopecia do not require an endocrinological workup unless there is evidence of virilism. They can be reassured that they will not become bald and that dyes, hair sprays, and permanents will not harm their hair.[2]

REFERENCES

1. Nielsen TA, Reichel M: Alopecia: diagnosis and management, *Am Fam Physician* 51:1513-1522, 1995.
2. Price VH: Treatment of hair loss, *N Engl J Med* 341:964-973, 1999.
3. Sinclair R: Male pattern androgenetic alopecia, *BMJ* 317:865-869, 1998.
4. Propecia and Rogaine Extra Strength for alopecia, *Med Lett* 40:25-27, 1998.
5. De Villez RL, Jacobs JP, Szpunar CA, et al: Androgenetic alopecia in the female: treatment with 2% topical minoxidil solution, *Arch Dermatol* 130:303-307, 1994.

CONTACT DERMATITIS

A common cause of contact dermatitis from earrings, watches, or eyeglass frames is nickel allergy. One method of preventing the contact is to coat the offending object with clear nail polish and let it dry. Repeat applications every 2 to 8 weeks are usually required.[1]

REFERENCES

1. Gore BQ: For nickel allergy, *Patient Care Can* 7(3):22, 1996.

FOLLICULITIS

Patients with recurrent staphylococcal skin infections tend to reinfect themselves through nasal carriage of the organism. In one study a monthly 5-day course of mupirocin (Bactroban) ointment applied to the nose over a 1-year period resulted in fewer recurrent skin infections than were seen in the placebo control group.[1]

REFERENCES

1. Raz R, Miron D, Colodner R, et al: A 1-year trial of nasal mupirocin in the prevention of recurrent staphylococcal nasal colonization and skin infection, *Arch Intern Med* 156:1109-1112, 1996.

HAND-FOOT-AND-MOUTH DISEASE

Hand-foot-and-mouth disease is caused by coxsackievirus A16. Outbreaks tend to occur in the late summer and fall. Vesicles in the mouth are usually the initial manifestation, followed by vesicles surrounded by erythema on the hands and feet. The buttocks may also be involved, and some children have fever. Lesions resolve in 3 to 7 days; treatment is symptomatic.[1]

REFERENCES

1. Adams SP: Dermacase: hand-foot-and-mouth disease, *Can Fam Physician* 44:985-993, 1998.

HIDRADENITIS SUPPURATIVA

Hidradenitis suppurativa, a chronic inflammatory condition of apocrine-bearing regions of the skin, most frequently affects the axillary, inguinal, buttock, or perineal regions. Women are more often affected than men. The disorder rarely occurs before puberty and often diminishes in severity at the time of menopause. Initially, small nodules may develop in the affected regions, and these sometimes drain spontaneously. With time numerous nodules and sinus tracts develop. Multiple open comedones (blackheads) may be seen. Treatment is difficult. Some patients respond to prolonged courses of topical or oral antibiotics. Clindamycin seems particularly useful. Isotretinoin has been tried, but the results of studies have been equivocal. In more severe cases wide surgical excision of the diseased area is the therapeutic option of choice.[1]

REFERENCES

1. Brown TJ, Rosen T, Orengo IF: Hidradenitis suppurativa, *South Med J* 91:1107-1114, 1998.

HIRSUTISM
(See also Cushing's syndrome; oral contraceptives; polycystic ovarian syndrome)

More than 95% of cases of hirsutism are idiopathic or secondary to polycystic ovarian syndrome.[1] Other causes include late-onset congenital adrenal hyperplasia, Cushing's syndrome, testosterone-secreting tumors, starvation, anorexia nervosa, obesity (sometimes), and drugs (progestins in some oral contraceptive pills, danazol, phenytoin, minoxidil).[1,2]

Source of Androgens
The ovary produces testosterone, androstenedione, and dehydroepiandrosterone (DHEA). The adrenal gland also produces these, as well as the sulfated form of DHEA (DHEA-S). Testosterone is 99% bound to sex hormone–binding globulin, and only the free portion is biologically active. In some obese women, sex hormone–binding globulin is decreased and hirsutism is related to weight gain.[2]

Investigations
The main purpose of investigating patients with hirsutism is to rule out ominous causes of the condition. In general, investigations are not indicated for patients whose clinical picture is associated with a benign cause of hirsutism. Such patients are usually between the ages of 15 and 25, have had hirsutism for more than a year (not a rapid new onset), and have no evidence of virilization. Investigations are required for the small group of women who do not have this clinical pattern. In particular, investigations should be carried out if the onset of hirsutism is rapid, if there are signs of virilism (frontal balding, voice deepening, increased muscle mass, clitoromegaly), or if Cushing's syndrome is suspected.[1]

It is not important clinically to distinguish among idiopathic hirsutism, polycystic ovarian syndrome, and late-onset congenital adrenal hyperplasia, all of which may be associated with mild elevations of testosterone level (usually less than twice the normal value). When indicated, initial investigations should include the following[1,2]:
1. Total testosterone. Levels greater than twice the normal value suggest a tumor.[2]
2. Dehydroepiandrosterone sulfate (DHEA-S). Levels greater than twice the normal value suggest a tumor.[2]
3. 17-Hydroxyprogesterone. Blood for this assay should be drawn in the early morning. The level is usually significantly elevated in patients with the more common and innocuous forms of congenital adrenal hyperplasia.[1]
4. Dexamethasone suppression test, urine and serum cortisol levels. If Cushing's syndrome is suspected, appropriate investigations should be undertaken (see discussion of Cushing's disease).

Treatment of Benign Forms of Hirsutism
Methods of treating benign forms of hirsutism include weight loss (if obese), electrolysis, birth control pills, and spironolactone (Aldactone). If birth control pills are chosen, they should have a low-androgen progestin, such as desogestrel or norgestimate, which are found in the third-generation oral contraceptives (see discussion of oral contraceptives). The usual dosage of spironolactone is 50 to 100 mg/day or even 200 mg/day in 2 divided doses. This drug may cause hyperkalemia. Androgen-suppressing drugs such as flutamide (Euflex) and finasteride (Proscar) have also been used to treat hirsutism.[2]

Electrolysis involves treating hair follicles one at a time, so treatment schedules may go on for weeks or years. A newly developed alternative for dark hairs is laser treatment. The melanin in dark hairs absorbs a spectrum of laser wavelengths, generating heat and selectively destroying the follicles. Fewer sessions are required than with electrolysis. As yet no large well-designed studies of this procedure have been completed.[3]

──────────── ◥ REFERENCES ◤ ────────────
1. McKennal TJ: Screening for sinister causes of hirsutism (editorial), *N Engl J Med* 331:1015-1016, 1994.
2. Kalve E, Klein J: Evaluation of women with hirsutism, *Am Fam Physician* 54:117-124, 1996.
3. Laser hair removal, *Med Lett* 41:68-69, 1999.

HYPERHIDROSIS PALMARIS
A solution of aluminum chloride hexahidride 20% (Drysol) may be used to treat sweaty palms. The usual regimen is to apply the medication to the palms qhs for 3 nights and to wear polyethylene gloves all night. The maintenance regimen is the same program once or twice a week.[1]

──────────── ◥ REFERENCES ◤ ────────────
1. Hurley HF: Questions and answers, *JAMA* 259:3325, 1988.

MELANOMA
(See also sun damage)

The risk of melanoma increases with increased sun exposure, either in adulthood[1] or in childhood.[2] A number of studies have found that unlike squamous cell carcinoma of the skin, intermittent sun exposure is a greater risk factor for melanoma than is regular prolonged exposure. The explanation for this is unknown. Sunburn has been called a risk factor for melanoma, but supporting evidence is tenuous. For outdoor activity, sunscreens should probably be applied even though they have not been proved to protect against melanoma. Sunscreens should not be used as an excuse for increasing the duration of sun exposure (see discussion of sun damage). Currently the best protection against melanoma is to limit one's exposure to harmful rays.[3]

Some types of nevi are risk factors for melanoma. Multiple small nondysplastic nevi are associated with a slight increase in risk, but the presence of 10 or more dysplastic nevi increases the risk 12 fold. Dysplastic nevi are flat and have a diameter greater than 5 mm, irregular poorly defined borders, an asymmetrical appearance, and variable color.[3]

REFERENCES

1. Elwood M, Jopson J: Melanoma and sun exposure: an overview of published studies, *Int J Cancer* 73:198-203, 1997.
2. Autier P, Doré J-F (EPIMEL and EORTC Melanoma Cooperative Group): Influence of sun exposures during childhood and during adulthood on melanoma risk, *Int J Cancer* 77:533-537, 1998.
3. Finkel E: Sorting the hype from the facts in melanoma, *Lancet* 351:1866, 1998.
4. Tucker MA, Halpern A, Holly EA, et al: Clinically recognized dysplastic nevi: a central risk factor for cutaneous melanoma, *JAMA* 277:1439-1444, 1997.

PEDICULOSIS PUBIS AND PEDICULOSIS CAPITIS

Transmission of head lice is usually by direct contact (head to head) and rarely if ever through fomites.[1] A 1% solution of permethrin (Nix Creme Rinse) is the pharmacological treatment of choice for pediculosis pubis and capitis.[2,3] After the area is shampooed, rinsed, and dried, the permethrin solution is applied in sufficient quantities to saturate the area and is left in place for 10 minutes before being rinsed off with water. Although a single treatment is sufficient to kill both the nits and the adult lice, many experts recommend a second treatment 7 to 10 days later as insurance.[1] Unfortunately, there is evidence that lice in the United States are becoming resistant to permethrin.[3] Although lindane (Kwellada) might be chosen as an alternative to permethrin, one systematic review concluded that there is insufficient evidence of benefit to justify using the drug.[4]

The policy of some schools that children must be free of nits before returning is not based on scientific evidence and should be discouraged. However, if the school insists on this policy, nits can be removed by applying a damp towel to the scalp for 30 to 60 minutes (or by applying a mixture of equal parts water and white vinegar to the scalp, which is then covered with a damp towel soaked in the same material for 15 minutes), followed by combing with a fine-toothed comb.[1]

Pesticides are not always needed to control pediculosis capitis. An alternative is to wash the hair with ordinary shampoo and then add conditioner. Immediately afterward, while the hair is still wet, it is combed thoroughly with a fine-toothed comb. The procedure is repeated every 3 or 4 days for a total of four shampoos and combings over a 2-week period. Wetting the hair slows down the lice, and conditioner makes the hair slippery so they have difficulty gripping the shafts. Thus the initial combing removes all adult and nymphal lice. Subsequent shampooing and combing remove further nymphal lice that have hatched from the nits (incubation period of 7 to 10 days) before they mature, mate, and lay still more eggs.[5]

REFERENCES

1. Infectious Diseases and Immunization Committee of the Canadian Paediatric Society: Head lice infestations: a persistent itchy "pest," *Paediatr Child Health* 1:237-240, 1996.
2. Drugs for parasitic infections, *Med Lett* 37:99-108, 1995.
3. Pollack RJ, Kiszewski A, Armstrong P, et al: Differential permethrin susceptibility of head lice sampled in the United States and Borneo, *Arch Pediatr Adolesc Med* 153:969-973, 1999.
4. Vander Stichele RH, Dezeure EM, Bogaert MG: Systematic review of clinical efficacy of topical treatments for head lice, *BMJ* 311:604-608, 1995.
5. Ibarra J, Hall DM: Head lice in schoolchildren, *Arch Dis Child* 75:471-473, 1996.

PHYTOPHOTODERMATITIS

Limes and lemons may be a cause of phytophotodermatitis. Erythema, vesicles, or bullae occur hours to days after contact with the fruit and may take weeks or months to resolve.[1]

REFERENCES

1. Goskowicz MO, Friedlander SF, Eichenfield LF: Endemic "lime" disease phytophotodermatitis in San Diego County, *Pediatrics* 93:828-830, 1994.

PORT-WINE STAINS

Vascular skin lesions, including port-wine stains, can often be treated effectively by lasers, but the recurrence rate is high.[1]

REFERENCES

1. Cosmetic surgery with lasers, *Med Lett* 39:10-11, 1997.

PSORIASIS
(See also psoriatic arthritis; topical steroids)

The common form of psoriasis is plaque psoriasis. Other variants are guttate, pustular, and arthritic psoriasis. Unless otherwise specified, this section deals with plaque psoriasis. Psoriasis affects between 1% and 3% of all individuals. The two peak ages of onset are the late teens to early twenties and the late fifties to early sixties. The natural history is one of exacerbations and remissions. Factors known to exacerbate psoriasis are trauma to the skin (physical, sunburn, or infection), psychological stress, and certain drugs. Drug classes to avoid prescribing, if possible, for patients with psoriasis are beta-blockers, ACE inhibitors, indomethacin, lithium, and antimalarials.[1]

A variety of treatment options are available for the control of psoriasis. Avoidance of precipitating factors is common to all of them. If lesions are sparse and do not bother the patient, no treatment is needed. If less than 20% of the body is involved, topical agents are often effective, but if more than 20% is involved, systemic therapy may be required from the onset.[1]

Frequently used topical agents are corticosteroids, the vitamin D analogue calcipotriene, which is also called calcipotriol (Dovonex), and the retinoid tazarotene (Tazorac). In general, medium-strength corticosteroids are used on the torso and extremities and low-potency drugs on the face, genitals, and flexural areas. High-potency corticosteroids should be used for only short periods on lesions of palms or soles or on individual plaques that do not respond to usual treatment. With continued use the efficacy of corticosteroids diminishes (tachyphylaxis), and sometimes a flare occurs when the drug is discontinued. Tachyphylaxis can be minimized by switching to less potent formulations as soon as possible or by using the corticosteroids intermittently. Lotions or gels should be used for scalp lesions. Calcipotriene is as effective as midpotency corticosteroids, and tachyphylaxis does not occur. It should not be applied to the face or groin. Tazarotene gives excellent results, often with an extended response, and it can be safely used on the face. It may be teratogenic, so strict precautions to prevent pregnancy are essential if it is used by women of childbearing age. Other topical agents that may be used are coal tar preparations and anthralin; both may stain the skin and clothes.[2]

Systemic therapies and phototherapies are usually administered by or in conjunction with a dermatologist. They include ultraviolet B phototherapy combined with topical tars or anthralin, ultraviolet A phototherapy combined with the photosensitizing drug methoxsalen, methotrexate, and in some cases cyclosporine.[1]

REFERENCES

1. Greaves MW, Weinstein GD: Treatment of psoriasis, *N Engl J Med* 332:581-588, 1995.
2. Federman DG, Froelich CW, Kirsner RS: Topical psoriasis therapy, *Am Fam Physician* 59:957-962, 1999.

ROSACEA

Acne rosacea has four classic phases. These are[1,2]:
1. Facial flushing
2. Persistent erythema with telangiectasias
3. Inflammatory lesions (papules, pustules, nodules)
4. Rhinophyma

Factors that aggravate acne rosacea include exposure to heat or cold, exposure to sunlight, and ingestion of alcohol and hot spicy foods. Patients with rosacea must avoid these precipitants.[1] Standard drug therapy is oral antibiotics, which are particularly effective in the papular and pustular phase of rosacea. First-line therapy is tetracycline (Achromycin) or tetracycline derivatives such as minocycline (Minocin) and doxycycline (Vibramycin). A suggested initial dosage of tetracycline is 1 g/day in divided doses for 2 to 3 weeks followed by 0.5 g/day for another 2 to 3 weeks. If a good response is not obtained, second-line drugs such as trimethoprim-sulfamethoxazole (Septra, Bactrim) or oral metronidazole (Flagyl) may be used.[2] Adding topical metronidazole to the oral antibiotic regimen is often advisable.[3]

Topical 0.75% metronidazole cream or gel applied twice a day may be used alone for the treatment of mild or even moderate rosacea. In more severe cases remission induced by antibiotics and topical metronidazole may be maintained by topical metronidazole alone. With this regimen both inflammatory lesions and erythema are lessened.[3]

REFERENCES

1. Thiboutot DM: Acne rosacea, *Am Fam Physician* 50:1691-1697, 1994.
2. Wilkin JK: Rosacea: pathophysiology and treatment (editorial), *Arch Dermatol* 130:359-362, 1994.
3. Dahl MV, Katz I, Krueger GG, et al: Topical metronidazole maintains remission of rosacea, *Arch Dermatol* 134:679-683, 1998.

SCABIES

Permethrin 5% (Nix Dermal Cream) is the treatment of choice for scabies, whereas Nix Creme Rinse is used for pediculosis capitis and pubis.[1] The usual way to apply Nix Dermal Cream is to wash and dry the skin and rub in the cream from head (except scalp) to toe over all parts of the body; 30 g will do for the average adult. It should be washed off after 12 to 14 hours. A single treatment is usually effective, but itch may persist for a significant period and does not mean treatment failure. All sexual contacts and close family members should be treated at the same time. All clothes and bedclothes used in the 48 hours before treatment should be machine washed. For children under age 2 years, 10% precipitated sulfur in petrolatum should be used. It should be left in place for 24 hours and the treatment repeated in 24 hours or 1 week. An alternative to topical permethrin is ivermectin (Stromectol) 200 µg/kg po once for both adults and children.[1]

REFERENCES

1. Drugs for parasitic infections, *Med Lett* 40:1-12, 1998.

SCALP LOTIONS, STEROID

Some of the available steroid-containing scalp lotions are betamethasone valerate 0.1% (Valisone, Betnovate), betamethasone dipropionate 0.05% plus salicylic acid (Diprosalic), and clobetasol-17-propionate 0.05% (Temovate, Dermovate).

SCALP SHAMPOOS, MEDICATED

The usual way of using medicated scalp shampoos is to shake the bottle thoroughly, rub the shampoo well into the scalp, leave it for 4 minutes, and then rinse it out. Some of the medicated scalp shampoos that are available are salicylic acid shampoo (Ionil, Sebcur), salicylic acid–tar shampoo (Ionil T, Sebcur/T), salicylic acid–sulfur shampoo (Sebulex), and salicylic acid–sulfur–tar shampoo (Sebutone).

SEABATHER'S ERUPTION
(See also swimmer's itch)

Seabather's eruption or sea lice is a pruritic dermatitis occurring mainly on body areas covered by the bathing suit in ocean swimmers. The eruption comes on 3 to 30 minutes after swimming. The condition is usually found in Florida and the Caribbean but has been reported as far north as Long Island. The probable cause is the planula larvae of *Edwardsiella lineata,* a sea anemone. Larvae of the thimble jellyfish *(Linuche unguiculata)* have also been implicated.[1] Treatment is antihistamines and topical steroids.

REFERENCES

1. Tomchik RS, Russell MT, Szmant AM, et al: Clinical perspectives on seabather's eruption, also known as "sea lice," *JAMA* 269:1669-1672, 1993.

SUN DAMAGE
(See also melanoma; seasonal affective disorder; wrinkles)

Solar radiation in the ultraviolet B (UVB) spectrum (290 to 320 nm) is a major cause of sunburn and skin cancers. UVB is blocked by window glass. Ultraviolet A (UVA) (320 to 400 nm) causes polymorphous light eruption and most photosensitivity reactions to drugs. It also contributes to chronic skin damage or photoaging, skin cancer, and to a lesser extent sunburn.[1-3] Tanning of any degree is a sign of sun damage.[1,2] Photoaging, especially wrinkling, and skin cancer are more prevalent in smokers than nonsmokers.[3]

Clouds give little protection against ultraviolet radiation, since they allow approximately 80% of it to be transmitted. Snow and beaches reflect almost all ultraviolet radiation, and immersion in water filters out only about 50%. Maximum exposure to ultraviolet radiation occurs between the hours of 10 AM and 3 PM. Aside from staying indoors, clothing and especially hats are probably the most effective protection against sun damage. However, wet clothes, loosely woven fabrics, and nylon stockings permit about 20% to 30% of ultraviolet rays to pass through to the skin.[1,2]

Some sunscreens protect only against UVB. This is no longer acceptable. Although UVA is only about 1/1000 as potent in producing skin erythema as UVB, between 10 and 100 times as much UVA reaches the earth's surface as UVB. Furthermore, UVA penetrates more deeply in the dermis and is a major contributor to photoaging and tumor promotion. Sunscreens should protect against both UVA and UVB, and indeed most of them now do; patients should be advised to buy only those stating on the labels that both UVA and UVB are screened. It is generally accepted that the sun protective factor (SPF) must be at least 15.[1,2]

Sunscreens are an essential adjunct to the primary prevention of photoaging and skin cancers, and they are also valuable for patients who have already sustained the ravages of ultraviolet radiation because they facilitate the repair of photoaging.[3] However, they will not work if they are used merely as a method of increasing the duration of sun exposure. In one randomized double-blind trial, individuals using sunscreens with an SPF factor of 30 stayed in the sun for considerably longer periods than did those using sunscreens with an SPF factor of 15.[4]

Various sunscreen formulations are available. The most frequently used are lotions or creams, but for persons exposed to dust, such as farmers, ranchers, and construction workers, gels may be better because the dirt will not stick to them as readily. Children sometimes prefer sprays. Some sunscreens are specifically formulated to be waterproof or water resistant, and these should be used by swimmers.[2] Ideally sunscreens should be applied liberally half an hour before exposure and reapplied after swimming or perspiring, as well as every 2 to 3 hours on a regular basis.[1] Even waterproof or very water-resistant preparations have a duration of action limited to about 80 minutes, so lovers of the water should come out at least every hour for a reapplication of sunscreen.[5] When sunscreens and DEET preparations are both applied, the SPF of the sunscreens is reduced by about one third. However, if a commercial preparation containing both products is used, the SPF is that recorded on the label.[6]

Although the dangers of sun exposure are well publicized in the medical literature, the frequency with which they occur is not, and the advantages of being in the sun are rarely mentioned. The most feared skin cancer, melanoma, is very rare, so even complete avoidance of sun exposure would save few lives. Sun exposure offers the benefits of increasing vitamin D production and probably improving mental health (see discussion of seasonal affective disorder). Sun exposure is an almost inevitable accompaniment of any outdoor exercise program, and the benefit of such exercise almost certainly outweighs the harm of UVA and UVB rays.[7] But wear a hat!

REFERENCES

1. Guercio-Hauer C: Photodamage, photoaging and photoprotection of the skin, *Am Fam Physician* 50:327-332, 1994.
2. Wentzell JM: Sunscreens: the ounce of prevention, *Am Fam Physician* 53:1713-1733, 1996.
3. Gilchrest BA: A review of skin ageing and its medical therapy, *Br J Dermatol* 135:867-875, 1996.
4. Autier P, Doré J-F, Négrier S, et al (European Organization for Research and Treatment of Cancer Melanoma Group): Sunscreen use and duration of sun exposure: a double-blind, randomized trial, *J Natl Cancer Inst* 91:1304-1309, 1999.
5. Farmer KC, Naylor MF: Sun exposure, sunscreens, and skin cancer prevention: a year-round concern, *Ann Pharmacother* 30:662-673, 1996.
6. Fradin MS: Mosquitoes and mosquito repellents: a clinician's guide, *Ann Intern Med* 128:931-940, 1998.
7. Ness AR, Frankel SJ, Gunnell DJ, et al: Are we really dying for a tan? *BMJ* 319:114-116, 1999.

SWIMMER'S ITCH
(See also seabather's eruption)

Swimmer's itch is caused by the penetration into the skin of the larval or cercarial form of an animal schistosome. (The usual natural cycle is duck-snail-duck.) Since humans are not the definitive host, the cercariae die after penetrating the skin and cause a delayed hypersensitivity reaction. The person often has a brief period of skin stinging when first exposed to the cercariae and perhaps a transient macular or urticarial rash. This is followed by a latent period of 1 to 14 days before the development of the maculopapular-vesicular rash, which is usually seen over body areas not protected by clothing. Resolution begins in a few days and is complete within 2 weeks. Treatment is symptomatic and includes antihistamines, topical antipruritics, and in severe cases corticosteroids.[1,2]

Most cases of swimmer's itch come from exposure in fresh water. The cercariae are most abundant in warm, shallow water.[1,2] Elimination of snails from the water eliminates swimmer's itch.

─────────── ◢ **REFERENCES** ◣ ───────────

1. Mulvihill CA, Burnett JW: Swimmer's itch: a cercarial dermatitis, *Cutis* 46:211-213, 1990.
2. Chapman A, Ekelund C, Tominaga J: Rash and pruritus after a camping trip, *Pediatr Infect Dis J* 12:966, 968-969, 1993.

TATTOOS

Professional tattoos can often be effectively treated by lasers that break down the ink particles into sufficiently small fragments to be removed by macrophages. Amateur and posttraumatic tattoos can be removed only by surgical excision.[1]

─────────── ◢ **REFERENCES** ◣ ───────────

1. Heoyberghs JL: Cosmetic surgery, *BMJ* 318:512-516, 1999.

TINEA
Tinea Pedis

Tinea pedis has generally been treated topically with one of the imidazoles such as clotrimazole (Lotrimin, Mycelex, Canesten), miconazole (Micatin, Monistat), ketoconazole (Nizoral), or oxiconazole (Oxistat, Oxizole). Some of the more recently introduced allylamines, such as terbinafine (Lamisil) or Naftifine (Naftin), and the benzylamine derivative butenafine (Mentax) appear to be more potent, at least in vitro.[1] Since the imidazoles are fungistatic, they must be applied continuously for 4 weeks, which is how long it takes for the infected layers of skin to be shed completely. In contrast, a fungicidal drug such as terbinafine can result in cure after 1 week of application.[2]

Some forms of tinea pedis, especially those caused by *Trichophyton rubrum,* have a "moccasin" distribution with chronic hyperkeratosis of the soles and heels. This form tends to be resistant to topical treatment but often responds to oral agents such as terbinafine (Lamisil) 250 mg/day for 2 to 6 weeks, itraconazole (Sporanox) 100 mg/day for 4 weeks, or fluconazole (Diflucan) 150 mg weekly for 2 to 6 weeks.[3]

Toe web intertrigo, which is usually secondary to tinea pedis, is a common site of entry for organisms causing cellulitis of the lower extremity. A search for and treatment of tinea pedis in patients with leg cellulitis should result in a decreased frequency of recurrent episodes of cellulitis.[4]

Tinea Versicolor

Like tinea pedis, tinea versicolor is traditionally managed with topical antifungal agents applied once or twice a day for 2 to 4 weeks,[5] or alternatively by the application of a 2.5% selenium sulfide solution (Selsun) for 10 minutes a day for 7 days or for 24 hours once a week for 4 weeks. In extensive or recurrent cases a single oral dose of 400 mg of fluconazole (Diflucan) may be effective.[6]

Onychomycosis

Fungal infections are only one cause of dystrophic nails, so it is important to obtain culture results or positive potassium hydroxide smears before initiating oral treatment for onychomycosis. The best specimens are obtained from the more proximal portions of the nail.[7] Onychomycosis probably cannot be cured by topical treatment,[5,6] but there no good trials dealing with this issue.[2] At present, oral agents should be used to treat onychomycosis.[2,7] Part of the reason for the efficacy of the newer oral agents such as terbinafine (Lamisil), itraconazole (Sporanox), and fluconazole (Diflucan) in curing onychomycosis is that these agents bind to nail keratin and persist in the nails for several weeks after oral therapy is discontinued.[7] Because of this an alternative to daily oral therapy is pulse therapy. Studies of pulse therapy for onychomycosis of the toenails with itraconazole (Sporanox) found that 200 mg of the drug given bid 1 week a month for two to four cycles was as effective as continuous therapy with daily doses of 100 to 200 mg/day for 3 to 4 months.[8,9]

A 1999 double-blind randomized trial of treatment for onychomycosis compared continuous terbinafine (250 mg/day for 16 weeks) with intermittent itraconazole (400 mg/day for 1 week in every 4 weeks for a total of 16 weeks). After 72 weeks the mycological cure rate was 81% for terbinafine and 49% for itraconazole.[10] In the opinion of one editorial writer, continuous oral terbinafine therapy is the current treatment of choice for onychomycosis.[2]

Tinea Capitis

Tinea capitis can be transmitted by humans *(Trichophyton tonsurans, Microsporum audouinii)* or animals *(Microsporum canis).* In the United States 96% of cases are caused by *T. tonsurans.* Tinea capitis is a disease of prepubertal children and occurs more frequently in blacks than in whites.[11]

Occipital and postauricular adenopathy are common findings in noninflammatory (no kerion) tinea capitis. The combination of either alopecia and adenopathy or scaling and adenopathy is almost pathognomonic of tinea capitis.[12] Treatment requires several weeks of oral agents; griseofulvin (Fulvicin) is the first choice, with ketoconazole, terbinafine, and itraconazole as alternatives.[11]

➤ REFERENCES ◄

1. Topical butenafine for tinea pedis, *Med Lett* 39:63-64, 1997.
2. Finlay AY: Skin and nail fungi—almost beaten (editorial), *BMJ* 319:71-72, 1999.
3. Noble SI, Forbes RC, Stamm PL: Diagnosis and management of common tinea infections, *Am Fam Physician* 58:163-174, 1998.
4. Dupuy A, Benchikhi H, Roujeau J-C, et al: Risk factors for erysipelas of the leg (cellulitis): case-control study, *BMJ* 318:1591-1594, 1999.
5. Kovacs SO, Hruza LL: Superficial fungal infections: getting rid of lesions that don't want to go away, *Postgrad Med* 98:61-75, 1995.
6. Faergemann J: Treatment of pityriasis versicolor with a single dose of fluconazole, *Acta Derm Venereol* 72:74-75, 1992.
7. Gupta AK, Shear NH: Onychomycosis: going for cure, *Can Fam Physician* 43:299-305, 1997.
8. De Doncker PRG, Scher RK, Baran RL, et al: Itraconazole therapy is effective for pedal onychomycosis caused by some nondermatophyte molds and in mixed infection with dermatophytes and molds: a multicenter study with 36 patients, *J Am Acad Dermatol* 36(2 Part 1):173-177, 1997.
9. Havu V, Brandt H, Heikkila H, et al: A double-blind, randomized study comparing itraconazole pulse therapy with continuous dosing for the treatment of toe-nail onychomycosis, *Br J Dermatol* 136:230-234, 1997.
10. Evans EG, Sigurgeirsson B (LION Study Group): Double blind, randomised study of continuous terbinafine compared with intermittent itraconazole in treatment of toenail onychomycosis, *BMJ* 318:1031-1035, 1999.
11. Temple ME, Nahata MC, Koranyi KI: Pharmacotherapy of tinea capitis, *J Am Board Fam Pract* 12:236-242, 1999.
12. Hubbard TW: The predictive value of symptoms in diagnosing childhood tinea capitis, *Arch Pediatr Adolesc Med* 153:1150-1153, 1999.

TOPICAL STEROIDS

A useful way of classifying topical steroids is by potency. The standard classification puts the most potent drugs in group I and the least potent in group VII. Selected products are listed this way in Table 23, which includes only creams. The same concentration of drug in a different vehicle such as an ointment might be more potent. The same drug (e.g., triamcinolone) in different concentrations would also have different potencies. It would take a large table indeed to cover all drugs, all doses, and all formulations. These can be found in standard textbooks of dermatology. Topical steroids should be applied as a thin film. In general, only the mildest steroids should be used on the face, axillae, or genitals.

Table 23   Selected Topical Steroid Creams

Generic names	Selected trade names
Group I	
Betamethasone dipropionate/propylene glycol 0.05%	Diprolene
Clobetasol 17-propionate 0.05%	Dermovate, Temovate
Group II	
Desoximetasone 0.25%	Topicort
Fluocinonide 0.05%	Lidex Regular
Halcinonide 0.1%	Halog-E
Group III	
Triamcinolone acetonide 0.5%	Aristocort "C"oncentrate
Group IV	
Amcinonide 0.1%	Cyclocort
Fluocinolone acetonide 0.2%	Synalar HP
Halcinonide 0.025%	Halog
Group V	
Betamethasone-17-valerate 0.1%	Betnovate, Celestoderm-V, Valisone
Fluocinolone acetonide 0.025%	Synalar Regular
Hydrocortisone valerate 0.2%	Westcort
Triamcinolone acetonide 0.1%	Aristocort "R"egular, Kenalog
Group VI	
Desonide 0.05%	Tridesilon
Triamcinolone acetonide 0.025%	Aristocort "D"ilute
Group VII	
Hydrocortisone 1%	Hytone, Synacort, Cortate
Methylprednisolone 0.25%	Medrol

ULCERS, DERMAL

(See also venous ulcers)

Staging of skin ulcers is as follows[1]:

Stage 1	Nonblanchable erythema of the intact skin
Stage 2	Partial thickness loss involving the epidermis or dermis or both; presents clinically as an abrasion, blister, or shallow crater
Stage 3	Full-thickness loss extending into the subcutaneous tissue, but not through the underlying fascia
Stage 4	Full-thickness loss extending to muscle, bone tendons, joint capsule, and so on

Occlusive Dressings

The modern treatment of skin ulcers often involves the use of occlusive dressings, and a confusingly large number of these are on the market. Occlusive dressings not only protect the area, but also maintain a moist wound surface that facilitates autolytic debridement and the formation of granulation tissue and increases the rate of reepithelialization. Pain is relieved, and the degree of scarring diminished. Although bacterial colonization takes place in this milieu, the rate of clinical infections is actually less than in wounds treated with gauze or other conventional dressings. However, occlusive dressings should not be used if the lesion is clearly infected.[1,2]

Occlusive dressings can be applied only if the surrounding skin is intact and healthy. The dressings should be large enough to give a 2.5-cm or 1-inch margin around the borders. They should be changed when they leak or look as if they are going to leak, or at least once a week. Patients wearing occlusive dressings can bathe or shower with them on. The dressings come in various sizes and shapes, so that the physician can keep a list handy to prescribe the specific size required or can tell the pharmacist the size and shape of the ulcer and let him or her dispense the appropriate product.

The following are some occlusive dressings and wound fillers that family physicians may use reasonably frequently[1,2]:

1. Transparent polymer films (e.g., Tegaderm Transparent Dressing, Duoderm Extra Thin Dressings and Border Dressings, Opsite Wound Dressing). In general these are used to cover first- and second-degree ulcers. They are impermeable to water and nonabsorbent, so serous fluid may accumulate. This is not in itself harmful, but if enough accumulates, it may break the seal and leak out.

2. Hydrocolloid dressings (e.g., Tegasorb Ulcer Dressing, Duoderm CGF [Controlled Gel Formulation] Dressings, IntraSite Wound Dressing). These dressings are used for third- and fourth-degree ulcers. They are self-adhering and contain gelling agents. Before application the wound should be cleaned with normal saline. When the dressing is removed, a viscous gel remains in the ulcer, but it can be easily removed by saline irrigations (not hydrogen peroxide or other antiseptic solutions).

3. Calcium alginate dressings (e.g., Kaltostat Wound Dressing, Algoderm calcium alginate wound packing, Sorbsan). Alginates are seaweed-derived polysaccharides that are useful for packing large exuding cavities because they are highly absorbent. Only half of the cavity should be gently packed because these products expand.[1]

4. Hydrocolloid pastes and polyurethane foam (e.g., Cutinova Cavity, Duoderm Hydroactive Paste or Hydroactive Granules, Allevyn Hydrophilic Polymer Foam Dressing, LYOfoam). These absorbent agents, like calcium alginate dressings, are used for large exuding cavities. About half the wound cavity should be gently packed.

⬥ REFERENCES ⬥

1. Findlay D: Practical management of pressure ulcers, *Am Fam Physician* 54:1519-1528, 1996.
2. Helfman T, Ovington L, Falanga V: Occlusive dressings and wound healing, *Clin Dermatol* 12:121-127, 1994.

URTICARIA AND ANGIOEDEMA
(See also antihistamines; insect stings)

Urticaria and angioedema are said to affect 15% to 25% of the population at least once in a lifetime. Among patients with these disorders, 40% have urticaria alone, 10% angioedema alone, and 50% a combination of the two. Urticaria involves swelling of the superficial dermal tissues, whereas angioedema is located in the deep dermal, subcutaneous, or submucosal tissues. The swelling of angioedema is usually found in the extremities, eyelids, and lips, but it may involve the gastrointestinal tract or the respiratory tract. In the latter instance respiratory obstruction is a real possibility. Patients with angioedema usually complain of burning or tingling rather than itching. Individual lesions of both urticaria and angioedema come on rapidly, usually resolve in 2 to 4 hours, and rarely last more than 24 hours.[1]

Common causes of acute urticaria are Hymenoptera insect stings; foods such as nuts, chocolate, shellfish, eggs, and milk; viral infections, including hepatitis B; and drugs, especially antibiotics.[1] Angioedema may develop months or even years after a patient starts taking ACE inhibitors. In one case the patient continued taking his enalapril because the initial episode of angioedema resolved, but it recurred several days later.[2]

Chronic urticaria is defined as the presence of widespread wheals daily or almost daily for at least 6 weeks. In about 75% of cases no etiological factor is found,[1,3] and about half of these patients will be symptom free after 1 year.[1] Physical urticarias such as cold, solar, pressure, and cholinergic (brought on by exercise or hot shower) should be considered in the differential diagnosis. One of the most important conditions to be ruled out is urticarial vasculitis. Urticarial vasculitis is associated with connective tissue diseases such as lupus and Sjögren's syndrome. In this condition the individual wheals last more than 24 hours, and often purpura and sometimes skin pigmentation are seen. Fever, arthralgia, nephritis, and abdominal pain may also be present. The diagnosis can be made with a skin biopsy. A rare condition causing recurrent episodes of urticaria or angioedema is deficiency of C1 esterase inhibitor. It is diagnosed by finding a low C4 complement level.[1,3]

Routinely ordering elaborate investigations for patients with chronic urticaria or angioedema in an attempt to determine the etiology is not necessary. In one study comparing a careful history plus a few selective investigations with a history plus an exhaustive investigative protocol, the minimal investigations missed only 6% of identifiable causative conditions. For example, all the patients whose urticaria was due to parasites had lived in or been born in tropical countries; these were the only persons who needed to have stools tested for ova and parasites.[4]

In one small U.S. study, patients with acute-onset urticaria, regardless of cause, had better itch control if given a 4-day course of prednisone 20 mg in addition to hydroxyzine (Atarax) 25 mg q4-8h prn compared with those given only hydroxyzine.[5]

Patients with chronic urticaria should avoid taking ACE inhibitors, aspirin, and other nonsteroidal antiinflammatory drugs.[3] For patients who fail to respond to H_1-receptor antagonists alone, the addition of an H_2 antagonist such as cimetidine or ranitidine may result in the control of symptoms.[6] The antidepressant doxepin (Sinequan) has significant H_1 antihistaminic activity and may be used in doses of 25 to 50 mg hs.[3]

⚓ REFERENCES ⚓

1. Kulp-Shorten CL, Callen J: Urticaria, angioedema, and rheumatologic disease: rheumatic disease, *Rheum Dis Clin North Am* 22:95-115, 1996.
2. Shionoiri H, Takasaki I, Hirawa N, et al: A case report of angioedema during long-term (66 months) angiotensin converting enzyme inhibition therapy with enalapril, *Jpn Circ J* 60:166-170, 1996.
3. Greaves MW: Chronic urticaria, *N Engl J Med* 332:1767-1772, 1995.
4. Kozel MM, Mekkes JR, Bossuyt PM, et al: The effectiveness of a history-based diagnostic approach in chronic urticaria and angioedema, *Arch Dermatol* 134:1575-1580, 1998.
5. Pollack CV, Romano TJ: Outpatient management of acute urticaria—role of prednisone, *Ann Emerg Med* 26:547-551, 1995.
6. Bleehen SS, Thomas SE, Greaves MW, et al: Cimetidine and chlorpheniramine in the treatment of chronic idiopathic urticaria: a multi-centre randomized double-blind study, *Br J Dermatol* 117:81-88, 1987.

WARTS

Between 5% and 10% of children and young adults have warts, which are lesions caused by the human papillomavirus.[1] The peak age is 12 to 16 years.[2] About 70% of warts resolve spontaneously within 2 years (most within 1 year), but because new lesions develop in a number of patients, only about 50% of patients are lesion free after 2 years if left untreated.[3]

Treatment of warts is not very effective, as indicated by the 23 or more therapeutic options listed by the American Academy of Dermatology.[4] Since many of the lesions resolve spontaneously, no treatment is often the preferred choice.[2,3] Specific indications for treatment include symptomatic warts, disfiguring or disabling lesions, large numbers of lesions, and an immunocompromised host.[4]

Topical treatments, which are usually accomplished with cantharidin (Cantharone) or salicylic acid, are as effective as more invasive therapies such as cryotherapy, laser treatment, or cautery.[1,3] Topical treatments have the disadvantage of often requiring considerable time to achieve complete resolution.

One of the frequently used topical agents is cantharidin, which is an extract of the blister beetle or "Spanish fly." The method of using cantharidin is as follows: Apply the liquid to the wart, allow it to dry, and cover the wart with nonporous tape for 24 hours. After 24 hours replace the tape with a loose bandage such as a Band-Aid. After 2 weeks reassess the wart and remove necrotic tissue. One treatment is usually effective for hand and body warts, but a second application may be given if necessary. Two or more treatments at 2-week intervals are usually required for plantar warts.

If salicylic compounds are used, the lesion should be soaked in water or a shampoo solution for 5 minutes before application. It should be rinsed and dried, and any debris should be mechanically removed from the lesion. The liquid should be applied to the lesion, with care not to include surrounding normal skin. Treatments should be repeated every 24 to 48 hours until the skin lines can be seen over the base of the lesion. Examples of the many available products are salicylic acid 17% (Compound W gel), salicylic acid 20% (Compound W liquid), salicylic acid 30% (Compound W plus), salicylic acid 16.7%–lactic acid 16.7% (Duofilm liquid), and salicylic acid 27% (Duoforte 27).

Salicylic acid compounds specifically formulated for plantar warts include 40% salicylic acid disks and plasters (Carnation Callous and Corn Caps, Clear Away Plantar Wart Remover, Scholl Corn Removers), and salicylic acid 25%, lactic acid 10%, and formalin 5% (Duoplant). Disks or plaster should be purchased or cut to fit the lesion exactly so that normal surrounding skin is not affected. The plaster should then be applied and covered with waterproof tape, and treatments should be repeated every 48 hours. Once skin lines can be seen across the base of the lesion, treatment can be stopped. Total duration of treatment varies but may be up to 12 weeks. Liquid salicylic acid products such as Duoplant may be applied to the wart and covered with a waterproof bandage.

Cryotherapy may require repeat treatments every 2 to 3 weeks until the lesions resolve. With cryotherapy a single freeze-thaw cycle lasting 5 to 30 seconds with white margins extending 1 to 3 mm beyond the lesion is usually adequate. Laser treatments probably offer no significant advantages over other therapeutic modalities.[3]

Numerous other therapeutic modalities have been reported, although many of these are anecdotal. There are reports that "magic" such as transferring the virus to a coin is effective for some children.[3] High-dose cimetidine (Tagamet) over a 3-month period has been reported to be effective for adults[5] and children[6] with multiple recalcitrant warts. Response to treatment may not be seen for 4 to 6 weeks.[6] The adult regimen is 30 to 40 mg/kg/day in 3 divided doses for 3 months with a maximum daily dose of 3.5 g,[5] and the dosage for children is 25 to 40 mg/kg/day in 3 or 4 divided doses.[6] In adults the treatment was found to be particularly efficacious for patients with plantar warts.[5] Cimetidine is thought to modulate the immune system. Immersing the affected area in a water bath at 45° C (113° F) for 30 minutes three times a week has been reported to be effective in immunocompromised patients with HIV who had widespread warts refractory to usual treatment modalities.[7] There are also anecdotal reports that recurrent applications of heat may be effective for plantar warts in nonimmunocompromised persons. The feet are soaked in hot water for 15 minutes once a week for 6 weeks.[8]

⚓ REFERENCES ⚓

1. Sterling J: Treating the troublesome wart, *Practitioner* 239:44-47, 1995.

2. Siegfried EC: Warts on children: an approach to therapy, *Pediatr Ann* 25:79-90, 1996.
3. Landow K: Nongenital warts: when is treatment warranted? *Postgrad Med* 99:245-249, 1996.
4. Committee on Guidelines of Care: Guidelines of care for warts: human papillomavirus, *J Am Acad Dermatol* 32:98-103, 1995.
5. Glass AT, Solomon BA: Cimetidine therapy for recalcitrant warts in adults, *Arch Dermatol* 132:680-682, 1996.
6. Orlow SJ, Paller A: Cimetidine therapy for multiple viral warts in children, *J Am Acad Dermatol* 28:794-796, 1993.
7. Kang S, Fitzpatrick TB: Debilitating verruca vulgaris in a patient infected with the human immunodeficiency virus: dramatic improvement with hyperthermia therapy, *Arch Dermatol* 130:294-296, 1994.
8. Larimore WL, Hartman JR: Family physician's notebook: diary from a week in practice, *Am Fam Physician* 47:1589-1590, 1993.

WRINKLES AND SKIN AGING

(See also sun damage)

Sun exposure and smoking are major risk factors for skin aging. Clinically aging skin is characterized by blotchy pigmentation, wrinkles, and in some cases actinic keratoses and skin cancer (see sun damage).[1]

A formulation of tretinoin (Renova) is available as a 0.05% cream for the treatment of facial wrinkles and mottled hyperpigmentation. For wrinkles it is applied lightly over the entire face once daily at bedtime. According to the manufacturer 6 months may be necessary for full effects to occur.

Laser resurfacing is an effective method for dealing with wrinkles present at rest. Exaggerated creases associated with facial expression such as crow's feet may be diminished by botulinum A toxin injections, which must usually be repeated every 3 to 4 months. Wrinkles caused by tissue sagging are best treated by face-lift (rhytidectomy).[2] Acceptance of wrinkling as a sign of character and wisdom is an attractive alternative.

◤ REFERENCES ◢

1. Farmer KC, Naylor MF: Sun exposure, sunscreens, and skin cancer prevention: a year-round concern, *Ann Pharmacother* 30:662-673, 1996.
2. Stratigos AJ, Arndt KA, Dover JS: Advances in cutaneous aesthetic surgery, *JAMA* 280:1397-1398, 1998.

EXERCISE

(Exercise has proven or putative influences on a wide variety of disorders. These are outlined in the ensuing sections but are often discussed in more detail under the relevant specific disease headings. Many of these are listed in the index under the heading "Exercise.")

EPIDEMIOLOGY

An analysis of self-reported leisure-time physical activity in the United States in 1991 indicated that 58.1% of adults did not participate in physical activity or did so only on an irregular basis.[1] In another U.S. study 22% of adults over the age of 20 reported no leisure-time physical activity. The rates were higher for the subgroups of Mexican Americans, black women, and the elderly.[2] In Britain the average annual walking distance has decreased by 22% in the last third of the twentieth century, largely because of increased car travel; one fourth of all car trips are shorter than 3.2 km (2 miles). In 1972 12% of children were driven to school; by 1994 the figure was 23%. Walking is likely to result in social interactions with other walkers, whereas driving is isolating and interactions with others may take the form of road rage.[3]

◤ REFERENCES ◢

1. Centers for Disease Control and Prevention: Prevalence of sedentary lifestyle, *MMWR* 42:576-579, 1993.
2. Crespo CJ, Keteyian SJ, Heath GW, et al: Leisure-time physical activity among US adults: results from the Third National Health and Nutrition Examination Survey, *Arch Intern Med* 156:93-98, 1996.
3. Roberts I: Reducing road traffic: would improve quality of life as well as preventing injury (editorial), *BMJ* 316:242-243, 1998.

AEROBIC EXERCISE EQUIVALENCIES

(See also nutrition)

The energy consumed by aerobic exercise depends on the individual's weight and the type of exercise. Compared with brisk walking (7.5 kph or 4.5 mph), swimming at 20 yards (or meters) per minute consumes one third less energy, bicycling at 21 kph or 13 mph one third more, and cross-country skiing or jogging at 13 kph or 8 mph a little more than twice as much.[1]

A study from Wisconsin measured energy expenditure in healthy volunteers at given ratings of perceived exertion for six indoor exercise machines (Airdyne, cross-country skiing simulator, cycle ergometer, rowing ergometer, stair stepper, and treadmill). The most energy was expended with the treadmill and the least with the Airdyne and cycle.[2]

◤ REFERENCES ◢

1. An amble a day, *Consumer Reports* 58(7):421, July 1993.
2. Zeni AI, Hoffman MD, Clifford PS: Energy expenditure with indoor exercise machines, *JAMA* 275:1424-1427, 1996.

BENEFITS OF EXERCISE

Proven and reputed benefits of exercise include a decreased risk of all-cause mortality,[1,2] coronary artery disease,[2,3] hypertension,[2,4] type 2 diabetes mellitus,[5] strokes,[6] osteoporosis,[7] colon cancer,[8] breast cancer,[9] and lung cancer.[10] Exercise increases mobility in the very elderly,[11] improves the functioning of patients with osteoarthritis of the knees,[12] is beneficial for depression,[14] anxiety,[14] and chronic fatigue syndrome,[15] appears to improve cognitive functioning in the elderly,[16] may decrease the incidence of serious gastrointestinal hemorrhages in the elderly,[17] and lowers intraocular pressure in patients with open angle glaucoma.[18] It is the cornerstone of the medical management of intermittent claudication,[19] and it improves insomnia in the elderly.[20] Men and women who exercise have lower body mass indices than do those who are sedentary,[21] and exercise appears to prevent some cases of symptomatic gallbladder disease.[22] Moderate exercise such as walking is associated with a decreased risk for the symptoms of benign prostatic hyperplasia,[23] and exercise during pregnancy decreases the risk of spontaneous abortion.[24] Most of these topics are discussed in more detail under the specific disease headings.

❧ REFERENCES ❧

1. Kujala UM, Kaprio J, Sarna S, et al: Relationship of leisure-time physical activity and mortality: the Finnish Twin Cohort, *JAMA* 279:440-444, 1998.
2. Shephard RJ, Balady GJ: Exercise as cardiovascular therapy, *Circulation* 99:963-972, 1999.
3. Manson JE, Hu FB, Rich-Edwards JW, et al: A prospective study of walking as compared with vigorous exercise in the prevention of coronary heart disease in women, *N Engl J Med* 341:650-658, 1999.
4. Hayashi T, Tsumura K, Suematsu C, et al: Walking to work and the risk for hypertension in men: the Osaka Health Survey, *Ann Intern Med* 130:21-26, 1999.
5. Hu FB, Sigal RJ, Rich-Edwards JW, et al: Walking compared with vigorous physical activity and risk of type 2 diabetes in women: a prospective study, *JAMA* 282:1433-1439, 1999.
6. Lee I-M, Hennekens CH, Berger K, et al: Exercise and risk of stroke in male physicians, *Stroke* 30:1-6, 1999.
7. Grisso JA, Kelsey JL, Strom BL, et al: Risk factors for hip fracture in black women, *N Engl J Med* 330:1555-1559, 1994.
8. Colditz GA, Cannuscio CC, Frazier AL: Physical activity and reduced risk of colon cancer: implications for prevention, *Cancer Causes Control* 8:649-667, 1997.
9. Rockhill B, Willett WC, Hunter DJ, et al: A prospective study of recreational physical activity and breast cancer risk, *Arch Intern Med* 159:2290-2296, 1999.
10. Lee I-M, Sesso HD, Paffenbarger RS: Physical activity and risk of lung cancer, *Int J Epidemiol* 28:620-625, 1999.
11. Fiatarone MA, O'Neill EF, Ryan ND, et al: Exercise training and nutritional supplementation for physical frailty in very elderly people, *N Engl J Med* 330:1769-1775, 1994.
12. Ettinger WH Jr, Burns R, Messier S, et al: A randomized trial comparing aerobic exercise and resistance exercise with a health education program in older adults with knee osteoarthritis: the Fitness, Arthritis, and Senior Trial (FAST), *JAMA* 277:25-31, 1997.
13. Blumenthal JA, Babyak MA, Moore KA, et al: Effects of exercise training on older patients with major depression, *Arch Intern Med* 159:2349-2356, 1999.
14. Petruzello SJ, Landers DM, Hatfield BD, et al: A meta-analysis on the anxiety-reducing effects of acute and chronic exercise, *Sports Med* 11:143-182, 1991.
15. Fulcher KY, White PD: Randomised controlled trial of graded exercise in patients with the chronic fatigue syndrome, *BMJ* 314:1647-1652, 1997.
16. Kramer AF, Hahn S, Cohen NJ, et al: Ageing, fitness and neurocognitive function, *Nature* 400:418-419, 1999.
17. Pahor M, Guralnik JM, Salive ME, et al: Physical activity and risk of severe gastrointestinal hemorrhage in older persons, *JAMA* 272:595-599, 1994.
18. Passo MS, Hunt SC, Elliot DL, et al: Regular exercise lowers intraocular pressure in glaucoma patients (abstract), *Invest Ophthalmol Vis Sci* 13(suppl):1254, 1994.
19. Gardner AW, Poehlman ET: Exercise rehabilitation programs for the treatment of claudication pain: a meta-analysis, *JAMA* 274:975-980, 1995.
20. King AC, Oman RF, Brassington GS, et al: Moderate-intensity exercise and self-rated quality of sleep in older adults: a randomized controlled trial, *JAMA* 277:32-37, 1997.
21. Thune I, Njølstad I, Løchen M-L, et al: Physical activity improves the metabolic risk profiles in men and women: the Tromsø study, *Arch Intern Med* 158:1633-1640, 1998.
22. Leitzmann MF, Giovannucci EL, Rimm EB, et al: The relation of physical activity to risk for symptomatic gallstone disease in men, *Ann Intern Med* 128:417-425, 1998.
23. Platz EA, Kawachi I, Rimm EB, et al: Physical activity and benign prostatic hyperplasia, *Arch Intern Med* 158:2349-2356, 1998.
24. Latka M, Kline J, Hatch M: Exercise and spontaneous abortion of known karyotype, *Epidemiology* 10:73-75, 1999.

Exercise as a Protection Against All-Cause Mortality

A study of both sexes by Blair and associates[1] with a mean follow-up period of 8.4 years found that moderate fitness as measured by maximal exercise testing was associated with decreased mortality regardless of whether the individuals were healthy, smokers, obese, hypercholesterolemic, or hypertensive or had strong family histories of coronary artery disease. The Harvard Alumni Study has also shown that an increase in physical activity reduces mortality.[2,3] The degree of benefit correlated with the total increase in energy expenditure per week.[2] A more recent report from the Harvard Alumni Study concluded that vigorous activities, but not nonvigorous activities, were associated with longevity. It is important to realize that the term "vigorous" included not only running, jogging, swimming laps, playing tennis, and shoveling snow, but also brisk walking.[3] The Iowa Women's Health Study documented decreased mortality in postmenopausal women participating in moderate activity,[4] and the Framingham Study found that current or recent physical activity decreased mortality rates in both men and women.[5]

Observational studies such as those discussed above clearly show that people who exercise have decreased mortality rates. This difference is not due merely to the fact that healthy people are more likely to exercise; studies have shown that even small improvements in physical fitness over time decrease the risk of death.[6]

❧ REFERENCES ❧

1. Blair SN, Kampert JB, Kohl HW III, et al: Influences of cardiorespiratory fitness and other precursors on cardiovascular disease and all-cause mortality in men and women, *JAMA* 276: 205-210, 1996.
2. Paffenbarger RS Jr, Kampert JB, Lee I-M, et al: Changes in physical activity and other lifeway patterns influencing longevity, *Med Sci Sports Exerc* 26:857-865, 1994.
3. Lee I-M, Chung-Cheng H, Paffenbarger RS Jr: Exercise intensity and longevity in men: the Harvard Alumni Health Study, *JAMA* 273:1179-1184, 1995.
4. Kushi LH, Fee RM, Folsom AR, et al: Physical activity and mortality in postmenopausal women, *JAMA* 277:1287-1292, 1997.
5. Sherman SE, D'Agostino RB, Silbershatz H, et al: Comparison of past versus recent physical activity in the prevention of premature death and coronary artery disease, *Am Heart J* 138:900-907, 1999.
6. Erikssen G, Liestøl K, Bjørnholt J, et al: Changes in physical fitness and changes in mortality, *Lancet* 352:759-762, 1998.

Exercise as a Protection Against Coronary Artery Disease

Protection against coronary artery disease is probably the most important health gain from exercise programs. Numerous studies have demonstrated this benefit in the prevention of both first-time events[1-4] and recurrences of myocardial infarction.[5] Results of the Harvard Alumni Study indicate that the quantitative benefit of exercise in reducing coronary artery mortality is as great as avoiding obesity, achieving good blood pressure control, or stopping smoking.[2]

A question of great clinical importance is the quantity of exercise that is necessary to produce a cardioprotective effect. An encouraging finding in recent years is that moderate exercise appears to be as or almost as beneficial as intense exercise in protecting against cardiovascular events.[1,3,4,6-9] Another important finding is that brief bouts of exercise are as beneficial as more prolonged exercise periods, provided the total amount of exercise is sufficient (30 minutes a day).[10] Although most exercise plans involve structured programs, life-style counseling leading to individualized programs has been found equally effective over the short term in reducing such risk factors as lipid levels and blood pressure. Some of the innovations that were developed included wearing a headset with a long cord while walking about during conference calls, scheduling 10-minute walking breaks at regular intervals throughout the day, or walking briskly around play areas while supervising children.[11]

Relatively few studies have evaluated the cardioprotective effects of exercise in women; those that have been done showed a significant decrease in the risk of coronary events.[3,7,9,12] For example, the Nurses' Health Study found that 3 hours of brisk walking a week was as beneficial as more vigorous exercise and led to a 30% to 40% reduction in the risk of coronary events, compared with sedentary women.[9] Few studies have evaluated the effect of exercise in smokers, but a Swedish prospective study found that vigorous physical activity decreased cardiovascular mortality in smokers by almost 40%.[13]

❧ REFERENCES ❧

1. Hakim AA, Petrovitch H, Burchfiel CM, et al: Effects of walking on mortality among nonsmoking retired men, *N Engl J Med* 338:94-99, 1998.
2. Paffenbarger RS Jr, Hyde RT, Wing AL, et al: The association of changes in physical-activity level and other lifestyle characteristics with mortality among men, *N Engl J Med* 328:538-545, 1993.
3. Kushi LH, Fee RM, Folsom AR, et al: Physical activity and mortality in postmenopausal women, *JAMA* 277:1287-1292, 1997.
4. Wannamethee SG, Shaper AG, Walker M: Changes in physical activity, mortality, and incidence of coronary heart disease in older men, *Lancet* 351:1603-1608, 1998.
5. Oldridge NB, Guyatt GH, Fischer ME, et al: Cardiac rehabilitation after myocardial infarction: combined experience of randomized clinical trials, *JAMA* 260:945-950, 1988.
6. Blair SN, Kohl HW III, Barlow CE, et al: Changes in physical fitness and all-cause mortality: a prospective study of healthy and unhealthy men, *JAMA* 273:1093-1098, 1995.
7. LaCroix AZ, Leveille SG, Hecht JA, et al: Does walking decrease the risk of cardiovascular disease hospitalizations and death in older adults? *J Am Geriatr Soc* 44:113-120, 1996.
8. Blair SN: Dose of exercise and health benefits (editorial), *Arch Intern Med* 157:153-154, 1997.
9. Manson JE, Hu FB, Rich-Edwards JW, et al: A prospective study of walking as compared with vigorous exercise in the prevention of coronary heart disease in women, *N Engl J Med* 341:650-658, 1999.
10. Pate RR, Pratt M, Blair SN, et al: Physical activity and public health: a recommendation from the Centers for Disease Control and Prevention and the American College of Sports Medicine, *JAMA* 273:402-407, 1995.
11. Dunn AL, Marcus BH, Kampert JB, et al: Reduction in cardiovascular disease risk factors: 6-month results from Project Active, *Prev Med* 26:883-892, 1997.
12. Rich-Edwards JW, Manson JE, Hennekens C, et al: The primary prevention of coronary heart disease in women, *N Engl J Med* 332:1758-1766, 1995.
13. Hedblad B, Ogren M, Isacsson S-O, et al: Reduced cardiovascular mortality risk in male smokers who are physically active: results from a 25-year follow-up of the Prospective Population Study Men Born in 1914, *Arch Intern Med* 157:893-899, 1997.

Exercise as a Protection Against Stroke

Two prospective observational studies published in 1999 documented a decreased risk of stroke in men over the age of 40 or 45 who exercised.[1,2] The Physicians' Health Study assessed only exercise that was vigorous enough to "work up a sweat" and found that those who exercised the most at baseline had the lowest risk of both ischemic and hemorrhagic strokes.[1] An Icelandic study found that moderate exercise such as walking and swimming was associated with a decreased risk of ischemic strokes.[2]

⊠ REFERENCES ⊾

1. Lee I-M, Hennekens CH, Berger K, et al: Exercise and risk of stroke in male physicians, *Stroke* 30:1-6, 1999.
2. Agnarsson U, Thorgeirsson G, Sigvaldason H, et al: Effects of leisure-time physical activity and ventilatory function on risk for stroke in men: the Reykjavík Study, *Ann Intern Med* 130: 987-990, 1999.

Exercise as a Protection Against Type 2 Diabetes Mellitus

A follow-up study of male alumni from the University of Pennsylvania found a significant protective effect of exercise against the development of type 2 diabetes.[1] The incidence was much lower in the most physically active compared with the least active, and a significant difference remained even after correction for obesity. The greatest protection was noted for men at highest risk for the disease (because of obesity, hypertension, and a family history of diabetes).[1] Similar results have been reported in a study of Finnish men.[2] Aside from a decrease in the level of obesity, the mechanism of protection is probably an increased insulin sensitivity induced by the exercise.[3]

⊠ REFERENCES ⊾

1. Helmrich SP, Ragland DR, Leung RW, et al: Physical activity and reduced occurrence of non-insulin-dependent diabetes mellitus, *N Engl J Med* 325:147-152, 1991.
2. Lynch J, Helmrich SP, Lakka TA, et al: Moderately intense physical activities and high levels of cardiorespiratory fitness reduce the risk of non-insulin-dependent diabetes mellitus in middle-aged men, *Arch Intern Med* 156:1307-1314, 1996.
3. Horton ES: Exercise and decreased risk of NIDDM (editorial), *N Engl J Med* 325:196-198, 1991.

Exercise as a Protection Against Osteoporosis

Although the relationship between exercise and osteoporosis has been well studied, this does not seem to be the case with major fractures. For example, a 1994 review of the various risk factors for hip fracture assessed many variables, including body weight, smoking, alcohol intake, thiazide use, and estrogen replacement therapy, but did not evaluate or even refer to exercise in the discussion of literature on the subject.[1]

The amount of physical activity in childhood seems to correlate directly with the adult bone density.[2] In addition, a number of reports indicate that exercise decreases the rate of bone density loss in postmenopausal women. This is discussed more fully under "Osteoporosis."

⊠ REFERENCES ⊾

1. Grisso JA, Kelsey JL, Strom BL, et al: Risk factors for hip fracture in black women, *N Engl J Med* 330:1555-1559, 1994.
2. McCulloch RG, Bailey DA, Houston S, et al: Effects of physical activity, dietary calcium intake and selected lifestyle factors on bone density in young women, *Can Med Assoc J* 142:221-227, 1990.

Exercise as a Protection Against Colon Cancer

A few studies have suggested that physical inactivity is associated with an increased risk of colon cancer.[1-4] A Swedish study covering a 14-year follow-up period found that the relative risk of colon cancer in the least physically active group was 3.6 times that of the most physically active group.[1] Rates of rectal cancer were unaffected. The Health Professionals Follow-up Study found that the colon cancer risk for men in the highest quintile of leisure-time physical activity was 0.53 that of those in the lowest quintile.[4] A possible explanation of this finding is that exercise decreases intestinal transit time and so diminishes exposure of the colonic mucosa to fecal carcinogens.

⊠ REFERENCES ⊾

1. Gerhardsson M, Floderus B, Norell SE: Physical activity and colon cancer risk, *Int J Epidemiol* 17:743-746, 1988.
2. Powell GE, Caspersen CJ, Hoplan JP, et al: Physical activity and chronic diseases, *Am J Clin Nutr* 49:999-1006, 1989.
3. Lee I, Paffenbarger RS, Hsieh C: Physical activity and risk of developing colorectal cancer among college alumni, *J Natl Cancer Inst* 83:1324-1329, 1991.
4. Giovannucci E, Ascherio A, Rimm EB, et al: Physical activity, obesity, and risk for colon cancer and adenoma in men, *Ann Intern Med* 122:327-334, 1995.

Exercise as a Protection Against Anxiety and Depression

Evidence supports the role of exercise as a protective factor against or therapeutic agent for anxiety and depression.[1-4]

⊠ REFERENCES ⊾

1. King AC, Taylor CB, Haskell WL, et al: Influence of regular aerobic exercise on psychological health, *Health Psychol* 8:305-324, 1989.
2. Taylor CB, Sallis JF, Needle R: The relationship of physical activity and exercise to mental health, *Public Health Rep* 100: 195-201, 1995.
3. Martinsen EW: Physical activity and depression: clinical experience, *Acta Psychiatr Scand* 377(suppl):23-27, 1994.
4. Byrne A, Byrne DG: The effect of exercise on depression, anxiety and other mood states: a review, *J Psychosom Res* 37:565-574, 1993.

Exercise in the Elderly

(See also geriatrics)

Men aged 64 to 84 who participated in moderate exercise such as walking or bicycling for 20 minutes a day three times a week were found to have lower all-cause and cardiovascular mortality than more sedentary control subjects.[1]

A study from the Hebrew Rehabilitation Center for the Aged in Roslindale, Massachusetts, has demonstrated a dramatic effect of resistance exercises in improving the mobility of the very elderly. The patients who were evaluated were residents of a nursing home. All were over 70 years of age, 38% were over 90 years of age, and the mean age was 87. The resisted exercise group underwent a regimen of high-intensity progressive resistance training of the hip and knee extensors lasting 45 minutes three times a week for 10 weeks. Muscle strength and mass increased significantly, but more important, the exercise intervention increased the habitual gait velocity, improved the ability to climb stairs, and produced an overall increase in physical activity. A liquid nutritional supplement did not improve the performance of either the exercising group or the nonexercising control group. The authors postulated that the failure of some other studies to show benefits in nursing home residents given endurance training (in contrast to resistance training) was because the patients had insufficient muscle strength to benefit from it.[2]

For the ambulatory elderly, Shephard[3] recommends endurance exercises plus 8 to 10 repetitions or resistance exercises twice a week for each set of major muscle groups. The degree of resistance should be enough to induce slight fatigue by the tenth repetition. The goal of such exercises is to maintain lean muscle mass.

A 1994 study of elderly patients in various U.S. communities found that the relative risk of severe gastrointestinal hemorrhage in elderly patients with a mean age of 77 was 0.7 for those who exercised at least three times per week compared with the nonexercising control group. Exercise was defined as walking, gardening, or "doing vigorous physical activity" three times a week or more. One theoretical explanation is that exercise decreases ischemia in the splanchnic circulation.[4]

Some aspects of cognitive functioning (executive functioning) in healthy elderly adults appear to be improved by moderate aerobic exercise in the form of walking. This is discussed under "Dementia."

❧ REFERENCES ❧

1. Bijnen FC, Caspersen CJ, Feskens EJ, et al: Physical activity and 10-year mortality from cardiovascular diseases and all causes: the Zutphen Elderly Study, *Arch Intern Med* 158:1499-1505, 1998.
2. Fiatarone MA, O'Neill EF, Ryan ND, et al: Exercise training and nutritional supplementation for physical frailty in very elderly people, *N Engl J Med* 330:1769-1775, 1994.
3. Shephard RJ: Physical activity, fitness and cardiovascular health: a brief counselling guide for older patients, *Can Med Assoc J* 151:557-561, 1994.
4. Pahor M, Guralnik JM, Salive ME, et al: Physical activity and risk of severe gastrointestinal hemorrhage in older persons, *JAMA* 272:595-599, 1994.

RISKS OF EXERCISE

(See also benefits of exercise; cardiac arrest; cardiopulmonary resuscitation; diarrhea and hematochezia in runners; exercise-induced hematuria; female athletes; preparticipation medical examinations; urinalysis-blood)

Exercise entails a number of risks, the most common of which are probably musculoskeletal problems. These are most likely to occur with high-intensity exercise.[1] Other important adverse effects in women come about when weight loss from the exercise is of such degree as to induce amenorrhea. This is associated with osteoporosis and an increased risk of infertility.[1] Cultural pressures on women athletes may also foster eating disorders and the so-called female athlete triad of an eating disorder, amenorrhea, and osteoporosis.[2]

The relative risk of sudden death is two to three times greater during the exercise period but is decreased by 50% for the remaining 23 hours of the day.[3] The relative risk of myocardial infarction during vigorous exercise (6 METS [metabolic equivalents of oxygen consumption]) is increased in sedentary individuals but not in physically active ones.[3,4] About 5% of myocardial infarctions are associated with heavy exercise. The mechanism is uncertain. Platelets are activated with exercise in sedentary individuals but not in those who are regularly physically active. Regular exercise increases the endogenous fibrinolytic system.[3] Vigorous exercise also alters mechanical forces on coronary arteries and may lead to plaque rupture.[4]

The risk of having cardiac events during exercise is 10 times greater in individuals with cardiovascular disease than in those without it. Therefore screening for cardiovascular disease before an exercise program is often recommended. Screening is probably best done by a short self-administered questionnaire such as the Revised Physical Activity Readiness Questionnaire (PAR-Q). If the answers to the questionnaire fail to raise any concern, no limitations to physical activity are needed; in all other cases further medical evaluation is indicated. For patients with heart disease, exercise prescriptions are based on a combination of clinical findings and the results of exercise tests. In general, patients are advised to monitor their heart rates and not to exceed the levels at which abnormalities were detected during the exercise tests.[5]

Acute exertional rhabdomyolysis is caused by damage to skeletal muscle with the release of myoglobin and other cellular constituents into the circulation. In severe cases there may be intravascular coagulation, renal failure, and even death. Mild to moderately severe cases may result in hyperkalemia, hypernatremia, hyperphosphatemia, hypocalcemia (from the deposition of calcium in necrotic muscle), and lactic acidosis. The condition should be suspected when the patient has a significant overuse syndrome involving pain and often swelling of muscles. Particular risk factors are high ambient temperature, high humidity, and inadequate fluid intake; the untrained exerciser is probably at greater risk than the trained athlete. A urine dipstick test will be positive for blood, but no red blood cells will be seen. Usually the serum creatine kinase level is markedly elevated. Fluid replacement is the cornerstone of treatment.[6]

⚓ REFERENCES ⚓

1. Manson JE, Lee I-M: Exercise for women—how much pain for optimal gain? (editorial), *N Engl J Med* 334:1325-1327, 1996.
2. Nattiv A, Agostini R, Drinkwater B, et al: The female athlete triad: the inter-relatedness of disordered eating, amenorrhea, and osteoporosis, *Clin Sports Med* 13:405-418, 1994.
3. Curfman G: Is exercise beneficial—or hazardous—to your heart? (editorial), *N Engl J Med* 329:730-731, 1993.
4. Giri S, Thompson PD, Kiernan FJ, et al: Clinical and angiographic characteristics of exertion-related acute myocardial infarction, *JAMA* 282:1731-1736, 1999.
5. Balady GJ, Chaitman B, Driscoll D, et al (American Heart Association/American College of Sports Medicine): Recommendations for cardiovascular screening, staffing, and emergency policies at health/fitness facilities, *Circulation* 97:2283-2293, 1998.
6. Line RL, Rust GS: Acute exertional rhabdomyolysis, *Am Fam Physician* 52:502-506, 1995.

EXERCISE GUIDELINES
Traditional Exercise Prescriptions

The traditional exercise prescription is aimed at developing cardiovascular fitness and, as discussed previously, is probably unnecessary for producing a cardioprotective effect. Traditional programs have aimed to increase the pulse rate to the following levels:

Healthy individuals	70%-85% of 220 − Age
Cardiovascular-compromised individuals	50%-70% of 220 − Age

The overall traditional exercise prescription is outlined below:

Frequency	3-5 times a week
Intensity	220 − Age etc. (see above)
Time	40-60 minutes
Type	Aerobic

Exercise Prescription Recommendations of U.S. Expert Panels

Some of the major recommendations of the 1996 NIH Consensus Conference on exercise are as follows[1]:

1. Children and adults should attempt to accumulate 30 minutes of moderate-intensity exercise on most and preferably all days of the week.
2. Several brief bouts of moderate activity are beneficial.
3. Types of exercise that are classified as moderate activity include many occupational functions or activities of daily living, as well as leisure-time activity: brisk walking, cycling, swimming, home repair, and yard work.
4. Persons already meeting these recommendations may gain further benefits through more exercise.
5. Exercise reduces all-cause mortality and cardiovascular mortality in patients with known cardiovascular disease. Patients with these conditions should participate in appropriately prescribed and supervised exercise training programs.

The preceding recommendations differ from many previous ones in that they are based on the principles that moderate exercise is effective in promoting health and that exercise does not have to be done in block periods to be beneficial, since intermittent short bouts of exercise are also efficacious.[2]

The 1996 U.S. Surgeon General's Report on Physical Activity and Health recommends moderate exercise such as brisk walking or raking leaves for 30 minutes a day, running 1.5 miles (2.5 km) in 20 minutes every day, swimming laps for 20 minutes a day, or playing basketball for 15 to 20 minutes a day. Additional exercise will lead to added health benefits.[3] Other ways of obtaining moderate exercise are walking up stairs rather than taking elevators, walking short distances instead of driving, pedaling a stationary bicycle while watching television, and housework or dancing at an intensity equivalent to brisk walking.[2]

In a Glasgow study a sign was placed beside the escalator in an underground station saying, "Stay Healthy, Save Time, Use the Stairs." Before the sign was posted, 8% of persons used the stairs. During the 3 weeks the sign was posted, stair use increased to an average of 21%. Twelve weeks after removal of the poster fewer people used the stairs but the rate was still higher than baseline. Both at baseline and after the placard was posted, twice as many men as women used the stairs.[4] Similar results were reported in a U.S. study using either a sign that said, "Your heart needs exercise, use the stairs" or one that said, "Improve your waistline, use the stairs."[5]

⚓ REFERENCES ⚓

1. Physical activity and cardiovascular health: NIH Consensus Development Panel on Physical Activity and Cardiovascular Health, *JAMA* 276:241-246, 1996.
2. Pate RR, Pratt M, Blair SN, et al: Physical activity and public health. a recommendation from the Centers for Disease Control and Prevention and the American College of Sports Medicine, *JAMA* 273:402-407, 1995.
3. Centers for Disease Control and Prevention: Surgeon General's report on physical activity and health, *JAMA* 276:522, 1996.
4. Blamey A, Mutrie N, Aitchison T: Health promotion by encouraged use of stairs, *BMJ* 311:289-290, 1995.
5. Andersen RE, Franckowiak SC, Snyder J, et al: Can inexpensive signs encourage the use of stairs? Results from a community intervention, *Ann Intern Med* 129:363-369, 1998.

ANAL AND ANORECTAL DISORDERS

(See also constipation)

Anal Fissures

Ninety percent of anal fissures are found in the posterior midline, and almost all the others are located in the anterior midline.[1,2] If fissures are detected in other locations, underlying diseases such as Crohn's disease or syphilis should be suspected.[1]

Conservative treatment of anal fissures is successful in most patients and consists of maneuvers to relieve spasm of the anal sphincter and avoid hard bulky stools. Stool management involves use of bulking agents such as fruits and vegetables and psyllium (Metamucil) with plenty of water.[1-3] Warm baths, 1% hydrocortisone ointment,[1-3] and if necessary 5% lidocaine applied to the anus just before bowel movements[3] are generally effective.

A prospective randomized placebo-controlled trial has shown that nitroglycerin (glyceryl trinitrate) ointment dramatically increases the healing rate of persistent anal fissures. In this study a 0.2% glyceryl trinitrate ointment was applied to the fissure twice a day for up to 8 weeks. Over half the patients treated with the ointment had headaches, which were short lived and mild in most. The drug is believed to relax the anal sphincter muscle. If prescribing this ointment, the physician should be sure to underline the dosage of 0.2%, since the concentration of nitroglycerin ointment used for angina is generally 2.0%.[4] An alternative method of relaxing the anal sphincter that has proved effective in a randomized controlled trial is the injection of botulinum toxin into the sphincter. In one randomized trial comparing two injections of botulinum toxin at the beginning of the study to 0.2% nitroglycerin ointment applications bid for 6 weeks, 96% of fissures had healed by 2 months in the botulinum-treated group while 60% had healed in the nitroglycerin group.[5]

If conservative treatment fails, surgery is probably indicated. The procedure of choice is a lateral internal sphincterotomy with the goal of breaking the cycle of internal sphincter spasm.[1-3] Digital stretching of the anal sphincter no longer has a role.[1,2]

In a few children under 6 years of age, anal fissures may be the result of cow's milk intolerance. The parents usually seek treatment for the child's chronic constipation, and in one double-blind crossover study, switching to soy milk caused the fissures and constipation to resolve.[6]

Hemorrhoids

Hemorrhoids may be external or internal. External hemorrhoids lie distal to the dentate line and are covered by skin; internal hemorrhoids are proximal to the dentate line and are covered by mucosa.[1]

External hemorrhoids become symptomatic when they become thrombosed. Pain peaks in 48 to 72 hours and then gradually resolves. If the patient has intense pain and is seen within 72 hours, incision and evacuation of the thrombus or excision of the lesion with overlying skin may be performed.[1,2] The usual conservative treatment consists of warm baths, increased fiber, and fluids.[2]

Four categories of internal hemorrhoids have been established. Grade I internal hemorrhoids are small and do not prolapse; grade II hemorrhoids prolapse with bowel movement but return spontaneously; grade III hemorrhoids prolapse but can be replaced manually; grade IV hemorrhoids prolapse and cannot be replaced manually. Internal hemorrhoids usually lie in the right anterior, right posterior, and left lateral positions.[1,2]

Anemia from rectal bleeding secondary to internal hemorrhoids is well documented. Among 43 patients with this condition reported from the Mayo Clinic, the mean hemoglobin concentration was 9.4 g/dl (94 g/L). Eighty-four percent of the patients gave a history of blood squirting from the anus or the passage of clots. Six of the 43 had coagulation defects.[7]

Conservative management of internal hemorrhoids is the initial treatment of choice for grade I to III lesions. This consists of avoiding straining at stool; increasing fiber in the form of fruit, vegetables, and fiber products such as psyllium; and maintaining a high fluid intake (six to eight glasses of caffeine-free fluid per day).[2] Interventional options include rubber band ligation, infrared photocoagulation, and injection sclerotherapy. Hemorrhoidectomy is indicated for grade IV lesions and for other cases that do not respond to less invasive procedures.[1,2]

Proctalgia Fugax

Proctalgia fugax is characterized by infrequent episodes of severe perianal pain. These episodes usually last only a few minutes and are sometimes relieved by defecation. In some patients the episodes are precipitated by orgasm. Proctalgia fugax is a disorder of adults and affects both sexes. No serious underlying diseases are associated with this condition, and when patients give a typical history, no investigations are required. Because the pain is brief and infrequent, there is generally no specific treatment, although digital dilatation of the anus by the patient has been reported to give relief, presumably by relaxing the sphincter. There are anecdotal reports that clonidine (Catapres) 0.15 mg bid or diltiazem (Cardizem) 80 mg bid is effective for very severe cases.[8]

Pruritus Ani

Pruritus ani has been estimated to occur in about 5% of the population, and men are four times more likely to be affected than women.[1] Most cases of pruritus ani are primary, but in some instances the condition is secondary to other benign or malignant anorectal or systemic disorders, including pinworms, hemorrhoids, fissures, fistulas, chronic dermatoses, diabetes, rectal carcinomas, Paget's disease, and Bowen's disease.[1-3] In children the most common cause is pinworms.[2] A thorough workup for secondary causes is indicated if suggested by the initial history or physical examination or if the patient fails to respond to treatment within a month or so.[2,3]

A variety of foods have been stated to cause or aggravate pruritus ani. Coffee seems to be high on the list of responsible agents; others are said to be tea, colas, beer, chocolate, tomatoes, and milk.[1-3] As far as I know, no good controlled studies have been published supporting these claims.

Treatment of primary pruritus ani consists of eliminating aggravating nutrients and potentially irritating local agents such as scented soaps and over-the-counter medications. If the area is acutely inflamed and weeping, warm baths may be helpful. Good perianal hygiene is important. After bowel movements or when washing, the perianal area may be gently cleansed and then dried by blotting with cotton balls or, even better, with the use of a hair dryer. Rubbing and scrubbing of the area should be avoided.[1,2] Although failure to clean the perianal region adequately after bowel movements may aggravate pruritus ani, excessive cleansing is equally detrimental.[2] As the condition improves, corn starch may be applied to keep the area dry; absorbent pads and loose undergarments also help keep moisture down.[1,2] In some cases a short course of 1% hydrocortisone cream hastens symptomatic relief.[1]

Anal Cancer

Squamous cell cancer of the anus is rare. An important risk factor for both men and women is receptive anal intercourse, which presumably allows transmission of the carcinogenic strains of human papillomavirus.[9]

--- ⚞ **REFERENCES** ⚟ ---

1. Fazio VW, Tjandra JJ: The management of perianal diseases, *Adv Surg* 29:59-78, 1996.
2. Nagle D, Rolandelli RH: Primary care office management of perianal and anal disease, *Primary Care* 23:609-620, 1996.
3. Mazier WP: Hemorrhoids, fissures, and pruritus ani, *Surg Clin North Am* 74:1277-1292, 1994.
4. Lund JN, Armitage NC, Scholefield JH: Use of glyceryl trinitrate ointment in the treatment of anal fissure, *Br J Surg* 83:776-777, 1996.
5. Brisinda G, Maria G, Bentivoglio AR, et al: A comparison of injections of botulinum toxin and topical nitroglycerin ointment for the treatment of chronic anal fissure, *N Engl J Med* 341:1100-1104, 1998.
6. Iacono G, Cavataio F, Montalto G, et al: Intolerance of cow's milk and chronic constipation in children, *N Engl J Med* 339:1100-1104, 1998.
7. Kluiber RM, Wolff BG: Evaluation of anemia caused by hemorrhoidal bleeding, *Dis Colon Rectum* 37:1006-1007, 1994.
8. Nidorf DM, Jamison ER: Proctalgia fugax, *Am Fam Physician* 52:2238-2240, 1995.
9. Frisch M, Glimelius B, van den Brule AJ, et al: Sexually transmitted infection as a cause of anal cancer, *N Engl J Med* 337:1350-1358, 1997.

BILIARY SYSTEM
Gallstones

Risk factors for the development of gallstones include obesity, a sedentary life-style, a diet high in refined sugars and animal fats but low in vegetable fats and fiber,[1] rapid voluntary weight loss by the obese, and weight cycling.[2] Diabetes has traditionally been considered a risk factor, but this association may be due to obesity and lack of physical activity rather than the disease itself.[1] A prospective cohort study of men over the age of 40 found that coffee consumption decreased the risk of symptomatic gallstone disease.[3]

Clear indications for cholecystectomy are acute cholecystitis and gallstone-associated pancreatitis. The presence of asymptomatic gallstones is not an indication for surgery because the incidence of biliary pain in such circumstances is only 1% to 2% per year and decreases over time; serious sequelae are 10 times less frequent in asymptomatic cases. A more difficult decision is whether a patient who has had one episode of biliary colic needs surgery. In 30% no more episodes of pain occur, but the overall risk of recurrent pain is 30% to 50% per year for a few years.[4]

The pain of gallbladder disease must be differentiated from other causes of abdominal pain. Biliary colic tends to be infrequent, episodic, and intense. Short or fleeting pain or continuous pain is usually not due to gallstones.[4] Meperidine (Demerol) has been considered preferable to morphine for controlling the pain of biliary colic on the grounds that morphine causes more constriction of the sphincter of Oddi. This is a myth; morphine is more effective, is less toxic, and does not increase the risk of pancreatitis.[5] A nonnarcotic alternative available in the United Kingdom is diclofenac (Voltaren) 75 to 150 mg given IV, intramuscularly, or rectally.[6]

Advantages of laparoscopic cholecystectomy are better cosmetic results and a more rapid return to work or full activity. In one study the mean time to full recovery was 2 weeks for the laparoscopic procedures versus 8 weeks for the open procedure.[6] Another advantage is that the procedure can be safely performed as day surgery with no need for hospital admission.[7] A concern about laparoscopic cholecystectomy is that the rate of injury to the common bile duct, although low (up to 0.3%), is two to three times the rate with open cholecystectomy.[8] This higher rate might result from a learning curve among surgeons who are adopting the procedure.[4]

Although diarrhea is frequently said to be a common complication of cholecystectomy, this has not been confirmed by prospective studies. At most, some patients have a slight increase in defecation frequency and a decrease in constipation.[9]

REFERENCES

1. Misciagna G, Centonze S, Leoci C, et al: Diet, physical activity, and gallstones—a population-based, case-control study in southern Italy, *Am J Clin Nutr* 69:120-126, 1999.
2. Syngal S, Coakley EH, Willett WC, et al: Long-term weight patterns and risk for cholecystectomy in women, *Ann Intern Med* 130:471-477, 1999.
3. Leitzmann MF, Willett WC, Rimm EB, et al: A prospective study of coffee consumption and the risk of symptomatic gallstone disease in men, *JAMA* 281:2106-2112, 1999.
4. Ransohoff DF, McSherry CK: Why are cholecystectomy rates increasing? (editorial), *JAMA* 273:1621-1622, 1995.
5. Lee F: Meperidine vs morphine in pancreatitis and cholecystis (letter), *Arch Intern Med* 158:2399, 1998.
6. Bateson M: Gallbladder disease, *BMJ* 318:1745-1748, 1999.
7. Keulemans Y, Eshuis J, de Haes H, et al: Laparoscopic cholecystectomy: day-care versus clinical observation, *Ann Surg* 228:734-740, 1998.
8. Fletcher DR, Hobbs MS, Tan P, et al: Complications of cholecystectomy: risks of the laparoscopic approach and protective effects of operative cholangiography; a population-based study, *Ann Surg* 229:449-459, 1999.
9. Hearing SD, Thomas LA, Heaton KW, et al: Effect of cholecystectomy on bowel function: prospective, controlled study, *Gut* 45:889-894, 1999.

Endoscopic Retrograde Cholangiopancreatography and Sphincterotomy

Endoscopic retrograde cholangiopancreatography (ERCP) is often combined with sphincterotomy. Indications include bile duct obstruction with secondary acute cholangitis, common bile duct stones, common bile duct strictures, and malignancy in the region of the sphincter of Oddi. The procedure is complicated by acute pancreatitis or retroperitoneal perforation in 5% to 10% of cases; endoscopists who perform few procedures have higher complication rates than those who perform many.[1]

Dysfunction of the sphincter of Oddi is largely an American disorder; in other parts of the world patients with similar symptoms are usually considered to have irritable bowel disease. Dysfunction of the sphincter of Oddi is an ill-defined condition in which the major symptoms are abdominal pain and, occasionally, transient elevations of liver enzyme levels. It is most frequently diagnosed in middle-aged women who have had previous cholecystectomies. Sphincterotomy relieves symptoms in less than 75% of cases and is associated with a complication rate of over 20%.[2]

REFERENCES

1. Brugge WR, Van Dam J: Pancreatic and biliary endoscopy, *N Engl J Med* 341:1808-1816, 1999.
2. Huibregtse K: Complications of endoscopic sphincterotomy and their prevention (editorial), *N Engl J Med* 335:961-963, 1996.

CELIAC DISEASE

Celiac disease may be diagnosed at any age but is most commonly found in childhood or in the third to fifth decades.[1-3] A variety of presenting symptoms have been described in the literature: diarrhea; weight loss; bone pain from fractures[1,2]; fatigue[2,3]; recurrent aphthous ulcers[2,4] or sore tongue and mouth[2]; unexplained hypocalcemia, anemia,[2] or folate deficiency[1]; and autoimmune thyroiditis.[1] In fact, many[1] if not most[2,3] patients have few or no gastrointestinal symptoms, only a small proportion are underweight, and a significant number are overweight.[5] Not surprisingly, the diagnosis is often missed or delayed by several years.[6] A primary care case-finding study selected 1000 patients with symptoms, signs, or laboratory findings that could be consistent with celiac disease and screened them for endomysial antibodies. When results were positive, small bowel biopsy was performed. Thirty cases of celiac disease were diagnosed: 70% had a current or past history of unexplained anemia (usually microcytic) and 30% were "tired all the time" (some patients had both findings). Looked at another way, 23% of male and 11% of female patients with anemia had celiac disease, whereas less than 3% of those with chronic fatigue had the disorder.[3]

Traditional screening tests for celiac disease are serum and red blood cell folate measurements because levels are reputed to low in nearly all cases.[7] More sophisticated tests, which are not available in all centers, are antigliadin antibodies (gliadin is a portion of the protein gluten)[8] or endomysial antibodies,[2,3] but definitive diagnosis is made with a small bowel biopsy.[2,3,8]

Major complications of celiac disease are osteoporosis, fractures, and small bowel lymphoma. A strict gluten-free diet not only relieves symptoms, but diminishes the risks of these complications.[2]

REFERENCES

1. Shaker JL, Brickner RC, Findling JW, et al: Hypocalcemia and skeletal disease as presenting features of celiac disease, *Arch Intern Med* 157:1013-1016, 1997.
2. Feighery C: Coeliac disease, *BMJ* 319:236-239, 1999.
3. Hin H, Bird G, Fisher P, et al: Coeliac disease in primary care: case finding study, *BMJ* 318:164-167, 1999.
4. Srinivasan U, Weir DG, Feighery C, et al: Emergence of classic enteropathy after longstanding gluten sensitive oral ulceration, *BMJ* 316:206-207, 1998.
5. Dickey W, Bodkin S: Prospective study of body mass index in patients with coeliac disease, *BMJ* 317:1290, 1998.
6. Dickey W, McConnell JB: How many visits dose it take before celiac sprue is diagnosed? *J Clin Gastroenterol* 23:21-23, 1996.

7. Ballinger AB, Cevallos AM, Clark ML: Patients with chronic diarrhea (letter), *N Engl J Med* 333:257, 1995.
8. Chartrand LJ, Agulnik J, Vanounou T, et al: Effectiveness of antigliadin antibodies as a screening test for celiac disease in children, *Can Med Assoc J* 157:527-533, 1997.

COLON

(See also inflammatory bowel disease; irritable bowel disease)

Colon Cancer

(See also anemia; hematochezia)

Epidemiology

About 15% of newly diagnosed cancers in both men and women occur in the colon and rectum. Colorectal cancer is the third most common cancer in the United States and has the third highest mortality rate. The incidence increases progressively with age; in North America the lifetime risk of having the disease is estimated to be 6% and the lifetime risk of dying of the disease is about 2.6%.[1] The median age at diagnosis is 70, and only 4% of cases occur in persons under 50.

The distribution of cancers within the colon has changed over the past few decades so that more lesions are now found on the right side and fewer on the left side. At present at least half of all colonic polyps and cancers are within 60 cm of the anus and so are at least theoretically within reach of the long flexible sigmoidoscope.[2]

A number of recognized risk factors have been recognized or postulated for colon cancer:

1. Familial polyposis syndrome[1]
2. Personal history of large adenomatous colonic polyps or colon cancer[1]
3. Personal history of endometrial, ovarian, or breast cancer[1]
4. Family history of colon cancer. The relative risk is much higher for persons under 45 years of age (5.37) and is negligible for those 60 and older.[3]
5. Family history of adenomatous polyps. The risk is particularly great if the polyps are diagnosed in patients under the age of 50.[4]
6. Inflammatory bowel disease. Ulcerative colitis and to a lesser extent Crohn's disease are risk factors. In the case of ulcerative colitis the risk is greatest if the patient has had extensive colonic involvement for over 7 years. The risk is higher with right-sided colonic involvement but is not increased if the disease is limited to the sigmoid colon and rectum.[5]
7. Cigarette smoking. The induction period appears to be on the order of 35 years.[6,7]
8. Diet. Epidemiological evidence points to an increased risk of colon cancer among those whose diet is high in fat and meat and a decreased risk among those who eat a lot of fruits and vegetables[8] or bread and pasta.[9] High-fiber diets (mainly cereals) have long been thought to protect against colon cancer,

and this view is supported by an international prospective cohort study published in 1999.[10] However, a prospective cohort study of nurses, also published in 1999, failed to find such a correlation.[11]

9. Vitamins. A diet high in folate or vitamin E[10] or the long-term use of multivitamins containing folate is associated with a lower risk of colon cancer.[12]
10. Activity and obesity. Both sedentary life-style[13] and obesity[13-15] increase the risk of colorectal cancer, whereas leisure-time physical activity decreases the risk.[13]
11. Diabetes. In the Nurses' Health Study, women with type 2 diabetes were found to be at increased risk for colorectal cancer.[16]
12. Constipation. A case-control trial found constipation to be a risk factor.[17]

The overall mortality rate for cancer of the large bowel is 50%. The rate depends on the stage of the cancer. For stage I disease (Dukes' stages A and B-1) in which invasion is limited to the muscularis propria without nodal involvement, the cure rate is 90%. For stage II (Dukes' stage B-2) in which cancer has invaded through the muscularis to the serosa but nodes are not involved, the cure rate is 75%. For stage III disease (Dukes' stage C), in which the disease has metastasized to the regional nodes, the cure rate is 35%.[18]

◢ REFERENCES ◣

1. US Preventive Services Task Force: *Guide to clinical preventive services,* ed 2, Baltimore, 1996, Williams & Wilkins, pp 89-103.
2. Lieberman D, Smith F: Screening asymptomatic subjects for colon malignancy with colonoscopy, *Am J Gastroenterol* 86:946-951, 1991.
3. Fuchs CS, Giovannucci EL, Colditz GA, et al: A prospective study of family history and the risk of colorectal cancer, *N Engl J Med* 331:1169-1174, 1994.
4. Ahsan H, Neugut AI, Garbowski GC, et al: Family history of colorectal adenomatous polyps and increased risk for colorectal cancer, *Ann Intern Med* 128:900-905, 1998.
5. Donald JJ, Burhenne HJ: Colorectal cancer: can we lower the death rate in the 1990s? *Can Fam Physician* 39:107-114, 1993.
6. Giovannucci E, Rimm EB, Stampfer MF, et al: A prospective study of cigarette smoking and risk of colorectal adenoma and colorectal cancer in U.S. men, *J Natl Cancer Inst* 86:183-191, 1994.
7. Giovannucci I, Colditz GA, Stampfer MJ, et al: A prospective study of cigarette smoking and risk of colorectal adenoma and colorectal cancer in U.S. women, *J Natl Cancer Inst* 86:162-164, 1994.
8. Potter JD: Nutrition and colorectal cancer, *Cancer Causes Control* 7:127-146, 1996.
9. Chatenoud L, Tavani A, La Vecchia C, et al: Whole grain food intake and cancer risk, *Int J Cancer* 77:24-28, 1998.
10. Jansen MC, Bueno-de-Mesquita HB, Buzina R, et al: Dietary fiber and plant foods in relation to colorectal cancer mortality: the Seven Countries Study, *Int J Cancer* 81:174-179, 1999.

11. Fuchs CS, Giovannucci EL, Colditz GA, et al: Dietary fiber and the risk of colorectal cancer and adenoma in women, *N Engl J Med* 340:169-176, 1999.

12. Giovannucci E, Stampfer MJ, Colditz GA, et al: Multivitamin use, folate, and colon cancer in women in the Nurses' Health Study, *Ann Intern Med* 129:517-524, 1998.

13. Martinez ME, Giovannucci E, Spiegelman D, et al: Leisure-time physical activity, body size, and colon cancer in women: Nurses' Health Study Research Group, *J Natl Cancer Inst* 89:948-955, 1997.

14. Schoen RE, Tangen CM, Kuller LH, et al: Increased blood glucose and insulin, body size, and incident colorectal cancer, *J Natl Cancer Inst* 91:1147-1154, 1999.

15. Ford ES: Body mass index and colon cancer in a national sample of adult US men and women, *Am J Epidemiol* 150:390-398, 1999.

16. Hu FB, Manson JE, Liu S, et al: Prospective study of adult on-set diabetes mellitus (type 2) and risk of colorectal cancer in women, *J Natl Cancer Inst* 91:542-547, 1999.

17. Jacobs EJ, White E: Constipation, laxative use, and colon cancer among middle-aged adults, *Epidemiology* 9:385-391, 1998.

18. Moertel CG: Chemotherapy for colorectal cancer, *N Engl J Med* 330:1136-1142, 1994.

Primary prevention of colon cancer

(See also exercise; healthy user effect)

Diet, exercise, and smoking. In view of the risk factors enumerated in the previous section, a diet containing plenty of vegetables, fruit, bread, and pasta would probably be beneficial, as might taking a multivitamin containing folate. Every effort should be made to be physically active and to refrain from smoking.

One study found that a daily supplement of 3 g of calcium carbonate (1200 mg of elemental calcium) decreased the risk for colonic adenomas. At least in theory this might also decrease the risk of colon cancer.[1]

Hormone replacement therapy. A number of observational studies have shown a decreased risk of colon cancer[2,3] and adenomatous polyps[3] in women on hormone replacement therapy. No randomized controlled trials have been published, so whether these findings represent a "healthy user" effect is not known.

Nonsteroidal antiinflammatory drugs. Several prospective studies involving men and women have shown a significant decrease in the incidence[4-6] and mortality[5] of colon cancer in individuals taking 325 mg of aspirin at least four to six times a week; this benefit may not become obvious until 10 years has elapsed.[6] However, a 12-year follow-up of the Physicians' Health Study failed to show such a relationship.[7] A retrospective population-based cohort study found that long-term use of nonaspirin NSAIDs also provided protection against colon cancer. No one class of drugs was better than another, and low doses appeared to be as effective as high ones.[8] NSAIDs reduce the incidence of adenomas in humans, and various NSAIDs inhibit carcinogenesis in the colon in experimental animals.[4,5] One editorial writer has recommended that patients at elevated risk of colon cancer take an aspirin a day. Elevated risk is defined as having a past history of colonic adenoma or cancer; a family history of colorectal cancer or adenoma; inflammatory bowel disease; or breast, ovarian, or endometrial cancer.[9]

──────────── ❧ **REFERENCES** ❧ ────────────

1. Baron JA, Beach M, Mandel JS, et al: Calcium supplements for the prevention of colorectal adenomas, *N Engl J Med* 340:101-107, 1999.

2. Paganini-Hill A: Estrogen replacement therapy and colorectal cancer risk in elderly women, *Dis Colon Rectum* 42:1300-1305, 1999.

3. Grodstein F, Martinez E, Platz EA, et al: Postmenopausal hormone use and risk for colorectal cancer and adenoma, *Ann Intern Med* 128:705-712, 1998.

4. Peleg II, Lubin MF, Cotsonis GA, et al: Long-term use of non-steroidal antiinflammatory drugs and other chemopreventors and risk of subsequent colorectal neoplasia, *Dig Dis Sci* 41:1319-1326, 1996.

5. Thun MJ, Namboodiri MM, Heath CW Jr: Aspirin use and risk of fatal cancer, *Cancer Res* 53:1322-1327, 1993.

6. Giovannucci E, Egan KM, Hunter DJ, et al: Aspirin and the risk of colorectal cancer in women, *N Engl J Med* 333:609-614, 1995.

7. Stürmer T, Glynn RJ, Lee IM, et al: Aspirin use and colorectal cancer: post-trial follow-up data from the Physicians' Health Study, *Ann Intern Med* 128:713-720, 1998.

8. Smalley W, Ray WA, Daugherty J, et al: Use of nonsteroidal anti-inflammatory drugs and incidence of colorectal cancer: a population-based study, *Arch Intern Med* 159:161-166, 1999.

9. Marcus AJ: Aspirin prophylaxis against colorectal cancer (editorial), *N Engl J Med* 333:656-657, 1995.

Secondary prevention of colon cancer

(See also hematochezia; informed consent; positive predictive value; prevention; relative risk reduction)

Fecal occult blood screening. In a study by Mandel and associates[1] from the University of Minnesota, mortality from colon cancer was decreased by a relative rate of 33% over 13 years by annual Hemoccult testing. (On average each patient submitted samples for 8 years; each test consisted of six specimens obtained from three different stool samples.) The number of individuals who had to be screened over 13 years to prevent one colon cancer death was 360, or put another way, screened individuals decreased their risk of dying of colon cancer by 0.3%.[1,2] There was no reduction in total mortality. This relative mortality reduction rate of 33% translates into an absolute mortality reduction rate of 3:1000 or 0.3%. The positive predictive value of the Hemoccult testing for cancer was 2.2%, but for cancer and polyps combined it was 30%.[1] After 18 years of follow-up the absolute reduction in cancer mortality in this group of patients was 5:1000 or 0.5% and there was still no reduction in total mortality; analysis of 3200 stool samples for occult blood was required to save one life.[3]

Fecal occult blood testing in the Minnesota trial triggered large numbers of colonoscopies. Among the 15,000 patients in the annual Hemoccult testing group, 4500 had colonoscopies.[4] The reported complications of colonoscopy in this study were four perforations requiring surgery and 11 episodes of serious bleeding, three of which required surgery.[1]

Two large prospective studies of fecal occult blood screening were published in the *Lancet* in 1996, one from Great Britain[5] and one from Denmark.[6] Both screened patients every 2 years, and both showed a small but significant decline in colon cancer–related mortality (but not total cohort mortality) in the screened group. In the British study the 15% relative reduction in colon cancer deaths over 8 years of follow-up meant that 747 patients had to be screened to prevent one colon cancer death,[2] while in the Danish study the 18% relative reduction of colon cancer deaths over 10 years of follow-up meant that 470 patients had to be screened to prevent one colon cancer death.[2] Both these studies are notable in that only about 4% of the screened cohort had full colonoscopies.[5,6] Six major complications of colonoscopy (a rate of 0.5%) were reported in the British study; only one occurred during diagnostic endoscopy, and the other five were associated with therapeutic interventions.[2]

The study by Mandel and associates from the University of Minnesota also analyzed a group of patients screened biennially. At 13 years of follow-up no decrease in colon cancer mortality was found,[1] but after 18 years there was a 21% relative reduction in cancer mortality. Screening 1000 patients led to three fewer colon cancer deaths after 18 years.[3]

A systematic review of five major Hemoccult screening studies concluded that Hemoccult screening of 10,000 people every second year for 10 years would result in 8.5 fewer cancer deaths than would occur in a nonscreened population of equal numbers (relative reduction of 16%; number needed to screen to prevent one cancer death = 1176).[7]

Fecal occult blood screening for colon cancer or adenomas is neither sensitive (few adenomas bleed and even advanced cancers tend to bleed intermittently) nor specific (most positive occult blood tests are associated with innocuous conditions). In prospective studies of asymptomatic populations comparing fecal occult blood screening to colonoscopy, only 26% of cancers and 12% of large adenomas were associated with positive Hemoccult tests. The low sensitivity explains why two thirds of colon cancers are not detected, and the low specificity why many colonoscopies (50 in the Minnesota trial) are required to detect one cancer. The decreased colon cancer mortality seen with fecal occult blood screening is probably due to the detection of early cancers rather than to the detection and removal of adenomas—adenomas rarely bleed and the incidence of colon cancer is not decreased in screened populations.[8]

Fecal occult blood screening is not innocuous. The high false-negative rate may falsely reassure patients and lead them to ignore symptoms of cancer, and many patients without cancer are subjected to colonoscopy with its attendant complications (see later discussion). It is even possible that deaths caused by screening cancel out the decreased mortality from colon cancer.[8]

The Canadian Task Force on Preventive Health Care gives fecal occult blood testing a "C" recommendation,[9] while the U.S. Preventive Services Task Force gives annual fecal occult blood testing (with or without sigmoidoscopy, time interval not specified) a "B" recommendation.[10] In 1997 guidelines for screening for colorectal cancer were issued by a multidisciplinary expert panel administered by the American Gastroenterological Association under the auspices of the Agency for Health Care Policy and Research (AHCPR). These guidelines were endorsed by a number of other organizations, including the American Cancer Society. They recommend that average-risk men and women 50 years and over undergo screening. Although the only screening programs that have been proved to decrease colon cancer mortality in randomized controlled studies are those using fecal occult blood testing, the new guidelines offer several screening options to be selected by individual patients and their physicians. These are annual fecal occult blood testing, flexible sigmoidoscopy every 5 years, flexible sigmoidoscopy every 5 years plus fecal occult blood testing annually, barium enema every 5 to 10 years, and full colonoscopy every 10 years.[11]

In 1999 the Centers for Disease Control and Prevention, the Health Care Financing Administration, and the National Cancer Institute launched a campaign called "Screen for Life" to educate people in the United States about the value of screening for colorectal cancer. The website (http://www.cdc.gov/cancer/screenforlife) does not mention the very small number of individuals who might benefit or the numerous adverse effects that are intrinsic to such a screening program.

Colonoscopy and sigmoidoscopy screening. No prospective randomized controlled trials have been published to show that screening sigmoidoscopy or colonoscopy decreases colon cancer mortality. However, case-control studies suggest a protective effect from sigmoidoscopy. Selby and co-workers[12] from the Kaiser Permanente Program in Oakland, California, studied a group of patients who died of colon cancer and compared them with a series of matched control subjects who did not have colon cancer. When cancers within reach of the sigmoidoscope were evaluated, 8.8% of the cancer patients had had one or more previous rigid sigmoidoscopies, compared with 24.2% of the control group. In contrast, when cancers above the reach of the sigmoidoscope were assessed, the rates of previous sigmoidoscopies were equal in the cancer patients and the control subjects. The protective effect of sigmoidoscopy was apparent even when it had been performed as much as 10 years previously.

In another study suggesting a protective effect of sigmoidoscopy, Atkin and associates[13] in Great Britain found that removal of tubular adenomas at sigmoidoscopy was associated with a low cancer rate at follow-up. Similar results were reported from a case-controlled Veterans Administration study in the United States; the odds ratio of mortality for patients who had a diagnostic procedure of the large bowel was 0.41 compared with control subjects who did not have such procedures. This protective effect was most marked if tissue had been removed.[14]

For flexible sigmoidoscopy or colonoscopy to be used as a screening method for the detection of colon cancer, the frequency of examinations needs to be determined. As noted previously, the AHCPR recommends flexible sigmoidoscopy every 5 years or full colonoscopy every 10 years.[10] Another approach for which suggestive but not definitive evidence has been presented is selective colonoscopy for screening of high-risk patients such as those with a strong family history of colon cancer.[15]

Is the potential value of sigmoidoscopy screening decreased in the elderly? A Norwegian colonoscopy screening study of 193 asymptomatic men and women with a mean age of 67.4 years detected adenomas in 38% of the women and 47% of the men, and in almost half the cases the adenomas were proximal to the sigmoid colon and would not have been detected by sigmoidoscopy. However, since the average time for an adenoma to progress to malignancy is 10 to 15 years, most elderly patients would die of other causes before the development of colon cancer.[16]

The best known complications of colonoscopy are perforation, major hemorrhage, and death. Both perforation and hemorrhage are more common if a polypectomy is performed during the endoscopy. In 1996 Waye, Kahn, and Auerbach[17] analyzed the combined complication rates of the few prospective studies of colonoscopy complications reported between 1987 and 1994. The perforation rate was 1:2222, the rate of significant hemorrhage was 1:81 if a polypectomy had been performed and 1:1352 if it had not, and the mortality rate was 1:16,745. These rates were lower than those reported in previous decades, which the authors attributed to improved physician training and better instruments. They cautioned, however, that reports from centers with extensive experience in endoscopy may not reflect the experience of the broader medical community, since complication rates are known to be higher for inexperienced operators.[17]

Morbidity and mortality after colonoscopy are not limited to the complications of perforation and hemorrhage. The most common cause of death associated with colonoscopy is cardiac, possibly related to stress or to onerous preparatory regimens. The detection of cancers (or adenomas that cannot be resected during endoscopy) leads to surgical interventions—procedures with mortality rates of 1% to 7%. Some patients who die as a result of surgery harbor lesions that would never have manifested themselves clinically had they been left alone.[8]

A rare but serious complication of colonoscopy is found in the report of the transmission of hepatitis C infection to two patients as a result of inadequate cleaning of a colonoscope.[18] That more cases have not been reported may be due to the difficulty in identifying the disease in many cases (the incubation period is 30 to 90 days, and only 25% of affected persons become jaundiced).[19] Although following the established guidelines for cleaning colonoscopes should prevent such transmission of disease,[20] surveys suggest that inadequate disinfection is common in clinical practice.[21,22] One microbiology study found that 24% of "patient-ready" endoscopes were contaminated.[22]

Waye, Kahn, and Auerbach[17] were unable to find any randomized prospective trials reporting the complications of flexible sigmoidoscopy. Cohen and associates[23] quoted a perforation rate of 1:8795, and a 1996 Swedish report recorded a rate of 1:716.[24] The authors of the latter study attributed their high rate to the initial inexperience of the endoscopists.[24] A survey of British gastroenterologists reported a perforation rate of 1:16,810 for flexible fiberoptic sigmoidoscopy.[25]

A potential barrier to adopting population-based screening by flexible sigmoidoscopy is a lack of adequately trained endoscopists. Nonphysician endoscopists might be the answer; two trials comparing endoscopies performed by a nurse[26,27] or physician assistant[27] with those performed by a gastroenterologist found no difference between the groups in the detection of adenomatous polyps or in complications.

Strong evidence suggests that screening by flexible fiberoptic sigmoidoscopy may decrease the incidence and mortality of colon cancer, but whether these probable benefits outweigh the adverse effects remains in question. In considering these issues, both physicians and patients should be aware that the published complication rates of sigmoidoscopy and colonoscopy are mostly from centers with considerable experience in the use of these instruments. It is almost certain that complication rates are higher for practitioners who only occasionally perform these procedures; as far as I have been able to determine, such statistics are not currently available. Physicians should also realize that if such screening is undertaken, the value, if any, of repeat screening in negative cases and the time intervals at which it should be performed are unknown.

If screening sigmoidoscopy is to be undertaken, adequate bowel preparation is necessary. A prospective single-blinded randomized trial found that a light breakfast on the morning of the procedure followed by two Fleet phosphate enemas was as effective as more complex regimens involving oral laxatives, clear liquid dinner the previous evening, and nothing per os after midnight.[28]

Barium enema screening. Although no definitive studies have shown a decrease in colorectal mortality associated with double-contrast barium enema screening, the American Gastroenterological Association recommends this procedure every 5 to 10 years as an alternative to fecal occult blood or endoscopy screening (see previous discussion).[11] The rationale is that any procedure that can detect polyps and allow their removal should prevent colorectal cancer.

Virtual colonoscopy. An evolving technology that may play an important role in colon cancer screening is virtual colonoscopy. Bowel preparation is similar to that used for conventional colonoscopy. The empty colon is distended with air, and multiple two-dimensional thin-section images of the colon are rapidly obtained by means of helical computed tomography. The images are then reconstructed off line to create three-dimensional images simulating what is seen with conventional colonoscopy. In preliminary trials this technique has proved as effective as conventional colonoscopy in detecting lesions larger than 5 mm.[29]

❧ REFERENCES ❧

1. Mandel JS, Bond JH, Church TR, et al: Reducing mortality from colorectal cancer by screening for fecal occult blood, *N Engl J Med* 328:1365-1371, 1993.

2. Robinson MH, Hardcastle JD, Moss SM, et al: The risks of screening: data from the Nottingham randomised controlled trial of faecal occult blood screening for colorectal cancer, *Gut* 45:588-592, 1999.

3. Mandel JS, Church TR, Ederer F, et al: Colorectal cancer mortality: effectiveness of biennial screening for fecal occult blood, *J Natl Cancer Inst* 91:434-437, 1999.

4. Mandel JS, Church TR, Ederer F: Screening for colorectal cancer (letter), *N Engl J Med* 329:1353-1354, 1993.

5. Hardcastle JD, Chamberlain JO, Robinson MH, et al: Randomised controlled trial of faecal-occult-blood screening for colorectal cancer, *Lancet* 348:1472-1477, 1996.

6. Kronborg O, Fenger C, Olsen J, et al: Randomised study of screening for colorectal cancer with faecal-occult-blood test, *Lancet* 348:1467-1471, 1996.

7. Towler B, Irwig L, Glasziou P, et al: A systematic review of the effects of screening for colorectal cancer using the faecal occult blood test, Hemoccult, *BMJ* 317:559-565, 1998.

8. Ahlquist DA: Fecal occult blood testing for colorectal cancer: can we afford to do this? *Gastroenterol Clin North Am* 26:41-55, 1997.

9. Canadian Task Force on the Periodic Health Examination: *Clinical preventive health care,* Ottawa, 1994, Canadian Communication Group—Publishing, pp 798-809.

10. US Preventive Services Task Force: *Guide to clinical preventive services,* ed 2, Baltimore, 1996, Williams & Wilkins, pp 89-103.

11. Winawer SJ, Fletcher RH, Miller L, et al: Colorectal cancer screening and surveillance: clinical guidelines, evidence and rationale, *Gastroenterology* 112:594-642, 1997.

12. Selby JV, Friedman GD, Quesenberry CP Jr, et al: A case-control study of screening sigmoidoscopy and mortality from colorectal cancer, *N Engl J Med* 326:653-657, 1992.

13. Atkin WS, Morson BC, Cuzick J: Long-term risk of colorectal cancer after excision of rectosigmoid adenomas, *N Engl J Med* 326:658-662, 1992.

14. Mueller AD, Sonnenberg A: Protection by endoscopy against death from colorectal cancer: a case-control study among veterans, *Arch Intern Med* 155:1741-1748, 1995.

15. Chen TH-H, Yen M-F, Lai M-S, et al: Evaluation of a selective screening for colorectal carcinoma: the Taiwan Multicenter Cancer Screening (TAMCAS) Project, *Cancer* 86:1116-1128, 1999.

16. Thiis-Evensen E, Hoff GS, Sauar J, et al: Flexible sigmoidoscopy or colonoscopy as a screening modality for colorectal adenomas in older age groups? Findings in a cohort of the normal population aged 63-72 years, *Gut* 45:834-839, 1999.

17. Waye JD, Kahn O, Auerbach ME: Complications of colonoscopy and flexible sigmoidoscopy, *Gastrointest Endosc Clin North Am* 6:343-374, 1996.

18. Bronowicki J-P, Venard V, Botté C, et al: Patient-to-patient transmission of hepatitis C virus during colonoscopy, *N Engl J Med* 337:237-240, 1997.

19. Bronowicki J-P, Bigard M-A: Transmission of hepatitis C virus during colonoscopy (letter), *N Engl J Med* 337:1849, 1997.

20. American Society for Gastrointestinal Endoscopy Ad Hoc Committee on Disinfection: Reprocessing of flexible gastrointestinal endoscopes, *Gastrointest Endosc* 43:540-546, 1996.

21. Spach DH, Silverstein FE, Stamm WE: Transmission of infection by gastrointestinal endoscopy and bronchoscopy, *Ann Intern Med* 118:117-128, 1993.

22. Kaczmarek RG, Moore RM, McCrohan J, et al: Multi-state investigation of the actual disinfection/sterilization of endoscopes in health care facilities, *Am J Med* 92:257-261, 1992.

23. Cohen LB, Basuk PM, Waye JD: *Practical flexible sigmoidoscopy,* New York, 1995, Igaku-Shoin, pp 117-125.

24. Kewenter J, Brevinge H: Endoscopic and surgical complications of work-up in screening for colorectal cancer, *Dis Colon Rectum* 39:676-680, 1996.

25. Robinson RJ, Stone M, Mayberry JF: Sigmoidoscopy and rectal biopsy—a survey of current UK practice, *Eur J Gastroenterol Hepatol* 8:149-151, 1996.

26. Schoenfeld P, Lipscomb S, Crook J, et al: Accuracy of polyp detection by gastroenterologists and nurse endoscopists during flexible sigmoidoscopy: a randomized trial, *Gastroenterology* 117:312-318, 1999.

27. Wallace MB, Kemp JA, Meyer F, et al: Screening for colorectal cancer with flexible sigmoidoscopy by nonphysician endoscopists, *Am J Med* 107:214-218, 1999.

28. Manoucheri M, Nakamura DY, Lukman RL: Bowel preparation for flexible sigmoidoscopy: which method yields the best results? *J Fam Pract* 48:272-274, 1999.

29. Fenlon HM, Nunes DP, Schroy PC III, et al: A comparison of virtual and conventional colonoscopy for the detection of colorectal polyps, *N Engl J Med* 341:1496-1503, 1999.

Colonoscopy versus barium enema for investigation of suspected colon cancer

(See also secondary prevention of colon cancer)

If clinical findings indicate that a patient may have colon cancer, the major investigative techniques of choice are colonoscopy and barium enema. Fecal occult blood testing has little or no value in this context, since further investigation is required regardless of whether the test result is positive.

A complete colonoscopy and a well-performed barium enema are excellent means of detecting cancers and polyps. A double-contrast barium enema is thought to give a greater yield for polyps smaller than 1 cm than does a single-contrast study, but for polyps larger than 1 cm they are equally effective.[1] Both barium enema and colonoscopy detect a few cases that were missed by the other. One review of the radiological literature found that colorectal cancer was detected by barium enema in 90% to 99% of cases.[2] In general, rigid sigmoidoscopy detects about 25% of colonic polyps and flexible 60-cm fiberoptic sigmoidoscopy detects 50% to 60%.[3]

A clear advantage of colonoscopy is that a biopsy can be performed at once if a cancer is detected and that a polyp, if seen, can be removed during the procedure. Another advantage, according to one survey, is that patients prefer colonoscopy to a double-contrast barium enema, probably because of the sedating and analgesic medications given with the former.[4]

An important factor influencing the choice of any investigative procedure is the complication rates. For a barium enema the perforation rate is 1:10,000 and the mortality rate is 1:50,000.[3] For a full colonoscopy these numbers are higher (see discussion of secondary prevention of colon cancer).

⚐ REFERENCES ⚐

1. Donald JJ, Burhenne HJ: Colorectal cancer: can we lower the death rate in the 1990s? *Can Fam Physician* 39:107-114, 1993.
2. Levine R, Tenner S, Fromm H: Prevention and early detection of colorectal cancer, *Am Fam Physician* 45:663-668, 1992.
3. Gelfand DW, Ott DJ: The economic implications of radiologic screening for colonic cancer, *Am J Roentgenol* 156:939-943, 1991.
4. Van Ness MM, Chobanian SJ, Winters C Jr, et al: A study of patient acceptance of double-contrast barium enema and colonoscopy: which procedure is preferred by patients? *Arch Intern Med* 147:2175-2176, 1987.

Management of colorectal cancer

(See also oncology)

Adjuvant chemotherapy. A combination of fluorouracil and levamisole has been shown to decrease the rate of recurrence of stage III (Dukes' C) colon cancer by 40% and the death rate by 33%.[1] Chemotherapy also appears to provide a slight benefit in stage II (Dukes' B) disease, but whether it should be prescribed for all patients is not yet clear.[2]

Adjuvant radiation therapy. A randomized prospective study from Sweden compared surgery alone to preoperative radiation plus surgery for resectable rectal carcinoma. After 5 years the local recurrence rate among those who did not receive radiation therapy was 27% compared with 11% among those who were irradiated. The overall 5-year survival was 48% in the surgery-only group and 58% in the surgery plus radiation therapy group.[3]

Resection of hepatic metastases. Resection of hepatic metastases is associated with a 2-year survival rate of 65%. In one study the addition of hepatic arterial chemotherapy infusion combined with systemic chemotherapy led to a 2-year survival rate of 86%.[4]

Alcohol avoidance. A small Japanese study reported a higher rate of liver metastases in patients with colon cancer who consumed alcohol than among those who did not.[5]

Postoperative surveillance. The American Society of Clinical Oncology guidelines for postoperative surveillance advise that the following interventions be undertaken: history and physical examinations every 3 to 6 months for the first 3 years and annually thereafter (expert opinion), colonoscopy every 3 to 5 years, regular flexible sigmoidoscopy for those who had rectal cancer resected but who received no adjuvant radiation therapy, and carcinoembryonic antigen assays every 2 to 3 months for patients with stage II disease provided they would be suitable candidates for resection of hepatic metastases. The Society of Clinical Oncology advises against performing regular complete blood counts, liver function tests, fecal occult blood tests, chest x-ray examinations, computed tomography, and pelvic imaging.[6]

⚐ REFERENCES ⚐

1. Moertel CG, Fleming TR, Macdonald JS, et al: Fluorouracil plus levamisole as effective adjuvant therapy after resection of stage III colon carcinoma: a final report, *Ann Intern Med* 122:321-326, 1995.
2. Harrington DP: The tea leaves of small trials (editorial), *J Clin Oncol* 17:1336-1338, 1999.
3. Swedish Rectal Cancer Trial: Improved survival with preoperative radiotherapy in resectable rectal cancer, *N Engl J Med* 336:980-987, 1997.
4. Kemeny N, Huang Y, Cohen A, et al: Hepatic arterial infusion of chemotherapy after resection of hepatic metastases from colorectal cancer, *N Engl J Med* 341:2039-2048, 1999.
5. Maeda M, Nagawa H, Maeda T, et al: Alcohol consumption enhances liver metastasis in colorectal carcinoma patients, *Cancer* 83:1483-1488, 1998.
6. Desch CE, Benson AB III, Smith TJ, et al: Recommended colorectal cancer surveillance guidelines by the American Society of Clinical Oncology, *J Clin Oncol* 17:1312-1321, 1999.

Diverticulitis

In Western society, diverticula are found in 5% to 10% of individuals over 45 years of age and the vast majority of those over 80. Diverticulitis develops in only 20% of those with diverticula, and in 85% of cases the disease involves the descending or sigmoid colon. The most common presenting symptoms and signs are pain and tenderness in the left lower quadrant. If the affected bowel is near the bladder, the patient may have dysuria and frequency, and if it crosses the midline, tenderness may be detected in the right lower quadrant. Diarrhea or constipation may also occur; gross blood in the stool is rare.[1]

The imaging process of choice for diagnosing diverticulitis is computed tomographic (CT) scanning. Endoscopy may help rule out other conditions but is not useful for making a positive diagnosis of diverticulitis because the inflammatory process in this condition is in the pericolic region and the bowel mucosa is normal.[1]

Treatment of a mild first attack of diverticulitis in patients who can tolerate oral hydration is a 7- to 10-day course of a liquid diet combined with broad-spectrum oral antibiotics, such as ciprofloxacin and metronidazole, that cover both aerobic and anaerobic organisms. Sicker patients, or those who do not respond to outpatient management, require admission, nothing by mouth, and IV antibiotics. In many cases abscesses detected by CT scanning can be drained percutaneously with CT guidance. About 20% of patients with diverticulitis require surgery. Once the acute attack has resolved, the patients should be placed on a high-fiber diet.[1]

REFERENCES

1. Ferzoco LB, Raptopoulos V, Silen W: Acute diverticulitis, *N Engl J Med* 338:1521-1526, 1998.

Familial Polyposis

Presymptomatic diagnosis of adenomatous familial polyposis is possible in the majority of cases by a blood test involving molecular genetic diagnosis.[1] Both indomethacin (Indocin, Indocid) and sulindac (Clinoril) have been shown to cause regression of polyps in familial polyposis and are routinely prescribed for patients who have had a total colectomy with ileorectal anastomosis.[2]

REFERENCES

1. Powell SM, Petersen GM, Krush AJ, et al: Molecular diagnosis of familial adenomatous polyposis, *N Engl J Med* 329:1982-1987, 1993.
2. Hirota C, Iida M, Aoyagi K, et al: Effect of indomethacin suppositories on rectal polyposis in patients with familial adenomatous polyposis, *Cancer* 78:1660-1665, 1996.

CONSTIPATION
(See also anal fissures; pain, chronic)

Normally persons have between three bowel movements a day and three bowel movements a week.[1] A working definition accepted by many experts is the "Rome criteria." According to these criteria constipation is the presence of two or more of the following for at least 3 months[2]:
1. Two or fewer bowel movements a week
2. Stool weight of less than 35 g/day
3. Hard lumpy stool on more than 25% of occasions
4. Straining on more than 25% of occasions
5. Sensation of incomplete evacuation on more than 25% of occasions

Management of Constipation in the Community

Once organic disease is ruled out, most patients in the community who are truly constipated may be managed with exercise, good hydration, and fiber. Constipated patients should be started on regular supplements of bran or psyllium (Metamucil, Prodiem), beginning with 1 tbsp/day and working up as rapidly as possible to 3 tbsp/day. Each dose should be accompanied or followed by 8 oz of water or other fluid. If this does not resolve the problem, the patient should be given an osmotic laxative, such as lactulose (Lactulax) 30 to 60 ml hs or magnesium hydroxide (Milk of Magnesia) 15 to 30 ml hs. Use of other laxatives, including mineral oil, those that cause intestinal secretion (docusate [Colace, Regulex]), and stimulant laxatives (sennosides [Senokot], bisacodyl [Dulcolax], glycerin suppositories), should be avoided because they may lead to the laxative abuse syndrome. An important behavioral aspect of the treatment plan is instructing the patient to sit on the toilet for 15 to 20 minutes after breakfast without any distractions and to avoid straining during this time.[1]

Laxatives in Palliative Care

The discussion on the use of laxatives in this section applies primarily to immobilized patients and those receiving narcotics. Stool softeners and peristaltic stimulants take 6 to 9 hours to work, so they should be given at bedtime. The two should be administered together because using only a stool softener may cause soft stool to accumulate in the rectum. Suppositories work within the hour, so they should be given half an hour before breakfast or supper.[3] The suppositories should be pushed against rectal mucosa, not into stool. They should be inserted with the "base" and not the pointed end first.[4]

The following sequence of therapeutic interventions for constipation is one physician's guideline for palliative care.[3] Missing here is the osmotic laxative lactulose (Lactulax). In doses of 15 to 60 ml/day it is usually very effective.
1. Encourage fluids, fiber, and exercise.
2. Use one of these: standardized sennosides (Senokot) 1 to 2 tablets hs plus docusate sodium (Colace, Regulex) 100 mg bid; or bisacodyl (Dulcolax) 5 to 15 mg po hs plus docusate sodium (Colace, Regulex) 100 mg bid; or magnesium hydroxide (Milk of Magnesia) 15 to 30 ml hs plus docusate sodium (Colace, Regulex) 100 mg bid.
3. Increase docusate sodium (Colace, Regulex) to 200 to 300 mg bid and double the dose of one of the other three laxatives.
4. Add one glycerin suppository and one bisacodyl (Dulcolax) suppository before breakfast.
5. Prescribe a phosphate enema (Fleet enema).
6. Prescribe an oil enema if the stool is hard or a saline enema if the stool is soft.
7. Disimpact the bowel.

Constipation in Children

One definition of constipation in children is having one bowel movement every 3 to 15 days.[5] Usually the condition is self-limited and responds to increases in dietary fiber and a program encouraging regular bowel habits. If these are unsuccessful, a short trial of Milk of Magnesia in doses of 1 to 2 ml/kg may be tried.[6] In some cases changing from cow's milk to a protein-hydrolysate formula containing 100% whey protein[6] or to soy milk[5] resolves the problem (see discussion of anal fissures).

An essential examination in children with chronic constipation or encopresis (because encopresis is often secondary to fecal impaction) is a digital rectal examination (DRE). In a study of 128 children referred to a pediatric gastroenterology center for chronic constipation 77% had not had a DRE performed by the referring physicians and over half had fecal impaction. The treatment of severe fecal impaction is repeated phosphate enemas followed by laxative therapy.[7]

REFERENCES

1. Camilleri M, Thompson WG, Fleshman JW, et al: Clinical management of intractable constipation, *Ann Intern Med* 121:520-528, 1994.
2. Thompson WG, Creed F, Drossman DA, et al: Functional bowel disease and functional abdominal pain, *Gastroenterol Int* 5:75-91, 1992.
3. Van Tilburg EG: Constipation: a frequent iatrogenic complication in cancer patients receiving narcotics, *Can Fam Physician* 36:967-970, 1990.
4. Larimore WL, Hartman JR, Shupe TB: Diary from a week in practice, *Am Fam Physician* 50:1673-1674, 1994.
5. Iacono G, Cavataio F, Montalto G, et al: Intolerance of cow's milk and chronic constipation in children, *N Engl J Med* 339:1100-1104, 1998.
6. Loening-Baucke V: Constipation in children (editorial), *N Engl J Med* 339:1155-1156, 1998.
7. Gold DM, Levine J, Weinstein TA, et al: Frequency of digital rectal examination in children with chronic constipation, *Arch Pediatr Adolesc Med* 153:377-379, 1999.

DIARRHEA

(See also celiac disease; cryptosporidiosis; cyclosporiasis; food poisoning; giardiasis; irritable bowel syndrome; lactase deficiency; sports medicine; travelers' diarrhea)

Infectious Diarrhea

Many bacterial, viral, and parasitic organisms may cause diarrhea, and some of these are listed in Table 24. Diarrhea-causing toxins such as ciguatoxin and tetrodotoxin are discussed under "Food Poisoning."

Mild to moderate community-acquired acute infectious diarrhea in adults can be treated with the antimotility agent loperamide (Imodium) 4 mg stat and 2 mg after each loose stool to a maximum of 16 mg/day. Severe diarrhea and some cases of moderate diarrhea require the addition of a quinolone antibiotic such as ciprofloxacin 500 mg bid for 2 to 5 days.[1] However, if *Shiga* toxin–producing *E. coli* (*E. coli* O157:H7) is suspected as a cause of diarrhea, antibiotics are contraindicated because they increase the risk for hemolytic-uremic syndrome.[2]

Chronic Diarrhea

Chronic diarrhea is defined as persistent diarrhea lasting more than 4 weeks. Before being placed into this category, a patient should be on a lactose-free diet for several days, since lactase deficiency may be a result of an infectious agent and cause persistence of symptoms after the organisms themselves have been eradicated.[3]

Excluding irritable bowel disease, lactase deficiency, and diarrhea in HIV-positive patients, the following, in order of frequency, are the most common causes of chronic diarrhea treated by gastroenterologists[3]:

1. Infections (giardiasis, amebiasis, *Clostridium difficile,* cyclosporiasis)
2. Inflammatory bowel disease
3. Steatorrhea (greasy or bulky stools difficult to flush, bad odor, oil in toilet bowel requiring brush for removal, weight loss)
4. Medications (e.g., antibiotics, antihypertensives, magnesium-containing antacids), foods (ethanol, caffeine), sweeteners (sorbitol in gum or mints, fructose in corn syrup)
5. Previous gastrointestinal surgery
6. Endocrine (Addison's disease, diabetes mellitus, hyperthyroidism, hypothyroidism)
7. Laxative abuse (often concealed by patient or parent)
8. Ischemic bowel disease
9. Radiation enteritis or colitis
10. Colon cancer
11. Idiopathic (functional)

Symptomatic Therapy for Diarrhea

Loperamide (Imodium) and diphenoxylate (Lomotil) are the drugs most frequently used for the symptomatic control of diarrhea. The usual dose of loperamide is 4 mg (2 tablets) initially and then 2 mg after each subsequent loose stool. Maximum is 16 mg (8 tablets) per day. The usual dose of diphenoxylate is 5 mg (2 tablets) initially and then 2.5 to 5 mg tid or qid. Cholestyramine (Questran) is also an effective symptomatic treatment for many cases of chronic diarrhea. The usual dose is 2 to 4 g (a half to a full packet) one to six times a day. Antibiotic use is discussed under "Travelers' Diarrhea."

Table 24   Selected Infectious Diseases Causing Diarrhea

Bacterial	Viral	Parasitic
Salmonella	Rotaviruses	*Giardia lamblia*
Shigella	Norwalk viruses	*Entamoeba*
Campylobacter	Adenoviruses	*histolytica*
Yersinia	Astroviruses	*Cyclospora*
Enterotoxigenic *Eschericha coli*		*cayetanensis*
Enteroinvasive *E. coli*		Cryptosporidiosis
Verotoxin-producing *E. coli* (hamburger disease; hemorrhagic colitis)		
Clostridium difficile		
Clostridium perfringens		
Vibrio cholerae		
Vibrio parahaemolyticus		

REFERENCES

1. Gorbach SL: Treating diarrhoea (editorial), *BMJ* 314:1776-1777, 1997.
2. Wong CS, Jelacic S, Habeeb RL, et al: The risk of the hemolytic-uremic syndrome after antibiotic treatment of *Escherichia coli* O157:H7 infections, *N Engl J Med* 342:1930-1936, 2000.
3. Donowitz, Kokke FT, Saidi R: Evaluation of patients with chronic diarrhea, *N Engl J Med* 332:725-729, 1995.

ESOPHAGUS

(See also asthma; cough; esophageal candidiasis; peptic ulcer disease)

Achalasia

Achalasia is a rare disease caused by inadequate relaxation of the lower esophageal sphincter and aperistalsis of the esophageal smooth muscles. Initial symptoms are dysphagia and heartburn. Aspiration is a complication of the disorder. Patients also have a 16-fold relative increase in their risk for carcinoma of the esophagus. Surveillance endoscopy for carcinoma is not recommended because the absolute risk is low and because 681 annual endoscopies would be necessary to detect one cancer.[1]

Treatment modalities for achalasia include isosorbide dinitrate or calcium channel blockers, botulinum toxin injections into the sphincter (the effect lasts for less than a year), balloon dilatation, and surgery, which can be performed using a laparoscopic approach.[1]

Dysphagia

Dysphagia may be esophageal or oropharyngeal. If a patient has trouble getting the food bolus out of the mouth or has nasal regurgitation, choking, or coughing on swallowing, dysphagia is likely to be oropharyngeal, whereas a definite feeling of sticking in the retrosternum indicates esophageal dysphagia. The initial symptom of organic strictures is difficulty swallowing solids, whereas motor disorders such as may be associated with cerebrovascular accidents, amyotrophic lateral sclerosis, myasthenia gravis, or other neurological conditions may be associated with episodic difficulty in swallowing both liquids and solids from the beginning. Idiopathic oropharyngeal neuromuscular dysphagia is common in the elderly, and many such persons never seek medical help for the condition.[2]

Gastroesophageal Reflux Disease

Gastroesophageal reflux occurs because of transient relaxation of the lower esophageal sphincter, not because of a low resting sphincter pressure. An associated hiatus hernia enhances reflux.[3]

In North America gastroesophageal reflux disease (GERD) affects 20% of adults at least once a week and 4% to 9% on a daily basis.[4] In Asia GERD is rare, probably because of a high prevalence of chronic gastritis secondary to widespread *H. pylori* infection[5]; chronic gastritis decreases acid secretion and protects against GERD.[5,6]

Coronary artery disease may be difficult to differentiate from GERD. According to one study, coronary artery disease can be ruled out with reasonable certainty if symptoms are controlled by omeprazole (Prilosec, Losec) 40 mg bid for 7 days (omeprazole test). Lower doses of omeprazole and ranitidine are not effective for this purpose.[7]

A number of reports suggest that reflux sometimes induces "acid laryngitis," which manifests itself as persistent cough, hoarseness, and a continual need to clear the throat. The existence of this entity is controversial. Believers treat the patients with omeprazole for 2 months,[3] but no randomized controlled studies have been published documenting benefit from this therapy.[8] Other reports suggest that reflux has a role in causing some cases of asthma. This is discussed under "Asthma."

American College of Gastroenterology guidelines recommend that patients with mild symptomatic GERD be started on empirical therapy without prior endoscopy provided they have no ominous symptoms such as dysphagia, bleeding, weight loss, or choking.[9]

The initial treatment of symptomatic esophageal reflux involves life-style changes and over-the-counter medications,[8-10] although few of these measures have been established by well-controlled trials.[10] Most cases with mild symptoms can be successfully controlled by these measures,[8-10] which include the following:

1. Avoiding bedtime snacks
2. Avoiding foods that relax the lower esophageal sphincter, such as fats, whole milk, chocolate, orange juice, tomatoes, carminatives (peppermint), and ethanol
3. Discontinuing smoking
4. Raising the head of the bed by at least 14 cm
5. Taking alginic acids such as Gaviscon Heart Burn Relief Formula (there are Gaviscon products without alginic acid) or Gastrocote. The usual dose is 2 to 4 tablets well chewed tid or qid.
6. Use of antacids such as calcium carbonate (Tums) or aluminum hydroxide/magnesium hydroxide (Maalox)
7. Using over-the-counter H_2-blockers

For many patients a combination of antacids and alginic acid is more effective than either one alone. Antacids act more quickly than H_2-blockers, but their duration of action is shorter. Patients who can predict activities that are likely to induce reflux should self-medicate prophylactically.[9]

For patients who do not respond to the measures outlined above, the physician can start with low-potency drugs such as H_2-blockers and if necessary replace them with more potent proton pump inhibitors. Alternatively, therapy can begin with high doses of proton pump inhibitors, which are then titrated down to lower doses and then less potent agents provided the patient remains asymptomatic. Although some have recommended a combination of H_2-blockers and prokinetic agents, proton pump inhibitors are probably preferable in terms of cost, compliance, and safety (see later discussion). Over a period of time those with mild disease can often discontinue medications or use them only on demand; those with severe disease may require prolonged maintenance therapy.[10] One suggested protocol is to start patients with omeprazole 20 mg/day for 2 weeks or, if symptoms have not completely resolved, for 4 weeks. Thereafter, medications are given only if symptoms recur. Ranitidine 150 to 300 mg bid may be used instead of omeprazole, but symptom relief is not as rapid.[11]

Frequently used H$_2$-blockers are cimetidine (Tagamet) 800 mg bid or ranitidine (Zantac) 150 mg bid. Both omeprazole (Prilosec, <u>Losec</u>) 20 to 40 mg/day and lansoprazole (Prevacid) 30 mg/day are effective proton pump inhibitors for GERD. Until recently cisapride (Propulsid) in doses of 5 to 10 mg tid ac, or qid ac and hs, was the most commonly used prokinetic agent for this disorder, but because of serious drug interactions, it should probably be used only for refractory cases of heartburn.[12]

Surgical interventions should be considered when medical therapy fails.[9]

Barrett's Esophagus

Barrett's esophagus is the replacement of the squamous epithelium of the lower esophagus with the columnar epithelium of intestinal metaplasia.[4,13,14] It is strongly associated with GERD and is thought to develop as a metaplastic form of healing when the squamous epithelium has been eroded by acid reflux.[4] The importance of Barrett's esophagus is its association with an increased incidence of adenocarcinoma of the lower esophagus.[4,14-17] Two large prospective endoscopic surveillance studies of patients with Barrett's esophagus in the United States found an adenocarcinoma incidence of 1:208[15] and 1:285[16] patient years. A population-based case-control study in Sweden reported that the risk of esophageal adenocarcinoma was eight times higher in patients who had regurgitation, heartburn, or both at least once a week, and over 20 times higher for those with more frequent or severe symptoms. Although the relative risk is high, the absolute risk is low. The authors of this study calculated that among patients with heartburn and thus a 20-fold increased risk of cancer, only 1 in 1400 would be found to have malignancy over a 1-year period.[13]

In terms of cancer risk, management of patients with heartburn is controversial. Cohen and Parkman[4] recommend that if heartburn is severe enough to be a primary complaint, the patient be assessed by endoscopy and biopsies. According to these authors, aggressive long-term treatment of erosive lesions with medical therapy should be instituted. They also suggest that ablation of Barrett's tissue by use of laser or thermal techniques may be indicated.[4] Whether endoscopy is feasible or desirable for all patients with heartburn is open to question. Large numbers of patients would be subjected to the anxiety, discomfort, and danger of endoscopy for unproven benefit. As Lagergren and associates[13] point out, there is no proof that intensive medical management of GERD decreases the incidence of either Barrett's esophagus or adenocarcinoma of the esophagus.

Once Barrett's esophagus is diagnosed by endoscopy and biopsy, current guidelines recommend regular endoscopic and biopsy surveillance to detect dysplasia and early cancer.[14,17] Cancers detected by this means tend to be small and free of nodal metastases, but whether long-term survival is increased is unknown.[17] Identification of mild dysplasia has no clinical value because 73% of such lesions regress spontaneously.[16] Management of severe dysplasia is controversial; up to 25% of cases regress, but others are associated with undetected carcinomas.[14,17]

Whether long-term intensive acid suppression can lead to regression of Barrett's esophagus is uncertain. One 2-year trial comparing ranitidine 150 bid with omeprazole 40 mg bid found no regression with ranitidine and a slight but statistically significant regression with omeprazole.[18]

Adenocarcinoma of the Esophagus

The incidence of adenocarcinoma of the esophagus has been increasing dramatically in the Western world over the past two decades, especially among white men, in whom its frequency now equals that of squamous cell cancer.[4] This rise has coincided with a marked decrease in the rate of *Helicobacter pylori* infection of the stomach. Preliminary evidence suggests that some strains of *H. pylori* exert a protective effect against gastroesophageal reflux disease, Barrett's esophagus, and adenocarcinoma of the esophagus.[19] The relationship of Barrett's esophagus to adenocarcinoma of the esophagus is discussed in the preceding section.

Most adenocarcinomas of the esophagus have regional lymph node involvement at the time of diagnosis, and the 5-year survival rate after surgical resection is less than 10%. One study found that preoperative radiation therapy and chemotherapy increased the 3-year survival rate for resectable tumors from 6% to 32%.[20]

Esophageal Varices

The treatment of choice for acute variceal bleeding is endoscopic band ligation of the varices.[21] Both beta-blockers and endoscopic variceal ligation have been used to decrease the incidence of recurrent bleeding from esophageal varices; according to one editorial writer, management of first choice is a nonselective beta-adrenergic blocker such as propranolol.[22]

Patients with portal hypertension and esophageal bleeding who do not respond to other therapeutic modalities may be treated by creating a shunt between the portal and hepatic veins. This is done by interventional radiologists who introduce a catheter through the jugular vein and pass it through the liver into the portal vein. The procedure is called a transjugular intrahepatic portosystemic shunt (TIPS).[23]

────────────── 🖎 **REFERENCES** 🖍 ──────────────

1. Spiess AE, Kahrilas PJ: Treating achalasia: from whalebone to laparoscope, *JAMA* 280:638-642, 1998.
2. Paterson WG: Dysphagia in the elderly, *Can Fam Physician* 42:925-932, 1996.
3. Pope CE II: Acid-reflux disorders, *N Engl J Med* 331:656-660, 1994.
4. Cohen S, Parkman HP: Heartburn—a serious symptom (editorial), *N Engl J Med* 340:878-879, 1999.
5. Wu JC, Sung JJ, Ng EK, et al: Prevalence and distribution of *Helicobacter pylori* in gastroesophageal reflux disease: a study from the East, *Am J Gastroenterol* 94:1790-1794, 1999.

6. El-Serag HB, Sonnenberg A, Jamal MM, et al: Corpus gastritis is protective against reflux oesophagitis, *Gut* 45:181-185, 1999.

7. Schindlbeck NE, Klauser AG, Voderholzer WA, et al: Empiric therapy for gastroesophageal reflux disease, *Arch Intern Med* 155:1808-1812, 1995.

8. Kahrilas PJ: Gastroesophageal reflux disease, *JAMA* 276:983-988, 1996.

9. DeVault KR, Castell DO (Practice Parameters Committee of the American College of Gastroenterology): Updated guidelines for the diagnosis and treatment of gastroesophageal reflux disease, *Am J Gastroenterol* 94:1434-1442, 1999.

10. Galmiche JP, Letessier E, Scarpignato C: Treatment of gastro-oesophageal reflux disease in adults, *BMJ* 316:1720-1723, 1998.

11. Bardhan KD, Müller-Lissner S, Bigard MA, et al (European Study Group): Symptomatic gastro-oesophageal reflux disease: double blind controlled study of intermittent treatment with omeprazole, *BMJ* 318:502-507, 1999.

12. Josefson D: FDA warns about heartburn drug, *BMJ* 317:101, 1998.

13. Lagergren J, Bergström R, Lindgren A, et al: Symptomatic gastroesophageal reflux as a risk factor for esophageal adenocarcinoma, *N Engl J Med* 340:825-831, 1999.

14. Sampliner RE and the Practice Parameters Committee of the American College of Gastroenterology: Practice guidelines on the diagnosis, surveillance and therapy of Barrett's esophagus, *Am J Gastroenterol* 93:1028-1032, 1998.

15. Drewitz DJ, Sampliner RE, Garewal HS: The incidence of adenocarcinoma in Barrett's esophagus—a prospective study of 170 patients followed 4.8 years, *Am J Gastroenterol* 92:212-215, 1997.

16. O'Connor JB, Falk GW, Richter JE: The incidence of adenocarcinoma and dysplasia in Barrett's esophagus, *Am J Gastroenterol* 94:2037-2042, 1999.

17. Morales TG, Sampliner RE: Barrett's esophagus: update on screening, surveillance, and treatment, *Arch Intern Med* 159:1411-1416, 1999.

18. Peters FT, Ganesh S, Kuipers EJ, et al: Endoscopic regression of Barrett's oesophagus during omeprazole treatment; a randomised double blind study, *Gut* 45:489-494, 1999.

19. Blaser MJ: *Helicobacter pylori* and gastric diseases, *BMJ* 316:1507-1510, 1998.

20. Walsh TN, Noonan N, Hollywood D, et al: A comparison of multimodal therapy and surgery for esophageal adenocarcinoma, *N Engl J Med* 335:462-467, 1996.

21. Van Dam, Brugge WR: Endoscopy of the upper gastrointestinal tract, *N Engl J Med* 341:1738-1748, 1999.

22. Burroughs AK, Patch D: Primary prevention of bleeding from esophageal varices (editorial), *N Engl J Med* 340:1033-1035, 1999.

23. Miller-Catchpole R: Transjugular intrahepatic portosystemic shunt (TIPS): diagnostic and therapeutic technology assessment (DATTA), *JAMA* 273:1824-1830, 1995.

FLATUS

Alpha-galactosidase (Beano) is available as an over-the-counter tablet or liquid preparation. Its mode of action is to hydrolyze undigestible complex sugars (oligosaccharides) of certain vegetables into their digestible monosaccharides and disaccharides. Most cruciferous vegetables and most legumes have a high content of undigestible sugars. Examples are beans, chickpeas, peas, lentils, brussels sprouts, cabbage, broccoli, carrots, corn, leeks, squash, onions, parsnips, oats, and wheat.

In a study from San Diego, volunteers took 8 drops of Beano or 8 drops of placebo before a meal of meatless chili consisting of navy, pinto, and kidney beans. Beano decreased the numbers of farts.[1] No solid evidence has been presented that simethicone relieves the discomfort of "gas,"[2] and activated charcoal is ineffective in reducing the volume or odor of released intestinal gas.[3]

--------------------- ❧ REFERENCES ❧ ---------------------

1. Ganiats TG, Norcross WA, Halverson AL, et al: Does Beano prevent gas—a double-blind crossover study of oral alpha-galactosidase to treat dietary oligosaccharide intolerance, *J Fam Pract* 39:441-445, 1994.

2. Simethicone for gastrointestinal gas, *Med Lett* 38:57-58, 1996.

3. Suarez FL, Furne J, Springfield J, et al: Failure of activated charcoal to reduce the release of gases produced by the colonic flora, *Am J Gastroenterol* 94:208-212, 1999.

HEMATOCHEZIA

(See also anal and rectal disorders; anemia; colon cancer; sports medicine)

In a British community study 24% of respondents to a questionnaire reported at least one episode of rectal bleeding in their lifetimes, and 19% had had such bleeding within the past 12 months. Only 41% of those who had ever had rectal bleeding sought medical advice.[1] Such data suggest that most of these incidents were innocuous. That this might not be the case is indicated by a study of U.S. veterans (almost all male and 80% over the age of 40). They were specifically asked about a history of rectal bleeding and, if it had occurred in the past 3 months, were given a complete examination of the colon. Colon cancer was detected in 6.5%, polyps in 13%, and inflammatory bowel disease in 4.5%. The character of the bleeding (e.g., frequency of bleeding, on the toilet paper, mixed with stool) did not distinguish innocuous from severe disease. The only two clinical features that correlated with a diagnosis of cancer were age and duration of bleeding of less than 2 months.[2]

Fecal occult blood testing is neither sensitive nor specific. When it is used as a screening test for colon cancer, between 2% and 16% of patients have positive results, many of which are false positives. Oral iron supplements turn the stool dark green or black but do not cause positive fecal occult blood tests to become positive.[3]

Occult blood in the stool has been found in 20% of marathon runners immediately after the race. Frank blood in stools occurs in about 6% of marathon runners.[4]

In a study of 248 nonanemic patients whose stools were positive for occult blood the source of gastrointestinal bleeding was more often the upper than the lower gastrointestinal tract. In just over half the cases the source of bleeding could not be identified.[5] In such cases the prognosis is good.[3]

➥ REFERENCES ➥

1. Crosland A, Jones R: Rectal bleeding—prevalence and consultation behaviour, *BMJ* 311:486-488, 1995.
2. Helfand M, Marton KI, Zimmer-Gembeck MJ, et al: History of visible rectal bleeding in a primary care population: initial assessment and 10-year follow-up, *JAMA* 277:44-48, 1997.
3. Rockey DC: Occult gastrointestinal bleeding, *N Engl J Med* 341:38-46, 1999.
4. McCabe ME 3d, Peura DA, Kadakia SC, et al: Gastrointestinal blood loss associated with running a marathon, *Dig Dis Sci* 31:1229-1232, 1986.
5. Rockey DC, Koch J, Cello JP, et al: Relative frequency of upper gastrointestinal and colonic lesions in patients with positive fecal occult-blood tests, *N Engl J Med* 339:153-159, 1998.

INFLAMMATORY BOWEL DISEASE

(See also biliary cirrhosis; colon cancer; diarrhea; psoriatic arthritis)

Crohn's Disease

Crohn's disease can affect any age group but peaks in early and late adulthood. Important exacerbating factors are cigarette smoking and NSAIDs.[1] Management protocols vary according to whether the disease is active or in remission and, when active, according to the severity of disease.[1,2] First-line treatment of mild to moderate active disease is sulfasalazine (Azulfidine, Salazopyrin) 3 to 6 g/day or mesalamine (Asacol, Mesasal, Pentasa, Salofalk) 3.2 to 4.8 g/day in divided doses, with metronidazole 10 to 20 mg/kg/day as an alternative for those who fail to respond to sulfasalazine.[2] Metronidazole combined with ciprofloxacin is reported to be effective, while preliminary studies suggest that ciprofloxacin and a number of other antibiotics such as clarithromycin and rifabutin either alone or in combination are beneficial.[1] Moderate to severe disease usually requires corticosteroids such as prednisone 40 to 60 mg/day for 1 to 4 weeks followed by gradual tapering.[1,2] Budesonide controlled release capsules may be used instead of prednisone and have the advantage of causing less adrenocortical suppression.[1] Drugs used for patients who do not respond to standard therapy include the immunosuppressant agents azathioprine or 6-mercaptopurine[1,2] and the antitumor necrosis factor a antibody infliximab (Remicade).[1] Cholestyramine 4 g once to three times may be used for the symptomatic control of diarrhea.[1] Mesalamine has some effect in decreasing relapse rates and is the drug of choice for maintenance therapy.[2]

Ulcerative Colitis

Ulcerative colitis is found three to four times as frequently in whites as in other races. Both sexes are equally affected. About 5% of patients have severe disease manifested as fulminating hemorrhagic colitis, toxic megacolon, or severe diffuse colitis. Ulcerative colitis is more common in non-

smokers than in smokers. The onset of the disease often correlates with discontinuing smoking, and smoking may control the symptoms of the disease. These apparently beneficial effects are not seen in Crohn's disease.[3]

One of the long-term complications of ulcerative colitis is colon cancer; risk increases with duration and extent of the disease. After 8 to 10 years the risk of cancer in patients with pancolitis is 0.5% to 1% per year. For those with left-sided colitis the risk reaches 0.5% to 1% per year after 30 to 40 years. Patients with only proctosigmoiditis do not have an increased cancer risk. Clinical practice guidelines recommend annual surveillance colonoscopy with multiple biopsies starting after 8 to 10 years in patients at risk of cancer. If dysplasia is found on any pathological specimen, colectomy is indicated. These guidelines are based on opinion, since no randomized trials of surveillance have been reported.[4]

Mild and moderate cases of ulcerative colitis can be managed on an outpatient basis. If colitis involves any portions of the colon proximal to the splenic flexure, oral medications are required, whereas for left side lesions either oral or topical treatments may be used. If topical agents are chosen, enemas are required for disease in the descending colon, foam can be used if involvement is limited to the distal 15 to 20 cm of the large bowel, and suppositories are effective for isolated proctitis that does not extend proximally beyond 10 cm.[4] Oral aminosalicylates such as sulfasalazine, mesalamine, or olsalazine (Dipentum) are usually started at relatively low doses and increased to full therapeutic doses at a rate that is tolerable for the patient. Enemas containing steroids such as hydrocortisone (Cortenema) or 5-acetylsalicylic acid compounds such as mesalamine (Rowasa) are usually given hs, and the patient is instructed to try to retain the enema all night.[5,6] Some of the newer steroid enemas such as tixocortol (Rectovalone) are not readily absorbed and do not suppress the pituitary-adrenal axis.[5] Mesalamine may also be administered as a suppository,[6] and 10% cortisone is available as a foam.[4] Once active disease is controlled, maintenance therapy with oral or topical aminosalicylates should be instituted.[4]

Patients with mild to moderate extensive disease who do not respond to aminosalicylates or patients with severe disease are treated with corticosteroids and sometimes 6-mercaptopurine or azathioprine.[4]

Short-term, randomized, double-blind studies of patients with ulcerative colitis have demonstrated symptom reduction with the use of nicotine patches, but at the cost of significant side effects.[7] The use of nicotine patches to help maintain remission in ulcerative colitis has not shown any benefit.[8]

Extraintestinal Manifestations of Inflammatory Bowel Disease

Peripheral arthritis, involving primarily the hips and ankles, and ankylosing spondylitis are fairly common complications of inflammatory bowel disease. Ocular manifestations are also common and include episcleritis and uveitis.[9] Sclerosing cholangitis is a rare complication of inflammatory bowel disease. Some patients are asymptomatic, but others have fatigue and pruritus. Levels of aspartate aminotransferase (AST or SGOT) and alanine aminotransferase (ALT or SGPT) may be normal or elevated, whereas alkaline phosphatase and gamma-glutamyl transferase (GGT) levels are markedly elevated.[10]

REFERENCES

1. Rampton DS: Management of Crohn's disease, *BMJ* 319: 1480-1485, 1999.
2. Hanauer SB, Meyers S: Practice guidelines: management of Crohn's disease in adults, *Am J Gastroenterol* 92:559-566, 1997.
3. Hanauer SB: Nicotine for colitis—the smoke has not yet cleared (editorial), *N Engl J Med* 330:856-857, 1994.
4. Kornbluth A, Sachar DB: Ulcerative colitis practice guidelines in adults, *Am J Gastroenterol* 92:204-211, 1997.
5. Hanauer SB: Inflammatory bowel disease, *N Engl J Med* 334:841-848, 1996.
6. Botoman VA, Bonner GF, Botoman DA: Management of inflammatory bowel disease, *Am Fam Physician* 57:57-68, 1998.
7. Sandborn WJ, Tremaine WJ, Offord KP, et al: Transdermal nicotine for mildly to moderately active ulcerative colitis, *Ann Intern Med* 126:364-371, 1997.
8. Thomas GAO, Mani V, Williams GT, et al: Transdermal nicotine as maintenance therapy for ulcerative colitis, *N Engl J Med* 332:988-992, 1995.
9. Hastings GE, Wever RJ: Inflammatory bowel disease. I. Clinical features and diagnosis, *Am Fam Physician* 47:598-608, 1993.
10. Buckley SE, Dipalma JA: Recognizing primary biliary cirrhosis and primary sclerosing cholangitis, *Am Fam Physician* 53:195-200, 1996.

IRRITABLE BOWEL SYNDROME

(See also alternative medicine; constipation; diarrhea; fibromyalgia; functional somatic syndromes; lactase deficiency)

Although the cause of irritable bowel syndrome is unknown, a number of cases appear to be precipitated by an episode of acute bacterial gastroenteritis[1,2] and symptoms may be aggravated by stress.[2] Lactose intolerance (lactase deficiency) is not a constituent aspect of the irritable bowel syndrome, but because symptoms of irritable bowel syndrome overlap with those of lactase deficiency, the latter should always be considered in the differential diagnosis.[3] In many women symptoms of irritable bowel become worse during the premenstrual phase.[4] An overlap in symptoms between irritable bowel syndrome and fibromyalgia has been reported (see discussion of fibromyalgia).

The diagnosis of irritable bowel is based on positive clinical findings, and unless red flags such as weight loss or hematochezia are present, investigations are usually unnecessary in patients under the age of 50. For patients over 50 with new onset of symptoms a colonoscopy or barium enema is probably indicated.[2]

The Manning criteria for diagnosing irritable bowel consist of abdominal pain plus two or more of the following[2]:

1. Pain relieved by defecation
2. Pain associated with loose stools
3. Pain associated with more frequent stools
4. Abdominal distention
5. Feeling of incomplete evacuation
6. Mucus in stools

The first four symptoms are the most valuable for making the diagnosis.

Recurrent abdominal pain is reported to affect 10% to 20% of school-age children, and in many of these children the symptoms meet the criteria of irritable bowel syndrome.[5]

Traditional therapeutic regimens are based on symptom control.[2,6] A normal diet should be taken, and unless lactase deficiency has been proved, milk need not be limited. Some patients feel better if they cut down on sorbitol, caffeine, alcohol, or fat,[2] and those who are constipated may improve with gradually increasing fiber supplements[2,6] such as ½ to 1 cup per day of bran or ½ to 1 tablespoon of psyllium (Metamucil, Prodiem) one to four times a day taken with plenty of fluids.[6] Diarrhea can usually be controlled with loperamide 2 to 4 mg qid prn, and for some patients it can be given prophylactically before trips, social events, and other occasions.[2]

Pain may be treated with antispasmodics such as dicyclomine (Bentyl, Bentylol) 10 to 20 mg tid to qid, hyoscine butyl bromide (Buscopan) 10 mg tid or qid, or trimebutine (Modulon) 200 mg tid or with smooth muscle relaxants such as the calcium channel blocker pinaverium bromide (Dicetel) 50 mg tid with meals.[4] For some patients with frequent or continuous pain, tricyclic antidepressants such as amitriptyline (Elavil) 25 to 100 mg qhs appear to be effective. No medications have been shown to control bloating.[2]

REFERENCES

1. García Rodríguez LA, Ruigómez A: Increased risk of irritable bowel syndrome after bacterial gastroenteritis: cohort study, *BMJ* 318:565-566, 1999.
2. Paterson WG, Thompson WG, Vanner SJ, et al: Recommendations for the management of irritable bowel syndrome in family practice, *Can Med Assoc J* 161:154-160, 1999.
3. Tolliver BA, Gerrerea JL, DiPalma JA: Evaluation of patients who meet clinical criteria for irritable bowel syndrome, *Am J Gastroenterol* 89:176-178, 1994.
4. Case AM, Reid R: Effects of the menstrual cycle on medical disorders, *Arch Intern Med* 158:1405-1412, 1998.
5. Hyams JS, Burke G, Davis PM, et al: Abdominal pain and irritable bowel syndrome in adolescents: a community based study, *J Pediatr* 129:220-226, 1996.
6. Thompson WG: Irritable bowel syndrome: strategy for the family physician, *Can Fam Physician* 40:307-316, 1994.

LACTASE DEFICIENCY
(See also diarrhea; irritable bowel syndrome)

Within Europe the incidence of lactose intolerance is lowest in Scandinavia and other northwestern countries (3% to 8%) and highest in the southeastern regions (70% in southern Italy and Turkey). The incidence in black Africa is high except among cattle-raising nomads. In Southeast Asia the incidence is almost 100%.[1]

Lactase levels in the small intestine normally fall with increasing age. The levels in a 1-year-old are about 25% to 50% of those in a newborn. Levels continue to fall thereafter in populations subject to lactase deficiency, so that by the age of 20 the levels in these groups decrease to only about 10% of the neonatal levels. This process continues into old age, particularly among blacks.[2]

The major symptoms of lactase deficiency are abdominal pain, diarrhea, bloating, borborygmi, and flatulence. These symptoms are similar to those in patients with irritable bowel syndrome, who have been found in numerous reports to have an increased incidence of lactase deficiency. In one study about half the patients meeting the criteria for irritable bowel syndrome were lactase deficient.[3] Lactase deficiency is probably responsible for a number of cases of recurrent abdominal pain in children.[4]

Not all patients who claim to be milk intolerant are as intolerant as they think. A double-blind study of lactose-intolerant patients who claimed they had symptoms even if they added milk to coffee found that they were able to tolerate 240 ml of milk a day taken in the morning with breakfast.[5]

The standard investigation for lactase deficiency is the breath hydrogen test. According to Thompson and co-workers[6] a cheaper and equally effective method is to have the patient abstain from all milk products for 1 week and then drink a quart of milk. If significant symptoms result, the test is positive.

A simple treatment for lactase deficiency is the avoidance of milk and milk products containing lactose. Aged cheese does not contain lactose because it is destroyed during the fermentation process. However, processed cheeses such as cream cheese, cottage cheese, and ricotta cheese do contain lactose and should be avoided. The adverse effect of limiting dairy products may be an inadequate calcium intake, so supplementary calcium should often be prescribed.

An alternative to avoiding milk products is to have the patients buy milk that has had lactase added, add lactase enzyme (Lactaid) to ordinary milk, or take lactase enzymes before ingesting dairy products. Lactase enzyme is supplied as a liquid in dropper bottles and as tablets. The usual dose is ½ to 3 tablets just before the ingestion of lactose-containing milk products or 5 to 15 drops added to each liter or quart of refrigerated milk 24 hours before its use. Five drops of lactase will hydrolyze 70% of the lactose in 1 liter of milk in 24 hours at refrigerator temperature; 15 drops in a liter of milk will hydrolyze 99% of the lactose. The reaction is much faster at room temperature.

There is evidence that lactose-intolerant individuals can adapt to some extent if given gradually increasing amounts of lactose.[7]

❧ REFERENCES ❧

1. Gudmand-Hoyer E: The clinical significance of disaccharide maldigestion, *Am J Clin Nutr* 59(suppl 3):S735-S741, 1994.
2. Rao DR, Bello H, Warren AP, et al: Prevalence of lactose maldigestion: influence and interaction of age, race, and sex, *Dig Dis Sci* 39:1519-1524, 1994.
3. Tolliver BA, Gerrerea JL, DiPalma JA: Evaluation of patients who meet clinical criteria for irritable bowel syndrome, *Am J Gastroenterol* 89:176-178, 1994.
4. Gudmand-Hoyer E: The clinical significance of disaccharide maldigestion, *Am J Clin Nutr* 59(suppl 3):S735-S741, 1994.
5. Suarez FL, Savaiano DA, Levitt MD: A comparison of symptoms after the consumption of milk or lactose-hydrolyzed milk by people with self-reported severe lactose intolerance, *N Engl J Med* 333:1-4, 1995.
6. Thompson WG, Drossman DA, Whitehead WE: Approaching IBS with confidence, *Patient Care Can* 31:51-66, 1993.
7. Johnson AO, Semenya JG, Buchowski MS, et al: Adaptation of lactose maldigesters to continued milk intakes, *Am J Clin Nutr* 58:879-881, 1993.

LIVER
Alcoholic Hepatitis
(See also alcohol; hepatitis)

The spectrum of illness in patients with alcoholic hepatitis varies from mild nonspecific symptoms (fatigue, anorexia, and weight loss) through liver failure with jaundice, ascites, and hepatic encephalopathy. Alcoholic hepatitis is generally limited to persons who drink 80 g or more of ethanol per day. This is more than eight 12-ounce beers, 1 liter (one and a half bottles) of 12% wine, or a half pint of 80-proof whiskey.[1]

Patients may have macrocytic anemia and leukocytosis (white blood cell count usually higher than 15,000/mm^3, but 8% have leukopenia), elevated prothrombin time, elevated bilirubin level, and mild elevation of liver enzyme levels. Usually the AST (or SGOT) level is less than five times normal. The ALT (or SGPT) level is usually less than half the AST. An AST/ALT ratio greater than 2 virtually establishes the diagnosis of alcoholic hepatitis (about 60% of cases). In more than 90% of cases of alcoholic hepatitis the AST level is greater than the ALT.[1]

❧ REFERENCES ❧

1. Woods SE, Hitchcock M, Meyer A: Alcoholic hepatitis, *Am Fam Physician* 47:1171-1178, 1993.

Ascites

The drug of choice for ascites resulting from cirrhosis is spironolactone (Aldactone) because it counters the hyperaldosteronism of this condition. One regimen is to start with 50 mg once daily and increase the dose every 3 or 4 days to a maximum of 400 mg/day. If necessary, a thiazide or loop diuretic may be added.[1] A variant of this regimen is to start with 100 mg spironolactone po and 40 mg furosemide (Lasix) po with all pills given at once in the morning. If weight does not decrease in 2 to 3 days, both drug doses should be doubled. The maximum dose is 400 mg of spironolactone and 160 mg of furosemide. Amiloride (Midamor) may be used instead of spironolactone, starting with 10 mg qam and increasing to a maximum of 40 mg/day. Amiloride has a faster action and does not cause painful gynecomastia.[2]

✍ REFERENCES ✍

1. Brater DC: Diuretic therapy, *N Engl J Med* 339:387-395, 1998.
2. Runyon BA: Care of patients with ascites, *N Engl J Med* 330: 337-342, 1994.

Cirrhosis

(See also connective tissue diseases; hypothyroidism; inflammatory bowel disease)

Biliary cirrhosis

Ninety-five percent of patients with biliary cirrhosis are women, and most are middle aged. The usual clinical presentation is pruritus and fatigue, although many asymptomatic cases are detected when an unexpectedly elevated alkaline phosphatase level is discovered during biochemical screening procedures. AST and ALT concentrations may be normal or only slightly elevated, whereas alkaline phosphatase and GGT levels are markedly elevated. Most patients are found to have increased levels of antimitochondrial antibodies, and low titers of smooth muscle and antinuclear antibodies are common.[1,2] Serum lipid levels are often strikingly elevated, with total cholesterol levels as high as 1000 mg/dl (26 mmol/L). However, patients are not at increased risk of cardiovascular disease, probably because HDL cholesterol levels are markedly elevated.[2]

The median survival is between 10 and 16 years for asymptomatic patients and 7 years for symptomatic patients. Although symptoms develop after 2 to 4 years in most asymptomatic patients, approximately a third remain symptom free for many years. The most common symptom is pruritus, which can usually be controlled with cholestyramine (Questran) 4 g po tid.[2]

An association has been reported between biliary cirrhosis and immunological disorders such as lupus, rheumatoid arthritis, scleroderma, CREST syndrome (calcinosis, Raynaud's phenomenon, esophageal involvement, sclerodactyly, and telangiectasia), Sjögren's syndrome, and thyroiditis.[1,2] About one fifth of the patients are hypothyroid.[2]

Diet for patients with cirrhosis

Protein-restricted diets have long been prescribed for patients with hepatic encephalopathy or patients with cirrhosis considered to be at risk of hepatic encephalopathy. Recent research has conclusively shown that such a practice is not only valueless, but harmful.[3]

✍ REFERENCES ✍

1. Buckley SE, Dipalma JA: Recognizing primary biliary cirrhosis and primary sclerosing cholangitis, *Am Fam Physician* 53:195-200, 1996.
2. Kaplan MM: Primary biliary cirrhosis, *N Engl J Med* 335:1570-1580, 1996.
3. Soulsby CT, Morgan MY: Dietary management of hepatic encephalopathy in cirrhotic patients: survey of current practice in United Kingdom, *BMJ* 318:1391, 1999.

Hepatitis

(See also adoption; alcoholic hepatitis; biliary cirrhosis; colon cancer; hemochromatosis; immunization schedules for children; transfusions; vaccines)

The common forms of viral hepatitis seen in family medicine, hepatitis A, B, and C, are discussed below. Rare causes of hepatitis that should be ruled out when investigating for the cause of chronic hepatitis are hemochromatosis, alpha$_1$-antitrypsin deficiency, and primary biliary cirrhosis.

Terminology and clinical correlations of laboratory tests used in investigating hepatitis

A discussion of viral hepatitis requires a knowledge of a number of terms and abbreviations. Some important ones are given in Table 25.[1]

Hepatitis A

About 20% of patients with hepatitis A have a brief relapse after initial improvement. Fulminant hepatitis occurs in 0.1% of patients with this disease. The diagnosis of acute infection may be confirmed by elevated titers of IgM anti-HAV.[2]

Travelers from industrialized countries to developing nations are at risk of acquiring hepatitis A even if they stay in luxury hotels. The overall risk if unprotected by passive or active immunization is estimated to be 3 to 6 per 1000 travelers per month, with the risk increasing to 20 per 1000 per month among those eating and drinking under poor hygienic conditions. Less than 20% of persons from industrialized countries born after 1945 have acquired natural immunity.[2]

For travelers, passive immunization with intramuscular immune globulin (human) is effective for 3 to 5 months in 85% to 90% of cases. Active immunization with a two-dose series of inactivated HAV vaccine (Havrix, Vaqta) is available. (In Canada a combination vaccine against hepatitis A and hepatitis B called Twinrix is given as a three-dose course at 0, 1, and 6 months.) Hepatitis A vaccination is effective, and immunity is estimated to persist for 7 to 10 years or more.[2] Patients at risk of exposure to hepatitis A within 4 weeks of vaccination may be given immune globulin at the same time as they are vaccinated, but in a different body site.[3] The usual adult dose of immune globulin is 0.02 ml/kg for travel of less than 3 months and 0.06 ml/kg for travel of 3 to 5 months. For postexposure prophylaxis of household or sexual contacts the dose of immune globulin is 0.02 mg/kg given as soon as possible and no later than 2 weeks after exposure.[4]

Table 25   Hepatitis Terminology

Term or abbreviation	Definition and comments
Liver Enzymes	
Alanine aminotransferase	ALT = SGPT
Aspartate aminotransferase	AST = SGOT
Hepatitis A	
HAV	Hepatitis A virus
IgM anti-HAV	Acute hepatitis A infection
IgG anti-HAV	Previous hepatitis A infection
Hepatitis B	
HBV	Hepatitis B virus
HBsAg	Hepatitis B surface antigen. Elevated in acute infections and in the carrier state.
Anti-HBs	Anti–hepatitis B surface antigen. Develops 1-3 months after recovery from acute infection.
HBcAg	Hepatitis B core antigen.
IgM anti-HBc	Positive in the window phase of acute hepatitis B when HBsAg has declined but anti-HBs has not yet developed.
HBeAg	Hepatitis B e antigen. Present during acute hepatitis B infection and in chronic active hepatitis B infection.
Anti-HBe	Develops after acute infection. Not usually tested.
HBIG	Hepatitis B immune globulin
Hepatitis C	
HCV	Hepatitis C virus
Anti-HCV	May not develop until 3 months after infection.
Hepatitis D	
HDV	Hepatitis D virus. Occurs only in patients who are carriers of HBsAg.
Anti-HDV	Order only for patients who are HBsAg positive and have clinical symptoms of acute hepatitis.
Hepatitis E	
HEV	Hepatitis E virus. Clinical picture similar to hepatitis A. Uncommon in developed countries.

Immunization of the entire population is not generally recommended, but in view of the fact that both widespread and sporadic outbreaks of hepatitis A have been traced to imported foods, a good case could be made for universal vaccination of children.[5]

Hepatitis B

The prevalence of hepatitis B is high in China, Southeast Asia, and Africa. In these regions up to half the population has been infected and about 8% are chronic carriers. In developed countries most cases of hepatitis B are a result of sexual exposure or IV drug use; no clear risk factors are found in about one fourth of those affected, but this may be due to reticence in revealing high-risk activities.[6] About half of adults who acquire hepatitis B are asymptomatic, one fourth have jaundice, and one fourth have nonspecific symptoms. Complete cure occurs in 90% of cases, and the carrier state develops in about 10%. In a quarter of this 10%, cirrhosis, chronic hepatitis, or liver cancer will develop. Hepatocellular cancer is most likely to develop in patients whose liver biopsies show severe chronic active hepatitis, cirrhosis, or both.[7]

In patients with acute hepatitis B, detectable HBsAg usually develops about 3 weeks before the onset of clinical symptoms. HBsAg declines over the next few weeks as the patient recovers, and shortly thereafter anti-HBs develops. A "window phase" may occur in the recovery stage of hepatitis B when neither HBsAg nor anti-HBs is present; at that time tests for IgM anti-HBc are usually positive.[1]

A patient with clinical hepatitis who has anti-HBs does not have acute hepatitis B. HBeAg is present during acute hepatitis B infection and in chronic hepatitis B. If a patient from an endemic area has elevated liver enzyme levels and is HBsAg and HBeAg positive, he or she probably has chronic active hepatitis.[1]

A person is defined as a chronic carrier of hepatitis B if two samples of sera taken 6 months apart are both HBsAg positive or if a single serum sample is HBsAg positive and anti-HBc negative. The risk of development of the carrier state depends on the age of the patient at the time of infection. Specific risks are 90% to 95% in infants, 25% to 50% in children under 5, and 6% to 10% in adults.[8]

Immunization against hepatitis B and postexposure prophylaxis. See the section on immunization.

Treatment of chronic hepatitis B. Indications for treating patients with chronic hepatitis B are the presence of HBsAg, HBV DNA, and elevated serum ALT levels. Most patients are also HBeAg positive. Whether liver biopsies are of value in the management of chronic hepatitis B is uncertain. The usual treatment has been interferon alfa-2b (Intron A) given subcutaneously as either 5 million units daily or 10 million units three times a week over a 4- to 6-month period; histological improvement and biochemical resolution have been reported in 30% to 40% of patients treated in this manner. A newer treatment option is lamivudine (3TC, Epivir) given orally in doses of 100 mg/day. A response rate of about 75% has been reported with this regimen. Duration of therapy is uncertain, but discontinuation of the drug may be tried after a year.[9] Superinfection with hepatitis A in patients with chronic hepatitis B rarely results in fulminant hepatitis.[10]

Hepatitis C

Before the discovery and implementation of anti-HCV testing in blood banks in 1989, hepatitis C was responsible for 90% of transfusion-related cases of non-A, non-B hepatitis.[11] At present the risk of acquiring hepatitis C from transfusions is estimated to be 1 in 100,000 for each transfused unit.[12] Other recognized risk factors for hepatitis C are IV drug use, transfusions, accidental needle sticks by health care workers, and living in an endemic area. The risk of acquiring infection from an anti-HCV-positive patient via a needle stick is about 3%; there is no effective postexposure prophylaxis.[11] Between 50% and 80% of IV drug users become hepatitis C positive within a year of beginning usage.[12] In the United States more than 35% of cases of hepatitis C occur without known risk factors and are labeled as sporadic. Transmission of hepatitis C by colonoscopy has been reported (see discussion of secondary prevention of colon cancer).

Transmission of infection by close physical contact or through sexual relations may occur but is rare.[12] Both a German[13] and an Austrian[14] follow-up study of long-term monogamous marriages in which only one partner had hepatitis C found that the risk of sexual transmission was nonexistent[13] or extremely small.[14] On the other hand, studies from Asia have shown that the risk of a noninfected partner's acquiring hepatitis C increases with the duration of marriage[15]; Neumayr and associates[14] suggest that the frequent use of medical injections and acupuncture in Asia could account for this finding.

Vertical transmission of hepatitis C has been reported to occur in 5% to 36% of pregnancies, with the higher figures found in women who were coinfected with HIV. A multicenter Italian study of pregnant women who had antibodies to hepatitis C but who were HIV negative reported a transmission rate to the infant of 5%. Only women with detectable hepatitis C RNA in their blood transmitted the infection to their offspring. Although previous studies had suggested a diminution of transmission if delivery was by Cesarean section, such was not the case in this study. Hepatitis C is not transmitted through breast feeding.[16]

A systematic review of studies of hepatitis C transmission found that the risk of transmission is extremely low if hepatitis C RNA cannot be detected in the blood when tested by polymerase chain reaction methods. This may be of particular importance in advising patients about sexual practices (whether to use condoms) and risks of transmitting the disease through pregnancy. When the polymerase chain reaction is positive, the risk of transmission from occupational exposure (needle sticks) and pregnancy is about 6%, whereas the risk from blood transfusions is around 80%.[17]

The incubation period of hepatitis C is usually 6 to 7 weeks but varies from 2 weeks to 6 months. Only 20% to 30% of patients are jaundiced, 10% to 20% have nonspecific symptoms, and the rest are asymptomatic. Most symptomatic patients have anti-HCV antibody, but in some cases antibodies do not develop until 3 or more months after the onset of infection. More than 85% of infected adult patients will have persistent infection, 70% chronic hepatitis, 26% to 50% chronic active hepatitis, and 10% to 20% cirrhosis. Cirrhosis is a risk factor for hepatocellular cancer, a malignancy that affects between 1% and 4% of cirrhotic patients per year. The 20-year mortality rate from liver disease in patients with hepatitis C is 1.6% to 6%.[12] The outcome of children infected with hepatitis C through blood transfusions appears to be considerably better. In one study half the children had no detectable HCV RNA after 20 years and of those who had detectable HCV RNA all but one had normal levels of liver enzymes.[18]

It has generally been thought that if the liver enzyme levels are consistently normal for 6 months, the patient does not have chronic active hepatitis. Recent studies have shown this concept to be false. Anti-HCV-positive females who do not drink are particularly likely to have chronic hepatitis without elevated liver enzyme levels. Although the hepatic changes are minimal in most such patients, a few have more advanced changes.[19]

Treatment of chronic hepatitis C. If patients with chronic hepatitis C are superinfected with hepatitis A, fulminant hepatic failure is a common sequela. All patients with chronic hepatitis C should be immunized against hepatitis A.[9,10]

Hepatitis C patients who consume alcohol dramatically increase their risk of liver damage, cirrhosis, and hepatocellular carcinoma.[20] Abstention from alcohol is mandatory for patients with hepatitis C.[20,21]

Only selected patients with hepatitis C require active drug treatment. The risk of serious liver disease is low in patients with persistently normal ALT levels and liver biopsies showing minimal hepatocellular inflammation and fibrosis. Such patients probably do not require treatment because its efficacy in this form of the disease is uncertain, because progression of the disease is slow, and because treatments that are being developed and will be available in the future may be more effective and less toxic.[21] In line with this reasoning, a National Institutes of Health Consensus Conference recommends treatment for patients who have persistently elevated ALT levels, HCV viremia, and fibrosis and moderate inflammation on biopsy.[22] The need for liver biopsy is controversial; some experts claim that it does not alter outcome and should be reserved for treatment failures.[9]

Interferon alpha (interferon alfa-2a [Roferon-A] or interferon alfa-2b [Intron A]) has been used for the treatment of chronic active hepatitis C. The current recommendation is 3 million units of interferon subcutaneously three times a week for 6 to 12 months. Response ceases in many patients once the drug is stopped; the overall sustained response rate is 10% to 15%. More encouraging results have been obtained when ribavirin (Virazole) in doses of 1000 to 1200 mg/day po was combined with interferon therapy. Between one third and one half of patients remained free of HCV virus 24 weeks after completion of treatment.[23]

▧ REFERENCES ▰

1. Friedman G, Sherker AH: The ABCs of hepatitis, *Can J Diagn* 13:85-97, 1996.
2. Steffen R, Kane MA, Shapiro CN, et al: Epidemiology and prevention of hepatitis A in travelers, *JAMA* 272:885-889, 1994.

3. Public health: hepatitis A, *Can Med Assoc J* 156:545, 1997.
4. *Canadian immunization guide,* ed 5, Ottawa, 1998, Minister of Supply and Services Canada.
5. Koff RS: The case for routine childhood vaccination against hepatitis A (editorial), *N Engl J Med* 340:644-645, 1999.
6. Lee WM: Hepatitis B virus infection, *N Engl J Med* 337:1733-1745, 1997.
7. Curley SA, Izzo F, Gallipoli A, et al: Identification and screening of 416 patients with chronic hepatitis at high risk to develop hepatocellular cancer, *Ann Surg* 222:375-380, 1995.
8. Mahoney FJ, Burkholder BT, Matson CC: Prevention of hepatitis B virus infection, *Am Fam Physician* 47:865-874, 1993.
9. Koff RS: Advances in the treatment of chronic viral hepatitis, *JAMA* 282:511-512, 1999.
10. Vento S, Garofano T, Renzini C, et al: Fulminant hepatitis associated with hepatitis A virus superinfection in patients with chronic hepatitis C, *N Engl J Med* 338:286-290, 1998.
11. From the Centers for Disease Control and Prevention: recommendations for follow-up of health-care workers after occupational exposure to hepatitis C virus, *JAMA* 1056-1057, 1997.
12. Moyer LA, Mast EE, Alter MJ: Hepatitis C. I. Routine serologic testing and diagnosis, *Am Fam Physician* 59:79-88, 1999.
13. Meisel H, Reip A, Faltus B, et al: Transmission of hepatitis C virus to children and husbands by women infected with con taminated anti-D immunoglobulin, *Lancet* 345:1209-1211, 1995.
14. Neumayr G, Propst A, Schwaighofer H, et al: Lack of evidence for the heterosexual transmission of hepatitis C, *Q J Med* 92:505-508, 1999.
15. Kao JH, Hwang YT, Chen PJ, et al: Transmission of hepatitis C virus between spouses—the important role of exposure duration, *Am J Gastroenterol* 91:2087-2090, 1996.
16. Resti M, Azzari C, Mannelli F, et al: Mother to child transmission of hepatitis C virus: prospective study of risk factors and timing of infection in children born to women seronegative for HIV-1, *BMJ* 317:437-441, 1998.
17. Dore GJ, Kaldor JM, McCaughan GW: Systematic review of role of polymerase chain reaction in defining infectiousness among people infected with hepatitis C virus, *BMJ* 315:333-337, 1997.
18. Vogt M, Lang T, Frösner G, et al: Prevalence and clinical outcome of hepatitis C infection in children who underwent cardiac surgery before the implementation of blood-donor screening, *N Engl J Med* 314:866-870, 1999.
19. Gholson CF, Morgan K, Catinis G, et al: Chronic hepatitis C with normal aminotransferase levels: a clinical histologic study, *Am J Gastroenterol* 92:1788-1792, 1997.
20. Bellentani S, Pozzato G, Saccoccio G, et al: Clinical course and risk factors of hepatitis C virus related liver disease in the general population: report from the Dionysos study, *Gut* 44:874-880, 1999.
21. Levine RA: Treating histologically mild chronic hepatitis C: monotherapy, combination therapy, or tincture of time? *Ann Intern Med* 129:323-326, 1998.
22. National Institutes of Health Consensus Development Conference Panel statement: management of hepatitis C, *Hepatology* 26(suppl 1):2S-10S, 1997.
23. Liang TJ: Combination therapy for hepatitis C infection (editorial), *N Engl J Med* 339:1549-1550, 1998.

PANCREAS
Pancreatic Cancer

Diabetic patients who have had the disease for at least 5 years have double the risk of pancreatic carcinoma compared with nondiabetic control subjects.[1] Current smokers have a 2.5-fold increase in the relative risk for this malignancy,[2] and obesity also appears to be a risk factor.[3] Overall, 80% of patients with pancreatic cancer are dead within a year of diagnosis.[4] A multicenter study of 100 U.S. veterans' hospitals found that the operative mortality for the Whipple procedure was 8%. Patients who underwent the surgery for pancreatic cancer had a mean survival of 15 months and a projected 5-year survival of 9%.[5] Testosterone is probably a growth promotor for pancreatic cancer. In one trial the antiandrogen flutamide (Eulexin, Euflex) almost doubled the survival time in both men and women and was associated with very few adverse reactions.[6] Gemcitabine (Gemzar) is also well tolerated. It produces symptom improvement in about one in five patients and objective evidence of partial tumor regression in 12% of cases.[7]

◢ REFERENCES ◣

1. Everhart J, Wright D: Diabetes mellitus as a risk factor for pancreatic cancer: a meta-analysis, *JAMA* 273:1605-1609, 1995.
2. Fuchs CS, Colditz GA, Stampfer MJ, et al: A prospective study of cigarette smoking and the risk of pancreatic cancer, *Arch Intern Med* 156:2255-2260, 1996.
3. Silverman DT, Swanson CA, Gridley G, et al: Dietary and nutritional factors and pancreatic cancer: a case-control study based on direct interviews, *J Natl Cancer Inst* 90:1710-1719, 1998.
4. Taylor WF, Everhart JE: Pancreatic cancer. In Everhart JE, ed: *Digestive diseases in the United States: epidemiology and impact,* Washington, DC, 1994, US Dept of Health and Human Services, Public Health Service, National Institutes of Health, National Institute of Diabetes and Digestive and Kidney Diseases, NIH Pub No 94-1447, pp 247-270.
5. Wade TP, Elghazzawy AG, Virgo KS, et al: The Whipple resection for cancer in US Department of Veterans Affairs hospitals, *Ann Surg* 221:241-248, 1995.
6. Greenway BA: Effect of flutamide on survival in patients with pancreatic cancer: results of a prospective, randomised, double blind, placebo controlled trial, *BMJ* 316:1935-1938, 1998.
7. Storniolo AM, Enas NH, Brown CA, et al: An investigational new drug treatment program for patients with gemcitabine: results for over 3000 patients with pancreatic carcinoma, *Cancer* 85:1261-1268, 1999.

STOMACH AND DUODENUM
Nonsteroidal Antiinflammatory Drug Gastropathy
(See also *Helicobacter pylori,* hypertension; nonsteroidal antiinflammatory drugs; osteoarthritis; peptic ulcer; statistics)

NSAIDs are associated with many adverse gastrointestinal effects, including dyspepsia, peptic ulcers that may bleed or perforate, pill esophagitis, small bowel ulceration, small bowel stricture, colonic strictures, and diverticular disease. Dyspepsia affects 10% to 20% of persons taking NSAIDs, but only a small percentage of those with serious gastrointestinal lesions have antecedent dyspepsia.[1]

Major risk factors for gastrointestinal complications from NSAIDs are old age, high doses of NSAIDs, concomitant use of corticosteroids, past history of peptic ulcer or gastrointestinal bleeding, and serious coexisting diseases (such as heart, renal, or hepatic failure).[1] The presence of *H. pylori* does not appear to increase the risk for NSAID-induced gastropathy.[1-3] According to one systematic review, no good evidence is available to support serological screening of patients for *H. pylori* and eradication treatment for those with positive results before initiating NSAID therapy. However, if patients taking NSAIDs have proven peptic ulcers, it is probably worth screening for *H. pylori* and treating those who test positive.[3]

Two new NSAIDs, celecoxib (Celebrex) and rofecoxib (Vioxx), belong to a class of NSAIDs that inhibit cyclooxygenase 2 (COX-2) without inhibiting cyclooxygenase 1 (COX-1). COX-1 facilitates the production of protective prostaglandins in the stomach and kidneys, whereas COX-2 is found in joints and aggravates inflammation.[1,4] A 6-month randomized trial of patients with osteoarthritis compared rofecoxib 25 or 50 mg/day with ibuprofen (Advil, Motrin) 800 mg tid. On endoscopic assessment far fewer gastroduodenal ulcers (defined as lesions ≥3 mm in diameter) were identified in the rofecoxib group than in the ibuprofen group.[5] A 12-week comparison of celecoxib and naproxen (Naprosyn) in patients with rheumatoid arthritis also showed a marked decrease in endoscopically detected ulcers ≥3 mm in diameter.[6]

The important clinical question is not whether COX-2-selective NSAIDs decrease the incidence of tiny asymptomatic mucosal ulcers but whether they reduce the complications of ulcers—bleeding, perforation, and obstruction.[7] Pooled data from eight randomized controlled trials comparing rofecoxib to first-generation NSAIDs indicated a very small decrease in ulcer complications in patients taking rofecoxib,[8] but the practical significance of these findings is uncertain.[4] COX-2-selective drugs may be the agents of choice for older patients with multiple risk factors for gastrointestinal complications from NSAIDs, but they seem to offer no advantage for young, healthy individuals requiring short courses of treatment.[4]

Prophylactic use of misoprostol (Cytotec) or proton pump inhibitors such as omeprazole (Prilosec, Losec) can reduce the risk of NSAID-induced peptic ulcers.[1] In a comparative study of misoprostol 200 μg bid and omeprazole 20 mg/day, omeprazole was more effective.[9] H_2-receptor blockers are minimally effective for preventing peptic ulcers in patients taking NSAIDs.[1]

The optimal treatment of patients who develop gastrointestinal disorders when taking NSAIDs is to discontinue the NSAIDs. If this cannot be done, the gastrointestinal disorder should be treated with a proton pump inhibitor because this class of drugs is the most effective for treating both NSAID-induced dyspepsia[1] and NSAID-related gastroduodenal ulcers.[1,10] An additional strategy would be to switch to a COX-2 selective NSAID.[1]

◢ REFERENCES ◣

1. Wolfe MM, Lichtenstein DR, Singh G: Gastrointestinal toxicity of nonsteroidal antiinflammatory drugs, *N Engl J Med* 340:1888-1899, 1999.
2. Hawkey CJ, Tulassay Z, Szczepanski L, et al: Randomised controlled trial of *Helicobacter pylori* eradication in patients on non-steroidal antiinflammatory drugs: HELP NSAIDs study, *Lancet* 352:1016-1021, 1998.
3. Chiba N, Lahaie R, Fedorak RN, et al: *Helicobacter pylori* and peptic ulcer disease: current evidence for management strategies, *Can Fam Physician* 44:1481-1488, 1998.
4. Peterson WL, Cryer B: COX-1-sparing NSAIDs—is the enthusiasm justified? (editorial), *JAMA* 282:1961-1963, 1999.
5. Laine L, Harper S, Simon T, et al: A randomized trial comparing the effect of rofecoxib, a cyclooxygenase 2-specific inhibitor, with that of ibuprofen on the gastroduodenal mucosa of patients with osteoarthritis, *Gastroenterology* 117:776-783, 1999.
6. Simon LS, Weaver AL, Graham DY, et al: Anti-inflammatory and upper gastrointestinal effects of celecoxib in rheumatoid arthritis: a randomized controlled trial, *JAMA* 282:1921-1928, 1999.
7. Beejay U, Wolfe MM: Cyclooxygenase 2 selective inhibitors: panacea or flash in the pan? (editorial), *Gastroenterology* 117: 1002-1004, 1999.
8. Langman MJ, Jensen DM, Watson KF, et al: Adverse upper gastrointestinal effects of rofecoxib compared with NSAIDs, *JAMA* 282:1929-1933, 1999.
9. Hawkey CJ, Karrasch JA, Szczepanski L, et al (Omeprazole Versus Misoprostol for NSAID-Induced Ulcer Management [OMNIUM] Study Group): Omeprazole compared with misoprostol for ulcers associated with nonsteroidal antiinflammatory drugs, *N Engl J Med* 338:727-734, 1998.
10. Yeomans ND, Tulassay Z, Juhász L, et al (NSAID-Associated Ulcer Treatment [ASTRONAUT] Study Group): A comparison of omeprazole with ranitidine for ulcers associated with nonsteroidal antiinflammatory drugs, *N Engl J Med* 338:719-726, 1998.

Nonulcer Dyspepsia
(See also peptic ulcer)

Dyspepsia may be defined as persistent or recurrent upper abdominal pain. Associated symptoms include nausea, vomiting, distention, bloating, and early satiety. Forty percent of patients with dyspepsia have underlying organic conditions; the remainder have nonulcer dyspepsia.[1]

Various types of nonulcer dyspepsia have been described. One variant mimics the symptoms of peptic ulcer (ulcerlike dyspepsia), a second is the presence of upper abdominal pain and reflux symptoms (refluxlike dyspepsia), and a third is upper abdominal discomfort in association with early satiety, postprandial fullness, nausea, vomiting, and bloating (dysmotility-like dyspepsia). The clinical significance of these subdivisions is questionable, although some workers use them in determining which pharmacological agents might be most beneficial.[1]

The cause of nonulcer dyspepsia is unknown. Although claims have been made that *H. pylori* plays a pathogenic role in some cases, recent randomized controlled trials failed to find any benefit from eradicating *H.pylori* in patients with nonulcer dyspepsia.[2-4]

A major issue in clinical practice is distinguishing peptic ulcer from nonulcer dyspepsia. Should patients with symptoms of uncomplicated peptic ulcer disease have a barium swallow x-ray examination or endoscopy, or should they be treated on clinical grounds alone? Authorities agree that patients with symptoms suggesting serious disease, such as new onset of symptoms after age 55, weight loss, anemia, and gastrointestinal bleeding, need endoscopy, but whether the remainder require it is controversial.[1,5] Arguments favoring endoscopy are that many patients with dyspepsia have organic disease and that a negative result is reassuring and may decrease the long-term cost of care. However, since dyspepsia is so common, a reasonable alternative would be to test patients for *H. pylori* with serology (or the much more expensive urea breath test) and, if the findings are positive, treat them for *H. pylori* infection.[1] In a trial from Belfast, *H. pylori*–positive patients with ulcerlike dyspepsia were randomly assigned to have endoscopy or empirical eradication therapy. At 12 months those treated empirically had fewer dyspeptic symptoms and better quality of life.[6]

Symptomatic treatment with H_2-blockers, proton pump inhibitors, or prokinetic agents such as metoclopramide (Maxeran) or cisapride (Propulsid) may help some patients who are *H. pylori* negative.[1] Since smoking and the regular use of aspirin are associated with an increased risk of nonulcer dyspepsia, symptomatic patients should avoid these agents.[7]

◣ REFERENCES ◢

1. Fisher RS, Parkman HP: Management of nonulcer dyspepsia, *N Engl J Med* 339:1376-1381, 1998.
2. Talley NJ, Vakil N, Ballard ED II, et al: Absence of benefit of eradicating *Helicobacter pylori* in patients with nonulcer dyspepsia, *N Engl J Med* 341:1106-1111, 1999.
3. Talley NJ, Janssens J, Lauritsen K, et al (Optimal Regimen Cures Helicobacter Induce Dyspepsia [ORCHID] Study Group): Eradication of *Helicobacter pylori* in functional dyspepsia: randomised double blind placebo controlled trial with 12 months' follow up, *BMJ* 318:833-837, 1999.
4. Greenberg PD, Cello JP: Lack of effect of treatment for *Helicobacter pylori* on symptoms of nonulcer dyspepsia, *Arch Intern Med* 159:2283-2288, 1999.
5. Jones R: *Helicobacter pylori* and dyspepsia: trick or treat? (editorial), *Gut* 45:164-169, 1999.
6. Heaney A, Collins JS, Watson RG, et al: A prospective randomised trial of a "test and treat" policy versus endoscopy based management in young *Helicobacter pylori* positive patients with ulcer-like dyspepsia, referred to a hospital clinic, *Gut* 45:186-190, 1999.
7. Nandurkar S, Talley NJ, Xia H, et al: Dyspepsia in the community is linked to smoking and aspirin use but not to *Helicobacter pylori* infection, *Arch Intern Med* 158:1427-1433, 1998.

Peptic Ulcer

(See also esophagus; nonsteroidal antiinflammatory agent gastropathy; nonulcer dyspepsia; stomach cancer)

Bleeding peptic ulcers

Bleeding peptic ulcers account for 50% of upper gastrointestinal hemorrhages. In 80% of cases the bleeding stops spontaneously and recovery is uneventful. Rebleeding, when it occurs, usually takes place within the first 3 days. NSAIDs appear to be a major risk factor not only for the development of peptic ulcers, but also for bleeding from peptic ulcers (see later discussion).[1]

In patients with uncontrolled bleeding, immediate hemostasis can usually be achieved through endoscopic procedures,[1,2] although rebleeding occurs in 10% to 30% of cases.[2] Intensive therapy with H_2-blockers has not been effective in controlling acute upper intestinal bleeding, but in India a trial of omeprazole (Prilosec, Losec) 40 mg po bid for 5 days for endoscopically documented bleeding peptic ulcers showed a significant decrease in requirements for transfusion or surgery. No endoscopic therapeutic interventions were attempted in this study.[3] Omeprazole has also been shown to be effective in preventing rebleeding after endoscopic control of hemorrhage from peptic ulcers. In one study the drug was begun as a 40-mg IV bolus, was followed by a continuous IV infusion of 160 mg/day for 3 days, and then was given as 20 mg/day po for 2 months.[2]

Once a patient has stopped bleeding and is in a stable condition, medical treatment is aimed at healing the ulcer and preventing recurrences of the ulcer and bleeding. If possible, NSAIDs should be discontinued. If the patient is positive for *H. pylori* (as are about 75% of patients with bleeding peptic ulcers), the organisms should be eradicated (see later discussion). Healing is facilitated by omeprazole 20 mg/day for 6 to 8 weeks or by an H_2-receptor antagonist for 2 to 3 months.[1]

Helicobacter pylori

Excluding patients taking NSAIDs, more than 80% of those with gastric ulcers and more than 90% of those with duodenal ulcers are infected with *H. pylori*. However, ulcers develop in only 15% to 20% of those infected with the organism. The ulcer recurrence rate is markedly decreased in patients treated for *H. pylori*.[4]

H. pylori infection is recognized as a cause of gastric and duodenal ulcers, as well as gastric carcinoma.[4,5] An interesting observation is that the incidence of gastric cancer is decreased in patients with a history of duodenal ulcer.[6] The probable explanation is that *H. pylori* acquired in early childhood (as occurs frequently in developing countries) leads to atrophic gastritis, which is both a predisposing factor for malignancy and, because of decreased acid secretion, a defense against duodenal ulcer formation. However, when the infection is acquired later in life, atrophic gastritis is less likely to develop and so acid secretion is not inhibited.[5] Atrophic gastritis also protects against gastroesophageal reflux disease (see discussion of the esophagus).

Diagnostic procedures for *H. pylori* include gastric biopsies, breath urea tests, and serological tests.[4,7,8] Serological findings remain positive for many months or years after eradication of the organisms and cannot be used to measure the efficacy of therapy within the first few months of treatment.[4,8] However, in one small study serological findings reverted to normal after 18 months in 65% of patients who had documented cure of *H. pylori* infection. The clinical significance is that a negative serological test many months after treatment of *H. pylori* rules out persistent infection whereas a positive one has no clinical significance. If earlier documentation of cure is necessary, it can be established with breath urea tests or gastric biopsies.[7,8] An important caveat is that one third of patients who are taking proton pump inhibitors have false-negative results of breath urea tests (temporary suppression of *H. pylori* by the drug). Patients should not take proton pump inhibitors for at least a week, and preferably 2 weeks, before the test.[9]

Treatment of *H. pylori* infections leads to faster healing of ulcers and a marked reduction in the relapse rate.[4,5] Since 95% of duodenal ulcers that are not NSAID related are associated with *H. pylori* infection, a reasonable approach is to treat all such patients with antimicrobial therapy without testing them for the presence of the organism.[4] Whether treating patients with *H. pylori* but no evidence of peptic ulcers will prevent gastric carcinoma is unknown.[7,10] Although at least one editorial writer considers it to be a reasonable option,[10] others disagree because of the possibility that eliminating *H. pylori* from the stomach may increase the risk of adenocarcinoma of the lower esophagus and cardia of the stomach (see discussion of adenocarcinoma of the esophagus).[7]

Because *H. pylori* is difficult to eradicate, two or more antibiotics should be used. The adjunct use of a proton pump inhibitor such as omeprazole (Prilosec, Losec) or lansoprazole (Prevacid) augments the efficacy of the antibiotics. Most studies to date have used omeprazole 20 mg bid, but new data suggest that other proton pump inhibitors such as lansoprazole 30 mg bid or pantoprazole (Pantoloc) 40 mg bid are equally effective.[4]

A confusing variety of treatments for *H. pylori* have been used, and some of the more effective ones are listed below.[4,11,12] Cure rates with any of these regimens are on the order of 85% to 90%.[4] Most of the studies of bismuth have been with bismuth subcitrate, which is not available in North America; probably bismuth subsalicylate (Pepto-Bismol), which is the standard form in North America, is equally effective when given as combination therapy.[11,12] Although in vitro resistance to metronidazole (Flagyl) is fairly common, this does not appear to affect its efficacy when used as part of combination therapy.[12]

At present, triple therapy appears to be the optimal first option[12,13]:

1. Clarithromycin (Biaxin) 500 mg bid plus metronidazole (Flagyl) 500 mg bid plus omeprazole (Prilosec, Losec) 20 mg bid for 7 to 10 days[12]
2. Clarithromycin (Biaxin) 500 mg bid plus amoxicillin 1 g bid plus lansoprazole (Prevacid) 30 mg bid for 14 days[13]

If triple therapy fails, the next step should be a bismuth-based quadruple therapy regimen[12]: bismuth subsalicylate 524 mg (Pepto-Bismol, 2 tablets) qid or bismuth subcitrate 120 mg qid plus tetracycline 250 or 500 mg qid plus metronidazole 250 mg qid plus omeprazole 20 mg bid or lansoprazole 30 mg bid. Amoxicillin 1 g bid or tid can be substituted for the tetracycline.

A less expensive regimen uses bismuth, tetracycline, and metronidazole alone[4]: bismuth subsalicylate (Pepto-Bismol) 2 tablets (262 mg each) qid for 7 to 14 days plus metronidazole (Flagyl) 250 mg qid for 7 to 14 days plus tetracycline 500 mg qid for 7 to 14 days.

Stress

That *H. pylori* and NSAIDs are causally related to peptic ulcer formation does not mean that psychological stress is not a risk factor. The incidence of peptic ulcers is higher in populations and among individuals experiencing increased levels of stress. Numerous physiological changes could account for this, including decreased blood flow to the stomach that adversely affects the mucosal barrier and increased acid secretion that might counter the *H. pylori*–inhibiting effects of bile acids in the duodenum.[14]

Specific ulcer medications

Traditional medications used for the treatment of peptic ulcers are listed in Table 26.

────────── ⚑ **REFERENCES** ⚑ ──────────

1. Laine L, Peterson WL: Bleeding peptic ulcer, *N Engl J Med* 331:717-727, 1994.
2. Lin H-J, Lo W-C, Lee F-Y, et al: A prospective randomized comparative trial showing that omeprazole prevents rebleeding in patients with bleeding peptic ulcer after successful endoscopic therapy, *Arch Intern Med* 158:54-58, 1998.

Table 26 Peptic Ulcer Medications

Drug	Usual doses
H₂-Blockers	
Cimetidine (Tagamet)	800 mg qhs or 600 mg bid
Famotidine (Pepcid)	40 mg qhs
Nizatidine (Axid)	300 mg qhs
Ranitidine (Zantac)	300 mg qhs or 150 mg bid
Proton Pump Inhibitors	
Lansoprazole (Prevacid)	15 mg qam
Omeprazole (Prilosec, Losec)	20 mg qam
Pantoprazole (Pantoloc)	40 mg qam
Rabeprazole (Aciphex)	20 mg once daily
Prostaglandins	
Misoprostol (Cytotec)	200 μg qid or 400 μg bid
Cytoprotectives	
Sucralfate (Sulcrate)	1-2 g qid ac and hs

3. Khuroo MS, Yattoo GN, Javid G, et al: A comparison of omeprazole and placebo for bleeding peptic ulcer, *N Engl J Med* 336:1054-1058, 1997.
4. Veldhuyzen van Zanten SJ, Sherman PM, Hunt RH: *Helicobacter pylori:* new developments and treatments, *Can Med Assoc J* 156:1565-1574, 1997.
5. Parsonnet J: *Helicobacter pylori* in the stomach—a paradox unmasked (editorial), *N Engl J Med* 335:278-280, 1996.
6. Hansson L-E, Nyrén O, Hsing AW, et al: The risk of stomach cancer in patients with gastric or duodenal ulcer disease, *N Engl J Med* 335:242-249, 1996.
7. Blaser MJ: *Helicobacter pylori* and gastric diseases, *BMJ* 316:1507-1510, 1998.
8. Feldman M, Cryer B, Lee E, et al: Role of seroconversion in confirming cure of *Helicobacter pylori* infection, *JAMA* 280:363-365, 1998.
9. Laine L, Estrada R, Trujillo M, et al: Effect of proton pump inhibitor therapy on diagnostic testing for *Helicobacter pylori,* *Ann Intern Med* 129:547-550, 1998.
10. Axon A, Forman D: *Helicobacter* gastroduodenitis: a serious infectious disease; antibiotic treatment may prevent deaths in the decades ahead (editorial), *BMJ* 314:1430-1431, 1997.
11. Soll AH: Medical treatment of peptic ulcer disease: practice guidelines, *JAMA* 275:622-629, 1996.
12. Salcedo JA, Al-Kawas F: Treatment of *Helicobacter pylori* infection, *Arch Intern Med* 158:842-851, 1998.
13. Schwartz H, Krause R, Sahba B, et al: Triple versus dual therapy for eradicating *Helicobacter pylori* and prevention of ulcer recurrence: a randomized, double-blind, multicenter study of lansoprazole, clarithromycin, and/or amoxicillin in different dosing regimens, *Am J Gastroenterol* 93:584-590, 1998.
14. Levenstein S, Ackerman S, Kiecolt-Glaser JK, et al: Stress and peptic ulcer disease, *JAMA* 281:10-11, 1999.

Stomach Cancer
(See also peptic ulcer)

In the 1930s gastric carcinoma was the leading cause of cancer death in North America among men and the third leading cause among women; since then the incidence has dropped dramatically in that part of the world but continues to be high in Japan, China, South America, and Eastern Europe. A correlation exists between the incidence of gastric carcinoma and the prevalence of *H. pylori* infection (see preceding discussion of peptic ulcer). Surgery is the treatment of choice. The 5-year survival of stage I tumor that has not invaded the muscularis, spread to nodes, or metastasized is 50% to 60% in North America, but stage I accounts for less than 10% of North American cases. The 5-year survival for stage II (invasion of muscularis propria but no serosal involvement) is 30%, and stages III and IV have much lower survival rates. Overall survival is better in Japan, probably because screening has led to detection of earlier stage lesions. Chemotherapy and radiation therapy offer relatively little for this form of cancer.[1]

Case-control studies suggest that survival of gastric cancer is better in Japan than elsewhere, possibly because widespread x-ray screening has led to detection of earlier stage lesions.[1] However, preliminary data from a cohort study failed to find significant benefit from screening.[2]

Early gastric cancer is often manifested as an ulcer or as dyspepsia, and treatment with proton pump inhibitors can result in the resolution of dyspeptic symptoms and even healing of malignant ulcers. For this reason some experts recommend endoscopy for all dyspeptic patients over the age of 45 before proton pump inhibitors are prescribed.[3]

◥ REFERENCES ◤

1. Fuchs CS, Mayer RJ: Gastric carcinoma, *N Engl J Med* 333:32-41, 1995.
2. Inaba S, Hirayama H, Nagata C, et al: Evaluation of a screening program on reduction of gastric cancer mortality in Japan: preliminary results from a cohort study, *Prev Med* 29:102-106, 1999.
3. Griffin SM, Raimes SA: Proton pump inhibitors may mask early gastric cancer: dyspeptic patients over 45 should undergo endoscopy before these drugs are started (editorial), *BMJ* 317:1606-1607, 1998.

GERIATRICS

(See also dementia; elderly abuse; exercise; hip fractures; hypertension; motor vehicle accidents; nonsteroidal antiinflammatory drugs; osteoarthritis; osteoporosis; practice patterns; prescribing habits; pseudohypertension; urinary tract infections)

Topics covered in this section

Epidemiology
Caregivers
Delirium

EPIDEMIOLOGY

Persons who are 85 or older are often labeled as the "oldest old." Among this group half of the men are living with their wives (most wives are younger than their husbands), whereas only 10% of women are living with their husbands (most husbands are dead). About half have impaired hearing, and a third have some degree of dementia. In the United States 25% of women over the age of 84 and 15% of men of similar age live in nursing homes.[1] The average life expectancy of 80-year-old U.S. women is 9.1 years, while for 80-year-old U.S. men it is 7 years.[2] Among 85-year-olds in the United States the life expectancy is 6.4 years for women and 5.2 years for men.[1] Use of health services by people aged 65 to 74 is little different from that of the general adult population, but for those 75 and older it increases significantly.[3] Middle-aged individuals with low health risk factors (nonsmokers, nonsedentary, and nonobese) not only live longer than their counterparts who have these risk factors, but also have less lifetime disability.[4]

Although exercise is well known to decrease mortality rates in the elderly, it appears that social and productive activities also have a protective role. Typical social activities are church attendance; going to movies, sports events, or restaurants; taking short trips; playing cards or other games; and belonging to social groups. Productive activities include preparing meals; shopping; gardening; paid employment; and volunteer community work.[5]

CAREGIVERS

It is often stated that elderly patients with dementia or terminal illnesses are best looked after at home. Except for the very affluent, this means that family members or close friends must perform most of the care. Considerable literature shows that this process may adversely affect the emotional and even the physical health of the caregivers, but surprisingly little evidence supports the notion that home care is better than institutional care for either the patient or the family caregivers.[6]

DELIRIUM

Five important precipitating factors for delirium in elderly hospitalized patients are malnutrition, physical restraints, bladder catheterization, taking more than three medications, and any iatrogenic event.[7] Optimal treatment is control of precipitating factors. If medications are required, neuroleptics such as haloperidol or droperidol are the drugs of choice. Benzodiazepines as monotherapy are ineffective, although some reports state that they may have value when combined with neuroleptics.[8]

DRY MOUTH AND DRY EYES

In a population survey just over one fourth of elderly patients complained of dry eyes or dry mouth. In two thirds of these cases the probable cause was drying effects from a variety of classes of medications. Autoimmune diseases were not a significant cause of sicca symptoms.[9]

EXERCISE IN THE ELDERLY

Exercise emphasizing strength and balance decreases the risk of falls in the elderly.[10,11] In one such program for women over the age of 80, physiotherapists visited the home every 2 weeks for 2 months. The women were taught lower limb–strengthening exercises using 0.5- and 1-kg ankle weights, walking on toes and heels, knee squatting, rising from chairs, climbing stairs, walking backward, turning around, tandem walking, and active range of motion to increase flexibility such as maximum head turning or hip and knee extension. Patients were asked to follow this routine on their own at least three times per week.[11]

FALLS

Some of the medical risk factors for falls in the elderly are cardiovascular disorders such as postural hypotension, arrhythmias, and pacemaker failure; visual impairment; muscle weakness; and peripheral neuropathy.[12] Excessive medications in general[13] and the use of benzodiazepines in particular[14] are associated with increased rates of falling and fractures. Reputed environmental factors leading to falls are uneven outdoor surfaces, change in surface level, and inappropriate floor coverings and footwear.[12]

A thorough medical assessment and a home evaluation by occupational therapists followed by appropriate therapeutic interventions have been shown to reduce the number of falls in elderly patients when compared with control subjects receiving usual care.[12] One of the most effective interventions in preventing falls is an exercise program emphasizing strength, balance, and aerobic fitness.[10,11] Not only is the degree of osteoporosis minimized, but improved balance and gait decrease the frequency of falls. Whether such programs actually decrease the risk of hip fractures has not been established.[10]

LIVING ALONE

The risk that a person living alone will become helpless from an illness or die without help increases with age. The highest risk group is men over the age of 85 who are living alone. The longer the interval between the onset of helplessness and being found, the higher the mortality rate.[15] Suggested solutions are frequent checking on such individuals[15,16] and use of electronic alert devices.[16]

PRESCRIBING HABITS AND THE ELDERLY

Inappropriate prescription of drugs for the elderly is rampant. A study by Tamblyn and associates[17] determined that over a 1-year period about one third of elderly Quebec residents received prescriptions for benzodiazepines to be taken for more than 30 consecutive days. A similar type of survey in British Columbia found that over a 1-year period 17% of noninstitutionalized persons over the age of 65 received at least one prescription for benzodiazepines while 4% of elderly patients received a prescription for 20 mg of diazepam or its equivalent to be taken daily for more than 2 months.[18] A U.S. report found that 60% of individuals in the United States who take nonsteroidal antiinflammatory drugs (NSAIDs) are 60 years or older,[19] and in Alberta 27% of persons over the age of 65 received at least one NSAID prescription during a 6-month study period.[20] A Canadian study of the prescribing habits of New Brunswick physicians treating elderly patients showed that high prescribers ordered 45% more prescriptions than did low prescribers and that morbidity, hip fracture, and mortality rates were higher among patients of high-prescribing physicians than among those of low prescribers.[13]

Other important adverse consequences of polypharmacy in the elderly are delirium and incontinence.[21] The number of potentially inappropriate drug combinations that are prescribed for elderly patients increases with the number of prescribing physicians the patient sees.[22]

Although polypharmacy is clearly a major problem with drug prescriptions in the elderly, underuse is also important. Examples are failure to prescribe beta-blockers for elderly patients who have had a myocardial infarction,[21,23] anticoagulants for those in atrial fibrillation,[21] or adequate medications to control systolic hypertension[23] or fully control cancer pain.[23]

An important aspect of geriatric care is a careful review of medications with the goal of stopping those that are unnecessary. In most cases discontinuation is accomplished successfully, but in some the process results in adverse drug withdrawal events. A relatively infrequent type of adverse drug withdrawal event is the physiological withdrawal reaction, which is most frequently seen with beta-blockers, benzodiazepines, antipsychotics, antidepressants, and corticosteroids. The solution is to taper the drug reduction slowly. A more common adverse effect is recurrence of the condition for which the drugs were originally prescribed, such as angina, hypertension, or congestive heart failure. Recurrences may not manifest themselves for 3 or 4 months.[24]

RETIREMENT

According to Finnish studies, retirement is not associated with a deterioration of physical health and in many instances mental health improves.[25]

▰ REFERENCES ▰

1. Campion EW: The oldest old (editorial), *N Engl J Med* 30:1819-1820, 1994.
2. Manton KG, Vaupel JW: Survival after the age of 80 in the United States, Sweden, France, England, and Japan, *N Engl J Med* 333:1232-1235, 1995.
3. Rosenberg MW, Moore EG: The health of Canada's elderly population: current status and future implications, *Can Med Assoc J* 157:1025-1032, 1997.
4. Vita AJ, Terry RB, Hubert HB, et al: Aging, health risks, and cumulative disability, *N Engl J Med* 338:1035-1041, 1998.
5. Glass TA, de Leon CM, Marottoli RA, et al: Population based study of social and productive activities as predictors of survival among elderly Americans, *BMJ* 319:478-483, 1999.
6. Grunfeld E, Glossop R, McDowell I, et al: Caring for elderly people at home: the consequences to caregivers, *Can Med Assoc J* 157:1101-1105, 1997.
7. Inouye SK, Charpentier PA: Precipitating factors for delirium in hospitalized elderly persons: predictive model and interrelationship with baseline vulnerability, *JAMA* 275:852-857, 1996.
8. Trzepacz P, Breitbart W, Franklin J, et al: American Psychiatric Association Practice Guideline for the treatment of patients with delirium, *Am J Psychiatry* 156:S1-S20, 1999.
9. Schein OD, Hochberg MC, Munoz B, et al: Dry eye and dry mouth in the elderly: a population-based assessment, *Arch Intern Med* 159:1359-1363, 1999.
10. Kannus P: Preventing osteoporosis, falls, and fractures among elderly people: promotion of lifelong physical activity is essential (editorial), *BMJ* 318:205-206, 1999.
11. Campbell AJ, Robertson MC, Gardner MM, et al: Randomised controlled trial of a general practice programme of home based exercise to prevent falls in elderly women, *BMJ* 315:1065-1069, 1997.
12. Close J, Ellis M, Hooper R, et al: Prevention of falls in the elderly trial (PROFET): a randomised controlled trial, *Lancet* 353:93-97, 1999.
13. Davidson W, Molloy DW, Bédard M: Physician characteristics and prescribing for elderly people in New Brunswick: relation to patient outcomes, *Can Med Assoc J* 152:1227-1234, 1995.
14. Herings RM, Stricker BH, de Boer A, et al: Benzodiazepines and the risk of falling leading to femur fractures, *Arch Intern Med* 155:1801-1807, 1995.
15. Gurley RJ, Lum N, Sande M, et al: Persons found in their homes helpless or dead, *N Engl J Med* 334:1710-1716, 1996.
16. Campion EW: Home alone, and in danger (editorial), *N Engl J Med* 334:1738-1739, 1996.
17. Tamblyn RM, McLeod PJ, Abrahamowicz M, et al: Questionable prescribing for elderly patients in Quebec, *Can Med Assoc J* 150:1801-1809, 1994.
18. Thomson M, Smith WA: Prescribing benzodiazepines for noninstitutionalized elderly, *Can Fam Physician* 41:792-798, 1995.
19. Gurwitz JH, Avorn J: The ambiguous relation between aging and adverse drug reactions, *Ann Intern Med* 114:956-966, 1991.
20. Hogan DB, Campbell NRC, Crutcher R, et al: Prescription of nonsteroidal anti-inflammatory drugs for elderly people in Alberta, *Can Med Assoc J* 151:315-322, 1994.

21. Hogan DB: Revisiting the O complex: urinary incontinence, delirium and polypharmacy in elderly patients, *Can Med Assoc J* 157:1071-1077, 1997.

22. Tamblyn RM, McLeod PJ, Abrahamowicz M, et al: Do too many cooks spoil the broth? Multiple physician involvement in medical management of elderly patients and potentially inappropriate drug combinations, *Can Med Assoc J* 154:1177-1184, 1996.

23. Rochon PA, Gurwitz JH: Prescribing for seniors: neither too much nor too little, *JAMA* 282:113-115, 1999.

24. Graves T, Hanlon JT, Schmader KE, et al: Adverse events after discontinuing medications in elderly outpatients, *Arch Intern Med* 157:2205-2210, 1997.

25. Joukamaa M, Saarijarvi S, Salokangas RK: The TURVA project: retirement and adaptation in old age, *Ztschrft Gerontol* 26:170-175, 1993.

GYNECOLOGY

Topics covered in this section

Abortion
Amenorrhea
Cervix
Circumcision, Female
Contraception
Dysfunctional Uterine Bleeding
Dysmenorrhea
Ectopic Pregnancy
Endometrium
Endometriosis
Human Papillomavirus
Infertility, Female
Menopause
Ovaries
Pelvic Inflammatory Disease
Premenstrual Dysphoric Disorder
Sexual Dysfunction in Women
Vaginitis

ABORTION

(See also ectopic pregnancy; postcoital contraception)

Risk Factors

Cigarette smoking and cocaine use are both associated with an increased risk of spontaneous abortion.[1] In a case-controlled study measuring the caffeine metabolite paraxanthine, spontaneous abortion was increased in pregnant women who drank more than an estimated five to six cups of coffee a day; no increase in abortions occurred among moderate coffee drinkers.[2] Carriers of factor V Leiden also appear to be at increased risk of spontaneous abortion and fetal loss later in pregnancy, probably as a result of placental thrombosis.[3]

Mifepristone-Induced Abortion

Mifepristone, or RU 486, is an antiprogestin drug that has been used in many parts of the world for inducing abortion. Maximum efficacy is achieved if a prostaglandin such as misoprostol (Cytotec) is given po or intravaginally 48 hours after the administration of the mifepristone. In a 1998 multicenter U.S. study, 600 mg of mifepristone was given po followed 48 hours later by 400 μg of misoprostol po. Pregnancy termination was achieved in 92% of women with pregnancy durations of 49 days or less, 83% of those with pregnancy durations of 50 to 56 days, and 77% of those with pregnancy durations of 57 to 63 days.[4] A study from Rochester, New York, found that 200 mg of mifepristone po followed in 48 hours by 800 μg of intravaginal misoprostol was just as effective.[5] Mifepristone can also be used for postcoital contraception (see discussion of postcoital contraception). Misoprostol taken during pregnancy is associated with an increased incidence of Möbius' syndrome (congenital facial paralysis) in surviving infants.

Abortion Induced by Methotrexate plus Misoprostol

Methotrexate is known to be cytotoxic to trophoblast and is used in the treatment of trophoblastic neoplasms and ectopic pregnancies. In a New York study of 171 women, successful abortion was achieved in 86% with a single intramuscular dose of methotrexate 50 mg/m[2] followed in 5 to 7 days by the vaginal insertion of 800 μg of misoprostol. The 25 women who did not have an abortion with this protocol were given a second intravaginal dose of misoprostol; 18 aborted and 7 required suction curettage. Since misoprostol is not available in commercial form as vaginal suppositories, half the women were treated with four 200-μg suppositories made up by a pharmacist and the other half were treated with the intravaginal insertion of four 200-μg oral tablets held in place by a vaginal tampon.[6] An almost identical protocol at another center had equally good results; side effects were nausea (70%), diarrhea (46%), and vomiting (23%).[7]

Management of Spontaneous Abortion

Up to 20% of clinical pregnancies end in spontaneous abortion, and an estimated one fourth of women have at least one spontaneous abortion.[8] The standard treatment of incomplete abortion is dilatation and curettage. Randomized studies from Sweden and Britain suggest that in most cases this is unnecessary. Entrance requirements for these studies were that the patients be in good health, hemodynamically stable, and not anemic and that the estimated gestational age of the pregnancy be less than 13 weeks and the maximum anterior-posterior diameter of the retained products be 50 mm as determined by vaginal ultrasound. The randomly selected group of women who had no treatment were not different from those receiving curettage in terms of pain, duration of bleeding, time off work, and future fertility. In almost all cases pain and bleeding had stopped within 1 week.[8,9]

There is general agreement that D immune globulin or RH$_0$ (D) immune globulin (RhoGAM) should be given to Rh-negative women after elective abortions.[10-12] In Canada and the United States the recommended dose is 300 μg except for pregnancies before 13 weeks, in which 50 μg is sufficient.[10,11] Treatment should be given within 72 hours. Whether D immune globulin should be given for spontaneous abortions is uncertain (the Canadian Task Force gives it a "C" recommendation[11]). British guidelines recommend giving D immune globulin for any spontaneous abortion treated with instrumentation, any spontaneous abortion after 12 weeks, and any threatened abortion after 12 weeks.[12]

Grief and Depression After Abortion

Grief reactions among women who have had spontaneous abortions may be as intense as that which follows a neonatal death.[13-15] The male partners of women who abort may also have grief reactions.[16] Spontaneous abortion is a a risk factor for major depression, especially in women who are childless or who have a past history of depressive illness. In a case-controlled study the incidence of depression in the first 6 months after a spontaneous abortion was 11% compared with 4.3% among control subjects over the same period.[17]

Risk of Breast Cancer

Claims have been made that induced abortions are associated with an increased risk of breast cancer. This is almost certainly untrue (see discussion of breast cancer risk factors).

❧ REFERENCES ❧

1. Ness RB, Grisso JA, Hirschinger N, et al: Cocaine and tobacco use and the risk of spontaneous abortion, *N Engl J Med* 340:333-339, 1999.
2. Klebanoff MA, Levine RJ, DerSimonian R, et al: Maternal serum paraxanthine, a caffeine metabolite, and the risk of spontaneous abortion, *N Engl J Med* 341:1639-1644, 1999.
3. Meinardi JR, Middeldorp S, de Kam PJ, et al: Increased risk for fetal loss in carriers of the factor V Leiden mutation, *Ann Intern Med* 130:736-739, 1999.
4. Spitz IM, Bardin CW, Benton L, et al: Early pregnancy termination with mifepristone and misoprostol in the United States, *N Engl J Med* 338:1241-1247, 1998.
5. Schaff EA, Eisinger SH, Stadalius LS, et al: Low-dose mifepristone 200 mg and vaginal misoprostol for abortion, *Contraception* 59:1-6, 1999.
6. Hausknecht RU: Methotrexate and misoprostol to terminate early pregnancy, *N Engl J Med* 333:537-540, 1995.
7. Schaff EA, Eisinger SH, Franks P, et al: Combined methotrexate and misoprostol for early induced abortion, *Arch Fam Med* 4:774-779, 1995.
8. Chipchase J, James D: Randomised trial of expectant versus surgical management of spontaneous miscarriage, *Br J Obstet Gynaecol* 104:840-841, 1997.
9. Nielsen S, Hahlin M: Expectant management of first-trimester spontaneous abortion, *Lancet* 345:84-86, 1995.
10. US Preventive Services Task Force: *Guide to clinical preventive services,* ed 2, Baltimore, 1996, Williams & Wilkins, pp 425-432.
11. Canadian Task Force on the Periodic Health Examination: *Canadian guide to clinical preventive health care,* Ottawa, 1994, Canada Communication Group—Publishing, pp 116-124.
12. Howard HL, Martlew VJ, McFadyen IR, et al: Preventing rhesus D haemolytic disease of the newborn by giving anti-D immunoglobulin—are the guidelines being adequately followed? *Br J Obstet Gynaecol* 1045:37-41, 1997.
13. Cecil R, Leslie JC: Early miscarriage: preliminary results from a study in Northern Ireland, *J Reprod Infant Psychol* 15:347-352, 1993.
14. Lasker JN, Toedter LJ: Acute versus chronic grief: the case for pregnancy loss, *Am J Orthopsychiatry* 61:510-522, 1991.
15. Prettyman RJ, Cordle CJ, Cook GD: A three-month follow-up of psychological morbidity after early miscarriage, *Br J Med Psychol* 66:363-372, 1993.
16. Johnson MP, Puddifoot JE: The grief response in the partners of women who miscarry, *Br J Med Psychol* 69:313-327, 1996.
17. Neugebauer R, Kline J, Shrout P, et al: Major depressive disorder in the 6 months after miscarriage, *JAMA* 277:383-388, 1997.

AMENORRHEA

(See also anorexia nervosa; female athletes)

Amenorrhea is divided into primary and secondary forms.[1] Primary amenorrhea is rare and is defined as the absence of vaginal bleeding in a 14-year-old with no secondary sexual characteristics or in a 16-year-old with normal secondary sexual development. Primary amenorrhea in a woman with normal breast development but absence of pubic and axillary hair may be due to an androgen insensitivity syndrome (testicular feminization). Secondary amenorrhea is the absence of menstruation for 6 months in women who previously had normal periods or for 12 months in those who previously had oligomenorrhea. The overall prevalence rate of secondary amenorrhea is 1% to 3%, but the rate is 3% to 5% among college students, 5% to 60% among competitive athletes, and 19% to 44% among ballet dancers.[1]

The most common cause of secondary amenorrhea is pregnancy, and it must always be ruled out before any further investigations are undertaken. Home pregnancy tests have neither the sensitivity nor the specificity to be reliable for this purpose.[2] The following are other important causes of secondary amenorrhea[1,3]:

1. Hypothalamic dysfunction brought about by psychological stress
2. Anorexia nervosa
3. Strenuous exercise
4. Weight loss
5. Drugs such as oral contraceptives, antipsychotics, tricyclic antidepressants, and calcium channel blockers
6. Pituitary tumors, many of which are prolactinomas
7. Thyroid disorders
8. Hyperandrogenic disorders such as polycystic ovarian syndrome, adrenal hyperplasia, and Cushing's syndrome[1]

The essential elements in the initial evaluation of a patient with secondary amenorrhea are as follows[1,3]:

1. History. Drugs, exercise, weight loss, psychological stress, galactorrhea, thyroid disease, gynecological surgery, hot flashes, and androgenic symptoms such as hirsutism, acne, frontal balding, and lowering of the voice

2. Physical examination. Signs of thyroid disease, galactorrhea, androgen excess, or genital tract abnormalities

3. Laboratory investigations. Pregnancy test, thyroid-stimulating hormone, prolactin; if symptoms suggest that the patient is hypoestrogenic, follicle-stimulating hormone (FSH) and luteinizing hormone; testosterone measurement is not needed unless the patient shows clinical evidence of androgen excess

The normal maximum prolactin level is 20 ng/ml. If the level is elevated above 100 ng/ml (100 µg/L), a careful neurological examination and imaging of the sella turcica are indicated.[1]

The estrogen status of a nonpregnant amenorrheic woman may be evaluated by performing a progesterone challenge test.[1,3] The patient is given 10 mg of medroxyprogesterone acetate (Provera) orally for 5 days.[3] The test is positive if any vaginal bleeding occurs within 2 to 7 days of completion of the drug course. A failure to bleed indicates inadequate estrogen stimulation, an unresponsive endometrium, or outflow tract obstruction such as Asherman's syndrome (intrauterine adhesions).[1] In most young women who fail to bleed, the underlying disorder is hypothalamic amenorrhea caused by psychological stress, excessive exercise, or excessive weight loss. In this condition the FSH level is normal or low (with primary ovarian failure it would be high).[3]

If an amenorrheic woman is hypoestrogenic, she is at high risk for osteoporosis. If the amenorrhea persists for more than 6 months, she probably requires hormone replacement therapy. The potency of estrogen in the standard postmenopausal replacement dose of 0.625 mg of conjugated equine estrogen (Premarin) is only one fifth that in 30 to 50 µg of ethinyl estradiol, which is the estrogenic component of most low-dose birth control pills. A small prospective randomized controlled trial of amenorrheic young women found that over a 12-month period birth control pills containing 35 µg of ethinyl estradiol increased lumbar spine density and total body bone mineral compared with control subjects receiving placebo or medroxyprogesterone.[4]

─────────── ◤ **REFERENCES** ◢ ───────────

1. Kiningham RB, Apgar BS, Schwenk TL: Evaluation of amenorrhea, *Am Fam Physician* 53:1185-1194, 1996.

2. Bastian LA, Piscitelli JT: Is this patient pregnant? Can you reliably rule in or rule out early pregnancy by clinical examination? *JAMA* 278:586-589, 1997.

3. Davis A: A 21-year-old woman with menstrual irregularity, *JAMA* 277:1308-1314, 1997.

4. Hergenroeder AC, O'Brian Smith E, Shypailo R, et al: Bone mineral changes in young women with hypothalamic amenorrhea treated with oral contraceptives, medroxyprogesterone, or placebo over 12 months, *Am J Obstet Gynecol* 176:1017-1025, 1997.

CERVIX
Cervical Cancer and Cervical Cytology
(See also human papillomavirus; prevention; screening; sexually transmitted diseases)

Epidemiology

Risk factors for cervical cancer are early onset of sexual intercourse, multiple partners, a partner who has had multiple partners, HIV infection, and smoking. A number of varieties of human papillomavirus, such as types 16, 18, 31, 33, and 35, are associated with cervical intraepithelial neoplasia (CIN) II and III and invasive cancer, whereas other types such as 6 and 11 are associated with condylomata acuminata and not neoplasia (see discussion of human papillomavirus).[1]

Techniques of obtaining Papanicolaou smears

A systematic review of sampling devices used for obtaining cervical cytology smears concluded that extended tip spatulas are superior to the traditional Ayre's spatula for collecting endocervical cells and identifying abnormal squamous cells. The combined use of spatulas and Cytobrushes is an even better way of collecting endocervical cells, but data are insufficient to assess whether such combined sampling detects more premalignant conditions.[2]

Guidelines for cervical cytology screening

Randomized controlled trials demonstrating the effectiveness of cervical cytology screening have not been performed. However, a number of studies comparing cervical cancer mortality rates with screening rates point to decreased mortality as a result of screening.[3]

The U.S. Preventive Services Task Force gives an "A" recommendation to initiating Papanicolaou smears for all women who are or have been sexually active and a "B" recommendation to performing repeat examinations at least every 3 years. Women who have had a hysterectomy (including removal of the cervix) for benign disease do not need to be screened. The U.S. Preventive Task Force found insufficient evidence for recommending for or against an upper age limit of 65 for screening, although it accepted as reasonable discontinuing screening if the patient had had regular negative smears in the past.[4] The Canadian Task Force on Preventive Health Care gives a "B" recommendation to screening women every 3 years until the age of 69 if they are or have been sexually active. Women at high risk should probably be screened more frequently.[5]

If a patient has had a hysterectomy for cervical dysplasia or carcinoma in situ, she should have follow-up vaginal vault smears at regular intervals. If the hysterectomy was for benign disease, there is no need to perform routine pelvic examinations or vaginal Pap smears.[4,6] Despite the evidence that Pap smears in women who have had hysterectomies for benign disease are not beneficial, the 1995 guidelines of the American College of Obstetricians and Gynecologists recommend that they be obtained.[7]

Although current guidelines recommend that adolescent females begin having Pap smears when they become sexually active, reasons have been proposed for delaying this for a few years. The issue is discussed in the section on sexually transmitted diseases.

Classification of Papanicolaou smears

Several classifications for abnormal Pap smears have been developed. One of the common ones uses the terminology cervical intraepithelial neoplasia (CIN). CIN grade I is the equivalent of mild dysplasia, CIN grade II of moderate dysplasia, and CIN grade III of severe dysplasia or carcinoma in situ. The newer Bethesda System, which is achieving widespread use in the United States, has three categories: atypical squamous cells of undetermined significance (ASCUS); low-grade squamous intraepithelial lesions (LSIL), which is equivalent to CIN grade I; and high-grade squamous intraepithelial lesions (HSIL), which is equivalent to CIN grades II and III.[8]

Discrepancies often occur between the degree of cytological abnormalities reported and the underlying histological lesions. Between 17.5% and 40% of smear reports are said to underestimate the severity of the lesion.[9] Conversely, up to 75% of patients with smears reported as ASCUS are normal histologically, and in most cases these cytological abnormalities revert to normal spontaneously over the next few months.[8,10] When the Pap smear result is LSIL, two thirds to three fourths of the cases revert to normal spontaneously, most commonly because of regression of the underlying histological abnormalities. For these reasons follow-up cytological studies in 4 to 6 months, rather than immediate colposcopy, are recommended by many for low-grade abnormal cytology reports.[10]

Advancing technology in the identification of oncogenic HPV strains (hybrid capture HPV DNA assay) is opening the door for more selective management of patients with abnormal Pap smears. Women with ASCUS smears can be tested for HPV, and if oncogenic strains are detected, they should be referred for immediate colposcopy; if no oncogenic strains are found, they can receive regular follow-up Pap smears.[11]

Incidence of abnormal smears

The percentage of abnormal smears is generally reported as between 5% and 10%, and only about 5% of these show high-grade atypia.[12] It is generally agreed that less than 5% of smears classified by the Bethesda System should be reported as ASCUS,[10] but unfortunately in some centers up to 30% of smears are placed in this category.[8]

A study from Bristol, England, found that the rate of mild to moderate dyskaryosis (dysplasia) and borderline changes has increased markedly over the past decade while the rate of severe dyskaryosis has remained stable. In the latest screening round, 10% of young women were found to have some degree of abnormality and the rate of abnormalities for the entire population was 6.8%; 2.5% were referred for colposcopy. Although a true rise in CIN may account for the increased rate of abnormal smears, the authors believe that a more likely explanation is a tendency to overdiagnose cases to avoid litigation.[13]

Psychological consequences of abnormal Papanicolaou smears

Raffle and associates[13] state that the death rate for cervical cancer in Britain is about 10 per million women in their twenties and 40 per million women in their thirties. Since 10% of women were declared at risk on the basis of cytological findings, large numbers of women who would never have cancer were subject to persistent anxiety about cancer, the effect of treatment on their ability to bear children, and in some cases their ability to obtain life insurance.

Patients' responses to learning that they had abnormal smears have been documented by Posner and Vessey.[14] The women used such words as shocked, devastated, stunned, and petrified to describe their reactions.

Campion and associates[15] found that women had a statistically significant decrease in sexual functioning 6 months after they received a diagnosis of CIN compared with control subjects who did not have CIN. Specifically, they had decreased spontaneous interest in sex, decreased frequency of intercourse, less arousal, fewer orgasms, more dyspareunia, and more negative feelings about sex. The authors postulated that these reactions may be related to the widespread knowledge that CIN is an STD. Patients may be angry at their partners, fear that continued sexual intercourse could be harmful, or have a diminished sense of worth and body image. Posner and Vessey[16] reported that 43% of women referred to a colposcopy clinic experienced psychosexual disturbances as a result of the diagnosis, which were still present 6 to 9 months later in 14% of the women.

Informed consent for cervical smears

Because the benefits of cervical cytology accrue to few while many suffer the psychological and physical consequences of abnormal smears, ethical practice requires obtaining informed consent from any woman to whom screening is recommended. This is rarely done.[17,18]

Management of abnormal Papanicolaou smears

Experts generally agree that patients whose cervical cytological examination shows severe atypia (HSIL, CIN II or III, severe dysplasia or dyskaryosis, carcinoma in situ, or invasive carcinoma) require immediate colposcopic evaluation.[10] Management of lesser degrees of atypia (ASCUS or LSIL, mild dysplasia, CIN I, low-grade intraepithelial lesion) is more controversial. Since a high percentage of women with such reports subsequently have normal smears without any therapeutic intervention,[19] it is acceptable to manage cases of mild atypia without immediate colposcopy but with careful follow-up cytological smears.[10,19] The National Cancer Institute in the United States states that acceptable management of mild atypias is to repeat the Pap smear at 6-month intervals. If this results in three normal smears, the patient may revert to the normal screening interval. If any smear shows high-grade atypia, or if abnormalities persist for 24 months, the patient should be referred for colposcopy.[10]

Standard treatment methods for lesions detected by colposcopy are electrocautery, cryosurgery, and loop electrosurgical excision (LEEP). A randomized trial of these three modalities found no differences in cure rates (81% to 87%) or the adverse effects of infection, bleeding, and cervical stenosis (2% to 8%).[20]

Invasive cervical cancer

Very early "microinvasive" cancer is usually treated with hysterectomy or in some cases cone biopsy. For more extensive but potentially curable disease, radical hysterectomy and radiation therapy give equal results.[1] Sexual dysfunction is common after treatment of cervical cancer by surgery or radiation therapy; difficulties reported included inadequate lubrication, short vagina, inadequate vaginal elasticity, and dyspareunia.[21]

Inflammation found on Papanicolaou smears

A study from the University of Washington in Seattle correlated cytology reports of "dense inflammation," genital tract findings on examination, and cultures for *Neisseria gonorrhoeae, Chlamydia trachomatis,* herpes simplex virus, and *Trichomonas vaginalis.* Two cohorts were studied: women in an STD clinic and university students. Dense inflammation was found in 33% of the women attending the STD clinic and in 19% of the students. For the patients with STDs, half the smears showing dense inflammation were associated with *N. gonorrhoeae, C. trachomatis,* herpes simplex virus, or trichomoniasis, whereas in the student group only 10% were associated with positive cultures, which were almost always *C. trachomatis.* In both cohorts many women with dense inflammation had negative cultures but cervical ectopy on examination. Inflammation on the smears also correlated with cervical mucopus.[22]

I interpret these results to mean that a report of dense inflammation requires no specific action if the woman is in a low-risk group for STDs. If she is in a high-risk group, guidelines suggest that specimens should already have been cultured for STDs.[23,24] If not, she should be recalled so this can be done. If the cytopathologist's report suggests inflammation dense enough to obscure the epithelial cells and pre-

vent interpretation, the smear is unsatisfactory and should be repeated.

The presence of trichomonads may be noted in cytology reports. In asymptomatic women 20% to 30% of such findings represent false positives.[25]

❧ REFERENCES ❧

1. Cannistra SA, Niloff DIM: Cancer of the uterine cervix, *N Engl J Med* 334:1030-1038, 1996.
2. Martin-Hirsch P, Lilford R, Jarvis G, et al: Efficacy of cervical-smear collection devices: a systematic review and meta-analysis, *Lancet* 354:1763-1770, 1999.
3. Quinn M, Babb P, Jones J, et al (United Kingdom Association of Cancer Registries): Effect of screening on incidence of and mortality from cancer of cervix in England: evaluation based on routinely collected statistics, *BMJ* 318:904-908, 1999.
4. *Report of the U.S. Preventive Services Task Force: guide to clinical preventive services,* ed 2, Baltimore, 1996, Williams & Wilkins, pp 105-117.
5. Canadian Task Force on the Periodic Health Examination: *Canadian guide to clinical preventive health care,* Ottawa, 1994, Canada Communication Group—Publishing, pp 882-889.
6. Pearce KF, Haefner HK, Sarwar SF, et al: Cytopathological findings on vaginal Papanicolaou smears after hysterectomy for benign gynecologic disease, *N Engl J Med* 335:1559-1562, 1996.
7. *ACOG committee opinion: recommendations on frequency of Pap test screening,* no 152, Chicago, 1995, American College of Obstetricians and Gynecologists.
8. Zuber TJ: The minimally abnormal Pap smear: a conservative approach (editorial), *Am Fam Physician* 53:1042-1057, 1996.
9. Ferris DG: ASCUS and LSIL Pap smear results: triage considerations (editorial), *Am Fam Physician* 53:1057-1066, 1996.
10. Kurman RJ, Henson DE, Herbst AL, et al: Interim guidelines for management of abnormal cervical cytology: the 1992 National Cancer Institute Workshop, *JAMA* 271:1866-1869, 1994.
11. Apgar BS, Brotzman G: HPV testing in the evaluation of the minimally abnormal Papanicolaou smear, *Am Fam Physician* 59:2794-2800, 1999.
12. Nuovo GJ: *Cytopathology of the lower female genital tract: an integrated approach,* Baltimore, 1994, Williams & Wilkins.
13. Raffle AE, Alden B, Mackenzie EFD: Detection rates for abnormal cervical smears: what are we screening for? *Lancet* 345:1469-1473, 1995.
14. Posner T, Vessey M: *Prevention of cervical cancer: the patient's view,* London, 1988, King's Fund Publishing Office, pp 45-73.
15. Campion MJ, Brown JR, McCance DJ, et al: Psychosexual trauma of an abnormal cervical smear, *Br J Obstet Gynaecol* 95:175-181, 1988.
16. Posner T, Vessey M: Psychosexual trauma of an abnormal cervical smear (letter), *Br J Obstet Gynaecol* 95:729, 1988.
17. Raffle AE: Informed participation in screening is essential (letter), *BMJ* 314:1762-1763, 1997.
18. Foster P, Anderson CM: Reaching targets in the national cervical screening programme: are current practices unethical? *J Med Ethics* 24:151-157, 1998.

19. Nuovo J, Melnikow J, Paliescheskey M: Management of patients with atypical and low-grade Pap smear abnormalities, *Am Fam Physician* 52:2243-2250, 1995.

20. Mitchell MF, Tortolero-Luna G, Cook E, et al: A randomized clinical trial of cryotherapy, laser vaporization and loop electrosurgical excision for treatment of squamous intraepithelial lesions of the cervix, *Obstet Gynecol* 92:737-744, 1998.

21. Bergmark K, Avall-Lunqvist E, Dickman PW, et al: Vaginal changes and sexuality in women with a history of cervical cancer, *N Engl J Med* 340:1383-1389, 1999.

22. Eckert LO, Koutsky LA, Kiviat NB, et al: The inflammatory Papanicolaou smear—what does it mean? *Obstet Gynecol* 86:360-366, 1995.

23. Davies HD, Wang EE (Canadian Task Force on the Periodic Health Examination): Periodic health examination, 1996 update. 2. Screening for chlamydial infections, *Can Med Assoc J* 154:1631-1644, 1996.

24. US Preventive Services Task Force: *Guide to clinical preventive services,* ed 2, Baltimore, 1996, Williams & Wilkins Co, pp 325-334.

25. Weinberger MW, Harger JH: Accuracy of the Papanicolaou smear in the diagnosis of asymptomatic infection with *Trichomonas vaginalis, Obstet Gynecol* 82:425-429, 1993.

CIRCUMCISION, FEMALE

Female circumcision is practiced almost exclusively in Africa and among immigrants from Africa. Depending on the area, the prevalence rate varies from 5% to 99%. Female circumcision is practiced not only by those who espouse indigenous African religions, but also by Christians, Muslims, and Jews. It is a custom that involves all socioeconomic groups.[1]

Circumcision is usually performed by lay operators without the use of anesthesia on girls between the ages of 4 and 10. The procedure may involve removal of the clitoris alone ("Sunna circumcision") or the clitoris along with some of the labia minora, or it may include clitorectomy plus removal of the labia minora plus incisions on the labia majora that are stitched together for near-occlusion of the vaginal orifice (infibulation).[1]

REFERENCES

1. Toubia N: Female circumcision as a public health issue, *N Engl J Med* 331:712-716, 1994.

CONTRACEPTION

It is estimated that 41% of pregnancies are unplanned among women aged 35 to 39 and 51% among those aged 40 to 44.[1]

REFERENCES

1. Peterson HB: A 40-year-old woman considering contraception, *JAMA* 279:1651-1658, 1998.

Comparative Efficacy of Various Contraceptive Methods

Contraceptive efficacy can be calculated on the basis of theoretical effectiveness and real-use effectiveness. The typical pregnancy rate in 1 year when no contraception is used is 85%. This compares with typical-use first-year pregnancy rates of less than 5% for combined and progestin only oral contraceptives, about 2% for the progesterone T intrauterine device (IUD), and less than 1% for the copper T 380A IUD, levonorgestrel subdermal implants (Norplant), and medroxyprogesterone acetate (Depo-Provera) injections. Typical use of mechanical barrier methods is associated with first-year pregnancy rates of about 15% for the male condom and about 20% for the diaphragm, the cervical cap in nulliparous women (the rate is twice as high in parous women), and the female condom. Spermicides alone and periodic abstinence protocols have typical-use rates of around 25%. For some methods theoretical effectiveness is much better than are typical-use rates. For example, the theoretical effectiveness of the condom alone is 3%, and that of diaphragm plus spermicide is 6%. Figures given for efficacy are generally derived from studies of young women. The efficacy of all modes is better in older women, partly because of decreasing fertility and partly because of a lower frequency of intercourse.[1] In the United States contraceptive failure is very high in poor women and is higher in black and Hispanic women than in white women.[2]

REFERENCES

1. Peterson HB: A 40-year-old woman considering contraception, *JAMA* 279:1651-1658, 1998.

2. Fu H, Darroch JE, Haas T, et al: Contraceptive failure rates: new estimates from the 1995 National Survey of Family Growth, *Fam Plann Perspect* 31:56-63, 1999.

Natural Family Planning Methods

Calendar method

Women with fairly regular periods should keep a diary of their menstrual periods for several months. The beginning of the fertile period is determined by subtracting 20 days from the shortest cycle, and the end of the fertile period by subtracting 10 days from the longest cycle.[1]

Basal body temperature

A slight drop in temperature occurs at the time of ovulation.[2] Proof of ovulation is a subsequent persistent rise of at least 0.5° C (measured orally after at least 6 hours of sleep) that persists over 3 days. The infertile period begins 3 days after the temperature rise.[1]

Billings or ovulation method

Days on which a woman is considered infertile are during the menstrual period, the subsequent days when the vagina is dry, and the interval beginning 4 days after the onset of spinnbarkeit (see below) and lasting until the next menstrual period. The time of relative fertility is the days when vaginal secretions are wet and the first 4 days of spinnbarkeit. Spinnbarkeit is the phenomenon whereby the cervical mucus has become sufficiently sticky to allow it to be stretched out between thumb and fingers like an egg white. Samples of cervical mucus are obtained by placing the fingers in the lower vagina; touching the cervix is not necessary. Spinnbarkeit occurs 24 hours before the luteinizing hormone surge and 48 hours before ovulation.[2]

Symptothermal method

The symptothermal method combines the Billings method and basal body temperature measurements.[1,2]

─────────────── ▧ REFERENCES ▧ ───────────────

1. Rowe T, Boroditsky RS, Guilbert E, et al (Canadian Consensus Committee): The Canadian Consensus Conference on Contraception Part III, *J Soc Obstet Gynaecol Can* 20:667-692, 1998.
2. Geerling JH: Natural family planning, *Am Fam Physician* 52:1749-1756, 1995.

Barrier Contraceptives

(See also sexually transmitted diseases)

Condoms

Regular condom use decreases the transmission of all sexually transmitted diseases, including HIV. Aside from noncompliance, condom failures are usually due to breakage or slippage, and both of these events are more common among inexperienced users. Breakage is more likely if condoms are stored in a hot humid environment, exposed to light, or used with oil-based lubricants. The storage problem is particularly acute in developing countries.[1] Other specific causes of breakage are opening the condom package with a sharp object, such as a knife, scissors, pencil, or teeth, and unrolling the condom before application. Slippage is more common if the male withdraws after losing an erection or if the condom base is not held during withdrawal.[2] In one small survey of male college students in Georgia, slippage, breakage, or failure to use condoms throughout intercourse was reported in 13% of acts of vaginal intercourse. In a 1-month period one third of consistent condom users and their partners were potentially exposed to STD transmission or pregnancy.[3] Even more shocking was the finding of another study that one third of the men who experienced a condom breakage failed to inform their partners of this event.[4]

Diaphragms

The diaphragm may be inserted up to 6 hours before intercourse and should be left in place for 6 hours after intercourse. For repeated intercourse without removal of the diaphragm, contraceptive jelly should be placed in the vagina before each episode.

There have been reports that diaphragms are effective without use of a spermicide. In a nonrandomized trial of this method, 110 women were instructed to wear a "fit-free" (60-mm) diaphragm continuously, removing it only once a day for washing, but not within 6 hours of intercourse. The accidental pregnancy rate was 24.1% after 12 months.[5] In another study a diaphragm plus spermicide was compared

with a diaphragm alone. The pregnancy rates were lower with the diaphragm plus spermicide. Although the difference was not statistically significant, the authors point out this may have been because the study lacked sufficient power to prove a difference.[6]

The role of diaphragms in preventing STDs, especially HIV infection, is controversial. When compared directly with condoms, they are less effective, but evidence suggests that they provide some protection. Since their use is controlled by women, they may prevent more infections than condoms, which many men refuse to use.[1,7]

Female condoms

In an open study of the female condom as the only method of contraception for couples in monogamous relationships, the pregnancy rates after 6 months were 12.4% among U.S. users and 22.2% among Latin American users. The female condom would probably be an effective method of decreasing HIV transmission.[8]

─────────────── ▧ REFERENCES ▧ ───────────────

1. Faúndes A, Elias C, Coggins C: Spermicides and barrier contraception, *Curr Opin Obstet Gynecol* 6:552-558, 1994.
2. Spruyt A, Steiner MJ, Joanis C, et al: Identifying condom users at risk for breakage and slippage: findings from three international sites, *Am J Public Health* 88:239-244, 1998.
3. Warner L, Clay-Warner J, Boles J, et al: Assessing condom use practices: implications for evaluating method and user effectiveness, *Sex Transm Dis* 25:273-277, 1998.
4. Warner DL, Boles J, Goldsmith J: Disclosure of condom breakage to sexual partners (letter), *JAMA* 278:291-292, 1997.
5. Smith C, Farr G, Feldblum PJ, Spence A: Effectiveness of the non-spermicidal fit-free diaphragm, *Contraception* 51:289-291, 1995.
6. Bounds W, Guillebaud J, Dominik R, et al: The diaphragm with and without spermicide: a randomized, comparative efficacy trial, *J Reprod Med* 40:764-774, 1995.
7. Stein ZA: More on women and the prevention of HIV infection (editorial), *Am J Public Health* 85:1485-1488, 1995.
8. Farr G, Gabelnick H, Sturgen K, et al: Contraceptive efficacy and acceptability of the female condom, *Am J Public Health* 84:1960-1964, 1994.

Spermicidal Contraceptives

On the market are numerous spermicidal contraceptives, which come in the form of foams, creams, or gels applied with an applicator or of sponges or ovules inserted with a finger. The active agent in most is nonoxynol-9. In general, foams and creams should be inserted no more than an hour before intercourse, and if intercourse is to be repeated, further applications are required. Manufacturers of some of the newer products such as Advantage Gel claim that it can be applied up to 24 hours before intercourse, with further applications if intercourse is to be repeated. Sponges or ovules should be inserted at least 15 minutes before intercourse and should not be removed until 6 hours after intercourse. However, they should remain in place no longer than 12 hours because of the risk of toxic shock syndrome. Instructions for individual products should be followed. Although claims have been made that nonoxynol-9 may have some protective effect against HIV infection,[1] supporting evidence is tenuous at best.[2] Spermicides may predispose women to urinary tract infections (see discussion of urinary tract infections).

◼ REFERENCES ◼

1. Faúndes A, Elias C, Coggins C: Spermicides and barrier contraception, *Curr Opin Obstet Gynecol* 6:552-558, 1994.
2. Roddy RE, Zekeng L, Ryan KA, et al: A controlled trial of nonoxynol 9 film to reduce male-to-female transmission of sexually transmitted diseases, *N Engl J Med* 339:504-510, 1998.

Intrauterine Devices

Two major variants of intrauterine devices (IUDs) are the copper T 380A (ParaGard) and the progesterone T (Progestasert). The copper T 380A is effective for 10 years and the progesterone T for 1 year. The failure rate of the copper T is less than 1%, and it is as effective, if not more so, as tubal ligation. Although it has generally been taught that cultures for sexually transmitted disease should be obtained before inserting an IUD, this may not be necessary for all patients. IUDs may be inserted at any time during the menstrual cycle provided pregnancy is ruled out.[1]

The major complication of IUD insertion is sexually transmitted disease. This is rare in women who, along with their partners, have monogamous relationships. If pelvic inflammatory disease does supervene, it is usually within the 3 to 4 weeks after insertion.[1]

The copper IUD probably protects against pregnancy through its spermicidal properties; it does not function as an abortifacient.[1]

◼ REFERENCES ◼

1. Canavan TP: Appropriate use of the intrauterine device, *Am Fam Physician* 58:2077-2084, 1998.

Oral Contraceptives

(See also cerebrovascular accidents; dysfunctional uterine bleeding; migraines; thrombophlebitis)

Benefits

Aside from contraception, the use of oral contraceptive pills has a number of advantages. These include control of dysfunctional uterine bleeding and dysmenorrhea[1]; relief of hot flashes in perimenopausal women[2]; and reduced incidence of endometrial cancer,[1] ovarian cancer,[1] ectopic pregnancy,[3] iron deficiency anemia,[3] and possibly osteoporosis and endometriosis.[1]

Adverse effects

Mild adverse effects of oral contraceptives are well known and are not discussed here.

Cerebrovascular accidents. A number of studies in the 1960s and 1970s showed an increased incidence of ischemic strokes and subarachnoid hemorrhages in women who used oral contraceptives. This was particularly marked if the women were smokers and over the age of 35. Because of the concern about the cardiovascular complications of oral contraceptives during that era, both the FDA and the Health Protection Branch of Health and Welfare Canada recommended that oral contraceptive pills be stopped at the age of 35.

Only a few studies of the cardiovascular complications of oral contraceptives have been published since the advent of low-dose estrogen birth control pills. A pooled analysis of two U.S. case-control studies found no increased risk of ischemic or hemorrhagic stroke in women taking low-dose oral contraceptives even if they had additional risk factors such as smoking, obesity, hypertension, or being over the age of 35.[4] However, an increased risk of stroke in oral contraceptives users suffering from migraines has been reported.[4,5]

An evaluation of the risks of contraceptives should include the risks associated with pregnancy in the control group. For example, the annual mortality rates for oral contraceptive users aged 35 to 39 have been calculated as 4.5:100,000 for nonsmokers and 13.4:100,000 for smokers. In contrast the mortality rate for women in this age group using no contraceptive methods is 20.8:100,000 per year.[2] As a result of such evidence, official recommendations have changed in both Canada and the United States. Oral contraceptive use by nonsmoking women is now considered safe until the time of menopause. However, smokers should discontinue oral contraceptives at the age of 35 and substitute another form of contraception.

Venous thromboembolic events. Users of third-generation oral contraceptives containing desogestrel (Marvelon, Ortho-Cept) or gestodene (none marketed in North America) are at slightly increased risk of venous thromboembolic disease compared with users of second-generation oral contraceptives.[6,7] Death from thromboembolic events among oral contraceptive users is extremely rare; according to one estimate the risk is 5 per 1 million per year for non–pill users, 14 per million per year for users of second-generation products, and 20 per million per year for users of third-generation products.[8] O'Brien[6] suggests that third-generation products be reserved for women who have such problems as acne and who are willing to accept a very small increased risk of thrombosis to take a less androgenic oral contraceptive.

Women with thrombophilias are at increased risk of thromboembolic disease if they take oral contraceptives (see discussion of thrombophlebitis). Oral contraceptive users who are carriers of factor V Leiden have an eight times greater risk of thromboembolic events than noncarrier oral contraceptive users and a 30 times greater risk than women who are not taking oral contraceptives. However, the absolute risk is low—one event per 350 women per year.[9]

Whether women requesting oral contraceptives should be screened for thrombophilias is somewhat controversial. Protein C, protein S, and antithrombin II deficiencies are extremely rare, and most women who have these disorders give a family history of thromboembolic events; screening for these disorders is done by history.[9] About 5% of the white population are carriers of factor V Leiden, and most carriers do not have a family history of thromboembolic disorders.[9] Creinin and associates[10] argue that not only is screening for factor V Leiden not cost effective ($300 million in U.S. dollars to save one life) but such screening may be harmful. Only 0.1% of women who are carriers of factor V Leiden would have a thromboembolic event if they took oral contraceptives, so 99.9% would be deprived of the advantages of these drugs, which, aside from contraception, include a decreased incidence of dysmenorrhea, menorrhagia, iron deficiency anemia, endometrial carcinoma, and ovarian carcinoma. It is even possible that mortality would decrease in factor V Leiden carriers taking oral contraceptives because the decrease in ovarian cancer mortality might outweigh deaths caused by pulmonary embolism.[10] Palareti and associates[9] disagree; they believe that being a carrier is not a strict contraindication to the use of oral contraceptives and that knowledge of being a carrier allows women to make informed decisions not only about oral contraceptives, but also about other life events such as pregnancy or surgery. The cost of detecting one carrier is only $433. Palareti and associates recommend a once-in-a-lifetime screening for women requesting oral contraceptives.

Myocardial infarction. A 1998 comprehensive review of the literature concluded that the risk of myocardial infarction is higher in current oral contraceptive users who are smokers or have hypertension than in normotensive current users who are nonsmokers. Past oral contraceptive users are not at increased risk of myocardial infarction.[11]

Breast cancer. The risk of breast cancer is slightly increased among current pill users.[12,13] For example, a 1994 update of the Nurses' Health Study, which was begun in 1976, found no increase in breast cancer in women who had used oral contraceptives before 1976 but who were not using them at the beginning of the study; in contrast, women who were current users of the pill in 1976 had a 1.63 increase in the relative risk of dying of breast cancer within 12 years.[12] However, the overall total mortality and the total cancer mortality were not increased, in part because the ovarian cancer incidence was decreased. A 1996 systematic review of 54 case-controlled studies found that the odds ratio for development of breast cancer among current users of the pill was 1.24, whereas for women who had stopped the pill 1 to 4 years before it was 1.16. No increase in risk was found for women who had stopped the pill 10 years before.[13]

Carcinoma of the cervix. Women who take oral contraceptives have very small increased incidences of squamous cell carcinoma and adenocarcinoma of the cervix. Whether a causal relationship exists is not known.[14]

Total mortality. There is no increase in mortality in women who have ever used oral contraceptives compared with women who have not, nor is there evidence that prolonged use of oral contraceptives increases mortality.[12]

Contraindications to the use of oral contraceptives

A personal history of myocardial infarction, stroke, venous thromboembolism, or breast cancer is a contraindication to oral contraceptive use, as is smoking in the perimenopausal age range. A family history of cardiovascular disease or breast cancer is a relative, not an absolute, contraindication. Patients who have hypertension or become hypertensive when started on oral contraceptives should be advised to consider other forms of birth control. No evidence has shown that routine laboratory investigations have value before oral contraceptives are prescribed.[14]

Selection of product

Low-dose oral contraceptives containing estrogens and progestins are divided into three main classes: fixed dose products, phasic products, and "selective" progestins (third-generation oral contraceptives).

In theory, selective progestins and triphasics have fewer androgenic side effects. A number of the currently available oral contraceptives are listed in Table 27.

Table 27   Selected Oral Contraceptive Pills

Composition	Trade names
Fixed-Dose Products	
Norethindrone 0.5 mg plus ethinyl estradiol 35 μg	Brevicon 0.5/35, Ortho 10/11, Synphasic 0.5/35
Norethindrone 1 mg plus ethinyl estradiol 35 μg	Ortho 1/35, Synphasic 1/35
Levonorgestrel 100 μg plus ethinyl estradiol 20 μg	Alesse
Levonorgestrel 150 μg plus ethinyl estradiol 30 μg	Levlen, Min-Ovral, Nordette
Levonorgestrel 250 μg plus ethinyl estradiol 50 μg	Ovral
Norgestrel 300 μg plus ethinyl estradiol 30 μg	Lo/Ovral
Phasic Products	
Norethindrone in variable concentrations plus ethinyl estradiol 35 μg	Ortho 777
Levonorgestrel in variable concentrations plus ethinyl estradiol 32 μg	Tri-Levlen, Triphasil, Triquilar
Norethindrone 1 mg plus ethinyl estradiol in variable concentrations	Estrostep Fe
"Selective" Progestins (Monophasic and Triphasic)	
Norgestimate 0.25 mg plus ethinyl estradiol 35 μg	Cyclen
Norgestimate in variable levels plus ethinyl estradiol 35 μg	Tri-Cyclen
Desogestrel 0.15 mg and ethinyl estradiol 30 μg	Desogen, Marvelon, Ortho-Cept

No firm rules govern selection of a pill. All the low-estrogen pills are safe and effective. Patients with large, tender breasts or heavy bleeding and clots may benefit from a low-estrogen, full-progestin pill such as Ortho 1/35. Patients prone to acne, oily skin, hirsutism, and mood swings or premenstrual tension might benefit from selective progestin pills or triphasics.

Starting day

Different starting days may be used. Common ones are the first day of the cycle, the fifth day of the cycle, the first Sunday after the beginning of the cycle, or anytime during the first 6 days of the cycle. The last is acceptable for all products. If the starting day is after the fifth day of the cycle, contraceptive reliability is uncertain until seven daily consecutive tablets have been taken. For double assurance in this circumstance, an alternative form of contraception should be used during the first 7 days of taking the pill. Pills should be taken at the same time each day.

Missed pills

The protocol for missed pills varies with the number of pills missed and the time in the cycle when they were missed.

If one pill is missed at any time in the cycle, the missed pill should be taken as soon as it is remembered.

If two pills are missed during the first 2 weeks of the cycle, one should be taken as soon as it is remembered, as well as the regular pill for that day. The next day, two pills should be taken, one in the morning and one in the evening. Backup contraception should be used for the next 7 days.

If two pills are missed during the third week of the cycle and the patient is not on a Sunday start, she should begin a new package of pills immediately and use backup contraception for 7 days. If on a Sunday start, she should take one pill daily until the following Sunday, at which time another package should be started whether or not the menses has commenced. Backup contraception should be used until completion of the first 7 days of the new cycle.

If three or more pills are missed at any time in the cycle and the patient is not on a Sunday start, she should start a new package of pills immediately and use backup contraception for 7 days. If on a Sunday start, the patient should take one pill daily until the following Sunday, at which time another package should be started whether or not the menses has commenced. Backup contraception should be used until completion of the first 7 days of the new cycle.

Compliance

Compliance with taking oral contraceptives is poor. Only 50% to 75% of women who do not want to become pregnant and start the pill are still taking it after 1 year. In one survey almost half of all women on the pill missed one pill per cycle and nearly a quarter missed two or more pills per cycle.[15]

Antibiotics and oral contraceptives

No good evidence has been published that taking antibiotics decreases the efficacy of oral contraceptives.[16]

Discontinuing the pill in perimenopausal women

If a nonsmoking perimenopausal woman is taking an oral contraceptive pill on a regular basis, how does the physician know when menopause has occurred so that the birth control pill may be discontinued and hormone replacement therapy started (assuming the latter is clinically indicated)? Haney[17] suggests simply stopping oral contraceptives arbitrarily at age 51 or 52. If periods do not resume within 3 months, or if vasomotor symptoms develop, menopause has occurred and hormone replacement therapy may be started. If menses does recur, the physician can either wait for menopause to occur or restart oral contraceptives for another year. Steinberg[18] goes one step further and suggests simply stopping oral contraceptives at age 50 and switching to hormone replacement therapy immediately. Another alternative is to measure FSH levels at yearly intervals on the seventh day of a pill-free week. Levels of 30 to 40 U/ml or higher suggest menopause. This is not a sensitive method.[19]

REFERENCES

1. Peterson HB: A 40-year-old woman considering contraception, *JAMA* 279:1651-1658, 1998.
2. Reid R: Which contraceptive methods are suitable for the older women? *J SOGC* 15:933-944, 1993.
3. Peterson HB, Lee NC: The health effects of oral contraceptives: misperceptions, controversies and continuing good news, *Clin Obstet Gynecol* 32:339-355, 1989.
4. Schwartz SM, Pettitti DB, Siscovick DS, et al: Stroke and use of low-dose oral contraceptives in young women: a pooled analysis of two US studies, *Stroke* 29:2277-2284, 1998.
5. Chang CL, Donaghy M, Poulter N (World Health Organisation Collaborative Study of Cardiovascular Disease and Steroid Hormone Contraception): Migraine and stroke in young women: case-control study, *BMJ* 318:13-18, 1999.
6. O'Brien PA: The third generation oral contraceptive controversy: the evidence shows they are less safe than second generation pills (editorial), *BMJ* 319:795-796, 1999.
7. Walker AM: Newer oral contraceptives and the risk of venous thromboembolism, *Contraception* 57:169-181, 1998.
8. Spitzer WO, Lewis MA, Heinemann LA, et al (Transnational Research Group on Oral Contraceptives and the Health of Young Women): Third generation oral contraceptives and risk of venous thromboembolic disorders: an international case-control study, *BMJ* 312:83-88, 1996.
9. Palareti G, Legnani C, Frascaro M, et al: Screening for activated protein C resistance before oral contraceptive treatment: a pilot study, *Contraception* 59:293-299, 1999.
10. Creinin MD, Lisman R, Strickler RC: Screening for factor V Leiden mutation before prescribing combination oral contraceptives, *Fertil Steril* 72:646-651, 1999.
11. Petitti DB, Sidney S, Quesenberry CP: Oral contraceptive use and myocardial infarction, *Contraception* 57:143-155, 1998.

12. Colditz GA (Nurses' Health Study Research Group): Oral contraceptive use and mortality during 12 years of follow-up: the Nurses' Health Study, *Ann Intern Med* 120:821-826, 1994.

13. Collaborative Group on Hormonal Factors in Breast Cancer: Breast cancer and hormonal contraceptives: collaborative re-analysis of individual data on 53,297 women with and 100,239 women without breast cancer from 54 epidemiological studies, *Lancet* 347:1713-1727, 1996.

14. Hannaford PC, Webb AM (Participants at an International Workshop): Evidence-guided prescribing of combined oral contraceptives: consensus statement, *Contraception* 54:125-129, 1996.

15. Rosenberg MJ, Waugh MS, Burnhill MS: Compliance, counseling and satisfaction with oral contraceptives: a prospective evaluation, *Fam Plann Perspect* 30:89-92, 104, 1998.

16. Cerel-Suhl S, Yeager BF: Update on oral contraceptive pills, *Am Fam Physician* 60:2073-2084, 1999.

17. Haney AF: Hormonal needs of the perimenopausal woman, *J SOGC* 15:1-8, 1993.

18. Steinberg WM: Benefits of perimenopausal contraception: HRT when? *Patient Care Can* 7(6):8-10, 1996.

19. Creinin M: Laboratory criteria for menopause in women using oral contraceptives, *Fertil Steril* 66:101-104, 1996.

Emergency Contraception

The usual method of using the "morning after pill" is the Yuzpe regimen, consisting of 100 μg of ethinyl estradiol and 500 μg (0.5 mg) of levonorgestrel (two Ovral pills) repeated in 12 hours. Standard guidelines state that this must be started within 72 hours of intercourse; the failure rate is 2.5%.[1] This hormonal intervention is thought to prevent endometrial implantation.[2] Fifty percent of women have nausea, and 25% vomit[1]; an antiemetic, such as meclizine (Bonine, Bonamine) or dimenhydrinate (Dramamine, Gravol) should be prescribed, as well as extra Ovral pills in case the original ones are regurgitated.

Lower dose contraceptive pills containing 30 μg of ethinyl estradiol may also be used. A prescription of eight tablets containing the active ingredients (four initially and four in 12 hours) of any of the following brands is acceptable: Levlen, Levora, Lo/Ovral, Min-Ovral, Nordette, Tri-Levlen (yellow tablets only), Triphasil (yellow tablets only), Trivora (pink tablets only).[3] Alesse may also be used, but five tablets must be taken at each dose because each tablet contains only 20 μg of ethinyl estradiol.[3]

An emergency contraceptive kit called Preven was introduced in the United States in 1998 and in Canada in 1999. It contains a pregnancy test to rule out a preexisting pregnancy, as well as four tablets (two to be taken immediately and two in 12 hours), each of which contains 50 μg of ethinyl estradiol and 0.25 mg of levonorgestrel.[3]

An international multicenter randomized double-blind trial found that levonorgestrel given within 72 hours of intercourse as an oral dose of 0.75 mg and repeated once in 12 hours was slightly more effective than the Yuzpe regimen and caused less nausea.[4] Maximum efficacy was obtained when the drug was taken within 12 hours.[5] Levonorgestrel

0.75 mg is available in the United States under the trade name Plan B.

A review of nine published studies of the Yuzpe regimen found a high success rate that was unrelated to whether the pills were started immediately or 1, 2, or 3 days after intercourse. In view of this the authors suggest that the regimen might be effective even 4 or 5 days after intercourse.[2] However, randomized controlled studies have reported that although efficacy is good if the pills are taken within 3 days of intercourse, maximum protection occurs if they are taken within 24 hours.[4] An analysis of postcoital contraception among women using either levonorgestrel or the Yuzpe regimen found the pregnancy rate to be 0.5% when medications were begun within 12 hours of intercourse and 4.1% when they were taken 61 to 72 hours after intercourse.[5]

A practical difficulty with the Yuzpe regimen is that the pills are available only by prescription and this is not always easy to obtain when the need arises. A good case can be made for giving a supply of emergency pills to women who want to have them.[6]

Mifepristone (RU 486) as a single dose of 600 mg has been shown in Britain to be effective as an emergency contraceptive and to cause less nausea and vomiting than the Yuzpe regimen.[7] A 1999 trial compared 600-, 50-, and 10-mg doses of mifepristone and found all three to be equally effective.[8] Insertion of a copper IUD within 5 days of intercourse is also effective.[1]

───────── ❧ **REFERENCES** ❧ ─────────

1. After the morning after and the morning after that (editorial), *Lancet* 345:1381-1382, 1995.

2. Trussell J, Ellertson C, Rodriguez G: The Yuzpe regimen of emergency contraception: how long after the morning after? *Obstet Gynecol* 88:150-154, 1996.

3. An emergency contraceptive kit, *Med Lett* 40:102-103, 1998.

4. Task Force on Postovulatory Methods of Fertility Regulation: Randomised controlled trial of levonorgestrel versus the Yuzpe regimen of combined oral contraceptives for emergency contraception, *Lancet* 352:428-433, 1998.

5. Piaggio G, von Hertzen H, Grimes DA, et al: Timing of emergency contraception with levonorgestrel or the Yuzpe regimen, *Lancet* 353:721, 1999.

6. Glasier A, Baird D: The effects of self-administering emergency contraception, *N Engl J Med* 339:1-4, 1998.

7. Glasier A, Thong KJ, Dewar M, et al: Mifepristone (RU 486) compared with high-dose estrogen and progestogen for emergency postcoital contraception, *N Engl J Med* 327:1041-1044, 1992.

8. Task Force on Postovulatory Methods of Fertility Regulation: Comparison of three single doses of mifepristone as emergency contraception: a randomised trial, *Lancet* 353:697-702, 1999.

Progestin Only Contraceptives

Levonorgestrel implants

Levonorgestrel under the trade name Norplant is available for subcutaneous implantation.[1] The capsules are made of flexible Silastic and contain 36 mg of levonorgestrel. Contraception is achieved by the subcutaneous insertion of six capsules. The efficacy of this form of contraception is high and lasts for 5 years. The most common side effect is menstrual irregularities.[1,2]

Progestin only oral contraceptives

Progestin tablets containing 350 μg of norethindrone include Nor-QD and Micronor. This form of contraception is indicated when estrogen compounds may be contraindicated such as in smokers over the age of 35, breast-feeding women, and those with hypertension or breast cancer.[1]

Medroxyprogesterone Acetate Injections

Medroxyprogesterone acetate (Depo-Provera) for intramuscular use is available in the United States and Canada. The recommended dosage for contraception is 150 mg every 3 months injected deeply into the deltoid or gluteal muscle. Pregnancy must be ruled out, so the drug is often given only during the first 5 days of a normal menstrual period.

REFERENCES

1. Choice of contraceptives, *Med Lett* 37:9-12, 1995.
2. Baird DT, Glasier AF: Hormonal contraception, *N Engl J Med* 328:1543-1550, 1993.

Sterilization

(See also vasectomy; vasovasostomy)

Tubal sterilization

On a worldwide basis the most common form of contraception is tubal sterilization. The overall reported incidence of poststerilization regret is low but varies widely from one country to another and from one region to another within the same country.[1] A prospective cohort study in the United States found that 14 years after tubal sterilization regret was expressed by 20% of women who were 30 years of age or younger at the time of the procedure and 6% of women who were over 30 years of age at the time of the procedure. Among younger women the rate of regret did not plateau but continued to increase with time. Regret was not greater among women who were sterilized during the postpartum period than among those undergoing the procedure within 1 year after the birth of their last child.[2]

Most studies of the efficacy of tubal sterilization at the time of the puerperium have found that the pregnancy rate is slightly greater than in patients who have interval tubal sterilization.[1]

REFERENCES

1. Chi IC, Petta CA, McPheeters M: A review of safety, efficacy, pros and cons, and issues of puerperal tubal sterilization—an update, *Adv Contraception* 11:187-206, 1995.
2. Hillis SD, Marchbanks PA, Tylor LR, et al: Poststerilization regret: findings from the United States Collaborative Review of Sterilization, *Obstet Gynecol* 93:889-895, 1999.

DYSFUNCTIONAL UTERINE BLEEDING

(See also endometrial carcinoma; oral contraceptives)

Dysfunctional uterine bleeding is excessive menstrual bleeding in the absence of obvious other abnormalities.[1] It is common during the perimenopause (usually ages 40 to 50) and results in many surgical interventions. Hysterectomies are performed in 19% of North American women, and 40% of these are because of dysfunctional uterine bleeding.[2]

Dysfunctional uterine bleeding may be ovulatory or anovulatory; the cycle is regular if it is ovulatory and irregular if it is anovulatory. Aside from history and physical examination the only investigation required for women with this condition is a complete blood count to check for anemia. Although hypothyroidism is commonly said to be a cause of menorrhagia, little evidence supports this hypothesis. Bleeding disorders are an extremely rare cause of menorrhagia, and coagulation screens should be ordered only if indicated by the history. Endometrial sampling is unnecessary unless underlying organic disease is suspected (e.g., women over 40 with intermenstrual bleeding who have not responded to medical therapy).[1]

The traditional medical treatment of dysfunctional uterine bleeding has been the administration of progestins such as Provera 10 mg for 10 to 14 days every month or two. According to systematic reviews such treatment is ineffective.[1]

Oral contraceptive pills control menorrhagia.[1,2] For nonsmoking perimenopausal women a low-dose pill is effective and safe and may be used right up to the time of the menopause.[2] Methods of determining the advent of the menopause in perimenopausal women taking the pill are discussed in the earlier section on oral contraceptives. Alternatives to oral contraceptives are the antifibrinolytic agent tranexamic acid (Cyklokapron) in doses of 1000 to 1500 mg bid or tid or any nonsteroidal antiinflammatory drug (NSAID); these agents are given only during the period of menstruation. Tranexamic acid decreases menstrual blood loss by one half, and NSAIDs decrease it by one third. A levonorgestrel-releasing intrauterine system (Mirena), which is available in Great Britain, is also effective.[1]

When medical treatment of severe menorrhagia is unsuccessful, the standard surgical option has been hysterectomy. An alternative is hysteroscopic endometrial ablation. A 4-year follow-up study of women assigned at random to have either endometrial ablation or hysterectomy reported that 25% of those who had endometrial ablation required a subsequent hysterectomy for persistent dysfunctional uterine bleeding.[3]

Severe acute bleeding can be controlled by estrogens. A common regimen is three or four low-dose oral contraceptive tablets a day continued for about a week after the bleeding is controlled. When the medications are stopped, withdrawal bleeding occurs. Since many women become nauseated when taking this many oral contraceptives, antiemetics should be prescribed.[4]

☙ REFERENCES ❧

1. Prentice A: Medical management of menorrhagia, *BMJ* 319: 1343-1345, 1999.
2. Farrell SA: Contraception in the perimenopause, *J SOGC* 16(suppl):1-7, 1994.
3. Grant AM, Bhattacharya S, Mollison J, et al (Aberdeen Endometrial Ablation Trials Group): A randomised trial of endometrial ablation versus hysterectomy for the treatment of dysfunctional uterine bleeding: outcome at four years, *Br J Obstet Gynaecol* 106:360-366, 1999.
4. Chuong CJ, Brenner PF: Management of abnormal uterine bleeding, *Am J Obstet Gynecol* 175:787-792, 1996.

DYSMENORRHEA

Primary dysmenorrhea has a prevalence rate approaching 90%. Pain develops within hours of the onset of menstruation and peaks within the first 2 days. It is usually suprapubic in location but may radiate to the legs or lower back. Nausea, vomiting, diarrhea, and faintness may also occur. Dysmenorrhea usually develops within the first 3 years after the menarche, but rarely within the first 6 months. Full therapeutic doses of any of the NSAIDs is usually effective; if one drug does not work, another from a different class should be tried. Aspirin is rarely potent enough to control symptoms. Oral contraceptives are effective, but up to 3 months of use may be necessary before benefits are realized.[1]

☙ REFERENCES ❧

1. Coco AS: Primary dysmenorrhea, *Am Fam Physician* 60:489-496, 1999.

ECTOPIC PREGNANCY

(See also abortion; pelvic inflammatory disease; sexually transmitted diseases)

Women who douche are at increased risk of ectopic pregnancies, pelvic inflammatory disease, and bacterial vaginosis. Whether a causal relationship exists is undetermined, but since douching has no known benefits, the practice should be discouraged.[1]

A study from Boston City Hospital of women with ectopic pregnancies found that 9% had no pain and one third had no adnexal tenderness on examination.[2] Ectopic pregnancies do occur in women who have had previous tubal sterilization procedures, although this is rare.[3]

Use of abdominal ultrasound alone permits diagnosis of about 10% of ectopic pregnancies. Vaginal ultrasound finds about 25% of such cases. The diagnosis of ectopic pregnancy is facilitated by combining quantitative beta–human choriogonadotropin levels and abdominal or vaginal ultrasonography. With conventional abdominal ultrasonography the "discriminatory zone" (level at which a normal intrauterine pregnancy should be detected) is 6500 IU, whereas for vaginal ultrasound it is 2800 IU; 50% of normal intrauterine sacs can be detected at levels of 1000 IU.[4]

A single intramuscular dose of methotrexate proved to be a successful treatment for 86% of women with unruptured ectopic pregnancies that were 3.5 cm or less in maximum diameter as determined by transvaginal ultrasonography. The dose used was 50 mg/m^2.[5] An alternative approach that proved successful in 89% of ectopic pregnancies of 8 weeks' duration or less (regardless of size or the presence of fetal cardiac activity) was the injection of a single dose of 100 mg of methotrexate into the amniotic sac using an ultrasound-controlled transvaginal approach or, when this was unsuccessful, laparoscopy.[6]

☙ REFERENCES ❧

1. Merchant JS, Oh MK, Klerman LV: Douching: a problem for adolescent girls and young women, *Arch Pediatr Adolesc Med* 153:834-837, 1999.
2. Kaplan BC, Dart RG, Moskos M, et al: Ectopic pregnancy: prospective study with improved diagnostic accuracy, *Ann Emerg Med* 28:10-17, 1996.
3. Peterson HB, Xia Z, Hughes JM, et al (US Collaborative Review of Sterilization Working Group): The risk of ectopic pregnancy after tubal sterilization, *N Engl J Med* 336:762-767, 1997.
4. De Cherney AH: Case records of the Massachusetts General Hospital: Case 3-1996, *N Engl J Med* 334:255-260, 1996.
5. Glock JL, Johnson JV, Brumsted JR: Efficacy and safety of single-dose systemic methotrexate in the treatment of ectopic pregnancy, *Fertil Steril* 62:716-721, 1994.
6. Tzafettas JM, Stephanatos A, Loufopoulos A, et al: Single high dose of local methotrexate for the management of relatively advanced ectopic pregnancies, *Fertil Steril* 71:1010-1013, 1999.

ENDOMETRIUM

(See also dysfunctional uterine bleeding; oncology; sexual dysfunction in women; tamoxifen)

Endometrial Carcinoma

Endometrial carcinoma is primarily a disease of elderly women, although 25% of cases occur premenopausally and 5% of cases are reported in women under the age of 40. Major risk factors are obesity, diabetes, and unopposed estrogen therapy. Some increased risk is also associated with tamoxifen therapy, nulliparity, and menopause occurring after the age of 52. Smoking and taking combined oral contraceptives decrease the risk. Smoking probably accomplishes this feat by inactivating estrogen.[1,2] The four main stages of endometrial carcinoma are as follows[1]:

Stage I	Limited to endometrium or myometrium
Stage II	Spread to cervix
Stage III	Spread to serosa, peritoneum, regional lymph nodes, or pelvic organs
Stage IV	Distant metastases or invasion of bladder or rectal mucosa

The prognosis varies with the stage. The 5-year survival is 72% for stage I (almost 100% for stage IA, which is carcinoma limited to the endometrium), 56% for stage II, 32% for stage III, and 11% for stage IV. Most cases are stage I.

One of the major reasons for investigating postmenopausal bleeding is to rule out endometrial cancer. Office-based endometrial biopsies and endovaginal ultrasound that measures endometrial thickness are now the primary modalities for doing this. The sensitivity of endovaginal ultrasound for detecting endometrial abnormalities is as good as that reported for endometrial biopsies. The probability of endometrial cancer in a postmenopausal woman with vaginal bleeding who is not receiving hormone replacement therapy and who has a negative ultrasound is 1%, whereas if she is on hormone replacement therapy it is only 0.1%. The false-positive rate of endovaginal ultrasound is relatively high, especially among patients on hormone replacement therapy (23%). For women not taking hormones it is 8%.[3]

REFERENCES

1. Von Gruenigen VE, Karlen JR: Carcinoma of the endometrium, *Am Fam Physician* 51:1531-1536, 1995.
2. Rose P: Endometrial carcinoma, *N Engl J Med* 335:640-649, 1996.
3. Smith-Bindman R, Kerlikowske K, Feldstein VA, et al: Endovaginal ultrasound to exclude endometrial cancer and other endometrial abnormalities, *JAMA* 280:1510-1517, 1998.

ENDOMETRIOSIS

Major symptoms of endometriosis are pelvic pain, dysmenorrhea, dyspareunia, backache, and infertility. However, 30% of women with endometriosis have no pain. Adamson[1] advises treating all women with dysmenorrhea with NSAIDs and oral contraceptives and, if relief is not obtained within 3 to 6 months, proceeding to laparoscopy. The definitive diagnosis of endometriosis is established by biopsy.[1] At the time of initial laparoscopy all visible endometrial lesions should be ablated to decrease pain[1] and increase fertility.[1,2]

Medications used to control the pain of endometriosis include gonadotropin-releasing hormones such as leuprolide acetate (Lupron), oral contraceptives, danazol (Danocrine, Cyclomen), and medroxyprogesterone (Provera). None of these agents increases fertility. A frequently used agent is leuprolide 3.75 mg intramuscularly once a month for 3 to 6 months (3 months is probably as effective as 6 months), but many women have difficulty tolerating the adverse effects, such as hot flashes, decreased libido, and vaginal dryness. Symptoms commonly recur 6 to 18 months after the completion of treatment, and therefore multiple treatment courses may be necessary.[1]

Laparoscopic confirmation of the diagnosis of endometriosis may not be required before initiating therapy. In one study women were selected who had had moderate to severe pelvic pain for at least 6 months that was unrelated to menstruation and that was incompletely relieved by NSAIDs. Women with evidence of pelvic inflammatory disease or substance abuse were excluded. Patients were assigned randomly to receive depot leuprolide (Lupron) or placebo over a 3-month period. Pain relief was significantly greater in those receiving leuprolide. At the termination of the trial laparoscopy was performed on all patients, and in the vast majority the clinical diagnosis of endometriosis was confirmed.[3]

REFERENCES

1. Adamson GD: A 36-year-old woman with endometriosis, pelvic pain, and infertility, *JAMA* 282:2347-2354, 1999.
2. Marcoux S, Maheux R, Bérubé S (Canadian Collaborative Group on Endometriosis): Laparoscopic surgery in infertile women with minimal or mild endometriosis, *N Engl J Med* 337:217-222, 1997.
3. Ling FW (Pelvic Pain Study Group): Randomized controlled trial of depot leuprolide in patients with chronic pelvic pain and clinically suspected endometriosis, *Obstet Gynecol* 93:51-58, 1999.

HUMAN PAPILLOMAVIRUS
(See also cervical cancer)

Human papillomavirus can be found in close to 50% of normal cervixes in sexually active women when highly sensitive techniques such as the polymerase chain reaction are used.[1]

About 60 subtypes of human papillomavirus have been identified. Subtypes 6 and 11 and most of the 40s group are associated with anogenital warts of condylomata acuminata, and with the possible exception of the rare nonmetastasizing verrucous carcinomas of the genital tract these are nononcogenic.[2,3] Condylomata acuminata, especially those involving the vagina and cervix, are often not visible clinically and can be detected only by enhancing techniques such as the application of acetic acid. There are few clinical indications for doing this because the treatment of subclinical lesions has not been shown to prevent the spread of infection.[3] Women with condylomata acuminata are not at increased risk for cervical intraepithelial neoplasia.[2]

Human papillomavirus subtypes 16 and 18 and some of the 30s, 50s, and 60s groups are associated with intraepithelial neoplasia and are thought to be oncogenic and responsible for many cases of cervical cancer, as well as some anal, vulvar, and vaginal cancers.[4,5] There is no evidence that identifying these strains and instituting some form of treatment will alter morbidity or mortality.[4]

The Canadian Task Force on Preventive Health Care has evaluated screening for human papillomavirus and concluded that it should not be done ("D" recommendation).[4] The U.S. Preventive Services Task Force gives screening for human papillomavirus a "C" rating but adds that "recommendations against such screening can be made on other grounds, including poor specificity and costs."[6]

A number of treatment modalities are available for anogenital warts. One of the newer ones is the application three times a week of 5% imiquimod (Aldara) cream. Resolution of the lesions takes 1 to 3 months. Imiquimod is an immunomodulator.[3] Another agent that can be used is podofilox

(Condylox), which is available as a 0.5% topical solution or gel that is applied to the lesions bid.[7]

REFERENCES

1. Bauer HM, Ting Y, Greer CE, et al: Genital human papillomavirus infection in female university students as determined by a PCR-based method, *JAMA* 265:472-477, 1991.
2. Evans BA, Bond RA, MacRae KD: A colposcopic case-control study of cervical squamous intraepithelial lesions in women with anogenital warts, *Genitourinary Med* 68:300-304, 1992.
3. Baker GE, Tyring SK: Therapeutic approaches to papillomavirus infections, *Dermatol Clin* 15:331-340, 1997.
4. Johnson K (Canadian Task Force on the Periodic Health Examination): Periodic health examination, 1995 update. 1. Screening for human papillomavirus infection in asymptomatic women, *Can Med Assoc J* 152:483-493, 1995.
5. Frisch M, Glimelius B, van den Brule AJ, et al: Sexually transmitted infection as a cause of anal cancer, *N Engl J Med* 337:1350-1358, 1997.
6. US Preventive Services Task Force: *Guide to clinical preventive services,* ed 2, Baltimore, 1996, Williams & Wilkins, pp 105-117.
7. Tyring S, Edwards L, Cherry LK, et al: Safety and efficacy of 0.5% podofilox gel in the treatment of anogenital warts, *Arch Dermatol* 134:33-38, 1998.

INFERTILITY, FEMALE

(See also appendicitis; infertility, male; pelvic inflammatory disease; sexually transmitted diseases)

One definition of infertility is the inability to conceive after 1 year of adequately timed unprotected intercourse.[1] According to this definition, the incidence in developed countries is 10% to 15%.[2] A major problem with this definition is that it is inaccurate. For women around the age of 30 who have not conceived after 1 year the chances of conception over the next 12 months is about 40%.[1] Although early referral to a center specializing in infertility is probably advisable for woman who are 35 years of age or older and have been trying to become pregnant for 1 year, as well as for those with a history of pelvic inflammatory disease, amenorrhea, or oligomenorrhea, or whose partners have azoospermia, referral for most other cases is appropriate only 3 years or more after stopping contraception.[3]

A study of the timing of intercourse and pregnancy among 221 healthy women (no fertility problems) from North Carolina who wanted to become pregnant found that pregnancy occurred only if intercourse took place during a 6-day period that ended at the time of ovulation. Intercourse on the day of ovulation resulted in pregnancy in one third of cases, whereas intercourse 6 days before ovulation led to pregnancy in only 8% of cases. No evidence was found that timing intercourse in relation to ovulation affected the sex of the baby or the survival of the pregnancy or that frequent intercourse decreased fertility (even though closely spaced ejaculations have been shown to decrease motile sperm counts).[4] Although the data might suggest that infertile

couples should attempt to time intercourse to the ideal periods of the menstrual cycle, there is no evidence that this improves the chance of conception and it certainly increases psychic stress.[3]

Potentially reversible causes of decreased fecundity are smoking[5] and drinking alcohol.[6,7] Even five or fewer drinks per week, especially if taken around the time of ovulation, decrease fertility in women, but not in men.[6] In healthy women, abstention from alcohol during one menstrual cycle doubled the chances of conception.[7]

The basic workup for infertility includes a thorough history and careful physical examination of both partners. Some investigations that may be appropriate in the family practice setting are a complete blood count, thryoid-stimulating hormone measurement, prolactin measurement and basal body temperature charts for three cycles for women,[2] semen analysis for men (see discussion of male infertility),[2,3] and screening both partners for *Chlamydia.*[3]

A number of options are available for the management of infertility. For many couples the first-line approach is the induction of superovulation with a mild stimulation protocol that minimizes the risk of multiple pregnancies, coupled with intrauterine insemination. If the problem is known to be male subfertility, intrauterine insemination is all that is required.[1]

In vitro fertilization is another option. It is expensive, time consuming, uncomfortable, painful, and psychologically traumatic.[8] The overall success rate may reach 50% if the procedure is undertaken for three cycles.[3] When infertility is related to sperm dysfunction in the male, intracytoplasmic sperm injection of the ovum is used in many centers (see discussion of male infertility).

REFERENCES

1. Te Velde ER, Cohlen BJ: The management of infertility (editorial), *N Engl J Med* 340:224-226, 1999.
2. Trantham P: The infertile couple, *Am Fam Physician* 54:1001-1010, 1996.
3. Hargreave TB, Mills JA: Investigating and managing infertility in general practice, *BMJ* 316:1438-1441, 1998.
4. Wilcox AJ, Weinberg CR, Baird DD: Timing of sexual intercourse in relation to ovulation: effects on the probability of conception, survival of the pregnancy, and sex of the baby, *N Engl J Med* 333:1517-1521, 1995.
5. Bolumar F, Olsen J, Boldsen J (European Study Group on Infertility and Subfecundity): Smoking reduces fecundity: a European multicenter study on infertility and subfecundity, *Am J Epidemiol* 143:578-587, 1996.
6. Jensen TK, Hjollund NH, Henriksen TB, et al: Does moderate alcohol consumption affect fertility? Follow up study among couples planning first pregnancy, *BMJ* 317:505-510, 1998.
7. Hakim RB, Gray RH, Zacur H: Alcohol and caffeine consumption and decreased fertility, *Fertil Steril* 70:632-637, 1998.
8. McCall M: Pursuing conception: a physician's experience with in-vitro fertilization, *Can Med Assoc J* 154:1075-1079, 1996.

MENOPAUSE

(See also dysfunctional uterine bleeding; endometrial carcinoma; exercise; oral contraceptives; osteoporosis; sexual dysfunction in women)

In the later years of a woman's reproductive life the frequency of cyclical ovulation declines and the frequency of anovulatory cycles increases. This phenomenon is sometimes called the climacteric and occurs during the perimenopause, which usually covers the fifth decade of a woman's life.[1]

One of the major issues concerning menopause in the 1990s has been hormone replacement therapy. This is dealt with in several sections below. Although hormone replacement therapy has a number of proven or putative benefits, physicians should be aware that the widespread enthusiasm for its use has trivialized, or at least deemphasized, life-style methods of disease prevention such as exercise and discontinuation of smoking in postmenopausal women. From the evidence available, exercise and stopping smoking may save more lives than hormone replacement therapy; this is discussed in more detail below in the section "Life-Style Changes for Disease Prevention in Menopausal Women." The investigation of postmenopausal bleeding is discussed in the section on endometrial carcinoma.

---------------------- ◣ REFERENCES ◢ ----------------------

1. Haney AF: Hormonal needs of the perimenopausal woman, *J SOGC* 15:1-8, 1993.

Benefits of Hormone Replacement Therapy

(See also adverse effects of hormone replacement therapy; consensus conferences; informed consent; osteoporosis; sleep disturbances; statistics; urinary tract infections)

The major reasons for prescribing hormone replacement therapy are to prevent or control vasomotor symptoms and genital atrophy and to decrease long-term morbidity from cardiovascular disease and osteoporosis. Additional benefits may be a decrease in sleep disturbances, mood disorders, strokes, tooth loss, colon cancer, and cognitive decline and an improvement in libido.

Control of vasomotor symptoms

One of the initial symptoms of estrogen deficiency is hot flashes or vasomotor symptoms. These occur in 75% of postmenopausal women and persist for longer than 5 years in 25% of them. In a few women the symptoms are lifelong. Only about 30% of women seek medical help for these symptoms.[1] Women who smoke or whose mothers suffered from hot flashes are at increased risk of having hot flashes.[2] The standard treatment for hot flashes is estrogen replacement therapy; the choice of regimens is discussed below. Such therapy is effective, resulting in an 85% reduction in vasomotor hot flashes. The beneficial effect may not be noted in the first 2 to 3 weeks, but the effect may persist for weeks after the estrogen is discontinued.[3]

If women are unable to take estrogens, hot flashes may sometimes be controlled by megestrol acetate (Megace) 20 mg bid[4] or by clonidine (Catapres, Dixarit) 0.025 mg, 2 tablets bid.[5]

Control of vulvar and vaginal atrophy

Aside from hot flashes, a common problem of postmenopausal women is vulvar and vaginal atrophy, which often manifests itself subjectively as a feeling of vaginal dryness, vulvar itch, decreased lubrication during sexual arousal, and dyspareunia. In addition, atrophy of the urethra and base of the bladder may lead to urinary urgency and frequency and perhaps even to urethral stenosis. These symptoms are caused by estrogen deficiency and are usually relieved by estrogen hormonal replacement therapy.[1,6] If a woman already receiving estrogen replacement therapy still experiences vaginal dryness, she may use a topical estrogen cream such as vaginal Premarin cream 2 to 4 g intravaginally or applied to the vulva as necessary. Since Premarin cream is absorbed systemically, she should not use oral or transdermal estrogens on the days she uses the estrogen cream.

Control of sleep disturbances

Hot flashes may cause sleep disturbances. A randomized placebo-controlled trial found that hormone replacement therapy significantly diminished sleep disturbances in postmenopausal women.[7]

Control of dysphoria

Whether dysphoria is a true menopausal symptom and whether estrogen treatment improves either the mood or the quality of life is unclear. A 1996 review of 46 primary research papers on the relationship of menopause to depression found little evidence supporting the menopause as a cause of depression.[8]

Control of decreased libido

A number of reports have suggested that androgen plus estrogen replacement therapy is effective for women with decreased libido.[6] In Canada, replacement androgen is available only as an injectable testosterone-estradiol combination, Climacteron, which is given as 1 ml intramuscularly every 4 to 8 weeks.

Prevention of coronary artery disease

If lives are to be saved by hormone replacement therapy, the major reason will be a decreased incidence of coronary artery disease. This is because the cumulative risk of death for women between the ages of 50 to 94 is 31% from coronary artery disease and only 3% each from breast cancer and hip fractures.[9] These figures are somewhat deceptive because for U.S. women under the age of 70 the cancer mortality rates exceed the cardiovascular mortality rates. In other words, most of the cardioprotective effects of hormone replacement therapy are manifested in the elderly and most women who die of cancer will lose more years of life than women who die of coronary artery disease.[10]

Many observational studies have shown a decreased relative risk of cardiovascular disease of about 40% to 50% in women who have used, or are using, estrogens. In the Nurses' Health Study current estrogen users had coronary disease rates about half those of never users, while women who had previously taken estrogens but were no longer doing so had only a slight benefit compared with never users.[11,12] The 40% to 50% reduction in coronary artery disease quoted above represents a relative reduction. When expressed in terms of numbers of women who need to take estrogens for 1 year to prevent one coronary event, the figures are less impressive. According to data reported by Grodstein and associates,[11] the figures vary from about 1500 to 2700 depending on the age of the women. Along the same lines, a Finnish study reported a significant decrease in sudden cardiac death (but not cardiovascular morbidity) in women taking estrogen replacement therapy compared with never users or former users. Approximately 1500 women had to be treated for 1 year to prevent one death.[13]

While most studies have evaluated doses of conjugated estrogens (Premarin) of 0.625 mg/day, data from the Nurses' Health Study suggest that 0.3 mg may be equally effective in preventing coronary artery disease.[11]

Unfortunately, two caveats cast doubt on the long-term benefits of hormone replacement therapy. The first problem is that although a clear association exists between prolonged hormone replacement therapy and decreases in cardiovascular disease and total mortality, this does not prove that hormone replacement therapy is responsible for the decreased risk. The benefit noted in epidemiological studies may be due to selection bias: women who follow healthy life-styles are more likely to use hormone replacement therapy, and therefore all or much of the observed benefit may come from life-style activities rather than the hormones (healthy user effect).[14-16] For example, a Swedish prospective population study found that women who later chose hormone replacement therapy were less obese, had lower blood pressures, and came from a higher social class than women who did not choose hormone replacement therapy.[14]

Further evidence that hormone replacement therapy may not prevent coronary artery disease comes from the Heart and Estrogen/Progestin Replacement Study (HERS), in which 2763 postmenopausal women with known coronary artery disease were randomly divided into groups receiving conjugated equine estrogens (Premarin) plus medroxyprogesterone (Provera) or placebo. At follow-up averaging 4.1 years the two groups showed no difference in cardiovascular events, although the treated group had significant lowering of low-density lipoprotein (LDL) cholesterol and elevation of high-density lipoprotein (HDL) cholesterol. The treated group also had an increased incidence of venous thromboembolic disease and gallbladder disease.[17]

The other problem is that in the Nurses' Health Study mortality benefits from the prevention of cardiovascular disease were shown to be attenuated after 10 years of hormone use, primarily because of an increased mortality from breast cancer (see discussion of adverse effects of hormone replacement therapy). The overall benefit of hormone replacement therapy was most marked for women with risk factors for coronary artery disease and was least for those with no risk factors.[12] Thus it might be wise to consider individual risk factors when recommending hormone replacement therapy and to limit the period for which it is prescribed.[18]

There was concern in the past that the addition of progestogens to estrogens in hormone replacement therapy would attenuate the beneficial effects of the estrogens. This has proved not to be the case,[11,12] but of some concern is a 2000 report that progestins may increase the risk of breast cancer to a greater extent than is associated with estrogens alone.[19] The cardioprotective effects of the transdermal estrogen patches have not yet been proved; very large doses are necessary to lower LDL cholesterol.[1]

The mechanisms by which estrogens exert beneficial effects on vascular disease have not been fully worked out. The effect has long been thought to be secondary to improvements in lipid profiles, but an alternative or complementary explanation is that estrogens increase fibrinolytic activity.[20] The Postmenopausal Estrogen/Progestin Interventions (PEPI) Trial measured various surrogate outcomes in women taking combined estrogen-progestin products. HDL levels were increased, and LDL and fibrinogen levels were decreased. Little effect was seen on blood pressure or insulin measurements.[21]

Prevention of strokes

Conflicting reports have been published on the effects of hormone replacement therapy on strokes. Some studies have shown a decreased incidence,[22,23] whereas others have not found a significant effect.[10]

Prevention of osteoporosis and fractures

Good evidence demonstrates that estrogens decrease the rate of development of osteoporosis. In a Swedish study, use of these agents in daily doses of 0.625 mg (but not 0.3 mg) of Premarin or the equivalent was associated with a decreased hip fracture rate provided that the patients were current users and had been taking the drugs for several years. This beneficial effect occurred in women who started hormone replacement therapy several years after menopause, as well as those who began at the time of menopause. How much of this apparent benefit was due to the "healthy user effect" described previously is unknown.[24]

Since the death rate from breast cancer is significantly increased after 10 years of hormone replacement therapy (see discussion of adverse effects of hormone replacement therapy), other modalities for the primary prevention of osteoporosis such as exercise, avoidance of smoking and excessive alcohol intake, and calcium and vitamin D supplementation should be emphasized.[25] Secondary prevention rather than primary prevention might be considered for some individuals; elderly women who have sustained osteoporotic fractures can be effectively treated with alendronate (Fosamax).[26] The role of these interventions is discussed in more detail under "Osteoporosis."

Prevention of tooth loss

Hormone replacement therapy may help to prevent tooth loss and the need for dentures, presumably by decreasing the degree of osteoporosis in the alveolar bone of the jaw.[27]

Preservation of cognitive functioning

Possible but as yet unproven benefits of estrogen replacement therapy are improved cognitive functioning in nondemented women, prevention of Alzheimer's disease, and improved functioning of women who have Alzheimer's disease. Although a metaanalysis of 10 observational studies on the role of estrogens in preventing Alzheimer's disease found the intervention to be beneficial, the authors point out that many of the assessed trials had substantial methodological problems, so little weight can be given to these results. Trials showing benefits for women with Alzheimer's disease also had significant methodological problems, including small sample sizes, short follow-up periods, and inclusion of individuals with varying degrees of severity of dementia.[28] A prospective study of 9651 elderly white women failed to find evidence that hormone replacement therapy prevented cognitive decline, whereas high levels of formal education were associated with preserved mental functioning.[29] At present the evidence is insufficient to conclude that estrogens delay memory loss or the onset of dementia.[30]

Diminished risk of colon cancer

Epidemiological studies have reported a decreased incidence of colon cancer in women taking hormone replacement therapy.[31]

--- **REFERENCES** ---

1. Belchetz PE: Hormonal treatment of postmenopausal women, *N Engl J Med* 330:1062-1071, 1994.
2. Staropoli CA, Flaws JA, Bush TL, et al: Predictors of menopausal hot flashes, *J Women's Health* 7:1149-1155, 1998.
3. Haas S, Walsh B, Evans S, et al: The effect of transdermal estradiol on hormone and metabolic dynamics over a six-week period, *Obstet Gynecol* 71:671-676, 1988.
4. Loprinzi CL, Michalak JC, Quella SK, et al: Megestrol acetate for the prevention of hot flashes, *N Engl J Med* 331:347-352, 1994.
5. Goldberg RM, Loprinzi CL, O'Fallon JR, et al: Transdermal clonidine for ameliorating tamoxifen-induced hot flashes, *J Clin Oncol* 12:155-158, 1994.
6. Walling M, Andersen BL, Johnson SR: Hormonal replacement therapy for postmenopausal women: a review of sexual outcomes and related gynecologic effects, *Arch Sex Behav* 19: 119-137, 1990.
7. Polo-Kantola P, Erkkola R, Helenius H, et al: When does estrogen replacement therapy improve sleep quality? *Am J Obstet Gynecol* 178:1002-1009, 1998.
8. Nicol-Smith L: Causality, menopause, and depression: a critical review of the literature, *BMJ* 313:1229-1232, 1996.
9. Cummings SR, Black DM, Rubin SM, et al: Lifetime risks of hip, Colles', or vertebral fracture and coronary heart disease among white postmenopausal women, *Arch Intern Med* 149: 2445-2448, 1989.
10. Colditz GA: Relationship between estrogen levels, use of hormone replacement therapy, and breast cancer, *J Natl Cancer Inst* 90:814-823, 1998.
11. Grodstein F, Stampfer MJ, Manson JE, et al: Postmenopausal estrogen and progestin use and the risk of cardiovascular disease, *N Engl J Med* 335:453-461, 1996.
12. Grodstein F, Stampfer MJ, Colditz A, et al: Postmenopausal hormone therapy and mortality, *N Engl J Med* 336:1769-1775, 1997.
13. Sourander L, Rajala T, Räihä I, et al: Cardiovascular and cancer morbidity and mortality and sudden cardiac death in postmenopausal women on oestrogen replacement therapy (ERT), *Lancet* 352:1965-1969, 1998.
14. Rödström K, Bengtsson C, Lissner L, et al: Pre-existing risk factor profiles in users and non-users of hormone replacement therapy: prospective cohort study in Gothenburg, Sweden, *BMJ* 319:890-893, 1999.
15. Rossouw JE: Estrogens for prevention of coronary heart disease: putting the brakes on the bandwagon, *Circulation* 94: 2982-2985, 1996.
16. Grover SA: Estrogen replacement for women with cardiovascular disease: why don't physicians and patients follow the guidelines? (editorial), *Can Med Assoc J* 161:42-43, 1999.
17. Hulley S, Grady D, Bush T, et al (Heart and Estrogen/Progestin Replacement Study Research Group): Randomized trial of estrogen plus progestin for secondary prevention of coronary heart disease in postmenopausal women, *JAMA* 280:605-613, 1998.
18. Brinton LA, Schairer C: Postmenopausal hormone-replacement therapy—time for a reappraisal? (editorial), *N Engl J Med* 336:1821-1822, 1997.
19. Schairer C, Lubin J, Troisi R, et al: Menopausal estrogen and estrogen-progestin replacement therapy and breast cancer risk, *JAMA* 283:485-491, 2000.
20. Kwang KK, Mincemoyer R, Bui M, et al: Effects of hormone-replacement therapy on fibrinolysis in postmenopausal women, *N Engl J Med* 336:683-690, 1997.
21. Writing Group for the PEPI Trial: Effects of estrogen or estrogen/progestin regimens on heart disease risk factors in postmenopausal women: the Postmenopausal Estrogen/Progestin Interventions (PEPI) Trial, *JAMA* 273:199-208, 1995.
22. Finucane FF, Madans JH, Bush TL, et al: Decreased risk of stroke among postmenopausal hormone users, *Arch Intern Med* 153:73-79, 1993.
23. Falkeborn M, Persson I, Terent A, et al: Hormone replacement therapy and the risk of stroke: follow-up of a population-based cohort in Sweden, *Arch Intern Med* 153:1201-1209, 1993.

24. Michaëlsson K, Baron JA, Farahmand BY, et al: Hormone replacement therapy and risk of hip fracture: population based case-control study, *BMJ* 316:1858-1863, 1998.
25. Willett WC, Colditz G, Stampfer M: Postmenopausal estrogens—opposed, unopposed, or none of the above (editorial), *JAMA* 283:534-535, 2000.
26. Ensrud KE, Black DM, Palermo L, et al: Treatment with alendronate prevents fractures in women at highest risk: results from the Fracture Intervention Trial, *Arch Intern Med* 157:2617-2624, 1997.
27. Krall EA, Dawson-Hughes B, Hannan MT, et al: Postmenopausal estrogen replacement and tooth retention, *Am J Med* 102:536-542, 1997.
28. Yaffe K, Sawaya G, Lieberburg I, et al: Estrogen therapy in postmenopausal women: effects on cognitive function and dementia, *JAMA* 279:688-695, 1998.
29. Matthews K, Cauley J, Yaffe K, et al: Estrogen replacement therapy and cognitive decline in older community women, *J Am Geriatr Soc* 47:518-523, 1999.
30. Barrett-Connor E: Rethinking estrogen and the brain (editorial), *J Am Geriatr Soc* 46:918-920, 1998.
31. Grodstein F, Martinez E, Platz EA, et al: Postmenopausal hormone use and risk for colorectal cancer and adenoma, *Ann Intern Med* 128:705-712, 1998.

Adverse Effects of Hormone Replacement Therapy

(See also breast cancer; informed consent; thrombophlebitis)

Endometrial cancer

Long-term unopposed estrogen use, whether in the form of conjugated estrogens or estradiol, is known to increase the risk of endometrial cancer. This risk may persist for more than 5 years after estrogens are discontinued. Long-term use of estrogen plus cyclical progestins is associated with a small increase in the risk for endometrial cancer, but this risk does not persist beyond 5 years after discontinuation of the hormones. Women taking estrogens plus continuous progestins have a lower risk of endometrial cancer than women not taking hormone replacement therapy.[1]

Routine endometrial biopsies to rule out endometrial carcinoma before starting hormone replacement therapy are unnecessary for asymptomatic women.[2]

Breast cancer

Until 1995 the existence of an association between hormone replacement therapy and breast cancer was controversial. The publication in 1995 of the Nurses' Health Study made it clear that hormone replacement therapy of more than 5 years' duration is a risk factor for breast cancer. Women who were currently taking hormones and had been doing so for more than 5 years had a relative risk of acquiring breast cancer of 1.46. This risk was even greater in older women; those aged 60 to 64 who had been taking hormones for at least 5 years had a relative risk of 1.7. This study also found that progestogens had no protective effect on the incidence of breast cancer. The mortality rate from breast cancer was also increased by a relative rate of 1.45 among

women who had used hormone replacement for more than 5 years.[3] Although this study did not give absolute figures, the authors provided some in response to a letter to the editor. They calculated that the risk that a 60-year-old woman would have breast cancer within the next 5 years if she never had hormone replacement therapy was 1.8%; if she was taking hormones and had done so for at least 5 years, her risk was 3%.[4] A further evaluation of mortality in the Nurses' Health Study showed a relative increase in breast cancer mortality of 43% among women taking hormones for more than 10 years. As a result the overall mortality benefit, which depends on a decrease in cardiovascular disease, was seriously attenuated.[5]

Additional evidence that hormone replacement therapy increases the risk of breast cancer comes from a comprehensive analysis of 90% of the world's published and unpublished studies.[6] The relative risk of acquiring the disease among current users who had been taking hormone replacement medications for 5 or more years was 1.35, but women who had discontinued the drugs 5 or more years previously did not have an increased risk. The excess numbers of breast cancers among 1000 women starting hormone replacement therapy at age 50 compared with control subjects were 2 at 5 years, 6 at 10 years, and 12 at 15 years. No figures for mortality were given in this study.[6] The Iowa Women's Health Study also found an increased risk of breast cancer (breast cancer mortality was not assessed) in women taking hormone replacement therapy, but the increase was almost exclusively limited to such histological types as mucinous and tubular adenocarcinomas, which are associated with a good prognosis.[7]

A recent cohort study found that the risk of breast cancer in women taking hormone replacement therapy was greater in those receiving estrogen-progestin combinations than in those receiving only estrogens.[8]

For some perusers of the literature the risk of breast cancer with long-term hormone replacement therapy is of sufficient magnitude that prescriptions should be limited to short periods.[9] Regardless of the physician's personal views, all women should be apprised of the pros and cons of hormone replacement therapy so they can decide for themselves whether they want to take these drugs (see discussion of informed consent).

Current evidence suggests that the risk of breast cancer is not increased or is only minimally increased in women who take hormone replacement therapy for 5 years or less, a view supported by the Canadian Task Force on Preventive Health Care[10] and the U.S. Preventive Services Task Force.[11] This knowledge should allow both patients and physicians to feel more comfortable about short-term hormonal replacement therapy for such symptoms as hot flashes.

Thromboembolism

Two case-controlled studies published in 1996 found that the relative risk of thromboembolic disorders in women taking hormone replacement therapy was about three times greater than among nonusers.[12,13] However, the absolute rate was very low. The authors of one of these studies estimated that the number of excess cases of thromboembolic disorders in hormone users was 1:5000 users per year.[12]

❧ REFERENCES ❧

1. Weiderpass E, Adami H-O, Baron JA, et al: Risk of endometrial cancer following estrogen replacement with and without progestins, *J Natl Cancer Inst* 91:1131-1137, 1999.
2. Korhonen MO, Symons JP, Hyde BM, et al: Histologic classification and pathologic findings for endometrial biopsy specimens obtained from 2964 perimenopausal and postmenopausal women undergoing screening for continuous hormones as replacement therapy (Chart 2 Study), *Am J Obstet Gynecol* 176:377-380, 1997.
3. Colditz GA, Hankinson SE, Hunter DJ, et al: The use of estrogens and progestins and the risk of breast cancer in postmenopausal women, *N Engl J Med* 332:1589-1593, 1995.
4. Colditz GA, Willett WC, Speizer FE: Breast cancer and hormone-replacement therapy (letter), *N Engl J Med* 333:1357-1358, 1995.
5. Grodstein F, Stampfer MJ, Colditz A, et al: Postmenopausal hormone therapy and mortality, *N Engl J Med* 336:1769-1775, 1997.
6. Beral V, Bull D, Doll R, et al (Collaborative Group on Hormonal Factors in Breast Cancer): Breast cancer and hormone replacement therapy: collaborative reanalysis of data from 51 epidemiological studies of 52,704 women with breast cancer and 108,411 women without breast cancer, *Lancet* 350:1047-1059, 1997.
7. Gapstur SM, Morrow M, Sellers TA: Hormone replacement therapy and risk of breast cancer with a favorable histology: results of the Iowa Women's Health Study, *JAMA* 281:2091-2097, 1999.
8. Schairer C, Lubin J, Troisi R, et al: Menopausal estrogen and estrogen-progestin replacement therapy and breast cancer risk, *JAMA* 283:485-491, 2000.
9. Brinton LA, Schairer C: Postmenopausal hormone-replacement therapy—time for a reappraisal? (editorial), *N Engl J Med* 336:1821-1822, 1997.
10. Canadian Task Force on the Periodic Health Examination: *Canadian guide to clinical preventive health care,* Ottawa, 1994, Canada Communication Group—Publishing, p 623.
11. US Preventive Services Task Force: *Guide to clinical preventive services,* ed 2, Baltimore, 1996, Williams & Wilkins, pp 829-843.
12. Daly E, Vessey MP, Hawkins MN, et al: Risk of venous thromboembolism in users of hormone replacement therapy, *Lancet* 348:977-980, 1996.
13. Jick H, Derby LE, Myers MW, et al: Risk of hospital admission for idiopathic venous thromboembolism among users of postmenopausal oestrogens, *Lancet* 348:981-983, 1996.

Guidelines for Hormone Replacement Therapy

Although some organizations such as the Society of Obstetricians and Gynecologists of Canada (SOGC) strongly support the use of hormone replacement therapy for almost all postmenopausal women,[1] most evidence-based guidelines take a somewhat less interventionist position. Neither the Canadian Task Force on Preventive Health Care[2] nor the U.S. Preventive Services Task Force[3] has given a blanket recommendation for postmenopausal hormonal replacement therapy. Rather, they both give a "B" recommendation to the idea that all women should be counseled concerning the benefits and possible risks of estrogen replacement therapy.

An aspect of hormone replacement therapy that is rarely discussed but should be remembered is the possibility that the current emphasis on this mode of prevention may lead to a deemphasis of other preventive modalities, such as exercise, that may be just as useful (see "Life-Style Changes for Disease Prevention in Menopausal Women").[4]

❧ REFERENCES ❧

1. Canadian Menopause Consensus Conference, *J SOGC* 16:4-40, 1994.
2. Canadian Task Force on the Periodic Health Examination: *Canadian guide to clinical preventive health care,* Ottawa, 1994, Canada Communication Group—Publishing, pp 619-631.
3. US Preventive Services Task Force: *Guide to clinical preventive services,* ed 2, Baltimore, 1996, Williams & Wilkins, pp 829-843.
4. Marshall KG: Prevention. How much harm? How much benefit? 2. Ten potential pitfalls in determining the clinical significance of benefits, *Can Med Assoc J* 154:1837-1843, 1996.

Methods of Prescribing Hormone Replacement

Hormone replacement therapy can be administered in several ways. Most of the examples given below use conjugated estrogens (Premarin) or estrogen patches containing estradiol (Estraderm, Vivelle, Climara) plus medroxyprogesterone acetate (Provera) simply because these are the most frequently used drugs in practice. Progestogens are required only for women who have an intact uterus. Another option is to give regular combined estrogen-androgen injections, along with cyclical progestogen if the patient has an intact uterus.

Table 28 lists generic and selected trade names of some of the available agents used for hormonal replacement. Methods of prescribing most of them are discussed in the text.

Continuous estrogen and continuous progestogen

Premarin 0.625 mg po is taken daily, or Estraderm 50 is applied twice a week, and in addition Provera 2.5 mg is given daily. This protocol is followed continuously throughout the year. Spotting or bleeding is common in the first 6 months. In one trial 27% of women receiving continuous Provera 5 mg and 39% of women receiving continuous Provera 2.5 mg had breakthrough bleeding.[1] On the other hand, after 6 to 12 months of this kind of regimen, many women had become completely amenorrheic, which is said to increase compliance with this therapeutic modality.[2] A metaanalysis of 42 studies of combined continuous

Table 28   Selected Medications for Hormonal Replacement

Generic name	Selected trade names
Estrogens	
Conjugated estrogens, equine	Premarin, CES, Congest,
Conjugated estrogens, equine	Premarin vaginal cream
Conjugated estrogens, synthetic	Cenestin
Estradiol-17 ß skin patch	Estraderm, Vivelle, Climara, Oesclin
Estropipate	Ogen
Ethinyl estradiol	Estinyl
Dienestrol vaginal cream	Ortho Dienestrol
Estrogens plus Progestins	
Conjugated estrogens plus medroxy-progesterone tablets	Prempro, Premphase
Estradiol plus norethindrone skin patch	CombiPatch, Estragest
Estrogens plus Androgens	
Testosterone plus estradiol	Climacteron (for IM use)
Progesterone Derivatives	
Medroxyprogesterone acetate	Provera
Progesterone, micronized	Prometrium
Megestrol acetate	Megace
Other	
Clonidine	Dixarit

estrogen-progestin use found that after 6 months of therapy 75% or more of women were amenorrheic.[3] In the United States both an oral formulation containing conjugated estrogens 0.625 plus medroxyprogesterone acetate 2.5 mg (Prempro) and a transdermal system containing estradiol and norethindrone (CombiPatch) are available for this form of treatment.

Continuous estrogen and cyclical progestogen

The standard method of using a continuous estrogen and cyclical progestogen combination is to take Premarin 0.625 mg po daily or to apply Estraderm 50 twice a week throughout the year. Provera 5 or 10 mg is taken for the first or last 10 to 14 days of each calendar month or of each 28-day cycle. The progestin withdrawal leads to bleeding in most women. A package containing 14 tablets of 0.625 mg of conjugated estrogens, to be taken during the first 14 days, and 14 tablets of 0.625 mg of conjugated estrogens plus medroxyprogesterone acetate 5 mg, to be taken on days 15 to 28 (Premphase), is available in the United States. Skin patches may be used to deliver estrogen only in the first 2 weeks of the cycle (Estraderm, Vivelle) and estrogen plus progestogen in the second 2 weeks (CombiPatch, Estragest). In Canada, a monthly supply containing four Estraderm patches and four Estragest patches comes in a single package under the trade name Estracomb.

Cyclical estrogen and cyclical progestogen

Premarin 0.625 mg po is taken daily or Estraderm 50 is applied twice a week from days 1 to 25 of each month, and in addition, medroxyprogesterone acetate (Provera) 5 or 10 mg is taken daily from days 14 or 16 to 25 of each month. With cyclical estrogen and cyclical progestin about 80% of women have regular withdrawal bleeding. In addition, a number of women have a recurrence of hot flashes and perhaps sleep disturbances during the period of hormonal withdrawal at the end of the month.[1]

Estrogen-androgen injections and cyclical progestogen

Testosterone plus estradiol (Climacteron) is given as a 1-ml intramuscular injection deep in the gluteus muscles once every 4 to 8 weeks. If the woman has an intact uterus, Provera 5 to 10 mg should be given on days 12 to 25 of the cycle, counting the day of injection as day 1.

◢ REFERENCES ◣

1. Archer DF, Pickar JH, Bottiglioni F: Bleeding patterns in post-menopausal women taking continuous combined or sequential regimens of conjugated estrogens with medroxyprogesterone acetate, *Obstet Gynecol* 83:686-692, 1994.
2. Rosenfeld J: Update on continuous estrogen-progestin replacement therapy, *Am Fam Physician* 50:1519-1523, 1994.
3. Udoff L, Langenberg P, Adashi EY: Combined continuous hormone replacement therapy—a critical review, *Obstet Gynecol* 86:306-316, 1995.

Life-Style Changes for Disease Prevention in Menopausal Women
(See also alcohol; benefits of hormone replacement therapy; exercise; osteoporosis; smoking)

While long-term current estrogen replacement therapy is clearly associated with decreases in the risk for cardiovascular disease, osteoporosis, and total mortality in postmenopausal women, some of this benefit may be related to the fact that women choosing estrogen replacement therapy tend to have healthier life-styles (see the earlier discussion of the benefits of hormone replacement therapy).[1,2] Whether or not future randomized controlled trials prove this to be the case, life-style changes themselves are beneficial, although their worth tends to be overshadowed in the widespread enthusiasm for estrogen replacement therapy.[3]

Stopping smoking is one of the most important measures that can be taken. Another is increasing physical activity. The few studies that have specifically addressed the relationship between exercise and cardiac disease in women have shown that physical activity has a protective effect against coronary artery disease (see discussion of exercise).[4,5] Exercise alone, exercise plus calcium supplementation, or exercise plus hormone replacement therapy has been shown to decrease bone loss in postmenopausal women,[6-10] and exercise correlates with a decreased incidence of hip fractures.[11-13] These issues are discussed more fully under "Osteoporosis." Moderate alcohol intake has been shown to reduce cardiovascular mortality in both men and women.[14]

⚓ REFERENCES ⚓

1. Posthuma WF, Westendorp RG, Vandenbroucke JP: Cardioprotective effect of hormone replacement therapy in postmenopausal women: is the evidence biased? *BMJ* 308:1268-1269, 1994.
2. Cauley JA, Seeley DG, Browner WS, et al: Estrogen replacement therapy and mortality among older women: the Study of Osteoporotic Fractures, *Arch Intern Med* 157:2181-2187, 1997.
3. Willett WC, Colditz G, Stampfer M: Postmenopausal estrogens—opposed, unopposed, or none of the above (editorial), *JAMA* 283:534-535, 2000.
4. Rich-Edwards JW, Manson JE, Hennekens C, et al: The primary prevention of coronary heart disease in women, *N Engl J Med* 332:1758-1766, 1995.
5. Kushi LH, Fee RM, Folsom AR, et al: Physical activity and mortality in postmenopausal women, *JAMA* 277:1287-1292, 1997.
6. Reid IR, Ames RW, Evans MC, et al: Effect of calcium supplementation on bone loss in postmenopausal women, *N Engl J Med* 328:460-464, 1993.
7. Reid IR, Ames RW, Evans MC, et al: Long-term effects of calcium supplementation on bone loss and fractures in postmenopausal women: a randomized controlled trial, *Am J Med* 98: 331-335, 1995.
8. Aloia JF, Vaswani A, Yeh JK, et al: Calcium supplementation with and without hormone replacement therapy to prevent postmenopausal bone loss, *Ann Intern Med* 120:97-103, 1994.
9. Prince RL, Smith M, Kick IM, et al: Prevention of postmenopausal osteoporosis: a comparative study of exercise, calcium supplementation, and hormone-replacement therapy, *N Engl J Med* 325:1189-1195, 1991.
10. Nelson ME, Fiatarone MA, Morganti CM, et al: Effects of high-intensity strength training on multiple risk factors for osteoporotic fractures: a randomized controlled trial, *JAMA* 272: 1909-1914, 1994.
11. Perez Cano R, Galan Galan F, Dilsen G: Risk factors for hip fracture in Spanish and Turkish women, *Bone* 14(suppl 1): S69-S72, 1993.
12. Jaglal SB, Kreiger N, Darlington G: Past and recent physical activity and risk of hip fracture, *Am J Epidemiol* 138:107-118, 1993.
13. Paganini-Hill A, Chao A, Ross RK, et al: Exercise and other factors in the prevention of hip fracture: the Leisure World study, *Epidemiology* 2:16-25, 1991.
14. Ashley MF, Room R, Rankin F, et al: Moderate drinking and health: report of an international symposium, *Can Med Assoc J* 151:809-828, 1994.

OVARIES
Ovarian Cancer

(See also breast cancer; positive predictive value; prevention; screening)

Epidemiology

Ovarian cancer is the fifth most common malignancy among women in the United States and is the leading cause of death from gynecological cancers. Ovarian cancer is predominantly a disease of postmenopausal women in the sixth decade. In 70% of patients the disease is advanced at diagnosis. The most important risk factor is a family history, especially if two or more first-degree relatives are affected.[1] Between 5% and 10% of cases of ovarian cancer are hereditary, but among Ashkenazi Jews the rate may be as high as 30%.[2] Other risk factors are nulliparity and first birth after age 35. However, most women with the disease have no evident risk factors.[1] Oral contraceptives offer some degree of protection.[1,2]

Screening or case finding

There is no evidence that screening modalities such as regular pelvic examinations, transabdominal or transvaginal sonography, or CA-125 alter the mortality rate of ovarian cancer.[1,3,4] A large British study of postmenopausal women used a biphasic screening modality. Women with CA-125 levels of 30 U/ml or higher underwent pelvic ultrasonography, and if enlarged ovaries were found, surgical exploration was undertaken. Between 2% and 4% of women had elevated CA-125 levels, but among these only 1.3% had ovarian cancer. Compared with the control group the women with elevated CA-125 levels did not have a decrease in ovarian cancer mortality.[3] The degree of psychological distress experienced by the 98.7% of women with "false-positive" CA-125 tests was not discussed in the report.

The Canadian Task Force on Preventive Health Care advises against using any of the screening modalities for the general population ("D" recommendation),[5] as do the U.S. Preventive Services Task Force[6] and the American College of Physicians.[7]

Management

Chemotherapy is the treatment of choice for advanced ovarian cancer, and its efficacy is increased if the residual tumor mass is small. Therefore the first stage of treatment is often surgical "debulking."[8] For most women the chemotherapeutic regimen of choice is a combination of paclitaxel (Taxol) and a platinum compound such as cisplatin (Platinol) or carboplatin (Paraplatin-AQ).[9]

Hereditary ovarian cancer syndromes

The most common form of hereditary ovarian cancer is the hereditary breast-ovarian cancer syndrome that is associated with BRCA1 or BRCA2 mutations. The tumors are always serous carcinomas. BRCA1 mutations account for over 90% of these cases, and the disorder is particularly common in Ashkenazi Jews. The risk for ovarian cancer developing by age 70 is 20% to 50% for BRCA1 mutation carriers but is considerably lower for BRCA2 carriers. The mean age at onset is about 5 years younger than that found in sporadic cases; in very few women with the BRCA1 mutation does ovarian cancer develop before the age of 45.[2]

As yet no trials have been published on the optimal methods for preventing ovarian cancer in BRCA1 or BRCA2 carriers. Oral contraceptives would seem to be indicated whenever possible, and annual screening by pelvic examination, vaginal ultrasound, and annual or biannual measurements of CA-125 has been recommended.[2] Oophorectomy after age 45 is also frequently recommended, although even this is not foolproof because women with these mutations are at increased risk for primary peritoneal carcinoma, which is histologically indistinguishable from papillary serous ovarian cancer.[2,10]

Another form of hereditary ovarian cancer is that associated with hereditary nonpolyposis colorectal cancer. Women with this disorder are at increased risk for colon, ovarian, endometrial, stomach, small bowel, and urinary tract malignancies.[2]

❧ REFERENCES ❧

1. NIH Consensus Development Panel on Ovarian Cancer: Ovarian cancer: screening, treatment, and follow-up, *JAMA* 273: 491-497, 1995.
2. Kasprzak L, Foulkes WD, Shelling AN: Hereditary ovarian carcinoma, *BMJ* 318:786-789, 1999.
3. Jacobs IJ, Skates S, Davies AP, et al: Risk of diagnosis of ovarian cancer after raised serum CA 125 concentration: a prospective cohort study, *BMJ* 313:1355-1358, 1996.
4. Urban N: Screening for ovarian cancer: we now need a definitive randomised trial (editorial), *BMJ* 319:1317-1318, 1999.
5. Canadian Task Force on the Periodic Health Examination: *Clinical preventive health care,* Ottawa, 1994, Canadian Communication Group—Publishing.
6. US Preventive Services Task Force: *Guide to clinical preventive services: an assessment of the effectiveness of 169 interventions,* Baltimore, 1989, Williams & Wilkins, pp 81-85.
7. American College of Physicians: Screening for ovarian cancer; recommendations and rationale, *Ann Intern Med* 121: 142-143, 1994.
8. Cannistra S: Cancer of the ovary, *N Engl J Med* 329:1550-1558, 1993.
9. Adams M, Calvert AH, Carmichael J, et al: Chemotherapy for ovarian cancer—a consensus statement on standard practice (editorial), *Br J Cancer* 78:1404-1406, 1998.
10. Eisen A, Weber B: Primary peritoneal carcinoma can have multifocal origins: implications for prophylactic oophorectomy, *J Natl Cancer Inst* 90:797-799, 1998.

Polycystic Ovarian Syndrome

Between 5% and 10% of women in the reproductive age range are thought to have the polycystic ovarian syndrome. The usual clinical manifestations are menstrual dysfunction or infertility, caused by oligoovulation or anovulation, and acne and hirsutism, caused by elevated testosterone levels. Serum free testosterone levels are elevated, and in most patients ultrasound detects enlarged ovaries with multiple small peripheral follicles. Women with this disorder, particularly if they are obese, have insulin resistance. This leads to higher insulin levels, which not only stimulate the ovary to produce androgens, but also are associated with an increased risk of cardiovascular disease from the so-called metabolic syndrome or syndrome X.[1]

Treatment of polycystic ovarian syndrome has been traditionally directed at symptom control such as oral contraceptives for menstrual irregularities, clomiphene citrate (Clomid) for infertility, and antiandrogens such as spironolactone (Aldactone) or cyproterone (Androcur) for hirsutism. Weight loss, which reduces insulin resistance, is an essential part of treatment for obese patients with the syndrome. Preliminary data suggest that metformin may also be useful.[1]

❧ REFERENCES ❧

1. Hopkinson ZE, Sattar N, Fleming R, et al: Polycystic ovarian syndrome: the metabolic syndrome comes to gynaecology, *BMJ* 317:329-332, 1998.

PELVIC INFLAMMATORY DISEASE

(See also bacterial vaginosis; ectopic pregnancy; sexually transmitted diseases)

Women who douche are at increased risk of pelvic inflammatory disease (PID), ectopic pregnancy, and bacterial vaginosis (see ectopic pregnancy).

The organisms most frequently causing PID are *Chlamydia trachomatis* and *Neisseria gonorrhoeae.* However, in a substantial number of cases other organisms, particularly anaerobes, are responsible for the infection.[1]

The clinical diagnosis of PID is often difficult and imprecise. Because the sequelae may be so serious, early treatment is recommended for young, sexually active women who display the minimum criteria of lower abdominal tenderness, adnexal tenderness, and cervical motion tenderness, provided that no other cause of symptoms can be identified. Criteria that support but are not required for the diagnosis include an oral temperature greater than 38.3° C (101.8° F), abnormal cervical or vaginal discharge, and laboratory evidence of cervical infection with *N. gonorrhoeae* or *C. trachomatis.*[1]

In one study infertility rates after PID were 8% after one episode, 19.5% after two, and 40% after three or more.[2] Severe PID is more likely to result in infertility than is mild PID, and second episodes of PID are far more likely to decrease fertility in women whose initial infection was severe.[3] Other complications of PID are recurrent episodes in 20% to 25% of cases[4] and a greatly increased risk of ectopic pregnancies.[5]

Patients with PID who are not in a toxic or pregnant state and who can comply with an outpatient oral regimen do not require initial hospitalization and parenteral therapy. Recommended oral regimens that cover *N. gonorrhoeae, C. trachomatis,* and anaerobes are[1,6]:

1. Ofloxacin (Floxin) 400 mg po bid for 14 days *plus* metronidazole (Flagyl) 500 mg bid for 14 days, *or*
2. Ceftriaxone (Rocephin) 250 mg IM once, *or* cefoxitin (Mefoxin) 2 g IM *plus* probenecid 1 g po once, *or* an-

other parenteral third-generation cephalosporin once *plus* doxycycline (Vibramycin) 100 mg po bid for 14 days

Sexual partners of women with PID should be contacted and treated for *N. gonorrhoeae* and *C. trachomatis* if they have had sexual relations with the patient within the past 60 days.[1]

REFERENCES

1. Centers for Disease Control and Prevention: 1998 Guidelines for treatment of sexually transmitted diseases, *MMWR* 47 (RR-1):1-116, 1998.
2. Westrom L, Joesoef R, Reynolds G, et al: Pelvic inflammatory disease and fertility: a cohort study of 1,844 women with laparoscopically verified disease and 657 control women with normal laparoscopic results, *Sex Transm Dis* 19:185-192, 1992.
3. Lepine LA, Hillis SD, Marchbanks PA, et al: Severity of pelvic inflammatory disease as a predictor of the probability of live birth, *Am J Obstet Gynecol* 178:977-981, 1998.
4. Soper DE: Diagnosis and laparoscopic grading of acute salpingitis, *Am J Obstet Gynecol* 164(5 Pt 2):1370-1376, 1991.
5. Egger M, Low N, Davey Smith G, et al: Screening for chlamydial infections and the risk of ectopic pregnancy in a county in Sweden: ecological analysis, *BMJ* 316:1776-1780, 1998.
6. Drugs for sexually transmitted infections, *Med Lett* 41:85-90, 1999.

PREMENSTRUAL DYSPHORIC DISORDER
(See also depression)

The nature or even the existence of the premenstrual syndrome has been a subject of controversy. Since over 150 symptoms of the disorder have been described in the medical literature, such uncertainty is understandable.[1] Recently more rigorous studies have shed considerable light on the issue. Premenstrual syndrome does exist. It is one of the affective or "mood" disorders, and for this reason the current favored nomenclature is premenstrual dysphoric disorder.[2] It is thought to affect about 5% of menstruating women and is to be distinguished from the less severe disturbances of cognition, behavior, and mood that affect 20% to 80% of women during the premenstrual phase.[3] The condition is more common in women whose mothers were affected and in women who are suffering from a major depression. Evidence indicates that untreated premenstrual dysphoric disorder may progress to major depression.[3]

The major symptoms of premenstrual dysphoric disorder are depression, irritability, and anxiety, often associated with sleep disturbances, appetite changes, and fatigue. To meet the criteria for the diagnosis, symptoms must be severe enough to disrupt social and occupational functioning, occur during the second half of the menstrual cycle, and remit completely at the time of menstruation. Timing of symptoms must be documented by prospective diaries over two or three cycles.[3]

Many drugs have been tried for premenstrual syndrome, and most have shown little or no evidence of benefit. These include vitamins, minerals, herbal remedies, diuretics, and estrogens and progesterone, including oral contraceptives.[4,5] For example, although the main conclusion of a 1999 systematic review of vitamin B_6 was that most of the studies evaluated were of poor quality, it appeared possible that 50 to 100 mg of vitamin B_6 daily might be helpful.[6] A 1998 multicenter randomized placebo-controlled trial of elemental calcium 600 mg bid (calcium carbonate 1500 mg bid) for treatment of premenstrual dysphoric disorder found a significant amelioration of all symptoms, including mood dysfunction, in the group taking calcium.[7]

Alprazolam (Xanax) appears to be effective, but the danger of addiction militates against its use.[4] At present the drugs of choice are the tricyclic antidepressant clomipramine (Anafranil) or one of the selective serotonin reuptake inhibitors (SSRIs).[3-5] Among the SSRIs, fluoxetine (Prozac),[8] paroxetine (Paxil),[9] and sertraline (Zoloft)[4] have all proved efficacious when given throughout the cycle in antidepressant doses. A small randomized trial of sertraline 50 to 100 mg versus placebo given for the last 2 weeks of the menstrual cycle reported good control of moderate-to-severe premenstrual dysphoric disorder with sertraline.[10]

REFERENCES

1. Robinson G: Determining which patients have premenstrual syndrome, *Can J Diagn* 11:73-81, 1994.
2. American Psychiatric Association: *Diagnostic and statistical manual of mental disorders,* ed 4, Washington, DC, 1994, American Psychiatric Association, pp 715-718.
3. Parry BL: A 45-year-old woman with premenstrual dysphoric disorder, *JAMA* 281:368-373, 1999.
4. Yonkers KA, Halbreich U, Freeman E, et al: Symptomatic improvement of premenstrual dysphoric disorder with sertraline treatment: a randomized controlled trial, *JAMA* 278:983-988, 1997.
5. Gold JH: Premenstrual dysphoric disorder: what's that? (editorial), *JAMA* 278:1024-1025, 1997.
6. Wyatt KM, Dimmock PW, Jones PW, et al: Efficacy of vitamin B-6 in the treatment of premenstrual syndrome: systematic review, *BMJ* 318:1375-1381, 1999.
7. Thys-Jacobs S, Starkey P, Bernstein D, et al: Calcium carbonate and the premenstrual syndrome: effects on premenstrual and menstrual symptoms, *Am J Obstet Gynecol* 179:444-452, 1998.
8. Steiner M, Steinberg S, Stewart D, et al (Canadian Fluoxetine/Premenstrual Dysphoria Collaborative Study Group): Fluoxetine in the treatment of premenstrual dysphoria, *N Engl J Med* 332:1529-1534, 1995.
9. Eriksson E, Hedberg MA, Andersh B, Sundblad C: The serotonin re-uptake inhibitor paroxetine is superior to the adrenalin re-uptake inhibitor maprotiline in the treatment of premenstrual syndrome, *Neuropsychopharmacology* 12:167-176, 1995.
10. Jermain DM, Preece CK, Sykes RL, et al: Luteal phase sertraline treatment for premenstrual dysphoric disorder: results of a double-blind, placebo-controlled, crossover study, *Arch Fam Med* 8:328-332, 1999.

SEXUAL DYSFUNCTION IN WOMEN
(See sexual dysfunction in men)

Androgen Replacement

Decreased libido and sexual response in postmenopausal women are usually secondary to depression, but in a few instances they may be related to low free testosterone levels. If free testosterone levels are low, small replacement doses (not pharmacological doses) of testosterone may be helpful. This could be in the form of intramuscular testosterone enanthate or cypionate in doses of 25 mg monthly or 15 mg every 2 weeks. In Canada oral testosterone undecanoate (Andriol) is available and can be given as one 40-mg capsule every second day.[1]

Vaginismus

Vaginismus is caused by spasm of the levator muscles, which can be detected on pelvic examination. (Pelvic examination should not be performed if the patient is too frightened to allow it or it is too painful.) The essence of treatment is behavioral; the patient is first taught Kegel exercises (contraction of the levators) and then reverse Kegel exercises (relaxation of the levators). The goal of the latter is longer and longer periods of relaxation after the initial contraction. As the patient gains confidence, she may insert one lubricated finger into the vagina to sense the tightening and relaxation of the levators, and with time she may be able to insert two or three fingers.[2] The purpose of finger insertion is not to dilate the vagina manually, which is now an obsolete concept, but to monitor the efficacy of voluntary relaxation of the muscles.[2,3] Once the patient can accomplish these exercises effectively, she may get her partner to participate in introducing fingers[3] and eventually inserting the penis with the woman in control.[2,3] For many women this works best if the woman is in the superior position.[2]

Hysterectomy

Sexual functioning in women improves after a hysterectomy. The probable reason is relief of symptoms as a result of the surgery.[4]

⟍ REFERENCES ⟍

1. Basson R: Androgen replacement for women, *Can Fam Physician* 45:2100-2107, 1999.
2. Lamont JA: Vaginismus: reflex response out of control, *Patient Care Can* 7(2):75-78, 1996.
3. Butcher J: ABC of sexual health: female sexual problems. II. Sexual pain and sexual fears, *BMJ* 318:110-112, 1999.
4. Rhodes JC, Kjerulff KH, Langenberg PW, et al: Hysterectomy and sexual functioning, *JAMA* 282:1934-1941, 1999.

VAGINITIS
(See also drugs and chemicals in pregnancy; ectopic pregnancy; inflammatory Papanicolaou smears; pelvic inflammatory disease)

The differential diagnosis of vaginitis should include contact dermatitis of the vulva. This has been reported with some brands of sanitary napkins.[1]

Candidiasis

Candida is present in the vaginas of one fourth of all women, and at least half of these are asymptomatic. In candidiasis the vaginal pH is usually less than 4.5. Table 29 lists drugs commonly used in the treatment of vaginal yeast infections. Vaginal preparations are available as creams or vaginal tablets. The tablets vary in dose; the more potent preparations are generally given for 1 or 3 days and the less potent for a week. Single-dose intravaginal regimens are probably not as effective as longer treatment programs.[2] A single oral dose of 150 mg of fluconazole (Diflucan) is as effective as intravaginal treatments of vulvovaginal candidiasis.[3]

When a patient has recurrent vaginal yeast infections, underlying precipitants such as diabetes mellitus, antibiotic use, and HIV infection should be ruled out. In addition, the diagnosis should be reevaluated to make sure some unrelated condition such as vulvar lichen sclerosus et atrophicus has not been misdiagnosed as candidiasis. If the infection is always related to antibiotic therapy, a 3-day course of a vaginal anticandidal preparation or a single oral dose of 150 mg of fluconazole (Diflucan) may be given near or at the end of the antibiotic treatment.[4] Fluconazole may also be particularly useful if the patient has frequent relapses. In this circumstance one dose of 100 or 150 mg per week or per month may be tried.[2] Another option for recurrent infections is to use one of the vaginal preparations once or twice weekly for prophylaxis. Whether yogurt has any value is doubtful. According to one report the daily oral consumption of 8 oz of unpasteurized yogurt containing *Lactobacillus acidophilus* decreased the incidence of recurrent vaginal yeast infections.[5] However, placebo-controlled studies have not confirmed the efficacy of this agent.

Bacterial Vaginosis

Women who douche are at increased risk of bacterial vaginosis, as well as pelvic inflammatory disease and ectopic

Table 29 Vaginal Yeast Infections

Generic name	Trade names
Topical Imidazoles	
Clotrimazole	Gyne-Lotrimin, Mycelex, Canesten
Miconazole	Monistat
Terconazole	Terazol
Oral Agents	
Fluconazole	Diflucan

pregnancy (see discussion of ectopic pregnancy). Douching has no value and should be eschewed.

Bacterial vaginosis is polymicrobial. Some of the organisms associated with it are *Gardnerella vaginalis, Mycoplasma hominis,* and anaerobes.[6] *G. vaginalis* can be cultured from 50% of women with no symptoms of vaginal disease, so vaginal cultures are not clinically useful.[2] There is no proof that bacterial vaginosis is an STD, and treating the partners has no value.[7]

Bacterial vaginosis is present in 20% of pregnancies. A number of studies have shown that pregnant women with bacterial vaginosis have an increased risk of preterm deliveries, but therapeutic trials of antibiotics have not shown conclusive benefits.[6] At present no guidelines recommend screening of all pregnant women; many would screen those with a major risk of premature delivery and treat those who are positive.[8] Other reported complications in patients with bacterial vaginosis are an increased incidence of PID after first-trimester abortion, an increased incidence of postpartum endometritis, chorioamnionitis, and an increased rate of vaginal cuff cellulitis after vaginal hysterectomy.[7]

Classic diagnostic criteria for bacterial vaginosis (Amstel's criteria) are that a patient must demonstrate three of the following: homogeneous vaginal discharge, more than 20% clue cells, amine (fishy) odor when potassium hydroxide is added to vaginal secretions, pH greater than 4.5, and absence of normal vaginal lactobacilli.[7]

Symptomatic patients with bacterial vaginosis should be treated, and in general, asymptomatic patients should not. However, it may be advisable to screen women who are candidates for Cesarean section, first-trimester abortion, or hysterectomy and treat those who are positive before the procedures.[9] Three standard treatment modalities for bacterial vaginosis are oral metronidazole, intravaginal metronidazole gel, and intravaginal clindamycin cream. In a comparative study of these three regimens all were equally effective, although patient satisfaction was greatest with the intravaginal products.[10] Specific treatment regimens include metronidazole (Flagyl) tablets 500 mg bid for 7 days or, as an alternative that may be less effective, 2 g as a single dose; 0.75% metronidazole vaginal gel (MetroGel-Vaginal) one applicator full once or twice daily for 5 days; or 2% clindamycin vaginal cream (Cleocin, Dalacin), 1 application qhs for 7 days.[2,9] Clindamycin 300 mg bid po for 7 days is also effective.[9]

Trichomoniasis

The usual treatment of trichomoniasis is metronidazole (Flagyl) 500 mg po bid for 7 days or 2 g as a single oral dose.[2] A recent study found that a single dose of 1.5 g was as effective as the 2-g single-dose treatment.[11] Although metronidazole is generally considered contraindicated during the first trimester of pregnancy,[2] the evidence for this is tenuous. A metaanalysis of patients exposed to orally ad-

ministered metronidazole in the first trimester found no increased teratogenicity.[12]

―――――― **REFERENCES** ――――――

1. Eason EL, Feldman P: Contact dermatitis associated with the use of Always sanitary napkins, *Can Med Assoc J* 154:1173-1176, 1996.
2. Drugs for sexually transmitted diseases, *Med Lett* 37:117-122, 1995.
3. Sobel JD, Brooker D, Stein GE, et al: Single oral dose fluconazole compared with conventional clotrimazole topical therapy of candidal vaginitis, *Am J Obstet Gynecol* 172:1263-1268, 1995.
4. Steinberg WM: Avoiding recurrent yeast infections, *Patient Care Can* 5:11, 1994.
5. Hilton E, Isenberg HD, Alperstein P, et al: Ingestion of yogurt containing *Lactobacillus acidophilus* as prophylaxis for candidal vaginitis, *Ann Intern Med* 116:353-357, 1992.
6. Brocklehurst P: Infection and preterm delivery: there is not yet enough evidence that antibiotics help (editorial), *BMJ* 318: 548-549, 1999.
7. Majeroni BA: Bacterial vaginosis: an update, *Am Fam Physician* 57:1285-1289, 1998.
8. Ferris DG: Management of bacterial vaginosis during pregnancy (editorial), *Am Fam Physician* 57:1215-1216, 1218, 1228, 1998.
9. Society of Obstetricians and Gynaecologists of Canada: Clinical practice guidelines: committee opinion; bacterial vaginosis, *J SOGC* 19(5):528-533, 1997.
10. Ferris DG, Litaker MS, Woodward L, et al: Treatment of bacterial vaginosis—a comparison of oral metronidazole, metronidazole vaginal gel, and clindamycin vaginal cream, *J Fam Pract* 41:443-449, 1995.
11. Spence MR, Harwell TS, Davies MC, et al: The minimum single oral metronidazole dose for treating trichomoniasis: a randomized, blinded study, *Obstet Gynecol* 89:699-703, 1997.
12. Burtin P, Taddio A, Ariburnu O, et al: Safety of metronidazole in pregnancy: a meta-analysis, *Am J Obstet Gynecol* 172:525-529, 1995.

HEMATOLOGY

Topics covered in this section

Anemia
Anticoagulants
Bleeding Disorders
Leukemias
Lymphadenopathy
Lymphomas
Multiple Myeloma
Sedimentation Rate
Transfusions
Vitamin B_{12}

ANEMIA

(See also aspirin; fecal occult blood screening; hematochezia; hemorrhoids; leukemias; peptic ulcers; restless legs syndrome; sports medicine; vitamin B$_{12}$)

Microcytic Anemias

The differential diagnosis of microcytic anemias includes iron deficiency anemia, thalassemia, and the anemia of chronic disease (usually normocytic but microcytic in 20% to 30% of cases). Classic findings of these anemias on laboratory examination are as follows[1]:

Iron deficiency	Mean corpuscular volume (MCV) usually <80, red blood cell distribution width index (RDW) >15, decreased reticulocytes, decreased ferritin level, elevated iron binding capacity, low serum iron level
Thalassemia	MCV often <70, normal RDW, normal reticulocyte count, target cells in peripheral smear
Anemia of chronic disease	Hemoglobin level usually >90 g/L (9 g/dl), MCV normal or low but >72, ferritin level normal or elevated

Iron deficiency anemias

Sequence of laboratory changes. Iron deficiency usually develops in the following sequence of changes[1]:

1. Decreased ferritin
2. Decreased MCV
3. Decreased hemoglobin
4. Subjective symptoms (usually when the hemoglobin level reaches 8 g/dl [80 g/L])

Some patients with mild iron deficiency have normal red blood cell indices.[2] The most useful test for diagnosing iron deficiency is the serum ferritin level.[3] In one study of elderly patients, ferritin levels less than 18 μg/L (18 ng/ml) were almost pathognomonic of iron deficiency, while levels above 100 μg/L (100 ng/ml) virtually ruled it out.[4]

Ferritin is an acute-phase reactant that tends to rise in cases of inflammatory or neoplastic disease and is therefore usually elevated in the anemias associated with chronic diseases. Patients with iron deficiency anemias in addition to neoplastic or other chronic disease may have a normal or elevated ferritin level. In such situations a bone marrow examination may be necessary to assess iron stores.

Sources of gastrointestinal bleeding in iron deficiency anemia. Gastrointestinal lesions are a common cause of chronic iron deficiency anemia, although 38% of adults with this condition have no demonstrable gastrointestinal lesions. According to one review, if patients with chronic iron deficiency anemia have specific gastrointestinal symptoms, the physician should first investigate the area suggested by the symptoms, and if a lesion is found, further investigation is not warranted. If no localizing symptoms are present and the patient is old, the most useful initial investigation is colonoscopy; if a colon lesion is found, upper gastrointestinal endoscopy is not needed.[5] Others believe that both the upper and lower intestinal tracts should be investigated re-

gardless of what is found during the initial procedure. A review of this approach performed for iron deficiency anemia in 89 patients over the age of 60 found that close to half of the 13 with colon cancer also had "acceptable" upper gastrointestinal causes for their anemia.[6]

The investigation of patients who test positive for fecal occult blood but are not anemic is discussed in the section on hematochezia.

Symptoms. Does iron deficiency anemia cause symptoms? The literature on this subject is sparse, and the only community-based study I could find, done by the British Medical Research Council in Wales in the 1960s, was on 20- to 64-year-old women with hemoglobin levels between 8 and 12 g/dl (80 and 120 g/L) as a result of iron deficiency. Symptoms including fatigue, dizziness, and breathlessness did not correlate with levels of hemoglobin, and patients randomly assigned to receive iron therapy experienced no greater subjective improvement than those given placebo.[7] However, hemoglobin levels less than 7.5 g/dl (75 g/L) appear to be related to symptoms including fatigue and shortness of breath, at least in patients undergoing dialysis therapy; erythropoietin therapy significantly relieved symptoms in this group of patients.[8] The message for family physicians is that complaints of fatigue in mildly anemic but otherwise well patients may not be related to the anemia and may not resolve with iron therapy.

Iron therapy. Numerous formulations of oral iron preparations are available for the treatment of iron deficiency anemia. The three major ones are ferrous sulfate, ferrous fumarate, and ferrous gluconate. The amount of elemental iron varies among these products. In general elemental iron makes up 20% to 30% of ferrous sulfate, 30% of ferrous fumarate, and 11% of ferrous gluconate. Doses should be calculated on the basis of elemental iron. For the treatment of iron deficiency anemia, adults usually require elemental iron 100 to 200 mg/day in divided doses, and children 3 mg/kg/day in divided doses.

Upper gastrointestinal tract discomfort, constipation, and sometimes diarrhea are the most frequent adverse effects of iron therapy,[9] and their severity depends on the dose of elemental iron.[10] Methods of minimizing these effects are to take the medication with meals, to increase the dose gradually, and to keep the total daily dose as low as possible.[10] Ferrous gluconate has been said to be tolerated better than ferrous sulfate; this may simply be a dose-related phenomenon. A standard dose of ferrous sulfate is 300 mg tid, which gives a daily dose of elemental iron of approximately 200 mg, whereas 300 mg of ferrous gluconate tid gives approximately 100 mg of elemental iron per day. In general, treatment for iron deficiency anemia should be continued for 4 to 6 months or until the serum ferritin level reaches 50 μg/L (50 ng/ml).[11]

Treatment with iron should cause reticulocytosis to begin within 3 to 5 days. If no such response is seen, the patient is not being compliant or the diagnosis is wrong.[1] Treatment with ferrous sulfate should raise the hemoglobin level by 20 g/L (0.2 g/dl) per day if there is no continued blood loss.[11]

Macrocytic Anemias

The following are some of the more important causes of macrocytic anemia:

1. Vitamin B_{12} deficiency (pernicious anemia)
2. Folate deficiency (often nutritional in elderly; celiac disease in younger patients)
3. Liver disease (alcoholism)
4. Hypothyroidism
5. Myelodysplasia (refractory anemia, sideroblastic anemia)
6. Acute bleeding or hemolysis with reticulocytosis (reticulocytes are larger than mature red blood cells)

Myelodysplasia is a common cause of macrocytic anemia in the elderly and usually has little clinical import (see discussion of leukemia).

Megaloblastic anemias often have oval macrocytosis and an MCV greater than 115 fL (115 μm^3). In chronic liver disease the macrocytosis is generally between 100 and 110 fL and oval macrocytes are not seen in the peripheral smear.[1]

Pernicious anemia is an autoimmune disease and may be associated with other autoimmune conditions such as Hashimoto's thyroiditis, Graves' disease, Addison's disease, primary hypoparathyroidism, primary ovarian failure, myasthenia gravis, and vitiligo.[12] Over 25% of patients with pernicious anemia who have neurological symptoms have normal hematocrits or normal MCVs.[13]

Laboratory testing for pernicious anemia is complex because the sensitivity and specificity of many tests are low. Initial clues to the diagnosis often come from the incidental finding of anemia or an elevated MCV in the complete blood count and the presence of oval macrocytes or hypersegmented polymorphonuclear leukocytes on the peripheral smear. When pernicious anemia is suspected, serum cobalamin (vitamin B_{12}) levels should be ascertained. Although the lower limit of normal is usually considered to be 148 pmol/L (200 pg/ml), levels may be decreased in numerous other conditions, including folate deficiency, and many patients with cobalamin deficiency do not have decreased levels. However, if the levels are below 74 pmol/L (100 pg/ml), the odds are high that the patient has cobalamin deficiency. Other useful tests are measurements of serum methylmalonic acid and serum homocysteine levels. Both are usually elevated in patients with cobalamin deficiency, whereas only homocysteine is elevated in folate deficiency. Eighty-five percent of patients with pernicious anemia have antiparietal cell antibodies in the serum, and about 50% have anti–intrinsic factor antibodies. Antiparietal antibodies are not specific, since they are present in 3% to 5% of healthy persons and many individuals with autoimmune endocrinopathies, whereas anti–intrinsic factor antibodies are quite specific. Bone marrow analysis and the Schilling test are rarely indicated.[13]

Treatment of pernicious anemia consists of monthly injections of at least 100 μg of vitamin B_{12}.[12]

➷ REFERENCES ⚜

1. Yeo EL: Anemia: a practical approach, *Can J Diagn* 13:79-92, 1996.
2. Macdonald D: How to recognize real deficiencies of iron, folate, vitamin B_{12}, *Patient Care Can* 7:6, 1996.
3. Guyatt GH, Oxman AD, Ali M, et al: Laboratory diagnosis of iron-deficiency anemia: an overview, *J Gen Intern Med* 7:145-153, 1992.
4. Guyatt GH, Patterson C, Ali M, et al: Diagnosis of iron-deficiency anemia in the elderly, *Am J Med* 88:205-209, 1990.
5. Rockey DC: Occult gastrointestinal bleeding, *N Engl J Med* 341:38-46, 1999.
6. Till SH, Grundman MJ: Prevalence of concomitant disease in patients with iron deficiency anaemia, *BMJ* 314:206-208, 1997.
7. Elwood P, Water WE, Greene WJ, et al: Symptoms and circulating haemoglobin level, *J Chronic Dis* 21:615-628, 1969.
8. Canadian Erythropoietin Study Group: Association between recombinant human erythropoietin and quallity of life and excercise capacity of patients receiving hemodialysis, *BMJ* 300:573-578, 1990.
9. Swerdlow PS: A tradition of testing ironclad practices (editorial), *JAMA* 267:560-561, 1992.
10. Wingard RL, Parker RA, Ismail N, et al: Efficacy of oral iron therapy in patients receiving recombinant human erythropoietin, *Am J Kidney Dis* 25:433-439, 1995.
11. Swain RA, Kaplan B, Montgomery E: Iron deficiency anemia: when is parenteral therapy warranted? *Postgrad Med* 100:181-182, 185, 188-193, 1996.
12. Ban-Hock Toh, van Driel IR, Gleeson PA: Pernicious anemia, *N Engl J Med* 337:1441-1448, 1997.
13. Snow CF: Laboratory diagnosis of vitamin B_{12} and folate deficiency: a guide for the primary care physician, *Arch Intern Med* 159:1289-1298, 1999.

ANTICOAGULANTS

(See also atrial fibrillation; cerebrovascular accidents; dentistry; myocardial infarction; prosthetic valves; thrombophlebitis; transient ischemic attacks)

Both diet and drugs can influence warfarin (Coumadin) levels.[1,2] Vitamin K, which is found predominantly in green leafy vegetables and certain legumes, such as avocados, broccoli, brussels sprouts, and lettuce, antagonizes the action of warfarin. Individuals eating a lot of these vegetables are at low risk of having excessively high international normalized ratios (INRs), whereas those eating few vitamin K–containing foods are at high risk of having high INRs.[1]

Many drugs potentiate or antagonize the effects of warfarin. Some of the more common agents that tend to increase the INR are erythromycin, metronidazole (Flagyl), isoniazid, some nonsteroidal antiinflammatory drugs, cimetidine (Tagamet), and omeprazole (Prilosec, Losec).[2] Acetaminophen can also raise the INR and is of particular concern to family physicians because outpatients frequently take the drug without informing their doctors.[1] Drugs that tend to lower the INR include barbiturates, carbamazepine (Tegretol), chlordiazepoxide (Librium), cholestyramine (Questran), and sucralfate (Sulcrate).[2]

Desirable levels of INR for patients taking warfarin are shown in Table 30.[3,4] Approximate INR-PT ratios are listed in Table 31.

If a patient is to receive anticoagulatants as an outpatient, one common method is to start with warfarin 10 mg/day for 2 to 4 days, adjusted according to frequent INR or PT readings. Effective anticoagulation is achieved almost as quickly and with less risk if 5 mg of warfarin is used from the beginning of treatment.[5] Alternatively, the estimated maintenance dosage of warfarin (4 mg/day for those under 70 years and 3 mg/day for those 70 or older) can be used from the onset.[6]

Traditionally, initial INR readings have been obtained daily; this is illogical because the full effect of a change in a warfarin dose does not manifest itself for 36 to 72 hours.[7] A better system is to begin measuring the INR on day 2 and continue with readings every 48 hours until control is achieved. Thereafter the intervals between INR readings are increased.[8]

Management of excessively elevated INRs in patients who are taking anticoagulants and are not actively bleeding is controversial. The guidelines of the American College of Chest Physicians suggest that for patients who are not bleeding and whose INR is <6, warfarin be withheld for a few doses; for those with an INR between 6 and 10, warfarin should be withheld and 1 to 2 mg of vitamin K (phyto-

nadione) should be administered subcutaneously; for those with an INR >10, warfarin should be withheld and 3 mg of vitamin K should be administered subcutaneously.[4] Since few studies supporting these guidelines have been published, and since vitamin K administration can result in thromboembolic events or subsequent difficulty in reestablishing anticoagulation, many physicians treat INR elevations as high as 10 by simply withholding warfarin doses. This approach is supported by two retrospective studies.[9,10]

Anticoagulants do not have to be temporarily discontinued before dental surgery (see section on dentistry),[11] and aspiration or injection of joints of anticoagulated patients appears safe provided INR levels are not excessive.[12]

If anticoagulants have to be discontinued for surgery, Hirsch[13] suggests discontinuing the warfarin and starting subcutaneous injections of low-molecular-weight heparin in full therapeutic doses 4 days before the procedure. The low-molecular-weight heparin should be stopped 14 hours before surgery and restarted at prophylactic (not therapeutic) doses 12 hours after surgery. Warfarin should also be restarted 12 hours after surgery. The low-molecular-weight heparin is discontinued when INR readings have been between 2 and 3 for 2 consecutive days.

Low-molecular-weight heparins are discussed under "Thrombophlebitis."

Table 30 Desirable INR Levels for Anticoagulation with Warfarin

Desirable INR level	Clinical condition
0.8-1.2	Normal
2.1-3.0*	All other conditions including mechanical heart valves[3] (some authors recommend that for mechanical heart valves the levels be 2.5 to 3.5[4])

INR, International normalized ratio.
*As indicated, the therapeutic levels of warfarin for most conditions, including atrial fibrillation, are those that maintain an INR of 2 to 3. This is roughly equivalent to a PT of 1.3 to 1.5.

Table 31 Approximate INR–Prothrombin Time Equivalencies

INR	Prothrombin time ratio
2	1.3
3	1.5
4	2.0

INR, International normalized ratio.

✎ REFERENCES ✍

1. Hylek EM, Heiman H, Skates SJ, et al: Acetaminophen and other risk factors for excessive warfarin anticoagulation, *JAMA* 279:657-662, 1998.
2. Wells PS, Holbrook AM, Crowther NR, et al: Interactions of warfarin with drugs and food, *Ann Intern Med* 121:676-683, 1994.
3. Saour JN, Sieck JO, Mamo LA, et al: Trial of different intensities of anticoagulation in patients with prosthetic heart valves, *N Engl J Med* 322:428-432, 1990.
4. Hirsh J, Dalen JE, Deykin D, et al: Oral anticoagulants: mechanism of action, clinical effectiveness and optimal therapeutic range, *Chest* 102(suppl):312S-326S, 1992.
5. Crowther MA, Ginsberg JB, Kearon C, et al: A randomized trial comparing 5-mg and 10-mg warfarin loading doses, *Arch Intern Med* 159:46-48, 1999.
6. Ezekowitz MD, Levine JA: Preventing stroke in patients with atrial fibrillation, *JAMA* 281:1830-1835, 1999.
7. Brigden ML: Oral anticoagulant therapy, newer indications and an improved method of monitoring, *Postgrad Med* 91:285-296, 1992.
8. Hanna MM, Meuser J: Time to change: rationalizing the daily PT, daily Coumadin order, *Can Fam Physician* 42:513, 1996.
9. Glover JJ: Conservative treatment of overanticoagulated patients, *Chest* 108:987-990, 1995.
10. Lousberg TR, Witt DM, Beall DG, et al: Evaluation of excessive anticoagulation in a group model health maintenance organization, *Arch Intern Med* 158:528-534, 1998.
11. Wahl MJ: Dental surgery in anticoagulated patients, *Arch Intern Med* 158:1610-1616, 1998.

12. Thumboo J, O'Duffy JD: A prospective study of the safety of joint and soft tissue aspirations and injections in patients taking warfarin sodium, *Arthritis Rheum* 41:736-739, 1998.

13. Hirsch J: Anticoagulant therapy and soft tissue surgery, *Patient Care Can* 10(9):8, 1999.

BLEEDING DISORDERS

Bleeding disorders are suspected on the basis of personal and family history and confirmed by laboratory tests. Standard investigations are a complete blood count and smear, PT, partial thromboplastin time (PTT), thrombin time or fibrinogen level, and bleeding time.[1]

Hemophilia

Two types of hemophilia are recognized. The classic form, or hemophilia type A, is caused by factor VIII deficiency, and the type B form, or Christmas disease, is caused by factor IX deficiency. Between 80% and 85% of cases are type A. Laboratory tests show a prolonged PTT and a normal PT and bleeding time. Both variants of the disease are sex-linked recessive. For optimal treatment of bleeding episodes, therapy should be initiated at the immediate onset of each incident. This is best done with home therapy in which the parents, other caregivers, or the patients themselves are trained to give replacement therapy preparations. The effective organization of such a program usually requires a specialized team.[2]

Thrombocytopenia

A low platelet count as reported by an automated counter may be an artifact caused by platelet clumping. This is easily determined by ordering a smear. If present, the platelet clumps will be seen.[3]

Immune thrombocytopenic purpura (ITP), which is also called idiopathic thrombocytopenic purpura, may occur as an acute (acute ITP) or chronic (chronic ITP) disorder. The chronic form is more common in adults and is often detected incidentally when a low platelet count is reported in a complete blood count.[3,4] Splenomegaly is rare. About three fourths of adult cases are in women, and most are in persons under 40.[4] The prognosis for adult cases is excellent.[5]

A harmless, self-limited form of thrombocytopenia is incidental thrombocytopenia of pregnancy. It occurs in the third trimester and does not cause maternal or fetal bleeding.[3]

Other causes of thrombocytopenia include drugs, some viral infections, hypersplenism, thrombotic thrombocytopenic purpura, autoimmune diseases such as lupus, lymphoproliferative disorders, and myelodysplasia.[4]

Bleeding after trauma or surgery may occur with platelet counts less than 50×10^9/L (50,000/mm^3), and serious spontaneous bleeding develops at levels less than 20×10^9 (20,000/mm^3).[1] Massive gastrointestinal bleeding and intracerebral bleeding are most often seen with levels less than 5×10^9/L (5000/mm^3).[6]

Treatment of chronic ITP is necessary only if the platelet count decreases to dangerous levels, which are somewhere around 20 to 30×10^9/L (20,000 to 30,000/mm^3). Prednisone at a dose of 1 mg/kg is the first line of therapy. Some patients require a splenectomy.[4] Nonbleeding patients rarely require platelet transfusions if platelet counts are above 5×10^9/L (5000/mm^3).[6]

A patient with thrombocytopenia must never be given aspirin.[6]

Von Willebrand's disease

Von Willebrand's disease is the most common inherited coagulopathy, with an incidence of about 1%. It is caused by an abnormality or reduction of von Willebrand's factor, which has the dual function of stabilizing factor VIII levels and promoting normal platelet functioning. The disease has an autosomal dominant inheritance, and most cases are mild. Bruising, nosebleeds, profuse bleeding from cuts, and hemorrhage after dental extractions are common, but hemarthroses are rare. When hemarthroses do occur, the bleeding begins immediately, whereas with coagulation defects such as hemophilia it is often delayed 12 to 24 hours. Classically the bleeding time is prolonged, and levels of factor VIII and von Willebrand factor are low. Repeated testing may be necessary to detect these abnormalities.[1,2]

───────────── ⚑ REFERENCES ✍ ─────────────

1. Hampton KK, Preston FE: ABC of clinical haematology: bleeding disorders, thrombosis and anticoagulation, *BMJ* 314:1026-1029, 1997.

2. Association of Hemophilia Clinic Directors of Canada: Hemophilia and von Willebrand's disease. 1. Diagnosis, comprehensive care and assessment, *Can Med Assoc J* 153:19-25, 1995.

3. Goldstein KH, Abramson N: Efficient diagnosis of thrombocytopenia, *Am Fam Physician* 53:915-920, 1996.

4. George JN, el-Harake MA, Raskob GE: Chronic idiopathic thrombocytopenic purpura, *N Engl J Med* 331:1207-1211, 1994.

5. Kirchner JT: Acute and chronic immune thrombocytopenic purpura: disorders that differ in more than duration, *Postgrad Med* 92:112-118, 125-126, 1992.

6. Beutler E: Platelet transfusion: the 20,000/microL trigger, *Blood* 81:1411-1413, 1993.

LEUKEMIAS
Childhood Leukemias

Acute lymphoblastic leukemia (ALL) accounts for 85% of childhood leukemias, and the peak age of incidence is 3 to 4 years.[1] Although claims have been made that long-term exposure to magnetic fields from high-tension power lines is a risk factor, a large case-control study failed to find such a correlation.[2] Over 97% of children with ALL have complete remission after initial therapy, and the cure rate approaches 80%. Late sequelae in cured children include brain tumors, acute myeloid leukemia, cardiomyopathy, short stature, and obesity. Brain tumors, short stature, and obesity are particularly prevalent among children who have had cranial irradiation. In most instances intensive systemic chemotherapy or intrathecal chemotherapy (or both) successfully eradicates leukemic cells from the central nervous system, so cranial radiation is rarely necessary. [3]

Acute Myeloid Leukemia

The overall 4-year survival rate for acute myeloid leukemia in adolescents and adults is 35%. Induction chemotherapy leads to complete remission in 70%. Whether bone marrow transplant is more effective than chemotherapy alone as postremission treatment is controversial. A 1998 study found that it was not.[4]

Chronic Lymphocytic Leukemia

The median age of persons with chronic lymphocytic leukemia (CLL) is 65 years, and only 10% to 15% of patients are younger than 50. The prognosis of CLL is variable. The median survival is 9 years. Patients with early stable disease do not require treatment.[5,6] When the disease is more advanced, chlorambucil is usually the drug of first choice.[5]

Chronic Myeloid Leukemia

Chronic myeloid leukemia usually affects middle-aged adults. Nearly half of all patients are asymptomatic at the time of diagnosis, and the disease is detected only because of an abnormal blood count. An initial stable chronic phase is followed within 3 to 5 years by a rapidly fatal blastic phase. Optimal treatment of the blastic phase is high-dose chemotherapy and allogeneic bone marrow transplantation from a suitable donor, who is usually a sibling. With this treatment up to 70% of patients are alive after 10 years, but unfortunately only 20% to 30% of patients are candidates for bone marrow transplantation.[7]

The chronic phase is usually treated with interferon, although bone marrow transplant may be considered for a few patients. About 30% of patients in the advanced phase revert to the chronic phase after treatment with hydroxyurea (Hydrea) or busulphan (Myleran).[7]

Myelodysplasia

Myelodysplasia (refractory anemia, sideroblastic anemia) is considered a preleukemic condition, although leukemia is by no means an inevitable outcome of the disorder. Bone marrow cellularity is normal or increased, but because of defects in cell maturation patients may have anemia, neutropenia, or thrombocytopenia. Although some patients have such initial symptoms as dyspnea, infections, bleeding, or bruising, many are clinically well and the disorder is detected as a result of abnormal routine complete blood counts. Most patients with myelodysplasia are elderly. The prognosis is extremely variable and depends in part on the percentage of blast cells in the marrow. Patients with fewer than 5% blasts are likely to remain well for many years and die of other causes, whereas those with more than 5% blasts

have a 30% to 75% chance of bone marrow failure or the development of acute myelogenous leukemia.[8]

REFERENCES

1. Liesner RJ, Goldstone AH: The acute leukaemias, *BMJ* 314: 733-736, 1997.
2. Linet MS, Hatch EE, Kleinerman RA, et al: Residential exposure to magnetic fields and acute lymphoblastic leukemia in children, *N Engl J Med* 337:1-7, 1997.
3. Pui C-H: Childhood leukemias, *N Engl J Med* 332:1618-1630, 1995.
4. Cassileth PA, Harrington DP, Appelbaum FR, et al: Chemotherapy compared with autologous or allogeneic bone marrow transplantation in the management of acute myeloid leukemia at first remission, *N Engl J Med* 339:1649-1656, 1998.
5. Rozman C, Montserrat E: Chronic lymphocytic leukemia, *N Engl J Med* 333:1052-1057, 1995.
6. Dighiero G, Maloum K, Desablens B, et al: Chlorambucil in indolent chronic lymphocytic leukemia, *N Engl J Med* 338:1506-1514, 1998.
7. Sawyers CL: Chronic myeloid leukemia, *N Engl J Med* 340: 1330-1340, 1999.
8. Heaney ML, Golde DW: Myelodysplasia, *N Engl J Med* 340: 1649-1660, 1999.

LYMPHADENOPATHY

The causes of most cases of lymphadenopathy in primary care are easily diagnosed. Unexplained lymphadenopathy is of more concern, but in the primary care setting only 1% turn out to be malignant.[1]

If lymphadenopathy is present in two or more noncontiguous areas, it is classified as generalized. If it is limited to one region, it is localized. In general, patients with localized lymphadenopathy of undetermined etiology who are otherwise well may be observed for 3 to 4 weeks. If improvement is noted, no further action is needed. Patients with generalized adenopathy of undetermined etiology usually require further investigation. Red flags for malignancy include the presence of supraclavicular nodes, stony hard nodes, and constitutional symptoms. Painful or tender nodes may be a manifestation of either an inflammatory or a neoplastic process.[1]

REFERENCES

1. Ferrer R: Lymphadenopathy: differential diagnosis and evaluation, *Am Fam Physician* 58:1313-1320, 1998.

LYMPHOMAS

The Ann Arbor staging system for lymphomas is as follows[1]:

Stage I	Single lymphoid or extranodal site
Stage II	Two lymphoid or extranodal sites on the same side of the diaphragm
Stage III	Lymphoid areas (including spleen) on both sides of the diaphragm
Stage IV	Diffuse involvement of extranodal organs (e.g., bone marrow, liver)

Symptoms of lymphomas are categorized as A if the patient has no systemic symptoms or B if the patient has weight loss, fever, or drenching night sweats.[1]

Hodgkin's Disease

Localized Hodgkin's disease is generally treated with radiation therapy, and more widespread disease with chemotherapy. The overall cure rate is 70% to 80%.[1]

Second tumors are common among children treated for Hodgkin's disease.[1-3] In one study the cumulative risk was 7% by 15 years.[1] The incidence of leukemia reached a plateau by 14 years, but such a leveling off was not seen with solid tumors. Breast cancer was the most common solid tumor, with a relative risk 75 times that of the normal population. The risk was related to radiation and was greatest in girls treated between the ages of 10 and 16 (when breast tissue was proliferating). Other solid tumors were thyroid cancers, basal cell carcinomas of the skin, brain tumors, bone tumors, and colorectal cancers.[1-3]

Non-Hodgkin's Lymphoma

Low-grade non-Hodgkin's lymphoma is a disease of the elderly. Ninety percent of patients are over the age of 50. Most of the follicular lymphomas fall into the non-Hodgkin's lymphoma group. These neoplasms have a similar epidemiology and natural course to chronic lymphocytic leukemia. The tumors are often widespread but indolent with slow progression over many years. The median survival is 5 to 8 years, and cure is rarely possible. Patients without symptoms do not necessarily require treatment. As the disease progresses, chemotherapy may be offered, often in the form of chlorambucil (Leukeran),[1,4] cyclophosphamide (Cytoxan), or fludarabine (Fludara). A new therapy that is effective for some patients is the monoclonal antibody rituximab (Rituxan).[4]

Intermediate-grade non-Hodgkin's lymphoma affects all age groups. The most common form is a diffuse large cell lymphoma that is a B cell neoplasm. These tumors are rapidly progressive, are often associated with type B symptoms, and require therapy.[1] The usual regimen involves several courses of chemotherapy, including doxorubicin (Adriamycin, Rubex) plus other agents such as vincristine (Oncovin, Vincasar), cyclophosphamide (Cytoxan), and prednisone. Chemotherapy may be combined with radiation therapy. The overall 5-year survival is about 40%,[1] but it exceeds 64% for those with stage I and II disease.[5]

High-grade non-Hodgkin's lymphomas make up only 5% of the non-Hodgkin's lymphomas. The high-grade form is primarily a disease of children and young adults.[1] The cure rate for non-Hodgkin's lymphoma in children is about 70%.[6]

◤ REFERENCES ◢

1. Mead GM: ABC of clinical haematology: malignant lymphomas and chronic lymphocytic leukaemia, *BMJ* 314:1103-1106, 1997.
2. Bhatia S, Robison LL, Oberlin O, et al: Breast cancer and other second neoplasms after childhood Hodgkin's disease, *N Engl J Med* 334:745-751, 1996.
3. Donaldson SS, Hancock SL: Second cancers after Hodgkin's disease in childhood (editorial), *N Engl J Med* 334:792-793, 1996.
4. Rituximab for non-Hodgkin's lymphoma, *Med Lett* 40:65-66, 1998.
5. Miller TP, Dahlberg S, Cassady R, et al: Chemotherapy alone compared with chemotherapy plus radiotherapy for localized intermediate- and high-grade non-Hodgkin's lymphoma, *N Engl J Med* 339:21-26, 1998.
6. Sandlund JT, Downing JR, Crist WM: Non-Hodgkin's lymphoma in childhood, *N Engl J Med* 334:1238-1248, 1996.

MULTIPLE MYELOMA
(See also metastatic breast cancer; osteoporosis)

Multiple myeloma is more common in whites than blacks and is rare in persons of Asian descent.[1]

In multiple myeloma the neoplastic plasma cells may grow diffusely in the bone marrow or, less commonly, form neoplastic tumors within the bone. They generally produce monoclonal peaks of IgG or IgA. The tumor induces osteoclastic activity, which results in diffuse osteoporosis, lytic lesions, and fractures. Bone pain is the initial complaint of about 60% of patients, and lassitude is another important symptom. The latter is thought to be due to anemia, hypercalcemia, or dehydration. Dehydration is a frequent complication of the disease and is due to proximal tubular dysfunction caused by damage from light chain excretion. Bacterial infections are common.[2]

Frequent laboratory abnormalities include normocytic anemia, elevated creatinine and calcium levels, and the presence of monoclonal bands (paraproteins) as determined by electrophoretic evaluations of blood or urine.[1] Bone scans are often negative in multiple myeloma. This is because the lesions are predominantly lytic and new bone formation is necessary for a bone scan to be positive.[3]

A major differential diagnosis of patients with serum M-protein peaks is benign monoclonal gammopathy or monoclonal gammopathy of undetermined significance (MGUS).[2] Monoclonal gammopathy of undetermined significance is characterized by an M-protein level less than 3 g/dl (30 g/L) that stays stable over time, less than 10% plasma cells in the bone marrow, no or very little M-protein in the urine (Bence Jones proteinuria), and absence of other clinical or laboratory findings typical of multiple myeloma. A 20- to 35-year follow-up of 241 patients with MGUS at the Mayo Clinic found that serious hematological disorders developed in one fourth of the patients (multiple myeloma in most cases, but also Waldenström's macroglobulinemia and other lymphoproliferative disorders) after a median follow-up of 22 years. The actuarial rate of the development of hematological malignancies was 17% after 10 years and 33% after 20 years. Patients with MGUS require no treatment but should have follow-up examinations at regular intervals.[4]

Patients experience considerable anxiety when told they have something wrong with their plasma cells that is not really serious but could become cancer after many years. The physician should not look for M-proteins without a good reason to suspect that the patient has multiple myeloma.

The treatment of myeloma depends on the symptoms and laboratory findings. Patients who are asymptomatic and who do not have significant anemia, renal failure, or severe bone lesions on x-ray examination are classified as having "smoldering" disease that may be followed without treatment. Other patients are treated with a high fluid intake of 3 L/day plus a chemotherapy regimen. The traditional regimen is melphalan (Alkeran) plus prednisone. Other protocols include combinations of multiple chemotherapeutic agents[1,2] or, according to one small trial, thalidomide (Thalomid).[5] The median survival of patients receiving active treatment is 3 years[1] with less than one third surviving 5 years.[5]

Berenson and associates[6] in a study of patients with multiple myeloma who had at least one lytic bone lesion reported that 90 mg of pamidronate (Aredia) given as an IV infusion over 4 hours every 4 weeks for nine cycles decreased pain significantly compared with control subjects. Few adverse effects were reported.

◣ REFERENCES ◤

1. George ED, Sadovsky R: Multiple myeloma: recognition and management, *Am Fam Physician* 59:1885-1892, 1999.
2. Bataille R, Harousseau J-L: Multiple myeloma, *N Engl J Med* 336:1657-1664, 1997.
3. Jacobson AF: Musculoskeletal pain as an indicator of occult malignancy: yield of bone scintigraphy, *Arch Intern Med* 157:105-109, 1997.
4. Kyle RA: Monoclonal gammopathy of undetermined significance, *Blood Rev* 8:135-141, 1994.
5. Raje, N, Anderson K: Thalidomide—a revival story (editorial), *N Engl J Med* 341:1606-1609, 1999.
6. Berenson JR, Lichtenstein A, Porter L, et al (Myeloma Aredia Study Group): Efficacy of pamidronate in reducing skeletal events in patients with advanced multiple myeloma, *N Engl J Med* 334:529-530, 1996.

SEDIMENTATION RATE
(See also connective tissue diseases; polymyalgia rheumatica)

Various reference values have been proposed for the upper limits of normal for sedimentation rates (Westergren method). Higher normal ranges are usually between 20 and 30 mm/hr. The sedimentation rate rises with age and is higher in women than men. It is also increased by anemia, pregnancy, obesity, and renal failure. Most cases of elevated sedimentation rates are not associated with significant disease,[1,2] and these elevations may persist for prolonged periods.[1]

The sedimentation rate is not an appropriate screening test for asymptomatic individuals and has no value in identifying serious disease in patients with nonspecific symptoms. Elevated sedimentation rates have diagnostic significance for only two diseases: polymyalgia rheumatica and temporal arteritis. Only 1% to 2% of patients with temporal arteritis have a normal sedimentation rate[2] compared with one fourth of patients with polymyalgia rheumatica.[3]

Sedimentation rates are claimed to be useful in following the course of four diseases: polymyalgia rheumatica, temporal arteritis, rheumatoid arthritis, and possibly Hodgkin's disease. In no case are these laboratory results as reliable as good clinical evaluations.[1,2]

◣ REFERENCES ◤

1. Zlonis M: The mystique of the erythrocyte sedimentation rate: a reappraisal of one of the oldest laboratory tests still in use, *Clin Lab Med* 13:787-800, 1993.
2. Brigden ML: Clinical utility of the erythrocyte sedimentation rate, *Am Fam Physician* 60:1443-1450, 1999.
3. Helfgott SM, Kieval RI: Polymyalgia rheumatica in patients with a normal erythrocyte sedimentation rate, *Arthritis Rheum* 39:304-307, 1996.

TRANSFUSIONS

A 1996 paper calculated that in the United States the risk of acquiring viral infections from transfusions was 1:493,000 for HIV, 1:103,000 for hepatitis C, and 1:63,000 for hepatitis B.[1] A 1997 estimate for HIV 1 infection from a single unit of blood was 1:641,000.[2] In looking at risk figures such as this, the practitioner must be aware of the variation in risk between urban and rural areas. In one Canadian study the risk of HIV transmission from a single unit of blood in a large urban area (Montreal) was calculated to be about 1:400,000, whereas for Canada as a whole it was assessed as about 1:1,000,000.[3] A 1998 study from Italy that prospectively measured HIV conversion rates in a group of patients with beta-thalassemia who received multiple transfusions found that the risk of acquiring HIV from a single unit of blood was 1:190,000.[4]

In 1999 the U.S. Food and Drug Administration and the Canadian Blood Service decreed that anyone who had spent more than 6 months in Great Britain between 1980 and 1997 could not be a blood donor because of the theoretical risk that they might transmit variant Creutzfeldt-Jakob disease.[5]

Since erythropoietin was synthesized by recombinant DNA technology, it has become commercially available for subcutaneous or IV use in the form of epoetin alfa (Epogen, Procrit, Eprex). It has numerous uses, including short courses for patients before elective surgery either alone or in combination with donating blood for autologous blood transfusions.[6]

◣ REFERENCES ◤

1. Schreiber GB, Busch MP, Kleinman SH, Korelitz JJ (Retrovirus Epidemiology Donor Study): The risk of transfusion-transmitted viral infections, *N Engl J Med* 334:1685-1690, 1996.

2. Guidelines for red blood cell and plasma transfusion for adults and children: report of the Expert Working Group, *Can Med Assoc J* 156(suppl 11):S1-S24, 1997.

3. Remis RS, Delage G, Palmer RW: Risk of HIV infection from blood transfusion in Montreal, *Can Med Assoc J* 157:375-382, 1997.

4. Prati D, Capelli C, Rebulla P, et al: The current risk of retroviral infections transmitted by transfusion in patients who have undergone multiple transfusions, *Arch Intern Med* 158:1566-1569, 1998.

5. Gottlieb S: FDA bans blood donation by people who have lived in UK, *BMJ* 319:535, 1999.

6. Goodnough LT, Monk TG, Andriole GL: Erythropoietin therapy, *N Engl J Med* 336:933-938, 1997.

VITAMIN B$_{12}$
(See also dementia; macrocytic anemia)

Low serum vitamin B$_{12}$ or cobalamin levels have been reported to have a positive predictive value for cobalamin deficiency of only 22%.[1] An evaluation of nondemented persons 75 to 85 years of age showed that low vitamin B$_{12}$ levels were common in this age group but that persons with these findings were no more likely to become demented than were those with normal levels.[2] Large numbers of patients are being inappropriately treated with intramuscular cyanocobalamin. Continued treatment of these patients seems appropriate if they have had megaloblastic anemia, intrinsic factor antibodies, a positive Schilling test, or neuropsychiatric symptoms. Treatment might be discontinued in others, remembering that if a patient has a true deficiency of B$_{12}$, it may take months or years for body stores to become depleted and for symptoms to declare themselves.[3]

─────────── ◼ REFERENCES ◣ ───────────

1. Matchar DB, McCrory DC, Millington DS, et al: Performance of the serum cobalamin assay for diagnosis of cobalamin deficiency, *Am J Med Sci* 308:276-283, 1994.

2. Crystal HA, Ortof E, Frishman WH, et al: Serum vitamin B-12 levels and incidence of dementia in a healthy elderly population—a report from the Bronx longitudinal aging study, *J Am Geriatr Soc* 42:933-936, 1994.

3. Delva MD: Vitamin B$_{12}$ replacement: to B$_{12}$ or not to B$_{12}$? *Can Fam Physician* 43:917-922, 1997.

IMMUNIZATIONS

(See also adoption; hepatitis; infectious diseases; meningococcal disease; pediatrics; tropical medicine)

Topics covered in this section

Storage and Shipping of Vaccines
Immunization Schedules for Children
Haemophilus b Immunization
Hepatitis B Immunization
Influenza Immunization
Measles-Mumps-Rubella Immunization
Pertussis Immunization
Pneumococcal Immunization
Polio Immunization
Rabies Immunization
Rubella Immunization
Tetanus Immunization
Typhoid Fever Immunization
Varicella Immunization

STORAGE AND SHIPPING OF VACCINES

Many vaccines are inactivated if they are exposed to high temperatures or if they are frozen. The jargon for the former phenomenon is "breaking the cold chain." Vaccine inactivation through breaking the cold chain probably occurs frequently in physicians' offices and may also occur during shipping, especially to remote regions. Apparently the Sabin oral polio vaccine can be frozen and thawed without affecting its potency. Some of the specific recommendations for maintaining the cold chain are as follows[1]:

1. Most vaccines should be stored between 2° and 8° C.
2. Refrigerators containing vaccines should have temperature monitors.
3. Refrigerators containing vaccines should not be used for other purposes.
4. The temperature in the refrigerator should be monitored and recorded twice a day.
5. Only vaccines should be kept in the refrigerator; food should be in another refrigerator so that temperature variations from frequent opening and closing of the door are avoided.
6. Vaccines should not be kept in the refrigerator door.
7. There should be space between vaccine vials to allow air circulation.
8. Vaccines should be removed from the refrigerator only to draw up a dose and should be returned to the refrigerator immediately.

─────────── ◼ REFERENCES ◣ ───────────

1. Laboratory Centre For Disease Control: National guidelines for vaccine storage and transportation, *Can Med Assoc J* 154:3534-3554, 1996.

IMMUNIZATION SCHEDULES FOR CHILDREN
(See also *Haemophilus* b immunization; hepatitis immunization; measles-mumps-rubella immunization; pertussis immunization; polio immunization; rabies immunization; tetanus immunization; typhoid fever immunization; varicella immunization)

The recommended immunization schedules for children in Canada and the United States differ in only minor details, many of which involve the exact timing of booster doses.[1,2] Three organizations in the United States—the Advisory Committee on Immunization Practices, the American Academy of Family Physicians, and the American Academy of Pediatrics—issue common annual recommendations for childhood immunizations.[2,3] Some of the important points in the 2000 U.S. recommendations[2] and the way they differ from Canadian recommendations[1] are as follows:

1. Hepatitis B immunizations. For infants born to hepatitis B surface antigen (HBsAg)-negative mothers, three vaccinations are recommended, the first within 12 months of birth, the second at least 1 month after the first dose, and the third at least 4 months after the first dose and at least 2 months after the second but not before 6 months of age. If the mother is HBsAg positive, the infant should receive hepatitis B immune globulin (HBIG) as well as an initial vaccination within 12 hours of birth. The second dose should be given at 1 to 2 months of age and the third dose at 6 months of age.[2] An additional recommendation is that children or adolescents who have not previously been vaccinated for hepatitis B should receive such immunizations whenever they are seen for routine medical care.[2] In Canada hepatitis B immunization may be given in infancy to children who were born of HBsAg-negative mothers, but many jurisdictions recommend that it be given in elementary school instead. This is because the risk of acquiring the infection becomes significant only in adolescence and because of concern that immunizations given in infancy may not be fully effective by the time the child passes through puberty.[1]

2. Diphtheria-tetanus-pertussis (DTP) or diphtheria–tetanus–acellular pertussis (DTaP). Acellular pertussis vaccine combined with DT (DTaP) is now preferred to DTP in both Canada and the United States because it has fewer side effects. The fourth dose may be given anytime between 15 and 18 months, but if there is reason to believe that the child will not be brought in at that time, it may be given as early as 12 months provided that 6 months has elapsed since the third dose. In Canada the fourth dose is given at 18 months. If a series was started with DTP, it may be completed with DTaP.

3. Booster tetanus-diphtheria toxoid (Td). The booster Td dose may be given anytime between 11 and 16 years (preferably between 11 and 12 years provided 5 years has elapsed since the last Td dose). In Canada it is given between 14 and 16 years.

4. *Haemophilus influenzae* type b (Hib). The three Hib vaccines licensed for infant vaccinations in the United States are considered interchangeable. If immunization is started with one brand, a different one may be used for booster doses. This is also acceptable in Canada, but use of the same brand for the entire series is preferred. If Hib conjugate vaccine (PRP-OMP) (PedvaxHIB or ComVax) is given at ages 2 and 4 months, a booster dose at 6 months is not required. Combinations of Hib vaccine and DTaP are not recommended for the 2-, 4-, and 6-month vaccinations in the United States because some studies have shown a lower immune response to Hib components when the combination was used.

5. Measles-mumps-rubella (MMR). An initial MMR dose may be given anytime between 12 and 15 months, and a second dose is recommended between 4 and 6 years. In Canada the initial dose is given at 12 months and a second dose is recommended at 18 months or 4 to 6 years.

6. Polio. U.S. guidelines for polio vaccinations changed in 1999. Except under unusual circumstances inactivated polio vaccine (IPV) should be used for all doses. In Canada IPV is recommended for all doses. The reason is to prevent the rare cases of paralytic polio that may follow administration of oral polio vaccine.

7. Rotavirus. Rotavirus immunization was included for the first time in the 1999 U.S. guidelines. However, this recommendation was withdrawn later in the year because of an association between rotavirus immunization and intussusception.[2]

8. Varicella. Varicella immunization is recommended as a routine vaccination of children anytime after age 12 months.[2] In 1999 the Canadian National Advisory Committee on Immunization added varicella to the recommended vaccinations for children aged 12 months or older.

9. Hepatitis A. Certain regions and states in the United States are now recommending hepatitis A immunization of children. Information about this is available from local health authorities.[2]

Adolescents who have not had a primary series of vaccinations may need catch-up immunizations, usually for hepatitis B, MMR, or varicella.[3]

Specific vaccines are discussed in more detail below.

──────────── ⚑ **REFERENCES** ⚑ ────────────

1. *Canadian immunization guide,* ed 5, Ottawa, 1998, Minister of Supply and Services Canada.
2. Recommended childhood immunization schedule—United States, 2000, *MMWR* 49:35-47, 2000.
3. Zimmerman RK: The 2000 harmonized immunization schedule, *Am Fam Physician* 61:232-239, 2000.

HAEMOPHILUS b IMMUNIZATION
(See also immunization schedules for children)

Until the introduction of immunization programs, *Haemophilus influenzae* type b (Hib) was the most common cause of bacterial meningitis in infants and young children. The case-fatality rate for meningitis was about 5%. Severe neurological sequelae occurred in 10% to 15% of survivors and deafness in 15% to 20%. Other diseases caused by Hib are acute epiglottitis, pneumonia, bacteremia, cellulitis, and septic arthritis.[1]

Three varieties of Hib conjugated vaccines that are available in the United States and Canada for infant immunizations are Hib TITER, PedvaxHIB, and Act HIB. Several of these are available in combination with other vaccines. Thus TETRAMUNE is Hib TITER combined with DTP, Penta is Act HIB combined with DPT and polio vaccines,[2] and

ComVax is PedvaxHIB combined with the hepatitis B vaccine Recombivax HB.[3] Combinations of *Haemophilus* b and DTaP include Acel-Immune and Tripedia. Because some studies have shown a decreased immune response to the Hib component of combined Hib/DTaP vaccines, such combinations are not recommended in the United States for the 2-, 4-, and 6-month vaccinations.[4] ProHIBiT is an Hib vaccine used as a single injection without boosters in children 15 months or older.

The recommended schedules for the different vaccine brands vary somewhat. If Hib conjugate vaccine (PRP-OMP) (PedvaxHIB or ComVax) is given at ages 2 and 4 months, a booster dose at 6 months is not required.[4] Between 15 months and 5 years of age, nonimmunized children require only one dose of Hib vaccine for adequate protection. Children older than 5 years of age do not require immunization.[1]

Rifampin prophylaxis is not required for contacts of Hib infection who are over the age of 5 years or for those under 5 if they have been adequately immunized for their age. If one or more contacts under the age of 5 have not been adequately immunized for age or are immunocompromised, rifampin prophylaxis is usually indicated not only for the children who have not been immunized but also for those who have, since vaccinated children may still be carriers of the organism. In situations of this nature, consultation with local public health units is advisable.[1]

The usual rifampin regimen for prophylaxis against Hib infections is a 4-day course of 600 mg q12h for adults, 20 mg/kg/day in 2 divided doses for children over the age of 1 month, and 10 mg/kg/day in 2 divided doses for children under the age of 1 month.

⚓ REFERENCES ⚓

1. *Canadian immunization guide,* ed 5, Ottawa, 1998, Minister of Supply and Services Canada.
2. Supplementary statement on newly licensed *Haemophilus influenzae* type B (HIB) conjugated vaccines in combination with other vaccines recommended for infants. From *Canada Communicable Disease Report* 20:157-160, 1994, *Can Med Assoc J* 152:527-529, 1995.
3. Centers for Disease Control and Prevention: FDA approval for infants of a *Haemophilus influenzae* type b conjugate and hepatitis B (recombinant) combined vaccine, *JAMA* 277:620-621, 1997.
4. Zimmerman RK: The 2000 harmonized immunization schedule, *Am Fam Physician* 61:232-239, 2000.

HEPATITIS B IMMUNIZATION

(See also hepatitis; immunization schedules for children)

Primary Immunization

Two recombinant DNA hepatitis B vaccines are available in Canada and the United States (Recombivax HB and Engerix-B), and a combined hepatitis B–*Haemophilus* b vaccine (Comvax) is available in the United States. Comvax is a combination of the Hib conjugated vaccine Pedvax HIB and the hepatitis B recombinant vaccine Recombivax HB (see discussion of immunization schedules for children).[1]

The two hepatitis B vaccines Recombivax HB and Engerix-B can be used interchangeably. Following the primary dose, boosters should be given after 1 and 6 months. If the schedule is interrupted, it can be taken up again where it was left off. The dosage should be checked for each product and varies with age. Injections are given intramuscularly into the deltoid of adults and into the anterolateral thigh of children. Gluteal injections should be avoided because in this location the vaccine may be inadvertently deposited in the fat, resulting in lower effectiveness.[2] Comvax should be given at 2, 4, and 12 to 15 months and should not be given before 6 weeks.[1] Evaluation of antibody and antigen status before immunization against hepatitis B is not necessary. A combined hepatitis A–hepatitis B vaccine called Twinrix is available in Canada (see discussion of hepatitis A).

Response rates to hepatitis B immunization vary with age. For those under 2 years it is 95%, for those 2 to 19 the rate is 99%, and for those over the age of 60 it is 50% to 70%.[2] Protection against both clinical disease and the carrier state has been documented to persist for 10 years, but whether such immunity will persist for longer periods is unknown at present. Response rates are lower in immunocompromised persons, and booster doses may be indicated. However, the timing and frequency of such boosters have not been established.[2]

In Canada routine immunization of children against hepatitis B is generally recommended during the elementary school years. In the United States immunization is usually given in early childhood (see immunization schedules for children).[2]

Postexposure Prophylaxis for Hepatitis B

All pregnant women should be screened for hepatitis B surface antigen (HBsAg). If a pregnant woman is HBsAg negative but is at high risk of acquiring hepatitis B, she should be immunized. Infants born to HBsAg-positive mothers should receive 0.5 ml hepatitis B immunoglobulin (HBIG, HyperHep, H-BIG) at birth plus a course of active immunization.[2]

Sexual contacts of a person with acute hepatitis B should receive active immunization. If prophylaxis can be started within 14 days, a single dose of HBIG should also be given. Household contacts need not be immunized except for infants under 1 year of age when the index case is the caretaker. HBIG in doses of 0.06 ml/kg and active immunization can be given at the same time but at different sites.[2]

All health care workers should receive a primary hepatitis B immunization series and document their postimmunization antibody levels. If the levels are above 10 IU/L, long-term protection is likely even if the levels subsequently fall below 10 IU/L. If a health care worker is subject to a percutaneous or mucosal exposure to blood or other body fluids, the risk level for hepatitis B and the HBsAg status of the source should be determined, as well as the anti–hepatitis B surface antigen (anti-HBs) level of the exposed health care worker. If the source is HBsAg negative or is known to be at negligible risk, the only treatment for the health care worker is completion of regular primary immunizations if this has not already been done. If the HBsAg status of the source is unknown, management depends on the vaccination and immune status of the health care worker[2]:

1. If the health care worker has been fully immunized and has had protective levels of antibodies documented, no further action is required.

2. If the health care worker has had two or more doses of vaccine but the worker's anti-HBs status is unknown, his or her anti-HBs status should be determined as soon as possible. If the risk of exposure was high, the worker should receive one vaccination dose immediately. If it was low, the worker may wait for the results of the anti-HBs status determination and then receive vaccination only if it is negative. HBIG is rarely indicated in these situations.

3. If the health care worker has not been vaccinated, has received only one dose, or has not developed antibodies from a full vaccination course, HBIG should be given at once concomitantly with a full course of immunization.

Complete protocols covering a variety of other permutations should be referred to as necessary.

_____ ❧ **REFERENCES** ❧ _____

1. Centers for Disease Control and Prevention: FDA approval for infants of a *Haemophilus influenzae* type b conjugate and hepatitis B (recombinant) combined vaccine, *JAMA* 277:620-621, 1997.

2. *Canadian immunization guide,* ed 5, Ottawa, 1998, Minister of Supply and Services Canada.

INFLUENZA IMMUNIZATION

(See also serotonin syndrome)

Vaccines

Whole virus and split virus influenza vaccines are available. The split virus has fewer side effects and should be used for children 13 years of age or younger. Doses of whole and split viruses are 0.5 ml intramuscularly except for children between the ages of 6 and 35 months, who should receive 0.25 ml. Children under age 9 years receiving influenza vaccine for the first time should be given two shots separated by at least 1 month. Vaccination of pregnant women is safe and probably indicated, since pregnancy increases the risk of complications from the disease.[1] The vaccine strains for 2000-2001 are A/Moscow/10/99 (H3N2)-like, A/New Caledonia/20/99 (H1N1)-like, and B/Beijing/184/93-like antigens.

In general, influenza outbreaks in North America occur from December through March. The optimal time for vaccination is between the beginning of October and the middle of November. Protection from the vaccine begins 1 to 2 weeks after injection and generally lasts 6 months. Protection lasts for shorter periods in some elderly patients. The peak influenza season in the Southern Hemisphere is April through September. In the Caribbean and other tropical regions outbreaks occur throughout the year. Outbreaks have been identified in cruise ships going to Alaska during the summer months.[1]

A randomized placebo-controlled study of healthy working adults found that the only adverse effect occurring more frequently in the cohort receiving the flu vaccine was arm soreness. About one third of both the placebo and flu vaccine cohorts reported fever, myalgias, fatigue, malaise, or headaches.[2]

Evidence indicates that influenza immunization decreases the incidence of pneumonia, hospitalization, and all-cause mortality in both high- and low-risk individuals who are 65 years of age or older.[3] A 3-year randomized prospective double-blind controlled trial found influenza vaccination to be effective in health care professionals.[4] The recommendations of the Canadian Task Force on Preventive Health Care[5] and the U.S. Preventive Services Task Force[6] for immunization with influenza vaccine are as follows:

1. High-risk groups (persons who are over 65 years, are institutionalized, have chronic debilitating diseases, or are immunocompromised) ("B" recommendation)

2. Health care providers in general in Canada and health care providers of high-risk patients in the United States ("B" recommendation)

3. General population under 65 years in Canada ("C" recommendation); no recommendations for this age group in the United States

Chronic diseases for which influenza vaccination is recommended include chronic cardiopulmonary disorders, diabetes, hemoglobinopathies, renal failure, and immunosuppression.[6] The *Medical Letter* suggests that vaccination of healthy people who are not in high-risk categories may also be beneficial,[1] and in 1999 the American Academy of Family Physicians recommended vaccinating all adults 50 years and over.[7]

Antiviral Drugs

Prophylaxis against influenza with amantadine (Symmetrel) or rimantadine (Flumadine) is 70% to 90% effective against influenza A when started before exposure.[8] It is recommended for all patients in nursing homes during outbreaks of influenza in the institution whether or not they have been vaccinated. For prophylaxis the drug is given for the duration of the outbreak or until 2 weeks after active immunization has been administered.[9] Both drugs may also be used to treat influenza A infections if given with 24 to 48 hours of the onset of the disease. For adults the usual dosage of either drug for prophylaxis or treatment is 200 mg/day as a single dose or 100 mg bid.[8]

The newest class of antiviral agents for influenza are the neuraminidase inhibitors Zanamivir (Relenza) and oseltamivir (Tamiflu), which are effective against both influenza A and influenza B. Zanamivir has poor oral bioavailability and so is given by inhalation using a Diskhaler. Zanamivir has been reported to be effective both in prophylaxis and, if given within 30 hours of the onset of symptoms, in treatment. The usual prophylactic dose is 2 inhalations (2 blisters of 5 mg each) daily while the therapeutic dose is 10 mg bid for five days. Oseltamivir is given orally. The prophylactic dose is 75 to 150 mg once daily and the therapeutic dose (starting within 36 hours of the onset of symptoms) is 75 to 150 mg bid for 5 days.[10]

The Canadian Task Force on Preventive Health Care gives an "A" recommendation for treating unimmunized high-risk patients exposed to an index case of influenza disease with amantadine.[5] The U.S. Preventive Services Task Force gives a "B" recommendation for this intervention using either amantadine or rimantadine.[6]

✎ REFERENCES ✎

1. Influenza vaccine, 1998-1999, *Med Lett* 40:91-92, 1998.
2. Nichol KL, Margolis KL, Lind A, et al: Side effects associated with influenza vaccination in healthy working adults: a randomized, placebo-controlled trial, *Arch Intern Med* 156:1546-1550, 1996.
3. Nichol KL, Wuorenma J, von Sternberg T: Benefits of influenza vaccination for low-, intermediate-, and high-risk senior citizens, *Arch Intern Med* 158:1769-1776, 1998.
4. Wilde JA, McMillan JA, Serwint J, et al: Effectiveness of influenza vaccine in health care professionals: a randomized trial, *JAMA* 281:908-913, 1999.
5. Canadian Task Force on the Periodic Health Examination: *Canadian guide to clinical preventive health care,* Ottawa, 1994, Canada Communication Group—Publishing, pp 743-751.
6. US Preventive Services Task Force: *Guide to clinical preventive services,* ed 2, Baltimore, 1996, Williams & Wilkins, pp 791-814.
7. Zimmerman RK: Lowering the age for routine influenza vaccination to 50 years: AAFP leads the nation in influenza vaccine policy, *Am Fam Physician* 60:2061-2070, 1999.
8. Drugs for non-HIV viral infections, *Med Lett* 39:69-76, 1997.
9. Canada communicable disease report: statement on influenza vaccination for the 1995-96 season, *Can Med Assoc J* 153:591-597, 1995.
10. Two neuraminidase inhibitors for treatment of influenza, *Med Lett* 41:91-93, 1999.

MEASLES-MUMPS-RUBELLA IMMUNIZATION
(See also immunization schedules for children)

Giving MMR to children who have proven egg allergy appears to be safe, but this should be done in a setting where they can be observed for 90 minutes and treated appropriately if necessary.[1] In 1996 a combined attenuated measles-rubella vaccine free of egg protein (MoRu-Viraten) became available in Canada.

To eliminate measles from the population, more than a single early childhood vaccination is necessary. According to one study, maximum antibody levels are obtained if the initial immunizations are not given before 1 year of age and if booster doses are given before entry to elementary school (ages 4 to 6) rather than before entry to middle school (ages 11 to 12).[2]

✎ REFERENCES ✎

1. James JM, Burks W, Roverson PK, Sampson HA: Safe administration of the measles vaccine to children allergic to eggs, *N Engl J Med* 332:1262-1266, 1995.
2. Poland GA, Jacobson RM, Thampy AM, et al: Measles reimmunization in children seronegative after initial immunization, *JAMA* 277:1156-1158, 1997.

PERTUSSIS IMMUNIZATION
(See also pertussis)

Immunization of infants against pertussis produces immunity in 80% to 90% of recipients. However, the acquired immunity wanes in time. Loss of protection begins within 3 to 5 years, and no antibodies are detectable after 10 to 12 years. New acellular pertussis vaccines have been developed that are at least as effective as whole-cell vaccines and have fewer side effects.[1] Acellular pertussis vaccines combined with tetanus and diphtheria vaccines (DTaP) are available under the trade names Acel-Imune, Infanrix, Tripedia, and Tripacel. In Canada a quadrivalent acellular pertussis vaccine that also contains inactivated polio is Quadricel, and this combined with Act-Hib is the pentavalent acellular pertussis vaccine Pentacel.[2]

✎ REFERENCES ✎

1. Edwards KM, Decker MD: Acellular pertussis vaccines for infants (editorial), *N Engl J Med* 334:391-392, 1996.
2. Halperin SA: Acellular pertussis vaccine has arrived in Canada, finally, *Can Fam Physician* 43:1581-1582, 1997.

PNEUMOCOCCAL IMMUNIZATION

The efficacy of pneumococcal vaccine in preventing pneumonia in immunocompetent middle-aged and elderly people is unknown; in most trials no benefit has been demonstrated.[1] In contrast, epidemiological evidence suggests that pneumococcal vaccination is effective in preventing pneumococcal bacteremia.[1,2] This alone is a good reason to give pneumococcal vaccine.

Specific recommendations vary tremendously. The 1997 guidelines of the Centers for Disease Control and Prevention for immunization with 23-valent pneumococcal polysaccharide vaccine (Pneumovax 23) are as follows[1]:

1. All persons 65 years or older
2. All persons aged 2 to 64 years with chronic diseases such as congestive heart failure, chronic obstructive

pulmonary disease, liver disease, alcoholism, and diabetes mellitus.

3. All persons aged 2 to 64 years with anatomical or functional asplenia (sickle cell anemia is a leading example)
4. All persons aged 2 to 64 years living in high-risk situations
5. All immunocompromised persons, including those with HIV disease; the efficacy of the vaccine may be less than in immunocompetent persons, but benefits are still achieved

Despite frequently published warnings against revaccination, the procedure is safe, although local reactions are more common than with initial vaccination.[1,3] The following are indications for one revaccination (it is not known if more than one is beneficial)[1]:

1. Patients 65 years or older who were immunized more than 5 years previously and were younger than 65 years of age when immunized
2. Persons who are functionally or anatomically asplenic after 5 years if over 10 years of age, and perhaps after 3 years if under 10 years of age
3. Immunocompromised patients after 5 years if over 10 years of age, and perhaps after 3 years if under 10 years of age

Individuals whose pneumococcal vaccination status is unknown should be vaccinated.[1]

REFERENCES

1. Prevention of pneumococcal disease: recommendations of the Advisory Committee on Immunization Practices (ACIP), *MMWR* 46(No. RR-8):1-24, 1997.
2. Pneumococcal vaccine, *Med Lett* 41:84, 1999.
3. Jackson LA, Benson P, Sneller V-P, et al: Safety of revaccination with pneumococcal polysaccharide vaccine, *JAMA* 281: 243-248, 1999.

POLIO IMMUNIZATION

(See also immunization schedules for children; postpolio syndrome)

One of the fears concerning poliomyelitis (polio) immunization is that the live virus vaccine may itself cause paralytic polio. This complication has been particularly common in Romania in the latter part of the twentieth century. The reason appears to be intramuscular injections of other drugs, usually antibiotics, within 30 days of receiving oral live polio vaccine.[1,2] This phenomenon was noted in the pre–polio vaccine era when it was known that polio developing in a child after tonsillectomy and adenoidectomy was likely to be bulbar, whereas polio striking a child who had had intramuscular injections was likely to cause paralysis of the limb in which the injection was given.[2]

Polio vaccines have been extraordinarily effective in eradicating the disease. No cases of wild polio infection have been reported in the Americas since October 1991, and

the disease was declared eradicated from this area by the World Health Organization.[3] The incidence of polio has dropped dramatically in the rest of the world, and since 1996 the Pacific countries have been free of the disease.[4] Africa remains the continent with the highest incidence.[4]

Since wild polio has been eliminated in North and South America, the only cases of paralytic polio in these regions are the extremely rare cases of paralytic polio secondary to the live Sabin polio vaccines (about 1 case per 2.6 million vaccinations). To avoid this complication many health authorities are recommending that henceforth all polio immunization, or at least the initial two immunizations, be done with the enhanced Salk vaccine, which gives high antibody titers against all three strains of wild polio vaccine. In June 1999 the American Advisory Committee on Immunization Practices recommended that with a few exceptions only inactivated polio vaccines should be used.[5] In Canada polio vaccine is available not only as a single agent, but also in the combination DPT-polio-Hib under the trade name Penta.

REFERENCES

1. Strebel PM, Ion-Nedelcu N, Baughman AL, et al: Intramuscular injections within 30 days of immunization with oral poliovirus vaccine—a risk factor for vaccine-associated paralytic poliomyelitis, *N Engl J Med* 332:500-506, 1995.
2. Wright PF, Karzon DT: Minimizing the risks associated with the prevention of poliomyelitis (editorial), *N Engl J Med* 332:528-529, 1995.
3. Expanded programme on immunization: certification of poliomyelitis eradication—the Americas, 1994, *Wkly Epidemiol Rec* 69:293-295, 1994.
4. Foege WH: Polio eradication—how near? (editorial), *JAMA* 275:1682-1683, 1996.
5. Centers for Disease Control and Prevention: Revised recommendations for routine poliomyelitis vaccination, *JAMA* 282: 522, 1999.

RABIES IMMUNIZATION

(See also immunization schedules for children)

Almost all cases of human rabies acquired from animals in the United States have resulted from bites of dogs, skunks, or foxes or from contact with bats. Rabies can also be transmitted by wolves, bobcats, bears, and groundhogs. Rabies frequently infects raccoons in the eastern United States and rarely affects cows, sheep, or horses; there are no reports of transmission of the disease to humans from any of these sources.[1] Bites from squirrels, chipmunks, rabbits, hares, rats, mice, hamsters, guinea pigs, and gerbils rarely require postexposure prophylaxis. However, local public health authorities should be consulted.

Rabies can be acquired only if a person has direct contact with saliva through a bite or scratch or through mucous membrane contact. With the exception of bats (see below), almost all reported cases are from bites. The risk of contracting the disease after a bite is 50 to 100 times greater than after a scratch.[1] The virus cannot be transmitted by petting a rabid animal or through contact with its blood, urine, or feces.[2]

Between 1980 and 1997, 21 documented cases of rabies were acquired from bats in the United States; in only one instance was there a clear history of being bitten. Even casual contact with bat variants of rabies may lead to infection, and therefore postexposure immunization should be considered for all bat contacts unless the bat is collected safely and proved to be rabies free. Such contacts include individuals sleeping in a room where a bat is discovered.[3] A study from Colorado emphasizes the risk posed by bats; 30% of bats that bit humans had rabies, compared with 14% of bats that did not bite humans.[4]

Immediate management of a bite from a potentially rabid animal is thorough washing with copious amounts of soap and water, a process that markedly reduces the risk of infection.[1,2] If a dog, cat, or ferret is responsible for the bite and has rabies, it will become ill within 10 days. If the animal appears healthy, it should be confined and watched for this period, but if it is behaving in an erratic or wild fashion, it should be killed and its brain evaluated for rabies.[2,5] Withholding postexposure vaccination for 10 days is safe except in cases of bites on the head or neck, in which instance the incubation period of rabies may be so short that immediate postexposure prophylaxis must be given. The immunization status of the animal is not a determining factor, since the degree of protection offered by animal rabies vaccines is less than that given by human vaccines.[1]

Three rabies vaccines are available in the United States: human diploid cell vaccine (HDCV; Imovax), rabies vaccine adsorbed (RVA), or purified chick embryo cell vaccine (PCEC; RabAvert). Standard injection technique is intramuscularly in the deltoid in adults or the anterolateral thigh in children. Postexposure vaccination in nonimmunized individuals consists of five 1-ml injections given on days 0, 3, 7, 14, and 28. In addition, human rabies immune globulin (HRIG; Imogam Rabies-HT; BayRab) should be given at a dose of 20 IU/kg.[2,6] Although it has been traditionally recommended that half the dose of HRIG be infiltrated around the wound and the other half given intramuscularly in the gluteal region or thigh, the U.S. Advisory Committee for Immunization Practices (ACIP) advises injecting as much of the HRIG as possible in and around the wound and then injecting any residual volume intramuscularly at a different site.[2,3] Postexposure immunization of previously immunized individuals consists of two doses of rabies vaccine on days 0 and 3.[1,2,6]

Preexposure vaccination is given to high- risk individuals as a series of three shots on days 0, 7, and either 21 or 28.[2,6] Individuals at risk include veterinarians and other animal handlers, spelunkers, and individuals traveling to regions where rabies is endemic (Asia, Africa, and Latin America) if they are unlikely to receive adequate medical care and postexposure prophylaxis within 2 days of exposure to a possibly rabid animal.[1] Persons who have been immunized and are at continued high risk should either have their titers checked or receive a booster dose every 2 years.[2,6]

⚓ REFERENCES ⚓

1. Basgoz N: Case Records of the Massachusetts General Hospital, Case 21-1998, N Engl J Med 339:105-112, 1998.
2. Human rabies prevention—United States, 1999: recommendations of the Advisory Committee on Immunization Practices (ACIP), MMWR 48(RR-1):1-21, 1999.
3. Centers for Disease Control and Prevention: Human rabies—Texas and New Jersey, 1997, JAMA 279:421-422, 1998.
4. Pape WJ, Fitzsimmons TD, Hoffman RE: Risk for rabies transmission from encounters with bats, Colorado, 1977-1996, Emerg Infect Dis 5:433-437, 1999.
5. Fleisher GR: The management of bite wounds (editorial), N Engl J Med 340:138-140, 1999.
6. A new rabies vaccine, Med Lett 40:64-65, 1998.

RUBELLA IMMUNIZATION

Acute arthralgias occur in about one fourth of women receiving rubella vaccination.[1] Reports have suggested an increased incidence of chronic arthritis after such vaccination, but recent studies have not verified this risk.[1,2]

⚓ REFERENCES ⚓

1. Ray P, Black S, Shinefield H, et al: Risk of chronic arthropathy among women after rubella vaccination, JAMA 278:551-556, 1997.
2. Tingle AJ, Mitchell LA, Grace M, et al: Randomised double-blind placebo-controlled study on adverse effects of rubella immunisation in seronegative women, Lancet 349:1277-1281, 1997.

TETANUS IMMUNIZATION
(See also immunization schedules for children)

Tetanus immunization of children is widely done. Booster doses for adults are not so widely performed. Only about one fourth of persons in the United States over the age of 70 were found to have protective antibodies against tetanus.[1]

⚓ REFERENCES ⚓

1. Gergen PJ, McQuillan GM, Kiely M, et al: A population-based serologic survey of immunity to tetanus in the United States, N Engl J Med 332:761-766, 1995.

TYPHOID FEVER IMMUNIZATION
(See also immunization schedules for children)

Immunization for typhoid fever is often indicated for travelers, especially those to the Indian subcontinent.[1] The traditional typhoid vaccines (Typhoid Vaccine H-P or AKD) are given as two subcutaneous doses 1 month apart with boosters every 3 years as needed. Two new vaccines, Typhim VI and Vivotif Berna, have recently become available. Both have a low incidence of side effects; their efficacy is about 70%.[2] Typhim VI is an inactivate vaccine given as a single intramuscular injection. Booster doses are recommended every 2 years in the United States and every 3 years in Canada. Vivotif Berna is a live oral attenuated vaccine. The usual regimen is a total of four capsules with one given every second day (days 1, 3, 5, 7). This vaccine is known to be efficacious for 7 years. Vivotif Berna should not be given to pregnant women or immunocompromised patients. The timing of booster doses has not been established, but a working recommendation is every 5 years.

Since antimicrobial resistance of *Salmonella typhi* is increasing in isolates obtained from U.S. patients, the current treatment of choice for typhoid fever is probably a quinolone or a third-generation cephalosporin.[1]

REFERENCES

1. Mermin JH, Townes JM, Gerber M, et al: Typhoid fever in the United States, 1985-94: changing risks of international travel and increasing antimicrobial resistance, *Arch Intern Med* 158: 633-638, 1998.
2. Keystone JS: Typhoid vaccination—update, *Can J Infect Dis* 6:231, 1995.

VARICELLA IMMUNIZATION
(See also immunization schedules for children; infectious diseases in pregnancy; varicella; varicella in children)

A live varicella vaccine (Varivax) became available in the United States in 1995; it must be stored in a freezer until reconstituted.[1] U.S. guidelines recommend immunization of children with a single dose at any visit on or after the first birthday. Children over the age of 13 who have not been immunized and who have not had chickenpox require two doses administered at least 4 weeks apart.[2]

An adult who gives a history of chickenpox is likely to be seropositive,[3] although the person may be seronegative if the original diagnosis was erroneous.[4] Most adults who give no history of chickenpox or who have an uncertain history of the disease are also seropositive. If vaccination is being considered for persons in this category, a serological test to determine whether they have had the disease is probably cost effective, since the test is usually less expensive than the two doses of vaccine.[3]

A specific indication for varicella vaccination may be family members of an index case. If given within 3 days of the onset of symptoms of the index case, vaccination prevents or markedly ameliorates disease.[5]

REFERENCES

1. Varicella vaccine, *Med Lett* 37:55-56, 1995.
2. Recommended childhood immunization schedule—United States, 2000, *MMWR* 49:35-47, 2000.
3. Ventura A: Varicella vaccination guidelines for adolescents and adults, *Am Fam Physician* 55:1220-1224, 1997.
4. Wallace MR, Chamberlin CJ, Sawyer MH, et al: Reliability of a history of previous varicella infection in adults, *JAMA* 278: 1520-1522, 1997.
5. Salzman MB, Garcia C: Postexposure varicella vaccination in siblings of children with active varicella, *Pediatr Infect Dis J* 17:256-257, 1998.

IMMUNOLOGY

Topics covered in this section

Allergic Rhinitis
Vasomotor Rhinitis
Food Allergies
Insect Stings and Bites
Drug Allergy
Connective Tissue Diseases
HIV and AIDS

ALLERGIC RHINITIS
(See also topical ophthalmic medications)

Environmental Control

Some ways of decreasing exposure to airborne pollens are to avoid cutting the grass, going camping, or going on picnics, to wear wraparound sunglasses, and to close the car and bedroom windows.[1]

Pharmacotherapy

The two major drug classes used for treating allergic rhinitis are topical nasal corticosteroids (Table 32) and oral antihistamines (Tables 33 and 34).[1-4] Maximum efficacy for both is seen if they are started before contact with the offending allergen and are given continuously throughout the period of exposure; they are less effective as "rescue" medications.[5] Both antihistamines and corticosteroids are effective in controlling nasal itching and sneezing. Antihistamines are reasonably effective for rhinorrhea but are not effective for nasal obstruction. Nasal steroids (Table 32) are very effective for rhinorrhea and moderately effective for nasal obstruction; their maximum efficacy is seen only after 1 to 2 weeks of treatment.[1] In general, topical steroids are slightly more effective than antihistamines,[1] but most investigators have found that many patients require a combination of drugs from both groups to control symptoms.[2] In contrast,

Table 32 Topical Nasal Steroids

Drug	Usual adult dose
Beclomethasone dipropionate (Beconase, Vancenase)	Two sprays each nostril bid
Budesonide (Rhinocort)	Two doses each nostril bid or four sprays each nostril once daily
Flunisolide (Nasarel, Nasalide, Rhinalar)	Two sprays each nostril bid
Fluticasone propionate (Flonase)	Two sprays each nostril once daily or one spray each nostril bid
Mometasone furoate (Nasonex)	Two sprays each nostril once daily
Triamcinolone acetonide (Nasacort)	Two sprays each nostril once daily

Table 33 First-Generation Antihistamines

Class and drug	Usual adult dose
Alkylamines	
Chlorpheniramine (Chlor-Trimeton, Chlor-Tripolon)	4-8 mg qhs as single daily dose[7]
Dexchlorpheniramine (Polaramine)	2 mg qid
Ethanolamines	
Diphenhydramine (Benadryl)	25-50 mg tid-qid
Ethylenediamines	
Tripelennamine (Pyribenzamine, PBZ)	25-50 mg qid
Piperazine derivatives	
Hydroxyzine (Atarax)	10-50 mg tid-qid
Piperidine derivatives	
Azatadine (Optimine)	1-2 mg bid

Table 34 Second-Generation Antihistamines

Drug	Usual adult dose
Cetirizine (Zyrtec, Reactine)	10 mg/day
Loratadine (Claritin)	10 mg/day
Fexofenadine (Allegra)	60 mg bid

one study found that adding loratadine (Claritin) 10 mg/day to 200 μg of fluticasone (Flonase) insufflated nasally once daily did not increase the benefit over that obtained with fluticasone alone.[3]

For patients with rhinorrhea who do not respond adequately to inhaled corticosteroids, the addition of ipratropium bromide (Atrovent Nasal), two sprays per nostril tid, may result in significant improvement.[1,6]

Intranasal cromolyn (sodium cromoglycate, Rynacrom) controls nasal itching, sneezing, or rhinorrhea in some patients but is not as potent as the antihistamines or nasal steroids.[1] This drug is also available as ophthalmic drops (Crolom, Opticrom).

A number of studies have shown that antileukotriene drugs such as zafirlukast (Accolate) in doses of 20 mg bid or montelukast (Singulair) in doses of 10 mg once daily may be beneficial for some patients with allergic rhinitis. At present they should probably be used for patients who do not respond adequately to antihistamines or nasal steroid sprays.[4]

As a group, first-generation antihistamines tend to be dismissed as unsuitable because they are more sedative than second-generation agents and may be hazardous for persons involved in occupational or recreational activities requiring optimal cognitive or psychomotor functioning.[5] However, sedation is not always a problem, especially with children and young adults, and drugs such as chlorpheniramine (Chlor-Trimeton, Chlor-Tripolon) are usually well tolerated, effective, and inexpensive.[2] The usually recommended dose for chlorpheniramine is 4 mg q4-6h, but 4 to 8 mg once

daily qhs is equally effective in most cases and causes less sedation.[7] There are several classes of first-generation antihistamines (Table 33); if a drug from one class is ineffective, it is worth trying one from another class.

Second-generation antihistamines are listed in Table 34. Terfenadine was withdrawn from the U.S. market in 1997 because of reports of arrhythmias and deaths attributed to the drug. Its active metabolite, fexofenadine (Allegra), does not induce arrhythmias. Astemizole may stimulate the appetite and has also been associated with arrhythmias.[8] The manufacturer discontinued production of astemizole in 1999.

Two antihistamines that are formulated as a nasal spray are azelastine (Astelin) and levocabastine (Livostin). The *Medical Letter* reviewed azelastine and concluded that corticosteroid sprays or nonsedating antihistamines were preferable.[9] A number of antihistamine-vasoconstrictor ophthalmic drops can be used as adjuncts to nasal steroids or antihistamines in the treatment of allergic rhinitis. These include antazoline-naphazoline (Vasocon-A), pheniramine-naphazoline (Naphcon-A), and pheniramine-phenylephrine (Ak Vernacon). Use of such topical ophthalmic agents has caused acute and chronic conjunctivitis.[10]

The long-term use of topical nasal vasoconstrictors has no role in the treatment of vasomotor or allergic rhinitis. However, they may be useful for a few days during the initiation of topical steroid therapy if the nose is completely blocked. The vasoconstrictor may be given a few minutes before the steroid to open up the nasal passages. Prolonged use may lead to rhinitis medicamentosa.[1] A short-acting topical decongestant is pheniramine-phenylephrine (Dristan Nasal Mist/Spray), and longer acting products include oxymetazoline HCl (Dristan Long Lasting Nasal Mist/Spray) and xylometazoline HCl (Otrivin).

Administration of nasal sprays
The proper way of administering nasal sprays is as follows:
1. Blow the nose to clear the nasal passages.
2. Point the nozzle straight toward the back of the head.
3. Press down on the canister or squeeze the pump bottle as you begin to inhale slowly.
4. Try to avoid blowing or sneezing for a few minutes after instillation of the medication.

Immunotherapy
Guidelines of the Canadian Society of Allergy and Clinical Immunology state that immunotherapy for seasonal allergic rhinitis caused by the pollens of trees, grasses, or ragweed is a third-line treatment to be undertaken only if an intensive program of allergen avoidance and symptomatic control with medications has been unsuccessful over a 2-year period.[11] Adverse reactions to immunotherapy vary from minimal local reactions to death. Risk factors for serious adverse reactions include patients with

asthma, immunotherapy during the season when pollens to which the patient is allergic are present, and first doses from a new vial.[12]

Short preseasonal courses of immunotherapy using absorbed serum have been developed for allergies to trees, grasses, and ragweed. Only six to 11 shots are required.[4]

REFERENCES

1. Parikh A, Scadding A: Seasonal allergic rhinitis, *BMJ* 314: 1392-1395, 1997.
2. Freedman SO: First-line treatment of hay fever: what is the best option? (editorial), *Can Med Assoc J* 156:1141-1143, 1997.
3. Ratner PH, van Bavel JH, Martin BG, et al: A comparison of the efficacy of fluticasone propionate aqueous nasal spray and loratadine, alone and in combination, for the treatment of seasonal allergic rhinitis, *J Fam Pract* 47:118-125, 1998.
4. Tkachyk SJ: New treatments for allergic rhinitis, *Can Fam Physician* 45:1255-1260, 1999
5. Kay GG, Berman B, Mockoviak SH, et al: Initial and steady-state effects of diphenhydramine and loratadine on sedation, cognition, mood, and psychomotor performance, *Arch Intern Med* 157:2350-2356, 1997.
6. Dockhorn R, Aaronson D, Bronsky E, et al: Ipratropium bromide nasal spray 0.03% and beclomethasone nasal spray alone and in combination for the treatment of rhinorrhea in perennial rhinitis, *Ann Allergy Asthma Immunol* 82:349-359, 1999.
7. Simons FE, Simons KJ: The pharmacology and use of H_1-receptor-antagonist drugs, *N Engl J Med* 330:1663-1670, 1994.
8. Fexofenadine, *Med Lett* 38:95-96, 1996.
9. Azelastine nasal spray for allergic rhinitis, *Med Lett* 39:45-47, 1997.
10. Soparkar CN, Wilhelmus KR, Koch DD, et al: Acute and chronic conjunctivitis due to over-the-counter ophthalmic decongestants, *Arch Ophthalmol* 115:34-48, 1997.
11. Canadian Society of Allergy and Clinical Immunology: Guidelines for the use of allergen immunotherapy, *Can Med Assoc J* 152:1413-1419, 1995.
12. Craig T, Sawyer AM, Fornadley JA: Use of immunotherapy in a primary care office, *Am Family Physician* 57:1888-1894, 1998.

VASOMOTOR RHINITIS

For vasomotor rhinitis, topical steroids are generally the drugs of choice unless the major symptom is a dripping nose, in which case a nasal spray of ipratropium bromide (Atrovent Nasal) may prove effective.[1,2] An 8-week placebo-controlled trial of ipratropium bromide nasal spray found the drug to be effective and to have no systemic adverse effects or nasal rebound symptoms in the week after discontinuation of the medication.[2] For some patients a combination of topical nasal steroids and nasal ipratropium bromide (two sprays tid) gives improved results.[3]

REFERENCES

1. Proceedings of the Canadian Rhinitis Symposium: assessing and treating rhinitis; a practical guide for Canadian physicians, *Can Med Assoc J* 151(suppl):S1-S27, 1994.

2. Georgitis JW, Banov C, Boggs PB, et al: Ipratropium bromide nasal spray in non-allergic rhinitis: efficacy, nasal cytological response and patient evaluation on quality of life, *Clin Exp Allergy* 24:1049-1055, 1994.
3. Dockhorn R, Aaronson D, Bronsky E, et al: Ipratropium bromide nasal spray 0.03% and beclomethasone nasal spray alone and in combination for the treatment of rhinorrhea in perennial rhinitis, *Ann Allergy Asthma Immunol* 82:349-359, 1999.

FOOD ALLERGIES
(See also insect stings and bites)

One study found that 20% of adults claimed to have a food allergy, but when these reports were investigated, the actual number turned out to be 1.4%. True food allergy is an IgE-mediated reaction. Symptoms usually come on within minutes of eating the offending agent, and only one food, or at most a few, provokes the reaction. Common symptoms are itching and swelling of the mouth and pharynx, often associated with symptoms of anaphylaxis such as urticaria, wheezing, nausea, vomiting, diarrhea, and in some cases faintness and syncope. Foods likely to induce food allergy in children are cows' milk, eggs, and peanuts, and in adults the offending foods are fish, shellfish, nuts, and fruits. Food additives such as salicylates, sulfites, tartrazine, and benzoates may also cause allergic reactions. By the age of 3 years 90% of children allergic to milk and 50% of those allergic to eggs have outgrown the reactivity.[1] Only a very few lose their sensitivity to peanuts.[2]

The most important tool for making a diagnosis is the history. When the history is suggestive, the next step is skin testing, and if this is positive, the third step is a diagnostic diet in which the suspected allergen is eliminated. The final and definitive test is an oral food challenge, which is often useful because 50% of those with positive skin tests are not allergic. Oral food challenges can be dangerous and should be undertaken only in carefully controlled situations.[1] Treatment of acute food allergy, as for any anaphylactic reaction, is epinephrine. Patients with food allergies not only must be very careful to avoid the offending foods, but should never be without an epinephrine syringe (see discussion of insect stings and bites).

Among the many nonallergic reaction to foods are lactose intolerance, flushing from monosodium glutamate, migraines secondary to tyramine in cheese or red wine, and contact urticaria in the perioral region of children eating citrus fruits. The most common reaction is simply "food aversion" in which patients experience nonspecific symptoms from a variety of foods and wrongly attribute this as a manifestation of food allergy.[1]

REFERENCES

1. Bindslev-Jensen C: Food allergy, *BMJ* 316:1299-1302, 1998.
2. Hourihane J O'B, Roberts SA, Warner JO: Resolution of peanut allergy: case-control study, *BMJ* 316:1271-1275, 1998.

INSECT STINGS AND BITES

(See also allergic rhinitis; food allergies; tropical medicine; urticaria and angioedema)

Types of Stinging Insects

Most stinging insects are members of the Hymenoptera order of the class Insecta. They include yellow jackets, hornets, wasps, honeybees, and bumblebees. The fire ant, *Solenopsis invicta,* is also a member of the Hymenoptera order but does not have wings. Only the females of these species sting. In the United States yellow jackets are responsible for most stings. The stingers of the honeybees have multiple barbs and tend to detach and remain in the skin, while the stingers of other insects do not remain in the skin. The venom of Africanized honeybees or "killer bees" is no more toxic and no more likely to induce anaphylaxis than is the venom of other members of the Hymenoptera order. However, the Africanized honeybee is more aggressive and more likely to sting than its docile cousin. Anaphylaxis may result from stinging insects but rarely from biting insects.[1]

Removal of Bee Stingers

Traditional advice for the immediate management of bee stings is to scrape out the embedded stinger rather than to pluck it out with fingers or forceps. The reason for this is the fear that plucking will compress the stinger and inject more venom into the victim. In fact, this is not so. The longer the stinger remains in the skin, the more venom is liberated. Therefore the stinger should be plucked out as rapidly as possible.[2]

Local Reactions to Insect Stings

Reactions to stings vary. In most cases localized pain, swelling, and erythema develop and then subside in a few hours. More extensive localized reactions are common, may reach a maximum size after 48 hours, and may last for up to a week. Extensive erythema is also common and may be mistaken for cellulitis, which in fact is a rare complication of stings.[1]

Treatment of large local reactions is acetylsalicylic acid 650 mg q4h prn plus an antihistamine. If the reaction is disabling, prednisone 40 mg/day may be given for 2 or 3 days. Persons who have had large local reactions are likely to have similar reactions if stung again; their risk of anaphylaxis with a future sting is 5% per episode. They are not candidates for immunotherapy and therefore are not candidates for venom skin tests. Tetanus prophylaxis is not necessary for insect stings.[1]

Anaphylactic Reactions

Anaphylactic reactions most often occur in persons under 20 and are twice as common in males, probably because they have greater exposure to stings. The most common symptoms are generalized urticaria, flushing, and angioedema. More serious reactions are upper airway edema, bronchospasm, and circulatory collapse. Most deaths occur in adults. Among unselected patients who have had an anaphylactic reaction and are subsequently stung (without having had venom immunotherapy), only 50% to 60% have a second anaphylactic reaction. The incidence of second anaphylactic reactions is much lower in children, particularly if the initial manifestation was dermal.[1]

Treatment of an acute anaphylactic reaction is 0.2 to 0.5 ml of 1:1000 epinephrine subcutaneously repeated every 30 minutes prn. If necessary, aerosolized bronchodilators and IV fluids should be added. In most cases acute symptoms subside in 30 minutes. In the rare cases in which they persist, IV steroids should be given followed by oral prednisone 60 mg/day for 2 days.[1]

Prophylaxis Against Insect Stings

Clothes that cover the body, including gloves when gardening, are helpful. Clothes should be dark colored. Perfumes, cosmetics, and hair sprays should be avoided. Food odors attract yellow jackets.[1]

If patients who have had a large local reaction or a mild generalized reaction are stung again, they should take a rapidly absorbed antihistamine such as one of the newer nonsedative varieties as soon as possible. Backup medication for these patients is epinephrine (Adrenaline). Epinephrine is first-line treatment for individuals who have had serious generalized reactions in the past.[3]

Epinephrine is available in kit form either as an EpiPen or as an ANA-Kit. Epinephrine is relatively unstable; it should be stored in the dark and not used after its expiration date.[4] The EpiPen comes as preloaded syringes of epinephrine. The adult form contains 2 ml of epinephrine 1:1000, and the children's version (EpiPen Jr) contains 2 ml of epinephrine 1:2000. The ANA-Kit contains a preloaded syringe of epinephrine, a tourniquet, alcohol swabs, and two 4-mg chewable chlorpheniramine tablets (Chlor-Trimeton, Chlor-Tripolon). Antihistamines are useful in controlling hives and angioedema.

Venom immunotherapy is indicated for patients who have had severe symptoms of anaphylaxis and have positive venom skin tests. It is not indicated for children (or probably for adults) who have had only dermal reactions, and it is probably not indicated for individuals with relatively mild symptoms such as urticaria plus some shortness of breath.[3,5] The Canadian Society of Allergy and Clinical Immunology currently recommends that immunotherapy be given every 4 to 6 weeks for 5 years.[5] According to a position statement of the American Academy of Allergy, Asthma and Immunology, individuals who have had a mild or moderate reaction may discontinue immunotherapy after 3 to 5 years. Those who have had a severe reaction may be able to safely discontinue treatment after 5 years, although the physician may choose to treat them for longer periods.[6] Recommendations from Britain state that 3 years is long enough for treatment but that this form of therapy should take place only in specialist centers with facilities for resuscitation. Patients must be observed for 1 hour after each dose.[3]

Mosquito Bites

Since mosquitoes breed in standing water, such as in old tires, birdbaths, clogged gutters, and empty containers, elimination of these sources may decrease the number of insects in the area. Ultrasonic electronic devices and bug "zappers" are ineffective and citronella candles only moderately effective. Symptomatic relief of bites may be obtained with topical corticosteroids or oral antihistamines.[7] The use of DEET and permethrin is discussed in the section on tropical medicine.

≈ REFERENCES ≈

1. Reisman RE: Insect stings, *N Engl J Med* 331:523-527, 1994.
2. Visscher PD, Vetter RS, Camazine S: Removing bee stings, *Lancet* 348:301-302, 1996.
3. Ewan PW: Venom allergy, *BMJ* 316:1365-1368, 1998.
4. Stability of drugs in solution, *Med Lett* 38:90, 1996.
5. Canadian Society of Allergy and Clinical Immunology: Guidelines for the use of allergen immunotherapy, *Can Med Assoc J* 152:1413-1419, 1995.
6. Graft DF, Golden DF, Reisman RE, et al: Position statement: the discontinuation of Hymenoptera venom immunotherapy; report from the Committee on Insects, *J Allergy Clin Immunol* 101:573-575, 1998.
7. Fradin MS: Mosquitoes and mosquito repellents: a clinician's guide, *Ann Intern Med* 128:931-940, 1998.

DRUG ALLERGY

True allergic reactions to drugs make up only a small proportion of all adverse drug reactions.[1,2] The more usual ones are toxicity, expected side effects, and drug interactions. Although urticaria is often a manifestation of drug allergy, it is also a common sequel to a variety of infectious diseases.[2] Patients who are taking drugs and experience angioedema, urticaria, or bronchospasm are likely to be having an anaphylactic reaction. On the other hand, the etiology of maculopapular rashes is uncertain. Cross-reactivity between penicillins and cephalosporins is well recognized; in most cases cephalosporins do not have an adverse effect if the original reaction to penicillin was a maculopapular rash, not an urticarial one.[1]

When a patient gives a history of drug allergy, an alternative drug class can often be prescribed.[1] However, skin testing for type I or immediate hypersensitivity reactions can be done safely for a number of drugs, particularly penicillin, provided prescribed protocols are followed. In the case of suspected penicillin allergy, skin tests have an excellent negative predictive value (if the test is negative, the patient is unlikely to be sensitive). Desensitization protocols for penicillin and sulfonamides, which have particular value for HIV-positive patients who require prophylaxis against *Pneumocystis carinii* and are allergic to trimethoprim-sulfamethoxazole, are generally safe and effective.[2]

≈ REFERENCES ≈

1. Segreti J, Trenholme GM, Levin S: Antibiotic therapy in the allergic patient, *Med Clin North Am* 79:935-942, 1995.
2. Rieder MJ: In vivo and in vitro testing for adverse drug reactions, *Pediatr Clin North Am* 44:93-111, 1997.

CONNECTIVE TISSUE DISEASES

(See also arthritis; biliary cirrhosis; polymyalgia rheumatica; rheumatology; sedimentation rate; thrombophlebitis)

Classification

The following disorders are usually included in the classification of connective tissue disorders[1]:

1. CREST syndrome (calcinosis, Raynaud's phenomenon, esophageal dysfunction, sclerodactyly, and telangiectasia)
2. Dermatomyositis
3. Mixed connective tissue disease
4. Overlap syndromes
5. Polymyositis
6. Progressive systemic sclerosis (scleroderma)
7. Rheumatoid arthritis
8. Sjögren's syndrome
9. Systemic lupus erythematosus (SLE)
10. Vasculitis

In some ways listing vasculitis as a separate entity is artificial because vasculitis is an element of many "connective tissue diseases," such as rheumatoid arthritis, Sjögren's syndrome, and SLE.

Laboratory Investigations

A welter of laboratory investigations are available for patients with suspected connective tissue disorders. For the family physician a complete blood count (CBC) and urinalysis are probably the two most important tests to order. In some cases a physician may order measurement of the erythrocyte sedimentation rate (ESR) simply because a normal ESR is rare in the presence of active polymyositis or vasculitis. However, false positives are common (see discussion of sedimentation rate).[1]

Other useful tests are creatine phosphokinase if polymyositis or dermatomyositis is suspected, rheumatoid factor if rheumatoid arthritis, Sjögren's syndrome, SLE, vasculitis, or dermatomyositis is being considered, thyroid-stimulating hormone to rule out thyroid disease that may be associated with myalgias, myositis, and muscle weakness, and antinuclear antibody (ANA) for any of the connective tissue diseases.[1]

False-positive results are common with ANA tests, especially in the elderly. In one study the positive predictive value as assessed in 1010 inpatients and outpatients in a teaching hospital was only 11% for both lupus and other rheumatic diseases.[2] Antineutrophil cytoplasmic autoantibodies (ANCA) are found in the blood of about 90% of patients with Wegener's granulomatosis or microscopic polyangiitis and 70% of those with the Churg-Strauss syndrome.[3]

Sjögren's Syndrome

The definition of Sjögren's syndrome is controversial; some workers require typical histological findings on biopsies of minor salivary glands to make the diagnosis, whereas others do not. As a result of inconsistencies in defining the entity, its epidemiology is uncertain. Major symptoms include dry eyes and dry mouth, but these in themselves are nonspecific and may be due to a variety of conditions, including drugs with anticholinergic side effects. Sjögren's syndrome is classified into primary and secondary forms. The primary form may involve only the salivary and lacrimal glands or may be associated with a small vessel vasculitis causing nephritis, cutaneous rashes, or pulmonary lesions. The secondary forms are usually associated with rheumatoid arthritis, SLE, scleroderma, polymyositis, or biliary cirrhosis.[4]

Systemic Lupus Erythematosus

The prevalence of SLE is generally stated to be about 40 per 100,000 in Europe and North America. More than 80% of cases occur in women during the childbearing years, and in this population the prevalence rate is close to 1:1000.[5]

Arthritis is the most common clinical manifestation of systemic lupus erythematosus, and tendinitis is also common. The arthritis tends to be oligoarticular and migratory, and pain is disproportionate to any signs of inflammation. Arthritis in SLE does not involve the spine.[5] Small joints of the hand are affected in 95% of cases, but deformities such as those seen in rheumatoid arthritis are rare.[2] Dermatitis is the second most common clinical feature of SLE, but the classic malar butterfly erythema is present in only one third of patients.[5] Clinically significant renal disease occurs in 40% to 75% of cases.[5,6]

Patients with lupus are at increased risk for the antiphospholipid-antibody syndrome, which is characterized by arterial and venous thrombosis, thrombocytopenia, and recurrent fetal loss (see discussion of thrombophlebitis).[5,6]

A variety of treatments are used for SLE, depending on the organ systems involved and the severity of the disease. Most joint inflammation is managed with nonsteroidal anti-inflammatory drugs, but care must be taken that these do not aggravate renal disease. Hydroxychloroquine (Plaquenil) may be used for some patients. Cutaneous manifestations are dealt with primarily by strict sun blocking. Renal manifestations are treated with drugs, such as azathioprine (Imuran), cyclophosphamide (Cytoxan), or corticosteroids. Lupus patients with the antiphosphlipid-antibody syndrome are given warfarin except during pregnancy (see discussion of antiphospholipid-antibody syndrome).[7]

Vasculitis

Vasculitis can be divided into large vessel vasculitis, which includes giant cell arteritis and Takayasu's arteritis; medium-sized vessel arteritis, which includes polyarteritis nodosa and Kawasaki disease; and small vessel vasculitis, which includes cutaneous leukocytoclastic angiitis (hypersensitivity vasculitis), Behçet's disease, Henoch-Schönlein purpura, Goodpasture's syndrome, serum sickness, and the three entities usually associated with ANCA in the blood, namely Wegener's granulomatosis, Churg-Strauss syndrome, and microscopic polyangiitis.[3] The dividing line between small and medium-sized arteries is not always well defined, and some of the listed disorders are not strictly limited to vessels of a particular size. Giant cell and Takayasu's arteritides are always limited to large vessels; hypersensitivity vasculitis, Henoch-Schönlein purpura, and the vasculitis of cryoglobulinemia are limited to small vessels; the remainder may affect both medium-sized and small vessels.[8]

Giant cell arteritis

Giant cell or temporal arteritis is primarily a disease of elderly whites. Headaches, jaw claudication, weight loss, malaise, and fever are common symptoms. About 15% of patients seek treatment for fever of unknown origin. Visual symptoms, which can include partial or complete visual loss, diplopia, and ptosis, are less common but are important harbingers of complete vision loss. Between one fourth and one half of the patients have symptoms of polymyalgia rheumatica. An association between temporal arteritis and the later development of thoracic aneurysms has been described.[9]

The diagnosis of giant cell arteritis is usually confirmed by temporal artery biopsy, although other cranial arteries may be chosen as the biopsy site. If the biopsy cannot be performed before the start of steroid therapy, it may still be done within the next 2 weeks with reasonable expectation of showing positive results if the patient actually has the disease.[9]

Treatment of giant cell arteritis is prednisone, usually starting with 40 to 60 mg/day. In most cases the daily dose may be decreased by about 10 mg after 2 weeks and by another 10 mg 2 weeks later. Thereafter it may be lowered by a maximum of 10% every 1 to 2 weeks, depending on symptoms and the sedimentation rate or C-reactive protein levels. As the dose of prednisone decreases, the frequency and magnitude of further decrements diminish. Many patients can be weaned from prednisone within 2 years.[9]

Takayasu's arteritis

Takayasu's arteritis or pulseless disease involves inflammation and stenosis of large and intermediate-sized arteries, especially in the region of the aortic arch. Most affected are women in their teens or early twenties.[8]

Kawasaki disease

The highest incidence of Kawasaki disease is in Asians, and the vast majority of cases are in children under age 5. The most serious sequelae of the disease are cardiac and include myocarditis and pericarditis during the acute phase of the illness and, more important, coronary artery aneurysms and thrombosis in the later stages. The following clinical manifestations are needed to make the diagnosis[10]:

1. Fever of at least 5 days' duration plus at least four of the other five findings
2. Changes in the extremities (erythema and edema of hands and feet in the acute phase and desquamation of fingertips in the convalescent phase)
3. Polymorphous rash over the body
4. Bilateral conjunctival injection that usually involves the bulbar conjunctiva and is not associated with exudate
5. Changes in lips and oral cavity (fissuring and erythema of lips, erythema of pharynx and oral mucosa, strawberry tongue)
6. Cervical adenopathy with at least one lymph node 1.5 cm in diameter or greater

In patients with fever the diagnosis can be based on fewer criteria if echocardiography or angiography demonstrates coronary artery disease.[10]

Long-term sequelae are diminished by adequate treatment. Recommended therapy is a single IV infusion of immune globulin 2 g/kg plus high-dose aspirin (80 to 100 mg/kg/day). High-dose aspirin is continued until several days after defervescence and is then reduced to 3 to 5 mg/kg as a single daily dose for 6 to 8 weeks if no coronary artery abnormalities are detected. If coronary artery abnormalities are detected, low-dose aspirin therapy should be continued indefinitely.[10]

Polyarteritis nodosa

Although polyarteritis nodosa is usually idiopathic, it may be associated with cryoglobulinemia, hairy cell leukemia, rheumatoid arthritis, Sjögren's syndrome, or hepatitis B.[8]

Cutaneous leukocytoclastic angiitis

Cutaneous leukocytoclastic angiitis, or hypersensitivity vasculitis, is a small vessel angiitis that affects primarily the skin of the lower legs and is manifested as purpura and sometimes focal areas of necrosis. The word "leukocytoclastic" refers to the fact that on histological examination the nuclei of white blood cells infiltrating the dermis are found to be broken up. The condition can be idiopathic, drug induced (in about 10% of cases), or rarely a manifestation of a systemic vasculitis. If no clinical evidence of systemic disease is found and possible provoking drugs have been discontinued, the condition resolves spontaneously over several weeks or months. Symptomatic treatment with antihistamines or topical corticosteroids is sufficient in most cases, although a few patients with severe disease require oral steroids.[3]

Behçet's disease

Behçet's disease is common in the eastern Mediterranean (particularly Turkey, Iran, and Saudi Arabia), China, Korea and Japan. It is rare in Western countries. Small vessel vasculitis results in a varied clinical picture. Recurrent oral ulceration is the most common initial symptom and is present in almost all cases; recurrent genital ulcers are also common. Other clinical manifestations include ocular inflammation, arthritis, dermatitis, and gastrointestinal and central nervous system symptoms.[11]

Henoch-Schönlein purpura

Henoch-Schönlein purpura is a small vessel vasculitis of children that is characterized by IgA immune complexes in the vessels. The peak age is 5 years, and common manifestations are purpura, arthralgias, and colicky abdominal pain. About half the patients have hematuria and proteinuria. The prognosis is excellent, and in most cases no specific treatment is required. About 5% of cases progress to end-stage renal failure, and the optimal management of this subgroup is uncertain.[3]

Churg-Strauss syndrome

The Churg-Strauss syndrome is a vasculitis with numerous eosinophils in the inflammatory infiltrate. Initial symptoms are those of allergic rhinitis and asthma, but after a few years or even several decades symptoms related to vasculitis such as eosinophilic (Loeffler's) pneumonia develop. Gastroenteritis, myocarditis, neuropathy, and in some cases nephritis may also be present. Almost all patients have eosinophilia, and 70% have ANCA.[3] A number of cases of Churg-Strauss syndrome have been reported in asthmatic patients taking leukotriene inhibitors such as zafirlukast (Accolate) or montelukast (Singulair) for the treatment of asthma. Because the leukotriene inhibitors improved asthma control, the treating physicians withdrew corticosteroids, an action that appears to have unmasked preexisting Churg-Strauss syndrome.[12]

Wegener's granulomatosis

Wegener's granulomatosis is a granulomatous vasculitis that involves the upper and lower respiratory tracts. About 20% of patients have evidence of glomerulonephritis at presentation, but as the disease evolves, this condition develops in about 80%. The typical clinical presentation is persistent inflammation of the nasal passages or sinuses in conjunction with fever, malaise, and migratory arthritis. ANCA is found in 90% of cases. Therapy for Wegener's granulomatosis is generally steroids and cyclophosphamide, which produce good remissions. Hemorrhagic cystitis and bladder cancer are complications of cyclophosphamide therapy. Once remission is achieved, some patients may be maintained on methotrexate alone; whether daily trimethoprim-sulfamethoxazole (Septra, Bactrim) decreases the relapse rate is uncertain.[3]

Microscopic polyangiitis

Microscopic polyangiitis exists to confuse family physicians. Some authors consider it to be a variant of Wegener's granulomatosis,[3] whereas others describe it as a variant of polyarteritis nodosa.[8]

❧ REFERENCES ❧

1. Moore PM, Pope J: Investigating connective tissue disease. I. An overview, *Can J CME* 6:39-49, 1994.
2. Slater CA, Davis RB, Shmerling RH: Antinuclear antibody testing: a study of clinical utility, *Arch Intern Med* 156:1421-1425, 1996.
3. Jennette JC, Falk RJ: Small-vessel vasculitis, *N Engl J Med* 337:1512-1523, 1997.
4. Fox RE, Saito I: Criteria for diagnosis of Sjögren's syndrome, *Rheum Dis Clin North Am* 20:391-407, 1994.
5. Mills JA: Systemic lupus erythematosus, *N Engl J Med* 330:1871-1879, 1994.
6. Cockwell P, Savage CO, Owen JJ, et al: Systemic lupus erythematosus complicated by lupus nephritis and antiphospholipid antibody syndrome, *BMJ* 314:292-295, 1997.
7. Petri M: Treatment of systemic lupus erythematosus: an update, *Am Fam Physician* 57:2753-2760, 1998.
8. Roane DW, Griger DR: An approach to diagnosis and initial management of systemic vasculitis, *Am Fam Physician* 60:1421-1430, 1999.
9. Hunder GG: Giant cell arteritis and polymyalgia rheumatica, *Med Clin North Am* 81:195-219, 1997.
10. Taubert KA: Epidemiology of Kawasaki disease in the United States and worldwide, *Prog Pediatr Cardiol* 6:181-185, 1997.
11. Sakane T, Takeno M, Suzuki N, et al: Behçet's disease, *N Engl J Med* 341:1284-1291, 1999.
12. D'Cruz DP, Barnes NC, Lockwood CM: Difficult asthma or Churg-Strauss syndrome? (editorial), *BMJ* 318:475-476, 1999.

HIV AND AIDS

(See also adoption; cervical cancer; poverty; sexually transmitted diseases)

Hotlines

Keeping up to date on human immunodeficiency virus (HIV) disease is difficult for most physicians. To answer physicians' questions about HIV patients, the San Francisco General Hospital has established a "warmline" at (800) 933-3413, which is available during weekday working hours.[1] A resource for advice on managing individuals after exposure is the National Clinicians' Postexposure Hotline at (888) 488-4911. In Canada help is available by calling the Canadian HIV and AIDS Mentorship Program (CHAMP) at (800) 773-5575.[2] Several resources are available on the World Wide Web, including Clinical Care Options for HIV (http://www.healthcg.com/hiv), Guidelines for the Use of Antiretroviral Agents in HIV-Infected Adults and Adolescents (http://www.hivatis.org), the HIV InSite of the University of California–San Francisco (http://hivinsite.ucsf. edu), and the American Foundation for AIDS Research (amFAR) HIV/AIDS Treatment Directory (http://www.amfar.org/td).

History

The first case of acquired immunodeficiency syndrome (AIDS) was reported in 1981,[3,4] and the virus was isolated in 1984.[4] However, archival serum samples reveal that the disease existed before that time. Perhaps the first European to be infected was a Norwegian merchant sailor who died of AIDS in 1976; probably he acquired the disease in Cameroon, West Africa, in 1962.[5]

HIV-1 has now been determined to be a zoonotic infection originating in the common chimpanzee, whose natural range is in West-Central Africa. Chimpanzees carry the virus but do not become clinically ill.[3,6] Transmission from chimpanzees to humans probably occurred when blood from a chimpanzee being butchered for food contaminated an open wound.[3]

Distribution of HIV Infection

In the United States HIV was originally a disease largely limited to gay men. At present most infections in the United States result from IV drug use or heterosexual contacts, and the incidence is increasing in women and minority groups. Worldwide, 33 million people (44% women) are infected, 95% of whom are in developing countries.[3]

HIV-1 Virus Strains

Over 99% of cases in the current pandemic of AIDS are caused by the group M strain of the HIV-1 virus.[5]

Prognosis

The median elapsed time from the acquisition of HIV infection to the development of AIDS is 10 to 11 years.[7] The rate of progression seems to be the same for men and women,[8] and pregnancy does not appear to accelerate it.[9] A Swedish study of HIV-positive homosexual men determined that progression was significantly faster in those who had a glandular fever (infectious mononucleosis) type of illness at the time of seroconversion than in those who had no or only minor symptoms at seroconversion. The authors estimated that a glandular fever–type syndrome is present in about half of men who become HIV positive.[10]

A surrogate measure of HIV progression is the CD4+ lymphocyte count.[11,12] On average the cell count decreases by 50 to 100/μl per year. Opportunistic infections usually develop in individuals with CD4+ counts less than 200/μl.[11]

An important prognostic factor is the plasma viral load in the early months or years of infection, as has been documented in hemophiliacs,[13] black IV drug users in the United States,[14] and HIV-positive patients living in the community in Switzerland.[12] In the hemophiliac study, for example, progression to AIDS at 10 years correlated with the viral load measured between 12 and 36 months after seroconversion. In patients with fewer than 1000 copies per milliliter, no progression was found at 10 years.[13]

The survival time of patients with AIDS correlates directly with the experience of their physicians in managing this disease. In a study published in 1996 the median survival of patients looked after by inexperienced physicians was 14 months compared with 26 months for those cared for by experienced physicians.[15] Health professionals inexperienced in the care of HIV-positive patients may obtain help from the various hotlines and warmlines or by accessing appropriate sites on the world wide web (see earlier discussion).

Another factor that determines the prognosis of patients with AIDS is the nature of the initial AIDS-defining illness. Survival is longer for those with esophageal candidiasis or Kaposi's sarcoma and shorter for those with *Pneumocystis carinii* pneumonia or other illness such as cytomegalovirus disease. In one series the median survival from the onset of an AIDS-defining illness was 20 months.[16] However, in developed countries survival has increased dramatically in the last few years because of the introduction of highly active antiretroviral therapy, which includes combinations of three or four drugs (see below).[3]

The frequency of specific opportunistic infections varies with geographical location. *P. carinii* pneumonia is common in the developed world, whereas tuberculosis is a far more frequent event in developing nations. Furthermore, because patients in the industrialized world are surviving longer, infections associated with more advanced degrees of immunosuppression such as cytomegalovirus retinitis and *Mycobacterium avium* complex infection are becoming more common.[17]

◣ REFERENCES ◢

1. Voelker R: Rural communities struggle with AIDS, *JAMA* 279:5-6, 1998.
2. Klein A: Beyond biases and outdated perceptions: HIV prevention and mentoring (editorial), *Can Fam Physician* 43:133-134, 1997.
3. Fauci AS: The AIDS epidemic: considerations for the 21st century, *N Engl J Med* 341:1046-1050, 1999.
4. Centers for Disease Control and Prevention: Identification of HIV-1 group O infection—1996, *JAMA* 276:521-522, 1996.
5. Hooper E: Sailors and star-bursts, and the arrival of HIV, *BMJ* 315:1689-1691, 1997.
6. Gao F, Bailes E, Robertson DL, et al: Origin of HIV-1 in the chimpanzee *Pan troglodytes troglodytes* (letter), *Nature* 397:436-441, 1999.
7. Pezzotti P, Phillips AN, Dorrucci M, et al: Category of exposure to HIV and age in the progression to AIDS: a longitudinal study of 1199 individuals with known dates of seroconversion, *BMJ* 313:583-586, 1996.
8. Lepri AC, Pezzotti P, Dorrucci M, et al: HIV disease progression in 854 women and men infected through injecting drug use and heterosexual sex and followed for up to nine years from seroconversion, *BMJ* 309:1537-1542, 1994.
9. Alliegro MB, Dorrucci M, Phillips AN, et al: Incidence and consequences of pregnancy in women with known duration of HIV infection, *Arch Intern Med* 157:2585-2590, 1997.
10. Lindback S, Brostrom C, Karlsson A, et al: Does symptomatic primary HIV-1 infection accelerate progression to CDC stage IV disease, CD4 count below 200 × 10 (6)/1, AIDS, and death from AIDS? *BMJ* 309:1535-1537, 1994.
11. Goldschmidt RH, Moy A: Antiretroviral drug treatment for HIV/AIDS, *Am Fam Physician* 54:574-580, 1996.
12. Yerly S, Perneger TV, Hirschel B, et al: A critical assessment of the prognostic value of HIV-1 RNA levels and CD4+ cell counts in HIV-infected patients, *Arch Intern Med* 158:247-252, 1998.
13. O'Brien TR, Blattner WA, Waters D, et al: Serum HIV-1 levels and time to development of AIDS in the Multicenter Hemophilia Cohort Study, *JAMA* 276:105-110, 1996.
14. Viahov D, Graham N, Hoover D, et al: Prognostic indicators for AIDS and infectious disease death in HIV-infected injection drug users: plasma viral load and CD4+ cell count, *JAMA* 279:35-40, 1998.
15. Kitahata MM, Koepsell TD, Deyo RA, et al: Physicians' experience with the acquired immunodeficiency syndrome as a factor in patients' survival, *N Engl J Med* 334:701-706, 1996.
16. Mocroft A, Youle M, Morcinek J, et al (Royal Free/Chelsea and Westminster Hospitals Collaborative Group): Survival after diagnosis of AIDS: a prospective observational study of 2625 patients, *BMJ* 314:409-413, 1997.
17. Beiser C: Recent advances: HIV infection—2, *BMJ* 314:579-583, 1997.

Transmission and Epidemiology of HIV Infection
(See also transfusions)

In 1995 one third of reported AIDS cases in the United States were directly or indirectly (through heterosexual contact or pregnancy) associated with IV use of illicit drugs.[1] Worldwide, 75% to 85% of HIV infections are sexually transmitted.[2]

Acute retroviral syndrome

In 40% to 90% of persons with HIV an infectious mononucleosis–like syndrome called acute human immunodeficiency virus type 1 infection, acute retroviral syndrome, or seroconversion syndrome develops. The incubation period is 4 to 11 days, and the illness usually lasts less than 2 weeks. Progression to AIDS is more rapid among patients who have a prolonged acute retroviral syndrome.[3]

Symptoms and signs of the acute retroviral syndrome may include fever, fatigue, myalgia, headache, a maculopapular rash, lymphadenopathy, and in some cases oral or genital ulcers or a stiff neck (aseptic meningitis). Acute retroviral syndrome is often misdiagnosed simply because physicians fail to include it in the differential diagnosis. Laboratory findings may include lymphopenia and thrombocytopenia, a reduction in CD4+ counts, and high levels of viral plasma load. The usual HIV serological tests (ELISA) are negative; they become positive 2 to 3 weeks, at the earliest, after the onset of illness. The only investigations that can confirm the diagnosis during the acute phase are blood samples for HIV-1 RNA testing or p24 antigen testing.[3]

Making a specific diagnosis of the acute retroviral syndrome is important for three reasons. First, preliminary evidence suggests that aggressive treatment of the disease at this stage may be beneficial. Second, identification of the disease during the acute phase when it is highly contagious may prevent further spread by the patient if he or she is made aware of the risks. Third, early contact tracing may also decrease spread of disease.[3]

Occupational exposure

The risk of HIV infection from a needlestick injury is estimated to be 0.36%. The risk is greater if the exposure is from an object visibly contaminated with blood of the HIV-positive patient, the needlestick was caused by an intravascular device, and the injury is a deep one. The risk is also higher if the patient is in a terminal phase of AIDS and thus has a higher titer of HIV in the blood. When none of these added risk factors is present, the risk of infection is less than 0.3%.[4] Postexposure use of zidovudine (ZDV) in doses of approximately 1000 mg/day for 3 to 4 weeks appears to decrease the risk by about 80%.[5]

Recommendations of the Centers for Disease Control and Prevention (CDC) on the management of occupational exposure include the following[6]:

1. Contaminated skin areas should be washed immediately with soap and water, and mucous membranes should be flushed with water.

2. When possible, an expert on retroviral diseases should be consulted. Resources include the National Clinicians' Postexposure Hotline, (888) 488-4911.

3. A detailed risk assessment should be performed; algorithms for doing so are included in the CDC report that is referenced here. Factors leading to the characterization of highest risk include deep injury, visible blood on the injuring device, injury from an intravascular needle, exposure from a patient thought to have a high HIV titer, prolonged or massive exposure to the skin, and exposure to portions of the skin whose integrity has been compromised.

4. Postexposure prophylaxis should be offered to persons exposed to body fluids or tissues known or suspected to be infectious. Blood is the most infectious, but other fluids associated with risk are semen, vaginal secretions, cerebrospinal fluid, and body cavity and joint fluids. Urine, feces, saliva, and sweat are not included in this category unless they are contaminated with blood. Although breast milk is associated with vertical transmission of HIV, it is not a risk factor for health care workers.

5. Postexposure prophylaxis should be started as soon as possible after exposure, preferably within 1 to 2 hours, and is probably not effective if started after 24 to 36 hours. However, in a case of high-risk exposure, treatment may be worth attempting if started within 2 weeks.

6. All prophylactic regimens include zidovudine (Retrovir) because this drug has been shown to be beneficial in such cases.

7. Two postexposure prophylactic regimens are recommended. The basic regimen is suitable for most exposures, and the expanded regimen for high-risk exposures. Both regimens are administered for 4 weeks.

8. The basic regimen consists of two nucleoside reverse transcriptase inhibitors—zidovudine (Retrovir) 600 mg/day in divided doses and lamivudine (3TC, Epivir) 150 mg bid.

9. The expanded regimen consists of the basic regimen plus a protease inhibitor, either indinavir (IDV, Crixivan) 800 mg q8h or nelfinavir (Viracept) 750 mg tid.

Sexual transmission

A variety of factors affect the risk of acquiring HIV through sexual contacts. Infectivity is greatest in the few weeks after HIV is acquired (before HIV serological tests become positive) and again in the late stages of the disease. In both these situations, viral blood titers are high. Chances of acquiring HIV are greater for persons with genital ulcers or other sexually transmitted diseases such as gonorrhea, Chlamydia infection, and trichomoniasis. Intercourse during menstruation increases the risk of infection for both men and women. Circumcised men are less likely to acquire HIV or transmit it to their partners than are uncircumcised men. Condoms offer good protection, but whether nonoxynol-9 affects transmission of HIV is unknown.[2] Male-to-female transmission occurs at about twice the rate of female-to-male transmission,[7] but because many more males than females in the North American population are HIV infected, the overall risk that a North American female will be infected through heterosexual intercourse has been estimated to be 12 times greater than the risk that a male will be infected in this manner.[8] A few persons appear to have a genetic resistance to infection.[2]

The risk of acquiring HIV from a single act of unprotected vaginal intercourse has been estimated as less than 1%.[9] Among 124 couples in which only one partner was HIV positive, no HIV transmission was recorded after 15,000 episodes of intercourse using condoms. In a similar situation in which condoms were used only intermittently, there was about a 5% conversion rate after 1 year with an estimated cumulative conversion rate of 13% at 2 years.[10]

A study of male homosexual and bisexual men found unprotected receptive anal intercourse to be the highest risk sexual activity, with an estimated per-contact risk of 0.82% if the partner was known to be HIV positive and 0.27% when partners of unknown serostatus were included in the analysis. The per-contact risk for unprotected insertive anal intercourse with HIV-positive or unknown serostatus partners was 0.06% and for unprotected receptive oral sex was 0.04%.[11]

Should postexposure treatment be given to individuals exposed to HIV through an isolated sexual or shared needle exposure? No data are available on which to base an answer; Katz and Gerberding[9] argue that treatment should be provided if continued exposure is unlikely and that such treatment can be started within 24 hours. Treatment is the same as for occupational exposure. This approach is generally supported by Lurie and associates,[10] with the proviso that if the risk of infection is low, postexposure prophylaxis may cause more harm than benefit. No data are available on the risk of acquiring HIV infection as a result of sexual assault or on the benefit of postexposure treatment. Current consensus is that treatment (following the protocol for occupational exposure) should be offered to all victims. It should be started within 72 hours and continued for 28 days.[12]

Blood transfusions

A 1996 U.S. paper calculated the risk of acquiring HIV from a single unit of blood as 1:493,000 (see discussion of transfusions).[13]

Household contacts

HIV transmission through household contacts is rare. As of May 1994, eight such cases in the United States had been reported to the CDC. These were probably the result of contact with blood or body fluids.[14]

Pregnancy

High maternal levels of HIV-1 RNA are a major risk factor for vertical transmission of HIV; in one study no transmission occurred with levels below 500 copies per milliliter.[15] Evidence is increasing that short courses of zidovudine given at the time of delivery or even to the newborn within 48 hours of delivery may be effective. In a retrospective cohort study from New York, Wade and associates[16] reported that HIV transmission from HIV-positive mothers to their infants was 26.6% if no zidovudine prophylaxis was given. If a standard three-part regimen of zidovudine was begun prenatally, continued during labor and delivery, and then given to the newborn, the transmission rate was 4.1%. If a two-part regimen was used beginning during labor, the transmission rate was 10%. When only the infant was treated, beginning within 48 hours of birth, the rate was 9.3%. Infants who began to receive treatment after 48 hours had a transmission rate of 18.4%. Although all HIV-positive pregnant women should receive zidovudine, potent combination therapy including zidovudine is probably preferable, especially in the second and third trimesters.[17] A prospective cohort study of uninfected children born to HIV mothers who were treated with zidovudine during pregnancy found no long-term adverse effects after up to 5.6 years of follow-up.[18]

A metaanalysis of 15 prospective American and European studies found that elective Cesarean section before rupture of membranes or onset of labor decreased the vertical transmission rate of HIV from 19% to 10% when the mothers did not receive antiretroviral therapy and from 7% to 2% when they did. Nevertheless, the clinical benefit of Cesarean section is uncertain. HIV-positive women have a higher complication rate from Cesarean section than do those who are not infected with the virus. In addition, most of the women who received antiretroviral therapy in the studies evaluated in the metaanalysis were treated with zidovudine alone; whether combination retroviral therapy would lower the vertical transmission rate enough that Cesarean section would not add further benefit is unknown.[19]

A decision analysis concluded that in the United States mandatory HIV testing of pregnant women would deter a significant number of women from prenatal care and therefore that a policy of voluntary testing is preferable.[20]

Breast feeding

HIV can be transmitted to newborns through breast feeding. An international (Europe and Africa) pooled analysis estimated that the overall risk of such transmission was 3.2% per year of breast feeding. The authors concluded that if breast feeding had been discontinued by 4 months, none of the 902 infants in the study would have been infected, and if it had been stopped at 6 months, three would have been infected.[21] A study from Malawi found the annual transmission rate of HIV through breast feeding to be a little over 7%, with the highest risk occurring in the first few months. Early weaning would decrease transmission rates, but in much of Africa such a practice would probably result in increased infant mortality from other diseases.[22]

◣ REFERENCES ◢

1. Centers for Disease Control and Prevention: AIDS associated with injecting-drug use—United States, 1995, *JAMA* 275: 1628-1629, 1996.
2. Royce RA, Sena A, Cates W Jr, et al: Sexual transmission of HIV, *N Engl J Med* 336:1072-1078, 1997.
3. Kahn JO, Walker BD: Acute human immunodeficiency virus type 1 infection, *N Engl J Med* 339:33-39, 1998.
4. Cardo DM, Culver DH, Ciesielski CA, et al: A case-control study of HIV seroconversion in health care workers after percutaneous exposure, *N Engl J Med* 337:1485-1490, 1997.
5. Centers for Disease Control and Prevention: Case-control study of HIV seroconversion in health-care workers after percutaneous exposure to HIV-infected blood—France, United Kingdom, and United States, January 1988–August 1994, *JAMA* 275:274-275, 1996.
6. Centers for Disease Control and Prevention: Public Health Service guidelines for the management of health care worker exposures to HIV and recommendations for postexposure prophylaxis, *MMWR* 47(no RR-7):1-33, 1998.
7. Nicolosi A, Leite ML, Musicco M, et al: The efficiency of male-to-female and female-to-male sexual transmission of the human immunodeficiency virus: a study of 730 stable couples, *Epidemiology* 5:570-575, 1994.
8. Padian NS, Shiboski S, Jewell N: The effect of the number of exposures on the risk of heterosexual HIV transmission, *J Infect Dis* 161:883-887, 1990.
9. Katz MH, Gerberding JL: Postexposure treatment of people exposed to the human immunodeficiency virus through sexual contact or injection-drug use, *N Engl J Med* 336:1097-1100, 1997.

10. Lurie P, Miller S, Hecht F, et al: Postexposure prophylaxis after nonoccupational HIV exposure: clinical, ethical, and policy considerations, *JAMA* 280:1769-1773, 1998.

11. Vittinghoff E, Douglas J, Judson F, et al: Per-contact risk of human immunodeficiency virus transmission between male sexual partners, *Am J Epidemiol* 150:306-311, 1999.

12. Bamberger JD, Waldo CR, Gerberding JL, et al: Postexposure prophylaxis for human immunodeficiency virus (HIV) infection following sexual assault, *Am J Med* 106:323-326, 1999.

13. Schreiber GB, Busch MP, Kleinman SH, et al (Retrovirus Epidemiology Donor Study): The risk of transfusion-transmitted viral infections, *N Engl J Med* 334:1685-1690, 1996.

14. Human immunodeficiency virus transmission in household settings—United States, *MMWR* 43:347, 353-356, 1994.

15. Mofenson LM, Lambert JS, Stiehm ER, et al: Risk factors for perinatal transmission of human immunodeficiency virus type 1 in women treated with zidovudine, *N Engl J Med* 341:385-393, 1999.

16. Wade NA, Birkhead GS, Warren BL, et al: Abbreviated regimens of zidovudine prophylaxis and perinatal transmission of the human immunodeficiency virus, *N Engl J Med* 339:1409-1414, 1998.

17. Carpenter CC, Fischl MA, Hammer SM, et al: Antiretroviral therapy for HIV infection in 1998: updated recommendations of the International AIDS Society—USA Panel, *JAMA* 280:78-86, 1998.

18. Culnane M, Fowler MG, Lee SS, et al: Lack of long-term effects of in utero exposure to zidovudine among uninfected children born to HIV-infected women, *JAMA* 281:151-157, 1999.

19. International Perinatal HIV Group: The mode of delivery and the risk of vertical transmission of human immunodeficiency virus type 1, *N Engl J Med* 340:977-987, 1999.

20. Nakchbandi IA, Longenecker JC, Ricksecker A, et al: A decision analysis of mandatory compared with voluntary HIV testing in pregnant women, *Ann Intern Med* 128:760-767, 1998.

21. Leroy V, Newell M-L, Dabis F, et al: International multicentre pooled analysis of late postnatal mother-to-child transmission of HIV-1 infection, *Lancet* 352:597-600, 1998.

22. Miotti PG, Taha TE, Kumwenda NI, et al: HIV transmission through breastfeeding: a study in Malawi, *JAMA* 282:744-759, 1999.

HIV Testing

After infection with HIV a serological window occurs during which HIV antibodies are not detectable. Among infected persons 95% become seropositive within 3 months and 99% within 6 months. The traditional screening test is ELISA. If it is positive, the serum is tested twice more with ELISA and, if positive, is further tested with Western blot, immunoblot, radioimmunoprecipitation, or immunofluorescence. Most results are positive or negative, but a few are indeterminate; in the latter situation the patient should be retested no sooner than 6 weeks after the initial blood was obtained.[1] Antibodies can be detected in saliva, and a commercially available system for doing this is OraSure. It has good sensitivity and specificity. Urine tests are not as sensitive or specific.[2] One of the latest technological advances is rapid HIV test kits that give results in 10 minutes and can be used in the offices of health professionals. Although positive tests require verification, rapid preliminary results may facilitate counseling. Many commercial kits are available, but the sensitivity and specificity with wide-scale use are uncertain. Early studies indicate that for most brands sensitivity and specificity are only slightly less than for standard enzyme immunoassays but that for a few brands results are unacceptable.[3]

False-positive results from HIV testing occur but are rare. In one study of blood transfusion donors 1 in 250,000 had a false-positive Western blot test. Of all positive Western blot tests, 5% turned out to be false positives when currently acceptable laboratory procedures were used.[4]

A controversial aspect of testing is the use of home sample collection tests. Patients buy a kit, obtain a fingerstick blood sample that they collect on a filter paper, and send the sample to the laboratory. Identification is with an anonymous code number. Patients call for results, and if the test is positive, they are given telephone counseling. If they do not have a physician, they are offered referrals. Preliminary data suggest that this system attracts a number of individuals who would otherwise not receive testing and that most of those who test positive have sources for medical care or appear willing to accept referrals. Whether they use these resources is unknown.[5]

❧ REFERENCES ❧

1. Expert Working Group on HIV Testing, Canadian Medical Association: *Counselling guidelines for HIV testing,* Ottawa, 1995, Canadian Medical Association.

2. Diagnostic tests for HIV, *Med Lett* 39:81-83, 1997.

3. Giles RE, Perry KR, Parry JV: Simple/rapid test devices for anti-HIV screening: do they come up to the mark? *J Med Virol* 59:104-109, 1999.

4. Kleinman S, Busch MP, Hall L, et al: False-positive HIV-1 test results in a low-risk screening setting of voluntary blood donation, *JAMA* 280:1080-1085, 1998.

5. Branson BM: Home sample collection tests for HIV infection, *JAMA* 280:1699-1701, 1998.

Initial Laboratory Investigations for Patients with HIV

Initial laboratory investigations of a patient who is found to be HIV positive should include the following:

1. CBC and differential, smear, platelets (drugs that may be used can affect the hemogram)
2. Absolute CD4 lymphocyte count
3. Plasma viral load
4. Vitamin B_{12} and folate (AZT may cause macrocytosis)
5. Blood urea nitrogen, creatinine, liver function, electrolytes
6. Hepatitis B and C screening
7. *Toxoplasma* titer
8. Chest x-ray examination (as a screening for tuberculosis)
9. Tuberculin skin test (repeated annually)

10. Papanicolaou smear
11. Swabs and serological tests for sexually transmitted diseases

Immunizations for HIV-Positive Patients

With the possible exception of measeles-mumps-rubella vaccine, patients with AIDS should not receive live vaccines such as oral polio, oral typhoid, or yellow fever. Asymptomatic HIV-positive patients with normal lymphocyte counts may receive such vaccines if they are clinically indicated.[1] Regular immunizations for HIV-positive patients should include the following:

1. Inactivated polio vaccine (IPV, Salk) every 10 years
2. Diphtheria-tetanus vaccine (Td) every 10 years
3. Influenza vaccine annually
4. Pneumococcal vaccine
5. Hepatitis B vaccine for patients at risk
6. Measles-mumps-rubella (MMR) vaccine (if serologically negative for these agents)
7. *Haemophilus* b vaccine (optional)

For travel, patients may receive, as indicated:

1. Inactivated polio vaccine
2. Inactivated typhoid vaccine
3. Gamma globulin
4. Japanese encephalitis vaccine
5. MMR vaccine

◣ REFERENCES ◤

1. Canadian communicable disease report: statement on travellers and HIV/AIDS, *Can Med Assoc J* 152:379-380, 1995.

Antiretroviral Strategies

Classes of antiretroviral drugs

The three main classes of antiretroviral drugs are nucleoside analogue reverse transcriptase inhibitors (nRTIs), protease inhibitors (PIs), and nonnucleoside reverse transcriptase inhibitors (NNRTIs).[1] A fourth class is nucleotide reverse transcriptase inhibitors (Table 35).[2]

Is there a cure for HIV?

Although treatment of asymptomatic HIV positive patients with highly active antiretroviral therapy (HAART) may appear to cause complete viral suppression, cure is unlikely.[1,3,4] A small pool of long-lived memory CD4+ cells continues to harbor replication-competent HIV for at least 2 years,[3] and ultrasensitive techniques reveal the continued presence of low-level replication in both peripheral blood monocytes and the peripheral plasma.[4]

Initiation of therapy

The goal of HIV therapy is to maintain or improve immunological function without inducing intolerable adverse effects. Aggressive treatment of asymptomatic HIV-infected individuals often reconstitutes immune function, but such treatment rarely restores immune function in persons with AIDS. The immunological benefits of early treatment have

Table 35   Antiretroviral Drugs

Drug	Usual adult dose
Nucleoside Reverse Transcriptase Inhibitors (nRTIs)	
Abacavir (ABC) (Ziagen)	300 mg bid
Didanosine, dideoxyinosine (ddl) (Videx)	200 mg bid (varies with weight)
Lamivudine, 3TC (Epivir)	150 mg bid
Stavudine (Zerit)	40 mg bid
Zalcitabine, dideoxycytidine (ddC) (Hivid)	0.375-0.750 mg tid
Zidovudine (ZDV), azidothymidine (AZT) (Retrovir)	200 mg tid or 300 mg bid
Nucleotide Reverse Transcriptase Inhibitors	
Adefovir (Preveon)	120 mg/day
Protease Inhibitors (PIs)	
Amprenavir (Agenerase)	1200 mg bid
Indinavir (Crixivan)	800 mg tid on empty stomach
Nelfinavir (Viracept)	750 mg tid or 1250 bid with food
Ritonavir (Norvir)	600 mg bid with food
Saquinavir (Invirase)	600 mg tid with food (poor bioavailability)
Saquinavir soft-gel capsules (Fortovase)	1200 mg tid or 1800 mg bid with food (good bioavailability)
Nonnucleoside Reverse Transcriptase Inhibitors (NNRTIs)	
Delavirdine (Rescriptor)	400 mg tid
Efavirenz (EFV) (Sustiva)	600 mg/day
Nevirapine (Viramune)	200 mg bid

to be balanced against the many adverse effects induced by current multiple drug protocols.[1]

The 2000 guidelines of the U.S. panel of the International AIDS Society recommend starting therapy if the plasma HIV RNA level is above 30,000 copies/ml, regardless of the CD4+ cell count, or if the CD4+ cell count is less than 350×10^6 /L (350/μl) regardless of the HIV RNA level. Treatment is also advised if the HIV RNA level is between 5000 and 30,000 copies/ml and the CD4+ cell count is between 350 and 500×10^6/L. Whether patients with CD4+ cell counts above 500×10^6/L and HIV RNA levels below 5000 copies/ml require treatment is uncertain; progression over a 3-year period is unlikely, so careful monitoring may be acceptable. Decisions about treatment should always be based on at least two measurements of HIV RNA levels and CD4+ counts.[1]

Combination therapy

Treatment of HIV-positive patients involves combination therapy not only to prevent the emergence of viral resistance but also to maintain or enhance immunological function. The most common regimen is HAART, which comprises at least three drugs, one of which is a PI. When effective viral suppression is achieved, the risk of opportunistic infections is dramatically decreased.[5] Ideally viral load should be reduced to fewer than 50 copies per milliliter (standard current tests cannot detect levels below 50 copies/ml) within 16 to 24 weeks of starting therapy, but whether patients who achieve suppression to fewer than 500 or even 5000 copies per milliliter with initial treatment should be considered treatment failures and switched to another regimen is unknown.[1] Recently published studies suggest that the combination of two nRTIs plus an NNRTI are as effective as two nRTIs plus a PI in lowering viral load. NNRTIs have the advantage of requiring fewer daily doses and having fewer side effects than PIs.[6]

Six nRTIs, one nucleotide reverse transcriptase inhibitor, four PIs, and three NNRTIs are either approved for use in North America or available through "expanded access programs" (Table 35).[2] Initial formulations of the protease inhibitor saquinavir (Invirase) had poor bioavailability, but a new formulation under the trade name Fortovase appears to have resolved that problem and is the variant that should be used.[1]

A large number of three- or four-drug combinations are acceptable for the treatment of HIV. First choices for initial therapy are two nRTIs plus one or two PIs, or two nRTIs plus one NNRTI. Other regimens that are being evaluated include three nRTIs, and one PI plus one NNRTI plus one nRTI.[1] If the treatment goal is long-term suppression of viral replication, maintaining intensive three- or four-drug treatment for prolonged periods appears necessary. Three 1998 studies evaluating a switch from a three- or four-drug initiation phase to a two-drug maintenance regimen found that two drugs did not maintain viral suppression in significant numbers of patients.[7]

The management of HIV infections is complex and rapidly changing. Consultation or referral to experts in the field is advisable in most instances (see discussion of hotlines and web sites).

⚔ REFERENCES ⚔

1. Carpenter CC, Fischl MA, Hammer SM, et al: Antiretroviral therapy for HIV infection in 1998: recommendations of the International AIDS Society—USA Panel, *JAMA* 280:78-86, 1998.
2. Amprenavir: a new HIV protease inhibitor, *Med Lett* 41:64-66, 1999.
3. Zhang L, Ramratnam B, Tenner-Racz K, et al: Quantifying residual HIV-1 replication in patients receiving combination antiretroviral therapy, *N Engl J Med* 340:1605-1613, 1999.
4. Dornadula G, Zhang H, VanUitert B, et al: Residual HIV-1 RNA in blood plasma of patients taking suppressive highly active antiretroviral therapy, *JAMA* 282:1627-1632, 1999.
5. Ledergerber B, Egger M, Erard V, et al: AIDS-related opportunistic illnesses occurring after initiation of potent antiretroviral therapy: the Swiss HIV Cohort Study, *JAMA* 282:2220-2226, 1999.
6. Clumeck N: Choosing the best initial therapy for HIV-1 infection (editorial), *N Engl J Med* 341:1925-1926, 1999.
7. Cooper DA, Emery S: Therapeutic strategies for HIV infection—time to think hard (editorial), *N Engl J Med* 339:1319-1321, 1998.

Prophylaxis of Opportunistic Infections

In 1995 the U.S. Public Health Service issued guidelines for the prophylaxis of opportunistic infections in HIV patients,[1] and these were revised in 1997.[2] The recommendations are evidence based and classified in A to E levels such as those found in publications of the U.S. Preventive Services Task Force and Canadian Task Force on Preventive Health Care. "A" represents strong evidence for implementing, "C" insufficient evidence to support a recommendation, and "E" good evidence for lack of efficacy or overwhelming adverse effects of an intervention.[1,2] The 1997 recommendations give "A" ratings for chemoprophylaxis against *Pneumocystis carinii* pneumonia (PCP), toxoplasmic encephalitis, tuberculosis, and disseminated *Mycobacterium avium* complex (MAC) disease among HIV-positive patients meeting specified criteria. An "A" rating is also given to vaccinating all adult and adolescent patients who are HIV positive with pneumococcal vaccine. "B" recommendations (moderate evidence of efficacy) are given to hepatitis B and influenza immunizations of HIV-positive patients.[2]

Pneumocystis carinii pneumonia

No way of preventing exposure to *P. carinii* is known. Evidence is insufficient ("C" rating) to support a recommendation that a patient with HIV not share a room with someone who has PCP.[2]

PCP prophylaxis is recommended for all HIV-positive patients with a CD4+ count less than 0.2×10^9/L (200/µl), signs of immunosuppression such as thrush or hairy leukoplakia, or an unexplained fever (higher than 37.7° C or 100° F) of at least 2 weeks' duration. The drug of choice is trimethoprim-sulfamethoxazole (Bactrim, Septra) one double-strength (DS) tablet daily or, if it is poorly tolerated, one regular strength tablet daily. In some cases one DS tablet may be given three times a week. These regimens give cross-protection against toxoplasmosis and other bacterial infections.[2]

An evolving issue with respect to prophylaxis of opportunistic infections is the feasibility of discontinuing drugs if the patient's CD4 counts have risen as a result of effective combination antiretroviral therapy. An uncontrolled observational study from Switzerland reported that discontinuing prophylaxis against PCP among patients whose CD4 counts had risen and remained above 200/µl for 12 weeks after antiretroviral therapy did not increase their risk of acquiring PCP pneumonia or toxoplasmic encephalitis.[3] Whether such an approach has widespread applicability remains to be determined.[4]

Alternatives to trimethoprim-sulfamethoxazole are dapsone (Avlosulfon) 50 mg bid or 100 mg/day plus pyrimethamine (Daraprim) 50 mg po once weekly plus leucovorin (Wellcovorin) 25 mg po once weekly or aerosolized pentamidine (NebuPent) 300 mg monthly via Respirgard.[2]

Toxoplasmosis

Patients who are HIV positive, especially those who do not have antibodies to *Toxoplasma,* should be advised to wash their hands after handling raw meat and to avoid eating rare (pink) or raw meat, especially lamb, pork, or venison. After gardening or other contact with soil, hands should be thoroughly washed. Cats can transmit the organisms. Strays should be avoided, and pet cats should be kept indoors, never be fed raw or rare meat, and have their kitty litter changed daily, preferably by someone who is HIV negative (see discussion of toxoplasmosis in pregnancy).[2]

AIDS-related *Toxoplasma* encephalitis is usually caused by reactivation of the disease. Patients who are seropositive for *Toxoplasma* and have a CD4+ count below 0.10×10^9 (100/μl) should receive prophylactic trimethoprim-sulfamethoxazole or dapsone-pyrimethamine-leucovorin in the regimens recommended for PCP prophylaxis (see earlier discussion).[2]

Tuberculosis

All patients who are HIV positive, have a purified protein derivative test showing an induration greater than 5 mm, and do not have active tuberculosis are at high risk for active disease.[5] They should receive antituberculosis prophylaxis for 12 months in the form of isoniazid (INH) 300 mg/day plus pyridoxine 50 mg/day, or INH 900 mg twice a week plus pyridoxine 50 mg twice a week (see discussion of tuberculosis).[2]

Mycobacterium avium-intracellulare

Mycobacterium avium is omnipresent in soil and water, and there are no known means of preventing exposure.[2] About half of North American patients with AIDS acquire *M. avium* infection.[6] *M. avium* complex prophylaxis should be given to all HIV patients when the CD4+ count drops below 0.05×10^9 (50/ml). The drugs of choice are clarithromycin (Biaxin) 500 mg bid or azithromycin (Zithromax) 1200 mg once weekly.[2]

Esophageal candidiasis

Fluconazole (Diflucan) 200 mg/day is an effective agent for the prevention of esophageal candidiasis in patients with advanced HIV disease.[7] However, prophylaxis is not recommended save in exceptional cirumstances because the acute disease can be easily treated, whereas continued prophylaxis may lead to drug interactions and resistant organisms.[2] If prophylaxis is given, it should be with fluconazole 100 to 200 mg/day po in selected patients with a CD4+ count less than 0.50×10^9/L (50/μl).[2]

Cytomegalovirus

Cytomegalovirus (CMV) infection is the leading cause of blindness in patients with AIDS.[8] The risk of CMV infection approached 50% in HIV-positive patients before the introduction of protease inhibitors,[9] but since then the rate has fallen because of partial immune recovery induced by these agents.[8] One study in the pre–protease inhibitor era found that oral prophylaxis with ganciclovir (Cytovene) 1000 mg tid in patients with advanced AIDS decreased the incidence of CMV.[9] A trial published in 1999 compared AIDS patients with unilateral CMV retinitis treated with intraocular ganciclovir implants plus high doses (4.5 g/day) of oral ganciclovir against patients treated with implants plus placebo. Patients who were not taking protease inhibitors and who received high doses of oral ganciclovir had a decreased risk of acquiring retinitis in the unaffected eye. Patients who were taking protease inhibitors had a low incidence of retinitis in the unaffected eye, and no additional benefit was obtained with oral ganciclovir.[8]

Kaposi's sarcoma

A trial of high-dose oral ganciclovir prophylaxis (4.5 g/day) decreased the risk of Kaposi's sarcoma in AIDS patients by 75%.[8]

⬛ REFERENCES ⬛

1. USPHS/IDSA Prevention of Opportunistic Infections Working Group: USPHS/IDSA guidelines for the prevention of opportunistic infections in persons infected with human immunodeficiency virus: disease-specific recommendations, *Clin Infect Dis* 2(suppl):S32-S43, 1995.
2. USPHS/IDSA Prevention of Opportunistic Infections Working Group: USPHS/IDSA guidelines for the prevention of opportunistic infections in persons infected with human immunodeficiency virus, *MMWR* 46(RR-12):1-46, 1997.
3. Furrer H, Egger M, Opravil M, et al: Discontinuation of primary prophylaxis against *Pneumocystis carinii* pneumonia in HIV-1-infected adults treated with combination antiretroviral therapy, *N Engl J Med* 340:1301-1306, 1999.
4. Masur H, Kaplan J: Does *Pneumocystis carinii* prophylaxis still need to be lifelong? (editorial), *N Engl J Med* 340:1356-1358, 1999.
5. Girardi E, Antonucci G, Ippolito G, et al: Association of tuberculosis risk with the degree of tuberculin reaction in HIV-infected patients, *Arch Intern Med* 157:797-800, 1997.
6. Beiser C: Recent advances: HIV infection-2, *BMJ* 314:579-583, 1997.
7. Powderly WG, Finkelstein DM, Feinberg J, et al: A randomized trial comparing fluconazole with clotrimazole troches for the prevention of fungal infections in patients with advanced human immunodeficiency virus infection, *N Engl J Med* 332:704-705, 1995.
8. Martin DF, Kuppermann BD, Wolitz RA, et al: Oral ganciclovir for patients with cytomegalovirus retinitis treated with a ganciclovir implant, *N Engl J Med* 340:1063-1070, 1999.
9. Spector SA, McKinley GF, Lalezari JP, et al: Oral ganciclovir for the prevention of cytomegalovirus disease in persons with AIDS, *N Engl J Med* 334:1491-1497, 1996.

Treatment of Specific AIDS-Related Disorders

The treatment of specific AIDS-related disorders is a vast topic, and only a few entities are covered here.

Aphthous ulcers

Aphthous ulcers in patients with AIDS can become progressively larger and deeper, causing severe pain and difficulty eating. A randomized prospective trial found that thalidomide 200 mg/day po ameliorated or healed these lesions. This effect is thought to be mediated through the drug's immune-modulating capacity.[1]

Diarrhea

Diarrhea in patients with AIDS has many causes. Aside from the usual organisms to which everyone is subject, these include *M. avium,* cytomegalovirus, *Clostridium difficile, Cryptosporidium, Isospora belli* (requiring acid-fast staining of stool for diagnosis), and *Microsporidia* (requiring a modified trichrome stain of stool for diagnosis). In clinical practice, if the diarrhea is mild or moderate without blood, investigations may be limited to a routine stool culture and symptomatic treatment may be instituted. Further investigations can be deferred unless the patient's condition deteriorates. Symptomatic treatment consists of short-term bowel rest with clear fluids, bulking agents such as psyllium, and drugs such as diphenoxylate (Lomotil), loperamide (Imodium), or codeine alone or in combination. For patients with uncontrolled profuse diarrhea, octreotide (Sandostatin) in subcutaneous doses of 50 to 100 mg tid may be effective.

Esophageal candidiasis

The initial treatment of eosphageal candidiasis may be instituted on the basis of clinical suspicion. Endoscopy is reserved for patients who do not respond. The most effective medication at present appears to be fluconazole (Diflucan) 100 to 200 mg/day as a single dose for 3 weeks or for 2 weeks after symptoms have resolved; alternatives are itraconazole (Sporanox) 200 mg/day for 2 to 3 weeks and ketoconazole (Nizoral) 200 to 400 mg/day for 2 to 3 weeks.[2]

Weight loss

HIV wasting is relatively rare in patients who are receiving highly active combination antiretroviral therapy. Aside from providing optimal antiretroviral drug therapy, interventions that may be helpful for patients with AIDS wasting include nutritional evaluation, drugs, and possibly exercise programs. Appetite-stimulating drugs such as megestrol (Megace) in doses of 800 mg/day may be useful when weight loss is clearly due to reduced food intake; any weight gain achieved is due primarily to increased fat. If androgen deficiency is shown by low levels of serum free testosterone in HIV-infected men, testosterone therapy may lead to an increase in lean body mass.[3] One study found that a combination of progressive resistance exercise combined with intramuscular administration of testosterone 100 mg per week plus the oral anabolic steroid oxandrolone (Hepandrin, Oxandrin) 20 mg/day increased lean body mass in men with HIV-associated weight loss.[4]

❧ REFERENCES ❧

1. Jacobson JM, Greenspan JS, Spritzler J, et al: Thalidomide for the treatment of oral aphthous ulcers in patients with human immunodeficiency virus infection, *N Engl J Med* 336:1487-1493, 1997.
2. Drugs for AIDS and associated infections, *Med Lett* 37:87-94, 1995.
3. Corcoran C, Grinspoon S: Treatments for wasting in patients with the acquired immunodeficiency syndrome, *N Engl J Med* 340:1740-1750, 1999.
4. Strawford A, Barbieri T, Van Loan M, et al: Resistance exercise and supraphysiologic androgen therapy in eugonadal men with HIV-related weight loss: a randomized controlled trial, *JAMA* 281:1282-1290, 1999.

INFECTIOUS DISEASES

(See also bites; HIV and AIDS; immunizations; malaria; pets; tropical medicine)

Topics covered in this section

Cat Scratch Disease
Common Cold
Ehrlichiosis
Food Poisoning
Hantavirus
Herpes Simplex
Herpes Zoster
Histoplasmosis
Infectious Mononucleosis
Lyme Disease
Meningitis
Meningococcal Disease
Necrotizing Fasciitis
Parasitology
Pertussis
Polio
Sexually Transmitted Diseases
Streptococcal Infections
Tuberculosis
Varicella

CAT SCRATCH DISEASE

(See also pets)

Cat scratch disease usually occurs in children. The disease is transmitted by cat (or more often kitten) scratches, licks, or bites. A localized papule is found 2 to 3 days after the contact, and within a week or two, tender regional adenopathy develops that may persist for weeks or months. In about 6% of cases the site of the inoculum is the conjunctiva and the initial sign is a polypoid lesion of the palpebral conjunctiva, often associated with preauricular adenopathy. This is called Parinaud's oculoglandular syndrome. Rarely patients have central nervous system involvement, often manifested as seizures.[1] The organism responsible for most cases is *Bartonella henselae* (previously called *Rochalimaea henselae*) of the order Rickettsiales, although *Afipia felis* may account for some.[1,2] Serological methods are available in some laboratories to detect *R. henselae,* but the significance of positive results has not been fully elucidated.[2] The disease is self-limited, and antibiotic treatment is usually not required.[1,2] Cats need not be treated because they are merely carriers of the organism.[1]

REFERENCES

1. Smith DL: Cat-scratch disease, *Am Fam Physician* 55:1785-1789, 1997.
2. Adal KA, Cockerell CJ, Petri WA Jr: Cat scratch disease, bacillary angiomatosis, and other infections due to *Rochalimaea, N Engl J Med* 330:1509-1516, 1994.

COMMON COLD
(See also antibiotic resistance; rhinitis)

Aside from virus exposure, proven or reputed risk factors for acquiring colds are psychological stress,[1] social isolation, lack of exercise, decreased quality of sleep, and smoking.[2]

As of 1998, 10 placebo-controlled trials of zinc for the treatment of adults with common colds had been reported. Five showed benefit, and five no benefit. A similar trial in children and adolescents found no benefit.[3] Ipratropium bromide (Atrovent Nasal) has been shown to reduce the amount of nasal secretions during upper respiratory infections, but not the degree of nasal congestion.[4]

Over-the-counter products that have been shown in some studies to give symptomatic relief of colds in adults but not in children include first-generation (but not second-generation) antihistamines and ephedrine or related alkaloids such as phenylpropanolamine and pseudoephedrine.[5] Serious adverse reactions, including psychoses, seizures, and stroke, may occur with ephedrine-containing products.[6] The role of vitamin C in the treatment of the common cold is uncertain; metaanalyses have given conflicting results. Studies of steam inhalation have also given conflicting results. Antibiotics are not indicated but are commonly prescribed,[5] and 2% buffered hypertonic saline nasal insufflations have no value.[7]

REFERENCES

1. Herbert TB, Cohen S: Stress and immunity in humans: a meta-analytic review, *Psychosom Med* 55:364-379, 1993.
2. Cohen S, Doyle WJ, Skoner DP, et al: Social ties and susceptibility to the common cold, *JAMA* 277:1940-1944, 1997.
3. Macknin ML, Piedmonte M, Calendine C, et al: Zinc gluconate lozenges for treating the common cold in children: a randomized controlled trial, *JAMA* 279:1962-1967, 1998.
4. Hayden FG, Diamond L, Wood PB, et al: Effectiveness and safety of intranasal ipratropium bromide in common colds—a randomized, double-blind, placebo-controlled trial, *Ann Intern Med* 125:89-97, 1996.
5. Mossad SB: Treatment of the common cold, *BMJ* 317:33-36, 1998.
6. Centers for Disease Control and Prevention: Adverse events associated with ephedrine-containing products—Texas, December 1993–September 1995, *JAMA* 276:1711-1712, 1996.
7. Adam P, Stiffman M, Blake RL Jr, et al: A clinical trial of hypertonic saline nasal spray in subjects with the common cold or rhinosinusitis, *Arch Fam Med* 7:39-43, 1998.

EHRLICHIOSIS

Ehrlichiosis is a tick-borne, *Rickettsia*-like bacterial disease with cases reported from 30 U.S. states. Infection usually develops between April and September with the peak incidence from May through July. More than 80% of patients report a tick bite within 3 weeks before the onset of illness. Symptoms are those of a generalized febrile illness and most commonly include fever, chills, malaise, headache, and myalgia. Upper respiratory tract symptoms are rare, and rash is uncommon and often evanescent. Inclusion bodies or morulae may be found in the cytoplasm of monocytes or granulocytes.[1]

REFERENCES

1. Weinstein RS: Human ehrlichiosis, *Am Fam Physician* 54:1971-1976, 1996.

FOOD POISONING
(See also cryptosporidiosis; cyclosporiasis; giardiasis; infectious diarrhea; travelers' diarrhea)

Only a few causes of food poisoning are discussed here. Some of the other causes are dealt with elsewhere in the text.

Ciguatera Fish Poisoning

Ciguatera fish poisoning is the most common illness caused by the ingestion of finned fish. The principal toxin is ciguatoxin-1, which is not inactivated by cooking or freezing. The toxin is produced by single-celled free-swimming dinoflagellates and is concentrated as it goes up the food chain. The disease is particularly prevalent in the Caribbean and the South Pacific islands but can also occur in temperate climates from the ingestion of affected imported fish.[1,2]

Fish most likely to cause ciguatera fish poisoning in North America and the Caribbean are grouper, red snapper, jack, and barracuda. Large fish are far more likely to harbor the toxin than are small ones. Of the fish listed above, barracuda are the worst offenders and should never be eaten.[1]

Major symptoms of ciguatera fish poisoning are gastrointestinal and neurological. A few patients also have cardiovascular symptoms such as arrhythmias, including bradycardia, and hypotension unrelated to hypovolemia. Gastrointestinal symptoms are usually the first to appear. Within 3 to 6 hours of eating affected fish, patients often have abdominal cramps, watery diarrhea, and vomiting. The gastrointestinal symptoms usually last 1 to 2 days. Typical neurological symptoms are paresthesias of the extremities and peroral region, a reversal of the sensations of hot and cold, perception of having loose teeth, ataxia, generalized or localized pruritus, and sometimes pain in the extremities, penis, or teeth and dysuria. These symptoms usually persist for 2 to 3 weeks but in some unfortunate persons last for months.[1,2] Since the concentration of toxin varies from one part of the fish to another, not everyone who has eaten portions of the same fish is necessarily symptomatic.[2]

An IV infusion of mannitol 1 g/kg over 30 to 45 minutes given within 24 hours of the onset of symptoms is said to be a specific treatment for ciguatera fish poisoning.[1,2] Lower doses are ineffective. Patients who have diarrhea or vomiting must be rehydrated before receiving mannitol.[2] The efficacy of mannitol is based on uncontrolled trials and therefore is uncertain. Patients with ciguatera fish poisoning should avoid nuts and alcohol, which exacerbate symptoms.[3]

Tetrodotoxin Poisoning

Tetrodotoxin poisoning is common in Japan but rare elsewhere. It has been reported in the United States from eating illicitly imported fugu, or puffer fish. The toxin is heat stable. Symptoms come on rapidly and include paresthesias, lightheadedness, and weakness. An ascending paralysis leads to death in about 60% of cases.[4]

Shellfish Food Poisoning

Shellfish can cause food poisoning with the usual bacterial and viral organisms such as *Salmonella, Shigella, Campylobacter, Vibrio,* hepatitis A, and Norwalk-like viruses. Cooking does not always prevent viral infections of this nature.[5] In addition, a number of forms of shellfish intoxication affect the central nervous system. Shellfish-borne toxins come from marine dinoflagellates (a significant component of plankton). Toxin levels rise during rapid multiplication of the dinoflagellates ("red tides"). Paralytic shellfish poisoning causes circumoral paresthesias, numbness of the tongue, paresthesias of the fingers and toes, a feeling of floating, and weakness of the limbs. The case-fatality rate (related to respiratory failure) is 8% to 10%. Symptoms of neurotoxic shellfish poisoning include circumoral paresthesias, paresthesias of the fingers, reversal of hot and cold sensation, ataxia, nausea, and vomiting. No deaths have been reported.

Escherichia coli O157:H7

Infection with *E. coli* O157:H7, which is also called hamburger disease and hemorrhagic colitis, is caused by a *Shiga* toxin produced by the organism. The incubation period is 1 to 9 days. Many cases involve hamburgers prepared at home. Although eating undercooked meat explains some of the cases, others may have resulted from contamination of other foods or utensils by the person who prepared the hamburgers.[6] A widespread outbreak of *E. coli* O157:H7 infection in the United States has also been reported to result from the ingestion of contaminated lettuce,[7] and in the spring of 2000 over 1000 persons were infected in Ontario as a result of a contaminated municipal water system. A rare but important complication of infection with *E. coli* O157:H7 is hemolytic-uremic syndrome; those most likely to be affected are children who have had bloody diarrhea.[8] Antibiotics should not be given to persons with *E. coli* O157:H7 infection because they increase the risk of the hemolytic-uremic syndrome.[9]

Mushroom Poisoning

Most cases of mushroom poisoning are caused by species of *Amanita.* The toxin, which results in hepatitis, is not destroyed by cooking and is tasteless. Symptoms develop after a latent period of 6 to 12 hours and consist of severe diarrhea and vomiting followed by hepatic and renal failure.[10]

◣ REFERENCES ◢

1. Lange WR: Ciguatera fish poisoning, *Am Fam Physician* 50: 579-584, 1994.
2. Beadle A: Ciguatera fish poisoning, *Milit Med* 162:319-322, 1997.
3. Caplan CE: Ciguatera fish poisoning, *Can Med Assoc J* 159: 1394, 1998.
4. Centers for Disease Control and Prevention: Tetrodotoxin poisoning associated with eating puffer fish transported from Japan—California, 1996, *JAMA* 275:1631, 1996.
5. McDonnell S, Kirkland KB, Hlady G, et al: Failure of cooking to prevent shellfish-associated viral gastroenteritis, *Arch Intern Med* 157:111-116, 1997.
6. Mead PS, Finelli L, Lambert-Fair MA, et al: Risk factors for sporadic infection with *Escherichia coli* O157:H7, *Arch Intern Med* 157:204-208, 1997.
7. Hilborn ED, Mermin JH, Mshar PA, et al: A multistate outbreak of *Escherichia coli* O157:H7 infections associated with consumption of mesclun lettuce, *Arch Intern Med* 159:1758-1764, 1999.
8. Fitzpatrick M: Haemolytic uraemic syndrome and *E coli* O157 (editorial), *BMJ* 318:684-685, 1999.
9. Wong CS, Jelacic S, Habeeb RL, et al: The risk of the hemolytic-uremic syndrome after antibiotic treatment of *Escherichia coli* O157:H7 infections, *N Engl J Med* 342:1930-1936, 2000.
10. Hoey J, Todkill AM: Gather ye rosebuds while ye may—but avoid the mushrooms, *Can Med Assoc J* 157:431, 1997.

HANTAVIRUS

The hantavirus has been known for many years to cause an epidemic hemorrhagic fever with renal failure. The mortality rate associated with this form of the disease is about 10%. Another syndrome caused by the organism is the hantavirus pulmonary syndrome (HPS), which was first described in 1993. Symptoms are fever, myalgia, and acute respiratory difficulties. The death rate is about 60%.[1] Hantavirus infection is found predominantly in the American Southwest, but cases have been reported from 24 U.S. states, Canada, Argentina, and Brazil.[2] The mean age of U.S. patients with HPS is 35 years.[2] The natural habitat for the virus is rodents (in most cases deer mice), and it is found in their urine and saliva. It is spread to humans through direct contact or inhalation.[1] As of 1995 five cases of hantavirus pulmonary syndrome had been reported in Canada; all the cases were in Alberta or British Columbia, and those affected had had contact with mice.[3]

REFERENCES

1. CDC update: hantavirus pulmonary syndrome—United States, *JAMA* 270:2287-2288, 1993.
2. Centers for Disease Control and Prevention: Hantavirus pulmonary syndrome—United States, 1995-1996, *JAMA* 275:1395-1397, 1996.
3. From the CCDR: hantavirus pulmonary syndrome in Canada; update, *Can Med Assoc J* 153:1303-1305, 1995.

HERPES SIMPLEX

(See also sexually transmitted diseases)

Herpes Simplex Type 1

A randomized double-blind placebo-controlled trial of patients with herpes labialis found that the topical application of 1% penciclovir (Denavir) commencing at the onset of symptoms and continuing every 2 hours while awake significantly improved pain relief and reduced time to healing and duration of viral shedding.[1]

A randomized double-blind placebo-controlled study of primary herpetic gingivostomatitis in young children found an excellent response to oral acyclovir in doses of 15 mg/kg five times daily for 7 days. Oral lesions resolved in a median of 4 days versus 10 days in the control group, and fever and difficulty drinking and eating also lasted for a shorter period.[2]

Herpes Simplex Type 2

The incidence of herpes simplex type 2 has been increasing in the United States over the past decade and now affects about 20% of individuals older than age 12. Only 10% of those who are seropositive give a history of genital ulcers.[3]

Transmission of herpes simplex is common and in one study was close to 10% per year. Transmission from male to female was more frequent than the reverse, and most incidents of transmission occurred when no clinical lesions were evident.[4] In a study from the University of Washington, women with genital herpes simplex were taught to take daily viral cultures from the vulva, cervix, and rectum and to record the presence or absence of symptoms for about a 3-month period. About one third of the episodes of viral shedding were subclinical.[5] A subsequent study from the same institution found that daily acyclovir (Zovirax) in doses of 400 mg bid suppressed subclinical shedding.[6] However, no studies have documented that taking acyclovir actually decreases transmission rates.[7] Patients should be advised that most persons with herpes do not know they have it, that asymptomatic transmission occurs, and that the efficacy of condoms for protection is uncertain, probably because the sites of viral shedding are often not in areas protected by condoms.[3]

In most patients the frequency of recurrences of genital herpes decreases gradually with time, but in one study more than a third showed no reduction over a 5-year period. The rate decrease in most patients suggests that if prophylactic therapy is prescribed, its continued need should be reassessed from time to time.[8] In one study 239 immunocompetent patients with a history of recurring genital herpes simplex virus infections (more than 12 episodes per year) received acyclovir (Zovirax) continuously for 6 or more years. During the year after stopping therapy, 86% had at least one infection. After 6 years of therapy the frequency of infection decreased in 72% of the patients.[9]

The usual dose of acyclovir for the prevention of recurrent herpes infections is 400 mg bid. The standard dose for initial infections is 400 mg tid for 7 to 10 days and for recurrent infections is 400 mg tid for 5 days.[10] Acyclovir is the drug of choice for primary herpetic infection during pregnancy because it has been used longer than other drugs and appears to be safe.[11]

Valacyclovir (Valtrex) and famciclovir (Famvir) are other drugs effective against herpes simplex. Valacyclovir is given as 1 g bid for 7 to 10 days for an initial infection and 500 mg bid for recurrent infections and prophylaxis. Famciclovir dosages are 250 mg tid for 5 to 10 days for an initial infection, 125 mg bid for 5 days for recurrent infections, and 250 mg bid for prophylaxis.[10]

REFERENCES

1. Spruance SL, Rea TL, Thoming C, et al: Penciclovir cream for the treatment of herpes simplex labialis: a randomized, multicenter, double-blind, placebo-controlled trial, *JAMA* 277:1374-1379, 1997.
2. Amir J, Harel L, Smetana Z, et al: Treatment of herpes simplex gingivostomatitis with acyclovir in children: a randomised double blind placebo controlled study, *BMJ* 314:1800-1803, 1997.
3. Fleming DT, McQuillan GM, Johnson RE, et al: Herpes simplex virus type 2 in the United States, 1976 to 1994, *N Engl J Med* 337:1105-1111, 1997.
4. Mertz GJ, Bemedetto JK, Ashley R, et al: Risk factors for the sexual transmission of genital herpes, *Ann Intern Med* 116:197-202, 1992.
5. Wald A, Zeh J, Selke S, et al: Virologic characteristics of subclinical and symptomatic genital herpes infections, *N Engl J Med* 333:770-775, 1995.
6. Wald A, Zeh J, Barnum G, et al: Suppression of subclinical shedding of herpes simplex virus type 2 with acyclovir, *Ann Intern Med* 124:8-15, 1996.
7. Patel R, Cowan FM, Barton SE: Advising patients with genital herpes: acyclovir reduces asymptomatic viral shedding, but effect on transmission is unclear (editorial), *BMJ* 314:85-86, 1997.
8. Benedetti JK, Zeh J, Corey L: Clinical reactivation of genital herpes simplex virus infection decreases in frequency over time, *Ann Intern Med* 131:14-20, 1999.

9. Fife KH, Crumpacker CS, Mertz GJ, et al: Recurrence and resistance patterns of herpes simplex virus following cessation of greater-than-or-equal-to-6 years of chronic suppression with acyclovir, *J Infect Dis* 169:1338-1341, 1994.

10. Drugs for non-HIV viral infections, *Med Lett* 39:69-76, 1997.

11. Balfour HH Jr: Antiviral drugs, *N Engl J Med* 340:1255-1268, 1999.

HERPES ZOSTER

(See also diabetic neuropathy; neuropathy; varicella; viral diseases in pregnancy)

Epidemiology

The incidence of herpes zoster is low in children and adolescents, about 0.5 to 1.6:1000 for persons under 20, whereas it is 11:1000 in adults over 80.[1] The incidence is high in HIV-positive patients and those with cancer, including childhood leukemia.[1]

Postherpetic neuralgia is defined in various ways, but a good working definition is persistence of pain for more than a month after the onset of the rash. It is rare in children but occurs in approximately 70% of persons over 70. The pain of postherpetic neuralgia may last for months or years.[1]

Clinical Presentation

The prodromal pain of herpes zoster may last for a few days or weeks.[1] The distribution of the lesions is as follows[2]:

Location	Percentage of cases
Thorax	55
Fifth cranial nerve	15
Lumbar roots	14
Neck	12
Sacral roots	3

Crusting occurs in 7 to 10 days, and resolution of the lesions takes 3 to 4 weeks. The area affected is usually hyperesthetic. The pain may be burning or lancinating and is sometimes precipitated by trivial stimuli. Paresthesias and hypesthesia commonly extend beyond the boundaries of the initial skin lesions.[1]

Treatment of Acute Illness

Antiviral agents that have been used for the treatment of herpes zoster include acyclovir (Zovirax), famciclovir (Famvir), and valacyclovir (Valtrex). Administration of these drugs within 72 hours of the onset of the rash is associated with a decrease in the herpetic pain of the acute disease. The standard dose of acyclovir for this purpose is 800 mg q4h (five times daily) for 7 to 10 days, that of famciclovir 500 mg tid for 7 days, and that of valacyclovir 1 g tid for 7 days. Famciclovir and valacyclovir may diminish the incidence of postherpetic neuralgia, although this has not been conclusively proved.[1] For example, in one randomized trial, famciclovir was started within 72 hours of the rash at doses of 500 mg or 750 mg tid and given for 7 days. It decreased the time until healing of the lesions and also decreased the median duration of postherpetic neuralgia by about 2 months.[3] Similar results have been reported in a study in which valacyclovir 1 g tid was used for 7 days.[4] Whether acyclovir started within 72 hours can decrease the severity or duration of postherpetic neuralgia is uncertain.[1] A recent metaanalysis concluded that by 6 months the incidence of residual pain was reduced by 46% in treated patients.[5]

The role of steroids in the management of herpetic pain has been controversial. A systematic review concluded that the combination of steroids and acyclovir decreases pain during the acute phase of illness (first month) but has no effect on postherpetic neuralgia.[6]

Treatment of Postherpetic Neuralgia

Aside from analgesics, a number of drugs have been recommended for the treatment of established postherpetic neuralgia. Aspirin and acetaminophen generally have little value. Narcotics are often ineffective in neuropathic pain, although some patients do obtain relief with these drugs.[1]

Two topical treatments that have been assessed are lidocaine gel and capsaicin (Zostrix). In a double-blind trial, 5% lidocaine gel was applied to cranial areas without occlusion for 8 hours and to trunk or limb areas under occlusion for 24 hours. This treatment resulted in significant pain relief.[7] Blinded studies using capsaicin are impossible because of the burning experienced during application of the drug. In a study of 143 patients with postherpetic neuralgia treated with either a 0.075% concentration of the drug or a placebo, significant pain relief was reported in the treated cohort.[8] However, an overview of the literature on capsaicin suggests that although the occasional patient receives significant relief, for most it is minor and for many the burning experienced on applying the drug is unacceptable.[1,9]

The tricyclic antidepressants amitriptyline (Elavil) and desipramine (Norpramin, Pertofrane) have been shown to be effective for the burning neuropathic pain of postherpetic neuralgia, while the anticonvulsant carbamazepine (Tegretol) is useful for lancinating but not continuous pain.[1] Although tricyclics are generally thought to be ineffective for lancinating pain, this is probably not true. The dose of tricyclics for pain relief is usually about half that required for depression, and the effect is seen within days rather than weeks. With amitriptyline and desipramine the dose would be about 75 mg/day.[10] Little or no benefit is obtained from selective serotonin reuptake inhibitors.[1,11]

The anticonvulsant gabapentin (Neurontin) titrated upward to doses of 1200 to 3000 mg/day has been shown to decrease postherpetic neuralgic pain and has been recommended as first-line therapy.[11]

REFERENCES

1. Kost RG, Straus SE: Postherpetic neuralgia—pathogenesis, treatment, and prevention, *N Engl J Med* 335:32-42, 1996.

2. Mamdani FS: Pharmacologic management of herpes zoster and postherpetic neuralgia, *Can Fam Physician* 40:321-332, 1994.

3. Tyring S, Barbarash RA, Nahlik JE, et al (Collaborative Famciclovir Herpes Zoster Study Group): Famciclovir for the treatment of acute herpes zoster: effects on acute disease and postherpetic neuralgia; a randomized, double-blind, placebo-controlled trial, *Ann Intern Med* 123:89-96, 1995.

4. Beutner KR, Friedman DJ, Forszpaniak C, et al: Valaciclovir compared with acyclovir for improved therapy for herpes zoster in immunocompetent adults, *Antimicrob Agents Chemother* 39:1546-1553, 1995.

5. Jackson JL, Gibbons R, Meyer G, et al: The effect of treating herpes zoster with oral acyclovir in preventing postherpetic neuralgia: a meta-analysis, *Arch Intern Med* 157:909-912, 1997.

6. MacFarlane LL, Simmons MM, Hunter MH, et al: The use of corticosteroids in the management of herpes zoster, *J Am Board Fam Pract* 11:224-228, 1998.

7. Rowbotham MC, Davies PS, Fields HL: Topical lidocaine gel relieves postherpetic neuralgia, *Ann Neurol* 37:246-253, 1995.

8. Watson CP, Tyler KL, Bickers DR, et al: A randomized vehicle-controlled trial of topical capsaicin in the treatment of postherpetic neuralgia, *Clin Ther* 15:510-526, 1993.

9. Watson CP: Topical capsaicin as an adjuvant analgesic, *J Pain Symptom Manage* 9:425-433, 1994.

10. McQuay HJ, Moore RA: Antidepressants and chronic pain: effective analgesia in neuropathic pain and other syndromes (editorial), *BMJ* 314:763-764, 1997.

11. Rowbotham M, Harden N, Stacey B, et al: Gabapentin for the treatment of postherpetic neuralgia, *JAMA* 280:1837-1842, 1998.

HISTOPLASMOSIS

Histoplasmosis is endemic in the Mississippi and Ohio river valleys, including the states of Kentucky, Illinois, Indiana, Missouri, Ohio, and Tennessee. Infection is acquired from inhaling the spores of the fungus *Histoplasma capsulatum.* Most cases are asymptomatic, many present as a mild flulike syndrome, some have evidence of pulmonary involvement, and in rare cases the disease is disseminated (in the very young, the very old, and the immunocompromised). A recognized source of outbreaks is bird droppings and bat guano.[1]

─────────────── ✒ **REFERENCES** ✑ ───────────────

1. Centers for Disease Control and Prevention: Histoplasmosis—Kentucky, 1995, *JAMA* 274:1189, 1995.

INFECTIOUS MONONUCLEOSIS

Infectious mononucleosis is primarily a disease of relatively affluent adolescents and young adults. In developing countries and in lower socioeconomic groups within developed countries, viral spread is common among young children so that most are infected by the age of 4; in this young group the disease is mild or asymptomatic. Infectious mononucleosis is rare after age 40.[1-3] Patients who have had infectious mononucleosis acquire lifelong immunity. Although they may acquire other mononucleosis-like illnesses in their lives, these are usually caused by other organisms.[2]

The incubation period of infectious mononucleosis is 1 to 2 months. For most patients the disease is self-limited. The major findings are the classic ones of fever, pharyngitis, and generalized lymphadenopathy. Lymphadenopathy and splenomegaly may persist for weeks,[1,2] and virus can be recovered from throat washings for up to 18 months.[3] Complications of infectious mononucleosis are rare but may be serious: encephalitis, myelitis, Guillain-Barré syndrome, Bell's palsy, cerebellar ataxia, uveitis, thrombocytopenia, hemolytic anemia, and pharyngeal obstruction from enlarged tonsils.[1,2] In over 95% of patients with infectious mononucleosis, a widespread maculopapular rash will develop if they are treated with ampicillin.[3]

Laboratory abnormalities include elevated numbers of white blood cells (in the range of 10 to 15×10^9/L [10,000 to 15,000/mm^3]) with a relative lymphocytosis. About 10% to 30% of the lymphocytes are atypical; these are not specific for infectious mononucleosis and may be seen in cytomegalovirus infections and other viral illnesses. The traditional serological investigation is the heterophile or Paul-Bunnell test or its more modern variant, the Monospot latex agglutination test. About 10% to 20% of adults with infectious mononucleosis and a higher percentage of very young children do not have a positive Monospot test. Conversely, 5% to 15% of positive results are false positives caused by other infections such as cytomegalovirus or adenovirus infections and toxoplasmosis.[1,2] Heterophile antibodies begin to develop after a week and peak between weeks 2 and 5.[3] The Monospot test remains positive for several months after the onset of infectious mononucleosis but usually reverts to negative within a year. More specific serological tests for infectious mononucleosis are available, but these are performed principally in reference laboratories.[1,2]

Treatment of infectious mononucleosis is generally symptomatic. Strenuous exercises should be avoided for 3 to 4 weeks and contact sports until splenomegaly has resolved; ultrasonography is often necessary to assess splenic size. Prednisone 60 to 80 mg/day for 5 to 7 days followed by tapering so that the drug is discontinued by 14 days is used for upper airway obstruction and severe hemolytic anemia and thrombocytopenia.[1-3]

─────────────── ✒ **REFERENCES** ✑ ───────────────

1. Bailey RE: Diagnosis and treatment of infectious mononucleosis, *Am Fam Physician* 49:879-888, 1994.

2. Strauss SE, Cohen JI, Tosato G, Meier J: NIH conference: Epstein-Barr virus infections; biology, pathogenesis and management, *Ann Intern Med* 118:45-58, 1993.

3. Auwaerter PG: Infectious mononucleosis in middle age, *JAMA* 281:454-459, 1999.

LYME DISEASE

(See also fibromyalgia; functional somatic syndromes)

Etiology and Epidemiology

Lyme disease was initially recognized in 1975.[1,2] The name comes from the initial cluster of cases in children around Lyme, Connecticut. The etiological agent of the disease is the spirochete *Borrelia burgdorferi*. It is transmitted by the *Ixodes ricinus (scapularis)* group of ticks. In North America these are *I. dammini* and *I. scapularis* along the Eastern Seaboard and in the Midwest and *I. pacificus* along the Pacific coast. The larval and nymph forms feed on white-footed mice, and the adult forms on white-tailed deer. It is the larval form that acquires the spirochetes from white-footed mice, and in 90% of cases the nymph form infects humans. Human infections may occur from May to November, but the majority occur from May to July.

In the United States Lyme disease has been reported in almost all states but is found predominantly in New England, the Mid-Atlantic region, the Southeast, small endemic areas of Wisconsin and Minnesota, and to a lesser extent on the Pacific coast.[1,2] In 1995, 92% of reported cases were from eight states, which in order of frequency were Connecticut, Rhode Island, New York, New Jersey, Pennsylvania, Maryland, Wisconsin, and Minnesota.[3] The disease is infrequent even in states reporting the highest incidence.[2] The only areas in Canada where Lyme disease is endemic are Long Point, Ontario (a peninsula in Lake Erie), and Vancouver Island and the Gulf Islands in British Columbia.[4] The disease is widespread in northern and central Europe and has also been described in Asia.[2]

Early Clinical Manifestations

Erythema migrans occurs in 50% to 80% of patients with Lyme disease[2]; in one prospective study of children 90% had one or more of these lesions.[5] Multiple lesions occur in about half of patients, and nonspecific viral-like symptoms also occur in about half the patients in the early stage of the illness. Erythema migrans is an expanding, annular, erythematous lesion at least 5 cm in diameter with central clearing. It is usually not pruritic or tender. It generally occurs 3 to 30 days after the tick bite (less than one fourth of patients recall this event), although it may develop after an interval of months, and it usually lasts for 3 to 4 weeks. Serological tests for Lyme disease are often negative at this stage of the disease and should not be ordered; the diagnosis of erythema migrans is a clinical one.[6] Lesions occurring within 48 hours of exposure are hypersensitivity reactions, not erythema migrans.[1,2]

The standard treatment of erythema migrans is a 2- to 4-week course of oral antibiotics. Common regimens for adults are doxycycline 100 mg bid, tetracycline 250 to 500 mg qid, or amoxicillin 250 to 500 mg qid.[2] Common regimens for children are amoxicillin 40 mg/kg/day in divided doses, erythromycin 30 mg/kg/day in divided doses, or penicillin V 25 to 50 mg/kg/day in divided doses.[2]

With rare exceptions appropriate antibiotic treatment of early Lyme disease prevents the development of late clinical manifestations.[2,5]

Late Clinical Manifestations

The late manifestations of Lyme disease may affect the joints, the central nervous system, and the heart.[1,2]

In 50% of untreated persons with Lyme disease, recurrent brief attacks (weeks to months) of swelling of one or a few large joints develop. The course may also be chronic progressive arthritis preceded by brief attacks. The onset occurs a few weeks to 2 years after the person is infected. In areas of the country where awareness of Lyme disease is high, many cases that elsewhere would be called fibromyalgia are misdiagnosed as Lyme disease.[1,2]

Between 15% and 20% of persons with untreated Lyme disease have central nervous system involvement. This may be lymphocytic meningitis, cranial neuritis, facial palsy, radiculopathy, and rarely encephalomyelitis.[1]

The cardiovascular system is affected in 4% to 8% of patients. This usually involves acute onset of atrioventricular conduction defects that resolve in days or weeks.[1]

Some patients who claim to have chronic Lyme disease probably are somatizing and suffer from what Barsky[7] calls a functional somatic syndrome (see discussion of functional somatic syndromes).

Laboratory Investigations

Serology is used to help confirm a diagnosis of Lyme disease. When the clinical picture is typical, the positive predictive value of the serological test is high. It is important to remember that the serological test is not positive until 6 to 8 weeks after a tick bite and that about 3% to 5% of uninfected persons also test positive. Test findings can remain positive long after a patient has been cured. A positive serological test in an asymptomatic person has no clinical significance.[1,2] Serology may be of some help in patients seeking treatment because of a recent tick bite if the physician plans simply to observe the patient and obtain a second serology specimen after several weeks.[8] Serological tests should not be ordered for patients with nonspecific symptoms of myalgias, arthralgias, and fatigue because a positive result does not increase the probability that the patient has Lyme disease.[6]

Prophylaxis After Tick Bites

Prophylactic antibiotic therapy is probably not indicated after tick bites even in endemic areas because of the low transmission rate. In a metaanalysis of three trials of 600 adults and children no cases of Lyme disease developed in patients given prophylactic antibiotics whereas the rate of infection in the placebo groups was 1.4%. None of the patients who became infected had serious sequelae.[9]

Overdiagnosis and Overtreatment

Most patients diagnosed as having late manifestations of Lyme disease do not, in fact, have that disorder. Correct diagnoses in these cases include fatigue-arthritis-myalgia syndrome (fibromyalgia), depression, rheumatoid arthritis, osteoarthritis, peripheral neuropathy, and myasthenia gravis. The harmful results of such misdiagnoses include adverse reactions to unnecessary antibiotic regimens and physical and mental distress resulting from failure to treat the correct clinical condition.[10]

Vaccinations

A vaccine against Lyme disease called LYMErix has been marketed and is administered intramuscularly, 30 μg (0.5 ml) in the deltoid at 0, 1, and 12 months. According to the *Medical Letter* it is 76% effective. Frequent booster doses will probably be required, and long-term safety is unknown. Since antibiotics are effective for treating early disease, use of the vaccine should be limited.[11] It is important to remember that vaccinated persons will have positive serological tests for Lyme disease.[6]

◾ REFERENCES ◾

1. Verdon ME, Sigal LH: Recognition and management of Lyme disease, *Am Fam Physician* 56:427-436, 1997.
2. Sigal LH: The Lyme disease controversy: social and financial costs of misdiagnosis and mismanagement, *Arch Intern Med* 156:1493-1500, 1996.
3. Centers for Disease Control and Prevention: Lyme disease—United States, 1995, *JAMA* 276:274, 1996.
4. Hamilton J: Zoonotic diseases in Canada: an interdisciplinary challenge, *Can Med Assoc J* 155:413-418, 1996.
5. Gerber MA, Shapiro ED, Burke GS, et al (Pediatric Lyme Disease Study Group): Lyme disease in children in southeastern Connecticut, *N Engl J Med* 335:1270-1274, 1996.
6. Wormser GP, Aguero-Rosenfeld ME, Nadelman RB: Lyme disease serology: problems and opportunities (editorial), *JAMA* 282:79-80, 1999.
7. Barsky AJ, Borus JF: Functional somatic syndromes, *Ann Intern Med* 130:910-921, 1999.
8. Barbour AG: Expert advice and patient expectations: laboratory testing and antibiotics for Lyme disease (editorial), *JAMA* 279:239-240, 1998.
9. Warshafsky S, Nowakowski J, Nadelman RB, et al: Efficacy of antibiotic prophylaxis for prevention of Lyme disease, *J Gen Intern Med* 11:329-333, 1996.
10. Reid MC, Schoen RT, Evans J, et al: The consequences of overdiagnosis and overtreatment of Lyme disease: an observational study, *Ann Intern Med* 128:354-362, 1998.
11. Lyme disease vaccine, *Med Lett* 41:29-30, 1999.

MENINGITIS
(See also meningococcal disease)

Before the introduction of conjugate vaccines against *Haemophilus influenzae* type b, meningitis was predominantly a disease of young children and the organism most frequently responsible was *H. influenzae*. At present few cases of meningitis are due to *Haemophilus,* and the median age for the disease is now 25 years rather than 5 years. In the United States the bacteria responsible for meningitis vary with age. In the first month of life, group B *Streptococcus* is the most common organism, followed by *Listeria monocytogenes*. From 1 month to 2 years, *Streptococcus pneumoniae* accounts for most cases with *Neisseria meningitidis* running second. From 2 to 18 years *N. meningitidis* is the most common pathogen (59%) with *S. pneumoniae* second, and after the age of 18, *S. pneumoniae* takes the lead. In the geriatric population there is a relative increase in the incidence of *L. monocytogenes*. The fatality rates for meningitis are 21% for disease caused by *S. pneumoniae* and 3% for *N. meningitidis*. However, with meningococcal bacteremia the fatality rate is 17%.[1]

Fever, lethargy, and seizures are the main findings in meningitis in the newborn; nuchal rigidity and meningeal signs are found more often in older children.[2]

A broad-spectrum IV cephalosporin such as cefotaxime (Claforan) or ceftriaxone (Rocephin) is used for all immunocompetent patients with bacterial meningitis, but for infants under 1 year of age and adults over 50 years of age IV ampicillin is given as well.[3] In one study of children with meningitis, IV meropenem (Merrem) was found to be as effective as IV cefotaxime.[4]

An area of controversy is whether all patients with suspected bacterial meningitis should have cranial computed tomography before lumbar puncture. In the view of some workers this is unnecessary except for patients with papilledema or focal neurological signs. If it is to be done, empirical antibiotic therapy should be started first.[3]

Although the evidence is inconclusive, adjunctive dexamethasone therapy is probably useful in children over the age of 2 months.[3,5]

◾ REFERENCES ◾

1. Schuchat A, Robinson K, Wenger JD: Bacterial meningitis in the United States in 1995, *N Engl J Med* 337:970-976, 1997.
2. Pohl CA: Practical approach to bacterial meningitis in childhood, *Am Fam Physician* 47:1595-1603, 1993.
3. Quagliarello VJ, Scheld WM: Treatment of bacterial meningitis, *N Engl J Med* 336:708-716, 1997.
4. Odio CM, Puig JR, Feris JM, et al: Prospective, randomized, investigator-blinded study of the efficacy and safety of meropenem vs. cefotaxime therapy in bacterial meningitis in children, *Pediatr Infect Dis J* 18:581-590, 1999.
5. McIntyre PB, Berkey CS, King SM, et al: Dexamethasone as adjunctive therapy in bacterial meningitis: a meta-analysis of randomized clinical trials since 1988, *JAMA* 278:925-931, 1997.

MENINGOCOCCAL DISEASE
(See also meningitis)

Of the 13 serogroups of *N. meningitidis,* A, B, C, Y, and W-135 are the most common. Meningococcal disease is largely a disorder of small children and young adults. The age-specific incidence in Canada per 100,000 during the period 1986-1992 was 18.8 for children under 1 year, 5.8 for those 1 to 4, 1.9 for those 5 to 19, and 0.5 for those over 20.[1] In some localized outbreaks the incidence is highest in teenagers.[2]

Since meningococcal infections are often rapidly fatal, starting treatment as early as possible is essential. Any physician who suspects the disease is present should administer penicillin G (benzylpenicillin) intramuscularly at once; investigations and consultations follow.[2-4] A hemorrhagic rash, usually on the legs or buttocks, is classic, but only half of the children with the disease manifest this sign before hospitalization. Other symptoms that should raise suspicion of the disease are lack of eye contact, unwillingness to interact, and altered mental status.[4]

If penicillin has been given, blood and cerebrospinal fluid (CSF) cultures may be negative even in proven cases of meningococcal disease; however, in a substantial number of patients treated with penicillin, nasopharyngeal smears and aspirates from the skin rash are still positive. Lumbar puncture is not always necessary in suspected cases of meningococcal disease. The procedure places the patient at risk of brainstem herniation and death, the presence of a clear CSF with no cells does not rule out meningitis, and in the presence of other clinical symptoms and signs such as a hemorrhagic rash, full treatment must be given regardless of CSF results.[2,3]

Management of Close Contacts

Close contacts of patients with meningococcal disease are defined as follows[1]:
1. Household members
2. Persons who share sleeping arrangements
3. Day care and nursery school contacts
4. Anyone whose nose or mouth has had direct contact with oral or nasal secretions from the patient with the disease

Chemoprophylaxis is recommended for close contacts because they have a 300 to 400 times increased relative risk of acquiring the infection. Chemoprophylaxis is not recommended for school contacts, transportation and workplace contacts, or casual social contacts.[1]

Chemoprophylaxis is ideally given within 24 hours of the contact and is unlikely to have any value if given after 10 days. It should be used only if the contact occurred during the infectious period, which is from 7 days before the onset of symptoms to 24 hours after the start of treatment. The prophylactic regimen of choice for close contacts of a patient with meningococcal disease is four doses of rifampin (Rifadin, Rimactane) given at 12-hour intervals. Each dose is usually 600 mg for adults, 10 mg/kg for children, and 5 mg/kg for infants younger than 1 month. Rifampin is contraindicated in pregnancy. Alternatives for patients who cannot take rifampin are ceftriaxone (Rocephin) or ciprofloxacin (Cipro).[1]

Vaccines

The standard meningococcal vaccine is quadrivalent and contains serogroups A, C, Y, and W-135. No vaccine against the B strain is available. Vaccination is indicated for adults and children over the age of 2 who are asplenic, populations at increased risk such as military recruits, travelers to areas where incidence of the disease is high, and selected populations during outbreaks of the disease. Meningococcal epidemics are particularly prevalent in sub-Saharan Africa.[5] A strong case can be made for immunizing university students, since the rate of meningococcal carriage in this popu-

lation increases from 7% at the beginning of the school term to 31% a month later.[6] For children over 6 years of age and for adults, protection from the group A virus lasts about 5 years and from group C virus 2 to 4 years. The duration of efficacy of group Y and W-235 vaccines is uncertain.[5]

⚐ REFERENCES ⚑

1. Laboratory Centre for Disease Control: Guidelines for control of meningococcal disease, *Can Med Assoc J* 150:1825-1831, 1994.
2. Wylie PA, Stevens D, Drake W III, et al: Epidemiology and clinical management of meningococcal disease in west Gloucestershire: retrospective, population based study, *BMJ* 315:774-779, 1997.
3. Cartwright K: Optimising the investigation of meningococcal disease: early treatment with benzylpenicillin is important and doesn't jeopardise diagnosis, *BMJ* 315:757-758, 1997.
4. Granier S, Owen P, Pill R, et al: Recognising meningococcal disease in primary care: qualitative study of how general practitioners process clinical and contextual information, *BMJ* 316:276-279, 1998.
5. *Canadian immunization guide,* ed 4, Ottawa, 1993, Minister of Supply and Services, Canada.
6. Neal KR, Nguyen-Van-Tam JS, Jeffrey N, et al: Changing carriage rate of *Neisseria meningitidis* among university students during the first week of term: cross sectional study, *BMJ* 320:846-849, 2000.

NECROTIZING FASCIITIS
(See also streptococcal infections)

Necrotizing fasciitis, or necrotizing myositis, became well known to Canadians in late 1994 when Lucien Bouchard, leader of the Bloc Québecois party and now premier of Quebec, fell victim to it and had a leg amputation. The disease has been known since the time of Hippocrates. Otherwise healthy individuals may be affected, and the mechanism of entry of the organism is uncertain.[1] An associated toxic shock syndrome is present in about half the cases.[2] The causative organisms are often beta-hemolytic streptococci alone or with staphylococci, but in other instances mixed aerobic and anaerobic organisms of gut origin are responsible.[3] Case reports suggest that the use of nonsteroidal antiinflammatory drugs may mask the symptoms and delay diagnosis, as well as alter the immune response to the detriment of the patient.[4] Treatment involves antibiotics, surgery, and in a few cases massive doses of IV immune globulins.[5]

Rare cases of secondary infection have been reported in close contacts,[2] but whether contacts should receive antibiotic prophylaxis is uncertain.[6] A prospective study of household contacts of patients with invasive group A *Streptococcus* infections found that one fourth of household contacts who had spent 24 hours or more with the index patient in the week before the onset of the illness carried the same strain of *Streptococcus* as the patient, whereas only 1.8% of household contacts who had spent 12 to 24 hours with the index patient during the same time period were carriers.

Based on these results prophylaxis (if indicated at all) is probably useful only for those whose contact with the patient exceeded 24 hours during the week before the illness developed.[7]

REFERENCES

1. Barza MJ: Case Records of the Massachusetts General Hospital. Case 21-1995, *N Engl J Med* 333:113-119, 1995.
2. Bisno AL, Stevens DL: Streptococcal infections of skin and soft tissues, *N Engl J Med* 334:240-245, 1996.
3. Kingston D, Seal DV: Current hypotheses on synergistic microbial gangrene, *Br J Surg* 77:260-264, 1990.
4. Browne BA, Holder EP, Rupnick L: Nonsteroidal anti-inflammatory drugs and necrotizing fasciitis, *Am J Health Syst Pharm* 53:265-269, 1996.
5. Lamothe F, Damico P, Ghosn P, et al: Clinical usefulness of intravenous human immunoglobulins in invasive group A streptococcal infections—case report and review, *Clin Infect Dis* 21: 1469-1470, 1995.
6. Working Group on Prevention of Invasive Group A Streptococcal Infections: Prevention of invasive group A streptococcal disease among household contacts of case-patients: is prophylaxis warranted? *JAMA* 279:1206-1210, 1998.
7. Weiss K, Laverdière M, Lovgren M, et al: Group A *Streptococcus* carriage among close contacts of patients with invasive infections, *Am J Epidemiol* 149:863-868, 1999.

PARASITOLOGY

(See also diarrhea; food poisoning; malaria; travelers' diarrhea; tropical medicine)

Ascaris lumbricoides

The *Medical Letter* recommends that *Ascaris lumbricoides,* or round worm, infestation be treated with mebendazole (Vermox) 100 mg bid for 3 days or 500 mg once for both children and adults. Alternatives are pyrantel pamoate (Combantrin) 11 mg/kg as a single dose or albendazole (Albenza) 400 mg once for adults and children.[1]

Babesiosis

Babesiosis is transmitted by the same tick that transmits Lyme disease, *Ixodes dammini.* The bite is usually by the nymph, which measures only 3 mm in diameter when fully engorged, so most persons are unaware of being bitten. The pathogen is *Babesia microti,* usually found in white-footed mice and voles. *B. microti* is an intraerythrocytic parasite. The disease has a high prevalence on Nantucket Island and in the 1970s was called "Nantucket fever." Babesiosis is limited to the northeastern United States and a small endemic area in Wisconsin. Cases peak in July. The incubation period is 3 to 5 weeks or longer. Patients with severe illness have fever, shaking chills, myalgia, fatigue, and sometimes hemoglobinuria,[2] but in many cases patients are asymptomatic or only mildly ill.[3] Silent infection may persist for many months. Treatment is required only for ill patients and usually consists of IV clindamycin plus oral quinine.[1,3] About half of treated patients have significant adverse effects from the quinine.[3]

Cryptosporidiosis

Cryptosporidiosis, which is caused by the parasitic organism *Cryptosporidium parvum,* is a common cause of diarrhea and vomiting in immunocompetent children and adults. The diarrhea lasts 1 to 20 days, with an average of 10.[4] Oocysts are relatively resistant to water purification programs. Transmission has been reported to occur from animals, other people, food, and contaminated water.[5] Laboratory diagnosis of this disease requires specific techniques, such as acid-fast staining, that are not part of most investigations for ova and parasites. If cryptosporidiosis is suspected, the laboratory should be specifically asked to check for it.[6] In immunocompetent patients symptoms are self-limited and treatment is rarely required; if treatment is given, the drug of choice is paromomycin (Humatin) 25 to 35 mg/kg/day in 3 or 4 divided doses.[1]

Cutaneous Larva Migrans

Cutaneous larva migrans results from erratic migration in the skin of the larvae of the dog or cat hookworm. These cause serpiginous inflammatory skin lesions that change shape from day to day. The larvae hatch from ova eliminated with the feces of dogs or cats and lie in the soil or sand waiting to invade the skin of their definitive hosts. Humans are accidental hosts, and in Canada and the northern United States most cases occur in travelers returning from beach holidays in southern climes. The treatment of choice is topical thiabendazole (Mintezol). Alternatives are ivermectin (Stromectol) 150 to 200 μg/kg once or albendazole (Albenza) 400 mg/day for 3 days for adults and children.[1]

Cyclosporiasis

Cyclosporiasis is a diarrheal disease caused by the parasitic organism *Cyclospora cayetanensis.* It is rare in North America and is usually reported in patients who have traveled to developing countries or in some cases in those who have eaten fruits imported from such countries. Transmission is through contaminated food or water. The incubation period is days to weeks, and the duration of symptoms if untreated is 1 to 7 weeks.[7] The drug of choice is trimethoprim-sulfamethoxazole (Bactrim, Septra) given as trimethoprim 160 mg, sulfamethoxazole 800 mg bid for 7 days or for children trimethoprim 5 mg/kg, sulfamethoxazole 25 mg/kg bid for 7 days.[1] As with cryptosporidiosis, laboratory diagnosis requires special techniques and skills that are not part of a routine investigation for ova and parasites.

Cysticercosis

Cysticercosis results from ingestion of the eggs of *Taenia solium,* the pork tapeworm, in food or water or through hand to mouth contamination from infested persons. The larval forms migrate preferentially to muscle and brain. The most common clinical presentation is one of central nervous system symptoms (neurocysticercosis), since the muscle cysts are usually asymptomatic. The disease is common in Mexico, South America, Africa, India, Asia, and Eastern Europe.[8] In New York, religious Jews acquired the disease from Central American servants in their employ who were infested with the *T. solium* tapeworm as a result of eating infected pork.[9] Computed tomography is the imaging procedure of choice for diagnosing the late granulomatous and calcified forms of the disorder. Magnetic resonance imaging is the optimal tool for detecting the earlier forms.[10]

The value of antihelminthic therapy with drugs such as praziquantel (Biltricide) or albendazole (Albenza) plus steroids is controversial. If drug treatment is used, albendazole is probably the drug of choice.[1] One randomized trial found more short- and long-term sequelae in patients receiving antihelminthic therapy than in control subjects who received only prednisolone.[8] However, other workers interpret the literature as indicating that treatment should be given to patients with numerous viable cysts (in contrast to inactive disease manifested by calcified cysts), solitary cysts and seizures, or meningitis.[11]

Enterobius vermicularis

The *Medical Letter* recommendation for treatment of pinworms is pyrantel pamoate (Combantrin) 11 mg/kg once, repeated after 2 weeks. Alternatives are mebendazole (Vermox) 100 mg as a single dose or albendazole (Albenza) 400 mg as a single dose repeated after 2 weeks for both children and adults.[1]

Giardiasis

Giardia duodenalis (G. lamblia) has a worldwide distribution and infects wild animals, domestic animals, including cows, and humans. A colloquial synonym is "beaver fever" because beavers (and muskrats) are frequently infected.[12] Water is a common source of human infection. Cysts are not killed by chlorination but are generally eliminated if the water supply is filtered.[13] The *Medical Letter* recommends metronidazole (Flagyl) 250 mg tid for 5 days. The pediatric dose is 15 mg/kg/day in 3 divided doses for 5 days.[1]

⚞ REFERENCES ⚟

1. Drugs for parasitic infections, *Med Lett* 40:1-12, 1998.
2. Case Records of the Massachusetts General Hospital: weekly clinicopathological exercises. Case 28-1993. A 63-year-old man with fever, sweats, and shaking chills, *N Engl J Med* 329: 194-199, 1993.
3. Krause PJ, Spielman A, Telford SR III, et al: Persistent parasitemia after acute babesiosis, *N Engl J Med* 339:160-165, 1998.
4. Centers for Disease Control and Prevention: Outbreak of cryptosporidiosis at a day camp—Florida, July-August 1995, *JAMA* 275:1790, 1996.
5. Centers for Disease Control and Prevention: Foodborne outbreak of diarrheal illness associated with *Cryptosporidium parvum*—Minnesota, 1995, *JAMA* 276:1214, 1996.
6. Navin TR: Detecting cryptosporidiosis as a cause of diarrheal illness: implications for clinicians (letter), *JAMA* 277:1355-1356, 1997.
7. Brennan MK, MacPherson DW, Palmer J, et al: Cyclosporiasis: a new cause of diarrhea, *Can Med Assoc J* 155:1293-1296, 1996.
8. Carpio A, Santillán F, León P, et al: Is the course of neurocysticercosis modified by treatment with antihelminthic agents? *Arch Intern Med* 155:1982-1988, 1995.
9. Schantz PM, Moore AC, Munoz JL, et al: Neurocysticercosis in an orthodox Jewish community in New York City, *N Engl J Med* 327:727-728, 1992.
10. Salgado P, Rojas R, Sotelo J: Cysticercosis: clinical classification based on imaging studies, *Arch Intern Med* 157:1991-1997, 1997.
11. Liu LX, Weller PF: Antiparasitic drugs, *N Engl J Med* 334: 1178-1184, 1996.
12. Hamilton J: Zoonotic diseases in Canada: an interdisciplinary challenge, *Can Med Assoc J* 155:413-418, 1996.
13. Juckett G: Intestinal protozoa, *Am Fam Physician* 53:2507-2516, 1996.

PERTUSSIS

(See also cough; immunization schedules for children; pertussis vaccines)

The classic clinical picture of pertussis is a cough lasting 2 weeks or longer that is often paroxysmal and that may end in vomiting or an apneic episode. There may also be an inspiratory "whoop," especially in infants. The usual clinical course of uncomplicated disease is 6 to 10 weeks. According to the World Health Organization definition a paroxysmal cough lasting at least 21 days is required as a basis for the diagnosis.[1]

Adults usually have an initial catarrhal phase lasting 1 to 2 weeks and indistinguishable from the common cold. This is followed by paroxysmal coughing lasting 2 to 4 weeks, but rarely is there associated whooping or cyanosis.[2] In one series choking or vomiting following paroxysms of coughing was reported in about half the adult cases.[3] In the third or convalescent phase, coughing gradually improves over several weeks. The total duration of the disease may be as long as 3 months.[2]

Because immunity acquired from vaccination wanes fairly rapidly, infection with *Bordetella* organisms is common. In one enhanced surveillance study of adults and children from Finland in which the major inclusion criterion was paroxysms of uncontrollable coughing of any duration, one fourth of the patients were found to harbor *B. pertussis* or *B. parapertussis* organisms.[4] Adults are thus a major reservoir of the disease, infecting both other adults and children.[2]

Laboratory diagnosis of *B. pertussis* is traditionally based on nasopharyngeal aspirations or a nasopharyngeal swab made with a calcium alginate swab. Cotton swabs are not effective, and oropharyngeal swabs are useless.[1] Polymerase chain reaction assays of the specimens are far more sensitive than cultures.[2,4]

Standard treatment of affected patients and prophylaxis of contacts (see below) is with erythromycin 40 to 50 mg/kg/day for 10 days,[1] although recent evidence has shown that treatment for 7 days is equally effective.[2] For those unable to tolerate erythromycin, trimethoprim-sulfamethoxazole may be used. Whether antibiotics shorten or ameliorate clinical symptoms is questionable, but they do kill the organisms and so limit the spread of the disease. There is no point giving antibiotics after 21 days of illness because by that time the organisms have cleared spontaneously.[1] A recent study from Japan found that clarithromycin (Biaxin) 10 mg/kg/day in 2 divided doses for 7 days or azithromycin (Zithromax) 10 mg/kg/day as a single dose for 5 days was as effective as erythromycin in eradicating the organism from infants and children with culture-proven pertussis.[5]

Patients with pertussis should be kept home until they have had the disease for 3 weeks, have stopped coughing, or have completed 5 days of a 10-day course of antibiotics. Close contacts should be kept away from day care for 14 days. Keeping close contacts away from regular schools is pointless because that milieu almost certainly contains many other unrecognized sources of infection.[1]

Chemoprophylaxis is generally reserved for nonimmunized contacts and infants under 1 year of age. It should be started within 14 days of initial contact with the primary case. In most cases decisions about chemoprophylaxis and exclusion from school or work should be made in conjunction with public health authorities.[1]

REFERENCES

1. National Advisory Committee on Immunization, Advisory Committee on Epidemiology, Canadian Paediatric Society: Statement on management of persons exposed to pertussis and pertussis outbreak control, *Can Med Assoc J* 152:712-716, 1995.
2. Wright SW, Edwards DM, Decker MD, Zeldin MH: Pertussis infection in adults with persistent cough, *JAMA* 273:1044-1046, 1995.
3. Postels-Multani S, Schmitt HJ, Wirsing von Konig CH, et al: Symptoms and complications of pertussis in adults, *Infection* 23:139-142, 1995.
4. He Q, Viljanen MK, Arvilommi H, et al: Whooping cough caused by *Bordetella pertussis* and *Bordetella parapertussis* in an immunized population, *JAMA* 280:635-637, 1998.
5. Aoyama T, Sunakawa K, Iwata S, et al: Efficacy of short-term treatment of pertussis with clarithromycin and azithromycin, *J Pediatr* 129:761-764, 1996.

POLIO
(See also immunization schedules for children; polio vaccines)

Postpolio Syndrome
Late-onset sequelae of polio, the postpolio syndrome, is characterized by increasing musculoskeletal symptoms compared with those during the stable period that follows recovery from the acute illness. After 40 or more years over 50% of polio survivors have such symptoms (primarily weakness), which often lead to deteriorating gait and occupational and social handicaps.[1]

Fatigue, muscle pain, muscle cramps, and muscle twitches are common during the stable period after recovery from polio, but increasing muscle weakness is not characteristic of this phase. Specific risk factors for increased muscle weakness are increasing age and the presence of muscle complaints and disabilities during the stable phase. Chronic overuse of muscles has been suggested as a pathogenetic factor in postpolio syndrome.[1]

REFERENCES

1. Ivanyi B, Nollet F, Redekop WK, et al: Late onset polio sequelae: disabilities and handicaps in a population-based cohort of the 1956 poliomyelitis outbreak in the Netherlands, *Arch Phys Med Rehabil* 80:687-690, 1999.

SEXUALLY TRANSMITTED DISEASES
(See also condoms; herpes simplex; HIV and AIDS; human papillomavirus; infertility, female; Papanicolaou smears; pelvic inflammatory disease; Reiter's syndrome; septic arthritis; vaginitis)

Gonorrhea
Single-dose therapy is effective for the treatment of gonococcal urethritis, cervicitis, and proctitis. Choices are cefixime (Suprax) 400 mg po once; ciprofloxacin (Cipro) 500 mg po once; ofloxacin (Floxin) 400 mg po once; or ceftriaxone (Rocephin) 125 mg intramuscularly once. If the patient is pregnant and allergic to beta-lactams, spectinomycin (Trobicin) 2 g may be given as a single intramuscular dose. Cefixime, ciprofloxacin, ofloxacin, and ceftriaxone are effective against pharyngeal gonorrhea, but spectinomycin is not. All patients with gonorrhea should also receive treatment for *Chlamydia* infection as outlined in the next section.[1]

Sexually transmitted diseases are hyperendemic in many parts of the developing world, and penicillin-resistant strains of gonorrhea are found in about 50% of isolates in some studies from Africa and Asia. Condoms are said to have a protective efficacy of 40% to 70%.[2] Whether the use of spermicides in addition to condoms gives additive protection against sexually transmitted diseases is unknown.[3]

DNA amplification techniques that can detect both *Neisseria gonorrhoeae* and *Chlamydia trachomatis* in urine samples are now available. The clinical implications of this technology are discussed in the next section.

Chlamydia Infection
Chlamydia is the most frequent cause of sexually transmitted diseases in North America. Chlamydial infection outstrips

gonorrhea by a ratio of 2:1 to 5:1. Between 60% and 80% of cases in females are asymptomatic, but serious consequences of the disease, particularly pelvic inflammatory disease, infertility, and ectopic pregnancy, are well known.[4,5] Ectopic pregnancies occur not only because of disruption of tubal architecture from past infections, but also from tubal ciliary damage during active chlamydial infection.[6] The prevalence of asymptomatic male carriers has been reported to be as high as 25%.[5] Risk factors for chlamydial infection include the following[4]:

1. Being sexually active and less than 25 years of age
2. Having a new partner or having had two or more partners in the last year
3. Not using barrier contraception
4. Having symptoms or signs of chlamydial infection

A study of sexually active females aged 12 to 19 from inner-city Baltimore found that no predictors successfully discriminated between those at high and low risk—all were at high risk. Reinfections after treatment were common, with a median interval of 6.3 months.[7]

Screening for *Chlamydia* has been shown to reduce the incidence of pelvic inflammatory disease[8] and ectopic pregnancies.[6] The U.S. Preventive Services Task Force recommends screening all sexually active adolescents and other women at high risk ("B" recommendation) but gives a "D" recommendation to the screening of low-risk adults. For pregnant women it recommends screening only those at high risk, which includes all women under 25.[5] The current recommendations of the Canadian Task Force on Preventive Health Care are that all women at high risk and all pregnant women in the first trimester be screened ("B" recommendations) but that screening of the general population should not be undertaken ("D" recommendation).[4] Burstein and associates[7] recommend that the screening interval for high-risk adolescents be 6 months.

Although screening for *Chlamydia* and gonorrhea has traditionally involved a pelvic examination to obtain cervical specimens in female patients and urethral swabs in males, equal or superior results are obtained by assessing urine specimens using amplified DNA tests that do not require the presence of viable organisms. Not only would use of this technology be cost effective,[9] but it would almost certainly increase the number of adolescents who would agree to be screened.[9-11]

Is it safe to omit pelvic examinations and Papanicolaou (Pap) smears for asymptomatic sexually active adolescent girls? Some argue that such examinations can be delayed for a limited number of years because the incidence of abnormal Pap smears is low in adolescents and most abnormalities that are found are low grade. Even if high-grade lesions develop in a few individuals, the rate of progression to invasive cancer usually takes many years, so a limited delay in cervical cytology screening is unlikely to result in an increase in invasive cervical cancer.[10,11] However, proponents

of pelvic examinations for this age range point out that the incidence of high-grade squamous intraepithelial lesions (HGSILs) in adolescents is almost as high as in women 20 to 29 years of age and therefore pelvic examinations and Pap smears should be mandatory.[12-14] A review of 10,296 Pap smears obtained from New England adolescents aged 10 to 19 reported that HGSILs were found in seven of every 1000 smears; no invasive cancers were detected.[14] This controversy has no clear resolution; as usual, family physicians will have to decide what is best for each patient.

Chlamydia is highly infectious; in one study, polymerase chain reaction testing for *Chlamydia* was positive in two thirds of both the male and female partners of infected patients. On this basis contact tracing and treatment for all partners of *Chlamydia*-infected individuals seem appropriate.[15]

Recommendations for the treatment of chlamydial infections in nonpregnant patients are azithromycin (Zithromax) 1 g as a single dose or doxycycline 100 mg bid for 7 days. Alternatives are ofloxacin 300 mg po bid for 7 days or erythromycin 500 mg qid for 7 days.[1] In pregnancy the recommended regimen is amoxicillin 500 mg po tid for 10 days or as an alternative azithromycin 1 g po as a single dose or erythromycin base 500 mg po qid for 7 days or amoxicillin 500 mg po tid for 7 days.[1]

Epididymitis

The usual cause of acute epididymitis in men under the age of 35 is *N. gonorrhoeae* or *C. trachomatis*, but in older men the infection may be caused by enteric gram-negative bacilli. Both sexually and nonsexually transmitted infections may be treated with ofloxacin 300 mg po bid for 10 days or alternatively ceftriaxone (Rocephin) 250 mg intramuscularly as a single dose followed by doxycycline 100 mg po bid for 10 days. Minocycline 100 mg po bid or tetracycline 500 mg po qid may be substituted for doxycycline.[1]

Syphilis

Recommended treatment regimens for early syphilis, defined as primary, secondary, or latent of less than 1 year's duration, are benzathine penicillin G 2.4 million units intramuscularly as a single dose. An alternative is doxycycline 100 mg po bid for 14 days.[1] Penicillin is recommended for the prevention of syphilis in exposed individuals,[3] and in one small study azithromycin 1 g po as a single dose was equally effective.[16]

Prevention of Sexually Transmitted Diseases in Adolescents

Two approaches are commonly taken to decrease the risk of sexually transmitted diseases in adolescents: abstinence counseling and safer sex (condom use) counseling. In a randomized controlled trial comparing these two methods to each other and to a control group, those receiving abstinence counseling reported a diminution of frequency of sexual intercourse at 3 months but not at 6 and 12 months, while those receiving safer sex counseling reported not only a decreased frequency of unprotected intercourse at all follow-up periods, but also a decreased frequency of sexual intercourse. Eight hours of counseling (two 4-hour periods) were given to all three groups (general life-style counseling to the control group) by highly trained and experienced counselors.[17]

The effectiveness of shorter interventions in some situations is shown by a study of patients in sexually transmitted disease clinics. Two 20-minute interactive counseling sessions were as effective in improving condom use and in reducing subsequent sexually transmitted disease incidence as four interactive sessions lasting a total of 3 hours and 20 minutes. Both of these "client-centered" interventions were far more effective than two brief didactic sessions on how to prevent sexually transmitted disease.[18]

There are wide discrepancies in what individuals mean by "having sex." In one survey 59% of male and female college students from the Midwest did not consider oral-genital contact to be "having sex."[19] Risk assessment and preventive counseling must be very specific.

❧ REFERENCES ❧

1. Drugs for sexually transmitted infections, *Med Lett* 41:85-90, 1999.
2. Canadian communicable disease report: statement on travellers and sexually transmitted diseases, *Can Med Assoc J* 152: 1826-1828, 1995.
3. Centers for Disease Control and Prevention: 1998 guidelines for treatment of sexually transmitted diseases, *MMWR* 47(No RR-1):1-116, 1998.
4. Davies HD, Wang EE (Canadian Task Force on the Periodic Health Examination): Periodic health examination, 1996 update. 2. Screening for chlamydial infections, *Can Med Assoc J* 154:1631-1644, 1996.
5. US Preventive Services Task Force: *Guide to clinical preventive services,* ed 2, Baltimore, 1996, Williams & Wilkins, pp 325-334.
6. Egger M, Low N, Davey Smith G, et al: Screening for chlamydial infections and the risk of ectopic pregnancy in a county in Sweden: ecological analysis, *BMJ* 316:1776-1780, 1998.
7. Burstein GR, Gaydos CA, Diener-West M, et al: Incident *Chlamydia trachomatis* infections among inner-city adolescent females, *JAMA* 280:521-526, 1998.
8. Scholes D, Stergachis A, Heidrich FE, et al: Prevention of pelvic inflammatory disease by screening for cervical chlamydial infection, *N Engl J Med* 334:1362-1366, 1996.
9. Shafer M-A B, Pantell RH, Schachter J: Is the routine pelvic examination needed with the advent of urine-based screening for sexually transmitted diseases? *Arch Pediatr Adolesc Med* 153:119-125, 1999.
10. Joffe A: Amplified DNA testing for sexually transmitted diseases: new opportunities and new questions (editorial), *Arch Pediatr Adolesc Med* 153:111-113, 1999.
11. Shafer MB: Annual pelvic examination in the sexually active adolescent female: what are we doing and why are we doing it? *J Adolesc Health* 23:68-73, 1998.
12. Perlman SE, Kahn JA, Emans SJ: Should pelvic examinations and Papanicolaou cervical screening be part of preventive health care for sexually active adolescent girls? *J Adolesc Health* 23:62-67, 1998.
13. Kahn JA, Emans SJ: Pap smears in adolescents: to screen or not to screen? (editorial), *Pediatrics* 103:673-674, 1999.
14. Mount SL, Papillo JL: A study of 10,296 pediatric and adolescent Papanicolaou smear diagnoses in northern New England, *Pediatrics* 103:539-545, 1999.
15. Quinn TC, Gaydos C, Shepherd M, et al: Epidemiologic and microbiologic correlates of *Chlamydia trachomatis* infection in sexual partnerships, *JAMA* 276:1737-1742, 1996.
16. Hook EW III, Stephens J, Ennis DM: Azithromycin compared with penicillin G benzathine for treatment of incubating syphilis, *Ann Intern Med* 131:434-437, 1999.
17. Jemmott JB III, Jemmott LS, Fong GT: Abstinence and safer sex HIV risk-reduction interventions for African American adolescents: a randomized controlled trial, *JAMA* 279:1529-1536, 1998.
18. Kamb ML, Fishbein M, Douglas JM, et al: Efficacy of risk-reduction counseling to prevent human immunodeficiency virus and sexually transmitted diseases: a randomized controlled trial, *JAMA* 280:1161-1167, 1998.
19. Sanders SA, Reinisch JM: Would you say you "had sex" if . . .? *JAMA* 281:275-277, 1999.

STREPTOCOCCAL INFECTIONS
(See also antibiotic resistance; glomerulonephritis; necrotizing fasciitis; tonsillectomy)

The incidence of strep throat is relatively low over the age of 35 and under the age of 3. The positive predictive value of clinical criteria for the diagnosis of group A beta-hemolytic streptococcal tonsillitis or pharyngitis varies with the prevalence of disease in the community, but even under the best of circumstances it is not very good. Criteria are less specific for young children. The main criteria are as follows[1,2]:

1. Fever or history of documented fever of over 38° C (101° F)
2. Tonsillar exudate
3. Swollen tender anterior cervical nodes
4. Absence of cough

Observational studies have found that in general practice about half of patients with a sore throat have none or only one of these criteria; the chance that these patients will have a positive culture is less than 10%. In contrast, 10% to 15% of patients have all four criteria, and about 50% of them will have a positive culture. Among those with two or three of the criteria, only about 30% will have positive cultures. McIsaac and associates[2] recommend no cultures or antibiotic treatment for patients with no or one criterion, cultures and delayed treatment as needed for those with two or three of the criteria, and cultures and immediate treatment for those with all four criteria. Perkins[3] suggests treating without culture all patients with four criteria, as well as patients with sore throats who have been in contact with individuals with proven streptococcal infections.

Rapid streptococcal screening tests have a sensitivity of about 50% to 90% but a specificity of 90%.[4] The false-negative rate of a single throat culture sent to a capable microbiology laboratory is about 5%. Between 15% and 20% of children and 5% to 10% of adults are carriers of beta-hemolytic streptococci, as are up to 25% of patients adequately treated with penicillin. Carriers do not appear to be a source of transmission and are not at risk for the complications of streptococcal disease. Further cultures are not needed after treatment.[4]

Treatment of strep throat with antibiotics prevents about 75% of the cases of rheumatic fever that would otherwise follow this infection. However, the actual numbers prevented by such a strategy are low because, except in epidemics, in which the risk of rheumatic fever is higher, rheumatic fever would be expected to develop in only about 3 to 4 persons per 1000 with untreated group A beta-hemolytic streptococcal pharyngitis. Furthermore, since many patients with streptococcal sore throats do not seek medical attention, only a small percentage of cases of rheumatic fever in the community could be prevented, even if every case of streptococcal pharyngitis seen by a physician were diagnosed and treated. Treating streptococcal disease does not prevent glomerulonephritis.[5]

Prospective placebo-controlled double-blind randomized trials in general practice have confirmed that antibiotic treatment of strep throat hastens symptom improvement by about 1 to 2 days.[6,7] Whether this gain is worth the possible risk of adverse effects from penicillin, the possible failure to develop immunity (there is some evidence that treating infection early rather than delaying treatment by 48 to 72 hours leads to more recurrent strep throats by preventing the initial immune response), the risk of facilitating bacterial resistance to antibiotics in the community, and the reinforcement in patients' minds that antibiotics are necessary to treat sore throats is debatable.[4,5,8]

Antibiotics take about 24 hours to eradicate the organisms. A good working rule is to keep children home from school for 24 hours after beginning antibiotics.[9] Although standard treatment of streptococcal pharyngitis is penicillin V given three times a day, amoxicillin 750 mg taken once daily has been shown to be equally effective in children.[10]

⚓ REFERENCES ⚓

1. Centor RM, Witherspoon JM, Dalton HP, et al: The diagnosis of strep throat in adults in the emergency room, *Med Decis Making* 1:239-246, 1981.
2. McIsaac WJ, Goel V, Slaughter PM, et al: Reconsidering sore throats. 2. Alternative approach and practical office tool, *Can Fam Physician* 43:495-500, 1997.
3. Perkins A: An approach to diagnosing the acute sore throat, *Am Fam Physician* 55:131-138, 1997.
4. Kiselica D: Group A beta-hemolytic streptococcal pharyngitis: current clinical concepts, *Am Fam Physician* 49:1147-1154, 1994.
5. McIsaac WJ, Goel V, Slaughter P, et al: Reconsidering sore throats. 1. Problems with current clinical practice, *Can Fam Physician* 43:485-493, 1997.
6. De Meyere M, Mervielde Y, Verschraegen G, et al: Effect of penicillin on the clinical course of streptococcal pharyngitis in general practice, *Eur J Clin Pharmacol* 43:581-585, 1992.
7. Dagnelie CF, van der Graaf Y, Melker RA: Do patients with sore throat benefit from penicillin? A randomized double-blind placebo-controlled clinical trial with penicillin V in general practice, *Br J Gen Pract* 46:589-593, 1996.
8. Little P, Williamson I, Warner G, et al: Open randomised trial of prescribing strategies in managing sore throat, *BMJ* 314:722-777, 1997.
9. Snellman LW, Stang HJ, Stang JM, et al: Duration of positive throat cultures for group A streptococci after initiation of antibiotic therapy, *Pediatrics* 91:1166-1170, 1993.
10. Feder HM Jr, Gerber MA, Randolph MF, et al: Once-daily therapy for streptococcal pharyngitis with amoxicillin, *Pediatrics* 103:47-51, 1999.

TUBERCULOSIS
Epidemiology

In the period 1986 to 1994 about one fourth of clinical cases of tuberculosis diagnosed in the United States were among immigrants from Latin America, Haiti, and Southeast Asia. The incidence of tuberculosis in this group is high not only in recent arrivals, but also in those who have lived in the United States for many years. Nearly half the cases were diagnosed in those under 35 years of age.[1]

Method of Transmission

Pulmonary tuberculosis is transmitted in airborne particles. The number of airborne bacteria produced by an individual with active disease is relatively low, so infection is almost never spread through outdoor contact. Transmission occurs most commonly among persons living in cramped quarters with infected individuals. Tuberculosis that does not involve the lungs or larynx is rarely contagious.[2]

Risk Factors for Spreading Infection

The risk of secondary infection is four to six times greater if the smear of the index case is positive for acid-fast bacilli. Contagiousness is also increased if the index patient is young, if the patient has a frequent cough or laryngeal tuberculosis, or if the x-ray examination shows extensive cavitation.[2]

Purified Protein Derivative

The Mantoux test is performed by injecting 0.1 ml of a liquid containing 5 tuberculin units (TU). The reaction is read

Table 36　Purified Protein Derivative Readings and Clinical Circumstances Determining the Need for Chemoprophylaxis with Isoniazid in Patients with No Evidence of Active Tuberculosis[2,4]

PPD	Indications for chemoprophylaxis
Negative	Children and adolescents who are close contacts[2,4]: treat for 3 months and repeat PPD. If negative after 3 months of treatment, discontinue treatment.[4]
5-9 mm	Close contacts, HIV positive, upper lobe fibrotic lesion
10-14 mm	High-incidence groups, IV drug users, high medical risk groups
15 mm+	Low-risk group

after 48 to 72 hours, and the degree of induration (not erythema) is measured in millimeters. The criteria for a positive test are outlined in Table 36.[2] If the initial PPD test is negative, it should be repeated in 1 week to assess the "booster effect." If patients are truly tuberculin positive but reactivity has waned over the years, they could have an initially negative PPD test; this would become positive if a second PPD were planted a week or more after the first one. Repeated PPD testing cannot by itself induce sensitization.[3] A negative PPD test does not rule out tuberculosis in an individual who has recently been exposed to an active case of tuberculosis because the PPD test takes 3 to 12 weeks to become positive.[3]

Between 20% and 30% of patients with newly diagnosed tuberculosis have a negative PPD because of anergy. This is particularly likely in individuals who are immunosuppressed because of HIV infection or chronic corticosteroid use. Anergy can also be induced by recent live virus vaccinations, chronic renal failure, and malnutrition.[2]

Bacille Calmette-Guérin (BCG) vaccinations do not prevent infection but are reasonably effective in preventing clinical disease. Thus they are widely used in many parts of the world. Such vaccinations usually lead to a positive PPD reaction, but this tends to wane with time, although readings of 10 mm or greater may be seen in some individuals even after 25 years. Current guidelines consider a positive PPD test as evidence of present or past tuberculous infection regardless of BCG vaccination status.[2] Nontuberculous mycobacteria, which are predominantly found in tropical and subtropical regions, may lead to false-positive PPD reactions, but since tuberculosis is a far more common cause of positive reactions in individuals from these areas, a positive PPD test is considered evidence of tuberculous infection.[2]

Individuals at particularly high risk of tuberculous infection are the very young, the very old, those with HIV infection or other immunosuppressive conditions, long-term corticosteroid users, and patients with silicosis, renal failure,

diabetes mellitus, or malnutrition. Populations at high risk include immigrants, aboriginals, the urban poor, and health care workers.[2] The risk of active infection after PPD conversion is greatest in the first 2 years.[3]

The definition of a positive PPD reading depends on risk factors and varies from 5 to 15 mm of induration measured in the greatest diameter (Table 36). Anyone with a positive PPD needs a complete medical assessment and a chest x-ray examination to rule out active disease.[2]

Adults over the age of 35 who are PPD positive but otherwise healthy, who have normal chest x-ray findings, and who are not known to have seroconverted within 2 years do not require INH prophylaxis. Management in adults between 20 and 35 years of age presenting a similar scenario is controversial; some experts recommend treatment and others do not. Anyone under the age of 20 years who is PPD positive requires INH prophylaxis, as does anyone who is a recent (within 2 years) converter.[2]

Chemoprophylaxis

The usual method of administering chemoprophylaxis is to give isoniazid at a dose of 300 mg/day for adults and 10 mg/kg to a maximum of 300 mg/day for children. Hepatitis and peripheral neuropathy are important side effects of isoniazid therapy. Patients over the age of 35 or any patients who have a history of alcoholism, liver disease, or IV drug use should have liver function studies at the initiation of therapy and monthly for the first 2 to 4 months of treatment and should be advised to avoid alcohol and acetaminophen. A doubling of the alanine aminotransferase or aspartate aminotransferase level is a reason for considering discontinuation of therapy. Peripheral neuropathy is often manifested as paresthesias of the hands or feet, and patients should be advised to report these symptoms. Some workers recommend giving prophylactic pyridoxine (vitamin B_6) in doses of 6 to 25 mg/day for all patients taking isoniazid.[4]

Treatment of Active Disease

All patients with active tuberculosis should be initially treated with a three-drug regimen of isoniazid, rifampin (Rifadin, Rimactane, Rofact), and pyrazinamide. In addition, patients at high risk of multidrug-resistant disease should receive ethambutol (Myambutol) or streptomycin. After 8 weeks of treatment with three of four drugs the regimen may be cut to isoniazid and rifampin provided that cultures have not shown resistance to these drugs. These two medications should be continued for another 16 weeks for a total treatment time of 24 weeks or approximately 6 months.[4] If compliance is uncertain, minor modifications of the preceding regimen may be made so that all medications can be given while a health care worker observes the patient swallowing the medications.[5]

Many workers suggest adding pyridoxine with the hope of decreasing the risk of neuropathy caused by isoniazid.

Monthly red/green color discrimination and visual acuity testing is advised for patients taking ethambutol. Regular liver function tests are indicated for the other drugs.[4]

◢ REFERENCES ◣

1. Zuber PL, McKenna MT, Binkin NJ, et al: Long-term risk of tuberculosis among foreign-born persons in the United States, *JAMA* 278:304-307, 1997.
2. Menzies D, Tannenbaum TN, FitzGerald JM: Tuberculosis. 10. Prevention, *Can Med Assoc J* 161:717-724, 1999.
3. Pennie RA: Mantoux tests: performing, interpreting, and acting upon them, *Can Fam Physician* 41:1025-1029, 1995.
4. McCollister P, Neff NE: Outpatient management of tuberculosis, *Am Fam Physician* 53:1579-1594, 1996.
5. Hershfield E: Tuberculosis. 9. Treatment, *Can Med Assoc J* 161:405-411, 1999.

VARICELLA

(See also herpes zoster; infectious diseases in pregnancy; varicella in children; varicella vaccine)

Varicella is transmitted via the respiratory route, and the usual incubation period is 10 to 21 days. The disease is infectious for 48 hours before the onset of the rash until the last vesicles crust over (about 1 week). The secondary attack rate among susceptible individuals within a family is 70% to 90%. Varicella infection during the first 20 weeks of pregnancy results in congenital anomalies in about 2% of cases.[1] It is extremely rare for an individual to get chickenpox twice; in most reported cases the original diagnosis was erroneous.[2]

Treatment of varicella in otherwise healthy children with acyclovir (Zovirax) is controversial. If medication is started within 24 hours of the onset of rash, defervescence may occur 1 to 2 days earlier than in untreated persons and fewer skin lesions develop. However, treatment does not decrease the rate of transmission of the infection within the household, decrease complications, or cause less scarring.[3] Theoretical objections to treatment are that it might foster the development of viral resistance to the drugs used and that either humoral or cellular immunity might be inhibited by treatment. To date, no evidence has been presented that either of these has occurred.[3,4] One factor that may influence the decision about treatment is the probable severity of the disease. It is greater in adolescents and in secondary household contacts (probably as a result of larger inocula of virus).[3]

Treatment of varicella in otherwise healthy adults with acyclovir (Zovirax) starting within 24 hours of the onset of the rash decreases the time to complete crusting by 1.5 to 2 days, as well as reducing the duration of fever by about the same amount. The usual dosage is 800 mg po 5 times a day for 5 to 7 days.[5,6]

The value of treating uncomplicated chickenpox in immunocompetent individuals is controversial. At present there is no consensus.[3,7,8]

◢ REFERENCES ◣

1. Pastuszak AL, Levy M, Schick B, et al: Outcome after maternal varicella infection in the first 20 weeks of pregnancy, *N Engl J Med* 330:901-905, 1994.
2. Wallace MR, Chamberlin CJ, Sawyer MH, et al: Reliability of a history of previous varicella infection in adults, *JAMA* 278: 1520-1522, 1997.
3. Feldman S: Acyclovir therapy for varicella in otherwise healthy children and adolescents, *J Med Virol* 1(suppl):85-89, 1993.
4. Levin MJ, Rotbart HA, Hayward AR: Immune response to varicella-zoster virus 5 years after acyclovir therapy of childhood varicella (letter), *J Infect Dis* 171:1383-1384, 1995.
5. Wallace MR, Bowler WA, Oldfield EC 3d: Treatment of varicella in the immunocompetent adult, *J Med Virol* 1(suppl):90-92, 1993.
6. Choo DC, Chew SK, Tan EH, et al: Oral acyclovir in the treatment of adult varicella, *Ann Acad Med Singapore* 24:316-321, 1995.
7. Balfour HH Jr: Acyclovir for childhood chickenpox: no reason not to treat, *BMJ* 310:109-110, 1995.
8. McKendrick MW: Acyclovir for childhood chickenpox: cost is unjustified, *BMJ* 310:108-109, 1995.

LOCOMOTOR SYSTEM

Topics covered in this section

Muscle Relaxants
Nonsteroidal Antiinflammatory Drugs
Orthopedics
Rheumatology

MUSCLE RELAXANTS

Whether muscle relaxants are useful in low back pain is controversial. One systematic review concluded they had value for acute low back pain.[1] Some of the drugs available in this class are listed in Table 37.

Table 37　Muscle Relaxants

Drugs	Usual doses
Chlorzoxazone (Paraflex, Parafon Forte DSC)	250-500 mg tid-qid
Chlorzoxazone + acetaminophen (Parafon Forte)	1-2 tablets tid-qid
Chlorzoxazone + acetaminophen + codeine (Parafon Forte C8)	1-2 tablets tid-qid
Cyclobenzaprine HCl (Flexeril)	10 mg tid po
Methocarbamol (Robaxin)	1-2 g tid-qid
Methocarbamol + acetaminophen (Robaxacet)	1-2 tablets tid-qid
Methocarbamol + acetaminophen + codeine (Robaxacet-8)	1-2 tablets tid-qid
Orphenadrine citrate (Norflex)	100 mg bid
Orphenadrine HCl (Disipal)	50 mg tid

REFERENCES

1. Van Tulder MW, Koes BW, Bouter LM: Conservative treatment of acute and chronic nonspecific low back pain: a systematic review of randomized controlled trials of the most common interventions, *Spine* 22:2128-2156, 1998.

NONSTEROIDAL ANTIINFLAMMATORY DRUGS

(See also chronic renal failure; colon cancer; dementia; hypertension; nonsteroidal antiinflammatory drug gastropathy; ophthalmology; prescribing habits and the elderly; renal colic)

A practical reason for dividing nonsteroidal antiinflammatory drugs (NSAIDs) into their different chemical classes is that if a drug from one class is ineffective, replacing it with one from another class is often better than using another from the same class (Table 38). So far, studies have failed to show any consistent evidence that one NSAID is superior to another.[1]

In theory drugs that selectively inhibit cyclooxygenase 2 (COX-2) and have little or no effect on cyclooxygenase 1 (COX-1) should have fewer adverse effects. This is because COX-2 is the enzyme that leads to the production of inflammation-producing prostaglandins in joints, whereas COX-1 leads to the production of protective prostaglandins in the stomach and kidney.[2,3] Two drugs that inhibit COX-2 more than COX-1 are etodolac (Ultradol, Lodine) and nabumetone (Relafen). A third group of drugs that includes celecoxib (Celebrex) and rofecoxib (Vioxx) is reputed to inhibit only COX-2. These drugs are discussed in the section on NSAID gastropathy.

The elderly are at particular risk for the gastrointestinal[4] and renal complications of NSAIDs.[4,5] If this class of drugs must be prescribed to geriatric patients, it should be for limited periods using the lowest possible doses.[4]

Patients who require NSAIDs but who have had an allergic reaction to them such as angioedema or asthma may be able to take salsalate (Disalcid).

Pain, not inflammation, is the primary indication for ketorolac (Toradol).

Table 38   Nonsteroidal Antiinflammatory Drugs

Drugs	Usual doses
Indolacetic Acids (Acetic Acid Derivatives)	
Indomethacin (Indocin, Indocid)	25-50 mg bid to tid
Ketorolac tromethamine (Toradol)	10 mg q4-6h; 10-30 mg IM
Sulindac (Clinoril)	200 mg bid
Tolmetin sodium (Tolectin)	400 mg tid
Phenylacetates	
Diclofenac sodium (Voltaren)	25-50 mg tid
Diclofenac sodium + misoprostol (Arthrotec)	1 tablet bid or tid
Oxicams	
Piroxicam (Feldene)	10 mg bid or 20 mg/day
Tenoxicam (Mobiflex)	20 mg/day
Propionic Acid Derivatives	
Fenoprofen calcium (Nalfon)	50-100 mg tid-qid
Flurbiprofen (Ansaid, Froben)	50-100 mg tid-qid
Ibuprofen (Motrin, Advil)	400-600 mg tid-qid
Ketoprofen (Orudis, Oruvail, Actron)	50 mg tid-qid
Naproxen (Naprosyn)	250-500 mg tid-qid
Naproxen sodium (Anaprox, Aleve, Naprelan)	275-550 mg tid-qid
Oxaprozin (Daypro)	1200 mg once daily
Tiaprofenic acid (Surgam)	100-200 mg tid
Salicylic Acids	
Acetylsalicylic acid, ASA (aspirin)	325-650 mg qid
Diflunisal (Dolobid)	500 mg bid
Salsalate (Disalcid)	500-750 mg bid
Fenamates	
Mefenamic acid (Ponstan)	250 mg qid
Alkanone Derivatives	
Nabumetone (Relafen)	1000 mg/day as a single dose
Pyranocarboxylic Acid	
Etodolac (Ultradol, Lodine)	200-300 mg bid
Diaryl Substituted Pyrazole	
Celecoxib (Celebrex)	100-200 mg bid
Rofecoxib (Vioxx)	12.5-25 mg/day

REFERENCES

1. Bellamy N: Treating musculoskeletal disease with NSAIDs: practitioner's guide, *Can Fam Physician* 42:482-492, 1996.
2. Tannenbaum H, Davis P, Russell AS, et al: Canadian NSAID Consensus Participants: an evidence-based approach to prescribing NSAIDs in musculoskeletal disease: a Canadian Consensus, *Can Med Assoc J* 155:77-88, 1996.
3. Celecoxib for arthritis, *Med Lett* 41:11-12, 1999.
4. Gutthann SP, Rodriguez LA, Raiford DS, et al: Nonsteroidal anti-inflammatory drugs and the risk of hospitalization for acute renal failure, *Arch Intern Med* 156:2433-2439, 1996.
5. Field TS, Gurwitz JH, Glynn RJ, et al: The renal effects of nonsteroidal anti-inflammatory drugs in older people: findings from the Established Populations for Epidemiologic Studies of the Elderly, *J Am Geriatr Soc* 47:507-511, 1999.

ORTHOPEDICS

(See also anticoagulants; dentistry)

Stress Fractures

Most stress fractures occur in the lower extremities, most commonly at the necks of the second and third metatarsals.[1] In athletes the tibia and tarsal bones head the list, followed by the metatarsals and shaft of the femur.[2] The reported incidence varies considerably from one report to another and is higher in more recent publications, probably because bone scans were used to make the diagnosis. In some reports of military recruits the incidence during basic training was as high as 31%.[1] Women are more likely to develop stress fractures than are men, and an incidence of 49% has been reported in oligomenorrheic runners.[2] The incidence is lower in blacks and Hispanics.[1] A change in exercise pattern or training often precedes the onset of symptoms by a few weeks.[1] Stress fractures are rare in children.[3]

Pain is the complaint of patients with stress fractures. Initially pain comes on after physical activity or late during the activity, but as the condition worsens, it begins earlier. There may be some swelling, but point tenderness is the most common physical finding. X-ray films usually fail to reveal the lesions early in the course of the disease and are often normal even after several weeks or months. The gold standard for making a specific diagnosis is the bone scan, which can be positive within a few days of the onset of symptoms. However, the specificity of this test is relatively low.[1]

Among athletes stress fractures may involve any portion of the tibia. In the case of the metatarsals, the shaft and neck of the second and third metatarsals are the usual sites.[1] Most stress fractures of the femur involve the upper shaft, but a small percentage occur in the femoral neck. The usual symptom of a femoral neck stress fracture is groin pain with exercise. Physical examination may reveal pain or limitation of motion on internal rotation of the hip. Making the correct diagnosis and obtaining appropriate consultations are important because of the high rate of progression to complete femoral neck fractures.[2]

Management of stress fractures involves rest, pain control, and exercises to prevent deconditioning. These are followed by gradual reintroduction of the causative exercise activity.[1]

⚓ REFERENCES ⚓

1. Monteleone GP Jr: Stress fractures in the athlete, *Orthop Clin North Am* 26:423-432, 1995.
2. Boden BP, Speer KP: Femoral stress fractures, *Clin Sports Med* 16:307-317, 1997.
3. Griffin LY: Common sports injuries of the foot and ankle seen in children and adolescents, *Orthop Clin North Am* 25:83-93, 1994.

Hip

(See also apophyseal injuries, foot; apophyseal injuries, knee; geriatrics; osteoarthritis; osteoporosis; septic arthritis; stress fractures)

Apophyseal injuries

Apophyseal injuries similar to Osgood-Schlatter disease occur in the region of the hip and are most likely to be seen in young athletes. Common sites are the anterior superior iliac spine, anterior inferior iliac spine, iliac crest, and ischial tuberosity. Rest, ice, and NSAIDs are usually effective.[1]

Developmental dysplasia of the hip

Developmental dysplasia of the hip is the term currently preferred over congenital dislocation of the hip because it is more inclusive and includes poorly developed acetabula without true dislocation. The single biggest risk factor is a family history of the condition; other risk factors are female sex, primiparity, oligohydramnios, breech presentations, and foot deformities. Standard screening techniques for detecting hip dysplasia are the Ortolani and Barlow maneuvers, but sensitivity is relatively low. In older infants limitation of hip abduction is the most sensitive sign of a dislocation.[2]

In the United States the usual treatment of hip dysplasia is splinting with a Pavlik harness for 2 to 3 months; the brace keeps the hips in flexion and abduction. In Europe abduction pillows are usually the initial treatment.[2]

Hip fractures

Many but not all of the risk factors for hip fracture parallel those for osteoporosis. Current alcohol use is a risk factor for hip fracture,[3] as are long- and short-acting benzodiazepines.[4] High rates of prescription medication use also correlate with hip fractures.[4,5] A prospective multicenter U.S. study of hip fractures in white women found that most had multiple risk factors; weight gain after the age of 25 was protective.[6]

The type of surgery selected for hip fractures depends on a number of variables. Nondisplaced femoral neck fractures in patients over 70 or even displaced fractures in those under 70 may be treated with internal fixation. The rate of nonunion and femoral head necrosis in displaced femoral neck fractures in patients over 70 is high, and such fractures are usually treated with a prosthesis. Intertrochanteric fractures are usually managed by internal fixation.[7]

Mortality rates after hip fractures are reported to be between 14% and 36%. Between 50% and 65% of patients regain their previous ambulatory status, 10% to 15% can ambulate only in the home, and 20% become nonambulatory. Recovery of ambulation is more likely among patients who are male, nondemented, and relatively young.[7] In many cases mortality associated with hip fractures appears to be due to serious underlying conditions that in themselves contribute to the fractures; it is doubtful that measures to prevent fractures (such as hormone replacement therapy) would significantly affect the mortality of this group of patients.[8]

The long-term results of hip prostheses are excellent even after 20 years.[9,10] One of the original problems with hip arthroplasty was aseptic loosening of the femoral component, but with advances in cementing techniques this is now a rare complication.[10]

Transient synovitis

Transient synovitis of the hip is the most common cause of hip pain in children aged 3 to 10 years. It affects males twice as often as females. The most important differential diagnosis is septic arthritis. Clues to septic arthritis are severe hip pain and spasm, fever, tenderness, and an elevated sedimentation rate. However, the absence of these criteria does not rule out infection. Patients with transient synovitis have usually improved spontaneously within a week to 10 days. Other joints may also be affected by transient synovitis; after the hip, the knee is the most frequently involved joint.[11]

────────────── ◣ **REFERENCES** ◢ ──────────────

1. Peck DM: Apophyseal injuries in the young athlete, *Am Fam Physician* 51:1891-1895, 1995.
2. French LM, Dietz FR: Screening for developmental dysplasia of the hip, *Am Fam Physician* 60:177-184, 1999.
3. Grisso JA, Kelsey JL, Strom BL, et al: Risk factors for hip fracture in black women, *N Engl J Med* 330:1555-1559, 1994.
4. Gerings RM, Stricker BH, de Boer A, et al: Benzodiazepines and the risk of falling leading to femur fractures: dosage more important than elimination half-life, *Arch Intern Med* 155: 1801-1807, 1995.
5. Davidson W, Molloy DW, Bédard M: Physician characteristics and prescribing for elderly people in New Brunswick: relation to patient outcomes, *Can Med Assoc J* 152:1227-1234, 1995.
6. Cummings SR, Nevitt MC, Browner WS, et al: Risk factors for hip fracture in white women, *N Engl J Med* 332:767-773, 1995.
7. Zuckerman JD: Hip fracture, *N Engl J Med* 334:1519-1525, 1996.
8. Browner WS, Pressman AR, Nevitt MC, Cummings SR (Study of Osteoporotic Fractures Research Group): Mortality following fractures in older women, *Arch Intern Med* 156:1521-1525, 1996.
9. Schulte KR, Callaghan JJ, Kelley SS, Johnston RC: The outcome of Charnley total hip arthroplasty with cement after a minimum twenty-year follow-up: the results of one surgeon, *J Bone Joint Surgery [Am]* 75:961-975, 1993.
10. Mulroy RD, Harris WH: The effect of improved cementing techniques on component loosening in total hip replacement, *J Bone Joint Surg [Br]* 72:757-760, 1990.
11. Hart JJ: Transient synovitis of the hip in children, *Am Fam Physician* 54:1587-1591, 1996.

Knee

(See also ankle trauma; apophyseal injuries, foot; apophyseal injuries, hip; foot trauma; osteoarthritis)

Apophyseal injuries

Osgood-Schlatter disease of the tibial tuberosity is the best known apophyseal disorder in the knee region. A similar phenomenon about the inferior patella is called the Sindig-Larsen-Johansson syndrome.[1]

Knee trauma

Clinical decision rules for ordering knee x-ray studies after trauma (Ottawa knee rules) are any of the following[2]:
1. Age greater than 55
2. Inability to walk four consecutive steps immediately after injury or in the emergency room (two steps on each limb)
3. Inability to flex 90 degrees
4. Tenderness over the head of the fibula
5. Isolated tenderness over the patella (no tenderness of bone elsewhere on knee)

Use of these rules was 100% sensitive for detecting fractures and had the potential for decreasing the number of radiographs by 28%.[2]

Patellofemoral pain syndrome

The patellofemoral syndrome is characterized by retropatellar pain and often crepitus that are brought on by such activities as squatting or going up and down stairs. Adolescents and young adults are most frequently affected. Although the condition has been reported to be more common in individuals with malalignment of the knee-extensor mechanism, trauma, overuse, immobilization, and excessive weight gain, the etiology is unknown. Some patients have demonstrable chondromalacia on arthroscopy but most do not, and many patients with chondromalacia have no pain. The treatment of choice is intensive quadriceps exercises. After such a program two thirds of patients become symptom free within 6 months and maintain this improvement for at least 7 years.[3]

────────────── ◣ **REFERENCES** ◢ ──────────────

1. Peck DM: Apophyseal injuries in the young athlete, *Am Fam Physician* 51:1891-1895, 1995.
2. Stiell IG, Greenberg GH, Wells GA, et al: Prospective validation of a decision rule for the use of radiography in acute knee injuries, *JAMA* 275:611-615, 1996.
3. Kannus P, Natri A, Paakkala T, et al: An outcome study of chronic patellofemoral pain syndrome: seven-year follow-up of patients in a randomized, controlled trial, *J Bone Joint Surg [Am]* 81:355-363, 1999.

Ankle

(See also foot trauma; knee trauma; stress fractures)

Ankle trauma

Refined clinical decision rules for ordering ankle radiographs apply only if there is pain in the region of either malleolus plus one of the following[1-3]:
1. Inability to bear weight both immediately after the injury and for four steps in the emergency department
2. Bone tenderness at the tip of either malleolus or over the posterior tibia or fibula in the regions 6 cm proximal to the tips of the malleoli

With use of these guidelines sensitivity for detecting fractures was virtually 100%.[1-3] Approximately 20% fewer radiographs are required, patient costs are lower, and time spent in the emergency room is less.[2]

The initial treatment for an ankle sprain is the standard RICE (relative rest, ice, compression, and elevation) therapy, but this should be followed in short order by an active rehabilitation program. The ankle should be iced before any exercise is tried. One set of recommendations that should be instituted on a progressive basis is as follows[4]:

1. Alphabet drawing. Have the patient draw the alphabet on the floor with the foot.
2. Towel exercises. Have the patient place the foot on a towel that has been laid out on the floor. Keeping the heel on the floor, the patient should move the towel back and forth with inversion and eversion movements of the ankle and foot.
3. Stretching exercises of the gastrocnemius and soleus. Initially this is done by having the patient sit on the floor with the legs extended. A towel is looped around the sole of the forefoot of the affected side, and the two ends are held in the patient's two hands. Gentle pulling on the ends of the towel causes dorsiflexion of the ankle. As the patient improves, he or she can stretch the calves by standing facing a wall and then leaning toward it while keeping the heels on the floor.
4. Proprioception or balance exercises. The patient stands on one foot and then extends the other one forward, laterally, backward, and back down. This should be repeated 10 times.

Long-term recovery from ankle sprains may be delayed. A U.S. population survey found that 6 to 18 months after an ankle sprain, 40% of patients reported at least one moderate to severe symptom that interfered with long walks, jumping, or pivoting. Few patients had participated in physiotherapy-type rehabilitation programs, which may be one reason for the prolonged duration of symptoms.[5]

─────────── ◤ **REFERENCES** ◢ ───────────

1. Stiell IG, Greenberg GH, McKnight RD, et al: Decision rules for the use of radiography in acute ankle injuries: refinement and prospective validation, *JAMA* 269:1127-1132, 1993.
2. Stiell IG, Wells K, Laupacis A, Brison R, et al (Multicentre Ankle Rule Study Group): Multicentre trial to introduce the Ottawa ankle rules for use of radiography in acute ankle injuries, *BMJ* 311:594-597, 1995.
3. Stiell I: Ottawa ankle rules, *Can Fam Physician* 42:478-480, 1996.
4. Vopicka AA: Acute ankle sprain: getting patients back on their feet, *Can J Diagn* 11:57-71, 1994.
5. Braun BL: Effects of ankle sprain in a general clinic population 6 to 18 months after medical evaluation, *Arch Family Med* 8:143-148, 1999.

Foot

(See also ankle trauma; apophyseal injuries, knee; apophyseal injuries, hip; knee trauma; stress fractures)

Plantar fasciitis

Most patients with plantar fasciitis complain of pain and tenderness over the medial plantar aspect of the calcaneus. Pain is generally most severe when the patient first steps with the affected foot in the morning. Plantar fasciitis is thought to be precipitated by excessive pronation of the foot (medial border down and lateral border up). Heel spurs have nothing to do with the disorder.[1]

Recommended management of plantar fasciitis includes icing the tender area at bedtime for 15 to 20 minutes over a 2-week period and in some cases taking NSAIDs for several weeks. Corticosteroid injections are reserved for intractable cases. Athletic shoes with prominent medial arches are advised, and orthotic devices that correct pronation might be prescribed. Night splints that prevent plantar flexion (and contraction of the plantar fascia) help some patients.[1] Stretching exercises for the plantar fascia are performed by gradually putting weight on the foot, which is positioned with the heel on the floor and the toes against a wall.[2] Achilles tendon stretching exercises are also advised—the heels are kept flat on the floor as the patient leans forward.[1] As far as I can determine, few of these recommendations are evidence based.

Freiberg's disease

Freiberg's disease is an osteochondritis of bone involving the distal portion of one of the metatarsals. It is seen most often in girls between the ages of 12 and 15. Two thirds of the cases involve the second metatarsal, most of the remainder the third, and about 5% the fourth. Patients have pain, swelling, and tenderness, and the x-ray picture is typical. Treatment involves metatarsal pads or orthotics to decrease weight bearing on the area.[3]

Sever's disease

Sever's disease is a traction apophysitis of the posterior calcaneus and is thus similar to Osgood-Schlatter disease of the knee. The disease usually affects girls between the ages of 8 and 10 and boys between 10 and 12. The patients complain of unilateral or bilateral heel pain that comes on after weight bearing and often after starting a new sport. They usually have no pain on arising in the morning, and the pain, when present, is relieved by rest. On examination there may be tenderness both over the posterior insertion of the Achilles tendon to the calcaneus and along the medial and lateral borders of the calcaneus near its posterior border (the line of junction of the posterior epiphysis of the calcaneus and the body of the calcaneus). The maneuver that reveals this pain is called the squeeze test. Initial treatment is ice, rest, and heel lifts. These are followed by heel cord, calf, and hamstring stretching exercises, as well as ankle dorsiflexion strengthening exercises. Sever's disease is not associated with long-term sequelae.[4]

Foot trauma

Adhering to refined clinical decision rules for foot radiographs is necessary only if the patient has pain in the midfoot plus either inability to bear weight immediately after the injury and for four steps in the emergency department or bone tenderness at the navicular or the base of the fifth metatarsal.[5] One study using these criteria found them to be 100% sensitive for 19 foot fractures.[5]

REFERENCES

1. Barrett SL, O'Malley R: Plantar fasciitis and other causes of heel pain, *Am Fam Physician* 59:2200-2206, 1999.
2. Singh D, Angel J, Bentley G, et al: Plantar fasciitis, *BMJ* 315: 172-175, 1997.
3. Griffin LY: Common sports injuries of the foot and ankle seen in children and adolescents, *Orthop Clin North Am* 25:83-93, 1994.
4. Madden CC, Mellion MB: Sever's disease and other causes of heel pain in adolescents, *Am Fam Physician* 54:1995-2000, 1996.
5. Stiell IG, Greenberg GH, McKnight RD, et al: Decision rules for the use of radiography in acute ankle injuries: refinement and prospective validation, *JAMA* 269:1127-1132, 1993.

Shoulder

(See also investigations)

Dislocation

In a Swedish prospective study of 247 anterior dislocations the patients were assigned at random to three forms of initial treatment: immobilization for 3 to 4 weeks by binding the arm to the torso, sling for pain relief that was discontinued when the patient was comfortable, and immobilization for various durations. At 10 years recurrent dislocations requiring surgical treatment had occurred in about one fourth of the patients. Another 22% had had at least two recurrences in the first 2 to 5 years, but then the condition stabilized with no further recurrences. The rate of recurrent dislocations was unrelated to the initial treatment. In this study 18% of patients under 30 had a dislocation of the opposite shoulder whereas the rate of contralateral dislocation for those between 30 and 40 was only 3%.[1]

Imaging studies of the shoulder

Magnetic resonance imaging (MRI) of the dominant shoulder was conducted on 96 persons with no shoulder complaints and with normal findings on examination of the shoulder. Of the subjects over 60 years of age, 28% had complete rotator cuff tears and 26% had partial tears. Comparable figures for those between the ages of 40 and 60 were 4% and 24%.[2] This study reconfirms the fundamental clinical principle that abnormal results from investigative procedures may be irrelevant to the patient's clinical condition.

Treatment of soft tissue injuries of the shoulder

A 1997 systematic review of treatment for soft tissue shoulder disorders failed to find any benefit from ultrasound therapy. Other treatment modalities such as exercise, mobilization, heat or cold applications, low-level laser therapy, and electrotherapy were also reviewed; although a few trials reported benefits, methodological errors were so common that no conclusions could be drawn.[3] Another systematic review concluded that few good studies exist and that little evidence has been presented to support or refute many of the therapeutic interventions that are practiced. NSAIDs and subacromial corticosteroid injections are probably better than placebos in improving abduction in patients with rotator cuff tendinitis, but no additional benefit is obtained by adding steroid injections to NSAIDs.[4]

A 1999 randomized double-blind placebo-controlled trial looked at patients with calcific tendinitis. Relief of symptoms at the end of treatment was better in those who received ultrasound, but by 9 months no difference was detectable between the placebo and ultrasound groups.[5] Another 1999 trial enrolled individuals with soft tissue shoulder injuries that failed to respond to six sessions of exercise therapy given over 2 weeks; no benefit accrued from either bipolar interferential electrotherapy or pulsed ultrasound.[6]

A study of patients with frozen shoulder (adhesive capsulitis) compared corticosteroid injections given by family physicians (mean of 2.2 per patient) against physiotherapy. After 7 weeks those receiving corticosteroids did much better, but by 26 and 52 weeks little difference was found between the groups.[7]

REFERENCES

1. Hovelius L, Augustini BG, Fredin H, et al: Primary anterior dislocation of the shoulder in young patients—a ten-year prospective study, *J Bone Joint Surg [Am]* 78A:1677-1684, 1996.
2. Sher JS, Uribe JW, Posada A, et al: Abnormal findings on magnetic resonance images of asymptomatic shoulders, *J Bone Joint Surg [Am]* 77A:10-15, 1995.
3. Van der Heijden GJ, Van der Windt DA, de Winter AF: Physiotherapy for patients with soft tissue shoulder disorders: a systematic review of randomised clinical trials, *BMJ* 315:25-35, 1997.
4. Green S, Buchbinder R, Glazier R, et al: Systematic review of randomised controlled trials of interventions for painful shoulder: selection criteria, outcome assessment, and efficacy, *BMJ* 316:354-360, 1998.
5. Ebenbichler GR, Erdogmus CB, Resch KL, et al: Ultrasound therapy for calcific tendinitis of the shoulder, *N Engl J Med* 340:1533-1538, 1999.
6. Van der Heijden GJ, Leffers P, Wolters PJ, et al: No effect of bipolar interferential electrotherapy and pulsed ultrasound for soft tissue shoulder disorders: a randomised controlled trial, *Ann Rheum Dis* 58:530-540, 1999.
7. Van der Windt DA, Koes BW, Devillé W, et al: Effectiveness of corticosteroid injections versus physiotherapy for treatment of painful stiff shoulder in primary care: randomised trial, *BMJ* 317:1292-1296, 1998.

Elbow

Apophyseal injuries

A medial epicondylitis in the elbow region similar to Osgood-Schlatter disease of the tibial tuberosity occurs in adolescent pitchers.[1]

Supracondylar fractures

Supracondylar fractures are the most common elbow fractures of children. The mechanism of injury is a fall that causes hyperextension of the elbow, and most cases occur between the ages of 5 and 8. Neurovascular damage is an important complication. Splinting in 20 to 30 degrees of flexion often relieves brachial artery obstruction.[2]

Tennis elbow

In more than 95% of patients tennis elbow has nothing to do with tennis.[3] In most young persons it is caused by sports and in older persons by occupation.[4] A study of treatment by general practices in Britain, comparing a single steroid injection to naproxen 500 mg bid or an oral placebo, found that at 4 weeks patients who had received the injections were greatly improved compared with those in the other two groups. Naproxen was no more effective than placebo. By 1 year almost all patients had recovered and no differences among the three treatment groups were detectable.[5]

────────────── ≥ REFERENCES ≤ ──────────────

1. Peck DM: Apophyseal injuries in the young athlete, *Am Fam Physician* 51:1891-1895, 1995.
2. Townsend DJ, Bassett GS: Common elbow fractures in children, *Am Fam Physician* 53:2031-2041, 1996.
3. Chop WM Jr: Tennis elbow, *Postgrad Med* 86:301-304, 307-308, 1989.
4. Gellman H: Tennis elbow (lateral epicondylitis), *Orthop Clin North Am* 23:75-82, 1992.
5. Hay EM, Paterson SM, Lewis M, et al: Pragmatic randomised controlled trial of local corticosteroid injection and naproxen for treatment of lateral epicondylitis of elbow in primary care, *BMJ* 319:961-968, 1999.

Hand

Boxer's fracture

Treatment of boxer's fracture (fracture of the neck of the fourth or fifth metacarpal) varies from one surgeon to another. Unless the angulation of the distal fragment is greater than 45 degrees, reduction is usually unnecessary. Pain can be relieved with a tensor bandage.[1]

Skier's thumb

Skier's or gamekeeper's thumb is a laxity of the ulnar collateral ligament of the metacarpophalangeal ligament of the thumb. It is an occupational disorder resulting from repetitive strain such as occurs when killing snared small game by forcefully hyperextending their heads using the thumb and forefinger. At present most injuries to this ligament take place as a result as forced abduction during sports injuries, particularly skiing accidents. If the patient has a complete tear of the ligament, surgical repair is indicated because in at least 50% of cases the proximal end is trapped in such a way that healing cannot take place.[2]

It is important to distinguish ligamentous tears from avulsion fractures. Before stress is placed on the ligament, x-ray examination should be performed; if a small avulsion fracture is found and the displacement is less than 5 mm, conservative treatment with a short arm or even glove-type spica cast for 4 to 6 weeks will suffice. If the gap is greater than 5 mm or the fragment involves more than 25% of the joint surface, surgical repair is indicated.[2]

If no fracture is seen on the x-ray film, the joint should be stressed for the assessment of a complete ligamentous tear. This maneuver should not be performed if the patient has an avulsion fracture because it may cause displacement of the fragment. The ligament is at maximum tension when the metacarpophalangeal joint is fully flexed, so that is the correct position for stressing. If the degree of angulation exceeds 30 degrees, or if it is 15 degrees more than on the unaffected side, surgical consultation is indicated. In many cases local anesthesia is necessary so the physician can adequately stress the joint.[2]

────────────── ≥ REFERENCES ≤ ──────────────

1. Ford MH: What's best for "boxer's fracture," *Patient Care Can* 7:15, 1996.
2. Richard JR: Gamekeeper's thumb: ulnar collateral ligament injury, *Am Fam Physician* 53:1775-1780, 1996.

Cervical Spine

(See also functional somatic syndromes; head restraints)

Whiplash injury

Whiplash injury is characterized by neck, head, and upper thoracic pain, often in association with minor cognitive changes, dizziness, tinnitus, and blurred vision. Women are more often affected than men. The pathogenesis of symptoms is uncertain, but facet joint injury may be responsible for the pain in many cases.[1] A Swiss prospective study of outcome found that 56% of patients had recovered by 3 months, 69% by 6 months, and 76% by 12 months.[2] Risk factors for a more prolonged course include severe initial symptoms, rotated or inclined head position at the time of injury, being unprepared for the injury, and being in a stationary automobile that is struck from the rear.[1]

Whether litigation plays a role in prolonging recovery is uncertain. Most claims that this is the case come from studies of patients in tertiary referral centers who have prolonged pain, and such patients constitute a small proportion of those suffering whiplash injury. That patients with prolonged pain have psychological disturbances is unquestionable, but a number of studies have found that psychological symptoms resolve once the pain is relieved.[1] The possibility that compensation is a factor in prolonging symptoms is suggested by a Lithuanian prospective study of rear end automobile collisions. In Lithuania few drivers are insured and the population is unaware that whiplash can cause chronic pain and disability. In this study half of those involved in accidents suffered acute neck or head pain but after 3 weeks all patients were asymptomatic.[3] Chronic whiplash injury seems to be more of a cultural than a biomechanical phenomenon; in other European countries such as Germany and Greece, where drivers are insured and have access to litigation if they so desire, chronic pain and even short-term disability are extremely rare after whiplash injuries.[4] Barsky[5] classifies it as a functional somatic syndrome (see discussion of functional somatic syndromes).

Is there a role for MRI imaging in patients with whiplash injury? In a series of 100 patients with whiplash injury, no abnormality on neurological examination, and normal plain radiographs, MRI performed within 3 weeks of injury did not reveal clinically significant abnormalities.[6]

No good evidence-based trials of treatment of whiplash injury have been published, so management decisions must be based on expert opinion.[1] Carette[4] emphasizes the importance of a conservative approach focused on the maintenance of function. Although analgesic or antiinflammatory drugs are useful in the early stages, the use of a collar is counterproductive if continued for more than a few days. Patients should be encouraged to mobilize the neck in spite of pain and reassured that this will not aggravate the condition. Prolonged physiotherapy may simply reinforce patients' images of themselves as sick. Steroid injections into apophyseal joints have not been shown to be valuable.[7]

⚓ REFERENCES ⚓

1. Teasell RW, Shapiro AP: Whiplash injuries: an update, *Pain Res Manag* 3:81-90, 1998.
2. Radanov BP, Di Stefano G, Schnidrig A, et al: Role of psychosocial stress in recovery from common whiplash, *Lancet* 328: 712-715, 1991.
3. Obelieniene D, Schrader H, Bovim G, et al: Pain after whiplash: a prospective controlled inception cohort study, *J Neurol Neurosurg Psychiatry* 66:279-283, 1999.
4. Ferrari R: Whiplash cultures (letter), *Can Med Assoc J* 161:368, 1999.
5. Barsky AJ, Borus JF: Functional somatic syndromes, *Ann Intern Med* 130:910-921, 1999.
6. Ronnen HR, Dekorte PJ, Brink PR, et al: Acute whiplash injury—is there a role for MR imaging: prospective study of 100 patients, *Radiology* 201:93-96, 1996.
7. Carette S: Whiplash injury and chronic neck pain (editorial), *N Engl Med J* 330:1083-1084, 1994.

Lumbar Spine

Low back pain

(See also ankylosing spondylitis; detrimental effects of smoking; investigations; muscle relaxants)

Epidemiology. In developed countries the lifetime risk of low back pain is about 75%. In the vast majority of cases the disorder is self-limited, but it recurs in 40% to 80% of patients. The highest prevalence rate is in those aged 45 to 64. Frequent lifting of heavy objects and twisting are important risk factors. Being sedentary, driving a motor vehicle for prolonged periods, and smoking are also associated with an increased risk of low back pain. In most studies sports participation has not been found to be a risk factor.[1]

The likelihood in family medicine that patients with low back pain have underlying systemic or visceral disease is low. Figures vary but range from about 0.05% to 0.1% for neoplasms and about half that for infectious disorders.[2] Malignancy as a cause of low back pain is most likely to occur in those over the age of 50, whereas an infectious etiology is most often seen in IV drug abusers.[3]

Diagnosis. In about 85% of cases of low back pain a definite pathophysiological diagnosis (substantive diagnosis) cannot be made. Instead nominative diagnoses such as "lumbar strain," "nonspecific low back pain," or "mechanical disorder of the back" are given.[3]

Inflammatory back pain (ankylosing spondylitis) is a rare but important cause of low back pain in those under 40. Findings suggesting this diagnosis are discussed under "Ankylosing Spondylitis."[3]

Important diagnostic roles of the family physician faced with a patient who has low back pain include ruling out a visceral cause (e.g., malignancy, infection, aortic aneurysm), ruling out an acute cauda equina syndrome (incontinence of urine or stool, difficulty walking, bilateral lower limb neurological signs, saddle anesthesia, and decreased rectal tone), and determining whether there is objective evidence of nerve root irritation.

Imaging. X-ray examination should not be ordered for most patients with low back pain. Suggested indications are a history of trauma or the presence of neurological deficits, fever, and clinical findings suggestive of cancer.[1]

Disk bulging or disk protrusions are extremely common in individuals without back pain. In one MRI study of the lumbar spine in persons aged 20 to 80 (mean 42) with no back pain, 52% of the subjects had a bulge in at least one level, 27% had a protrusion, and 1% an extrusion.[4] The implication of this and other similar studies is that abnormalities found by imaging may mislead clinicians into thinking that what is detected is necessarily a cause of the patient's symptoms. The potential for unnecessary surgery is great in such situations.[1]

In most cases computed tomography or MRI should not be ordered by primary care physicians. These investigations are rarely indicated unless surgery is being seriously considered, and in that circumstance the patient should usually be referred to the surgeon, who will order the appropriate imaging tests.[1]

Prognosis. Most reports state that more than 90% of cases of low back pain resolve spontaneously within 3 months and that the vast majority of patients return to work within 6 weeks.[3] A 1998 British primary care study confirmed that 90% of patients with low back pain stopped consulting their physicians after 3 months, but follow-up assessment of these patients found that after 1 year only 25% had completely recovered in terms of pain and disability.[5]

Only 1% of patients with acute low back pain require surgery, and these are almost all patients who have proven disk protrusion with nerve root irritation that has not responded to conservative therapy. Of patients with proven disk protrusions causing neurological symptoms, only 5% to 10% require surgery.[3]

When surgery is undertaken for patients with proven sciatica and disk herniation, 90% have good results at 1 year compared with 60% among those followed conservatively. However, after 10 years of follow-up, results are similar in the two groups, with about one third having persistent motor or sensory abnormalities. Thus the prime indication for surgery (aside from the acute cauda equina syndrome) is immediate pain relief.[1]

Psychosocial factors are important issues in low back pain.[1,3,6,7] In a prospective study of industrial injury claims for low back pain, the only positive predictors were job dissatisfaction and distress as reported on Scale 3 (indicating tendencies to somatize and deny emotional distress) of the Minnesota Multiphasic Personality Inventory.[6] Among primary care patients with low back pain, important premorbidity factors correlating with long-term persistent pain and disability are psychological distress and dissatisfaction with employment. Patients with low back pain who also complain of pain in multiple other sites (fibromyalgia) also have a poor prognosis.[7]

Management. Optimal management of low back pain remains controversial. Waddell[3] summed up the nihilistic view of many when he stated that for the vast majority of patients there is no evidence that any form of treatment is better than time and placebo effect. Although bed rest was formerly an integral aspect of treatment, evidence shows that it has no value for nonspecific low back pain.[8] The value of physiotherapy for acute low back pain also remains uncertain; a Dutch study found that a physical therapy program did not shorten the time to return to work.[9]

A systematic review of randomized controlled trials of treatment modalities for acute (less than 6 weeks' duration) and chronic (longer than 12 weeks' duration) nonspecific low back pain came to the following conclusions.[8] Evidence indicates that for acute low back pain NSAIDs and analgesics are equally effective and that no one NSAID is better than another. Muscle relaxants are also effective. Little evidence supports the use of manipulation or traction, and no evidence supports back schools, transcutaneous electrical nerve stimulation (TENS), or behavior therapy for acute low back pain. Bed rest has no therapeutic value. For chronic back pain there is good evidence supporting exercise programs and moderate evidence that NSAIDs are effective (no one NSAID is better than another). Evidence for beneficial effects from analgesics and muscle relaxants is limited. Manipulation and back schools are clearly better than no treatment, and limited evidence suggests that they are superior to other treatment modalities. No good evidence supports antidepressants, TENS, behavior therapy, traction, or acu-

puncture. While epidural steroid injections are better than placebo treatments, they offer no advantage over other therapeutic modalities.

An important goal of exercise programs for chronic low back pain is to motivate patients to cope with their pain and not limit their movements or activities because of it. For this purpose a cognitive-behavioral oriented physiotherapy program appears beneficial.[10]

The value of bed rest for patients with nerve root compression (sciatica) has been a subject of controversy. Most practitioners advocate bed rest for at least a few days. A randomized trial of 2 weeks of bed rest compared with "being up and about whenever possible" demonstrated no benefit from bed rest.[11] Given time, a herniated nucleus pulposus shrinks; in a prospective MRI study substantial shrinkage was found in 36% of patients at 6 weeks and in 60% of patients at 6 months after presentation.[12]

An observational study from North Carolina found that for patients with low back pain who did not require surgery, the times to functional recovery, return to work, and complete recovery were identical for patients treated by primary care physicians, orthopedic surgeons, and chiropractors. The cost of care was highest for orthopedic surgeons and chiropractors (the latter because of multiple visits) and least for primary care physicians. However, patient satisfaction was greatest when patients were treated by chiropractors (see discussion of alternative medicine).[13]

Patients with root compression who do not respond to conservative therapy may be treated with a number of specific interventions. Some of the newer ones include laser disk decompression[14] and microlumbar diskectomy, a procedure that may be done on an outpatient basis.[15]

Prevention. A large-scale controlled trial of an educational program taught by physiotherapists (such as is used in back schools) failed to demonstrate any long-term benefits.[16] A randomized controlled study of an industrial population in the Netherlands found no preventive benefit from either an educational program or lumbar supports.[17]

───────────── ➤ REFERENCES ➤ ─────────────

1. Weinstein JN: A 45-year-old man with low back pain and a numb left foot, *JAMA* 280:730-736, 1998.
2. Deyo RA, Diehl AK: Lumbar spine films in primary care: current use and the effects of selective ordering criteria, *J Gen Intern Med* 1:20-25, 1986.
3. Waddell G: A new clinical model for the treatment of low-back pain (1987 Volvo Award in Clinical Sciences), *Spine* 12:632-644, 1987.
4. Jensen MC, Brant-Zawadzki MN, Obuchowski N, et al: Magnetic resonance imaging of the lumbar spine in people without back pain, *N Engl J Med* 331:69-73, 1994.
5. Croft PR, Macfarlane GJ, Papageorgiou AC, et al: Outcome of low back pain in general practice: a prospective study, *BMJ* 316:1356-1359, 1998.
6. Bigos SJ, Battie MC, Spengler DM, et al: A longitudinal, prospective study of industrial back injury reporting, *Clin Orthop Rel Res* 279:21-34, 1992.

7. Thomas E, Silman AJ, Croft PR, et al: Predicting who develops chronic low back pain in primary care: a prospective study, *BMJ* 318:1662-1667, 1999.

8. Van Tulder MW, Koes BW, Bouter LM: Conservative treatment of acute and chronic nonspecific low back pain: a systematic review of randomized controlled trials of the most common interventions, *Spine* 22:2128-2156, 1997.

9. Faas A, van Eijk JT, Chavannes AW, et al: A randomized trial of exercise therapy in patients with acute low back pain: efficacy on sickness absence, *Spine* 20:941-947, 1995.

10. Moffett JK, Torgerson D, Bell-Syer S, et al: Randomised controlled trial of exercise for low back pain: clinical outcomes, costs, and preferences, *BMJ* 319:279-283, 1999.

11. Vroomen PC, de Krom MC, Wilmink JT, et al: Lack of effectiveness of bed rest for sciatica, *N Engl J Med* 340:418-423, 1999.

12. Modic MT, Ross JS, Obuchowski NA, et al: Contrast-enhanced MR imaging in acute lumbar radiculopathy: a pilot study of the natural history, *Radiology* 195:323-324, 1995.

13. Carey TS, Garrett J, Jackman A, et al: The outcomes and costs of care for acute low back pain among patients seen by primary care practitioners, chiropractors, and orthopedic surgeons, *N Engl J Med* 333:913-917, 1995.

14. Ohnmeiss DD, Guyer RD, Hochschuler SH: Laser disc decompression: the importance of proper patient selection, *Spine* 19:2054-2058, 1994.

15. Zahrawi F: Microlumbar discectomy: is it safe as an outpatient procedure? *Spine* 19:1070-1074, 1994.

16. Daltroy LH, Iversen MD, Larson MG, et al: A controlled trial of an educational program to prevent low back injuries, *N Engl J Med* 337:322-328, 1997.

17. Van Poppel MN, Koes BW, van der Ploeg T, et al: Lumbar supports and education for the prevention of low back pain in industry: a randomized controlled trial, *JAMA* 279:1789-1794, 1998.

Scoliosis

Evidence is limited regarding the effectiveness of scoliosis screening and treatment, and the natural history of the disease is uncertain.[1-3] A Rochester, Minnesota, school scoliosis screening program found that to identify one child requiring treatment, 448 children had to be screened and 20 had to have further medical assessments.[3] Although in the short run bracing effectively straightens out many of the more severe curvatures, long-term studies have shown that much of the benefit is lost with time.[4] Because scoliosis screening programs benefit few participants and cause significant psychological morbidity, both the Canadian Task Force on Preventive Health Care[1] and the U.S. Preventive Services Task Force[2] have given screening of adolescents for scoliosis a "C" recommendation. In contrast, such organizations as the American Academy of Pediatrics and the American Academy of Orthopaedic Surgeons advocate screening,[1] and 26 U.S. states have enacted compulsory scoliosis screening laws.[3] As might be expected, the British Orthopaedic Association and the British Scoliosis Society advise against a national policy of screening.[1]

REFERENCES

1. Canadian Task Force on the Periodic Health Examination: *Clinical preventive health care,* Ottawa, 1994, Canadian Communication Group—Publishing, pp 345-354.

2. US Preventive Services Task Force: *Guide to clinical preventive services,* ed 2, Baltimore, 1996, Williams & Wilkins, pp 517-529.

3. Yawn BP, Yawn RA, Hodge D, et al: A population-based study of school scoliosis screening, *JAMA* 282:1427-1432, 1999.

4. Diguiseppi CG, Woolf SH: The family physician's role in adolescent idiopathic scoliosis (editorial), *Am Fam Physician* 53:2268-2272, 1996.

Reflex Sympathetic Dystrophy

Reflex sympathetic dystrophy is usually precipitated by trauma, but the severity of the trauma does not correlate with the incidence of reflex sympathetic dystrophy. Women are more commonly affected than men and whites more than other races. Symptoms occur more often in the lower than the upper extremity. The cardinal symptom is pain, and this is accompanied by tenderness of the affected limb. Some patients cannot tolerate light touch as occurs with bed clothing. In the early stages patients may have edema; later, dystrophic changes are found with smooth shiny skin and mottling and coolness of the extremity. The cornerstone of treatment is pain relief and physiotherapy. Some patients require sympathetic blockade or even a sympathectomy. Drugs that may be useful aside from analgesics or NSAIDs are calcium channel blockers or in some cases parenteral injections of calcitonin.[1]

REFERENCES

1. Drake WT, Anderson K: Reflex sympathetic dystrophy: what are the signs? *Can J Diagn* 12:67-81, 1995.

RHEUMATOLOGY

(See also anticoagulants; Behçet's disease; hemochromatosis; Lyme disease; nonsteroidal antiinflammatory drugs; nonsteroidal antiinflammatory drug gastropathy; rubella immunization; Sjögren's syndrome; systemic lupus erythematosus; transient synovitis)

Crystal-Induced Arthritis

For patients with crystal-induced arthritis who cannot take NSAIDs, prednisone 30 to 50 mg/day tapered over 7 to 10 days is effective.[1]

Gout

In gout the most frequently affected joints are the first metatarsophalangeal joints, ankles, midfoot joints, and knees. Put another way, gout usually involves the joints of the lower extremities, excluding the hips.[1-3] The wrists and fingers are also sometimes involved.[2] An initial attack usually comes on suddenly and involves only one joint.[1-3] Subsequent attacks may be polyarticular.[2] Males are affected more often than females, and gout is almost unheard of in premenopausal women.[2]

An acute attack of gout may be precipitated by minor trauma, systemic illnesses, surgery, or anything causing either a rapid rise in the uric acid level (thiazides, other diuretics, low-dose aspirin, and alcohol) or a rapid decrease in uric acid (high-dose aspirin, allopurinol [Zyloprim], probenecid [Benemid], or sudden cessation of alcohol).[4]

The risk of gout increases with increasing levels of serum urate. The risk is 5% per year for persons with a urate level of 9 mg/dl or 535 μmol/L (normal is 2 to 7 mg/dl or 120 to 420 μmol/L).[1] There is no clinical indication for treating asymptomatic hyperuricemia, but it would seem advisable to identify, and if possible modify, known causes of this condition such as myeloproliferative disorders, low-dose salicylates, thiazides, loop diuretics, excessive alcohol consumption, high-purine diets, and obesity.[1,2] Common foods with high purine content are all meats (including organ meats), gravies, meat extracts, seafood, yeast, yeast extracts, beer, other alcoholic beverages, asparagus, beans, cauliflower, lentils, mushrooms, oatmeal, peas, and spinach.[1]

The drugs of choice for acute gout are NSAIDs. The agent used most frequently is indomethacin (Indocin, Indocid) in doses of 150 to 300 mg/day (usually 50 mg tid or qid) with gradual reduction of the dose as symptoms resolve.[1-3] Other NSAIDs such as naproxen, ketoprofen, and ibuprofen have also been used starting with maximum doses and tapering as symptoms resolve.[2,3] Some degree of pain relief usually occurs within 2 to 4 hours if the drug is started reasonably soon after the onset of symptoms. Alternatives to NSAIDs are oral prednisone starting at 30 to 50 mg/day (0.5 mg/kg) and tapering gradually over 7 to 10 days or, if only one joint is involved, intraarticular injection of steroid. Colchicine can also be used. Best results are obtained if it is started within 24 hours; it is ineffective if started after 5 days. The initial dose is 0.5 to 1 mg, and this is followed by 0.5 or 0.6 mg every 1 to 2 hours until the patient has diarrhea or abdominal cramps or until a total of 6 to 8 mg has been administered.[1-3] Pain relief usually begins after an interval of 12 to 18 hours if the drug has been started reasonably soon after the onset of symptoms.[1,3] A few patients with recurrent episodes of gout are able to abort acute attacks if they recognize the initial symptoms and immediately take 1 to 1.2 mg of colchicine.[3]

Prophylaxis for gout is indicated if the patient has recurrent attacks or has tophi. Colchicine in doses of 0.5 to 1 mg/day is often effective in preventing recurrent attacks and should be continued for about a year after the last attack. If a patient with recurrent attacks is hyperuricemic or has tophi, urate-lowering drugs should also be used. The usual drug is allopurinol (Zyloprim). Allopurinol and other drugs that lower serum uric acid may precipitate acute attacks of gout, a risk that may be decreased by starting with low doses (allopurinol 50 to 100 mg/day, increasing weekly up to 300 mg/day in most cases but up to 600 mg/day[4] or even 800 mg/day[3] in a few), by avoiding use of these drugs until several weeks since the last acute attack, and by giving prophylactic medi-

cations such as low-dose colchicine (0.5 to 1 mg/day) before and concurrently with the allopurinol. Lifelong treatment is often needed, and the goal is to maintain the uric acid level below 6 mg/dl (360 μmol/L) unless there are tophi, in which case the target is less than 5 mg/dl (300 μmol/L).[1]

Pyrophosphate arthropathy

Pyrophosphate arthropathy (chondrocalcinosis, calcium pyrophosphate deposition disease [CPPD]) is also called pseudogout if the onset of the illness is acute and mimics gout. It is caused by the intraarticular precipitation of pyrophosphate dihydrate crystals. CPPD is usually a disease of the elderly, and the most commonly affected joint is the knee. Other joints that are commonly inflamed are the wrist, elbow, shoulder, ankle, and metacarpophalangeal joints. The disease may have an acute onset (pseudogout), affecting one or two joints. The onset of the acute disease is not quite as dramatic as that of gout but requires 2 hours to 3 days for the pain to reach maximum intensity.[5] As with gout, acute episodes of CPPD may be precipitated by minor trauma, surgery, or systemic illness.[4] A more common presentation of CPPD is that of chronic arthritis involving several joints and thus mimicking osteoarthritis.[4]

Acute CPPD can usually be controlled by NSAIDs. Other therapeutic modalities are IV colchicine (1 to 2 mg as a single dose IV on day 1 and 0.5 mg q6h IV on day 2 and sometimes day 3), oral colchicine (which is not as reliably effective as the IV route), aspiration of the joint without steroid instillation (to remove the crystals), and aspiration of the joint with steroid injection. For recurrent attacks prophylactic colchicine 0.6 mg bid is effective.[5]

───────────── ✄ REFERENCES ✄ ─────────────

1. Emmerson BT: The management of gout, *N Engl J Med* 334: 445-451, 1996.
2. Harris MD, Siegel LB, Alloway FA: Gout and hyperuricemia, *Am Fam Physician* 59:925-934, 1999.
3. Schumacher HR Jr: Crystal-induced arthritis: an overview, *Am J Med* 100(suppl 2A):46S-52S, 1996.
4. Joseph J, McGrath H: Gout or "pseudogout": how to differentiate crystal-induced arthropathies, *Geriatrics* 50:33-39, 1995.
5. Handy JR: Pyrophosphate arthropathy in the knees of elderly persons, *Arch Intern Med* 156:2426-2432, 1996.

Fibromyalgia

(See also chronic fatigue syndrome; depression; functional somatic syndromes; irritable bowel disease; multiple chemical sensitivities)

Fibromyalgia, chronic fatigue syndrome, and multiple chemical sensitivities are three conditions whose very existence is controversial. Believers search ever more intensely for organic causes, while unbelievers attribute the symptoms to psychiatric disorders. There is considerable overlap in the symptoms and epidemiology of the three conditions.[1] Many patients with fibromyalgia also meet the criteria of chronic fatigue syndrome,[2] 70% of patients with fibromyalgia meet the diagnostic criteria of irritable bowel syndrome,[3] and 65% of patients with irritable bowel syndrome meet the diagnostic criteria of fibromyalgia.[3] Barsky[4] considers fibromyalgia to be a functional somatic syndrome (see discussion of functional somatic syndromes).

In recent years even some of the original proponents of fibromyalgia as a specific disorder have begun to view the condition as a variant of a chronic pain syndrome and have acknowledged that many patients whose condition was diagnosed as fibromyalgia actually have major affective, somatization, or personality disorders.[5] Some argue that the very diagnosis of fibromyalgia is counterproductive and tends to foster somatization as a long-term character pattern.[2,6] Others claim that making a diagnosis is enabling because it reassures patients that they do not have a more serious progressive disease and that once a diagnosis is made, health care use and hospital admissions diminish.[7]

The detailed 1990 diagnostic criteria for fibromyalgia published under the auspices of the American College of Rheumatology include the following[8]:

1. History of widespread pain involving at least three sites, one of which must be the axial spine. The axial spine is defined as including the cervical, thoracic, or lumbar spine and the anterior chest.
2. Tenderness over 11 of 18 tender points. These points are all bilateral and include the following:
   a. Suboccipital
   b. Midpoint of sternocleidomastoid muscles
   c. Medial portion of supraspinatus muscles above spines of scapulae
   d. Midpoint of upper border of trapezius muscles
   e. Second costochondral junctions
   f. Lateral epicondyles
   g. Upper outer buttocks
   h. Greater trochanters
   i. Medial fat pad of knees proximal to joint line

The validity and specificity of these tender points are controversial.[2,6]

Fibromyalgia, like chronic fatigue syndrome and multiple chemical sensitivities, is predominantly a disorder of middle-aged[1,5-7] and elderly women.[7] Aside from the rheumatological symptoms and signs just listed, a variety of symptoms are found in patients with this diagnosis. In most series well over 50% have sleep disturbances, fatigue, muscle weakness, and cognitive changes such as memory loss.[1] Hudson and associates[9] reported in 1992 that at least two thirds of patients with fibromyalgia had been or were currently suffering from an affective or anxiety disorder. Furthermore, if the symptoms of fibromyalgia had been scored as symptoms of somatization disorder, 25% of patients would have fulfilled the criteria for that condition.[9] In a 1999 multicenter investigation of fibromyalgia patients, 48% were found to have a current psychiatric diagnosis; the lifetime prevalence of major depression was 68% and that

of panic disorder 16%. These patients also manifested high levels of neuroticism and hypochondriasis, both of which are associated with somatization.[10]

Fibromyalgia is a chronic but nonprogressive disease. Studies from specialized referral centers have reported gradual improvement over the years, and many patients who still have considerable pain can function well at work. Outcomes of patients treated in the community are generally better than for patients treated in tertiary referral centers.[7]

Tricyclic antidepressants have been recognized as effective over the short term for some patients with fibromyalgia. The usual doses given have been between 25 and 75 mg/day.[11] A 1996 crossover study compared 25 mg of amitriptyline (Elavil) daily, 20 mg of fluoxetine (Prozac) daily, a combination of the two antidepressants, and placebo, each given over a 4- to 6-week period. All of the regimens that included antidepressants caused improvement compared with placebo, but the combination of amitriptyline and fluoxetine worked best.[12] A small uncontrolled trial of venlafaxine (Effexor) titrated up to full antidepressant doses resulted in improvement in over half the patients.[13] NSAIDs and corticosteroids are not effective, but cognitive behavior therapy appears to be helpful.[7]

--- ⚓ **REFERENCES** ⚓ ---

1. Buchwald D, Garrity D: Comparison of patients with chronic fatigue syndrome, fibromyalgia, and multiple chemical sensitivities, *Arch Intern Med* 154:2049-2053, 1994.
2. Hadler NM: Fibromyalgia, chronic fatigue and other diagnostic algorithms: do some labels escalate illness in vulnerable patients? *Postgrad Med* 102:161-177, 1997.
3. Veale D, Kavanagh G, Fielding JF, et al: Primary fibromyalgia and the irritable bowel syndrome: different expressions of a common pathogenetic process, *Br J Rheumatol* 30:220-222, 1991.
4. Barsky AJ, Borus JF: Functional somatic syndromes, *Ann Intern Med* 130:910-921, 1999.
5. Wolfe F: The fibromyalgia problem (editorial), *J Rheumatol* 24:1247-1249, 1997.
6. Hadler NM: Fibromyalgia: La maladie est morte. Vive le malade! (editorial), *J Rheumatol* 24:1250-1251, 1997.
7. Goldenberg DL: Fibromyalgia syndrome a decade later: what have we learned? *Arch Intern Med* 159:777-785, 1999.
8. Wolfe F, Smythe HA, Yunus MB, et al: The American College of Rheumatology 1990 criteria for the classification of fibromyalgia: report of the multicenter criteria committee, *Arthritis Rheum* 33:160-172, 1990.
9. Hudson JI, Goldenberg DL, Pope HG, et al: Comorbidity of fibromyalgia with medical and psychiatric disorders, *Am J Med* 92:363-367, 1992.
10. Epstein SA, Kay G, Clauw D, et al: Psychiatric disorders in patients with fibromyalgia: a multicenter investigation, *Psychosomatics* 40:57-63, 1999.
11. Carette S, Bell MJ, Reynolds WJ, et al: Comparison of amitriptyline, cyclobenzaprine, and placebo in the treatment of fibromyalgia: a randomized, double-blind clinical trial, *Arthritis Rheum* 37:32-40, 1994.

12. Goldenberg D, Mayskiy M, Mossey C, et al: A randomized, double-blind crossover trial of fluoxetine and amitriptyline in the treatment of fibromyalgia, *Arthritis Rheum* 39:1852-1859, 1996.

13. Dwight MM, Arnold LM, O'Brien H, et al: An open clinical trial of venlafaxine treatment of fibromyalgia, *Psychosomatics* 39:14-17, 1998.

Osteoarthritis

(See also nonsteroidal antiinflammatory drugs; nonsteroidal antiinflammatory drug gastropathy; prescribing habits and the elderly)

Epidemiology

Osteoarthritis is a disease of the elderly, and the incidence of the disease in various joints varies with race. Osteoarthritis of the hips is common in whites but rare in Chinese and blacks. On the other hand, osteoarthritis of the knees is more common in black American women than white American women.[1] Risk factors for osteoarthritis include obesity and previous joint injury. In general, athletic activity has not been associated with the later development of osteoarthritis, although one study found a weak association between tennis and osteoarthritis of the hips.[2] An occupational history of heavy lifting has also been reported to be associated with an increased risk of osteoarthritis of the hip.[3] Smoking appears to have a protective role.[2]

Clinical presentation

Joints frequently and rarely involved by osteoarthritis are listed in Table 39.

Prognosis

Mild osteoarthritis in elderly patients rarely progresses to severe joint damage; severity of symptoms correlates more with depression and isolation than with degree of joint damage.[4] Osteoarthritis of the hands usually does not impair function except when the thumb joints are involved.[1]

Management

Management of osteoarthritis centers on pain control. Simple measures for those with hip pain include splitting heavy loads or carrying the load on the side of the affected hip. Physical activity is important because the health of cartilage depends on normal loads being applied to joints.[1] A 1997 investigation of 439 community-living elderly patients with osteoarthritis of the knees reported that aerobic exercises (walking) and to a lesser extent resistance exercises of major muscle groups decreased pain and increased mobility.[5] A 1999 systematic review of exercise treatments for osteoarthritis of the hip or knees concluded that exercise has a modest effect in ameliorating pain and disability.[6] Psychosocial issues augmenting the perception of pain should be identified and treated.[4]

No good evidence has shown that NSAIDs are better than simple analgesics, and theoretically some NSAIDs may actually damage cartilage (see discussion of NSAIDs below).[1] One set of evidence-based guidelines recommends starting with acetaminophen 4 g/day and, if that does not adequately control pain, substituting ibuprofen (Advil, Motrin) 1.2 g/day. If pain relief is still inadequate, acetaminophen 4 g/day may be added to the ibuprofen or the dose of ibuprofen may be doubled to 2.4 g/day. If pain still persists, other NSAIDs such as diclofenac (Voltaren) or naproxen (Anaprox) may be tried.[7]

Hyaluronic acid or its hylan derivatives have been available for treatment of joint injection in Europe for many years, in Canada since 1992, and in the United States since 1997. Synovial fluid in osteoarthritis has decreased viscosity, and hyaluronic acid injections are thought to restore normal viscosity to the joint fluid.[8] Some studies have found that injections give relief for several months,[9] while others have reported no benefit.[10] No long-term studies of efficacy have been published, and multiple joint injections carry risks.[11] Hylan G-F 20 is commercially available as Synvisc and Hyalgan.

Glucosamine has been shown in a few short-term controlled trials to relieve pain and increase range of motion in patients with osteoarthritis. In doses of 500 mg po tid it is about equivalent to 400 mg of ibuprofen tid. The product is available over the counter, but in North America purity and concentrations are not regulated.[12]

Joint replacement is usually indicated for patients with osteoarthritis who cannot function adequately after a reasonable trial of conservative management.[8]

Table 39   Joint Involvement in Osteoarthritis

Frequently involved	Rarely involved
Upper Extremity	
Distal interphalangeal joints of fingers (Heberden's nodes)	Metacarpophalangeal joints of fingers
Proximal interphalangeal joints of fingers (Bouchard's nodes)	Wrists
First carpometacarpal joints	Elbows
Acromioclavicular joints	Glenohumeral joints
Lower Extremity	
Hips	
Knees	
First metatarsophalangeal joints	Ankles (unless previous trauma)
Spine	
Cervical spine	Thoracic spine
Lumbar spine	

━━━━━━━━━━━━━━ ◤ **REFERENCES** ◣ ━━━━━━━━━━━━━━

1. Sack KE: Osteoarthritis: a continuing challenge, *West J Med* 163:579-586, 1995.
2. Cooper C, Inskip H, Croft P, et al: Individual risk factors for hip osteoarthritis: obesity, hip injury, and physical activity, *Am J Epidemiol* 147:516-522, 1998.

3. Coggon D, Kellingray S, Inskip H, et al: Osteoarthritis of the hip and occupational lifting, *Am J Epidemiol* 147:523-528, 1998.

4. Dieppe P: Osteoarthritis: time to shift the paradigm (editorial), *BMJ* 318:1299-1300, 1999.

5. Ettinger WH Jr, Burns R, Messier S, et al: A randomized trial comparing aerobic exercise and resistance exercise with a health education program in older adults with knee osteoarthritis: the Fitness Arthritis and Senior Trial (FAST), *JAMA* 277:25-31, 1997.

6. Van Baar ME, Assendelft WJ, Dekker J, et al: Effectiveness of exercise therapy in patients with osteoarthritis of the hip or knee, *Arthritis Rheum* 42:1361-1369, 1999.

7. Eccles M, Freemantle N, Mason J (North of England Non-Steroidal Anti-Inflammatory Drug Guideline Development Group): North of England evidence based guideline development project: summary guideline for non-steroidal anti-inflammatory drugs versus basic analgesia in treating the pain of degenerative arthritis, *BMJ* 317:526-530, 1998.

8. LaPrade RF, Swiontkowski MF: New horizons in the treatment of osteoarthritis of the knee, *JAMA* 281:876-878, 1999.

9. Lussier A, Cividino AA, McFarlane CA, et al: Viscosupplementation with hylan for the treatment of osteoarthritis: findings from clinical practice in Canada, *J Rheumatol* 23:1579-1585, 1996.

10. Henderson EB, Smith EC, Pegley F, et al: Intra-articular injections of 750 kD hyaluronan in the treatment of osteoarthritis: a randomised single centre double-blind placebo-controlled trial of 91 patients demonstrating lack of efficacy, *Ann Rheum Dis* 53:529-534, 1994.

11. Hyaluronan injections for osteoarthritis of the knee, *Med Lett* 40:69-70, 1998.

12. Glucosamine for osteoarthritis, *Med Lett* 39:91-92, 1997.

Paget's Disease

Paget's disease is common in Europe and North America and rare in Asia. Although it may be monostotic, multiple lesions are usually present. Sites of predilection are the axial skeleton, long bones, and skull. The vast majority of lesions are asymptomatic. Although the individual lesions of Paget's disease may cause pain, many of the symptoms result from complications of the disease. These include enlargement of the skull, hearing loss, bowing of long bones, pain from secondary osteoarthritis or fractures, osteosarcoma (in less than 1% of cases), and neurological deficits from entrapment of nerves or compression of the spinal cord. The serum alkaline phosphatase level is usually but not always elevated. Bone scans are the investigative procedure of choice.[1]

Treatment is indicated for patients with symptoms or for asymptomatic patients at risk of complications such as hearing loss (lesions at base of skull), spinal cord compression (lesions in vertebrae), and osteoarthritis or fractures (lesions in long bones).[1] In many cases the drug of choice is alendronate (Fosamax) in oral doses of 40 mg/day. Alternatives are etidronate (Didrocal), calcitonin (Calcimar, Miacalcin),[1] pamidronate (Aredia), risedronate (Actonel), and tiludronate (Skelid).[2]

━━━━━━━━━━━ ❧ **REFERENCES** ❧ ━━━━━━━━━━━

1. Delmas PD, Meunier PJ: The management of Paget's disease of bone, *N Engl J Med* 336:558-566, 1997.

2. Risedronate for Paget's disease of bone, *Med Lett* 40:87-88, 1998.

Palindromic Rheumatism

Palindromic rheumatism consists of recurrent attacks of arthritis that usually involve one or only a few joints. Patients can be quite incapacitated during the attacks, but once an attack resolves, they are asymptomatic without any evidence of residual joint damage. The natural course of palindromic rheumatism is variable. Some patients have lasting remissions, but some continue to have recurrent attacks. By 6 years after onset a little over one fourth will have rheumatoid arthritis and a very few will have lupus or other connective tissue diseases. Those at greatest risk of progression to connective tissue diseases are women with positive tests for rheumatoid factor and involvement of hand joints.[1]

━━━━━━━━━━━ ❧ **REFERENCES** ❧ ━━━━━━━━━━━

1. Gonzalez-Lopez L, Gamez-Nava JI, Jhangri GS, et al: Prognostic factors for the development of rheumatoid arthritis and other connective tissue diseases in patients with palindromic rheumatism, *J Rheumatol* 26:540-545, 1999.

Polymyalgia Rheumatica
(See also giant cell arteritis; sedimentation rate)

The onset of polymyalgia rheumatica can be indolent or sudden. In most cases aching and stiffness of proximal limb muscles, especially the shoulder girdle, are prominent symptoms. Morning stiffness and gelling after activities, as well as malaise and fatigue, are also common. The patient may have pain, especially at night, that makes getting out of bed or into and out of the bathtub difficult. Transient synovitis of joints may occur. Elevated sedimentation rates and a mild normocytic anemia are common findings; slight elevation of liver function tests may also occur.[1] It is important to realize that in one fifth of patients the sedimentation rate is normal (30 mm/hr or less).[2]

If biopsy specimens of temporal artery are obtained from patients with polymyalgia rheumatica, many of them will be found to have histological evidence of temporal arteritis. However, this finding is a poor predictor for the development of clinical temporal arteritis. Furthermore, temporal arteritis develops later in a number of patients with negative biopsies. Fortunately, severe sequelae such as vision loss are rarely if ever the initial manifestation of temporal arteritis. Therefore temporal artery biopsies should be reserved for patients with suggestive symptoms or signs such as jaw claudication, headaches, visual changes, or tender temporal arteries.[3]

The differential diagnosis of polymyalgia rheumatica includes fibromyalgia, paraneoplastic syndromes, endocarditis, hypothyroid myopathy, polymyositis, systemic lupus erythematosus, monoclonal gammopathies, and rheumatoid arthritis, particularly if it is seronegative. Investigations that may clarify the diagnosis are urinalysis (looking for hematuria), creatine kinase, rheumatoid factor, antinuclear antigen (ANA), thyroid-stimulating hormone, and serum and urine electrophoresis.[1]

An important diagnostic test for polymyalgia rheumatica is a response within 24 to 48 hours to low-dose steroids such as prednisone 10 mg/day. A few other conditions, most commonly seronegative rheumatoid arthritis, respond in the same way.[3]

The usual treatment of polymyalgia rheumatica is corticosteroids.[1,3] The initial dose, which is titrated to a level that gives complete symptom relief, is usually prednisone 10 to 20 mg/day. This is decreased every 2 to 4 weeks by 2.5 mg until a daily dose of 10 mg is achieved, and thereafter tapering continues by 1-mg decrements every 2 to 4 weeks until a maintenance dose of 5 to 7.5 mg is achieved. Total duration of treatment varies from 2 to 15 years. Between one fourth and one half of patients have a relapse after discontinuation of treatment.[3] Mild symptoms may be successfully managed with NSAIDs.[1] Adverse effects from both NSAIDs and corticosteroids are common and are dose related. Minimal doses should be used.[4]

Patients with polymyalgia rheumatica who have sedimentation rates lower than 40 mm/hr tend to have a milder clinical course. Fever, anemia, and weight loss are less common than in patients with higher sedimentation rates.[5]

◣ REFERENCES ◢
---

1. Hunder GG: Giant cell arteritis and polymyalgia rheumatica, *Med Clin North Am* 81:195-219, 1997.
2. Helfgott SM, Kieval RI: Polymyalgia rheumatica in patients with a normal erythrocyte sedimentation rate, *Arthritis Rheum* 39:304-307, 1996.
3. Brooks RC, McGee SR: Diagnostic dilemmas in polymyalgia rheumatica, *Arch Intern Med* 157:162-168, 1997.
4. Gabriel SE, Sunku J, Salvarani C, et al: Adverse outcomes of antiinflammatory therapy among patients with polymyalgia rheumatica, *Arthritis Rheum* 40:1873-1878, 1997.
5. González-Gay MA, Rodriguez-Valverde V, Blanco R, et al: Polymyalgia rheumatica without significantly increased erythrocyte sedimentation rate—a more benign syndrome, *Arch Intern Med* 157:317-320, 1997.

Rheumatoid Arthritis

(See also nonsteroidal antiinflammatory drugs; nonsteroidal antiinflammatory drug gastropathy; palindromic rheumatism)

Three times more women than men have rheumatoid arthritis, but among the elderly the ratio evens out.[1] Some studies have shown an association between smoking and rheumatoid arthritis.[2]

According to the American Rheumatism Association a diagnosis of rheumatoid arthritis can be made if the patient has four or more of the following findings[3]:

1. Morning stiffness for 1 hour or more persisting for at least 6 weeks
2. Soft tissue swelling (arthritis) in three or more locations for at least 6 weeks; the swelling has to be documented by a physician
3. Swelling of the wrist, metacarpophalangeal joints, or proximal interphalangeal joints for at least 6 weeks
4. Symmetrical joint involvement for at least 6 weeks
5. Rheumatoid nodules
6. Presence of rheumatoid factor
7. X-ray findings consistent with rheumatoid arthritis (erosion or osteopenia of wrist or hand joints)

It is now believed that "disease-modifying" drugs should be started as early as possible when rheumatoid arthritis is diagnosed (see later discussion). To achieve this goal primary care physicians must make the diagnosis without delay and, when indicated, arrange appropriate referral. Unfortunately, the diagnosis is rarely made until many months after onset.[4]

Nonsteroidal antiinflammatory drugs

Until recently NSAIDs were considered the first-line drugs for rheumatoid arthritis, with no one drug superior to another. The protocol for using NSAIDs involves starting with one and continuing it for 10 to 14 days before deciding whether it is effective. If the initial drug fails to control symptoms, another NSAID is chosen, and the process is continued until several different NSAIDs had been tried.[5] Some workers recommend choosing NSAIDs such as celecoxib (Celebrex) and rofecoxib (Vioxx), which selectively inhibit cyclooxygenase 2 (COX-2), but as yet no long-term studies of the efficacy or adverse effects of these agents are available (see discussions of nonsteroidal antiinflammatory drugs and NSAID gastropathy).[6]

Disease-modifying drugs. Traditional "disease-modifying," "antirheumatic," or "second-line" drugs for rheumatoid arthritis include methotrexate (Rheumatrex), sulfasalazine (Azulfidine), hydroxychloroquine (Plaquenil), azathioprine (Imuran), cyclosporine (Sandimmune), gold salts (Myochrysine, Solganal), and penicillamine (Cuprimine, Depen). Newer drugs of this nature are the pyrimidine synthesis inhibitor leflunomide (Arava) and the tumor necrosis factor inhibitors etanercept (Enbrel) and infliximab (Remicade). The rationale for using disease-modifying drugs is to alter the basic pathological processes responsible for the inflammation and through this mechanism to prevent deformities and disabilities. Evidence to date suggests that if treatment is started early, this goal can be achieved provided that patients continue to take their medications.[7,8] If medications are discontinued, relapses are frequent.[7]

No disease-modifying drug has been definitively shown

to have more beneficial effects than another, but at present methotrexate and hydroxychloroquine are preferred for single-drug therapy by most North American rheumatologists,[9] while the most popular drug in Great Britain is sulfasalazine.[10] There is growing evidence that combinations of disease-modifying drugs are more effective than single agents from this class.[7]

Several long-term studies of patients taking disease-modifying drugs have shown a high rate of discontinuation of the medications because of toxic side effects or perceived lack of beneficial effect.[11,12] Among all these drugs, methotrexate appears to have the lowest discontinuation rate.[12] In one 5-year study of methotrexate in rheumatoid arthritis, 36% of patients discontinued the medication, 7% because of adverse effects and 7% because of lack of efficacy. However, in the same study, more than two thirds of the patients showed a marked clinical improvement.[11] Mucosal and gastrointestinal side effects of methotrexate can be reduced by regular folate supplementation.[13]

When methotrexate is used, it is usually given in small weekly doses in the range of 7.5 to 25 mg. Methotrexate may be given orally or parenterally. The parenteral route is preferred for doses over 20 mg weekly, for patients who cannot tolerate oral medications because of gastrointestinal side effects, and for patients who have not responded to orally administered methotrexate.[11]

Minocycline (Minocin) may be beneficial in the treatment of early seropositive rheumatoid arthritis. In one double-blind placebo-controlled trial patients who had received 100 mg of minocycline bid for 3 to 6 months had a much higher remission rate when assessed 4 years later than did those who were given placebos.[14]

Corticosteroids

Corticosteroids in combination with disease-modifying agents were shown in one study to decrease erosion rates,[15] and they also improve symptoms.[15,16] Whether these benefits outweigh potential adverse effects is uncertain.[7]

⚓ REFERENCES ⚓

1. Akil M, Amos RS: Rheumatoid arthritis. I. Clinical features and diagnosis, *BMJ* 310:587-590, 1995.
2. Karlson EW, Lee I-M, Cook NR, et al: A retrospective cohort study of cigarette smoking and risk of rheumatoid arthritis in female health professionals, *Arthritis Rheum* 42:910-917, 1999.
3. Arnett FC, Edworthy SM, Bloch DA, et al: The American Rheumatism Association 1987 revised criteria for the classification of rheumatoid arthritis, *Arthritis Rheum* 31:315-324, 1988.
4. Weinblatt ME: Rheumatoid arthritis: treat now not later (editorial), *Ann Intern Med* 124:773-774, 1998.
5. Grondin C: L'arthrite rhumatoïde: approche thérapeutique, *Can Fam Physician* 36:487-490, 499, 1990.
6. Celecoxib for arthritis, *Med Lett* 41:11-12, 1999.
7. Brooks P: Rheumatology, *BMJ* 316:1810-1812, 1998.
8. Strand V, Tugwell P, Bombardier C, et al: Function and health-related quality of life: results from a randomized controlled trial of leflunomide versus methotrexate or placebo in patients with active rheumatoid arthritis, *Arthritis Rheum* 42:1870-1878, 1999.
9. Drugs for rheumatoid arthritis, *Med Lett* 36:101-106, 1994.
10. Emery P: Therapeutic approaches for early rheumatoid arthritis. How early? How aggressive? *Br J Rheumatol* 34(suppl 2):87-90, 1995.
11. Weinblatt ME, Kaplan H, Germain BF, et al: Methotrexate in rheumatoid arthritis: a five-year prospective multicenter study, *Arthritis Rheum* 37:1492-1498, 1994.
12. Pincus T: Long-term outcomes in rheumatoid arthritis, *Br J Rheumatol* 34(suppl 2):59-73, 1995.
13. Oritz Z, Shea B, Suarez-Almazor ME, et al: The efficiency of folic acid and folinic acid in reducing methotrexate gastrointestinal toxicity in rheumatoid arthritis: a meta-analysis of randomized controlled trials, *J Rheumatol* 24:36-43, 1998.
14. O'Dell JR, Paulsen G, Haire CE, et al: Treatment of early seropositive rheumatoid arthritis with minocycline: four-year followup of a double-blind, placebo-controlled trial, *Arthritis Rheum* 42:1691-1695, 1999.
15. Kirwan JR (Arthritis and Rheumatism Council Low-Dose Glucocorticoid Study Group): The effect of glucocorticoids on joint destruction in rheumatoid arthritis, *N Engl J Med* 333:142-146, 1995.
16. Boers M, Verhoeven AC, Markusse HM, et al: Randomised comparison of combined step-down prednisolone, methotrexate and sulphasalazine with sulphasalazine alone in early rheumatoid arthritis, *Lancet* 350:309-318, 1997.

Septic Arthritis

(See also gonorrhea; transient synovitis of hip)

The joints most commonly affected in nongonococcal septic arthritis are large joints such as the knees and hips. Between 80% and 90% of cases of septic arthritis are monarticular.

Gonococcal arthritis is two to three times more common in women than in men. Migratory tendinitis and arthritis often precede gonococcal monarthritis. One half to three fourths of patients with disseminated gonococcal infections have skin lesions, which usually number less than 30 and are located primarily on the extremities. Ninety percent of patients with disseminated gonococcal infections have arthritis.[1] Disseminated meningococcal disease must be considered in the differential diagnosis because it too can cause skin and joint disease.[2]

⚓ REFERENCES ⚓

1. Handsfield HH: Disseminated gonococcal infection, *Clin Obstet Gynecol* 18:131-142, 1975.
2. Rompalo AM, Hook WE 3d, Roberts PL, et al: The acute arthritis-dermatitis syndrome: the changing importance of *Neisseria gonorrhoeae* and *Neisseria meningitidis*, *Arch Intern Med* 147:281-283, 1987.

Seronegative Spondyloarthropathies
(See also sexually transmitted diseases)

The seronegative spondyloarthropathies are a group of inflammatory arthritides that are rheumatoid factor and ANA negative and that have a much greater frequency in HLA-B27-positive persons than in those who do not carry this histocompatibility antigen. Conditions included in this category are ankylosing spondylitis, psoriatic arthritis, Reiter's syndrome,[1] and arthritis associated with inflammatory bowel disease.[1] Some workers also place Whipple's disease and Behçet's disease into the category of seronegative spondyloarthropathies. Reiter's syndrome and the arthritis of inflammatory bowel disease are often called reactive arthritides.[1]

Frequent clinical findings in patients with seronegative spondyloarthropathies are involvement of the back and the sacroiliac joints, involvement of only a few peripheral joints, most often in an asymmetrical pattern in the lower extremities, and inflammatory reactions involving the entheses or sites of attachments of ligaments and tendons to bones (enthesopathy). Typical manifestations of enthesopathy are pain and tenderness over the plantar fascia where it inserts on the calcaneus or pain and tenderness over the region where the Achilles tendon inserts onto the calcaneus. Isolated arthritis and tenosynovitis of a single digit of the toes or fingers (dactylitis) occurring as a diffuse sausagelike swelling are particularly characteristic of Reiter's syndrome and psoriatic arthritis.[1]

Extraarticular manifestations are common with the seronegative spondyloarthropathies. Iritis or other inflammatory eye conditions may be seen in all of them, skin lesions in psoriatic arthritis and Reiter's syndrome, and urethritis in Reiter's syndrome even when precipitated by a dysenteric syndrome.[1]

Ankylosing spondylitis

Archaic synonyms for ankylosing spondylitis are rheumatoid spondylitis and Marie-Strumpell disease. It was formerly thought that males were affected 20 times as often as women. This is erroneous; women usually have fewer symptoms, and the diagnosis is often missed. The true sex ratio is probably about 5:1 in favor of males. Although some persons are disabled by the disease, the majority are not.[1] Ankylosing spondylitis is a rare but important cause of low back pain in persons under the age of 40. The following findings suggest this diagnosis[2,3]:

1. Insidious onset
2. Onset before age 40
3. Pain for more than 3 months
4. Morning stiffness longer than 30 minutes
5. Pain relief with activity
6. Pain forcing the patient from bed
7. History of psoriasis, Reiter's disease, uveitis, or colitis
8. Chest expansion of less than 2 inches
9. Peripheral joint disease

The first five criteria have a high sensitivity and specificity, but because of the low prevalence of the disorder the positive predictive value is on the order of only 0.04.[3]

The classic physical findings of ankylosing spondylitis are a positive Schober's test, a positive occiput to wall test, and decreased chest expansion (less than 5 to 6 cm or 2 inches).

Schober's test is performed as follows. With the patient standing vertically, the end of a measuring tape is placed over the spinous processes at the level of the posterior superior iliac spines and stretched proximally along the spine. A mark is placed on the skin at the 10-cm level. With the end of the tape kept in place, the patient is asked to flex as fully forward as possible. The distance to the skin mark is measured. Normally it is about 15 cm because of flexion of the lumbar spine. In patients with ankylosing spondylitis it is less because most or all flexion takes place at the hips.

In the occiput to wall test the patient stands with heels against the wall and tries to press the occiput against the wall. Many patients with ankylosing spondylitis cannot do this because of fixed flexion deformity of the spine.

Unfortunately, the defining signs are not usually present in the early stages of the disease. Testing for HLA-B27 is not usually helpful. If the clinical picture is convincing, this study is unnecessary (10% of patients with the disease are HLA-B27 negative), and if the diagnosis is unlikely on a clinical basis, the presence of a positive HLA-B27 adds little useful information.[1]

Reiter's syndrome

Reiter's syndrome may be initiated by either urethritis, which is usually chlamydial in origin, or a dysentery-like syndrome caused by a variety of organisms, including *Shigella, Salmonella, Campylobacter,* and *Yersinia.* The postvenereal form of Reiter's syndrome affects about five to nine times as many men as women, whereas the postdysentery form affects the sexes equally. The classic triad is urethritis, conjunctivitis, and arthritis, usually appearing in that order, but only one third of patients have all three entities. Symptoms of urethritis usually develop 2 to 4 weeks after either sexual exposure or a diarrheal illness. Ocular symptoms are reported in about half the cases and are usually the result of a short-lived mild conjunctivitis; some patients have iritis, uveitis, or keratitis. Arthritis develops last. The most frequently affected joints are the knees, ankles, and toes ("sausage" digits). Asymmetrical oligoarthritis is the rule. In half the patients the spine or sacroiliac joints are involved. Enthesopathy, circinate balanitis of the penis, and keratoderma blennorrhagicum of the palms and soles are common. About half of the patients have a prolonged course or recurrences over months or years, but only a few have functional disability.[1,4] Standard treatment is NSAIDs for symptom relief and antibiotics if active chlamydial infection is still present (see discussion of sexually transmitted diseases).[1,4,5] Antibiotics are not beneficial for Reiter's syndrome that results from enteric infections.[5]

Psoriatic arthritis

In 85% of patients with psoriatic arthritis, skin lesions develop before the arthritis. In some patients skin stigmata of psoriasis may not be obvious at first glance; patients may have pitting of nails, onycholysis, scalp lesions, or lesions between the buttocks or in the umbilicus. The arthritis is usually asymmetrical and involves only a few joints. Dactylitis of a toe or finger is characteristic of psoriatic arthritis or Reiter's syndrome.[1]

Enteropathic arthropathies

Seronegative arthropathies develop in about 8% of patients with ulcerative colitis and 14% of those with Crohn's disease. Larger joints of the lower extremities are usually involved, and the activity of the arthritis tends to parallel that of the bowel disease.[1]

──────────── ◁ **REFERENCES** ▷ ────────────

1. Osial TA Jr, Cash JM, Eisenbeis CH Jr: Arthritis-associated syndromes, *Primary Care* 20:857-882, 1993.
2. Calin A, Porta J, Fries JF, et al: Clinical history as a screening test for ankylosing spondylitis, *JAMA* 237:2613-2614, 1977.
3. Calin A, Kaye B, Sternberg M, et al: The prevalence and nature of back pain in an industrial complex: a questionnaire and radiographic and HLA analysis, *Spine* 5:201-205, 1980.
4. Kirchner JT: Reiter's syndrome: a possibility in patients with reactive arthritis, *Postgrad Med* 97:111-112, 115-117, 121-122, 1995.
5. Barth WF, Segal K: Reactive arthritis (Reiter's syndrome), *Am Fam Physician* 60:499-503, 1999.

METABOLIC

Topics covered in this section

ADRENAL DISORDERS
Adrenal Insufficiency

Addison's disease is a rare disease that is more common in females than males and is most frequently diagnosed in young and middle-aged adults. The three cardinal symptoms are weight loss, fatigue, and weakness. Gastrointestinal and psychiatric symptoms are common. Most patients have hyperpigmentation, and a number are hypotensive. Laboratory abnormalities include mild normocytic anemia, mild eosinophilia, hyponatremia, and hyperkalemia. In many cases an 8 AM cortisol determination can confirm or rule out the diagnosis. If the level is 83 nmol/L (3 μg/dl) or less, the diagnosis is confirmed, whereas if the concentration is 525 nmol/L (19 μg/dl) or more, it is ruled out (assuming a normal range to be 165 to 662 nmol/L [6 to 24 μg/dl]).[1]

The treatment of choice for chronic adrenal insufficiency is oral hydrocortisone or cortisol. Although the dosage is variable, most patents receive cortisone 25 to 37.5 mg/day. Usually two thirds of the daily dose is given in the morning and one third at night, although some patients feel better if the daily dose is given in equal amounts three times a day. In times of stress, such as intercurrent illnesses, injury, or surgery, the maintenance dose is usually doubled. Patients with primary adrenal insufficiency often lose salt and may need to take fludrocortisone (Florinef) 50 to 200 μg as a single daily dose; those with secondary adrenal insufficiency (caused by pituitary disorders) rarely require fludrocortisone.[1] Recent studies suggest that patients with adrenal insufficiency whose strength and well-being remain subnormal on standard maintenance therapy may benefit from the addition of a daily dose of 25 to 50 mg of dehydroepiandrosterone.[2]

Prednisone, prednisolone, and dexamethasone are not the drugs of choice for Addison's disease because they have little mineralocorticoid activity. Addison's disease may still develop in patients taking these drugs for other reasons.[3]

Cushing's Syndrome

Rapid weight gain is characteristic of Cushing's syndrome. The rounded "moon" facies is due to increased facial fat, and the florid complexion to telangiectasias. The buffalo hump is a common finding with any type of weight gain, whereas filling out of the supraclavicular fat pads is more specific for Cushing's syndrome. Muscle wasting leads to difficulty climbing stairs, getting out of a low chair, or rising from a squatting position.[4]

If Cushing's syndrome is suspected, a 24-hour urine study for free cortisol (plus creatinine to assess the adequacy of collection) should be performed and repeated on 1 or 2 consecutive days.[4] A dexamethasone suppression test is the standard alternative. This test is performed by giving 1 mg of dexamethasone at 11 PM and measuring the serum cortisol by 9 AM the next day. If the level is less than 135 nmol/L (5 μg/dl), the diagnosis of Cushing's syndrome is ruled out in 98% of cases. Unfortunately, the dexamethasone suppression test has a high false-positive rate. An alternative that can be used when standard investigations fail to give a specific diagnosis is to obtain a midnight cortisol measurement from a resting, fasting patient who has had an indwelling venous catheter inserted at least 2 hours before sampling; levels above 206 μmol/L (7.5 μg/dl) are highly specific for Cushing's syndrome.[5]

Incidentalomas

About 5% of patients who have an abdominal computed to-mographic scan are found to have an incidental adrenal mass; over 80% of these are benign and hormonally non-functional.[6] A long-term follow-up of incidentalomas vary-ing in diameter from 1 to 5.6 cm revealed no cases of ma-lignancy and a 10% rate of hyperfunctioning.[7] Most authorities advise surgical removal if the mass is over 6 cm because of an increased risk of malignancy. Some authors suggest that hormonal evaluation be performed in all cases; if needle aspiration is being considered, pheochromocytoma must first be ruled out.[6]

──────────── ◤ REFERENCES ◢ ────────────

1. Oelkers W: Adrenal insufficiency, *N Engl J Med* 335:1206-1212, 1996.
2. Oelkers W: Dehydroepiandrosterone for adrenal insufficiency (editorial), *N Engl J Med* 341:1073-1074, 1999.
3. Cronin CC, Callaghan N, Kearney PJ, et al: Addison disease in patients treated with glucocorticoid therapy, *Arch Intern Med* 157:456-458, 1997.
4. Orth DN: Cushing's syndrome, *N Engl J Med* 332:791-803, 1995.
5. Papanicolaou DA, Yanovski JA, Cutler GB Jr, et al: A single midnight serum cortisol measurement distinguishes Cushing's syndrome from pseudo-Cushing states, *J Clin Endocrinol Metab* 83:1163-1167, 1998.
6. Ooi TC: Adrenal incidentalomas: incidental in detection, not significance, *Can Med Assoc J* 157:903-904, 1997.
7. Barzon L, Scaroni C, Sonino N, et al: Risk factors and long-term follow-up of adrenal incidentalomas, *J Clin Endocrinol Metab* 84:520-526, 1999.

DIABETES MELLITUS

(See also endometrial carcinoma; screening)

Until recently the diagnosis of diabetes mellitus was made if two fasting glucose readings were greater than 7.8 mmol/L (140 mg/dl) or if two random glucose readings were greater than 11.1 mmol/L (200 mg/dl). In 1997 the American Diabetes Association recommended that the diag-nosis of diabetes be made if the fasting sugar level is 7 mmol/L (126 mg/dl) or over.[1] The Canadian Diabetes Asso-ciation followed suit in 1998.[2] Individuals with fasting plasma glucose levels between 6.1 and 7 mmol/L (109 mg/dl and 126 mg/dl) are not at increased risk for microvas-cular disease but are at increased risk for diabetes. They are classified as having "impaired fasting glucose."[2]

A variety of criticisms have been leveled against the changes. Davidson and associates[3] argue that 60% of indi-viduals with fasting plasma glucose levels between 7 mmol/L (126 mg/dl) and 7.7 mmol/L (139 mg/dl) have nor-mal HbA_{1c} and that they are not really diabetic but may be subject to negative psychological, social, employment, and insurance consequences because they are so labeled. An ac-companying editorial by Vinicor[4] strongly disagrees. A number of researchers have concluded that using only fast-ing sugar levels, even lower ones, misses many patients at increased risk of morbidity[5] and death[6] from diabetes-related macrovascular complications but that most of these could be detected by modified glucose tolerance tests. These authors advocate a return to the World Health Organization recommendation that glucose levels above 11.1 mmol/L (200 mg/dl) 2 hours after a 75-g glucose load be considered diagnostic of diabetes. Some of these issues are discussed in more detail in the section on prevention and screening.

To convert SI units (mmol/L) to traditional units (mg/dl), divide by 0.05551. To convert traditional units (mg/dl) to SI units (mmol/L), multiply by 0.05551.

──────────── ◤ REFERENCES ◢ ────────────

1. American Diabetes Association: Standards of medical care for patients with diabetes mellitus, *Diabetes Care* 20(suppl 1):S1-S70, 1997.
2. Meltzer S, Leiter L, Daneman D, et al: 1998 Clinical practice guidelines for the management of diabetes in Canada, *Can Med Assoc J* 159(suppl 8):S1-S29, 1998.
3. Davidson MB, Schriger DL, Peters AL, et al: Relationship be-tween fasting plasma glucose and glycosylated hemoglobin: po-tential for false-positive diagnoses of type 2 diabetes using new diagnostic criteria, *JAMA* 281:1203-1210, 1999.
4. Vinicor F: When is diabetes diabetes? (editorial), *JAMA* 281:1222-1224, 1999.
5. Barzilay JI, Spiekerman CF, Wahl PW, et al: Cardiovascular disease in older adults with glucose disorders: comparison of American Diabetes Association criteria for diabetes mellitus with WHO criteria, *Lancet* 354:622-625, 1999.
6. Tuomilehto J et al (DECODE study group on behalf of the Eu-ropean Diabetes Epidemiology Group): Glucose tolerance and mortality: comparison of WHO and American Diabetes Asso-ciation diagnostic criteria, *Lancet* 354:617-621, 1999.

Microvascular Complications of Diabetes Mellitus
Diabetic retinopathy

(See also eating disorders)

Classification. Three types of retinal abnormalities are common in diabetes: nonproliferative or background reti-nopathy, proliferative retinopathy, and macular edema. Vi-sual loss is caused by either macular edema or proliferative retinopathy. If untreated, half of all patients with prolifera-tive retinopathy will become blind within 5 years, but with argon laser photocoagulation the rate is less than 5%. Pho-tocoagulation is also effective in reducing visual loss in about half of diabetic patients with macular edema.[1] Patients with more severe degrees of retinopathy are at in-creased risk of death from cardiovascular disease.[2]

Nonproliferative retinopathy. The initial and most com-mon manifestation of diabetic retinopathy is microaneurysm formation. As the disease progresses, erythrocytes escape from the lesions, leading to dot and blot hemorrhages. Leak-age of serous fluid from the capillaries may lead to the for-mation of retinal or macular edema and is often associated with the presence of hard exudates and sometimes venous beading. Microaneurysms, dot and blot hemorrhages, and hard exudates are collectively termed "background retinopathy" or "nonproliferative retinopathy." Nonproliferative retinopathy does not lead to loss of vision unless it occurs near the maculae and causes macular edema.[1]

Proliferative retinopathy. As the diabetic retinal disease progresses, some vessels become occluded, leading to infarcts of the retinae seen as soft or "cotton wool" exudates. In response to ischemia, new vessels develop and proliferate out of the retina into the vitreous. This is "proliferative retinopathy." These attenuated fragile vessels tend to bleed, causing vitreous hemorrhages. Vitreous hemorrhages usually resorb in 1 to 3 months, but subsequent fibrous proliferation can lead to retinal detachment and loss of vision. Aspirin does not increase the frequency or severity of vitreous hemorrhages in patients with nonproliferative or early proliferative retinopathy, and since it is protective against cardiovascular disease, many diabetics should be taking it.[3]

Macular edema. Macular edema can rarely be detected by direct ophthalmoscopy, but its presence may be suspected if the macula is surrounded by hard exudates. Ophthalmologists detect macular edema by binocular slit lamp examination or by stereoscopic fundus photography.[1]

Prevalence and progression. Retinopathy is far more likely to develop in patients with type 1 diabetes than in those with type 2. If the onset of diabetes occurs before age 30, almost all patients will have some degree of diabetic retinopathy after 20 years and in half the cases it will be proliferative. In contrast, only 20% of patients with type 2 diabetes who do not require insulin will have some degree of diabetic retinopathy after 20 years and in only 5% will it be proliferative. Among elderly type 2 patients requiring insulin, 80% will display some degree of retinopathy and 20% will have proliferative retinopathy. After 15 to 20 years about 15% of all diabetics will have macular edema.[1]

In type 1 diabetes retinopathy rarely develops before puberty and usually only after the patient has had the disease for 3 to 5 years. After 7 years approximately 50% will have some degree of retinopathy.[3]

Although most studies of newly diagnosed type 2 diabetes have reported that about 20% of patients have early-stage retinopathy at the time of diagnosis, a 1998 report found an overall incidence of 39% in men and 35% in women. In 92% of the male cases and 95% of the female cases the disease was early background retinopathy (see above), and in about 20% of cases the retinopathy was so minimal that the diagnosis was based on the finding of three or fewer microaneurysms with no other detectable abnormalities.[4]

Pregnancy[5] and eating disorders[6] are recognized risk factors for the progression of diabetic retinopathy. Between one fourth and one third of adolescent girls with type 1 diabetes also have eating disorders. They tend to vomit, purge, and omit insulin doses, and their metabolic control is poor (some cases of "brittle diabetes" are probably due to this phenomenon). They have a greatly increased risk for retinopathy.[6]

Diabetic control and retinopathy

In both type 1 and type 2 diabetes the degree of retinopathy and the risk of progression correlate with the degree of elevation of the glycosylated hemoglobin level.[7] The Diabetes Control and Complications Trial (DCCT) showed that intensive treatment of type 1 diabetes significantly decreased the incidence of proliferative retinopathy. However, a small proportion of patients displayed "early worsening" of retinopathy. In about half of these patients recovery occurred by 18 months, but in the other half it did not. Because of the risk of worsening retinopathy, any diabetic patient starting a program of intensive diabetic control should be assessed by an ophthalmologist before treatment is initiated and should be monitored during the early treatment period.[8]

In the United Kingdom Prospective Diabetes Study (UKPDS) relatively tight control of patients with type 2 diabetes (HbA$_{1c}$ of 7% compared with less intensive treatment of control subjects with mean HbA$_{1c}$ levels of 7.9%) resulted in slower progression of retinopathy, but the groups did not differ in terms of decreased visual acuity. In this study 323 patients had to be treated intensively for 1 year to prevent one person from requiring retinal photocoagulation.[9]

Guidelines for ophthalmological care

The American Diabetes Association[10] recommends that initial ophthalmological evaluations be obtained for the following:

1. Patients with type 1 diabetes who are at the onset of puberty or older and have had diabetes for 5 or more years
2. Patients over the age of 30 whose diabetes has first been diagnosed
3. Diabetic patients with any other ocular pathological condition
4. Diabetic women in the first trimester of pregnancy
5. Women with type 1 diabetes who are planning a pregnancy

The initiation of a program of tight control also mandates ophthalmological surveillance. Patients with established retinopathy should have annual ophthalmological examinations.[10]

The Canadian Task Force on Preventive Health Care gives a "B" recommendation to funduscopy or retinal photography of diabetic patients during the periodic health examination.[11] The U.S. Preventive Services Task Force makes no specific recommendation on this issue.

❧ REFERENCES ❧

1. Ferris FL III, Davis MD, Aiello LM: Treatment of diabetic retinopathy, *N Engl J Med* 341:667-678, 1999.
2. Klein R, Klein BE, Moss SE: Epidemiology of proliferative diabetic retinopathy, *Diabetes Care* 15:1875-1891, 1992.
3. Nathan DM: Long-term complications of diabetes mellitus, *N Engl J Med* 328:1676-1685, 1993.

4. United Kingdom Prospective Diabetes Study, 30: diabetic retinopathy at diagnosis of non-insulin-dependent diabetes mellitus and associated risk factors, *Arch Ophthalmol* 116:297-303, 1998.

5. Klein BE, Moss SE, Klein R: Effect of pregnancy on progression of diabetic retinopathy, *Diabetes Care* 13:34-40, 1990.

6. Rydall AC, Rodin GM, Olmsted MP, et al: Disordered eating behavior and microvascular complications in young women with insulin-dependent diabetes mellitus, *N Engl J Med* 336:1849-1854, 1997.

7. Klein R, Klein BE, Moss SE, et al: Relationship of hyperglycemia to the long-term incidence and progression of diabetic retinopathy, *Arch Intern Med* 154:2169-2178, 1994.

8. Diabetes Control and Complications Trial Research Group: Early worsening of diabetic retinopathy in the Diabetes Control and Complications Trial, *Arch Ophthalmol* 116:874-886, 1998.

9. UK Prospective Diabetes Study (UKPDS) Group: Intensive blood-glucose control with sulphonylureas or insulin compared with conventional treatment and risk of complications in patients with type 2 diabetes (UKPDS 33), *Lancet* 352:837-853, 1998.

10. American Diabetes Association: Standards of medical care for patients with diabetes mellitus, *Diabetes Care* 20(suppl 1):S5-S13, 1997.

11. Canadian Task Force on the Periodic Health Examination: *Canadian guide to clinical preventive health care*, Ottawa, 1994, Canada Communication Group—Publishing, pp 932-942.

Diabetic nephropathy

(See also hypertension; microalbuminuria)

Although nephropathy has generally been considered a more common complication of type 1 than type 2 diabetes, this pattern appears to be changing as life expectancy of persons with type 2 diabetes increases. Twenty-five years after the diagnosis of diabetes approximately 50% of both type 1 and type 2 diabetic patients have nephropathy as manifested by proteinuria. Factors known to accelerate the progression of diabetic nephropathy are hypertension, proteinuria, poor glycemic control, and smoking. Whether high-protein diets or elevated lipid levels affect progression is uncertain.[1]

The first evidence of renal damage in diabetes is microalbuminuria, followed by manifest proteinuria. In the case of type 1 diabetes the mean duration of the disease from the onset of microalbuminuria to the development of proteinuria is 17 years. In half of diabetic patients with proteinuria, end-stage renal failure develops, and the mean time from the onset of proteinuria to azotemia is 5 years.[2] Blacks, Asians, and Native Americans are at greater risk of end-stage renal disease than are whites. The 5-year survival rate for type 2 diabetics with end-stage renal disease is at best 25%.[1]

Microalbuminuria is defined as albuminuria that is too little to be detected by standard urine dipsticks, as a urinary albumin excretion of 30 to 300 mg in 24 hours, or as 20 to 200 µg/ml or 20 to 200 µg/min. Type 2 diabetic patients with microalbuminuria are at very high risk for cardiovascular events.[1]

Good control of hypertension, especially with the use of angiotensin-converting enzyme (ACE) inhibitors, may ameliorate diabetic nephropathy or at least slow its progression. Because of this the American Diabetes Association recommends that the target level for blood pressure control in hypertensive diabetic patients be less than 130/85 mm Hg.[3] Support for controlling hypertension as a way of preventing nephropathy comes from a United Kingdom Prospective Diabetes Study Group (UKPDS) report of patients with type 2 diabetes and hypertension who were treated intensively with either a beta-blocker or an ACE inhibitor as first-line therapy (other drug classes were added if necessary). Both drug classes slowed the development of proteinuria compared with that in less intensively treated hypertensive diabetics (see discussion of hypertension).[4]

Even in normotensive diabetic patients ACE inhibitors may be valuable.[1,5-8] One study found that lisinopril (Prinivil, Zestril) given to normotensive patients with type 1 diabetes decreased the rate of progression of renal disease as measured by the degree of albuminuria.[5] Similar results in normotensive patients with type 2 diabetes were obtained with enalapril (Vasotec).[6] An expert panel of the U.S. National Kidney Foundation recommends that all diabetics with microalbuminuria be treated with ACE inhibitors.[7] A case can even be made for treating most type 2 diabetics with ACE inhibitors whether or not they have evidence of proteinuria or microalbuminuria.[8]

Tight control of type 1 diabetes has been shown to decrease the incidence of microalbuminuria and proteinuria,[9] but whether this will translate into a decreased incidence of end-stage renal failure is unknown.

Transplantation options for type 1 diabetics with renal failure are renal transplant alone or combined renal and pancreatic transplants. A comparative survey of these two modalities from the Netherlands found mortality rates to be significantly lower in patients who received combined transplants.[10]

The Canadian Task Force on Preventive Health Care recommends screening for microalbuminuria in patients with insulin-dependent diabetes ("A" recommendation),[11] whereas the U.S. Preventive Services Task Force makes no recommendation on the subject.[12] After a thorough literature review, Vijan and associates[13] recommend that patients with type 2 diabetes be screened regularly for microalbuminuria.

_____ ◣ **REFERENCES** ◤ _____

1. Ritz E, Orth SR: Nephropathy in patients with type 2 diabetes mellitus, *N Engl J Med* 341:1127-1133, 1999.

2. Nathan DM: Long-term complications of diabetes mellitus, *N Engl J Med* 328:1676-1685, 1993.

3. American Diabetes Association: Clinical practice recommendations 1996: diagnosis and management of nephropathy in patients with diabetes mellitus, *Diabetes Care* 19(suppl 1):S103-S106, 1996.

4. UK Prospective Diabetes Study Group: Tight blood pressure control and risk of macrovascular and microvascular complications in type 2 diabetes: UKPDS 38, *BMJ* 317:703-713, 1998.

5. EUCLID study group: Randomised placebo-controlled trial of lisinopril in normotensive patients with insulin-dependent diabetes and normoalbuminuria or microalbuminuria, *Lancet* 349:1787-1792, 1997.

6. Ravid M, Lang R, Rachmani R, et al: Long-term renoprotective effect of angiotensin-converting enzyme inhibition in non-insulin-dependent diabetes mellitus, *Arch Intern Med* 156:286-289, 1996.

7. Bennett PH, Haffner S, Kasiske BL, et al: Screening and management of microalbuminuria in patients with diabetes mellitus: recommendations to the Scientific Advisory Board of the National Kidney Foundation from an ad hoc committee of the Council on Diabetes Mellitus of the National Kidney Foundation, *Am J Kidney Dis* 25:107-112, 1995.

8. Golan L, Birkmeyer JD, Welch HG: The cost-effectiveness of treating all patients with type 2 diabetes with angiotensin-converting enzyme inhibitors, *Ann Intern Med* 131:660-667, 1999.

9. Diabetes Control and Complications Trial Research Group: The effect of intensive treatment of diabetes on the development and progression of long-term complications in insulin-dependent diabetes mellitus, *N Engl J Med* 329:977-986, 1993.

10. Smets YF, Westendorp RG, van der Pijl JW, et al: Effect of simultaneous pancreas-kidney transplantation on mortality of patients with type-1 diabetes mellitus and end-stage renal failure, *Lancet* 353:1915-1919, 1999.

11. Canadian Task Force on the Periodic Health Examination: *Clinical preventive health care,* Ottawa, 1994, Canadian Communication Group—Publishing, pp 436-445.

12. US Preventive Services Task Force: *Guide to clinical preventive services,* ed 2, Baltimore, 1996, Williams & Wilkins.

13. Vijan S, Stevens DL, Herman WH, et al: Screening, prevention, counseling, and treatment for the complications of type II diabetes mellitus: putting evidence into practice, *J Gen Intern Med* 12:567-580, 1997.

Diabetic neuropathy

(See also herpes zoster; neuropathy)

Diabetic peripheral neuropathy eventually develops in almost half of all diabetics.[1] Neuropathic pain is often treated with amitriptyline (Elavil) starting at doses of 25 mg hs and slowly building to 150 to 200 mg/day if necessary. Other tricyclic agents are also effective but perhaps less so than amitriptyline. Carbamazepine (Tegretol) and phenytoin (Dilantin) have been used for lancinating neuropathy,[2] but tricyclic drugs are also effective for this form of pain.[3] Capsaicin 0.075% cream (Zostrix H.P.) has also been reported to give pain relief.[2] A randomized placebo-controlled trial found that gabapentin (Neurontin) in daily doses of 900 to 3600 mg/day relieved neuropathic pain in diabetic patients, and the authors recommend it as a first-line agent.[1]

Focal motor neuropathies also occur in diabetic patients. These may be cranial or peripheral and usually resolve spontaneously in 2 to 12 months.

Autonomic neuropathies are common. The most frequent manifestation is impotence, which affects more than 50% of men with diabetes. Other features of autonomic neuropathy are diabetic gastroparesis, orthostatic hypotension, and diarrhea.[2]

Treatment options for gastroparesis include erythromycin 250 to 500 mg qid or metoclopramide (Maxeran) 10 mg tid ac. In a direct comparison of these two drugs erythromycin was more effective. However, a 1999 systematic review of erythromycin for gastroparesis found no evidence that erythromycin has a beneficial effect and concluded that it should not be used.[4] Domperidone (Motilium) and cisapride (Propulsid) have also been helpful in some cases. The dosage of cisapride is 10 to 20 mg po qid before meals.[2]

One treatment method for the diarrhea of autonomic neuropathy is one or two doses of tetracycline (200 or 500 mg) at the onset of symptoms. The mechanism of action is unknown. A more traditional treatment is diphenoxylate with atropine (Lomotil).[2]

Postural hypotension caused by autonomic neuropathy is difficult to treat; increasing salt intake, wearing elastic tights, and sleeping with the head of the bed elevated might be tried. In some cases fludrocortisone (Florinef) is indicated.[2]

The Diabetes Control and Complications Trial has shown that intensive insulin treatment of patients with type 1 diabetes decreases the incidence of peripheral neuropathy measured after 5 years (13% versus 5%).[5] Intensive treatment of patients with type 2 diabetes in the United Kingdom Prospective Diabetic Study (UKPDS) did not result in a lower rate of impotence than in the conventionally treated control subjects.[6]

⚓ REFERENCES ⚓

1. Backonja M, Beydoun A, Edwards KR, et al: Gabapentin for the symptomatic treatment of painful neuropathy in patients with diabetes mellitus: a randomized controlled trial, *JAMA* 280:1831-1836, 1998.

2. Clark CM Jr, Lee DA: Prevention and treatment of the complications of diabetes mellitus, *N Engl J Med* 332:1210-1217, 1995.

3. McQuay HJ, Moore RA: Antidepressants and chronic pain: effective analgesia in neuropathic pain and other syndromes (editorial), *BMJ* 314:763-764, 1997.

4. Prescrire: evidence-based drug reviews: erythromycin and gastroparesis? *Can Fam Physician* 45:1887-1891, 1999.

5. Diabetes Control and Complications Trial Research Group: The effect of intensive diabetes therapy on the development and progression of neuropathy, *Ann Intern Med* 122:561-568, 1995.

6. UK Prospective Diabetes Study (UKPDS) Group: Intensive blood-glucose control with sulphonylureas or insulin compared with conventional treatment and risk of complications in patients with type 2 diabetes (UKPDS 33), *Lancet* 352:837-853, 1998.

Macrovascular Complications of Diabetes Mellitus
(See also hypertension; secondary prevention of coronary artery disease)

Cardiovascular disease is the major cause of the increased morbidity and mortality associated with diabetes,[1] and the risk for both strokes and myocardial infarcts is greater in diabetic women than in diabetic men.[2,3] In type 2 diabetes the risk of cardiovascular disease is two to three times that of the nondiabetic population[1,3] and is equivalent to the risk of nondiabetics who have had a previous myocardial infarction.[4]

Specific risk markers for coronary artery disease in patients with type 2 diabetes include elevated levels of low-density lipoprotein (LDL) cholesterol, low levels of high-density lipoprotein (HDL) cholesterol, hypertension, and hyperglycemia.[1] Because diabetics are at high risk for myocardial infarctions and strokes, aggressive treatment of hypertension and lipid abnormalities is essential (see discussion of hypertension). Vijan and associates[5] advise daily aspirin in doses of 81 to 325 mg for all patients with type 2 diabetes over the age of 50, as well as for those under 50 who show evidence of cardiovascular disease. Fagan and Sowers[3] support the American Diabetes Association's view that any evidence of cardiovascular disease in a diabetic is an indication for aspirin therapy unless strictly contraindicated.[6] A large multicenter international study found that the ACE inhibitor ramipril (Altace) 10 mg once daily led to a decrease in both macrovascular and microvascular complications in diabetics that was greater than could be expected from the small decrease in blood pressure resulting from this treatment.[7] Haffner and associates,[4] underlining the importance of assiduously treating risk factors in diabetes, recommend that all patients with type 2 diabetes be managed in the same way as patients who have had myocardial infarctions.

The United Kingdom Prospective Diabetes Study (UKPDS) found no evidence that tight control of patients with type 2 diabetes treated with sulfonylureas or insulin decreased the incidence of macrovascular events,[8] although such a decrease was reported in a subgroup of obese patients treated with metformin.[9] Tight control does decrease microvascular disease (see earlier discussion).

◢ REFERENCES ◣

1. Turner RC, Millns H, Neil HA, et al: Risk factors for coronary artery disease in non-insulin dependent diabetes mellitus: United Kingdom Prospective Diabetes Study (UKPDS 23), *BMJ* 316:823-828, 1998.

2. Howard BV, Cowan LD, Go O, et al: Adverse effects of diabetes on multiple cardiovascular disease risk factors in women, *Diabetes Care* 21:1258-1263, 1998.
3. Fagan TC, Sowers J: Type 2 diabetes mellitus: greater cardiovascular risks and greater benefits of therapy (editorial), *Arch Intern Med* 159:1033-1034, 1999.
4. Haffner SM, Lehto S, Rönnemaa T, et al: Mortality from coronary heart disease in subjects with type 2 diabetes and in nondiabetic subjects with and without prior myocardial infarction, *N Engl J Med* 339:229-234, 1998.
5. Vijan S, Stevens DL, Herman WH, et al: Screening, prevention, counseling, and treatment for the complications of type II diabetes mellitus: putting evidence into practice, *J Gen Intern Med* 12:567-580, 1997.
6. American Diabetes Association: Aspirin therapy in diabetes, *Diabetes Care* 21(suppl 1):S45-S49, 1998.
7. Heart Outcomes Prevention Evaluation (HOPE) Study Investigators: Effects of ramipril on cardiovascular and microvascular outcomes in people with diabetes mellitus: results of the HOPE study and MICRO-HOPE substudy, *Lancet* 355:253-259, 2000.
8. United Kingdom Prospective Diabetes Study (UKPDS) Group: Intensive blood-glucose control with sulphonylureas or insulin compared with conventional treatment and risk of complications in patients with type 2 diabetes (UKPDS 33), *Lancet* 352:837-853, 1998.
9. United Kingdom Prospective Diabetes Study (UKPDS) Group: Effect of intensive blood-glucose control with metformin on complications in overweight patients with type 2 diabetes (UKPDS 34), *Lancet* 352:854-865, 1998.

Other Complications of Diabetes
Glucose toxicity

Prolonged hyperglycemia can in itself aggravate insulin resistance and impair insulin secretion from the pancreas.[1] Correction of the hyperglycemia by diet, oral agents, or insulin often rapidly improves glucose control.[2] This is why a simple change in diet, such as eliminating refined sugars or stopping the patient from drinking 2 or 3 L of fruit juice a day, can lead to a rapid decline in hyperglycemia without any weight loss. One symptom of marked hyperglycemia is transient decreased visual acuity. This is due to the hyperosmolar effect of high glucose levels on the shape of the crystalline lens. I had one patient who could always tell when his glucose levels were very high because at these times he could not read the channel numbers on his television screen.

◢ REFERENCES ◣

1. Rossetti L, Giacarri A, DeFronzo RA: Glucose toxicity, *Diabetes Care* 13:610-630, 1990.
2. Genuth S: Insulin use in NIDDM, *Diabetes Care* 13:1240-1264, 1990.

Diabetic foot

Foot ulcers develop in at least 15% of diabetics, and the underlying cause is almost always a sensory neuropathy.[1] Many diabetologists argue that if clinicians could detect sensory neuropathy in diabetic patients and institute appropriate preventive foot care, the incidence of foot ulcers would decrease.[2]

Three modalities recommended for detecting diabetic peripheral neuropathy are questionnaires, measurement of vibration perception thresholds by holding a biothesiometer to the large toe, and testing of patients' ability to perceive the application of a Semmes-Weinstein monofilament wire to various sites on the foot. In a case-control comparison of these three modalities (comparing diabetic patients who had ulcers or recently healed ulcers against a control group of diabetics without ulcers), all three techniques were sensitive and reasonably specific, and combining two modalities increased specificity.[2] Four questions were included in the questionnaire: Do your feet ever feel numb? Do your feet ever tingle, as if electricity were traveling into them? Do your feet ever feel as if insects were crawling on them? Do your feet ever burn? A positive answer to any one of these questions had a sensitivity of 100% but a specificity of about 65%.[2]

The Semmes-Weinstein monofilament is meant to buckle with a pressure of 10 g, although according to one report the buckling pressure varies considerably from one monofilament to another. The test is considered positive if the patient fails to feel the filament at the point where it buckles. There are no well-defined standards as to which locations on the foot should be tested or how many should be tested. McGill and associates[3] reported reasonable sensitivity and specificity if two sites were tested—the plantar surfaces of the first and fifth metatarsals (the test was considered positive if the patient was unable to detect the monofilament at either site).

Diabetic foot ulcers heal slowly. A systematic review of standard treatment of uninfected ulcers (avoidance of weight bearing, debridement if indicated, and saline-moistened gauze dressings) found that 24% had healed by 12 weeks and 31% by 20 weeks.[1]

Infected foot ulcers may be categorized into limb-threatening and non-limb-threatening infections. Non-limb-threatening infections are superficial, and the erythema extends less than 2 cm from the edge of the ulcer. Organisms causing non-limb-threatening infections are usually gram-positive cocci, such as streptococci or staphylococci, and these infections may be treated on an outpatient basis if the home situation is adequate and follow-up every 24 to 48 hours can be arranged. Weight bearing must be avoided, and in most cases oral antibiotics such as clindamycin (Cleocin, Dalacin), cephalexin (Keflex), dicloxacillin (Dycill, Dynapen, Pathocil), or cloxacillin (Tegopen, Orbenin) are effective as single agents. Limb-threatening infections are generally polymicrobial, involving gram-positive aerobes, gram-negative aerobes, and anaerobes, and patients with such a condition require hospitalization and IV antibiotics.[2]

With deep ulcers, the presence of an underlying osteomyelitis is often difficult to determine. If bone can be detected in the base of the ulcer by probing with a metal probe, the odds are high that osteomyelitis is present. If the infection is not limb threatening, bone cannot be detected on probing, and initial x-ray findings are negative, the duration of treatment can be that for soft tissue infection (10 to 14 days) with reassessment after it is completed.[4]

◢ REFERENCES ◣

1. Margolis DJ, Kantor J, Berlin JA: Healing of diabetic neuropathic foot ulcers receiving standard treatment, *Diabetes Care* 22:692-695, 1999.
2. Armstrong DG, Lavery LA, Vela SA, et al: Choosing a practical screening instrument to identify patients at risk for diabetic foot ulceration, *Arch Intern Med* 158:289-292, 1998.
3. McGill M, Molyneaux L, Spencer R, et al: Possible sources of discrepancies in the use of the Semmes-Weinstein monofilament, *Diabetes Care* 22:598-602, 1999.
4. Caputo GM, Joshi N, Weitekamp MR: Foot infections in patients with diabetes, *Am Fam Physician* 56:195-202, 1997.

Pregnancy in Women with Type 1 Diabetes

Patients with type 1 diabetes generally are at much higher risk of having children with congenital anomalies and fetal death than nondiabetic women.[1-4] In a clinical trial of tight control in both the pregestational and gestational period monitored by a highly specialized center, these rates decreased nearly to those of nondiabetic control subjects.[4] Unfortunately, such good results have not been achieved in some community settings.[2,3]

◢ REFERENCES ◣

1. Simmons D: Persistently poor pregnancy outcomes in women with insulin dependent diabetes (editorial), *BMJ* 315:263-264, 1997.
2. Casson IF, Clarke CA, Howard CV, et al: Outcomes of pregnancy in insulin dependent diabetic women: results of a five year population cohort study, *BMJ* 315:275-278, 1997.
3. Hawthorne G, Robson S, Ryall EA, et al: Prospective population based survey of outcome of pregnancy in diabetic women: results of the Northern Diabetic Pregnancy Audit, 1994, *BMJ* 315:279-281, 1997.
4. Diabetes Control and Complications Trial Research Group: Pregnancy outcomes in the diabetes control and complications trial, *Am J Obstet Gynecol* 174:1343-1353, 1996.

Initial and Annual Laboratory Investigations for Diabetic Patients

Initial and annual (and sometimes more frequent) laboratory investigations recommended by the expert committee of the Canadian Diabetes Advisory Board are as follows[1]:

1. Fasting glucose
2. Glycated hemoglobin
3. Fasting plasma lipid levels (total cholesterol, high- and low-density cholesterol, and triglycerides)
4. Serum creatinine

5. Urinalysis, including microscopy
6. Microalbuminuria (preferably at the time of diagnosis in patients without proteinuria, and then annually in patients without proteinuria who have had diabetes for more than 5 years)
7. 24-Hour urine protein excretion (in patients with proteinuria)
8. Creatinine clearance (in patients with proteinuria)
9. Electrocardiogram (if indicated)
10. Thyroid-stimulating hormone (for type 1 diabetes and, if indicated, for type 2)

➤ REFERENCES ➤

1. Expert Committee of the Canadian Diabetes Advisory Board: Clinical practice guidelines for diabetes mellitus in Canada, *Can Med Assoc J* 147:697-712, 1992.

Target Levels for Glucose in the Control of Diabetes Mellitus

Target levels for glucose control as set by various expert committees have become more stringent since the publication of the Diabetes Control and Complications Trial in 1993 (see below). According to the current position statement of the American Diabetes Association, the optimal preprandial glucose level is 4.4 to 6.7 mmol/L (80 to 120 mg/dl) and remedial action should be taken if values are above 7.8 mmol/L (140 mg/dl) or below 4.4 mmol/L (80 mg/dl). Bedtime glucose should be between 5.6 and 7.8 mmol/l (100 to 140 mg/dl), and remedial action is indicated if the levels are below 5.6 mmol/L (100 mg/dl) or above 8.9 mmol/L (160 mg/dl). The ideal HbA_{1c} level is below 7%, and action should be taken if it is over 8%.[1] Canadian guidelines are almost identical.[2]

Although the United Kingdom Prospective Diabetes Study (UKPDS) has shown that intensive treatment of type 2 diabetes lowers the rate of microvascular disease (see discussion of intensive treatment in preventing diabetic complications in type 2 diabetes below), the mean levels of HbA_{1c} did not fall below 7%. In the opinion of the authors of the UKPDS study, levels lower than 7% have been obtained only in small groups of obese patients receiving large doses of insulin in the context of intensive short-term trials and probably cannot be achieved in the community setting.[3]

➤ REFERENCES ➤

1. American Diabetes Association: Standards of medical care for patients with diabetes mellitus, *Diabetes Care* 20(suppl 1):S5-S13, 1997.
2. Meltzer S, Leiter L, Daneman D, et al: 1998 Clinical practice guidelines for the management of diabetes in Canada, *Can Med Assoc J* 159(suppl 8):S1-S29, 1998.
3. United Kingdom Prospective Diabetes Study (UKPDS) Group: Intensive blood-glucose control with sulphonylureas or insulin compared with conventional treatment and risk of complications in patients with type 2 diabetes (UKPDS 33), *Lancet* 352:837-853, 1998.

Intensive Treatment in Preventing Diabetic Complications in Type 1 Diabetes

A seminal article dealing with the beneficial effects of tight control in diabetes was the 1993 report of the Diabetes Control and Complications Trial Research Group (DCCT), published in the *New England Journal of Medicine*. It showed that after a mean follow-up of 6.5 years patients with insulin-dependent diabetes mellitus (type 1 diabetes) given intensive therapy had a significant diminution of retinopathy, neuropathy, proteinuria, and microalbuminuria. Specifically, intensive therapy slowed the progression of retinopathy by 54% and reduced the development of proliferative or severe nonproliferative retinopathy by 47%. Clinical neuropathy was reduced by 60%, albuminuria by 54%, and microalbuminuria by 39%. No statistically significant decline occurred in macrovascular disease, but because of the youth of the study population this was not unexpected.[1]

The improvements in microvascular complications were achieved at a cost. In the DCCT trial the incidence of severe hypoglycemic reactions increased threefold and patients had significant weight gain. The mean weight gain over 5 years was 4.6 kg (10 lb) greater than in the conventionally treated control subjects; 33% of the intensively treated group met the criteria for obesity (body mass index >27.8 kg/m^2 for men and >27.3 kg/m^2 for women) compared with 19% of the conventionally treated group.[2,3] Of particular concern was the finding that those in the intensively treated group who became obese met the criteria for the central obesity–insulin resistance syndrome ("syndrome X"). This syndrome, which includes insulin resistance, elevated blood pressure, increased abdominal obesity, and dyslipidemia, is associated with an increased risk of coronary artery disease.[3]

Evidence that establishing complete normoglycemia (a state not achieved by the DCCT trial) may reverse the lesions of diabetic nephropathy comes from a study of eight diabetic patients with this disorder who had pancreas transplants. No improvement was detectable after 5 years, but a reversal of the biochemical abnormalities and histological lesions was achieved by 10 years.[4]

➤ REFERENCES ➤

1. Diabetes Control and Complications Trial Research Group: The effect of intensive treatment of diabetes on the development and progression of long-term complications in insulin-dependent diabetes mellitus, *N Engl J Med* 329:977-986, 1993.
2. Diabetes Control and Complications Trial Research Group: Adverse events and their association with treatment regimens in the Diabetes Control and Complications Trial, *Diabetes Care* 18:1415-1427, 1995.
3. Purnell JQ, Hokanson JE, Marcovina SM, et al: Effect of excessive weight gain with intensive therapy of type 1 diabetes on lipid levels and blood pressure: results from the DCCT, *JAMA* 280:140-146, 1998.
4. Fioretto P, Steffes MW, Sutherland DE, et al: Reversal of lesions of diabetic nephropathy after pancreas transplantation, *N Engl J Med* 339:69-75, 1998.

Intensive Treatment in Preventing Diabetic Complications in Type 2 Diabetes

(See also attitudes, physician)

From the viewpoint of the family physician the practical significance of the DCCT findings is clear enough for patients with type 1 diabetes (see above), but whether the findings are relevant to those with type 2 whose disease cannot be controlled by diet and exercise alone is a critical question.

In 1995 a clinical trial of Japanese patients with type 2 diabetes managed with multiple insulin injections showed that after 6 years, lowering the HbA_{1c} to less than 6.5% was associated with a decrease in microvascular complications. The patients were extremely cooperative and relatively young and lean, and insulin requirements were modest.[1]

Of more direct clinical relevance to the North American and European populations are the results of the United Kingdom Prospective Diabetics Study (UKPDS) published in 1998. In the main study, which had a follow-up period averaging 10 years, close to 3000 patients with type 2 diabetes were treated intensively with sulfonylureas or insulin and a little over 1000 were treated primarily by diet and exercise. Over the 10-year period the HbA_{1c} was 7% in the intensively treated group and 7.9% in the conventionally treated group. Those in the intensively treated group had a significant reduction in microvascular endpoints, particularly retinopathy as assessed by ophthalmoscopy, although the actual numbers of patients who benefited was small—in a year about 250 patients had to receive intensive treatment to prevent one person from requiring retinal laser photocoagulation. The rate of deterioration of vision and the incidence of impotence did not differ between the groups. Perhaps most important, there was no difference in the rates of diabetes-related or all-cause mortality between the groups (tight control did not decrease the incidence of cardiovascular disease). The major adverse effect of tight control was weight gain (1.7 to 2.6 kg for those taking sulfonylureas and 4 kg for those taking insulin). However, intensive therapy did not increase the risk of macrovascular disease by increasing insulin resistance.[2] Thus "tight control" of type 2 diabetes using sulfonylureas or insulin appears to prevent microvascular complications in a small number of treated patients but not to have a beneficial effect on macrovascular complications, which are of course the major cause of morbidity and mortality in this disease.

A different set of results was reported for a subset of obese diabetic patients in the UKPDS who were treated with metformin alone. Compared with those treated conventionally, the metformin group demonstrated a decreased total and diabetes-related mortality because of a decrease in macrovascular complications. Metformin did not induce weight gain and was associated with few hypoglycemic reactions. However, patients who were treated with a combination of metformin and sulfonylureas had an increase in diabetes-related and all-cause mortality.[3] Although this may be a chance finding,[3] it is worrisome.

An important question that has been addressed only recently is whether good control of type 2 diabetes improves patients' quality of life. A randomized double-blind placebo-controlled trial lasting 12 weeks compared outcomes of patients treated with glipizide and those treated with placebo. At the end of 12 weeks the glipizide-treated group had a mean HbA_{1c} of 7.5% whereas it was 9.3% in the placebo group. Quality of life measurements, including cognitive functioning, general perceived health, and symptom distress, were significantly better in the glipizide group, as were work-related measurements such as degree of productivity and days absent.[4]

Should family physicians recommend tight control for their patients with type 2 diabetes? I believe that it would help many patients but that the decision should be made on an individual basis after full discussion of the benefits and harm of such an intervention. Even if a decision to try for tight control is not made, every patient deserves thorough assessment and management of risk factors for both the microvascular and macrovascular complications of diabetes.

◾ REFERENCES ◾

1. Ohkubo Y, Kishikawa H, Araki E, et al: Intensive insulin therapy prevents the progression of diabetic microvascular complications in Japanese patients with non-insulin-dependent diabetes mellitus: a randomized prospective 6-year study, *Diabetes Res Clin Pract* 28:103-117, 1995.
2. United Kingdom Prospective Diabetes Study (UKPDS) Group: Intensive blood-glucose control with sulphonylureas or insulin compared with conventional treatment and risk of complications in patients with type 2 diabetes (UKPDS 33), *Lancet* 352:837-853, 1998.
3. United Kingdom Prospective Diabetes Study (UKPDS) Group: Effect of intensive blood-glucose control with metformin on complications in overweight patients with type 2 diabetes (UKPDS 34), *Lancet* 352:854-865, 1998.
4. Testa MA, Simonson DC: Health economic benefits and quality of life during improved glycemic control in patients with type 2 diabetes mellitus: a randomized, controlled, double-blind trial, *JAMA* 280:1490-1496, 1998.

Type 1 Diabetes

(See also eating disorders)

Epidemiology

By 20 years of age between 1 in 300 and 1 in 600 individuals has type 1 diabetes. Type 1 comprises about 5% of cases of diabetes. The incidence varies with age and is lowest in infants and highest in adolescents. The incidence is increased in those who have a first-degree relative with type 1 diabetes (father 6%, mother 2%, sibling 5%, nonidentical twin 5%, identical twin 30% to 50%). In general, the farther from the equator, the higher the incidence of type 1 diabetes. The highest incidence in Europe is in Finland, and the lowest incidence in the world is in Japan. The disease most frequently becomes manifest in the spring and autumn. Type 1 diabetes is more common in children who have not been breast fed or who have been breast fed for only a short period.[1]

━━━━━━━━━━━ ◤ **REFERENCES** ◢ ━━━━━━━━━━━

1. Atkinson MA, Maclaren NK: The pathogenesis of insulin-dependent diabetes mellitus, *N Engl J Med* 331:1428-1436, 1994.

Insulin therapy for type 1 diabetes

(See also glucose monitoring for type 2 diabetes; hypoglycemia; insulin therapy for type 2 diabetes)

Classification of insulins. A variety of insulins are available in North America: ultra-short-acting, short-acting, and long-acting insulins; mixtures of long- and short-acting insulins; human insulins; pork insulins; insulins in vials; and insulins in pens.

Trade names of human insulins. Trade names of human insulins available in Canada or the United States are Humulin, Novolin, Velosulin, and Humalog. Humalog is the trade name for lispro, which is an analogue of human insulin. It is ultra-short acting (see below).

Trade names of pork insulins. The only pork insulin now being manufactured is Lilly's Iletin II. Pork-beef insulins are no longer being produced.

Choice of human or animal insulins. At present most physicians prescribe human insulin, and some go so far as to consider animal insulins to be of "historical interest only."[1]

Duration of action of insulins. Insulins are subclassified according to their duration of action (Table 40),[1,2] and the figures given vary from one source to another. The table gives a rough approximation of the time of onset, peak effect, and duration of action of various human insulins. One reason that the figures are "approximate" is that rates of absorption of insulin—and therefore their durations of action—vary widely from one patient to another.[2]

Human insulins have a slightly earlier onset and a slightly shorter duration of action than do animal insulins. As a result, patients taking human rather than animal intermediate-acting insulins before supper are more likely to have hyperglycemia before breakfast.[1]

Lispro (Humalog) is a synthetic analog of human insulin that is very rapidly absorbed. One of its main advantages is that it can be injected up to 15 minutes before a meal, which increases the flexibility of mealtimes.[3] (If regular insulin is used preprandially, the "lag time" between injection and eating is usually 20 to 30 minutes.[2]) Preprandial lispro does not lead to better control than preprandial regular insulin, but among patients with type 1 diabetes who are aiming for very tight control it decreases the frequency of nocturnal hypoglycemic reactions.[3]

Insulin vials, pens, cartridges, and syringes. All insulins, regardless of the format in which they are supplied and whether they are premixed, contain 100 units/ml.

Pork insulins are available only in 10-ml multidose vials containing 100 units/ml of unmixed insulins (e.g., regular, NPH, Ultralente). Human insulins are also available in this format but in addition come as premixed vials containing regular plus NPH insulin in various proportions. In Canada the figures given for mixtures have regular insulin first followed by NPH insulin. Thus 30/70 means 30% regular insulin and 70% NPH. In the United States the order is sometimes reversed so that the above mixture might be written 70/30. The practitioner can avoid confusion by remembering that except for a 50/50 mixture (in which the order does not matter), the smaller figure is always regular insulin and the larger one is NPH. In this text the convention of putting regular insulin first is used. In Canada a full range of mixtures of regular and NPH insulins from 10/90 to 50/50 is available, whereas in the United States only the 30/70 and 50/50 mixtures are marketed.

A variety of cartridges for dial-a-dose insulin pens that contain regular or NPH insulin or mixtures of regular and NPH insulin (as 30/70 in the United States and in various proportions from 10/90 to 50/50 in Canada) may be purchased. Pens take 1.5-ml cartridges (containing 150 units of insulin) or 3-ml cartridges (containing 300 units of insulin), and the correct dose can be dialed. Disposable pens are also available. Before using an insulin pen, patients should suspend the NPH insulin by tipping the pen 20 times.[4]

Only human regular insulin and human NPH insulin are available in premixed formats, whether as vials, insulin pen cartridges, or disposable dispensing devices. Patients who are receiving pork insulins or Lente or Ultralente insulins (human or animal) and require mixtures of regular and longer acting insulins have to mix their own.

Insulin syringes have a 1-ml capacity and are graduated in 0.01-ml portions. Since all commercial insulins are supplied as 100 units/ml, 0.01 ml = 1 unit.

Insulin injection sites. Intramuscular injections are more rapidly absorbed than subcutaneous ones. Injections into an extremity that has been exercising, massage of the injection site, or application of heat to the injection site increases the rate of insulin absorption and may lead to hypoglycemia.[2] It

Table 40   Classification of Human Insulins by Time of Action

Type of insulin	Time of action in hours		
	Onset	Peak	Duration
Very Short Acting			
Lispro (Humalog)	0.12-0.25	0.5-2	3-5
Short Acting			
Regular (CZI , Toronto)	0.5-1	2-4	5-8
Intermediate Acting	1-3	4-8	13-20
Isophane insulin (NPH)			
Insulin zinc suspension (Lente)			
Long Acting			
Extended insulin zinc suspension (Ultralente)	2-4	8-12	18-30+

CZI, Crystalline zinc insulin; *NPH,* neutral protamine Hagedorn.

is safe to exercise the muscles at the injection site after an elapsed period of half an hour.[5] Absorption of insulin varies with the anatomical site of injection; it is most rapid in the abdomen, intermediate in the arm, and slowest in the thigh or hip. Sites should be rotated in the same general anatomical area, such as the abdominal wall, rather than using the thigh one day, the arm the next, and so on.[2] Injecting insulin through clothes is both safe and convenient.[6]

Glucose monitoring. Numerous glucometers are available. Modern ones are compact reflectance meters that are operated in one step and that draw fingertip capillary blood onto the strips by osmosis. Glucose strips that are designed for a particular glucometer must be used. The patient must calibrate each package of glucose strips before use.

The technique of drawing blood for home glucose monitoring involves the following steps:

1. Wash and dry hands. Do not clean the area of fingerprick with alcohol.
2. Choose the lateral or medial side of the pulp of the fingers as the site for the fingerprick, not the volar surface.
3. Load an autolancet into its carrier, apply the tip of the carrier firmly to the finger, and release the spring.
4. Make sure the drop of blood is adequate to cover the glucose strip.

Until recently most patients with type 1 diabetes were treated with twice-daily mixtures of short- and long-acting insulins (see below). For such patients a common initial routine for home glucose monitoring was to test the blood glucose twice daily before breakfast and before supper with the aim of keeping the glucose levels between 4 and 10 mmol/L (70 and 180 mg/dl) before meals.[7] This protocol is now outmoded for type 1 diabetics. The new guidelines of the American[8] and Canadian[9] diabetes associations recommend preprandial glucose levels of 4.4 to 6.7 mmol/L (80 to 120 mg/dl), a goal that can be achieved only by monitoring glucose levels three to four times a day, usually before meals and at bedtime.[2] The bedtime measurement is particularly important as a check for hypoglycemia; nocturnal hypoglycemia may be unrecognized and lead to convulsions or coma.[10]

Preliminary studies of a new technology for continuous noninvasive glucose monitoring (Gluco Watch, Cygnus, Inc., Redwood City, Calif.) look promising.[11]

Glycosylated or glycated hemoglobin is monitored to assess the efficacy of diabetic control over a 2- to 3-month period, whereas fructosamine is used for a 2- to 3-week period. Glycated hemoglobin is measured either as HBA_{1C} or as total glycated hemoglobin.[7] Ideal levels are below 0.07 (7%).[8,9] Measurements should be taken every 3 months. An elevation of 0.01 (1%) corresponds to a rise of about 1.7 mmol/L (30 mg/dl) in the average glucose level.[7]

Initial insulin dose

The usual total daily dose of insulin for a patient with type 1 diabetes is 0.5 to 1 unit/kg. Patients are started on 0.2 to 0.6 unit/kg/day, and on the basis of frequent glucose readings the dose is increased gradually as necessary.[2]

Until recently the standard insulin regimen was to give two thirds of the daily dose 30 minutes before breakfast and one third 30 minutes before supper, with the injections given 10 to 12 hours apart. The usual mixture of each dose was 30% regular or Toronto insulin and 70% NPH or Lente insulin. Current guidelines aim for much tighter control than is possible with twice-daily doses.[8,9]

The usual protocol for tight control involves a morning and bedtime injection of NPH or Lente insulin to cover the basal insulin needs plus regular insulin or insulin lispro before each meal.[2,10] The evening dose of NPH is given at bedtime rather than suppertime to help prevent nocturnal hypoglycemia and to better control prebreakfast hyperglycemia.[2] Doses of preprandial insulin are determined by preprandial sugar levels and an estimation of the number of calories to be ingested. About 10 units of insulin is required for every 500 calories.[10] Variations of this basic insulin regimen are possible; a common one for patients who use regular insulin before meals is to omit the morning intermediate-acting insulin. If insulin lispro is used before meals, both morning and evening doses of intermediate insulin are required.[2]

An alternative to multiple insulin injections is continuous subcutaneous insulin infusion. Regular or lispro insulin is used, and infusion rates can be varied from hour to hour. In one small nonrandomized trial comparing multiple injections to continuous infusion of insulin, those receiving continuous infusion had better control and fewer severe hypoglycemic reactions.[12]

Adjusting insulin doses

The insulin dose may be increased or decreased at any time by 1 to 2 units (or for higher doses by 10%). The particular insulin to be modified is determined by the blood sugar levels at different times during the day.[13] Assuming a twice a day insulin regimen with a mixture of regular and NPH insulin at each dose, the theoretical relationship would be as shown in Table 41.

Before insulin doses are adjusted, it is important to ensure that some exogenous factor such as an intercurrent illness, unusual exercise, irregularity of meal and snack schedules, or noncompliance with the insulin doses is not responsible for the inadequate control.

Table 41 Relationship Between Glucose Levels and Insulin Dose Adjustments in Patients Taking Mixture of Regular and NPH Insulins

Glucose reading	Responsible insulin
Before lunch	Before breakfast: regular
Before supper	Before breakfast: NPH
Bedtime	Before supper: regular
Before breakfast	Before supper: NPH

Hypoglycemic reactions

Severe, asymptomatic, spontaneously resolving nocturnal hypoglycemia appears to be common in young diabetic children, but as far as can be determined, cognitive functioning is unaffected by these events.[14] Missed meals, exercise without a snack, and erroneous insulin doses are some of the causes of clinically evident hypoglycemic reactions.

First-line treatment of hypoglycemia is sugar by mouth if the patient is conscious or applied to the buccal mucosa if the patient is not. Alternatives are a glucagon injection (1 mg for adults and older children and 0.5 mg for children under 5) or IV glucose.

✒ REFERENCES ✒

1. Burge MR, Schade DS: Insulins, *Endocrinol Metabol Clin North Am* 26:575-598, 1997.
2. Hirsch IB: Type 1 diabetes mellitus and the use of flexible insulin regimens, *Am Fam Physician* 60:2343-2356, 1999.
3. Heller SR, Amiel SA, Mansell P (U.K. Lispro Study Group): Effect of the fast-acting insulin analog lispro on the risk of nocturnal hypoglycemia during intensified insulin therapy, *Diabetes Care* 22:1607-1611, 1999.
4. Jehle PM, Micheler C, Jehle DR, et al: Inadequate suspension of neutral protamine Hagedorn (NPH) insulin in pens, *Lancet* 354:1604-1607, 1999.
5. Fahey PF, Stallcamp ET, Kwatra S: The athlete with type I diabetes: managing insulin, diet and exercise, *Am Fam Physician* 53:1611-1617, 1996.
6. Fleming DR, Jacober SJ, Vandenberg MA, et al: The safety of injecting insulin through clothing, *Diabetes Care* 20:244-247, 1997.
7. Koch B: Glucose monitoring as a guide to diabetes management: critical subject review, *Can Fam Physician* 42:1142-1152, 1996.
8. American Diabetes Association: Standards of medical care for patients with diabetes mellitus, *Diabetes Care* 20(suppl 1):S1-S70, 1997.
9. Meltzer S, Leiter L, Daneman D, et al: 1998 Clinical practice guidelines for the management of diabetes in Canada, *Can Med Assoc J* 159(suppl 8):S1-S29, 1998.
10. Havas S: Educational guidelines for achieving tight control and minimizing complications of type 1 diabetes, *Am Fam Physician* 60:1985-1998, 1999.
11. Tamada JA, Garg S, Jovanovic L, et al: Noninvasive glucose monitoring, *JAMA* 282:1839-1844, 1999.
12. Boland EA, Grey M, Oesterle A, et al: Continuous subcutaneous insulin infusion, *Diabetes Care* 22:1779-1784, 1999.
13. Hirsch I: Intensive insulin therapy. II. Multicomponent insulin regimens, *Am Fam Physician* 45:2141-2147, 1992.
14. Matyka KA, Wigg L, Pramming S, et al: Cognitive function and mood after profound nocturnal hypoglycaemia in prepubertal children with conventional insulin treatment for diabetes, *Arch Dis Child* 81:138-142, 1999.

Diet and type 1 diabetes

Rigid diabetic meal planning has long been a cornerstone of the management of type 1 diabetes, and despite a lack of evidence that it is beneficial,[1,2] it is still being used in many centers.

The traditional dietary plan for patients with type 1 diabetes was to divide the daily food intake into three regular meals plus snacks at midmorning, at midafternoon, and just before bedtime. The timing and quantity of the meals were to be as consistent as possible in order to prevent large fluctuations in glucose levels.[3] The purpose of the snacks was to prevent hypoglycemia caused by either the regular or the intermediate-acting insulin the patient was taking. If the patient was taking a mixture of regular and NPH insulin twice a day (before breakfast and before supper), the midmorning snack countered the effect of the morning regular insulin, the afternoon snack countered that of the morning NPH, and the evening snack countered that of the before supper regular insulin. A substantial evening snack was also one way of obviating early morning hypoglycemia resulting from the before supper NPH.

The current view of diet in type 1 diabetes is that it should have as few restrictions as possible. Usual food intake should be assessed and used as a basis for adjusting insulin types and doses.[2,4] Sucrose need not be specifically restricted.[2] Patients should monitor glucose levels and use varying doses of short-acting insulins to cover meals (more for a big meal, less for a small meal). Using such an approach, patients have far more flexibility in the timing of meals and may even be able to miss meals safely.[2,4]

✒ REFERENCES ✒

1. Berger M, Mühlhauser I: Diabetes care and patient-oriented outcomes, *JAMA* 281:1676-1678, 1999.
2. Berger M: To bridge science and patient care in diabetes, *Diabetologia* 39:749-757, 1996.
3. Service FJ, Rizza RA, Hall LD, et al: Prandial insulin requirements in insulin-dependent diabetics: effects of size, time of day, and sequence of meals, *J Clin Endocrinol Metab* 57:931-936, 1983.
4. American Diabetes Association: Nutrition recommendations and principles for people with diabetes mellitus, *Diabetes Care* 22(suppl 1):S42-S48, 1999.

Exercise and type 1 diabetes

An exercise program is believed to be important for patients with insulin-dependent diabetes because it is thought to improve the quality of their lives and protect against macrovascular disease.[1] However, evidence supporting these hypotheses has not yet been published.[2]

Whenever possible, exercise should be done at regular times. The major risk is hypoglycemia, which may develop during, shortly after, or 6 to 12 hours after exercise. The patient may try to prevent this with a preexercise snack or, when exercising is done on a regular basis, by decreasing the appropriate insulin dose. For low- to moderate-intensity exercise of less than an hour's duration, a preexercise snack is usually not required unless the preexercise glucose level is less than 5.6 mmol/L (100 mg/dl). For high-intensity exercises, snacks are advised.[3]

Athletes with type 1 diabetes who exercise regularly should, at least initially, monitor their blood sugar before, during, and for several hours after the exercise. If the exercise is performed in the late afternoon or evening, this includes a 2 AM glucose measurement. In general a 30% to 50% reduction in the preprandial insulin dose before exercise is required. In hot weather lower doses may be required than in cold weather. To prevent postexercise nocturnal hypoglycemia, the patient should have only regular insulin before supper and NPH or, even better, Lente at bedtime.[3]

A danger signal for athletes is a preexercise glucose level greater than 13.9 mmol/L (250 mg/dl). In this situation exercise can aggravate hyperglycemia and even cause ketoacidosis. If the glucose level is between 13.9 mmol/L (250 mg/dl) and 16.7 mmol/L (300 mg/dl) and the urine is free of ketones, participation in the athletic event can proceed. If ketones are present or the glucose level is above 16.7 mmol/L (300 mg/dl), exercise should be postponed until better control is achieved.[3]

Exercise of the muscle that is the site of an insulin injection increases the rate of absorption and so the risk of hypoglycemia, but only if the exercise takes place within half an hour of the injection.[4] Absorption from the abdomen is greater than from the thigh, so switching from thigh to abdomen may result in hypoglycemia. The practical significance of these findings is that the athlete should rotate insulin injection sites around one anatomical area and not switch from one to another body site. If there is a choice, the abdomen is probably the preferable site.[3]

──────────── ⬎ **REFERENCES** ⬏ ────────────

1. Expert Committee of the Canadian Diabetes Advisory Board: Clinical practice guidelines for diabetes mellitus in Canada, *Can Med Assoc J* 147:697-712, 1992.
2. Berger M, Mühlhauser I: Diabetes care and patient-oriented outcomes, *JAMA* 281:1676-1678, 1999.
3. Fahey PF, Stallcamp ET, Kwatra S: The athlete with type I diabetes: managing insulin, diet and exercise, *Am Fam Physician* 53:1611-1617, 1996.
4. Kemmer FW: Prevention of hypoglycemia during exercise in type I diabetes, *Diabetes Care* 15:1732-1735, 1992.

Type 2 Diabetes

Epidemiology and prevention

Diabetes affects 4% to 6% of Canadians. About 90% of persons with diabetes are not insulin dependent (type 2) and 5% to 10% are insulin dependent (type 1).

The genetic propensity for type 2 diabetes is greater than for type 1. A person who has one first-degree relative with the disease has twice the risk, and if the person has two first-degree relatives with the condition, the risk is quadrupled. The concordance rate for identical twins is 60% to 80%.[1] Race is also a risk factor; the disease is twice as common in blacks[1] and two-and-one-half to three times as common in Mexican-Americans as in whites.[2] Diabetes among Native Americans was virtually unknown before 1940, but it now has a high prevalence rate.[3] This increase is almost certainly due to a marked increase in the incidence of obesity in this population. In the United States the incidence of diabetes in Native Americans is five times that of whites.[2] In the northern Canadian community of Sioux Lookout the prevalence of type 2 diabetes in adolescents under 16 was 2.5 : 1000. Most patients were asymptomatic obese females with a strong family history of type 2 diabetes.[4]

A major risk factor, which at least in theory can be controlled, is weight gain. In a prospective cohort study of American nurses, a weight gain after the age of 18 of 5 to 7.9 kg increased the risk of diabetes by 1.9 and a weight gain of 8 to 10.9 kg increased the risk by 2.7. A weight loss of more than 5 kg decreased the relative risk by 50%.[5] A 2-year study of nondiabetic obese Americans with a mean BMI of 36 compared four management protocols: no specific program (control group), diet, exercise, and diet plus exercise. The mean weight loss in both the diet and diet plus exercise groups was about 10 kg in the first 6 months (compared with 1 to 2 kg in the control and exercise groups), but by 2 years most of the weight had been regained. In this study 25% of all patients had a weight loss of 4.5 kg at 2 years and these patients decreased their relative risk of acquiring type 2 diabetes by 30%.[6]

Exercise, such as brisk walking, that leads to improved cardiorespiratory fitness results in a decreased risk of type 2 diabetes[7,8] and impaired fasting glucose.[8] Cigarette smoking[9] and hypertension[10] increase the risk of type 2 diabetes, whereas moderate alcohol intake appears to protect against it.[9]

An estimated 50% of cases of type 2 diabetes in the United States are undiagnosed.[11]

──────────── ⬎ **REFERENCES** ⬏ ────────────

1. Bennett PH: Epidemiology of diabetes mellitus. In Rifkin H, Porte D Jr, eds: *Ellenberg and Rifkin's diabetes mellitus,* New York, 1990, Elsevier, pp 363-377.
2. Harris MI, Hadden WC, Knowler WC, et al: Prevalence of diabetes and impaired glucose tolerance and plasma glucose levels in the US population, *Diabetes* 36:523-534, 1987.
3. Hall PF: Ironies most bittersweet (editorial), *Can Med Assoc J* 160:1315-1316, 1999.
4. Harris SB, Perkins BA, Whalen-Brough E: Non-insulin-dependent diabetes mellitus among First Nations children: new entity among First Nations people of northwestern Ontario, *Can Fam Physician* 42:869-876, 1996.
5. Colditz GA, Willett WC, Rotnitzky A, et al: Weight gain as a risk factor for clinical diabetes mellitus in women, *Ann Intern Med* 122:481-486, 1995.
6. Wing R, Venditti E, Jakicic J, et al: Lifestyle intervention in overweight individuals with a family history of diabetes, *Diabetes Care* 21:350-359, 1998.

7. Hu FB, Sigal RJ, Rich-Edwards JW, et al: Walking compared with vigorous physical activity and risk of type 2 diabetes in women: a prospective study, *JAMA* 282:1433-1439, 1999.

8. Wei M, Gibbons LW, Mitchell TL, et al: The association between cardiorespiratory fitness and impaired fasting glucose and type 2 diabetes mellitus in men, *Ann Intern Med* 130:89-96, 1999.

9. Rimm EB, Chan J, Stampfer MJ, et al: Prospective study of cigarette smoking, alcohol use, and the risk of diabetes in men, *BMJ* 210:545-546, 1995.

10. Hayashi T, Tsumura K, Suematsu C, et al: High normal blood pressure, hypertension, and the risk of type 2 diabetes in Japanese men: the Osaka Health Survey, *Diabetes Care* 22:1683-1687, 1999.

11. Harris MI: Undiagnosed NIDDM: clinical and public health issues, *Diabetes Care* 16:642-652, 1993.

Insulin resistance and the pathogenesis of type 2 diabetes

(See also role of intensive treatment in preventing diabetic complications in type 2 diabetes)

Insulin resistance seems to be a necessary, but not sufficient, condition for the development of type 2 diabetes. The theory is that individuals who develop insulin resistance but have good beta-cell reserves simply produce more insulin (hyperinsulinemia) to maintain normoglycemia. When the reserves of the beta-cells become inadequate, type 2 diabetes supervenes.

Hyperinsulinemia is thought to be responsible for type 2 diabetes, obesity, hypertension, dyslipidemia, and atherosclerotic vascular disease,[1-3] a group of conditions often lumped together as "central obesity–insulin resistance syndrome" or "syndrome X." This is one reason that many authorities are reluctant to treat type 2 diabetes with insulin. On the other hand, some workers think that elevated insulin levels are simply markers of insulin resistance and not pathogenetic factors for atherosclerosis.[4]

◣ REFERENCES ◢

1. De Fronzo RA, Ferrannini E: Insulin resistance: a multifaceted syndrome responsible for NIDDM, obesity, hypertension, dyslipidemia and atherosclerotic vascular disease, *Diabetes Care* 14:173-194, 1991.

2. Dagogo-Jack S, Santiago JV: Pathophysiology of type 2 diabetes and modes of action of therapeutic interventions, *Arch Intern Med* 157:1802-1817, 1997.

3. Purnell JQ, Hokanson JE, Marcovina SM, et al: Effect of excessive weight gain with intensive therapy of type 1 diabetes on lipid levels and blood pressure, *JAMA* 280:140-146, 1998.

4. Wingard DL, Barrett-Connor EL, Ferrara A: Is insulin really a heart disease risk factor? *Diabetes Care* 18:1299-1304, 1995.

Screening for type 2 diabetes

(See also prevention; screening)

Two expert panels that have reviewed the evidence for screening patients for fasting plasma glucose have come to similar conclusions. No evidence supports routine screening of the general population over 50.[1,2] However, screening may be considered for those with a family history of diabetes, a history of gestational diabetes, or marked obesity, even though early detection has not been shown to affect the ultimate outcome.[1] The Canadian Task Force on Preventive Health Care gives screening of the general population for diabetes a "D" recommendation,[1] whereas the U.S. Preventive Services Task Force gives it a "C."[2]

In 1997 the American Diabetes Association recommended screening all adults over the age of 45 for diabetes, as well as screening younger individuals if they are obese, have first-degree relatives with diabetes, are members of high-risk populations, have delivered infants weighing more than 4 kg (9 lb), have been found to have gestational diabetes, or have cardiovascular risk factors such as hypertension or lipid abnormalities.[3] The Canadian Diabetes Association published essentially the same recommendations in 1998, specifying that these were based on expert opinion, not evidence.[4]

An estimated 30% to 50% of cases of type 2 diabetes are undiagnosed.[4] The only reason for trying to detect affected individuals by screening would be to decrease morbidity and mortality. The therapeutic interventions of choice for the vast majority of patients with type 2 diabetes are diet and exercise to decrease body weight and insulin resistance. Since only a minuscule number of individuals are able to lose weight and maintain the loss,[5] a belief that screening for diabetes will make people change their life-styles is wishful thinking.

If diabetic patients identified by screening cannot lose weight, might they benefit from the institution of earlier intensive pharmacological therapy to decrease the risk of macrovascular and microvascular disease? No studies dealing with this issue have been published, but as discussed in the ensuing paragraphs, the probability of this happening is low.

The United Kingdom Prospective Diabetes Study (UKPDS) has documented that intensive treatment with insulin or sulfonylureas does not decrease morbidity or mortality from macrovascular disease—a rather discouraging result, since 60% of diabetics die as a result of macrovascular complications.[6] A ray of hope comes from another UKPDS report that intensive metformin treatment of obese persons with type 2 diabetes decreased the risk of macrovascular disease. Unfortunately, such patients treated with a combination of metformin and sulfonylureas had higher mortality rates than conventionally treated control subjects.[7]

The UKPDS reported a 25% reduction in microvascular disease with intensive treatment.[6] This was due primarily to a decrease in the progression of retinopathy as determined by ophthalmological examination; in addition, about 1 in 250 intensively treated patients was spared retinal photocoagulation. The rate of visual loss was not lower in those treated intensively than in conventionally treated control subjects, nor did intensive treatment prevent impotence.

According to the UKPDS reports, microvascular disease develops in 9% of type 2 diabetics within 9 years of diagnosis.[6] Harris and associates[8] claimed that 21% of diabetics in the United States and 10% in Australia had some degree of retinopathy at the time of diagnosis, and the UKPDS reported the rate to be 39% in men and 35% in women.[9] On the face of it, the high incidence of retinopathy found in the UKPDS could be interpreted as powerful indirect evidence that screening is useful in preventing visual loss. This is doubtful, however. The figures were in large part a result of using retinal photographs (rather than direct ophthalmoscopy as had been done in previous studies) to make the diagnosis, and in 20% of cases the only detected abnormalities were three or fewer microaneurysms. In over 92% of cases in men and 95% of cases in women the detected retinopathy was mild, and in the remaining cases it was moderate. In no case did patients have advanced retinopathy (preproliferative or proliferative), which is the type that requires retinal photocoagulation.[9] Further, many of the patients with moderate retinopathy had hypertension,[9] and if testing for diabetes were an integral part of the workup for hypertension, their disease could have been detected at the time hypertension was diagnosed.

In my review of the literature I saw no evidence that screening the entire adult population over the age of 45 for diabetes would decrease morbidity or mortality. What screening would accomplish is to label thousands of people as ill when they thought they were well.[10] Others hold contrary views.[11]

❧ REFERENCES ❧

1. Canadian Task Force on the Periodic Health Examination: *Clinical preventive health care,* Ottawa, 1994, Canadian Communication Group—Publishing, pp 602-609.
2. US Preventive Services Task Force: *Guide to clinical preventive services,* ed 2, Baltimore, 1996, Williams & Wilkins, pp 193-208.
3. American Diabetes Association: Standards of medical care for patients with diabetes mellitus, *Diabetes Care* 20(suppl 1):S1-S70, 1997.
4. Meltzer S, Leiter L, Daneman D, et al: 1998 Clinical practice guidelines for the management of diabetes in Canada, *Can Med Assoc J* 159(suppl 8):S1-S29, 1998.
5. Foreyt J, Goodrick K: The ultimate triumph of obesity (editorial), *Lancet* 346:134-135, 1995.
6. United Kingdom Prospective Diabetes Study (UKPDS) Group: Intensive blood-glucose control with sulphonylureas or insulin compared with conventional treatment and risk of complications in patients with type 2 diabetes (UKPDS 33), *Lancet* 352:837-853, 1998.
7. United Kingdom Prospective Diabetes Study (UKPDS) Group: Effect of intensive blood-glucose control with metformin on complications in overweight patients with type 2 diabetes (UKPDS 34), *Lancet* 352:854-865, 1998.
8. Harris MI, Klein R, Welbourn TA, et al: Onset of NIDDM occurs at least 4-7 years before clinical diagnosis, *Diabetes Care* 15:815-819, 1992.
9. United Kingdom Prospective Diabetes Study, 30: diabetic retinopathy at diagnosis of non-insulin-dependent diabetes mellitus and associated risk factors, *Arch Ophthalmol* 116:297-303, 1998.
10. Marshall KG: The folly of population screening for type 2 diabetes (editorial), *Can Med Assoc J* 160:1592-1593, 1999. (Rebuttal by Gerstein HC, Meltzer S: *Can Med Assoc J* 160:1596, 1999.)
11. Gerstein HC, Meltzer S: Preventive medicine in people at high risk for chronic disease: the value of identifying and treating diabetes (editorial), *Can Med Assoc J* 160:1593-1595, 1999. (Rebuttal by Marshall KG: *Can Med Assoc J* 160:1595-1596, 1999.)

Diet, exercise, and weight-lowering drugs in type 2 diabetes

(See also obesity)

Diet and exercise are essential components of the treatment of type 2 diabetes because of their value in controlling weight, reducing insulin resistance, and preventing coronary artery disease.[1,2] Except in a few symptomatic patients the initial treatment of patients with type 2 diabetes should be an intensive, individualized diet and exercise program. Only if it is unsuccessful after 6 months of persistent endeavor should pharmacological treatment be considered.[2]

The role of weight-lowering drugs in type 2 diabetes is uncertain. Anorexiants such as fenfluramine (Pondimin, Ponderal) and dexfenfluramine (Redux) have been associated with lethal adverse effects (see discussion of obesity) and have been taken off the market. A 1998 study of obese diabetics reported that orlistat (Xenical), which inhibits gastrointestinal lipases, given as 120 mg tid for 1 year resulted in a mean loss of 6.2% of initial body weight at 1 year compared with a loss of 4.3% in the placebo control group. The orlistat-treated patients also had improved glycemic control, as determined by HbA_{1c} levels and medication requirements, and improved lipid profiles.[3] However, no long-term trials of orlistat have been published, gastrointestinal side effects are common, and in clinical trials a statistically significant increase in breast cancer occurred among patients taking orlistat compared with those taking placebo.[4]

❧ REFERENCES ❧

1. Mayer-Davis EJ, D'Agostino R Jr, Karter AJ, et al: Intensity and amount of physical activity in relation to insulin sensitivity: the Insulin Resistance Atherosclerosis Study, *JAMA* 279:669-674, 1998.
2. Expert Committee of the Canadian Diabetes Advisory Board: Clinical practice guidelines for diabetes mellitus in Canada, *Can Med Assoc J* 147:697-712, 1992.
3. Hollander PA, Elbein SC, Hirsch IB, et al: Role of orlistat in the treatment of obese patients with type 2 diabetes, *Diabetes Care* 21:1288-1294, 1998.
4. Prescrire: orlistat; no hurry. . ., *Can Fam Physician* 45:2330-2338, 1999.

Pharmacological treatment of type 2 diabetes

(See also intensive treatment in preventing diabetic complications in type 2 diabetes; type 1 diabetes)

The pros and cons of intensive treatment of type 2 diabetes are discussed previously in the section on intensive treatment for preventing complications of type 2 diabetes.

Oral hypoglycemic agents. The target levels for glucose control set by the American[1] and Canadian[2] diabetes associations are stringent (see discussion of target levels for glucose control). The usual protocol for trying to reach these goals in patients with type 2 diabetes is to start with lifestyle changes, followed by oral hypoglycemic agents, then a combination of oral agents and insulin, and then insulin alone.

When oral therapy is indicated, the physician has the choice of starting with one of the sulfonylureas, a biguanide, an alpha-glucosidase inhibitor,[3] or even a thiazolidinedione (Table 42).[4] Since the United Kingdom Prospective Diabetes Study (UKPDS) has demonstrated that tight control with sulfonylureas or insulin does not decrease macrovascular complications of diabetes[5] whereas treating obese persons with type 2 diabetes with metformin alone does,[6] metformin might be the drug of first choice for obese patients. If metformin is chosen, the physician should bear in mind that in the UKPDS study, obese patients treated with a combination of metformin and a sulfonylurea had an increased rate of death from macrovascular disease.[6] Whether this represents a causal relationship or a statistical fluke is unknown.

The primary action of sulfonylureas is to increase insulin output from the pancreatic beta-cells. These agents may cause hypoglycemic reactions, weight gain, and hyperinsu-

Table 42   Oral Hypoglycemic Agents

Drugs	Usual doses
Sulfonylureas, Second Generation	
Glyburide (Diabeta, Glynase, Micronase)	5-10 mg qam or 10 mg bid
Gliclazide (Diamicron)	40-160 mg bid
Glimepiride (Amaryl)	1-8 mg qam
Glipizide (Glucotrol)	5-40 mg qam or 10-20 mg bid
Glipizide extended release	5-10 mg qam
Biguanides	
Metformin (Glucophage)	500 mg tid-qid or 850 mg bid-tid
Alpha-Glucosidase Inhibitors	
Acarbose (Precose, Prandase)	25-100 mg tid
Miglitol (Glyset)	50 mg tid at beginning of each meal
Thiazolidinediones	
Pioglitazone (Actos)	15-45 mg once daily
Rosiglitazone (Avandia)	4-8 mg once daily
Troglitazone (Rezulin)	Withdrawn from market
Meglitinides	
Repaglinide (GlucoNorm, Prandin)	0.5-4 mg tid-qid ac

linemia[3] and should not be given to patients who are allergic to sulfonamides.

The biguanides, of which the only one currently available in Canada and the United States is metformin (Glucophage), act primarily by decreasing glucose output from the liver but also by increasing the insulin sensitivity of muscle. Metformin leads to weight loss and decreases levels of triglycerides, total cholesterol, and LDL cholesterol.[7] Metformin is as effective as the sulfonylureas and rarely induces hypoglycemia.[3] Disadvantages of the drug are that it has to be given two or three times a day and that 5% to 20% of patients have transient gastrointestinal effects, usually diarrhea. Metformin should not be given to persons with impaired liver or renal function because of the risk of lactic acidosis. Specifically, physicians should be wary of prescribing the drug to someone with a creatinine level above 150 mmol/L (1.7 mg/dl).

Acarbose (Prandase, Precose) is an alpha-glucosidase inhibitor that is taken three times daily immediately before meals. It acts by inhibiting the hydrolysis of dietary disaccharides and thus inhibits the absorption of monosaccharides. It has been used for both type 1 and type 2 diabetes. The main adverse effects are flatulence, distention, cramps, and diarrhea, and these are of sufficient importance to cause many patients to discontinue the drug.[8]

Acarbose may be used as the only pharmacological agent for type 2 diabetes or may be given in conjunction with one or more oral agents or insulin. The UKPDS found that acarbose alone or added to other medications improved glycemic control in patients with type 2 diabetes.[8]

A second alpha-glucosidase inhibitor, miglitol (Glyset), became available in the United States in 1999.

A new class of agents is the thiazolidinediones, which include troglitazone (Rezulin), rosiglitazone (Avandia), and pioglitazone (Actos). These agents act by increasing insulin sensitivity so that liver and muscle cells increase their consumption of glucose. The first of these agents, troglitazone, has been associated with a number of cases of hepatotoxicity, and because of this the drug was withdrawn from the market in Great Britain in 1997. The FDA did not withdraw the drug from the U.S. market but issued new guidelines recommending that the drug not be used as monotherapy and that if it is used in combination with other agents, liver enzyme levels be obtained monthly for 12 months and every 3 months thereafter. However, because of increasing reports of liver failure associated with use of troglitazone, the manufacturer voluntarily withdrew the drug from the U.S. market in early 2000. Rosiglitazone and pioglitazone do not appear to lead to serious adverse hepatic effects, but long-term safety and benefits have not been determined.[9]

One of the newest nonsulfonylurea oral agents is repaglinide (Gluconorm, Prandin), which belongs to the meglitinide class.[10] It stimulates the release of insulin from the pancreas and can be used as monotherapy or in combination with metformin.

If adequate control of glucose cannot be obtained with one class of oral hypoglycemic medication, a member of another class can be added, or insulin can be added to or replace the oral agents (see below).[3] Most patients with type 2 diabetes require polytherapy if they are to achieve an HbA_{1c} below 7%. In the UKPDS study, 50% of patients required two or more pharmacological agents 3 years after diagnosis and 75% required multiple therapies after 9 years. This is undoubtedly a reflection of a progressive decline in beta-cell function over time.[11]

Temporary insulin therapy. Patients with type 2 diabetes often require temporary insulin therapy if they become pregnant, undergo surgery, or have intercurrent illnesses such as acute myocardial infarction or pneumonia. A widespread hospital practice in such cases is to use sliding insulin scales so that the patient is given regular insulin q6h with the doses changed frequently on the basis of regularly measured capillary blood glucose levels. The origin of this practice is unclear, and its net effect is poor control of glycemia.[12,13] Patients are far better off continuing with oral hypoglycemic agents or standard combinations of long- and short-acting insulins.[12-14]

Long-term insulin therapy. A common protocol when planning long-term insulin therapy for a patient with type 2 diabetes is to prescribe a single morning injection of an intermediate- or long-acting insulin in a low dose (0.3 unit/kg or about 15 to 25 units/day). The dose is adjusted according to glucose levels, and many patients require as much as 1 unit/kg/day, particularly if they are obese. If the patient is already taking oral agents, these are stopped on the morning insulin is begun. Doses are increased by 2 to 4 units once or twice a week as necessary.[15] Another method of attempting to improve control in type 2 diabetes is to give a single dose of an intermediate- or long-acting insulin at bedtime combined with oral agents during the day (see later discussion).[2,16]

Insulin plus oral hypoglycemic agents. A 1-year randomized controlled trial of obese patients whose type 2 diabetes was inadequately controlled with oral hypoglycemic agents alone compared bedtime isophane insulin (NPH) for all patients plus either glyburide and placebo, metformin and placebo, glyburide and metformin, or a second dose of isophane insulin given in the morning. In patients taking insulin plus metformin, glycosylated hemoglobin dropped from 9.7% to 7.2%, there was no weight gain, and hypoglycemic reactions were rare. All other groups gained weight and had poorer glycemic control and more hypoglycemic reactions. In this study patients adjusted their own insulin doses, starting with a dose equivalent to the fasting blood glucose level measured in millimoles per liter and increasing by 4 IU per day if the fasting levels exceeded 8 mmol/L on three consecutive measurements and by 2 IU per day if they exceeded 6 mmol/L. The dose of metformin was 1000 mg before breakfast and 1000 mg before supper and that of glyburide 3.5 mg before break-

fast and 7 mg before supper. Bedtime insulin was given at 9 PM.[16]

Unnecessary insulin. Even when rather strict criteria are used to define metabolic control, about half of obese diabetic patients who are receiving insulin can stop taking the drug and maintain glycemic control with diet and exercise alone. Reasons for this may be an initial misdiagnosis of type 1 diabetes, an inadequate trial of diet, exercise, or oral agents, significant weight loss since starting insulin, or a prescription of insulin that was ordered during a stressful illness and never discontinued.[17] It behooves all family physicians to remember this and, where appropriate, to try to discontinue insulin.

Home glucose monitoring. Home glucose monitoring of patients with type 2 diabetes does not lead to improved glycemic control. Although a few patients feel empowered when they use this technique, anxiety, helplessness, and guilt are much more common reactions.[18] A comparison of blood and urine glucose monitoring in patients with newly diagnosed type 2 diabetes found no difference between the two in glycosylated hemoglobin levels at 6 and 12 months, although urine testing was six times less expensive.[19]

White coat hyperglycemia. In a British study of patients with non-insulin-dependent diabetes, glucose levels monitored at home were often lower than those measured in the clinic even when technical errors in home readings were ruled out. The authors labeled this phenomenon "white coat hyperglycemia."[20]

⬧ REFERENCES ⬧

1. American Diabetes Association: Standards of medical care for patients with diabetes mellitus, *Diabetes Care* 20(suppl 1):S1-S70, 1997.

2. Meltzer S, Leiter L, Daneman D, et al: 1998 Clinical practice guidelines for the management of diabetes in Canada, *Can Med Assoc J* 159(suppl 8):S1-S29, 1998.

3. Dagogo-Jack S, Santiago JV: Pathophysiology of type 2 diabetes and modes of action of therapeutic interventions, *Arch Intern Med* 157:1802-1817, 1997.

4. Troglitazone for non-insulin-dependent diabetes mellitus, *Med Lett* 39:49-51, 1997.

5. United Kingdom Prospective Diabetes Study (UKPDS) Group: Intensive blood-glucose control with sulphonylureas or insulin compared with conventional treatment and risk of complications in patients with type 2 diabetes (UKPDS 33), *Lancet* 352:837-853, 1998.

6. United Kingdom Prospective Diabetes Study (UKPDS) Group: Effect of intensive blood-glucose control with metformin on complications in overweight patients with type 2 diabetes (UKPDS 34), *Lancet* 352:854-865, 1998.

7. Robinson AC, Burke J, Robinson S, et al: The effects of metformin on glycemic control and serum lipids in insulin-treated NIDDM patients with suboptimal metabolic control, *Diabetes Care* 21:701-705, 1998.

8. Holman RR, Cull CA, Turner RC, et al: A randomized double-blind trial of acarbose in type 2 diabetes shows improved glycemic control over 3 years (U.K. Prospective Diabetes Study 44), *Diabetes Care* 22:960-964, 1999.

9. Rosiglitazone for type 2 diabetes mellitus, *Med Lett* 41:71-73, 1999.

10. Repaglinide for type 2 diabetes mellitus, *Med Lett* 40:55-56, 1998.

11. Turner RC, Cull CA, Frighi V, et al: Glycemic control with diet, sulfonylurea, metformin, or insulin in patients with type 2 diabetes mellitus: progressive requirement for multiple therapies (UKPDS 49), *JAMA* 281:2005-2012, 1999.

12. Queale WS, Seidler AJ, Brancati FL: Glycemic control and sliding scale insulin use in medical inpatients with diabetes mellitus, *Arch Intern Med* 157:545-552, 1997.

13. Sawin CT: Action without benefit: the sliding scale of insulin use (editorial), *Arch Intern Med* 157:489, 1997.

14. Jacober SJ, Sowers JR: An update on perioperative management of diabetes, *Arch Intern Med* 159:2405-2411, 1999.

15. Shlossberg AH: Treating non-insulin-dependent diabetes: oral agents or insulin? *Can Fam Physician* 39:119-126, 1993.

16. Hannele Y-J, Ryysy L, Nikkilä K, et al: Comparison of bedtime insulin regimens in patients with type 2 diabetes mellitus: a randomized controlled trial, *Ann Intern Med* 130:389-396, 1999.

17. Genuth S: Insulin use in NIDDM, *Diabetes Care* 13:1240-1264, 1990.

18. Gallichan M: Self monitoring of glucose by people with diabetes: evidence based practice, *BMJ* 324:964-966, 1997.

19. Miles P, Everett J, Murphy J, et al: Comparison of blood or urine testing by patients with newly diagnosed non-insulin dependent diabetes: patient survey after randomised crossover trial, *BMJ* 315:348-349, 1997.

20. Campbell LV, Ashwell SM, Borkman M, et al: White coat hyperglycaemia: disparity between diabetes clinic and home blood glucose concentrations, *BMJ* 305:1194-1196, 1992.

ELECTROLYTES
Potassium

Fist clenching during phlebotomy, with or without the use of a tourniquet, raises the serum potassium level by as much as 1.6 mmol/L (1.6 mEq/L).[1]

◣ REFERENCES ◢

1. Don BR, Sebastian A, Cheitlin M, et al: Pseudohyperkalemia caused by fist clenching during phlebotomy, *N Engl J Med* 322:1290-1292, 1990.

HYPOGLYCEMIA
(See also diabetes; functional somatic syndromes)

A number of conditions may cause true hypoglycemia. Insulin reactions in diabetic patients are the most common. Factitious hypoglycemia from the self-injection of insulin is primarily a disorder of female health care workers. Insulinomas and drugs are other well-recognized causes of hypoglycemia, and Addison's disease, hypopituitarism, and gastric resection may also result in the syndrome.[1,2]

Functional, reactive, or alimentary hypoglycemia is a controversial entity.[1,2] It is characterized by a variety of nonspecific symptoms, such as weakness, palpitations, tremors, sweating, headaches, and hunger, that come on after meals and are relieved by eating.[1] Control has been said to be achievable with a high-protein, low-carbohydrate diet.[1] Little scientific evidence supports the existence of functional or alimentary hypoglycemia.[1,2] In studies of patients thought to have this disorder, glucose levels have almost always been normal (greater than 2.8 mmol/L or 50 mg/dl) during the period of symptoms.[1,2] The diagnosis should not be based on a glucose tolerance test, since it is neither sensitive nor specific.[1] The argument that the glucose level may be normal but have dropped rapidly, thereby causing symptoms, does not hold up because this phenomenon is never observed after insulin injections in volunteers.[2] Many patients come to physicians with a diagnosis of hypoglycemia that they have either made themselves or been given by health care workers. A better term for their problem would be idiopathic postprandial syndrome.[2]

◣ REFERENCES ◢

1. Service FJ: Hypoglycemic disorders, *N Engl J Med* 332:1144-1152, 1995.

2. Palardy J, Havrankova J, Lepage R, et al: Blood glucose measurements during symptomatic episodes in patients with suspected postprandial hypoglycemia, *N Engl J Med* 321:1421-1425, 1989.

LIPIDS
Conversion from Systéme International Units to Traditional Units

To convert cholesterol readings from Systéme International (SI) units (mmol/L) to traditional units (mg/dl), divide by 0.0259. To convert cholesterol readings from traditional units (mg/dl) to SI units (mmol/L), multiply by 0.0259.

Epidemiology of Lipid Disorders
(See also risk factors for coronary artery disease)

Wide variation is seen in the rates of coronary heart disease (CHD) in different geographical areas, and this is not fully explained by differences in cholesterol levels. For example, men with cholesterol levels in the range of 5.45 mmol/L (210 mg/dl) had CHD mortality rates varying from between 4% and 5% in Japan and Southern Europe to 12% in the United States and 15% in Northern Europe. Within any one culture, CHD risk correlates well with cholesterol levels.[1] The reasons for this discrepancy are unknown, but a reasonable hypothesis is that intimal dysfunction secondary to chemical (hyperhomocysteinemia?), physical, or biological (chlamydial pneumonia?) injury is the prime cause of atherosclerosis and that hyperlipidemia merely acts as a promoting factor.[2]

Elevated triglyceride levels have been shown to be a risk factor for ischemic heart disease,[3-5] but whether therapeutic interventions to lower triglycerides are beneficial is unknown because no published randomized controlled trials address this issue.[3,4]

Whether lipid levels are good predictors of CHD in the elderly is uncertain; several trials failed to find any correlation, although one study reported increased morbidity and mortality from CHD in persons over 70 who had low levels of HDL-C,[6] while another found that elevated LDL-C and total cholesterol levels were related to an increased incidence of CHD.[7] On the other hand, a Netherlands study of individuals over the age of 85 found that increasing levels of total cholesterol correlated with lower mortality rates.[8]

Even if abnormal lipid levels in the elderly represent true risk factors for CAD, whether drug therapy for primary prevention is indicated is unclear because no trials of cholesterol-lowering therapy have been directed at the elderly.[9,10] Secondary prevention with lipid-lowering agents seems reasonable.[10]

Low cholesterol in the elderly is associated with increased death rates (see discussion of adverse effects associated with low cholesterol).

REFERENCES

1. Verschuren WMM, Jacobs DR, Bloemberg M, et al: Serum total cholesterol and long-term coronary heart disease mortality in different cultures: twenty-five-year follow-up of the seven countries study, *JAMA* 274:131-136, 1995.
2. Moore S: Cholesterol revisited: prime mover or a factor in the progression of atherosclerosis? *Ann RCPSC* 32:198-204, 1999.
3. Sattar N, Packard CJ, Petrie JR: The end of triglycerides in cardiovascular risk assessment? Rumours of death are greatly exaggerated (editorial), *BMJ* 317:553-554, 1998.
4. Jeppesen J, Hein HO, Suadicani P, et al: Triglyceride concentration and ischemic heart disease: an eight-year follow-up in the Copenhagen Male Study, *Circulation* 97:1029-1036, 1998.
5. Coresh J, Kwiterovich PO Jr: Small, dense low-density lipoprotein particles and coronary heart disease risk: a clear association with uncertain implications (editorial), *JAMA* 276:914-915, 1996.
6. Corti M-C, Guralnik JM, Salive ME, et al: HDL cholesterol predicts coronary heart disease mortality in older persons, *JAMA* 274:539-544, 1995.
7. Frost PH, Davis BR, Burlando A, et al (Systolic Hypertension in the Elderly Research Program): Serum lipids and the incidence of coronary heart disease: findings from the Systolic Hypertension in the Elderly Program (SHEP), *Circulation* 94:2381-2388, 1996.
8. Weverling-Rijnsburger AW, Blauw GJ, Lagaay AM, et al: Total cholesterol and risk of mortality in the oldest old, *Lancet* 350:1119-1123, 1997.
9. Denke MA, Winker MA: Cholesterol and coronary heart disease in older adults: no easy answers (editorial), *JAMA* 274:575-576, 1995.
10. Grundy SM, Cleeman JI, Rifkind BM, et al: Cholesterol lowering in the elderly population, *Arch Intern Med* 159:1670-1678, 1999.

Variability of Cholesterol Levels

(See also prevention; screening)

A person's cholesterol levels vary substantially from one day to another independent of diet and laboratory testing procedures. In an Ontario study of cholesterol levels any patient whose initial total cholesterol level was greater than 6.2 mmol/L (240 mg/dl) was asked to give a second sample. On the basis of the initial results patients were divided into three risk categories[1]:

Normal risk	<6.2 mmol/L (240 mg/dl)
Moderate risk	6.2-6.9 mmol/L (240-266 mg/dl)
High risk	>6.9 mmol/L (266 mg/dl)

When a second sample was obtained, the two results were averaged and the patient's risk category was reassigned. The results were striking. Fifty percent of patients initially classified as at high risk were reclassified to moderate risk, 10.5% of those initially classified as at moderate risk were reclassified to the normal category, and 4.8% of those initially classified as at moderate risk were moved up to a high-risk category.[1] From the findings of this and other studies, no one should be treated for an elevated cholesterol reading on the basis of one sample. Unfortunately, obtaining a second reading may cause significant psychological morbidity, since the patient will know that the initial cholesterol measurement was "up." Even if subsequent readings are normal, that nagging doubt will not be easily dispelled.

REFERENCES

1. Speechley M, McNair S, Leffley A, Bass M: Identifying patients with hypercholesterolemia: more than one blood sample is needed, *Can Fam Physician* 41:240-245, 1995.

Cholesterol-Lowering Studies in Adults Without Known Coronary Artery Disease

(See also exercise; relative risk reduction)

Diet and exercise

The common belief that low-fat and low-cholesterol diets will lower LDL-C is based on observational studies, cross-sectional population-based studies, and metabolic ward–based studies.[1,2] No randomized controlled trial has shown that diet in ambulatory patients lowers coronary artery disease risk, and most studies have shown only small effects on cholesterol levels.[2] For example, a randomized prospective trial of ambulatory patients with elevated LDL-C and low HDL-C who were put on the National Cholesterol Education Program (NCEP) Step 2 diet found that diet alone did not alter lipid profiles. However, when this diet was combined with a regular aerobic exercise program, LDL-C levels fell and HDL-C levels rose. Exercise alone did not bring about these changes.[1]

Patients with elevated cholesterol levels are often advised to decrease their consumption of red meats and increase their consumption of white meats (poultry and fish). A 36-week trial in which hypercholesterolemic subjects were selected at random to eat 80% of their meat as lean pork, beef, or veal or to eat 80% as lean poultry or fish found no differences in LDL-C or HDL-C between the two groups.[3]

Table 43 Cholesterol-Lowering Drug Studies in Patients Without Coronary Artery Disease

Drug studies	Drug
Lipid Research Clinics Program trial (LRC)[4]	Cholestyramine (Questran)
Helsinki Heart Study (HHS)[5]	Gemfibrozil (Lopid)
World Health Organization (WHO)[6]	Clofibrate (Atromid-S)
Upjohn's Colestipol Study (UCS)[7]	Colestipol (Colestid)
West of Scotland Coronary Prevention Study Group (WOSCOPS)[8]	Pravastatin (Pravachol)
Air Force/Texas Coronary Atherosclerosis Prevention Study (AFCAPS/TexCAPS)[9]	Lovastatin (Mevacor)

Drugs

Table 43 lists six major cholesterol-lowering studies of the effects of lipid-lowering drugs in individuals with elevated cholesterol levels but without known coronary artery disease (CAD).[4-9] With the exception of the AFCAPS/TexCAPS, these studies enrolled primarily middle-aged men with high cholesterol levels but without clinical evidence of CAD. The AFCAPS/TexCAPS enrolled men (82%) and postmenopausal women (18%) with normal or only slightly elevated lipid levels. All of these studies showed a statistically significant decline in coronary events, but only the WOSCOPS demonstrated a statistically significant decrease in cardiovascular mortality. In the World Health Organization (WHO) clofibrate study, total mortality of the treated group was increased by a relative rate of 47%.

The two most relevant studies for current practice are those that used HMG-CoA reductase inhibitors (statins). In WOSCOPS approximately 3300 middle-aged men with very high cholesterol levels but without known CAD received pravastatin 40 mg/day for an average of 4.9 years, while an equal number in the control group received a placebo. Prominently presented figures in the abstract of this *New England Journal of Medicine* report were a relative reduction of 31% in definite nonfatal and fatal myocardial infarctions and a 22% relative reduction in death from all causes in the treated cohort. By careful reading of the text it is possible to calculate that the absolute reduction in definite nonfatal and fatal myocardial infarctions was 2.4% and that more than 200 men had to be treated for 1 year to prevent one such adverse event. The absolute reduction in total cohort mortality was 0.9%, and this required the treatment of 555 men for 1 year to prevent one death.[8] Although WOSCOPS is usually thought of as a primary prevention study, 5% of the men in both the placebo and treatment groups had stable angina.[8] Because of this, purists question whether a reduction in mortality through pharmacotherapy of hypercholesterolemic men without CAD can truly be claimed.

In the AFCAPS/TexCAPS study approximately 3300 middle-aged men and women without known CAD and with normal or slightly elevated lipid levels received lovastatin 20 to 40 mg/day for an average of 5.2 years while an equal number received placebos. Lipid entry requirements were a total cholesterol of 4.65 to 6.82 mmol/L (180 to 264 mg/dl), LDL-C of 3.36 to 4.91 mmol/L (130 to 190 mg/dl), and HDL-C of 1.16 mmol/L (45 mg/dl) or less for men and 1.22 mmol/L (47 mg/dl) or less for women. The reported relative reduction in total cardiac events in the treated group (fatal and nonfatal myocardial infarction, unstable angina, or sudden cardiac death) was 37%. The absolute reduction was 4.1 : 1000 or 0.4%, and 250 individuals had to be treated for 1 year to prevent one event.[9]

No long-term lipid-lowering studies of young adults have been published,[10] and therefore the value of screening young asymptomatic individuals for cholesterol and treating them if it is elevated is unknown. Hulley and associates[11] point out that the mortality rate from cardiovascular disease is so low in persons under 40 that treatment would be unlikely to have beneficial results, whereas the adverse effects of treatment would continue unabated. They argue that delaying treatment until after age 40 would be unlikely to do any harm.

Data on the effects of cholesterol-lowering programs on women are inconclusive; too few women have been studied to generate enough statistical power to give meaningful results.[12]

WOSCOPS and AFCAPS/TexCAPS clearly show that statins can reduce the incidence of cardiovascular events in asymptomatic middle-aged and elderly individuals. The WOSCOPS results prove that cardiovascular mortality can be reduced, while those of the AFCAPS/TexCAPS indicate that statins may be beneficial even in individuals whose LDL-C levels are below those recommended by the National Cholesterol Education Program for the initiation of treatment (treat anyone over 35 who has no additional risk factors and has an LDL-C ≥4.9 mmol/L [190 mg/dl] and anyone with two or more additional risk factors if the LDL-C is 4.1 to 4.9 mmol/L (160 to 190 mg/dl]). At present, little or no evidence has shown that statins are beneficial for asymptomatic young individuals (except those with inborn errors of lipid metabolism) or for women of any age.

Although primary prevention of coronary events in asymptomatic hypercholesterolemic men (and perhaps women) can be achieved with statins, large numbers of individuals must take these drugs while only very few may benefit. Whether benefits derived from statins surpass those of life-style changes is unknown, but unlikely.

◣ REFERENCES ◢

1. Stefanick ML, Mackey S, Sheehan M, et al: Effects of diet and exercise in men and postmenopausal women with low levels of HDL cholesterol and high levels of LDL cholesterol, *N Engl J Med* 339:12-20, 1998.
2. Steinberg D, Gotto AM Jr: Preventing coronary artery disease by lowering cholesterol levels, *JAMA* 282:2043-2050, 1999.

3. Davidson MH, Hunninghake D, Maki KC, et al: Comparison of the effects of lean red meat vs lean white meat on serum lipid levels among free-living persons with hypercholesterolemia, *Arch Intern Med* 1331-1338, 1999.

4. Lipid Research Clinics Coronary Prevention Trial. 1. Reduction in incidence of coronary heart disease, *JAMA* 251:351-374, 1984.

5. Frick MH, Elo O, Haapa K, et al: Helsinki Heart Study: primary prevention trial with gemfibrozil in middle-aged men with dyslipidaemia; safety of treatment, changes in risk factors, and incidence of coronary heart disease, *N Engl J Med* 317:1237-1245, 1987.

6. Heady JA, Morris JN, Oliver MF: WHO Clofibrate/Cholesterol Trial: clarifications, *Lancet* 340:1405-1406, 1992.

7. Dorr AE, Gundersen K, Schneider JC Jr, et al: Colestipol hydrochloride in hypercholesterolemic patients—effect on serum cholesterol and mortality, *J Chron Dis* 31:5-14, 1978.

8. Shepherd J, Cobbe SM, Ford I, et al: Prevention of coronary heart disease with pravastatin in men with hypercholesterolemia, *N Engl J Med* 333:1301-1307, 1995.

9. Downs JR, Clearfield M, Weis S, et al: Primary prevention of acute coronary events with lovastatin in men and women with average cholesterol levels: results of AFCAPS/TexCAPS, *JAMA* 279:1615-1622, 1998.

10. Sox HC Jr: Preventive health services in adults, *N Engl J Med* 330:1589-1595, 1994.

11. Hulley SB, Newman TB, Grady D, et al: Should we be measuring blood cholesterol levels in young adults? *JAMA* 269:1416-1419, 1993.

12. Rich-Edwards JW, Manson JE, Hennekens C, et al: The primary prevention of coronary heart disease in women, *N Engl J Med* 332:1758-1766, 1995.

Cholesterol-Lowering Studies in Patients with Coronary Artery Disease

(See also cerebrovascular accidents; cholesterol-lowering studies in adults without known coronary artery disease; cholesterol screening in children; cholesterol-lowering diets; coronary artery disease; exercise; myocardial infarction; prevention; smoking; treatment of elevated lipids)

Lipid-lowering strategies in patients with known CAD are effective, and far fewer patients need to be treated in order that one individual benefits than is the case with patients who have elevated lipid levels but no known CAD.

A Scandinavian randomized placebo-controlled trial of patients with a history of angina or myocardial infarction (Scandinavian Simvastatin Survival Study [4S]) treated patients with either simvastatin (Zocor) 20 to 40 mg or a placebo. There was a 30% relative and 3.3% absolute reduction in all-cause mortality (8.2% in the treated group versus 11.5% in the placebo group), which was due almost entirely to a 42% decrease in coronary events. Another way of looking at these figures is that 150 patients had to be treated for 1 year to prevent one death. The rates of noncardiovascular deaths were the same in the treatment and placebo groups (no increase in violent deaths occurred in the treated group).[1] A 1995 Dutch study of 885 men with angiographi-cally proven coronary artery disease compared treatment with pravastatin (Pravachol) to a placebo. At the end of 2 years 19% of patients in the placebo group had had vascular events compared with 11% in the treated group. More than twice as many in the placebo group as in the control group required angioplasty.[2]

In patients with known coronary artery disease, "normal" cholesterol levels may be too high. The Cholesterol and Recurrent Events (CARE) trial showed that cholesterol-lowering drugs were beneficial in post–myocardial infarction patients with "average" cholesterol and LDL-C levels. In a 5-year study of more than 4000 patients (mostly men), half were given pravastatin (Pravachol) 40 mg/day and half placebo. At the onset of the study all patients had a cholesterol level less than 240 mg/dl (6.2 mmol/L) with a mean of 209 mg/dl (5.4 mmol/L). At the end of the study the fatal coronary and nonfatal myocardial infarct rates were 10.2% in the pravastatin group and 13.2% in the placebo group for an absolute reduction of risk of 3% (relative risk reduction of 24%). The absolute reduction in the mortality rate of the treated group was 0.8%, which meant that 640 men had to be treated for 1 year to prevent one death. Fewer treated patients required angioplasty or coronary artery bypass surgery, and fewer had strokes.[3] Diabetic patients in the CARE study who received pravastatin experienced a greater absolute reduction in cardiovascular events than did nondiabetics.[4] The Long-Term Intervention with Pravastatin in Ischaemic Disease (LIPID) study, which enrolled patients who had had a myocardial infarction or who had unstable angina, also observed benefits in patients with a broad range of initial cholesterol levels.[5]

Data on the benefits of cholesterol-lowering programs in women with proven CAD are limited. On the basis of the information available, this treatment seems to be beneficial.[6]

The prime goal of lipid-lowering agents in patients with proven CAD is to reduce the LDL-C level, and the best drugs for this purpose are HMG CoA reductase inhibitors.[7] The goal of therapy is to lower the LDL-C to 2.6 mmol/L (100 mg/dl) if possible.[8] In some patients with CAD the LDL-C concentration is not elevated but the HDL-C level is low (1 mmol/L [40 mg/dl]). One double-blind placebo-controlled trial found that in these circumstances treatment with slow release gemfibrozil (Lopid SR) 1200 mg once daily increased HDL-C level, decreased triglyceride levels, and decreased the risk of myocardial infarctions, coronary artery deaths, and strokes.[9]

The efficacy of dietary interventions in patients with CAD is controversial. In a 4-year study a very small number of patients with proven CAD were treated with intensive life-style changes, including a vegetarian diet limited to a 10% fat intake. The treated group had a decrease in coronary events and a small degree of regression of coronary artery lesions (determined by angiography) compared with the control group.[10] That more palatable selective diets may be effective is suggested by a French study of 302 post–myocardial infarction patients placed on a Mediterranean diet (see discussion of treatment of elevated lipids) and 303 control patients following the usual post–myocardial infarction "prudent" diet. At the end of 2 years 59 control patients had died of cardiovascular causes, had had another myocardial infarction, or had been found to have unstable angina, stroke, heart failure, or thromboembolism. In the Mediterranean diet group only 14 patients experienced similar events. This represents a 76% relative reduction rate and a 15% absolute reduction rate. Between six and seven patients had to be treated for 2 years to prevent one event.[11] A 4-year follow-up of these patients found that the benefits of the Mediterranean diet were maintained.[12] These results are better than those reported in the 1994 Scandinavian simvastatin study of patients with known CAD. The nature of the Mediterranean diet is discussed below in the section on treatment of elevated cholesterol levels.

────────────── ◣ **REFERENCES** ◤ ──────────────

1. Scandinavian Simvastatin Survival Study Group: Randomised trial of cholesterol lowering in 4444 patients with coronary heart disease: the Scandinavian Simvastatin Survival Study (4S), *Lancet* 344:1383-1389, 1994.

2. Jukema JW, Bruschke AVG, Vanboven AJ, et al: Effects of lipid lowering by pravastatin on progression and regression of coronary artery disease in symptomatic men with normal to moderately elevated serum cholesterol levels: the Regression Growth Evaluation Statin Study (REGRESS), *Circulation* 91:2528-2540, 1995.

3. Sacks FM, Pfeffer MA, Moye LA, et al: The effect of pravastatin on coronary events after myocardial infarction in patients with average cholesterol levels, *N Engl J Med* 335:1001-1009, 1996.

4. Goldberg RB, Mellies MJ, Sacks FM, et al: Cardiovascular events and their reduction with pravastatin in diabetic and glucose-intolerant myocardial infarction survivors with average cholesterol levels: subgroup analyses in the Cholesterol and Recurrent Events (CARE) Trial, *Circulation* 98:2513-2519, 1998.

5. Long-Term Intervention with Pravastatin in Ischaemic Disease (LIPID) Study Group: Prevention of cardiovascular events and death with pravastatin in patients with coronary heart disease and a broad range of initial cholesterol levels, *N Engl J Med* 339:1349-1357, 1998.

6. Walsh JM, Grady D: Treatment of hyperlipidemia in women, *JAMA* 274:1152-1158, 1995.

7. Kantner T: HMG CoA reductase inhibitors for treatment of hyperlipidemia, *Am Fam Physician* 47:1623-1627, 1993.

8. National Cholesterol Education Program: *The second report of the Expert Panel on Detection, Evaluation, and Treatment of High Blood Cholesterol in Adults (Adult Treatment Panel II),* Bethesda, Md, 1993, National Heart, Lung, and Blood Institute, National Institutes of Health, NIH Pub No 93-3095.

9. Rubins HB, Robins SJ, Collins D, et al: Gemfibrozil for the secondary prevention of coronary heart disease in men with low levels of high-density lipoprotein cholesterol, *N Engl J Med* 341:410-418, 1999.

10. Ornish D, Scherwitz LW, Billings JH, et al: Intensive lifestyle changes for reversal of coronary heart disease, *JAMA* 280:2001-2007, 1998.

11. De Lorgeril M, Salen P, Martin J-L, et al: Effect of a Mediterranean type diet on the rate of cardiovascular complications in patients with coronary artery disease—insights into the cardioprotective effect of certain nutriments, *J Am Coll Cardiol* 28:1103-1108, 1996.

12. De Lorgeril M, Salen P, Martin J-L, et al: Mediterranean diet, traditional risk factors, and the rate of cardiovascular complications after myocardial infarction: final report of the Lyon Diet Heart Study, *Circulation* 99:779-785, 1999.

Cholesterol-Lowering Studies in Children Without Known Coronary Artery Disease
(See also obesity in childhood)

In 1992 an expert panel on blood cholesterol levels in children and adolescents convened by the National Heart, Lung, and Blood Institute recommended that all Americans over the age of 2 years reduce their dietary fat intake.[1] This same organization sponsored the Dietary Intervention Study in Children (DISC) with the goal of assessing the efficacy and safety of lowering LDL-C levels in pubescent children. The results of the study were reported in 1995.[2]

Dietary Intervention Study in Children

The children enrolled in the DISC study were between the ages of approximately 8 and 11.[2] They were initially assessed by capillary blood cholesterol measurement, and if it was above the 75th percentile, a fasting venous sample for LDL-C was obtained. If the LDL-C level was between the 70th and 99th age- and sex-specific percentiles, a second fasting venous sample was obtained. If the average of the LDL-C levels from the two venous samples was between the 70th and 99th percentiles, the children were randomly assigned to ordinary care or dietary intervention with a 3-year follow-up. The parents of children in both groups were told that their children's cholesterol levels were high, and in both groups body mass index was calculated and the hip, waist, and skinfold thickness at various sites were measured. In the dietary intervention group 28% of energy was obtained from fat of which 9% was polyunsaturated (Step 2–type diet). Over the 3-year study period children and families of the intervention group attended approximately 27 group and individual meetings and received monthly phone calls between meetings. Capillary blood cholesterol measurements were obtained periodically during individual meetings, and at the termination of the study venous samples were obtained for the measurement of a variety of parameters. The report does not mention the children's physical activities.[2]

The primary outcome of the DISC study was a decrease in LDL-C in both the intervention group and the ordinary care group. The reduction was 0.09 mmol/L (3.3 mg/dl) greater in the intervention group, which is a statistically significant difference. The intervention group showed no evidence of decreased growth or decreased ferritin levels, and in fact there was no difference in any of the anthropomorphic measurements, including sexual maturation, between the groups. Psychological measurements showed a lower adjusted mean depression score for the intervention children at 3 years.[2]

The clinical significance of the DISC trial is hard to comprehend. Normal children were labeled as having high cholesterol, and a vast amount of time and energy was devoted to altering the diets of the intervention group. One fact is obvious; even if the physician believes that measuring cholesterol levels in children and instituting a dietary program if they are high is desirable, this clinical trial has no applicability to ordinary clinical practice. What family physician or pediatrician could possibly offer 27 group and individual meetings plus interval phone calls over a 3-year period as a part of his or her regular practice?

Epidemiological data suggest that children of parents with early CAD are more likely to be obese than control subjects and that other indices of CAD risk such as elevated LDL levels appear as they grow older.[3] The benefits and drawbacks of life-style preventive interventions directed toward such children are unknown; one study reports success in controlling obesity in children with an intensive behavioral therapy program.[4]

Psychological harm of screening

Does screening children and finding them hypercholesterolemic cause psychological harm? Some studies have found that it does not.[2,5,6] However, a 1997 report from Montreal found a much higher rate of behavioral disturbances in children 12 months after they received the diagnosis of hyperlipidemia.[7]

Guidelines for cholesterol screening

The Expert Panel on Blood Cholesterol Levels in Children and Adolescents of the National Heart, Lung, and Blood Institute's National Cholesterol Education Program, the American Academy of Family Physicians, the American Academy of Pediatrics, and the American Medical Association do not recommend universal screening of cholesterol levels in children. However, if the child is over 2 and has a parent with a cholesterol level greater than 240 mg/dl (6.25 mmol/L) or if the parents or grandparents have a history of premature (under age 55) cardiovascular disease, screening is recommended.[8] Both the U.S. Preventive Services Task Force[9] and the Canadian Task Force on Preventive Health Care[10] give a "C" recommendation to general cholesterol screening of children and adolescents. The U.S. Preventive Services Task Force qualifies this by stating that a family history of very high cholesterol levels, premature coronary heart disease in a first-degree relative (before age 50 in males and before age 60 in females), or other major risk factors for coronary heart disease may be reasons for measuring cholesterol levels in adolescents or young adults.[9]

◭ REFERENCES ◮

1. Expert Panel on Blood Cholesterol Levels in Children and Adolescents: National Cholesterol Education Program report, *Pediatrics* 89(suppl):525-584, 1992.
2. Dietary Intervention Study in Children (DISC): Efficacy and safety of lowering dietary intake of fat and cholesterol in children with elevated low-density lipoprotein cholesterol, *JAMA* 273:1429-1435, 1995.
3. Bao W, Srinivasan SR, Valdez R, et al: Longitudinal changes in cardiovascular risk from childhood to young adulthood in offspring of parents with coronary artery disease: the Bogalusa Heart Study, *JAMA* 278:1749-1754, 1997.
4. Epstein LH, Valoski, Wing RR, et al: Ten-year follow-up of behavioral, family-based treatment for obese children, *JAMA* 264:2519-2523, 1990.
5. Hanna KJ, Ewart CK, Kwiterovich PO: Child problem solving competence, behavioral adjustment and adherence to lipid-lowering diet, *Patient Educ Couns* 16:119-131, 1990.
6. Rosenthal SL, Knauer-Black S, Stahl MP, et al: The psychological functioning of children with hypercholesterolemia and their families: a preliminary investigation, *Clin Pediatr* 32:135-141, 1993.
7. Rosenberg E, Lamping DL, Joseph L, et al: Cholesterol screening of children at high risk: behavioural and psychological effects, *Can Med Assoc J* 156:489-496, 1997.
8. US Public Health Service: Cholesterol screening in children, *Am Fam Physician* 51:1923-1927, 1995.
9. US Preventive Services Task Force: *Guide to clinical preventive services,* ed 2, Baltimore, 1996, Williams & Wilkins, pp 15-38.
10. Canadian Task Force on the Periodic Health Examination: *Canadian guide to clinical preventive health care,* Ottawa, 1994, Canada Communication Group—Publishing, pp 650-669.

Cholesterol-Lowering Studies and Stroke

An overview of randomized cholesterol-lowering studies involving more than 36,000 persons failed to detect a reduced incidence of strokes.[1] However, an overview of 16 randomized trials of HMG-CoA reductase inhibitors (which are among the most potent cholesterol-lowering agents) by the same authors found a 29% relative reduction in stroke rates.[2]

◭ REFERENCES ◮

1. Hebert PR, Gaziano M, Hennekens CH: An overview of trials of cholesterol lowering and risk of stroke, *Arch Intern Med* 155:50-55, 1995.
2. Hebert PR, Gaziano M, Chan KS, et al: Cholesterol lowering with statin drugs, risk of stroke, and total mortality, *JAMA* 278:313-321, 1997.

Adverse Effects Associated with Low Cholesterol Levels
Low cholesterol as a marker of increased mortality risk

A number of malignancies such as those of the lung, pancreas, rectum, bladder, liver, and kidney, as well as some nonmalignant diseases such as chronic lung disease and strokes, are associated with low cholesterol levels.[1-3] Total mortality in middle-aged and elderly patients is increased among those with the lowest cholesterol levels,[3,4] and this appears to be particularly so in those who have both a low albumin and a low cholesterol level.[5] The accepted explanation for these findings is that the disease processes themselves cause the cholesterol levels to drop even if the diseases have not yet manifested themselves clinically.[5]

Low cholesterol and aggression

A 1990 metaanalysis of controlled trials of cholesterol-lowering diets and medications by Muldoon and associates[6] showed that the incidence of cardiovascular deaths in the treated groups decreased, but not the overall mortality. In the treated groups significantly higher death rates from suicide, accidents, and violence were observed, a finding that was consistent across all studies. However, a number of more recent studies have found no such correlation.[7-9]

Carcinogenic potential of cholesterol-lowering drugs

A well-established but rarely discussed aspect of cholesterol-lowering agents is that many of them, including the fibrates such as gemfibrozil and clofibrate and the HMG-CoA reductase inhibitors such as lovastatin and pravastatin, are carcinogenic in rodents. This issue was put in the spotlight by a 1996 article in *JAMA* by Newman and Hulley.[10] They pointed out that almost all human carcinogens are also carcinogenic in rodents but that the specificity of this phenomenon is unknown. Since the latent period between exposure to a carcinogen and the development of cancer may be two decades or more, it will be a long time before it is known whether currently used statins and fibrates are carcinogenic for humans. Newman and Hulley[10] suggest that in the interval niacin or cholestyramine may be safer to use if lipid-lowering drugs are required. The concept that cholesterol-lowering drugs may be carcinogenic has been vehemently challenged in an editorial by Dalen and Dalton,[11] who point out that many cholesterol-lowering studies have not shown an increase in cancer deaths in follow-up periods of 4 to 9 years, that even if an increased rate were proved to exist, it would be small, and that animal experiments showing carcinogenicity of lipid-lowering drugs should not be taken too seriously because the doses were many times those used for humans.

Whether statins are carcinogenic in humans is not known. Even if they prove to be, their benefits will probably far outweigh this risk for patients with known CAD. Such may not be the case for asymptomatic persons whose only risk factor for CAD is an elevated cholesterol level.

------------------- ≈ **REFERENCES** ≈ -------------------

1. Wannamethee G, Shaper AG, Whincup PH, et al: Low serum total cholesterol concentrations and mortality in middle aged British men, *BMJ* 311:409-413, 1995.
2. Davey Smith G, Shipley MJ, Marmot MG, et al: Plasma cholesterol concentration and mortality: the Whitehall study, *JAMA* 267:70-76, 1992.
3. Manolio TA, Ettinger WH, Tracy RP, et al: Epidemiology of low cholesterol levels in older adults, *Circulation* 87:728-737, 1993.
4. Staessen J, Amery A, Birkenhager W, et al: Is a high serum cholesterol level associated with longer survival in elderly hypertensives? *J Hypertens* 8:755-761, 1990.
5. Reuben DB, Ix JH, Greendale GA, et al: The predictive value of combined hypoalbuminemia and hypocholesterolemia in high functioning community-dwelling older persons: MacArthur Studies of Successful Aging, *J Am Geriatr Soc* 47:402-406, 1999.
6. Muldoon MF, Manuck SB, Mathhews KA: Lowering cholesterol concentrations and mortality: a quantitative review of primary prevention trials, *BMJ* 301:309-314, 1990.
7. Scandinavian Simvastatin Survival Study Group: Randomised trial of cholesterol lowering in 4444 patients with coronary heart disease: the Scandinavian Simvastatin Survival Study (4S), *Lancet* 344:1383-1389, 1994.
8. Shepherd J, Cobbe SM, Ford I, et al: Prevention of coronary heart disease with pravastatin in men with hypercholesterolemia, *N Engl J Med* 333:1301-1307, 1995.
9. Downs JR, Clearfield M, Weis S, et al: Primary prevention of acute coronary events with lovastatin in men and women with average cholesterol levels: results of AFCAPS/TexCAPS, *JAMA* 279:1615-1622, 1998.
10. Newman TB, Hulley SB: Carcinogenicity of lipid-lowering drugs, *JAMA* 275:55-60, 1996.
11. Dalen JE, Dalton WS: Does lowering cholesterol cause cancer? (editorial), *JAMA* 275:67-69, 1996.

Guidelines for Cholesterol Screening
(See also coronary artery disease)

Many U.S. medical organizations recommend cholesterol screening for the general population of adults, whereas the recommendations of the Canadian Task Force on Preventive Health Care,[1] the U.S. Preventive Services Task Force,[2] and the American College of Physicians[3] are more restrictive. Examples of these guidelines are given in Table 44.

Ramsay, Haq, and associates[7] from Sheffield, England, have developed tables that calculate the risk of cardiovascular disease in asymptomatic patients based on sex, age, smoking, hypertension, left ventricular hypertrophy, and diabetes. According to their calculations, which are based primarily on the Framingham data,[8] even extremely high cholesterol levels in the absence of other risk factors pose relatively little threat to health (excluding cases of hereditary lipid abnormalities). Not only does this approach stringently limit the number of patients who would be screened or treated, but it also permits the selection of some patients with multiple risk factors who would merit lipid-lowering treatment even if their cholesterol levels were normal.[7]

The updated cholesterol screening recommendations of the American College of Physicians published in 1996 were based on a thorough review of the literature, which included the West of Scotland Coronary Prevention Study Group report. The College gave conditional approval to screening but stated clearly that there is no proof that lowering choles-

Table 44   Variability of Guidelines for Cholesterol Screening

Organization	Recommendation
American Academy of Family Physicians	Every 5 years starting at age 19[4]
American College of Obstetricians and Gynecologists	All women over 20 and selected high-risk adolescents[5]
American College of Physicians	Appropriate but not mandatory for men aged 35-65 and women aged 45-65; insufficient evidence for or against those 65-75; not recommended for those over 75[3]
National Cholesterol Education Program	At least once every 5 years after age 20[6]
U.S. Preventive Services Task Force	Men aged 35-65 and women aged 45-65 ("B" recommendation); interval of screening uncertain—probably 5 years[2]; insufficient evidence for or against screening those over 65 ("C" recommendation)[2]
Canadian Task Force on Preventive Health Care	Case finding in men 30-59 ("C" recommendation)[1]
Sheffield risk and treatment tables	Screening should be limited to patients with multiple risk factors—sex, age, smoking, hypertension, left ventricular hypertrophy, and diabetes[7]

terol prolongs life.[9] *A British Medical Journal* editorial points out that not only is there is no evidence proving that unselective population screening is beneficial, but labeling large numbers of people as ill may have deleterious effects.[10]

An elevated cholesterol level is unquestionably a risk factor for vascular disease. However, it is just one of many. Who should be screened and, if the cholesterol level is elevated, receive pharmacotherapy is a matter of controversy. As a family physician who wants to be sure that I am not doing more harm than good (see "Prevention"), I find the Sheffield risk and treatment tables appealing. Even if they are too restrictive for the taste of many of us, they emphasize that significant risk of coronary artery disease is related to multiple risk factors, not just to elevated cholesterol level.

⚓ REFERENCES ⚓

1. Canadian Task Force on the Periodic Health Examination: *Canadian guide to clinical preventive health care,* Ottawa, 1994, Canada Communication Group—Publishing, pp 650-669.
2. US Preventive Services Task Force: *Guide to clinical preventive services,* ed 2, Baltimore, 1996, Williams & Wilkins, pp 15-38.
3. American College of Physicians: Clinical guideline. I. Guidelines for using serum cholesterol, high-density lipoprotein cholesterol, and triglyceride levels as screening tests for preventing coronary heart disease in adults, *Ann Intern Med* 124:515-517, 1996.
4. American Academy of Family Physicians: *Age charts for periodic health examination,* Kansas City, Mo, 1994, American Academy of Family Physicians, Reprint No 510.
5. American College of Obstetricians and Gynecologists: The obstetrician-gynecologist in primary preventive health care: a report of the ACOG Task Force on Primary and Preventive Health Care, Washington, DC, 1993, American College of Obstetricians and Gynecologists.
6. Expert Panel on Detection, Evaluation, and Treatment of High Blood Cholesterol in Adults: Summary of the second report of the National Cholesterol Education Program (NCEP) Expert Panel on the Detection, Evaluation, and Treatment of High Blood Cholesterol in Adults (Adult Treatment Panel II), *JAMA* 269:3015-3023, 1993.
7. Ramsay LE, Haq IU, Jackson PR, et al: Targeting lipid lowering drug therapy for primary prevention of coronary disease: an updated Sheffield table, *Lancet* 348:387-388, 1996.
8. Anderson KM, Odell PM, Wilson PW, et al: Cardiovascular disease risk profiles, *Am Heart J* 121:293-298, 1991.
9. Garber AM, Browner WS, Hulley SB (American College of Physicians): Clinical guideline. II. Cholesterol screening in asymptomatic adults, revisited, *Ann Intern Med* 124:518-531, 1996.
10. Fahey T: Assessing heart disease risk in primary care: cholesterol lowering should be just one part of a multiple risk factor intervention, *BMJ* 317:1093-1094, 1998.

Treatment of Elevated Lipid Levels

(See also adverse effects associated with lowering cholesterol levels; antioxidants; cardiac arrest; cholesterol-lowering studies in patients with coronary artery disease; cholesterol-lowering studies in patients without coronary artery disease; prevention; risk factors for stroke)

Guidelines for who should be treated for elevated lipids

A variety of guidelines have been presented for the treatment of elevated lipids, four of which are listed below:

1. National Cholesterol Education Program II (NCEP II) treatment criteria. These guidelines recommend treating all adult males under the age of 35 and all adult premenopausal females if the LDL-C level is 5.7 mmol/L (220 mg/dl) or higher. For men aged 35 or over and for postmenopausal women treatment is recommended if the LDL-C is 4.9 mmol/L (190 mg/dl) or higher or if the LDL-C is 4.1 to 4.9 mmol/L (160 to 190 mg/dl) and the patient has two or more additional risk factors. Additional risk factors are age greater than 45 for men and 55 for women, family history of premature CAD (under 55 if male and 65 if female), current smoking, hypertension, diabetes mellitus, and HDL-C level less than 0.91 mmol/L (35 mg/dl). One point is subtracted from the total risk factors if the HDL-C is 1.6 mmol/L (60 mg/dl) or higher.[1]

2. Modified NCEP II treatment criteria. The guidelines are similar to those of the NCEP II except that every decade over 35 in men and over 45 in women is considered an additional risk factor, and an extra risk fac-

tor is added if the LDL-C level is 5.2 mmol/L (200 mg/dl) or higher.[2]

3. Sheffield risk and treatment tables. Multiple risk factors are assessed to determine which patients are likely to benefit from lipid-lowering protocols (see reference to obtain tables).[3]

4. Canadian nomogram for risk assessment and treatment. Multiple risk factors are assessed to determine which patients are likely to benefit from lipid-lowering protocols (see reference to obtain nomogram).[4]

An underlying principle of all these guidelines—but particularly emphasized by the Sheffield risk and treatment tables[3] and the Canadian nomogram[4]—is that single risk factors such as elevated cholesterol levels in the absence of other risk factors have relatively little import. McCormack and co-workers[4] also make the point that even if treatment decreases overall statistical risk of CAD, only a very small percentage of those treated will actually benefit (the number of patients that must be treated to prevent one clinical event is large).

Target lipid levels

For treatment of hypercholesterolemia the National Cholesterol Educational Program recommends the following target levels[1]:

No CAD and fewer than two risk factors	LDL <4.1 mmol/L (160 mg/dl)
No CAD and two risk factors	LDL <3.4 mmol/L (130 mg/dl)
Established CAD	LDL <2.6 mmol/L (100 mg/dl) and HDL-C >1 mmol/L (40 mg/dl)

Lipid levels in postmenopausal women who are undergoing cyclical hormone replacement therapy may fluctuate considerably from one phase of the cycle to another. If such women are treated with lipid-lowering agents, lipid levels should be monitored at consistent periods of the cycle.[5]

Diet

The usual protocol for lowering blood cholesterol is to begin with a 3- to 6-month trial of diet and to add drugs only if dietary changes are unsuccessful. As far as I know, until the publication of the effects of a Mediterranean diet on patients with known CAD (see discussion of cholesterol-lowering studies in patients with CAD),[6-8] no studies showed a total cohort decrease in mortality from diet alone. While studies from metabolic wards have shown that diet can lower cholesterol by 10% to 15%, dietary advice in outpatient settings usually results in only about a 5% decrease.[9]

The Mediterranean diet that was so effective in decreasing cardiovascular events and deaths in post–myocardial infarction patients did not change the serum concentration of total, low-density, or high-density cholesterol.[7,8] The diet

was high in linolenic and oleic acid, relatively low in saturated fatty acids and linoleic acid, and high in some antioxidant vitamins.[6,8] The reason for its efficacy is unknown, but constituents such as omega-3 fatty acids, oleic acid, and antioxidant vitamins may be cardioprotective (see discussion of antioxidants).[1,6]

A Mediterranean diet has a high content of oil, particularly olive oil or canola (rapeseed) oil, complex carbohydrates such as bread and pasta, fruits, vegetables, fish, and poultry. It has a low content of beef, pork, and other meats, and the amount of cheese and wine consumed is moderate. More specifically, patients on this diet are instructed to eat the following[7]:

1. More bread
2. More vegetables
3. More fish
4. Less beef, lamb, and pork (to be replaced with poultry)
5. Fruit daily
6. No butter or cream (in the study a special margarine based on canola oil was provided)
7. Olive oil or canola oil (rapeseed without erucic acid) to be used exclusively for preparing foods and salad dressings

A number of studies have shown that fish consumption (which does not lower LDL levels) is associated with a decreased rate of sudden cardiac death. This is discussed under "Cardiac Arrest."

Pharmacotherapy

The treatment of elevated lipids with any class of drugs is a lifelong undertaking. When medications are stopped, cholesterol levels almost always rise to pretreatment levels.[10] As discussed previously, many of the indications for treating lipid disorders are controversial in part because of possible or proven adverse effects. The bulk of evidence strongly supports the use of cholesterol-lowering drugs in patients with known CAD, and they are likely to be used more and more frequently for asymptomatic individuals with multiple risk factors for CAD. For better or worse, they will probably also be used with increasing frequency in asymptomatic patients whose only risk factor is hypercholesterolemia. The National Cholesterol Educational Program (NCEP II) estimated that if its recommendations were followed, 7% of U.S. adults would be taking cholesterol-lowering drugs and 30% would be following nonpharmacological regimens to lower cholesterol.[1]

Immediately after a myocardial infarction, lipid levels often drop significantly, so lipid-lowering treatment programs should be based on figures obtained 8 weeks after the event.[11]

A wide variety of lipid-lowering drugs are available (Table 45), and the choice depends on numerous variables. All the lipid-lowering drugs lower LDL-C, and niacin (nicotinic acid) and the fibrates such as gemfibrozil are particularly effective in lowering triglycerides. Whether lowering

Table 45   Lipid-Lowering Drugs

Drugs	Usual doses
Bile Acid Sequestrants	
Cholestyramine (Questran)	4 g 1-6 times per day
Fibrates	
Bezafibrate (Bezalip)	200 mg tid
Clofibrate (Atromid-S)	Not recommended
Fenofibrate (Lipidil)	100 mg tid with meals
Micronized fenofibrate (Tricor)	67-201 mg once daily with a meal
Gemfibrozil (Lopid)	600 mg bid
HMG-CoA Reductase Inhibitors	
Atorvastatin (Lipitor)	20-80 mg/day, with evening meal
Cerivastatin (Baycol)	0.2-0.3 mg/day in the evening
Fluvastatin (Lescol)	20-40 mg/day in the evening
Lovastatin (Mevacor)	20-80 mg/day with the evening meal
Pravastatin (Pravachol)	10-40 mg/day in the evening
Simvastatin (Zocor)	20-40 mg/day in the evening
Niacin Derivatives	
Niacin, nicotinic acid	1-6 g/day in 2-4 divided doses
Niacin extended release (Niaspan)	1-3 g hs
Other Lipid-Lowering Drugs	
Probucol (Lorelco)	500 mg bid
Psyllium (Metamucil)	5-15 g/day (1-3 rounded teaspoons)

triglycerides significantly reduces the morbidity or mortality of CAD is unknown. The HMG-CoA reductase inhibitors are potent and can be taken once daily, but they are more expensive than some of the other drugs. Nicotinic acid is inexpensive, available over the counter, and often effective. It not only lowers total cholesterol, LDL-C, and triglycerides, but also is more effective in raising HDL than any other drug.[10] However, for many patients its side effects are unacceptable for long-term treatment. In one study 43% of patients discontinued the drug for this reason.[12] The efficacy of nicotinic acid is related to the dose, but even doses as low as 1.5 g/day may be effective in raising HDL.[13] Flushing caused by nicotinic acid can be diminished by pretreatment with aspirin or ibuprofen (Advil, Motrin), and adverse effects may be diminished by using a newly marketed extended-release formulation (Niaspan).[10,14] Adaptation to side effects may be improved by initiating treatment with small doses and increasing them gradually.

Probucol (Lorelco) is a weak cholesterol-lowering agent and is no longer available in the United States, in part because it lowers HDL as well as LDL.[15] It is, however, a potent antioxidant that significantly decreases the rate of restenosis in patients undergoing angioplasty.[16]

Soluble fiber such as psyllium (Metamucil) in doses of 5 to 15 g/day (1 to 3 rounded teaspoons) may reduce cholesterol by a small amount.[17,18] The drug appears to be most effective if given with rather than between meals.[19]

REFERENCES

1. National Cholesterol Education Program: *The second report of the Expert Panel on Detection, Evaluation, and Treatment of High Blood Cholesterol in Adults.* (Adult Treatment Panel II.) Bethesda, Md, 1993, National Heart, Lung, and Blood Institute, National Institutes of Health, NIH Pub No 93-3095.
2. Avins AL, Browner WS: Improving the prediction of coronary heart disease to aid in the management of high cholesterol levels, *JAMA* 279:445-449, 1998.
3. Haq IU, Jackson PR, Yeo WW, et al: Sheffield risk and treatment table for cholesterol lowering for primary prevention of coronary heart disease, *Lancet* 346:1467-1471, 1995.
4. McCormack JP, Levine M, Rangno RE: Primary prevention of heart disease and stroke: a simplified approach to estimating risk of events and making drug treatment decisions, *Can Med Assoc J* 157:422-428, 1997.
5. Weintraub MS, Grosskopf I, Charach G, et al: Fluctuations of lipid and lipoprotein levels in hyperlipidemic postmenopausal women receiving hormone replacement therapy, *Arch Intern Med* 158:1803-1806, 1998.
6. De Lorgeril M, Salen P, Martin J-L, et al: Effect of a Mediterranean type of diet on the rate of cardiovascular complications in patients with coronary artery disease: insights into the cardioprotective effect of certain nutriments, *J Am Coll Cardiol* 28:1103-1108, 1996.
7. Renaud S, de Lorgeril M, Delaye J, et al: Cretan Mediterranean diet for prevention of coronary heart disease, *Am J Clin Nutr* 61(suppl):1360S-1367S, 1995.
8. De Lorgeril, Renaud S, Mamelle N, et al: Mediterranean alpha-linolenic acid-rich diet in secondary prevention of coronary heart disease, *Lancet* 343:1454-1459, 1994.
9. Tang JL, Armitage JM, Lancaster T, et al: Systematic review of dietary intervention trials to lower blood total cholesterol in free-living subjects, *BMJ* 316:1213-1220, 1998.
10. Choice of lipid-lowering drugs, *Med Lett* 38:67-70, 1996.
11. Dafoe W, Huston P: Current trends in cardiac rehabilitation, *Can Med Assoc J* 156:527-532, 1997.
12. Gibbons LW, Gonzalez V, Gordon N, et al: The prevalence of side effects with regular and sustained-release nicotinic acid, *Am J Med* 99:378-385, 1995.
13. Martin-Jadraque R, Tato F, Mostaza JM, et al: Effectiveness of low-dose crystalline nicotinic-acid in men with low high-density lipoprotein cholesterol levels, *Arch Intern Med* 156:1081-1088, 1996.
14. Guyton JR, Goldberg AC, Kreisberg RA, et al: Effectiveness of once-nightly dosing of extended-release niacin alone and in combination for hypercholesterolemia, *Am J Cardiol* 82:737-743, 1998.
15. Libby P, Ganz P: Restenosis revisited—new targets, new therapies (editorial), *N Engl J Med* 337:418-419, 1997.
16. Tardif J-C, Coté G, Lespérance J, et al (Multivitamins and Probucol Study Group): Probucol and multivitamins in the prevention of restenosis after coronary angioplasty, *N Engl J Med* 337:365-372, 1997.
17. Glore SR, Van Treeck D, Knehans AW, et al: Soluble fiber and serum lipids: a literature review, *J Am Dietetic Assoc* 94:425-436, 1994.

18. Wolever TM, Jenkins DJ, Mueller S, et al: Psyllium reduces blood lipids in men and women with hyperlipidemia, *Am J Med Sci* 307:269-273, 1994.

19. Wolever TM, Jenkins DJ, Mueller S, et al: Method of administration influences the serum cholesterol-lowering effect of psyllium, *Am J Clin Nutr* 59:1055-1059, 1994.

OSTEOPOROSIS

(See also celiac disease; female athletes; geriatrics; hip fractures; hormone replacement therapy; hyperparathyroidism; tamoxifen)

Epidemiology

(See also hip fractures)

Peak bone mass is reached at about age 25 and is about 20% less in women than in men. After age 35, bone mass declines by about 0.5% to 1% per year in both men and women. Between ages 50 and 80 a woman's bone density decreases 30%. In the first 10 years after menopause the decline is about 3% to 5% per year. Men lose about two thirds as much bone mass as women; their rate of bone loss increases after age 65.[1]

Osteoporotic fracture occurs in an estimated 25% of white women over the age of 60. The common sites are the distal radius, hip, ribs, and vertebral bodies. Vertebral fractures in women 50 to 60 years of age are 10 times as common as they are in men of similar age, and hip fractures occur twice as often in women as in men. Patients with osteoporotic hip fractures are usually over 75, and the median age for such fractures in postmenopausal women is 80.[2] Mortality from hip fractures is between 10% and 25% in the first year, many patients lose mobility, and up to 25% require nursing care.[3]

An assessment of proximal femur bone density in a sample of U.S. postmenopausal women who had never used exogenous hormones found 17% to be osteoporotic. Only 7% of the identified women were previously aware that they had osteoporosis.[4]

─────────── ◪ **REFERENCES** ◪ ───────────

1. Scientific Advisory Board, Osteoporosis Society of Canada: Clinical practice guidelines for the diagnosis and management of osteoporosis, *Can Med Assoc J* 155:1113-1133, 1996.

2. Lees B, Molleson T, Asnett T: Differences in proximal femur bone density over two centuries, *Lancet* 341:673-675, 1993.

3. Kelly PJ, Eisman JA, Sambrook PN: Interaction of genetic and environmental influences on peak bone density, *Osteoporosis Int* 1:56-60, 1990.

4. Osteoporosis among estrogen-deficient women—United States 1988-1994, *MMWR* 47:969-973, 1998.

Risk Factors for Osteoporosis

(See also anorexia nervosa; vitamin A)

Recognized risk factors for osteoporosis are listed in Table 46. There is a poor correlation between these risk factors and the bone density of individual patients. Some of these risk factors are discussed in more depth below.

Table 46   Risk Factors for Osteoporosis

Race	**Medical Conditions**
White	Surgically induced early
Asian	menopause
Age	Hypogonadism
Old age	Cushing's disease
Genetics	Thyrotoxicosis
Female sex	Hyperparathyroidism
Thin habitus	Anorexia nervosa
Early menopause	Multiple myeloma
Family history of osteoporosis	Intestinal malabsorption
Life-Style	Gastrectomy
Smoking	Rheumatoid arthritis
Excessive use of alcohol	**Medications**
Sedentary life-style	Long-term corticosteroid use
Excessive exercise causing	Anticonvulsant medications
amenorrhea	Long-term heparin therapy
Inadequate nutrition causing	Long-term oral anticoagulants
low weight	Long-term lithium use
Inadequate calcium intake	Chemotherapy
Inadequate vitamin D	Thyroid replacement?
(or sunlight)	
Excessive vitamin A	

Body weight

Thin women are at significantly greater risk of hip fracture than heavy women.[1,2]

Smoking

Smoking is associated with an increased fracture rate in postmenopausal women. On the basis of a metaanalysis, Law and Hackshaw[3] estimated that one in eight hip fractures was a result of smoking. The mechanism by which smoking aggravates osteoporosis is unknown.[3]

Corticosteroids

Patients on long-term oral corticosteroid treatment in doses equivalent to 7.5 mg/day or more lose bone density and have twice the risk of hip and radius fractures and four times the risk of vertebral fractures.[4]

Thyroid replacement therapy

A metaanalysis of numerous studies has shown substantial decreases in bone mass in patients treated with thyroxine.[5] However, the current view is that if the thyroid-stimulating hormone level is kept within normal limits, osteopenia does not occur.[6]

─────────── ◪ **REFERENCES** ◪ ───────────

1. Pruzansky ME, Tuarano M, Luckey M, et al: Low body weight as a risk factor for hip fracture in both black and white women, *J Orthop Res* 7:192-197, 1989.

2. Grisso JA, Kelsey JL, Strom BL, et al: Risk factors for hip fracture in black women, *N Engl J Med* 330:1555-1559, 1994.

3. Law MR, Hackshaw AK: A meta-analysis of cigarette smoking, bone mineral density and risk of hip fracture: recognition of a major effect, *BMJ* 315:841-846, 1997.
4. Lips P: Prevention of corticosteroid induced osteoporosis (editorial), *BMJ* 318:1366-1367, 1999.
5. Uzzan B, Campos J, Cucherat M, et al: Effects on bone mass of long term treatment with thyroid hormones: a meta-analysis, *J Clin Endocrinol Metab* 81:4278-4289, 1996.
6. Gharib H, Mazzaferri EL: Thyroxine suppressive therapy in patients with nodular thyroid disease, *Ann Intern Med* 128:386-394, 1998.

Bone Density

The following are some of the techniques for measuring bone density:

1. Dual photon absorptiometry (DPA)
2. Dual energy x-ray absorptiometry (DXA, DEXA); by use of a dual beam the absorption caused by soft tissues can be calculated and more accurate bone densities assessed; this is currently the standard technique
3. Quantitative computerized tomography (QCT); this is accurate but causes more radiation and costs more than DXA
4. Ultrasound; this is a new technology that may not yet be fully standardized

The evidence that bone densitometry can identify individuals who will sustain fractures is not well established.[1,2] The arguments against using bone density measurements as a screening tool are that a great overlap exists between the bone densities of those who have fractures and those who do not, compliance with such a screening program is unknown, and the effectiveness of preventive interventions for fractures is not well established.[2] Screening all perimenopausal women could be beneficial only if those with low bone densities were willing to comply with prophylactic interventions such as taking hormone replacement therapy or bisphosphonates (see discussion of prevention of osteoporosis).[3] The U.S. Preventive Services Task Force gives a "C" recommendation to bone density screening of all postmenopausal women,[4] while the Canadian Task Force on Preventive Health Care gives it a "D" recommendation.[5] The U.S. National Osteoporosis Foundation advises bone density studies for all women over the age of 65 and for postmenopausal women under the age of 65 who have additional risk factors for osteoporosis.[6]

In selected cases bone density measurements may be very useful. They should be ordered for all patients receiving long-term corticosteroid therapy and for young women with prolonged amenorrhea.[3,7] Bone density studies may help patients and physicians decide whether to initiate hormone replacement therapy after menopause, and they are essential for monitoring treatment programs for established osteoporosis. For the latter indication, follow-up measurements should not be obtained at intervals less than a year.[8]

Radiation exposure from DXA is low, about 300 times less than that received from a standard chest x-ray.[7]

◀ **REFERENCES** ▶

1. Wilkin TJ: Changing perceptions in osteoporosis, *BMJ* 318:862-865, 1999.
2. Marshall D, Johnell O, Wedel H: Meta-analysis of how well measures of bone mineral density predict occurrence of osteoporotic fractures, *BMJ* 312:1254-1259, 1996.
3. Fogelman I: Screening for osteoporosis: no point until we have resolved issues about long term treatment (editorial), *BMJ* 319:1148-1149, 1999.
4. US Preventive Services Task Force: *Guide to clinical preventive services,* ed 2, Baltimore, 1996, Williams & Wilkins, pp 509-516.
5. Canadian Task Force on the Periodic Health Examination: *Canadian guide to clinical preventive health care,* Ottawa, 1994, Canada Communication Group—Publishing, pp 620-631.
6. National Osteoporosis Foundation: *The physician's guide to prevention and treatment of osteoporosis,* Washington, DC, 1998, The Foundation.
7. Lips P: Prevention of corticosteroid induced osteoporosis (editorial), *BMJ* 318:1366-1367, 1999.
8. Sturtridge W, Lentle B, Hanley DA: The use of bone density measurement in the diagnosis and management of osteoporosis, *Can Med Assoc J* 155:924-929, 1996.

Prevention of Osteoporosis

(See also exercise; hip fractures; hormone replacement therapy; prevention of corticosteroid-induced osteoporosis; surrogate outcomes)

Any reversible medical or life-style risk factors for osteoporosis should be eliminated if possible; smoking and excessive alcohol use are high on the list. Other specific interventions that may be used are discussed in the ensuing paragraphs.

Calcium and vitamin D supplementation

Whether calcium supplementation inhibits the development of osteoporosis is controversial, but the bulk of the evidence suggests that it does. For example, Reid and associates[1] from Auckland, New Zealand, studied 122 healthy women who were at least 3 years postmenopausal and whose mean dietary calcium intake was 750 mg/day. They treated one cohort with calcium supplements of 1000 mg/day. At the end of 4 years the rate of appendicular and axial bone loss was significantly lower in the calcium-treated group.[1] There is also evidence that supplementation with both vitamin D and calcium may decrease the risk of osteoporosis.[2,3]

The National Institutes of Health has recommended the following daily allowances of calcium[4]:

Children 1-10 years	800-1200 mg/day
Adolescents and young adults 11-24	1200-1500 mg/day
Pregnant and lactating women	1200-1500 mg/day
Adult men ages 25-65	1000 mg/day
Adult women ages 25-50	1000 mg/day
Postmenopausal women 51-65 on estrogens	1000 mg/day
Postmenopausal women 51-65 not taking estrogens	1500 mg/day
Everyone over the age of 65	1500 mg/day

The basic North American diet without dairy products provides a daily intake of 300 to 400 mg of calcium. One 8-ounce (250-ml) glass of 1% or 2% milk contains 300 mg of calcium. Other good sources of calcium, supplying about 300 mg per serving, are firm cheeses (45 g or 1½ ounces), canned salmon (125 ml or ½ cup), and canned sardines (seven medium sized) if the bones are eaten. In addition, 125 ml or ½ cup of tofu has about 150 mg, 250 ml or 1 cup of cooked soy beans about 200 mg, and 125 ml or ½ cup of dry-roasted almonds about 200 mg.[5]

It would seem reasonable to recommend that all post-menopausal women, as well as all men over the age of 65, take daily supplements of 1000 to 1500 of "elemental" calcium and 400 to 800 IU of vitamin D (most multivitamins contain 400 IU of vitamin D). A large number of calcium products are available without prescription. Most of them are in the form of calcium carbonate. In choosing a product or prescribing a dose, it is important that the dose be based on the milligrams of "elemental calcium" in each tablet, not the milligrams of calcium carbonate. Absorption of calcium supplements is most effective if no more than 500 mg is taken at one time and if the tablets are taken with meals.[6] Calcium supplements are available in liquid form, as tablets to be dissolved in water, as chewable tablets, or as tablets or capsules to be swallowed. Some of the tablets are large, so many patients prefer chewable forms such as Tums, Os-Cal, and Caltrate.

Exercise

Femoral neck bone densities of the skeletons of premeno-pausal and postmenopausal women buried in the crypt of Christ Church, Spitalfields, London, between 1729 and 1852 were significantly greater than those of present-day women. The probable explanation was a greater degree of physical activity in these 18th- and 19th-century women.[7] Studies of living 20th-century women confirm that exercise correlates with a decrease in hip fractures.[8,9] High-intensity strength training has been shown to increase bone density, muscle mass, overall strength, overall physical activity levels, and dynamic balance.[8] Probably the observed decrease in hip fractures among physically active women is due not only to greater bone density, but also to improved balance, muscle strength, reaction time, and coordination.[9]

Hormone replacement therapy

Hormone replacement therapy with oral estrogens and progestins not only decreases the rate of bone loss but also increases bone density.[3,10,11] One study found that the combination of calcium, vitamin D, and low-dose hormone replacement therapy increased bone density to a greater extent than was seen with calcium and vitamin D supplementation alone,[3] while a systematic review of hormone replacement therapy and osteoporosis concluded that the addition of calcium supplements significantly augmented the beneficial effects of the hormones.[12]

Maintenance of good bone density through hormone replacement therapy might be expected to correlate with a decreased fracture risk, and this is actually the case, with certain provisos. The most important of these is that protection seems to be limited to women who are currently taking hormones. Women who have discontinued hormones, even after many years of use, appear to lose any benefit.[13-15] Although the Study of Osteoporotic Fractures Research Group found that women started taking hormones more than 5 years after menopause received little benefit,[13] a study of women aged 60 to 98 showed that those who initiated hormone replacement therapy after age 60 and who continued to take it had bone densities almost equal to women of similar ages who had been taking hormones continuously since the menopause.[14]

Although most studies documenting a decreased risk of osteoporosis in women on estrogen replacement therapy used doses of conjugate estrogen (Premarin) of 0.625 mg or the equivalent (1.25 mg of estropipate [Ogen], 1 mg of estradiol [Estrace], and 0.02 mg of ethinyl estradiol [Estinyl]), a 2-year study by Genant and associates[16] suggested that 0.3 mg might be almost as effective. Recker and associates[3] found that elderly women taking conjugated equine estrogen 0.3 mg/day and medroxyprogesterone (Provera) 2.5 mg/day plus calcium and vitamin D supplements had a significant increase in bone density.[3]

One study of hip fractures found that serious underlying medical conditions were often a major factor leading to the falls that caused the fractures. In these cases the mortality associated with the fractures was due largely to the underlying medical conditions and would probably not have been altered by preventive interventions such as hormone replacement therapy.[17]

Even if prolonged estrogen replacement therapy is desirable, it may be difficult to achieve. In one British study 39% of the women for whom hormone replacement therapy was recommended because of low bone density either stopped the therapy prematurely or never started it.[18]

One of the most important issues regarding hormone replacement therapy for preventing osteoporosis is the risk/benefit ratio. As noted in the discussion of hormone replacement therapy, far more postmenopausal women will die of cardiovascular disease than as a result of complications from hip fractures, so from the point of view of mortality the prevention of cardiovascular disease takes precedence. This does not appear to create a conflict, since observational studies have shown that hormone replacement therapy decreases the risks of both disorders. (Whether hormone replacement therapy actually decreases coronary artery disease is now being disputed—see section on hormone replacement therapy.) However, after 10 years of hormone use the risk of breast cancer mortality rises sufficiently to vitiate much of the apparent benefit achieved through a decrease in CAD (see discussion of hormone replacement therapy).[19] Therefore lifetime prescriptions for hormones may do more harm than good.[19,20] If this is so, exercise, calcium and vitamin D supplements, and in some cases bisphosphonates (see below) are the preventive measures of choice.

Bisphosphonates

Alendronate (Fosamax) in doses of 5 mg/day was found to prevent bone loss in healthy postmenopausal women under the age of 60 approximately as well as standard hormonal replacement therapy.[21] In elderly women who have already sustained one or more osteoporotic fractures, alendronate has been shown to increase bone density and markedly reduce the number of subsequent fractures.[22] Selectively treating only women at high risk (those who suffer fractures) may be a reasonable alternative to prolonged hormone replacement therapy.[22,23] The role of bisphosphonates in the treatment of corticosteroid-induced osteoporosis is discussed in the next section.

Selective estrogen receptor modulators

Selective estrogen receptor modulators include drugs such as tamoxifen (Nolvadex) and raloxifene (Evista) that have agonist effects on some tissues and antagonist effects on others. Raloxifene has been approved by the Food and Drug Administration for the prevention of osteoporosis. It has agonist effects on bones but antagonist effects on breast and endometrium. The usual dose for the prevention of osteoporosis is 60 mg/day. Long-term efficacy and the drug's relative value compared with other preventive measures have not yet been determined.[24]

❧ REFERENCES ❧

1. Reid IR, Ames RW, Evans MC, et al: Long-term effects of calcium supplementation on bone loss and fractures in postmenopausal women: a randomized controlled trial, *Am J Med* 98:331-335, 1995.
2. Dawson-Hughes B, Harris SS, Krall EA, et al: Effect of calcium and vitamin D supplementation on bone density in men and women 65 years of age or older, *N Engl J Med* 337:670-676, 1997.
3. Recker RR, Davies M, Dowd RM, et al: The effect of low-dose continuous estrogen and progesterone therapy with calcium and vitamin D on bone in elderly women: a randomized, controlled trial, *Ann Intern Med* 130:897-904, 1999.
4. NIH releases consensus statement on optimal calcium intake, *Am Fam Physician* 50:1385-1387, 1994.
5. Miller A: 10 practical answers in dietary counselling, *Patient Care Can* 6:22-49, 1995.
6. Calcium supplements, *Med Lett* 38:108-109, 1996.
7. Lees B, Molleson T, Asnett T: Differences in proximal femur bone density over two centuries, *Lancet* 341:673-675, 1993.
8. Nelson ME, Fiatarone MA, Morganti CM, et al: Effects of high-intensity strength training on multiple risk factors for osteoporotic fractures: a randomized controlled trial, *JAMA* 272:1909-1914, 1994.
9. Gregg EW, Cauley JA, Seeley DG, et al: Physical activity and osteoporotic fracture risk in older women, *Ann Intern Med* 129:81-88, 1998.
10. Writing Group for the PEPI Trial: Effects of hormone therapy on bone mineral density: results from the Postmenopausal Estrogen/Progestin Interventions (PEPI) Trial, *JAMA* 276:1389-1396, 1996.
11. Speroff L, Rowan J, Symons J, et al (CHART Study Group): The comparative effect on bone density, endometrium, and lipids of continuous hormones as replacement therapy (CHART Study), *JAMA* 276:1397-1403, 1996.
12. Nieves JW, Komar L, Cosman F, et al: Calcium potentiates the effect of estrogen and calcitonin on bone mass: review and analysis, *Am J Clin Nutr* 67:18-24, 1998.
13. Cauley JA, Seeley DG, Ensrud K, et al (Study of Osteoporotic Fractures Research Group): Estrogen replacement therapy and fractures in older women, *Ann Intern Med* 122:9-16, 1995.
14. Schneider DL, Barrett-Connor EL, Morton DJ: Timing of postmenopausal estrogen for optimal bone mineral density: the Rancho Bernardo Study, *JAMA* 277:543-547, 1997.
15. Michaëlsson K, Baron JA, Farahmand BY, et al: Hormone replacement therapy and risk of hip fracture: population based case-control study, *BMJ* 316:1858-1863, 1998.
16. Genant HK, Lucas J, Weiss S, et al: Low-dose esterified estrogen therapy: effects on bone, plasma estradiol concentrations, endometrium, and lipid levels, *Arch Intern Med* 2609-2615, 1997.
17. Browner WS, Pressman AR, Nevitt MC, et al (Study of Osteoporotic Fractures Research Group): Mortality following fractures in older women, *Arch Intern Med* 156:1521-1525, 1996.
18. Ryan PJ, Harrison R, Blake GM, et al: Compliance with hormone replacement therapy (HRT) after screening for post menopausal osteoporosis, *Br J Obstet Gynaecol* 99:325-328, 1992.
19. Grodstein F, Stampfer MJ, Colditz A, et al: Postmenopausal hormone therapy and mortality, *N Engl J Med* 336:1769-1775, 1997.
20. Brinton LA, Schairer C: Postmenopausal hormone-replacement therapy—time for a reappraisal? (editorial), *N Engl J Med* 336:1821-1822, 1997.
21. Hosking D, Chilvers CE, Christiansen C, et al: Prevention of bone loss with alendronate in postmenopausal women under 60 years of age, *N Engl J Med* 338:485-492, 1998.
22. Ensrud KE, Black DM, Palermo L, et al: Treatment with alendronate prevents fractures in women at highest risk: results from the Fracture Intervention Trial, *Arch Intern Med* 157:2617-2624, 1997.
23. Maricic M: Early prevention vs late treatment for osteoporosis (editorial), *Arch Intern Med* 1545-1546, 1997.
24. Raloxifene for postmenopausal osteoporosis, *Med Lett* 40:29-30, 1998.

Prevention of Corticosteroid-Induced Osteoporosis

According to one study, treatment with calcium carbonate 1000 mg/day plus 500 IU of vitamin D_3 to patients receiving long-term corticosteroids prevented bone loss.[1] A similar study showed equivocal benefits.[2] Regular use of a bisphosphonate, etidronate (Didronel)[3] or alendronate (Fosamax),[4] has increased bone density in patients receiving long-term corticosteroid therapy.

The 1996 American College of Rheumatology Task Force on Osteoporosis Guidelines recommended preventive therapy for all patients likely to be taking long-term corticosteroids in doses of 7.5 mg or more of prednisone daily. Bone density measurements are indicated for most patients. Everyone should take calcium and vitamin D supplements and maintain a program of weight-bearing exercises, and women should receive hormone replacement therapy, especially if their bone density is low. Thiazide diuretics increase the absorption of calcium from the gastrointestinal tract and decrease its urinary excretion. Therefore the addition of hydrochlorothiazide in doses of 25 mg or less may be helpful, especially in patients excreting more than 300 mg of calcium in their urine over a 24-hour period. The guidelines also suggested that if postmenopausal women were unable to take replacement hormones, consideration be given to a bisphosphonate such as etidronate or alendronate or to use of calcitonin (Calcimar).[5]

Recent guidelines from Great Britain also target individuals taking 7.5 mg of prednisone or the equivalent per day. Treatment is recommended for all patients over 65 years of age and anyone taking 15 mg or more of prednisone or the equivalent per day. Other patients require treatment if bone densities are decreased. The treatment of choice is bisphosphonates. The role of hormone replacement therapy is less clear; according to one editorial writer it should only be considered for women who do not respond to bisphosphonates.[6]

_____ ◢ **REFERENCES** ◣ _____

1. Buckley LM, Leib ES, Cartularo KS, et al: Calcium and vitamin D-3 supplementation prevents bone loss in the spine secondary to low-dose corticosteroids in patients with rheumatoid arthritis—a randomized, double-blind, placebo-controlled trial, *Ann Intern Med* 125:961-968, 1996.
2. Adachi JD, Bensen WG, Bianchi F, et al: Vitamin D and calcium in the prevention of corticosteroid induced osteoporosis—a 3 year follow-up, *J Rheumatol* 23:995-1000, 1996.
3. Adachi JD, Bensen W, Brown J, et al: Intermittent etidronate therapy to prevent corticosteroid-induced osteoporosis, *N Engl J Med* 337:382-387, 1997.
4. Saag KG, Emkey R, Schnitzer TJ, et al: Alendronate for the prevention and treatment of glucocorticoid-induced osteoporosis, *N Engl J Med* 339:292-299, 1998.
5. Hochberg MC, Prashker MJ, Rogers EN, et al: Recommendations for the prevention and treatment of glucocorticoid-induced osteoporosis: American College of Rheumatology Task Force on Osteoporosis guidelines, *Arthritis Rheum* 39:1791-1801, 1996.
6. Lips P: Prevention of corticosteroid induced osteoporosis (editorial), *BMJ* 318:1366-1367, 1999.

Treatment of Established Osteoporosis

(See also amenorrhea; metastatic breast cancer; multiple myeloma; prevention of osteoporosis)

Bisphosphonates

Bisphosphonates are probably the pharmacological agents of choice for the treatment of established osteoporosis. They bind to bone and inhibit osteoclast activity, thus decreasing bone removal. Postmenopausal women treated with alendronate (Fosamax)[1-3] or risedronate (Actonel)[4] have an increase in bone density and a decrease in vertebral and nonvertebral fracture rates.

The usual dose of alendronate (Fosamax) is 10 mg/day taken with water on an empty stomach 30 minutes before breakfast. Esophageal ulceration is a rare complication of swallowing alendronate pills. Taking the pill with a large glass of water and remaining vertical for half an hour afterward may help prevent this problem.[5] The recommended dose of risedronate for treating osteoporosis is 5 mg once daily.[4]

Calcitonin

Calcitonin has an analgesic effect and may give rapid pain relief from compression fractures.[1,6] The usual dose of the parenteral formulation (Calcimar) for the pain relief of osteoporotic vertebral fractures is 50 IU subcutaneously or intramuscularly daily, increasing to 100 IU daily if 50 IU is ineffective. Pain relief may be noted within a few days and almost always within 2 weeks. The dose can be tapered after 4 to 6 weeks, and in some cases pain relief persists for months after discontinuing the medication.[6] The nasal spray formulation (Miacalcin) is administered as one spray of 200 IU in one nostril daily (alternate nostrils each day).

Hormone replacement therapy

Estrogen treatment of postmenopausal women with established osteoporosis has been reported to increase bone density[7] and to decrease the incidence of vertebral fractures (see discussions of amenorrhea and prevention of osteoporosis).[8] According to some authorities, estrogens are the treatment of first choice.[1]

Selective estrogen receptor modulators

A randomized controlled trial of raloxifene (Evista) 60 mg/day for postmenopausal women with osteoporosis found that after 3 years the women had fewer radiologically evident vertebral fractures than in the control group. No difference in extremity fractures was observed, and most vertebral fractures were asymptomatic. Both the treated and control groups took supplemental calcium and vitamin D.[9]

Other treatment modalities

Important life-style changes in the treatment of established osteoporosis are stopping smoking, avoiding excessive alcohol intake, and walking for exercise. Calcium supplements of 1500 mg/day should be given, and for those who are housebound 800 mg vitamin D daily is essential.[1]

_____ ◢ **REFERENCES** ◣ _____

1. Eastell R: Treatment of postmenopausal osteoporosis, *N Engl J Med* 338:736-746, 1998.
2. Black DM, Cummings SR, Karpf DB, et al: Randomised trial of effect of alendronate on risk of fracture in women with existing vertebral fractures, *Lancet* 348:1535-1541, 1996.

3. Karpf DB, Shapiro DR, Seeman I, et al: Prevention of nonvertebral fractures by alendronate: a meta-analysis, *JAMA* 277:1159-1164, 1997.

4. Harris ST, Watts NB, Genant HK, et al: Effects of risedronate treatment on vertebral and nonvertebral fractures in women with postmenopausal osteoporosis: a randomized controlled trial, *JAMA* 282:1344-1352, 1999.

5. De Groen PC, Lubbe DF, Hirsch LJ, et al: Esophagitis associated with the use of alendronate, *N Engl J Med* 335:1016-1021, 1996.

6. Maksymowych WP: Managing acute osteoporotic vertebral fractures with calcitonin, *Can Fam Physician* 44:2160-2166, 1998.

7. Lindsay R, Tohme JF: Estrogen treatment of patients with established postmenopausal osteoporosis, *Obstet Gynecol* 76:290-295, 1990.

8. Lufkin EG, Wahner HW, O'Fallon WM, et al: Treatment of postmenopausal osteoporosis with transdermal estrogen, *Ann Intern Med* 117:1-9, 1992.

9. Ettinger B, Black DM, Mitlak BH, et al (Multiple Outcomes of Raloxifene Evaluation [MORE] Investigators): Reduction of vertebral fracture risk in postmenopausal women with osteoporosis treated with raloxifene, *JAMA* 282:637-645, 1999.

THYROID DISORDERS
Thyroid Tests

In outpatient practice a sensitive thyroid-stimulating hormone (sTSH) measurement is sufficient to screen for a hyperthyroid or hypothyroid state. Free thyroxine (FT$_4$) determinations are required only if the sTSH result is abnormal.[1]

---------------- ◤ **REFERENCES** ◢ ----------------

1. Bauer DC, Brown AN: Sensitive thyrotropin and free thyroxine testing in outpatients: are both necessary? *Arch Intern Med* 156:2333-2337, 1996.

Euthyroid Sick Syndrome

The euthyroid sick syndrome occurs in three forms. In all of them triiodothyronine (T$_3$) or thyroxine (T$_4$) concentrations are abnormal but the TSH level is normal or near normal. The normal TSH is the clue to the diagnosis.

Low T$_3$ Syndrome

Normally T$_4$ is converted in almost equal amounts to T$_3$ and reverse (inactive) T$_3$. In severe catabolic states or with carbohydrate restriction the enzyme catalyzing T$_3$ formation is inhibited, resulting in increased production of the metabolically inactive reverse T$_3$. This causes a state of functional hypothyroidism that helps to prevent nitrogen loss during stress. Hypothyroidism is rapidly reversible once the stress (illness, surgery) is removed. In the low T$_3$ syndrome, the T$_4$ level is normal and the T$_3$ level is low. The diagnosis is made by measuring TSH concentration, which is normal or near normal (except in the rare cases of pituitary or hypothalamic failure as the cause of low T$_3$).

Low T$_3$, Low T$_4$ Syndrome

The low T$_3$, low T$_4$ syndrome is seen in severely ill patients and indicates a poor prognosis. Both T$_3$ and T$_4$ levels are low, but the TSH level is normal.

High T$_4$ Syndrome

In the high T$_4$ syndrome the T$_4$ level is elevated because of excessive iodine intake, as occurs with recent gallbladder studies and occasionally from drugs such as amiodarone. The high iodine inhibits the conversion of T$_4$ to T$_3$, leading to a buildup of T$_4$. TSH concentrations are normal or near normal.

Hyperthyroidism

Smokers have an increased incidence of Graves' disease and particularly Graves' ophthalmopathy.[1] Lithium therapy, which is known to be a risk factor for hypothyroidism, may also be associated with an increased risk of hyperthyroidism.[1]

Subclinical hyperthyroidism

Subclinical hyperthyroidism may be defined as undetectable or extremely low sTSH level in association with normal levels of free thyroxine. It affects 1% of men and 1.5% of women over the age of 60. Patients with this condition are at increased risk for atrial fibrillation and possibly osteoporosis. Since no randomized trials have been performed to determine if treatment of subclinical hyperthyroidism ameliorates these risks, whether screening for or treating the disorder has value in unknown.[2]

Overview of the treatment of thyrotoxicosis

Therapy for hyperthyroidism is targeted at either immediate control of symptoms (adjunct treatment), usually with beta-blockers, or modification of the disease through the use of drugs or radioactive iodine.

Beta-blockers and calcium channel blockers. A number of beta-blockers can be used to control the symptoms of tachycardia and palpitations. Examples are propranolol (Inderal) 20 to 40 mg qid, nadolol (Corgard) 80 to 240 mg/day as a single dose, atenolol (Tenormin) 50 to 100 mg/day as a single dose, and metoprolol (Lopressor) 50 to 100 mg bid. Treatment usually starts with low doses that are increased as necessary. Symptomatic beta-blocker treatment should be continued for 4 to 6 weeks, overlapping with the definitive treatment. For patients who cannot take beta-blockers, the calcium channel blocker diltiazem (Cardizem) 30 to 120 mg tid is often effective.[3]

Radioactive iodine. The choice of radioactive iodine as the initial definitive treatment for hyperthyroidism is becoming more common in North America, but it is used much more often in Europe or Japan. [131]I is particularly indicated in patients with risk factors for relapse such as those with severe symptoms or a large goiter.[3]

Antithyroid drug therapy. The two major antithyroid drugs in use are propylthiouracil (Propyl-Thyracil) and methimazole (Tapazole). Methimazole is the active metabolite of a third antithyroid drug, carbimazole.[3,4]

The goals of antithyroid drug treatment in Graves' disease are the control of symptoms and the attainment of long-term remission.[3,4] Factors weakly associated with good remissions are small size of goiter and recent onset of hyperthyroidism.[1] More important is the duration of treatment. Long-term remissions have been reported to be much more common after 2 years of treatment than after 6 months of treatment.[5]

In North America antithyroid drugs remain the treatment of first choice in patients under 40 with a first episode of Graves' disease. Older patients, as well as younger ones with a relapse of Graves' disease after treatment with an antithyroid drug, are usually treated definitively with radioactive iodine. Even when use of radioactive iodine is selected, patients may initially be given antithyroid drugs for a short period to control symptoms.[4]

Standard protocol in North America is to treat patients with antithyroid drugs for 1 to 2 years, since attempts at longer treatment are associated with prolonged monitoring and poor compliance. Relapses are most likely to occur in the 6 months after discontinuing therapy but may take place after many years.[4]

The choice of antithyroid drug seems to be arbitrary. In North America propylthiouracil (Propyl-Thyracil) is used more often than methimazole (Tapazole) for unclear reasons. According to Franklyn,[4] methimazole has several advantages and should be the drug of choice. It requires only once a day dosage and in moderate doses is associated with a lesser risk of agranulocytosis.[4]

The major side effect of both propylthiouracil and methimazole is agranulocytosis. It is an idiosyncratic reaction that is slightly more common in patients over the age of 40. Since it comes on rapidly, routine blood counts are not helpful; instead patients should be warned to report fever or sore throat immediately.[4] A baseline complete blood count before the initiation of therapy may be helpful.[3]

Propylthiouracil is usually started with doses of 75 to 100 mg tid. After 4 to 6 weeks the dose should be decreased by about one third if the TSH has risen to a normal or above normal level or if the T_4 or T_3 level has returned to normal. After another 4 to 6 weeks the dose may have to be reduced again. The usual maintenance dose is about 50 mg tid. The patient should then be examined clinically and have TSH and T_4 determinations every 2 months for 6 months, then every 3 months for 6 months, then twice a year for 1 year, and then annually. Treatment is generally continued for 1 to 2 years.[3,4]

Treatment with methimazole is usually begun with 10 to 20 mg once a day. After 4 to 6 weeks the dose should be decreased by about one third if the T_4 or T_3 has returned to normal or if the TSH has risen to a normal or above normal level. Since the TSH level may take weeks or even months to return to normal, doses are usually adjusted according to the T_4 and T_3 levels. After another 4 to 6 weeks the dose

may have to be reduced once again. The usual maintenance dose is about 5 to 10 mg of methimazole a day. TSH and T_4 levels should be determined every 2 months for 6 months, then every 3 months for 6 months, then twice a year for 1 year, and then annually. Treatment is generally continued for 1 to 2 years.[3,4]

Ophthalmopathy. In patients with Graves' disease ophthalmopathy develops before thyroid disease in about 20% of patients, at the same time in 40%, and afterward in 40%. In most cases the disorder improves spontaneously. Ophthalmopathy is more likely to develop in smokers. Treatment of Graves' disease with radioiodine is associated with an increased incidence or a greater rate of progression of ophthalmopathy than is treatment with antithyroid drugs. However, only a few patients are so affected and for them the condition can be controlled with prednisone.[6,7] Prudence dictates avoiding the use of radioactive iodine for most patients with clinically apparent ophthalmopathy.[8]

REFERENCES

1. Prummel MF, Wiersinga WM: Smoking and risk of Graves' disease, *JAMA* 269:479-482, 1993.
2. Helfand M, Redfern CC: Clinical guideline. 2. Screening for thyroid disease: an update, *Ann Intern Med* 129:144-158, 1998.
3. Singer PA, Cooper DS, Levy EG, et al: Treatment guidelines for patients with hyperthyroidism and hypothyroidism, *JAMA* 273:808-812, 1995.
4. Franklyn JA: The management of hyperthyroidism, *N Engl J Med* 330:1731-1738, 1994.
5. Tamai H, Nakagawa T, Fukino O, et al: Thionamide therapy in Graves' disease: relation of relapse rate to duration of therapy, *Ann Intern Med* 92:448-490, 1980.
6. Bartalena L, Marcocci C, Bogazzi F, et al: Relation between therapy for hyperthyroidism and the course of Graves' ophthalmopathy, *N Engl J Med* 338:73-78, 1998.
7. Wiersinga WM: Preventing Graves' ophthalmopathy (editorial), *N Engl J Med* 338:121-122, 1998.
8. Walsh JP, Dayan CM, Potts MJ: Radioiodine and thyroid eye disease (editorial), *BMJ* 319:68-69, 1999.

Hypothyroidism

(See also biliary cirrhosis; celiac disease; smoking; thyroiditis)

Epidemiology

Lithium therapy is an important risk factor for hypothyroidism; 5% of patients receiving lithium have overt hypothyroidism, and 25% have subclinical hypothyroidism.[1] Smoking probably aggravates both the clinical and the biochemical effects of overt hypothyroidism.[2]

Hypercholesterolemia

Hypercholesterolemia may be a clue to hypothyroidism. In a retrospective analysis of hypercholesterolemic patients referred to a lipid clinic, 4.2% were hypothyroid; correction of the hypothyroidism lowered the lipid levels only if the TSH was at least 10 mU/L (10 μU/ml). Put another way, subclinical hypothyroidism is probably not a risk factor for atherosclerosis.[3]

Guidelines for screening

The Canadian Task Force on Preventive Health Care recognizes the high prevalence of hypothyroidism among perimenopausal and postmenopausal women but gives screening for this disorder with thyroid function tests a "C" recommendation,[4] and the U.S. Preventive Services Task Force gives screening of asymptomatic adults and children a "D" recommendation.[5] For high-risk groups, including the elderly, the U.S. Preventive Services Task Force gives screening a "C" recommendation.[5]

The 1998 guidelines of the American College of Physicians recommend screening of women over the age of 50 for thyroid disease using a sensitive TSH test. If the TSH is either undetectable or greater than 10 mU/L, a free thyroxine test should be ordered. If the TSH is above 10 mU/L and the free thyroxine level is low, the patient has overt hypothyroidism and should be treated; if the free thyroxine level is in the normal range, the patient has subclinical hypothyroidism (see below).[6]

Treatment

For patients over the age of 50 the usual starting dose of thyroxine (Synthroid, Eltroxin) is 50 μg/day, which is increased after an interval of 3 to 4 weeks to 100 to 150 μg/day. In patients under 50 years of age or those in whom hypothyroidism develops rapidly (postthyroidectomy or post–radioactive iodine treatment), the initial dose may be 100 μg/day.[7]

Thyroxine replacement therapy that does not suppress the TSH to below normal limits does not cause osteopenia. If the TSH is suppressed below the normal levels, there is an increased risk of osteopenia, but whether this will translate into an increased fracture rate is unknown.[8] The practical point for family physicians is that when hormone replacement therapy is prescribed for hypothyroidism, the TSH level should be kept in the normal rather than the subnormal range.

────────────── ⚞ **REFERENCES** ⚟ ──────────────

1. Prummel MF, Wiersinga WM: Smoking and risk of Graves' disease, *JAMA* 269:479-482, 1993.
2. Müller B, Zulewski H, Huber P, et al: Impaired action of thyroid hormone associated with smoking in women with hypothyroidism, *N Engl J Med* 333:964-969, 1995.
3. Diekman T, Lansberg PJ, Kastelein JJP, et al: Prevalence and correction of hypothyroidism in a large cohort of patients referred for dyslipidemia, *Arch Intern Med* 155:1490-1495, 1995.
4. Canadian Task Force on the Periodic Health Examination: *Canadian guide to clinical preventive health care,* Ottawa, 1994, Canada Communication Group—Publishing, pp 612-618.
5. US Preventive Services Task Force: *Guide to clinical preventive services,* ed 2, Baltimore, 1996, Williams & Wilkins, pp 209-218.
6. American College of Physicians: Clinical guideline. 1. Screening for thyroid disease, *Ann Intern Med* 129:141-143, 1998.
7. Singer PA, Cooper DS, Levy EG, et al: Treatment guidelines for patients with hyperthyroidism and hypothyroidism, *JAMA* 273:808-812, 1995.
8. Gharib H, Mazzaferri EL: Thyroxine suppressive therapy in patients with nodular thyroid disease, *Ann Intern Med* 128:386-394, 1998.

Subclinical hypothyroidism
(See also smoking; thyroiditis)

Subclinical hypothyroidism is diagnosed when the TSH is 6 mU/L or higher and the free thyroxine is in the normal range. Subclinical hypothyroidism is much more common than overt hypothyroidism and may affect up to 8% of women over the age of 35. In only a small percentage of detected cases is the TSH level 10 mU/L or higher, which is clinically important because the risks of complications are greatest in patients with higher levels of TSH.[1] Risk factors for progression to overt hypothyroidism are older age, TSH levels of 10 mU/L or higher, and the presence of positive microsomal antibody tests.[1,2] In some susceptible subjects, subclinical hypothyroidism may be precipitated by smoking.[3]

Whether treatment of subclinical hypothyroidism is indicated is controversial.[1,2] One argument for treatment is that mild reversible target organ damage has been reported with this condition, including impaired left ventricular function, reduced hearing, and increased capillary permeability to protein. Many patients with this disorder are reported to feel better when receiving treatment.[2] Although cholesterol levels may be slightly elevated in subclinical hypothyroidism, this does not seem to constitute a significant risk factor for atherosclerosis.[2,4] Treatment prevents progression to overt disease. According to some authorities treatment is probably indicated in the following circumstances[1,2]:

1. The TSH level is unequivocally elevated (greater than twice the upper limit of normal).
2. There are high levels of microsomal antibodies.
3. The cholesterol level is elevated.

────────────── ⚞ **REFERENCES** ⚟ ──────────────

1. Helfand M, Redfern CC: Clinical guideline. 2. Screening for thyroid disease: an update, *Ann Intern Med* 129:144-158, 1998.
2. Weetman AP: Hypothyroidism: screening and subclinical disease, *BMJ* 314:1175-1178, 1997.
3. Müller B, Zulewski H, Huber P, et al: Impaired action of thyroid hormone associated with smoking in women with hypothyroidism, *N Engl J Med* 333:964-969, 1995.
4. Diekman T, Lansberg PJ, Kastelein JJP, et al: Prevalence and correction of hypothyroidism in a large cohort of patients referred for dyslipidemia, *Arch Intern Med* 155:1490-1495, 1995.

Thyroid Nodules
(See also screening)

In most clinical series in which patients were examined for the presence of thyroid nodules, only 5% to 8% of patients were found to have clinically palpable nodules and less than 10% of these nodules were cancerous.[1] However, in one California study in which a special effort was made to look for thyroid nodules by palpation in asymptomatic patients, 9% were found to have solitary nodules and 12% had multiple nodules for a total of 21%. When assessed by ultrasound, 67% of these patients were found to have nodules; none was malignant.[2] A Mayo Clinic evaluation comparing palpation and ultrasonography found that nodules less than 1 cm in diameter were rarely palpable and that about 50% of glands thought to have a solitary nodule on palpation were actually multinodular on ultrasonography.[3]

If a low-functioning ("cold") nodule is found in a woman living in an iodine-deficient area, the chance that it is malignant is about 1.5%.[4] On the other hand, a solitary nodule in an elderly man has a greater than 50% chance of being malignant.[5] Thyroid nodules are four times as common in females as in males, and their incidence increases in direct proportion to age.[6]

The vast majority of thyroid cancers are relatively nonaggressive papillary or follicular carcinomas; papillary carcinomas are the more common. Although regional lymph node metastases are reasonably common with these forms of cancer, cure is usually possible with surgery, often in conjunction with therapeutic doses of radioactive iodine. Distant metastases occur in only 10% to 15% of patients with well-differentiated follicular or papillary carcinomas, and if these tumor deposits take up radioactive iodine, complete long-lasting remissions may be expected in close to 50% of cases.[7]

Fine needle aspiration is the investigative procedure of choice for clinically solitary thyroid nodules. When this technique is used, about 70% of nodules will be cytologically benign (with a false-negative rate of 1% to 2%), 4% are malignant, and the remainder either have insufficient cellular material for a diagnosis or are inconclusive.[8] The aspiration is done with a 10- or 25-ml syringe and a 22- to 27-gauge needle. Three to six passes with the needle are generally made to ensure adequate sampling.[1]

About 15% to 25% of aspirated nodules are found to be cysts. Most cysts are benign, but 15% have been reported to be necrotic papillary carcinomas.[6] If the nodule disappears permanently after aspiration, no further testing is required even if no cytological diagnosis has been made.[8]

If a thyroid nodule is smaller than 1 cm, the chances of its being malignant are very low. In this situation a reasonable management plan is simply follow-up observation.[9]

Hyperfunctioning (hot) nodules (detected by thyroid scan) are almost never malignant.[1]

Treatment of benign thyroid nodules with levothyroxine (Synthroid) to suppress thyroid nodule growth is controversial. Some studies have shown no benefit and others only slight benefit. Since this treatment is associated with decreased bone density and possibly an increased risk of atrial fibrillation, there seems little indication for using it.[8]

⊿ REFERENCES ⊾

1. Ridgway EC: Clinical review 30: clinician's evaluation of a solitary thyroid nodule, *J Clin Endocrinol Metab* 74:231-235, 1992.
2. Ezzat S, Sarti DA, Cain DR, Braunstein GD: Thyroid incidentalomas: prevalence by palpation and ultrasonography, *Arch Intern Med* 154:1838-1840, 1994.
3. Tan GH, Gharib H, Reading CC: Solitary thyroid nodule: comparison between palpation and ultrasonography, *Arch Intern Med* 155:2418-2423, 1995.
4. Belfiore A, La Rosa GL, La Porta GA, et al: Cancer risk in patients with cold thyroid nodules: relevance of iodine intake, sex, age and multinodularity, *Am J Med* 93:363-369, 1992.
5. Mazzaferri EL: Thyroid cancer in thyroid nodules: finding a needle in the haystack (editorial), *Am J Med* 93:359-362, 1992.
6. Mazzaferri EL: Current concepts: management of a solitary thyroid nodule, *N Engl J Med* 328:553-559, 1993.
7. Schlumberger MJ: Papillary and follicular thyroid carcinoma, *N Engl J Med* 338:297-306, 1998.
8. Hermus AR, Huysmans DA: Treatment of benign nodular thyroid disease, *N Engl J Med* 338:1438-1447, 1998.
9. Gharib H, James EM, Charboneau JW, et al: Suppressive therapy with levothyroxine for solitary thyroid nodules, *N Engl J Med* 317:70-75, 1987.

Thyroiditis

(See also hypothyroidism; subclinical hypothyroidism)

Classification

Thyroiditis can be classified as follows[1,2]:
1. Acute thyroiditis (bacterial, fungal, or parasitic)
2. Subacute thyroiditis (subacute granulomatous thyroiditis [de Quervain's or painful thyroiditis], painless thyroiditis, postpartum thyroiditis)
3. Chronic lymphocytic thyroiditis (Hashimoto's disease)
4. Riedel's thyroiditis (invasive fibrous thyroiditis or chronic sclerosing thyroiditis)

Acute thyroiditis and Riedel's thyroiditis are very rare. Symptoms of acute infectious thyroiditis are anterior neck pain, swelling, fever, dysphagia, and dysphonia. Riedel's thyroiditis is found in middle-aged or elderly women and consists of a fibrous replacement of the gland that turns the gland into a stony hard mass.

Subacute granulomatous thyroiditis

Subacute granulomatous thyroiditis was described by de Quervain in 1904. It is thought to be secondary to a viral infection. It affects women four times as often as men, most patients are middle aged, and cases are most likely to occur in the summer and fall.[1,2]

The usual symptoms are either those of thyrotoxicosis (about 50% of patients), resulting from the excessive release of thyroid hormone by the damaged gland, or anterior neck pain. Granulomatous thyroiditis is the most common cause of anterior neck pain in the region of the thyroid gland. Patients may have low-grade fever and general malaise. The thyroid gland tends to be firm and tender.[1,2]

The symptoms of granulomatous thyroiditis often develop rapidly, and this is a distinguishing point from Graves' disease. If the distinction between these two conditions is not obvious clinically, it can be resolved by measuring ^{131}I uptake. This is significantly increased in Graves' disease but very low (less than 5%) in granulomatous thyroiditis.[1,2]

The initial phase of inflammation and pain usually lasts 3 to 6 weeks. About one third of patients subsequently enter a hypothyroid stage that persists for several weeks before the euthyroid state is restored. Approximately 5% of patients become permanently hypothyroid.[1,2] A number of patients have elevated antithyroid antibody levels, which suggests the development of an autoimmune process during the disease.[1,2]

Treatment of granulomatous thyroiditis is symptomatic. Nonsteroidal antiinflammatory drugs are usually effective in relieving the neck pain, but sometimes prednisone 20 to 40 mg/day in divided doses and tapered over 2 to 4 weeks is required. Thyrotoxic symptoms can be controlled by beta-blockers (see discussion of hyperthyroidism), and the subsequent hypothyroid state may need temporary thyroid replacement therapy.[1,2] Antithyroid drugs such as propylthiouracil or methimazole have no role in treating any of the forms of subacute thyroiditis (granulomatous, painless, or postpartum), since the pathogenesis is leakage of preformed hormone, not its excessive production.[1,2]

Painless thyroiditis

Painless thyroiditis may be sporadic or postpartum. Both forms are believed to be autoimmune disorders, since thyroid antibodies are present in 50% of patients with painless thyroiditis and 80% of those with postpartum thyroiditis.[1,2]

The sporadic form of painless thyroiditis is concentrated in the Great Lakes region of North America and accounts for about one third of cases of thyrotoxicosis in this area. Outside of the Great Lakes region it constitutes only about 5% of thyrotoxicosis cases.[1,2]

Like granulomatous thyroiditis, painless thyroiditis affects women four times as often as men and most patients are 40 to 50 years of age. Symptoms are those of thyrotoxicosis and tend to come on abruptly. Patients do not have neck pain. The thyroid gland is slightly enlarged but nontender.[1,2]

Also like granulomatous thyroiditis, painless thyroiditis usually begins with a thyrotoxic phase, passes through a hypothyroid phase, and ends with a recovery phase. In a few patients only the hypothyroid phase is seen. About 6% of patients become permanently hypothyroid, but this may take years to develop. Thus annual TSH testing is indicated for all patients with painless thyroiditis.[1,2]

Painless thyroiditis can be differentiated from Graves' disease by radioactive iodine uptake (RAIU). It is high in Graves' disease and usually less than 3% in painless thyroiditis.[1,2]

Treatment of painless thyroiditis is directed at the symptoms. Some patients require no treatment, whereas others benefit from beta-blockers in the thyrotoxic phase and a temporary course of levothyroxine if symptomatic hypothyroidism ensues.[1,2]

Postpartum thyroiditis

As indicated previously, postpartum thyroiditis is a variant of painless thyroiditis. It occurs in 4% to 5% of women and is usually self-limited. The disorder begins with symptoms of hyperthyroidism, which are classically followed by a period of hypothyroidism and finally a return to the euthyroid state. The entire sine wave cycle may last 6 to 9 months. The syndrome is likely to recur with subsequent pregnancies,[1,2] and about 25% of those who have recovered from the disorder are found to be overtly hypothyroid 4 years later.[3,4]

RAIU scanning shows no or little uptake in patients with postpartum thyroiditis. The test should not be performed if the mother is nursing.[1,2]

Treatment of postpartum thyroiditis is symptomatic. Beta-blockers may be needed in the hyperthyroid stage and short-term levothyroxine in the hypothyroid stage.[1,2]

Chronic lymphocytic thyroiditis

Chronic lymphocytic thyroiditis was described by the Japanese physician Hashimoto in 1912. It is the most common cause of hypothyroidism. Up to 95% of patients are women,[1] and most are over the age of 45 when the diagnosis is made.[5] A small to medium-sized goiter is usually found. Antithyroid antibodies (antimicrosomal or antithyroglobulin) are present in 90% of patients, and the titers of these, particularly the antimicrosomal antibodies, are usually high. The usual replacement dose of levothyroxine (Synthroid, Eltroxin) is 75 to 150 μg/day. Initial doses are low (12.5, 25, and 50 μg), especially in the elderly or those with coronary artery disease. Increments, based on TSH levels, are made every 4 to 6 weeks (see discussion of hypothyroidism above).[1] If a patient with chronic lymphocytic thyroiditis becomes pregnant, she will probably require a dose increase of 25% to 50%.[5]

In one study 11% of patients with Hashimoto's thyroiditis had a spontaneous remission. Levothyroxine was withdrawn after 1 year of treatment, and thyroid function remained normal for up to a year.[6]

◤ REFERENCES ◢

1. Sakiyama R: Thyroiditis: a clinical review, *Am Fam Physician* 48:615-621, 1993.
2. Morrison A: Guidelines for the diagnosis of common thyroid disorders, *Can J CME,* May 1992, pp 79-85.
3. Othman S, Phillips DI, Parkes AB, et al: A long-term follow-up of postpartum thyroiditis, *Clin Endocrinol* 32:559-564, 1990.
4. Tachi J, Amino N, Tamaki H: Long-term follow-up and HLA association in patients with postpartum hypothyroidism, *J Clin Endocrinol Metab* 66:480-484, 1988.

5. Dyan CM, Daniels GH: Chronic autoimmune thyroiditis, *N Engl J Med* 335:99-107, 1996.

6. Comtois R, Faucher L, Lafleche L: Outcome of hypothyroidism caused by Hashimoto's thyroiditis, *Arch Intern Med* 155:1404-1408, 1995.

PARATHYROID DISORDERS

(See also osteoporosis; renal colic)

Ninety percent of patients with hyperparathyroidism have a parathyroid adenoma. The diagnosis is usually suspected because an elevated serum calcium level is detected in a "routine" biochemical screen, and it is confirmed by finding an elevated serum parathyroid hormone level. The major complications of hyperparathyroidism—hypercalcuria, nephrolithiasis, renal insufficiency, and osteopenia—are rare. Standard practice has been to avoid surgery for patients with no evidence of complications. However, a number of recent studies suggest that many "asymptomatic" patients have subtle physical and mental disabilities that are rectified when parathyroid surgery produces normocalcemia. Parathyroid surgery, which can be performed on an outpatient basis, has become less complex in recent years because radioactive imaging can localize hyperfunctioning parathyroid tissue and rapid parathormone assays can show that parathyroid tissue has been adequately resected while the patient is still anesthetized. A reasonable case can be made for operating on most patients with hyperparathyroidism.[1]

─────────────── ❧ **REFERENCES** ❧ ───────────────

1. Utiger RD: Treatment of primary hyperparathyroidism (editorial), *N Engl J Med* 341:1301-1302, 1999.

PITUITARY DISORDERS

(See also practice patterns; screening)

Acromegaly

The initial treatment of choice for acromegaly is surgical removal of the pituitary tumor. Results are vastly better if the operation is performed by a surgeon experienced in this subspecialty.[1]

Hypopituitarism

Pituitary adenomas, which may be secreting or nonsecreting, are the most common cause of hypopituitarism. Postpartum hemorrhage with hypovolemia may lead to hypopituitarism (Sheehan's syndrome) either immediately or after a delay of several years.[2]

Clinical manifestations

The clinical manifestations of hypopituitarism are often subtle and variable. The variability depends in large part on which target endocrine glands are deficient and whether the deficiency is mild or severe.[2]

Symptoms of corticotropin deficiency include weakness, headache, orthostatic hypotension, fatigue, anorexia, nausea, vomiting, abdominal pain, and weight loss. In long-standing cases patients may have thinning or loss of axillary and pubic hair. On examination the patient often appears pale because of decreased pigmentation, and this contrasts with the hyperpigmentation of Addison's disease. Deficiency of gonadotropins results in decreased libido and erectile function in men and menstrual irregularities or amenorrhea in women. In addition, women may have decreased libido and even hot flashes. Deficiency of TSH results in the symptoms of hypothyroidism. Adults with growth hormone deficiency have nonspecific symptoms such as decreased energy and decreased exercise tolerance. If the cause of the hypopituitarism is a prolactin-secreting adenoma, the patient may have galactorrhea.[2]

Laboratory investigations

If hypopituitarism is suspected, a family physician may order some initial blood tests as discussed below. Imaging of the pituitary gland and sella is the next level of investigation and is probably best done in conjunction with a consultant.[2]

The most important point about basal serum hormone measurements is that they may be entirely normal even in patients with symptomatic hypopituitarism. Test results are helpful only if they are abnormal, particularly with hormones secreted in pulsed fashion, such as luteinizing hormone, follicle-stimulating hormone, and growth hormone. Initial blood tests should include complete and differential blood cell counts, electrolytes, prolactin, morning serum cortisol, T_4 and TSH, and follicle-stimulating and luteinizing hormones. Some patients have normocytic normochromic anemia and eosinophilia because of corticotropin deficiencies. Hyponatremia may also be found, but not hyperkalemia as occurs in Addison's disease because the adrenocortical production of aldosterone is not dependent on corticotropin.[2]

Pituitary Incidentalomas

A pituitary incidentaloma is a lesion of the pituitary gland that is neurologically and endocrinologically inapparent and is discovered incidentally during magnetic resonance imaging or computed tomography. Almost all such diseases are adenomas, and if they are under 10 mm in diameter (microadenomas), only about 1 in 200 will eventually lead to neurological or endocrinological dysfunction. There is no consensus on the optimal investigation and management of asymptomatic patients with incidentally discovered pituitary microadenomas. Conclusions based on a decision analytical model are that the only endocrinological parameter that might be worth assessing is prolactin and that other endocrine panels or regular magnetic resonance imaging examinations would probably lead to more harm than good.[3]

The most common form of functioning pituitary adenoma is a prolactinoma; treatment of these lesions with bromocriptine leads to decrease in tumor size and control of endocrinologically mediated symptoms.[3]

━━━━━━━━━━ ◣ **REFERENCES** ◤ ━━━━━━━━━━

1. Clayton RN, Stewart PM, Shalet SM, et al: Pituitary surgery for acromegaly: should be done by specialists (editorial), *BMJ* 319:588-589, 1999.
2. Vance ML: Hypopituitarism, *N Engl J Med* 330:1651-1662, 1994.
3. King JT Jr, Justice AC, Aron DC: Management of incidental pituitary microadenomas: a cost-effectiveness analysis, *J Clin Endocrinol Metab* 82:3625-3632, 1997.

MISCELLANEOUS

Topics covered in this section

ALTERNATIVE MEDICINE
(See also physician-patient communications)

According to Angell and Kassirer,[1] the most important features distinguishing alternative or complementary medicine from conventional medicine are that the former has not been scientifically tested and that those who practice it see no need for such testing. Alternative medicine is based on unproven hypotheses and testimonials, whereas the underlying premise of conventional medicine is that it is, or should be, evidence based.

Many terms are encompassed by the term "alternative medicine." According to one classification an overall encompassing term is "complementary health care services"; synonyms are "unorthodox," "holistic," "unconventional," "questionable," and "new medicine." According to some authors the term "complementary medicine" should be used if such services are offered by qualified physicians, rather than the more encompassing term "complementary health care services," which may be administered by physicians or nonphysicians.[2]

Because alternative medicine has become so popular and has garnered such a plethora of descriptive names, conventional medicine has begun embracing its own set of rubrics: mainstream, orthodox, regular, scientific, evidence based, Western, modern, and allopathic.[3] Since the term "allopathic" was coined by Samuel Hanemann, the founder of homeopathy, to describe physicians who use harsh and abusive treatments, Gundling[4] suggests that those of us who are traditional physicians should not endorse it.

Segen[5] divides the various practices of alternative medicine them into three categories:
1. Formal therapeutic systems (alternative): chiropractic, homeopathy, osteopathy, classical Chinese medicine (including acupuncture), Indian Ayurvedic medicine, naturopathy, herbal medicine
2. Informal therapeutic systems (fringe): manual healing (e.g., massage, aromatherapy, reflexology), mind-body medicine (e.g., biofeedback, visual imagery, hypnosis, therapeutic touch, yoga, t'ai chi, music therapy, meditation, faith healing)
3. Quackery (unproven) (e.g., laetrile, snake oil)

Others would put pharmacological or biological therapies (e.g., chelation therapy for vascular disease) and nutritional therapy (macrobiotics, nutritional supplements) into their own separate categories.[2]

Whether physicians like it or not, alternative medicine plays a major role in the health care systems of the Western world. In 1990 at least 30% of Americans used some form of alternative therapy, and by 1997 the figure had risen to 40%. Most patients do not tell their physicians they are doing so.[6] From the patient's viewpoint, seeing an alternative medical practitioner does not preclude conventional medical treatment; many receive both concurrently.[2]

Evidence of Efficacy

Many randomized controlled trials of alternative medicine have been published (Tang and associates found approximately 10,000 such trials dealing with traditional Chinese medicine), but virtually all of them suffer from serious methodological errors.[7] With few exceptions, alternative medicine is not evidence based.

Appeal of Alternative Medicine

Various reasons have been given to explain why patients seek alternative therapies. Patients may feel they can take control of their disease with this form of treatment, or they may think they will be given more time, be listened to with more respect, and be treated more as a whole person than would be the case with traditional practitioners. Some with chronic diseases such as cancer or AIDS may believe that they have exhausted the potential of traditional medicine.[2,8] A national survey in the United States found that variables predicting the use of alternative care included having a higher level of education and an active interest in environmentalism, feminism, spirituality, or growth psychology. For these patients alternative care appeared to be congruent with their spiritual and philosophical beliefs. Dissatisfaction with conventional medicine was not a predictor for choosing alternative therapies, and over 95% of those who used alternative therapies continued to obtain conventional medical care.[9]

For many, alternative medicine is religion or magic. For them alternative medicine is a belief system that depends on faith and testimonials. Priestly healing has much deeper roots in our culture than does scientific medicine, and it is unlikely to disappear.[10] Looking at alternative medicine in this way, physicians who categorically reject its unscientifically tested premises may at least understand why patients turn to it.

Cancer and Alternative Medicine

An estimated half of all cancer patients seek some form of alternative medicine, and close to half of these do so in the early stages of the disease; approximately 75% fail to inform their conventional physicians of these activities, and about 40% discontinue conventional treatments. Most alternative medicine practitioners are presentable and well educated, and many have medical or osteopathic degrees. Testimonials are almost always the only form of evidence used to support alternative therapies for cancer, so patients are informed only of successes. Although some forms of alternative therapy are innocuous, others cause significant physical, economic, social, or psychological harm. For example, one powerful argument given for alternative regimens is that they offer the patient autonomy and a sense of control. This may be, but such a benefit can backfire badly if individual patients are told that psychological discipline can cure their disease and, when this proves unsuccessful, are led to believe that the reason for the failure was their inadequate commitment to a prescribed regimen.[8]

A survey of 480 women with early-stage breast cancer found that 28% used alternative medicine while continuing standard medical therapy. As a group, women who chose to use alternative medicine after the diagnosis of breast cancer was made reported a worse quality of life (more fear of cancer recurrence, more depression, less sexual satisfaction, and more physical symptoms) than did women who did not

choose alternative medicine. The use of alternative medicine by cancer patients may thus be seen as a marker of psychological distress necessitating further investigation and management by the physician.[11]

HIV-Infected Patients

A survey of HIV-infected patients found that two thirds used various herbs or dietary supplements and close to one half regularly visited alternative medicine practitioners. The goal of alternative therapies was symptom relief rather than hope for an HIV cure, and in the majority of instances patients reported that they benefited from these interventions. Most of the patients informed their regular physicians that they were also obtaining alternative therapies.[12]

Adverse Effects

Few systematic studies of the adverse effects of alternative medicine therapies have been published, but indirect evidence suggests that the incidence of such effects is much higher than has been reported.[13] Specific adverse effects are discussed in more detail in the sections dealing with specific forms of alternative medicine.

Attitudes of Physicians to Alternative Medicine

A 1998 literature survey found that many physicians refer patients to alternative practitioners, particularly chiropractors and acupuncturists. Approximately half of the surveyed physicians believed that acupuncture, chiropractic, and massage were efficacious, 26% believed in homeopathy, and 13% believed in herbal medicine. These rates varied widely from one study to another.[14]

Marketing Strategies

A technique some alternative medicine and health food proponents use to promote their products is to impress the consumer with obfuscating scientific jargon lauding the scientific breakthrough of antioxidants, chromium, chelated minerals, and so on. This approach is most successful when one of the many items advocated has some preliminary or proven credibility in the scientific community. A current example is vitamin E and its antioxidant effects.

⚓ REFERENCES ⚓

1. Angell M, Kassirer JP: Alternative medicine—the risks of untested and unregulated remedies (editorial), *N Engl J Med* 339:839-841, 1998.
2. Gordon JS: Alternative medicine and the family physician, *Am Fam Physician* 54:2205-2212, 1996.
3. Dalen JE: "Conventional" and "unconventional" medicine: can they be integrated? (editorial), *Arch Intern Med* 158:2179-2181, 1998.
4. Gundling KE: When did I become an "allopath"? *Arch Intern Med* 158:2185-2186, 1998.
5. Segen JC: *Dictionary of alternative medicine,* Stamford, Conn, 1998, Appleton & Lange.

6. Eisenberg DM, Davis RB, Ettner SL, et al: Trends in alternative medicine use in the United States, 1990-1997: results of a follow-up national survey, *JAMA* 280:1569-1575, 1998.

7. Tang J-L, Zhan S-Y, Ernst E: Review of randomised controlled trials of traditional Chinese medicine, *BMJ* 319:160-161, 1999.

8. Brigden ML: Unproven cancer therapies: a multi-headed Hydra, *Ann RCPSC* 31:9-14, 1998.

9. Astin JA: Why patients use alternative medicine: results of a national study, *JAMA* 279:1548-1553, 1998.

10. Levin S: The religions of medicine, *Ann RCPSC* 31:219, 1998.

11. Burstein HJ, Gelber S, Guadagnoli E, et al:. Use of alternative medicine by women with early-stage breast cancer, *N Engl J Med* 340:1733-1739, 1999.

12. Fairfield KM, Eisenberg DM, Davis RB, et al: Patterns of use, expenditures, and perceived efficacy of complementary and alternative therapies in HIV-infected patients, *Arch Intern Med* 158:2257-2264, 1998.

13. Abbot NC, Hill M, Barnes J, et al: Uncovering suspected adverse effects of complementary and alternative medicine, *Int J Risk Safety Med* 11:99-106, 1998.

14. Astin JA, Marie A, Pelletier KR, et al: A review of the incorporation of complementary and alternative medicine by mainstream physicians, *Arch Intern Med* 158:2303-2310, 1998.

Dietary Supplements and Herbal Products

(See also antioxidants; dementia; nutrition; vegetarians; vitamins)

Dietary supplements

A wide variety of agents, including almost all vitamins and many minerals, are sold in health food stores as dietary supplements.

Dehydroepiandrosterone (DHEA) has become an extremely popular "dietary supplement" sold by health food stores. It is reputed to do many things, including improve libido; increase muscle mass; strengthen the immune system; prevent type 2 diabetes mellitus, cancer, and heart disease; slow down the process of memory loss; and help in the treatment of Parkinson's disease and Alzheimer's disease. None of these benefits has been demonstrated in large randomized placebo-controlled trials, and the long-term safety of the product is unknown.[1] As is the case with herbal products, DHEA is poorly regulated. One analysis of 16 randomly chosen commercial preparations found that fewer than half contained the quantity of DHEA listed on the label. One sample contained none, one only a trace, and one 150% of the labeled amount.[2]

Gamma-butyrolactone (GBL) has been marketed as a dietary supplement in the United States under a variety of trade names, including "Revivarant." Among the claims for GBL are that it can enhance sexual activity and athletic performance, induce sleep, and prolong life. Severe toxicity, including coma, seizures, and death, has been reported with use of this product.[3] Contaminated plantain has caused digitalis toxicity.[4] Androstenedione is discussed in the section on sports medicine.

Herbal products

Herbal products are widely used in the United States and Canada, and in North America these products are poorly regulated. Their degree of benefit, optimal doses, and adverse effects are largely unknown because of lack of adequate studies.[5-7] In many cases no human trials have been performed, and when they have, methodology has often been poor. Furthermore, even if benefits are proved for some agents, standardization of the products is unlikely under current regulatory systems because of biological differences in soil and growth conditions and diverse methods of collection, extraction, and storage of the products.[5,6] Some of the more popular products and their usual indications are listed in Table 47; several of these are discussed elsewhere in the text in discussion of the diseases they are reputed to ameliorate.

Adverse effects. Although many herbal products are harmless, serious and even fatal adverse effects may occur.[6-18] The alkaloid ephedrine, which is found in a number of remedies, has been reported to cause paranoid psychosis, hypertension, coronary spasm, convulsions, coma, and death. Such adverse effects are not necessarily dose related.[9] Hepatotoxicity has been reported with germander,[10] jin bu huan,[11] and chaparral (creosote bush, grease-wood),[12] and Chinese herbal remedies for eczema have led to chronic renal failure requiring dialysis and renal transplantation.[13] Severe gastrointestinal toxicity has followed the ingestion of "American" mandrake (containing podophyllotoxin), which was taken under the mistaken belief that it was the usual an-

Table 47   Selected Herbal Products

Product	Purported Benefits*
Alfalfa	Cholesterol reduction
Bee pollen	Enhance energy; tonic
Blue-green algae *(Spirulina)*	Weight loss; nutritional supplement
Chamomile tea	Sedative
Devil's claw	Rheumatoid arthritis
Echinacea	Common cold
Evening Primrose Oil	Mastodynia; premenstrual syndrome
Feverfew	Migraines
Garlic	Cholesterol reduction; hypertension
Ginkgo Biloba	Alzheimer's disease
Ginseng	Enhance energy; tonic
Green tea	Prevention of gastrointestinal cancers
Kelp	Weight loss
Milk thistle	Cirrhosis
Royal jelly	Increased longevity; enhanced energy; skin tonic
Saw palmetto	Benign prostatic hyperplasia
St. John's wort	Depression
Valerian	Sedative

Modified from Cadario B: *Patient Care Can* 9:64-89, 1998.
*Multiple benefits are claimed for many of these products; only a few are listed here.

ticholinergic and hallucinatory form of mandrake.[14] An herbal product promoted as nonestrogenic had potent estrogenic activity,[15] and tablets of "Indian plants" have caused lead poisoning.[16] In addition to direct toxicity, numerous interactions have been reported between conventional drugs and herbal remedies.[17] Chemical analysis of a number of Chinese herbal creams that were supposed to be steroid free found them to contain high concentrations of dexamethasone; in blissful ignorance patients had been applying the cream to their own or their infants' faces and flexural surfaces as often as several times a day.[18]

Benefits. As noted previously, few good trials have been published assessing the benefits of herbal products, although more are being undertaken. Some of the products that have demonstrated benefit in one or more clinical trials are Ginkgo Biloba for dementia,[19] St. John's wort for depression,[20] glucosamine for osteoarthritis,[21] Chinese herbal medicines for irritable bowel syndrome,[22] and saw palmetto for benign prostatic hyperplasia.[23] The quality of these studies is variable, and in many cases the chosen controls were placebos, not standard pharmacological agents that have been proved effective.

In view of the unproven benefits of most herbal remedies and the risk of serious adverse effects, Drs. Marcia Angell and Jerome Kassirer recommend that the scientific community "stop giving alternative medicine a free ride."[24]

--- **⚓ REFERENCES ⚓** ---

1. Skolnick AA: Medical news & perspectives: scientific verdict still out on DHEA, *JAMA* 276:1365-1367, 1996.
2. Parasrampuria J, Schwartz K, Petesch R: Quality control of dehydroepiandrosterone dietary supplement products (letter), *JAMA* 280:1565, 1998.
3. Adverse events associated with ingestion of gamma-butyrolactone—Minnesota, New Mexico, and Texas, 1998-1999, *MMWR* 48:137-140, 1999.
4. Slifman NR, Obermeyer WR, Aloi BK, et al: Contamination of botanical dietary supplements by *Digitalis lanata*, *N Engl J Med* 339:806-811, 1998.
5. Winslow LC, Kroll DJ: Herbs as medicines, *Arch Intern Med* 158:2192-2199, 1998.
6. Kozyrskyj A: Herbal products in Canada: how safe are they? *Can Fam Physician* 43:697-702, 1997.
7. Cadario B: Replace misinformation with facts about herbal medicine, *Patient Care Can* 9(1):64-89, 1998.
8. Eisenberg DM: Advising patients who seek alternative medical therapies, *Ann Intern Med* 127:61-69, 1997.
9. Centers for Disease Control and Prevention: Adverse events associated with ephedrine-containing products—Texas, December 1993–September 1995, *JAMA* 276:1711-1712, 1996.
10. Larry D, Vial T, Pauwels A, et al: Hepatitis after germander (*Teucrium chamaedrys*) administration: another instance of herbal medicine hepatotoxicity, *Ann Intern Med* 117:129-132, 1992.
11. Woolf GM, Petrovic LM, Rojter SE, et al: Acute hepatitis associated with the Chinese herbal product jin bu huan, *Ann Intern Med* 121:729-735, 1994.
12. Sheikh NM, Philen RM, Love LA: Chaparral-associated hepatotoxicity, *Arch Intern Med* 157:913-919, 1997.
13. Lord GM, Tagore R, Cook T, et al: Nephropathy caused by Chinese herbs in the UK, *Lancet* 354:481-482, 1999.
14. Frasca T, Brett AS, Yoo SD: Mandrake toxicity: a case of mistaken identity, *Arch Intern Med* 157:2007-2009, 1997.
15. DiPaola RS, Zhang H, Lambert GH, et al: Clinical and biologic activity of an estrogenic herbal combination (PC-SPES) in prostate cancer, *N Engl J Med* 339:785-789, 1998.
16. Beigel Y, Ostfeld I, Schoenfeld N: A leading question, *N Engl J Med* 339:827-830, 1998.
17. Miller LG: Herbal medicinals: selected clinical considerations focusing on known or potential drug-herb interactions, *Arch Intern Med* 158:2200-2211, 1998.
18. Keane FM, Munn SE, Du Vivier AW, et al: Analysis of Chinese herbal creams prescribed for dermatological conditions, *BMJ* 318:563-564, 1999.
19. LeBars PL, Katz MM, Berman N, et al: A placebo-controlled, double-blind, randomized trial of an extract of Ginkgo Biloba for dementia, *JAMA* 278:1327-1332, 1997.
20. Linde K, Ramirez G, Mulrow CD, et al: St John's wort for depression—an overview and meta-analysis of randomised clinical trials, *BMJ* 313:253-258, 1996.
21. Glucosamine for osteoarthritis, *Med Lett* 39:91-92, 1997.
22. Bensoussan A, Talley NJ, Hing M, et al: Treatment of irritable bowel syndrome with Chinese herbal medicine: a randomized controlled trial, *JAMA* 280:1585-1589, 1998.
23. Wilt TJ, Ishani A, Stark G, et al: Saw palmetto extracts for treatment of benign prostatic hyperplasia, *JAMA* 280:1604-1609, 1998.
24. Angell M, Kassirer JP: Alternative medicine—the risks of untested and unregulated remedies (editorial), *N Engl J Med* 339:839-841, 1998.

Chiropractic, Homeopathy, Acupuncture, and Therapeutic Touch

Chiropractic

According to one reviewer the few randomized controlled trials of chiropractic manipulation for chronic low back pain are methodologically flawed and as a result whether the procedure is beneficial is unknown. Serious adverse effects from lumbar manipulation appear to be rare, although fractures and the cauda equina syndrome have been reported. Cervical manipulation has resulted in vertebrobasilar accidents and paralysis. Most patients consulting chiropractors are subject to a number of x-rays, but whether this is harmful is unknown.[1]

In a 1998 study of patients from primary care practices with low back pain that had persisted for 1 week, the subjects were randomly assigned to three treatment groups: receipt of an educational booklet, a physical therapy exercise program using the McKenzie approach, and chiropractic manipulation. No differences in outcomes were detectable between the physiotherapy and chiropractic groups, and these two groups had marginally better outcomes in terms of pain and function than the group that received the educational booklet. However, patients who received active treatment were more satisfied with their care than were those whose only treatment was being given an educational booklet.[2] Patient satisfaction with chiropractic treatment is well documented in many studies and is almost certainly related to positive therapist-patient relationships.[3]

Claims are often made that chiropractic manipulations of the spine improve other medical conditions such as hypertension, asthma, and otitis media.[4] A randomized trial of active and simulated chiropractic manipulation in asthmatic children found no benefit from active treatment.[5] A somewhat similar study failed to demonstrate any benefit for the control of episodic tension-type headaches.[6]

Homeopathy

A large metaanalysis of placebo-controlled trials of homeopathy concluded that the overall odds ratios slightly favored homeopathy.[7] However, even if this result is valid, which according to one editorialist is questionable,[8] it is of no clinical significance because no evidence has shown that any specific homeopathic treatment is clearly efficacious for any one clinical entity.[9]

Homeopathy was founded by Samuel Hahnemann in Germany in the late 18th century. Its popularity has waxed and waned over the years. At present it is on the upswing in North America but even more so in Europe, where many conventional physicians also use homeopathic treatment.[9]

Two of the principles of homeopathic therapy are[9]:

1. An effective drug will produce in normal individuals symptoms similar to those experienced by the patient (law of similars).
2. Before use a drug should be diluted in water and shaken many times (succussion) so the concentration is minuscule. In some cases no molecules of the original drug remain, but to homeopathists this does not matter because in some undefined way the message of the drug is passed on in the water, the so-called memory of water.

In view of the unscientific basis for such therapeutic regimens, many physicians attribute the reported successes of homeopathy, as well as its popularity, to a powerful placebo effect. This is probably brought about in part by the taking of a long and sympathetic history, a procedure that many patients find contrasts sharply with their experience in conventional medical settings.[9]

Acupuncture

There are few high-quality studies of the efficacy of acupuncture. At present there is reasonable evidence that it may be beneficial for the nausea and vomiting of chemotherapy and for postoperative surgical and dental pain. No evidence has shown that it helps smoking cessation. Evidence is insufficient to determine whether it is useful for a wide variety of other conditions, including addictions, menstrual cramps, headaches, tennis elbow, fibromyalgia, osteoarthritis, carpal tunnel syndrome, asthma, and stroke rehabilitation.[10]

Therapeutic touch

Therapeutic touch is widely practiced in North America, particularly by nurses. No touching of the patient is involved. The theory is that by placing the hands close to the patient's body, the practitioner can "feel" his or her "energy field" and then "repattern" it. Therapeutic touch is reputed to be useful in many situations, from increasing infant-maternal bonding to treating measles and cancer. An experiment to validate this premise was devised by a 9-year-old fourth-grade student for her science fair and published in *JAMA* in 1998. Experienced therapeutic touch practitioners who were prevented from viewing the "patient" were asked to hold out their hands so they could detect "energy fields." The experimental subject held one of her hands close to one or the other of the practitioners' hands and asked the practitioner to indicate which of her hands detected the "energy field." The practitioners were correct in 44% of cases.[11]

REFERENCES

1. Ernst E, Assendelft WJ: Chiropractic for low back pain: we don't know whether it does more good than harm (editorial), *BMJ* 317:160, 1998.
2. Cherkin DC, Deyo RA, Battié M, et al: A comparison of physical therapy, chiropractic manipulation, and provision of an educational booklet for the treatment of patients with low back pain, *N Engl J Med* 339:1021-1029, 1998.
3. Kaptchuk TJ, Eisenberg DM: Chiropractic: origins, controversies, and contributions, *Arch Intern Med* 158:2215-2224, 1998.
4. Shekelle PG: What role for chiropractic in health care? (editorial), *N Engl J Med* 339:1074-1075, 1998.
5. Balon JB, Aker PD, Crowther ER, et al: A comparison of active and simulated chiropractic manipulation as adjunctive treatment for childhood asthma, *N Engl J Med* 339:1013-1020, 1998.
6. Bove G, Nilsson N: Spinal manipulation in the treatment of episodic tension-type headache, *JAMA* 280:1576-1590, 1998.
7. Linde K, Clausius N, Ramirez G: Are the clinical effects of homeopathy placebo effects? A meta-analysis of placebo controlled trials, *Lancet* 350:834-843, 1997.
8. Vandenbroucke JP: Homeopathy trials: going nowhere (editorial), *Lancet* 350:824, 1997.
9. Ernst E, Kaptchuk TJ: Homeopathy revisited (editorial), *Arch Intern Med* 156:2162-2164, 1996.
10. NIH Consensus Development Panel on Acupuncture: *JAMA* 280:1518-1524, 1998.
11. Rosa L, Rosa E, Sarner L: A close look at therapeutic touch, *JAMA* 279:1005-1010, 1998.

ASPIRIN

(See also anemia; angina; asthma; asthma in children; atrial fibrillation; cerebrovascular accidents; colon cancer; coronary artery disease; gout; migraines; myocardial infarction; niacin; nonsteroidal antiinflammatory drugs; peptic ulcer; thrombophlebitis; transient ischemic attacks)

Aspirin has multiple reputed and proven benefits. It is also well known to have adverse effects on the gastrointestinal tract and to precipitate asthma in susceptible persons. Only a few of these topics are discussed here; others can be found elsewhere in the text.

Prevention of Neoplasms

Evidence suggests that regular aspirin use decreases the risk of several types of cancer. The most striking is colon cancer (see discussion of colon cancer). Other cancer sites where regular aspirin use is said to reduce risk are the esophagus, stomach, rectum, lung, and breast.[1,2] The absolute reduction rates are low, and whether potential benefits outweigh risks has not been established.

Pathophysiology of Antithrombotic Effect

Aspirin acetylates platelet prostaglandin G/H synthase, causing an irreversible loss of its cyclooxygenase activity. Cyclooxygenase is necessary for the formation of thromboxane A_2, which in turn causes platelet aggregation. This effect is produced within 1 hour by the oral ingestion of 100 mg of aspirin. However, aspirin also reversibly inhibits endothelial cell prostacyclin, a potent inhibitor of platelet aggregation. Some workers have hypothesized that lower doses of acetylsalicylic acid given at longer intervals may be the most effective prophylactic program against thromboembolic phenomena because they will cause less inhibition of endothelial prostacyclin.[3]

Gastrointestinal Bleeding

One of the major adverse effects of aspirin is an increased incidence of gastrointestinal bleeding. An increased incidence of clinically significant bleeding episodes has been documented even with daily doses as low as 75[4] or 100 mg.[5] The 100-mg study emanating from Australia enrolled 400 men and women with an age range of 70 to 90 years.[5] Over a 1-year period the total percentage of overt bleeding episodes was 3% in treated patients versus none in the control group. In addition, the hemoglobin concentration of the treated group dropped by a mean of 0.33 g/dl (33 g/L), which was statistically significant, but more important, 17.4% of the aspirin-treated group had a reduction of 1 g/dl (100 g/L) or more compared with 9.3% of the control subjects. The mean corpuscular volume increased in the treated group compared with the placebo group, perhaps because of an increase in reticulocytes. Gastrointestinal symptoms were reported by 18% of those taking aspirin and by 12.5% of those given placebo.[5] Similar results have been reported in a Canadian study.[6]

In a British case-controlled study the odds ratio for bleeding peptic ulcer disease in patients taking regular doses of aspirin was 2.3 for 75 mg/day, 3.2 for 150 mg/day, and 3.9 for 300 mg/day. For enteric-coated aspirin it was only 1.1.[7]

Hemorrhagic Stroke

A 1998 metaanalysis found that aspirin was associated with an absolute increase in hemorrhagic strokes of $12:10,000$

users.[8] In view of this it seems prudent to use aspirin prophylactically for individuals at high risk of cardiovascular disease but to refrain from using it as a primary preventive measure for those at low risk.[9]

Aspirin Sensitivity

Aspirin sensitivity with bronchospasm that is not allergic or IgE mediated occurs in about 20% of persons with asthma.[10]

⚓ REFERENCES ⚓

1. Thun MJ, Namboodiri MM, Calle EE, et al: Aspirin use and risk of fatal cancer, *Cancer Res* 53:60-74, 1993.
2. Schreinemachers DM, Everson RB: Aspirin use and lung, colon, and breast cancer incidence in a prospective study, *Epidemiology* 5:138-146, 1994.
3. Patrono C: Aspirin as an antiplatelet drug, *N Engl J Med* 330:1287-1294, 1994.
4. SALT Collaborative Group: Swedish aspirin low-dose trial (SALT) of 75 mg aspirin as secondary prophylaxis after cerebrovascular ischaemic events, *Lancet* 338:1345-1349, 1991.
5. Silagy CA, McNeil JJ, Donnan GA, et al: Adverse effects of low-dose aspirin in a healthy elderly population, *Clin Pharmacol Ther* 54:84-89, 1993.
6. Leibovici A, Lavi N, Wainstok S, et al: Low-dose acetylsalicylic acid use and hemoglobin levels: effects in a primary care population, *Can Fam Physician* 41:64-68, 1995.
7. Weil J, Colinjones D, Langman M, et al: Prophylactic aspirin and risk of peptic ulcer bleeding, *BMJ* 310:827-830, 1995.
8. He J, Whelton PK, Vu B, et al: Aspirin and risk of hemorrhagic stroke: a meta-analysis of randomized controlled trials, *JAMA* 280:1930-1935, 1998.
9. Boissel J-P: Individualizing aspirin therapy for prevention of cardiovascular events (editorial), *JAMA* 280:1949-1950, 1998.
10. Manning ME, Stevenson DD: Aspirin sensitivity: a distressing reaction that is now often treatable, *Postgrad Med* 90:227-233, 1991.

ATTITUDES, PHYSICIAN

(See also consensus conferences; gestational diabetes mellitus; informed consent; investigations; practice patterns; prevention; risk analysis; risk assessment in pregnancy; screening; skepticism; uncertainty)

In their attitudes toward case finding and screening procedures physicians have been categorized by Stephenson as maximalists ("If in doubt, screen") or minimalists ("If in doubt, don't screen").[1] A third category, ritualists ("I was taught it, so I do it") has been added by Jeyapragasan and Morris.[2]

According to Stephenson,[1] the Maximum School is based on three concepts:

1. One must prevent the worst possible eventuality.
2. Interventions are beneficial and do not have serious side effects.
3. The anxiety provoked in physicians by uncertainty can be relieved by accepting protocols or courses of action that by implication guarantee successful outcomes.

The Minimum School is based on three different tenets[1]:

1. Patient care must be based on evidence.
2. "Above all, do no harm," or in more technical terms, avoid malfeasance. In other words, consider the detrimental effects of any intervention.
3. Management should be individualized, and this takes precedence over following protocols.

A similar division was made by Sackett and Holland[3] in 1975; they divided physicians into "advocates" and "methodologists" or, as they later referred to them, "evangelists" and "snails." As Davidoff[4] put it in the context of the cholesterol screening debate, evangelists believe it would be wrong to withhold a preventive program that might be beneficial and that has not demonstrated harm, whereas snails believe it would be wrong to impose an intervention that has undemonstrated benefits and has the potential for harm. There is no right answer here; it is a difference in values that is an inevitable result of scientific uncertainty.[4]

"Practice style" is a term that often reflects physicians' attitudes. An example is the tendency of obstetricians to perform Cesarean deliveries on women with gestational diabetes even when no evidence of macrosomia is present.[5] In some cases it seems that "practice style" is a euphemism for "ritualistic behavior."

The training of young physicians in hospitals where errors of omission are considered much more serious than those of commission may foster the attitude that many investigations are better than few and that investigations do no harm.[6] This relates to what Johnson calls the "uncertainty principle"—subspecialists with narrow referral practices (who are the prime mentors in teaching hospitals) are obligated to eliminate uncertainty, whereas generalists cannot function unless they accept uncertainty with equanimity (see discussion of uncertainty). Because of these ingrained attitudes, a subspecialist has great difficulty embracing a dual role as both expert consultant and generalist.[7]

--- ### ✎ REFERENCES ✎ ---

1. Stephenson MJ: Gestational diabetes mellitus (editorial), *Can Fam Physician* 39:745-748, 1993.
2. Jeyapragasan M, Morris B: Are you a maximalist, a minimalist, or a ritualist? (letter), *Can Fam Physician* 39:1878, 1881, 1993.
3. Sackett DL, Holland WW: Controversy in the detection of disease, *Lancet* 2:357-359, 1975.
4. Davidoff F: Evangelists and snails redux: the case of cholesterol screening, *Ann Intern Med* 124:513-514, 1996.
5. Naylor CD, Sermer M, Chen E, Sykora K (Toronto Trihospital Gestational Diabetes Investigators): Cesarean delivery in relation to birth weight and gestational glucose tolerance: pathophysiology or practice style? *JAMA* 275:1165-1170, 1996.
6. Woolf SH, Kamerow DB: Testing for uncommon conditions: the heroic search for positive test results, *Arch Intern Med* 150:2451-2458, 1990.
7. Johnson W: Comparing apples with oranges (editorial), *Arch Intern Med* 158:1591-1592, 1998.

AVIATION MEDICINE

(See also cardiac arrest; insomnia; middle ear effusion)

Aerotitis Media

In a study of aerotitis media, 250 adult volunteers with a history of recurrent ear discomfort when flying were selected at random to receive 120 mg of oral pseudoephedrine (Sudafed) or placebo 30 minutes before departure. Ear discomfort was reported by 32% of those taking pseudoephedrine but 62% of those given placebo.[1] In contrast, a placebo-controlled double-blind trial of children aged 6 months to 6 years found no benefit from pseudoephedrine taken 30 to 60 minutes before flight departure.[2] A common belief is that a warm wet towel placed over the ear during descent will relieve pain by decreasing the "ambient" pressure in the external canal. As far as I know, no studies evaluating this intervention have been published.

Infectious Diseases on Aircraft

One of the concerns about air travel is the possiblity of increased risk of infection in the cabin environment. An evaluation of the concentration of organisms in the cabin air of domestic and international flights found the levels to be much lower than those in city locations such as buses, shopping centers, or airline terminals.[3]

The number of air exchanges per hour in an aircraft cabin varies with cruise conditions and ranges from 5 to 42. This compares favorably with the 6 air exchanges per hour recommended for hospital isolation rooms housing patients with active tuberculosis.[4] In first-generation jet passenger aircraft all air exchanges used outside compressed air that was heated by the engines to 250° C, compressed, and cooled. In aircraft built since the mid-1980s half of cabin air is fresh and half recirculated, but it is passed through high-efficiency particulate filters.[5]

Many organisms that infect the respiratory tract are spread by large droplets that fall rapidly to the floor. Examples are streptococci, meningococci, and even hemorrhagic fever viruses such as Ebola. Of more concern regarding air travel are organisms spread by tiny aerosol droplets, which in theory could circulate and recirculate in the cabin air for prolonged periods. Examples are measles, influenza, and tuberculosis.[5]

Studies of actual transmission of infections in the aircraft cabin environment are few. One dramatic example was an outbreak of influenza affecting 59% of the occupants of an early model Boeing 737. The aircraft was delayed on the runway for 3 hours before takeoff, and the ventilation system was defective.[6]

In 1994 a 32-year-old Korean woman with advanced pulmonary tuberculosis that led to her death 2 weeks later flew from Chicago to Honolulu on a Boeing 747 100 aircraft. She was seated at the back of the rear cabin for the flight, which lasted 8 hours and 45 minutes. Intensive follow-up of the passengers and crew showed no purified protein derivative

(PPD) conversion among individuals sitting in other cabin sections. Among those who had been in the same section, six individuals with no other risk factors for tuberculosis had positive PPD tests and four of these were passengers who had sat within two rows of the index case. This study makes it clear that the transmission of the disease was not through the aircraft's recirculation system.[7] As far as I can see, infectious disease transmission as described above could have occurred in many other locations and there is no reason to consider an aircraft cabin a particularly risky environment.

Food poisoning is another uncommon infectious disease risk in commercial air travel. Most cases are caused by *Salmonella* species, and the chances of being affected are much greater among first-class or Concorde (supersonic) passengers than among tourist-class passengers.[8] Bugs as well as people like first-class food.

Flight Emergencies

Major medical emergencies aboard commercial aircraft are rare. A survey of nine U.S. airlines found that the rate was 1:58,000 passengers. The most frequent problems were faintness, loss of consciousness, trauma, respiratory problems, chest pain, seizures, and nausea and vomiting.[9]

As of mid-1998, emergency medical kits on U.S. airlines must include four drugs: 50% dextrose, nitroglycerin tablets, injectable diphenhydramine (Benadryl), and epinephrine 1:1000. An Aerospace Medical Association Task Force has recommended adding other drugs, including albuterol (salbutamol, Proventil, Ventolin), oxymetazoline (Dristan), diazepam (Valium) injectable, glucagon injectable, ketorolac (Toradol) injectable, acetylsalicylic acid, acetaminophen, and meclizine (Antivert).[9]

Automatic external defibrillators (AEDs) that can identify ventricular fibrillation or tachycardia and apply appropriate shocks are available on some airlines; cabin crew are trained to operate them. Qantas Airlines has been carrying AEDs since 1991, and American Airlines on over-water flights since 1997. Delta Airlines planned to install this equipment in 1998. Virgin Atlantic and Air Zimbabwe also carry AEDs.[9]

Jet Lag

Jet lag is a common result of crossing five or more time zones. Adjustment to a new time zone takes longer after an eastward than after a westward flight. Suggested preventive and management protocols are a good night's sleep before the flight, avoidance of alcohol during the flight, ingestion of plenty of fluids to avoid dehydration, and immediate adjustment to the time cycle of the destination. Exposure to several hours of bright outdoor light on arrival seems beneficial.[10]

Whether melatonin is effective in controlling jet lag is controversial.[10,11] A placebo-controlled trial of several different concentrations of melatonin given to 257 Norwe-gian physicians who flew from New York to Oslo found no benefit from the drug.[11]

Preexisting Medical Conditions and Air Travel[12]
Chronic obstructive pulmonary disease
Patients with severe but stable chronic obstructive lung disease or heart disease may require supplemental oxygen during flight. The pressurization of commercial aircraft maintains a relative altitude of 8000 feet or lower. If a person's arterial partial pressure of oxygen (Pao_2) is below 68 to 70 mm Hg at sea level, supplemental oxygen will probably be required during flight. Commercial carriers will generally provide oxygen, but arrangements have to be made in advance and in most cases additional charges are levied.

Pneumothorax
Pneumothorax is a strict contraindication to air travel.

Myocardial infarction
Patients who have had an uncomplicated myocardial infarction may fly 2 weeks after the event.

Thrombophlebitis
Individuals at risk of thromboembolism should have an aisle seat, walk around frequently, perform isometric exercises of the legs, wear support stockings, and drink plenty of fluids to maintain adequate hydration in the face of the low relative humidity of the cabin air. Low-molecular-weight heparin may be indicated in high-risk patients.

Diabetes mellitus
Persons with diabetes who require insulin will have to modify their doses if crossing several time zones. Traveling eastward means a short day and lower insulin doses, whereas traveling westward means a long day and larger doses. Frequent glucose self-monitoring is probably the easiest way of adjusting the doses.

Surgery
No one should fly within 7 to 10 days after surgery involving procedures, such as laparoscopy, that introduce air into the body. The air expands as cabin altitude decreases. Recently applied casts should be bivalved.

Scuba Diving
Scuba divers who make only one dive on the day of or before a flight should wait 12 hours before flying; those who make several dives or who require decompression stops during ascent should wait 24 hours.[12]

Mortality in General Aviation Accidents
Mortality rates of general aviation pilots who are involved in crash landings are lower among those who use both lap and shoulder restraints.[13]

Radiation Exposure

Cosmic ray exposure is significantly increased at the altitudes flown by commercial jet aircraft. For occasional recreational travelers (pregnant or not) the increased risk is minimal, but for air crew and frequent flyers, the radiation exposure may be greater than that experienced by radiation workers in ground-based industries.[14]

REFERENCES

1. Csortan E, Jones J, Haan M, et al: Efficacy of pseudoephedrine for the prevention of barotrauma during air travel, *Ann Emerg Med* 23:1324-1327, 1994.
2. Buchanan BJ, Hoagland J, Fischer PR: Pseudoephedrine and air travel—associated ear pain in children, *Arch Pediatr Adolesc Med* 153:466-468, 1999.
3. Wick RL Jr, Irvine LA: The microbiological composition of airliner cabin air, *Aviat Space Environ Med* 66:220-224, 1995.
4. Centers for Disease Control: Guidelines for preventing the transmission of tuberculosis in health-care settings with special focus on HIV-related issues, *MMWR* 39:1-29, 1990.
5. Wenzel RP: Airline travel and infection (editorial), *N Engl J Med* 334:981-982, 1996.
6. Moser MR, Bender TR, Margolis HS, et al: An outbreak of influenza aboard a commercial airliner, *Am J Epidemiol* 110:1-6, 1979.
7. Kenyon TA, Valway SE, Ihle WW, et al: Transmission of multidrug-resistant *Mycobacterium tuberculosis* during a long airplane flight, *N Engl J Med* 334:933-938, 1996.
8. Tauxe RV, Tormey MP, Mascola L, et al: Salmonellosis outbreak on transatlantic flights: foodborne illness on aircraft: 1947-1984, *Am J Epidemiol* 125:150-157, 1987.
9. Rayman RB: Aerospace medicine, *JAMA* 280:1777-1778, 1998.
10. Canada communicable disease report: travel statement on jet lag, *Can Med Assoc J* 155:61-63, 1996.
11. Spitzer RL, Terman M, Williams JB, et al: Jet lag: clinical features, validation of a new syndrome-specific scale, and lack of response to melatonin in a randomized, double-blind trial, *Am J Psychiatry* 156:1392-1396, 1999.
12. Bettes TN, McKenas DK: Medical advice for commercial air travelers, *Am Fam Physician* 60:801-808, 1999.
13. Rostykus PS, Cummings P, Mueller BA: Risk factors for pilot fatalities in general aviation airplane crash landings, *JAMA* 280:997-999, 1998.
14. Barish RJ: In-flight radiation: counseling patients about risk, *J Am Board Fam Pract* 12:195-199, 1999.

BED REST COMPLICATIONS

The following are some of the important complications of bed rest[1,2]:

1. Musculoskeletal
   a. Muscle weakness and atrophy. A muscle at complete rest loses 10% to 15% of its strength each week. Nearly 50% of normal strength is lost in 3 to 5 weeks. Strength is recovered at a rate of only 6% per week. Associated with weakness is decreased endurance, manifested as fatigue and muscle atrophy.
   b. Contractures
   c. Disuse osteoporosis
2. Cardiovascular
   a. Increased heart rate. The heart rate increases by 1 beat per minute every 2 days during bed rest. The maximum heart rate resulting from bed rest alone is about 80 beats per minute.
   b. Decreased cardiac output
   c. Orthostatic hypotension. Orthostatic hypotension develops after 3 weeks of bed rest in most adults and sooner in the elderly.
   d. Thromboembolism
3. Respiratory
   a. Decreased ventilation
   b. Atelectasis and pneumonia
4. Metabolic
   a. Glucose intolerance. Glucose intolerance in patients confined to bed is due to increased insulin resistance.
   b. Decreased metabolic rate
   c. Negative nitrogen balance
   d. Hypercalcemia and renal stones (usually with coma or quadriplegia)
5. Gastrointestinal
   a. Anorexia
   b. Constipation
6. Dermatological
   a. Pressure sores
7. Central nervous system
   a. Decreased balance and coordination. Decreased balance and coordination are due not only to muscle weakness but also to deficits in neural control.
8. Social
   a. Social isolation
   b. Dependency

A systematic literature review found almost no evidence supporting bed rest as a therapeutic treatment and much evidence of its potential harm. Bed rest has no value after spinal anesthesia, and 2 to 4 hours is the maximum period required after cardiac catheterization. No bed rest is required for uncomplicated low back pain, 12 hours of bed rest is all that is currently recommended after a myocardial infarction, and early ambulation is the norm after surgery.[3]

REFERENCES

1. Dittmer DK, Teasell R: Complications of immobilization and bed rest. I. Musculoskeletal and cardiovascular complications, *Can Fam Physician* 39:1428-1432, 1435-1437, 1993.
2. Teasell R, Kittmer DK: Complications of immobilization and bed rest. II. Other complications, *Can Fam Physician* 39:1440-1442, 1445-1446, 1993.
3. Allen C, Glasziou P, Del Mar C: Bed rest: a potentially harmful treatment needing more careful evaluation, *Lancet* 354:1229-1233, 1999.

BITES
Animal Bites
(See also human bites; rabies)

Epidemiology

Bites account for about 1% of emergency room visits. The incidence varies from one institution to another. Dog bites are responsible for 80% to 90% of all bites assessed by physicians, cat bites for 5% to 15%, and human bites for 3% to 20%.[1] It has been estimated that in the United States each year 2% of the population is bitten by dogs.[2]

In about 90% of dog bite cases the animal belongs to or is known to the victim. Most dog bites involve the extremities except in children under 4, who most commonly have bites to the head and neck. Rates of infection from dog bites are low, between 2% and 20%.[1]

Prevention of animal bites begins by selecting only appropriate animals as pets. Ferrets should be banned from homes where infants and small children are present. Nonhuman primates should be banned from all homes because these animals are prone to vicious attacks on humans. Numerous breeds of dogs are considered dangerous in the presence of small children, but identifying them is difficult because of lack of published data; 40 dangerous breeds were listed in one authoritative book on dogs in 1997, but because of protests from breeders the book was recalled.[3]

Attacks by dogs are considerably decreased by neutering or spaying them and by giving them intensive socialization training between the ages of 7 and 12 weeks. Preventing dogs from roaming free clearly decreases the risk of bites; chaining dogs in the yard or restraining them with buried electric fences is inadequate because such measures do not prevent children from approaching the animal.[3] Infants and toddlers should never be left alone with a dog. Children should be trained to avoid approaching an unknown dog, to stand still and not to scream if approached by a dog, to avoid eye contact with a dog, and if knocked down by a dog, to roll up into a ball and stay perfectly still.[4]

Cat bites are much more likely than dog bites to become infected; the infection rate is 30% to 50%. One reason is that cat bites are often puncture wounds and involve the hands, which are more susceptible to infection than many other parts of the body.[1]

Management principles

Animal bites are managed with meticulous wound irrigation and if indicated debridement, as well as assessment for risk of tetanus and rabies. Facial lacerations from cat or dog bites can generally be sutured if this is possible within 12 to 24 hours of the injury. Hand wounds and puncture wounds should not be sutured, but bites to the arms or legs may be sutured if this can be done within 6 to 12 hours.[5]

Microbiology of cat and dog bites

Most infections caused by cat or dog bites are polymicrobial. On average five different organisms are cultured from infected wounds. The most frequently isolated aerobes are *Pasteurella* species (*P. multocida* from cats and *P. canis* from dogs), *Streptococcus* species, *Staphylococcus* species, *Corynebacterium, Moraxella,* and *Neisseria*. In over half of infected wounds a variety of anaerobes are found, almost always in conjunction with aerobes. Most of the anaerobes and many of the aerobes are β-lactamase producers.[6]

Antibiotic treatment of infected cat and dog bites

Antibiotics chosen for treatment should be effective against *Pasteurella,* streptococci, staphylococci, and anaerobes and should have activity against β-lactamase-producing organisms.[6] In most cases this can be accomplished by giving a β-lactam antibiotic such as amoxicillin combined with a β-lactamase inhibitor such as clavulanate (Augmentin, Clavulin).[5] Other options are a second-generation cephalosporin, a combination of penicillin and a first-generation cephalosporin, or a combination of clindamycin and a fluoroquinolone. In vitro sensitivities suggest that azithromycin (Zithromax) given alone may be effective. Drugs that should not be used as sole treatment are erythromycin, first-generation cephalosporins, antistaphylococcal penicillins, or clindamycin.[6]

Capnocytophaga canimorsus is a rare source of infection after dog bites. It should be suspected if fever develops in an immunocompromised patient after a dog bite. The organism is sensitive to penicillin.[5]

Antibiotic prophylaxis of cat and dog bites

Although a 1994 metaanalysis showed that antibiotic prophylaxis after dog bites reduced the relative risk of infection by 44%, this translated into an absolute risk reduction of only 4%. In other words, 25 patients would have to be treated for one patient to benefit.[7] Antibiotic prophylaxis is unnecessary for minor wounds, but most experts recommend it for high-risk bites such as deep puncture wounds (a common form of injury in cat bites) and bites involving the hands. Broad coverage for most cases of dog or cat bites may be achieved with amoxicillin-clavulanate (Augmentin, Clavulin) 500 mg tid.[1,5] An acceptable alternative is cefuroxime (Ceftin) 500 mg bid.[1]

Snake bites

There are only two families of poisonous snakes in North America. Pit vipers belong to the family Crotalidae and include rattlesnakes, cottonmouths, and copperheads. The Elapidae family includes the coral snakes, which are found only in the southern United States. In Canada, the only poisonous snakes are rattlesnakes. The term "pit viper" comes from the presence of a heat-sensitive pit located between the eyes and the nostrils. Other identifying features of pit vipers are their vertically elliptical pupils (cat's eye pupils) which contrast with the round pupils of nonvenomous snakes, and in the case of rattlesnakes, the presence of a rattle on the tail.[8]

Up to 30% of proven snake bites are "dry bites" in which no envenomation occurs. Symptoms and signs of pit viper envenomation are severe pain and burning followed by increasing edema, ecchymosis, and constitutional symptoms.[8]

Dead snakes are not safe snakes. There are several reports of serious envenomation occurring when foolhardy individuals picked up the heads of decapitated rattlesnakes.[9]

Field therapy of poisonous snake bites consists of immobilization of the bitten appendage, which should be kept below heart level, and removal of the patient to an emergency room as quickly as possible. Constricting bands such as elastic bandages should be applied 5 to 10 cm proximal to the bite and kept sufficiently loose to allow the fifth finger to be slipped between the bands and the skin without causing discomfort. The bands should be periodically loosened and readjusted as edema evolves. The purpose of the bands is to decrease lymph flow without obstructing venous return. Incision and suction of the wound in the field is not recommended.[8]

Hospital treatment consists of supportive care, antibiotics, tetanus booster if necessary, and the IV administration of 4 to 20 vials of antivenin. Antivenin is made from immune horse serum, so skin testing is mandatory before administration. Wyeth's Crotalidae antivenin covers copperheads, cottonmouths, and rattlesnakes, but not coral snakes.

───────────── ◥ REFERENCES ◤ ─────────────

1. Griego RD, Rosen T, Orengo IF, et al: Dog, cat, and human bite: a review, *J Am Acad Dermatol* 33:1019-1029, 1995.
2. Voelker R: Dog bites recognized as public health problem, *JAMA* 277:278-280, 1997.
3. Hoff GL, Brawley J, Johnson K: Companion animal issues and the physician, *South Med J* 92:651-659, 1999.
4. Centers for Disease Control and Prevention: Dog-bite-related fatalities—United States, 1995-1996, *JAMA* 278:278-279, 1997.
5. Fleisher GR: The management of bite wounds (editorial), *N Engl J Med* 340:138-140, 1999.
6. Talan DA, Citron DM, Abrahamian FM, et al: Bacteriologic analysis of infected dog and cat bites, *N Engl J Med* 340:85-92, 1999.
7. Cummings P: Antibiotics to prevent infection in patients with dog bite wounds: a meta-analysis of randomized trials, *Ann Emerg Med* 23:535-540, 1994.
8. Forks TP: Evaluation and treatment of poisonous snakebites, *Am Fam Physician* 50:123-130, 1994.
9. Suchard JR, Lo Vecchio F: Envenomations by rattlesnakes thought to be dead (letter), *N Engl J Med* 340:1930, 1999.

Human Bites
(See also animal bites)

One study found that the infection rate of simple human bites sustained in an institution for developmentally disabled persons was about 18% compared with a rate of 13% for simple lacerations occurring in the same population.[1]

Although this infection rate is not very high, the situation is different with bites to the hand. Hand bites may be categorized as clenched fist injuries sustained by punching someone in the teeth or as simple bites. Any bite to the hand carries a greater risk of infection than bites elsewhere on the body, but this is particularly so with clenched fist injuries.[2] The actual skin laceration in hand bites may be small, but in many cases the teeth have penetrated closed hand spaces, tendons, or joints.[3] In clenched fist injuries the laceration is often only a 3- to 8-mm puncture wound on the dorsum of the hand or over the third metacarpophalangeal joint.[2] In view of the high incidence of infection and the complexity of the hand, most human bites of the hand require assessment and management by a hand surgeon.[2,3]

Microbiology of human bites

Like cat and dog bites, infections from human bites are almost always polymicrobial. On average, five different organisms are cultured.[2] The organisms from human bites are those of the oral flora and include alpha-hemolytic streptococci, beta-hemolytic streptococci, *Staphylococcus aureus, Staphylococcus epidermidis, Eikenella corrodens,* and anaerobes.

E. corrodens is a gram-negative facultative anaerobe that can be cultured from about 25% of human bite wounds. It causes serious indolent infections. The organism is sensitive to penicillin, amoxicillin-clavulanate (Augmentin, Clavulin), tetracycline, trimethoprim-sulfamethoxazole (Septra, Bactrim), and ciprofloxacin. It is usually resistant to erythromycin, dicloxacillin, cloxacillin, nafcillin, and first-generation cephalosporins.

Anaerobes can be cultured from nearly 50% of human bite wound infections. Many produce beta-lactamase and are penicillin resistant.

Antibiotic prophylaxis

Whether all human bites (except the most minimal injuries) require prophylactic antibiotics is controversial. However, if the bite involves the hand, prophylactic antibiotics should certainly be given.[1,4] This approach is supported by a prospective study of uncomplicated human bites of the hand that were treated with mechanical wound care alone or accompanied by prophylactic antibiotics. No infections occurred in those who received antibiotics, whereas the infection rate was 47% in those who did not.[4] Other indications for prophylactic antibiotics are similar to those for cat and dog bites.[1]

Broad coverage for most cases of human bites may be achieved by amoxicillin-clavulanate (Augmentin, Clavulin) 500 mg tid or cefuroxime (Ceftin) 500 mg bid. Alternatives are penicillin 500 mg qid (covers *E. corrodens*) plus dicloxacillin (Dycill, Dynapen, Pathocil) 500 mg qid (covers *S. aureus*) or, for those allergic to penicillin, doxycycline 100 mg bid. Erythromycin is not a good choice because *E. corrodens* tends to be resistant to it. When given prophylactically, these drugs should be used for 3 to 5 days.[1]

⚓ REFERENCES ⚓

1. Lindsay D, Christopher M, Hollenbach J, et al: Natural course of the human bite wound: incidence of infection and complications in 434 bites and 803 lacerations in the same group of patients, *J Trauma* 27:45-48, 1987.
2. Griego RD, Rosen T, Orengo IF, et al: Dog, cat, and human bite: a review, *J Am Acad Dermatol* 33:1019-1029, 1995.
3. Kelly IP, Cunney RJ, Smyth EG, et al: The management of human bite injuries of the hand, *Injury* 27:481-484, 1996.
4. Zubowicz VN, Gravier M: Management of early human bites of the hand: a prospective randomized study, *Plast Reconstr Surg* 88:111-114, 1991.

CHRONIC FATIGUE SYNDROME

(See also celiac disease; fibromyalgia; functional somatic syndromes; multiple chemical sensitivities)

Chronic fatigue syndrome, fibromyalgia, and multiple chemical sensitivities are three conditions whose existence is controversial, and the symptoms and epidemiology of the three entities overlap. Believers search ever more intensely for organic causes such as occult infections or subtle immunological dysfunctions, while unbelievers attribute the symptoms to a variety of functional somatic symptoms that may or may not fit into well-defined psychiatric disorders such as depression, somatoform disorder, or one of the personality disorders.[1,2] Many skeptics are loath to make a diagnosis of "chronic fatigue syndrome," not only because of the lack of scientific evidence supporting its existence, but also because of fear that such a diagnosis would become a self-fulfilling prophecy. On the other hand, many patients who receive the diagnose feel enabled rather than disabled; being labeled as having chronic fatigue syndrome affirms for them that their illness is genuine.[3] Barsky[4] considers chronic fatigue syndrome to be a functional somatic syndrome (see functional somatic syndromes).

Whether chronic fatigue syndrome is a new disorder or simply a new name for "neurasthenia," which was a frequently diagnosed condition in the latter half of the 19th and early decades of the 20th century, is unknown. Abbey and Garfinkel[2] point out striking similarities in the epidemiology and clinical descriptions of the two conditions, and Ware and Kleinman[5] suggest that in both conditions symptoms serve as a metaphor for unacceptable social stresses.

Chronic fatigue syndrome has a variety of definitions. One current example is unexplained (recognized organic and psychiatric disorders having been ruled out) new-onset persistent or recurring fatigue that lasts 6 months or more and substantially reduces the functional level, plus four of the following symptoms, which must not have predated the onset of the illness[6]:

1. Self-reported decrease in short-term memory or concentration
2. Sore throat
3. Tender cervical or axillary lymph nodes
4. Muscle pains
5. Multiple arthralgias without swelling or redness
6. Headaches
7. Unrefreshing sleep
8. Postexertional malaise lasting over 24 hours

Patients who have been suffering from fatigue for more than 6 months but do not meet the criteria for chronic fatigue syndrome are said to have "idiopathic chronic fatigue." The term "chronic fatigue" includes both the "chronic fatigue syndrome" and "idiopathic chronic fatigue."[6,7] In one British study of patients in primary care practices the prevalence of "chronic fatigue" was 11.3%, "idiopathic chronic fatigue" 9%, and "chronic fatigue syndrome" 2.6%. However, when patients with comorbid psychological disorder were eliminated, the figures were 4.1%, 3.6%, and 0.5%.[7] Most patients in whom the chronic fatigue syndrome is diagnosed are middle-aged women.[1,8]

Although many workers believe that chronic fatigue syndrome is an infectious illness, others consider psychiatric disorders to be responsible for the symptoms in many patients. A British investigation found that 80.6% of patients meeting the criteria of chronic fatigue syndrome had probable depression. In this study a linear correlation was seen between the mean number of somatic symptoms and the degree of psychological symptoms.[8] A community-based American study reported that 55% of patients with chronic fatigue syndrome had at least one current and 81% at least one lifetime Axis I psychiatric diagnosis. (According to the authors this high rate of psychiatric morbidity was probably secondary to chronic fatigue syndrome and its social consequences, not a cause of it.[9]) Another evaluation of patients with chronic fatigue syndrome found that 27% met the clinical criteria of somatoform disorder.[10]

The natural history of chronic fatigue syndrome has not been fully defined. An 18-month follow-up of 298 self-referred patients meeting the criteria of chronic fatigue syndrome found that 3% reported complete recovery and 17% had improvement.[11] In children and adolescents the prognosis is much better, with 95% improved or cured after 1 to 4 years of follow-up.[12]

As would be expected, optimal treatment for a condition of unknown etiology is uncertain. A 1996 study from the Netherlands found no benefit from an 8-week treatment regimen of fluoxetine (Prozac) 20 mg.[13] On the other hand, a series of 13[14] or 16[15] weekly or biweekly sessions of cognitive therapy was associated with a satisfactory outcome in about three fourths of treated patients compared with about one fourth of the control subjects who received either relaxation therapy[14] or general medical care from their general practitioners.[15] A randomized controlled trial of graded aerobic exercises versus flexibility exercises and relaxation therapy found a marked improvement with aerobic exercises,[16] while a trial comparing graded aerobic exercises with fluoxetine resulted in improvement in fatigue and work capacity with exercise but not with fluoxetine.[17] A placebo-controlled crossover trial found no benefit from fludrocortisone (Florinef),[18] whereas a randomized crossover trial of patients with no comorbid psychiatric conditions reported subjective benefit from hydrocortisone 5 or 10 mg/day, a benefit that rapidly attenuated when the drug was discontinued.[19]

❧ REFERENCES ❧

1. Buchwald D, Garrity D: Comparison of patients with chronic fatigue syndrome, fibromyalgia, and multiple chemical sensitivities, *Arch Intern Med* 154:2049-2053, 1994.
2. Abbey S, Garfinkel P: Neurasthenia and chronic fatigue syndrome: the role of culture in the making of a diagnosis, *Am J Psychiatry* 148:1638-1646, 1991.
3. Woodward RV, Broom DH, Legge DG: Diagnosis in chronic disease: disabling or enabling; the case of chronic fatigue syndrome, *J R Soc Med* 88:325-329, 1995.
4. Barsky AJ, Borus JF: Functional somatic syndromes, *Ann Intern Med* 130:910-921, 1999.
5. Ware NC, Kleinman A: Culture and somatic experience: the social course of illness in neurasthenia and chronic fatigue syndrome, *Psychosom Med* 20:35-53, 1992.
6. Fukuda K, Straus SE, Hickie I, et al (International Chronic Fatigue Syndrome Study Group): The chronic fatigue syndrome: a comprehensive approach to its definition and study, *Ann Intern Med* 121:953-959, 1994.
7. Wessely S, Chalder T, Hirsch S, et al: The prevalence and morbidity of chronic fatigue and chronic fatigue syndrome: a prospective primary care study, *Am J Public Health* 87:1449-1455, 1997.
8. Wessely S, Chalder T, Hirsch S, et al: Psychological symptoms, somatic symptoms and psychiatric disorder in chronic fatigue and chronic fatigue syndrome: a prospective study in primary care, *Am J Psychiatry* 153:1050-1059, 1996.
9. Jason LA, Richman JA, Rademaker AW, et al: A community-based study of chronic fatigue syndrome, *Arch Intern Med* 159:2129-2137, 1999.
10. Hickie I, Lloyd A, Hadzi-Pavlovic D, et al: Can the chronic fatigue syndrome be defined by distinct clinical features? *Psychol Med* 25:923-925, 1995.
11. Vercoulen JH, Swanink CM, Fennis JF, et al: Prognosis in chronic fatigue syndrome—a prospective study on the natural course, *J Neurol Neurosurg Psychiatry* 60:489-494, 1996.
12. Krilov LR, Fisher M, Friedman SB, et al: Course and outcome of chronic fatigue in children and adolescents, *Pediatrics* 102:360-366, 1998.
13. Vercoulen JH, Swanink CM, Zitman FG, et al: Randomised, double-blind, placebo-controlled study of fluoxetine in chronic fatigue syndrome, *Lancet* 347:858-861, 1996.
14. Deale A, Chalder T, Marks I, et al: Cognitive behavior therapy for chronic fatigue syndrome: a randomized controlled trial, *Am J Psychiatry* 154:408-414, 1997.
15. Sharpe M, Hawton K, Simkin S, et al: Cognitive behaviour therapy for the chronic fatigue syndrome: a randomized controlled trial, *BMJ* 312:22-26, 1996.
16. Fulcher KY, White PD: Randomised controlled trial of graded exercise in patients with the chronic fatigue syndrome, *BMJ* 314:1647-1652, 1997.
17. Wearden A, Morriss R, Mullis R, et al: A double-blind, placebo-controlled treatment trial of fluoxetine and graded exercise for chronic fatigue syndrome, *Br J Psychiatry* 172:485-490, 1998.
18. Peterson PK, Pheley A, Schroeppel J, et al: A preliminary placebo-controlled crossover trial of fludrocortisone for chronic fatigue syndrome, *Arch Intern Med* 158:908-914, 1998.
19. Cleare AJ, Heap E, Malhi GS, et al: Low-dose hydrocortisone in chronic fatigue syndrome: a randomised crossover trial, *Lancet* 353:455-458, 1999.

CLINICAL PRACTICE GUIDELINES

(See also attitudes, physician; evidence-based medicine; informed consent; periodic health examination; screening)

Principles

Ideally clinical practice guidelines should do the following[1]:
1. Result in improved health care
2. Not be so rigid that they inhibit the judgment of individual physicians
3. Be evidence based and cite the appropriate references
4. Be reviewed by both experts and users and field tested before implementation

Categories of Evidence and Strength of Recommendations

The quality of evidence in the medical literature and therefore the strength of guideline recommendations are variable. One widely used hierarchical classification lists four levels for quality of evidence (I to IV), from randomized controlled trials to opinion. These four levels of evidence directly correlate with four levels for strength of evidence (A to D). Thus a level A recommendation is based on evidence from randomized controlled trials (evidence category I), whereas a level D recommendation is based on opinion only (evidence category IV).[2]

Controversy over Validity of Guidelines

A variety of publications have expressed concern about the quality or the intended use of clinical practice guidelines.[3-9]

Guidelines as tools for controlling physicians

The raison d'être of guidelines is to improve the quality and consistency of patient care, but some authors fear that health care administrators will use them as cost containment measures[3] or as inflexible norms for judging the competence of physicians during clinical audits[4] or malpractice suits.[5]

Quality of evidence supporting guideline recommendations

A review of 279 guidelines published from 1985 to 1997 found that only half of them followed the established standards for formulating guidelines and that the major common deficit was inadequate identification, evaluation, and synthesis of evidence.[9]

Relevance of the guidelines to a specific practice population

An important concern about guidelines is that rigidly adhering to them could cause harm even if they are based on well-done randomized controlled trials—the complex and idiosyncratic problems presented by one patient may not match the medical problems of the highly selected populations that are evaluated in developing guidelines.[5]

Development of guidelines: consensus conferences

Clinical practice guidelines are produced by consensus conferences. Because the guidelines deal with subjects that tend to be controversial, members of consensus conference committees find it difficult or impossible to settle the issues, no matter how good their intentions. Just because specific recommendations are published does not mean that unanimity was achieved. When opinions differ, recommendations are often those of a majority vote—a laudable democratic procedure, but one that fails to instill confidence in the scientific validity of the conclusions.

The fallibility of expert bodies is underlined by the number of occasions on which initial recommendations have been reversed. In one recent instance this was associated with political pressure. In January 1997 a majority report of a consensus conference convened by the National Institutes of Health stated evidence was insufficient to recommend universal mammographic screening of women aged 40 to 49. This caused a political furor, and a few months later the National Cancer Institute decreed that women in this age bracket should have screening every 1 to 2 years.[10]

Membership is an important factor influencing the recommendations of consensus conferences. Participants are usually chosen for their expertise; their views are well known and are unlikely to change during the conference. Does the membership include a balance of disciplines? Have known dissenters or skeptics been invited? If so, do they have a real voice or are they token representatives?[6] Specialists tend to be biased in favor of procedures in which they have a vested interest, and this can be countered only by an effective multidisciplinary representation at the conference table.[2]

Could funding for consensus conferences influence recommendations? Does the fact that financial support for a Canadian Menopause Consensus Conference came from five pharmaceutical companies—all of which market hormonal products—make any difference, or does it not?[11] According to Sheldon and Davey Smith,[12] some so-called consensus conferences are nothing but a front for drug promotional activities of the sponsoring pharmaceutical industries.

Conflicting guidelines

Since numerous organizations produce guidelines, practitioners are faced with a plethora of often contradictory recommendations. Family physicians looking for evidence-based recommendations would be wise to follow those issued by the U.S. Preventive Services Task Force or the Canadian Task Force on Preventive Health Care rather than those provided by specialty societies (e.g., the American Urological Association or the Society of Obstetricians and Gynecologists of Canada) or disease-specific advocacy groups (e.g., the American Cancer Society).[13] The National Guideline Clearinghouse Internet web site is a source of evidence-based clinical guidelines (www.guideline.gov). It has been developed under the auspices of the U.S. Agency for Health Care Policy and Research (AHCPR), the American Association of Health Plans (AAHP), and the American Medical Association (AMA). Canadian clinical practice guidelines (CPG Infobase) can be found at www.cma.ca/cpgs.

Efficacy of practice guidelines in improving patient outcomes

Little research has been devoted to assessing whether clinical practice guidelines actually improve patient outcomes. From what has been published so far, there is little evidence that they have made any difference in the primary care setting,[14] probably because few physicians implement guidelines in their practice (see following paragraphs).[15]

Implementing Practice Guidelines in Clinical Practice

Numerous barriers to implementing clinical practice guidelines in everyday clinical practice have been identified.

Lack of awareness of guidelines

Family physicians are overwhelmed with guidelines.[16-18] Hibble and associates[17] collected all the guidelines that were available in 22 general practices in Great Britain. They ended up with 855, which formed a pile 68 cm (27 inches) high and weighing 28 kg (61 lb). No wonder few physicians are aware of all the guidelines that might be applicable to their practices.[15]

Lack of familiarity with guidelines

More common than unawareness of guidelines is lack of familiarity with their contents.[15] This is an inevitable consequence not only of the number of guidelines, but in many instances of their complexity; some are so detailed that they are presented in booklet format.[17] As Gray[16] put it, "The present position is intolerable" and a major effort has to be directed toward managing "knowledge and know how." Slawson and Shaughnessy's goal of "Patient Oriented Evidence That Matters (POEM)" would seem to be the ideal for busy primary care practitioners.[18]

Lack of agreement with guidelines

Disagreement with some guidelines is inevitable when two or more give contradictory recommendations; the

American Cancer Society and the American Urological Association recommend annual prostate specific antigen screening, whereas the U.S. Preventive Services Task Force and the Canadian Task Force on Preventive Health Care recommend against it (see discussion of prostate specific antigen).

Lack of confidence in having the ability to implement the guidelines

If physicians feel inadequate to counsel patients or answer questions about certain topics, they are unlikely follow guidelines related to those topics.[15]

Lack of confidence in the successful outcome of implementing guidelines

Physicians who fail to see positive responses to certain interventions may stop performing them. It is difficult to keep telling patients to stop smoking if only 2% to 3% comply.[15]

Inertia

Old habits are hard to change.[15] Some physicians simply prefer to obtain their medical information from traditional sources rather than from guidelines.[19]

External barriers

Lack of time or reminder systems may inhibit full implementation of guidelines.[15]

Patient preferences

Patients may not consider the guidelines important or relevant.[15]

Guidelines for Patients

A recent innovation is the publication of lay or consumer versions of clinical practice guidelines. The idea behind these is to empower patients to make informed decisions.[4]

≫ REFERENCES ≪

1. National Partnership for Quality in Health: *Guidelines for Canadian clinical practice guidelines,* Ottawa, 1994, Canadian Medical Association.
2. Shekelle PG, Woolf SH, Eccles M, et al: Developing guidelines, *BMJ* 318:593-596, 1999.
3. Berger JT, Rosner F: The ethics of practice guidelines, *Arch Intern Med* 156:2051-2056, 1996.
4. Woolf SH, Grol R, Hutchinson A, et al: Potential benefits, limitations, and harms of clinical guidelines, *BMJ* 318:527-530, 1999.
5. Hurwitz B: Legal and political considerations of clinical practice guidelines, *BMJ* 318:661-664, 1999.
6. Woolf SH: Practice guidelines: what the family physician should know, *Am Fam Physician* 51:1455-1463, 1995.
7. Weingarten S: Practice guidelines and prediction rules should be subject to careful clinical testing (editorial), *JAMA* 277:1977-1978, 1997.
8. Lewis S: Paradox, process and perception: the role of organizations in clinical practice guidelines development, *Can Med Assoc J* 153:1073-1077, 1995.
9. Shaneyfelt TM, Mayo-Smith MF, Rothwangl J: Are guidelines following guidelines? The methodological quality of clinical practice guidelines in the peer-reviewed medical literature, *JAMA* 281:1900-1905, 1999.
10. Marwick C: Final mammography recommendation? *JAMA* 277:1181, 1997.
11. Canadian Menopause Consensus Conference, *J SOGC* 16:4-40, 1994.
12. Sheldon TA, Davey Smith G: Consensus conferences as drug promotion, *Lancet* 341:100-102, 1993.
13. Czaja R, McFall SL, Warnecke RB, et al: Preferences of community physicians for cancer screening guidelines, *Ann Intern Med* 120:602-608, 1994.
14. Worrall G, Chaulk P, Freake D: The effects of clinical practice guidelines on patient outcomes in primary care: a systematic review, *Can Med Assoc J* 156:1705-1712, 1997.
15. Cabana MD, Rand CS, Powe NR, et al: Why don't physicians follow clinical practice guidelines? *JAMA* 282:1458-1465, 1999.
16. Gray JA: Where's the chief knowledge officer? To manage the most precious resource of all (editorial), *BMJ* 317:832, 1998.
17. Hibble A, Kanaka D, Pencheon D, et al: Guidelines in general practice: the new tower of Babel? *BMJ* 317:862-863, 1998.
18. Slawson DC, Shaughnessy AF: Obtaining useful information from expert based sources, *BMJ* 314:947-949, 1997.
19. Hayward RS, Guyatt GH, Moore K-A, et al: Canadian physicians' attitudes about and preferences regarding clinical practice guidelines, *Can Med Assoc J* 156:1715-1723, 1997.

CONSULTATIONS

(See also practice patterns)

A common form of consultation between primary care physicians and specialists is the "curbside" or "corridor" consultation. Generalists usually consult specialists and are more enthusiastic than the specialists about the value of such a process. Consultants tend to worry that the information they receive may be incomplete and that as a result their advice may be inappropriate.[1,2] This is particularly likely if the clinical problem is complex. A good curbside consultation deals with brief simple issues, a bad one with complex issues.[3]

Some of the reputed advantages of curbside consultations for the primary care physician are saving of time, verification of correctness of data obtained from manuals or texts, a "free" consultation for the patient, and no fear that the consultant will "steal" the patient. Two advantages for the consultant are a sense of satisfaction in helping colleagues and improving care and the intellectual stimulation of being asked difficult but pertinent questions. For full-time salaried consultants a third advantage is in time management, since curbside consultations take far less time than formal ones.[3]

Whether curbside consultations actually improve patient care is unknown because the subject has not been formally studied.[2]

⚓ REFERENCES ⚓

1. Keating NL, Zaslavsky AM, Ayanian JZ: Physicians' experiences and beliefs regarding informal consultation, *JAMA* 280:900-904, 1998.
2. Kuo D, Gifford DR, Stein MD: Curbside consultation practices and attitudes among primary care physicians and medical subspecialists, *JAMA* 280:905-909, 1998.
3. Manian FA, Janssen DA: Curbside consultations: a closer look at a common practice, *JAMA* 275:145-147, 1996.

EVIDENCE-BASED MEDICINE

(See also attitudes, physician; clinical practice guidelines; medical education; periodic health examination; screening)

Good physicians are skeptical about much of what they do and most of what they read, including this text. Being skeptical helps keep us attuned to new evidence and probably keeps us from harming our patients by either prematurely endorsing new investigative or therapeutic procedures or rigidly sticking to outmoded interventions. Skepticism is one of the driving forces behind "evidence-based medicine" and is well exemplified by the critical approach taken by the Canadian Task Force on Preventive Health Care[1] and the U.S. Preventive Services Task Force.[2] However, skepticism carried to extremes leads to diagnostic and therapeutic paralysis.

Evidence-based data are only part of what physicians require to care adequately for their patients. They need easy access to accurate information that is relevant to everyday practice; as Slawson and Shaughnessy[3] put it, they are looking for "Patient Oriented Evidence That Matters (POEM)." Finding what we need among the 6 million medical articles which are published annually requires us all to develop some understanding of how to perform critical appraisals of the medical literature.[4]

Although randomized controlled trials are the gold standard for evidence-based medicine, they are not always applicable to the patients seen in family medicine. Controlled trials often enroll patients from referral centers, and women, elderly patients, and patients with comorbid illnesses are commonly excluded from such trials. Drug trials may give good information about when to start medications but no evidence-based data on when to stop them.[5]

Randomized controlled trials and critical appraisals apply to populations of patients, not to individual patients. To practice high-quality medicine, family physicians must use evidence-based guidelines but at the same time recognize the physical, psychological, ethical, spiritual, and social uniqueness of each patient. When patient individuality is incorporated into management decisions, "evidence-based" recommendations must often be abandoned.[6]

Expert opinion, whether verbal or in the form of a review article, is a common but sometimes unreliable source of information for generalists. Antman and associates[7] compared current written reviews of "experts" in the specific content area of myocardial infarction with current metaanalyses on the same subject. The reviews of the "experts" often con-

tained potentially harmful recommendations and omitted newer beneficial therapeutic modalities. (On the other hand, metaanalyses may lead to erroneous conclusions compared with large randomized controlled trials.[8-10]) Oxman and Guyatt[11] analyzed the methodological rigor of a number of review articles and concluded that the greater the expertise of the authors, the poorer the quality of the reviews. It may be that some "experts" are consciously or unconsciously biased because they have vested interests in certain viewpoints or,[11] to put it more bluntly, they value their personal experience more than randomized controlled trials.[3]

It has often been stated that only 10% to 20% of medical interventions are evidence based. When this hypothesis was tested on inpatients on general medical services in Oxford, England,[12] and Ottawa, Canada,[13] 82% of the decisions made in the English study and 84% of those in the Canadian study were evidence based.

Classification of categories of evidence and strength of recommendations is discussed in the section on clinical practice guidelines.

⚓ REFERENCES ⚓

1. Canadian Task Force on the Periodic Health Examination: *Canadian guide to clinical preventive health care,* Ottawa, 1994, Canada Communication Group—Publishing.
2. US Preventive Services Task Force: *Guide to clinical preventive services,* ed 2, Baltimore, 1996, Williams & Wilkins.
3. Slawson DC, Shaughnessy AF: Obtaining useful information from expert based sources, *BMJ* 314:947-949, 1997.
4. Miser WF: Critical appraisal of the literature, *J Am Board Fam Pract* 12:315-333, 1999.
5. Knottnerus JA, Dinant GJ: Medicine based evidence, a prerequisite for evidence based medicine: future research methods must find ways of accommodating clinical reality, not ignoring it (editorial), *BMJ* 315:1109-1110, 1997.
6. Tonelli MR: The philosophical limits of evidence-based medicine, *Acad Med* 73:1234-1240, 1998.
7. Antman EM, Lau J, Kupelnick B, et al: A comparison of results of meta-analyses of randomized control trials and recommendations of clinical experts: treatments for myocardial infarction, *JAMA* 268:240-248, 1992.
8. LeLorier J, Grégoire G, Benhaddad A, et al: Discrepancies between meta-analyses and subsequent large randomized, controlled trials, *N Engl J Med* 337:536-542, 1997.
9. Bailar JC III: The promise and problems of meta-analysis (editorial), *N Engl J Med* 337:559-561, 1997.
10. DerSimonian R, Levine RJ: Resolving discrepancies between a meta-analysis and a subsequent large controlled trial, *JAMA* 282:664-670, 1999.
11. Oxman AD, Guyatt GH: The science of reviewing research, *Ann NY Acad Sci* 703:125-133, 1993.
12. Ellis J, Mulligan I, Rowe J, Sackett DL (A-Team, Nuffield Department of Clinical Medicine): Inpatient general medicine is evidence based, *Lancet* 346:407-410, 1995.
13. Michaud G, McGown JL, van der Jagt R, et al: Are therapeutic decisions supported by evidence from health care research? *Arch Intern Med* 158:1665-1668, 1998.

FEVER

(See also febrile seizures; fever in children)

Normal Temperature Values

In young adults rectal temperatures exceeded oral readings by 0.4° C (0.7° F) and these in turn exceeded tympanic readings by 0.4° C (0.7° F). Smoking and mastication have been found to increase oral readings, and this effect persists for longer than 20 minutes. Drinking ice water causes a short-term diminution in temperature readings.[1]

What is a normal temperature, and what is the normal range? Mackowiak and associates[2] studied this in a group of healthy young adult men and women between the ages of 18 and 40. The mean oral temperature was 36.8° C (98.2° F), and 37.7° C (99.9° F) was the upper limit of normal. A diurnal variation with an amplitude of variability of about 0.5° C (0.9° F) was normal with the nadir at 6 AM and the zenith at 4 to 6 PM.[2]

Taking Temperatures

Whether axillary temperatures are accurate is controversial. Shann and Mackenzie[3] from Australia studied temperatures taken by various routes in 120 children of different ages. They concluded that axillary temperatures were accurate. In children over 1 month of age the rectal temperature was very close to 1° C higher than the axillary temperature. During the first 5 weeks of life rectal temperature exceeded axillary temperature by 0.2° C for every week of life. Forehead temperatures were not as accurate as axillary temperatures.[3] However, most other studies have found the axillary route to have a low sensitivity but a high specificity.[4,5] In other words, if the axillary temperature is elevated, the child is febrile, but if it is not, fever cannot be ruled out.

In the past few years noncontact tympanic or external auditory canal thermometers that detect infrared radiation from the tympanic membrane have come into widespread use. How accurate are they? In an emergency room study of children under 4 years the readings of noncontact tympanic thermometers in both the rectal-equivalent mode and the actual-ear mode were compared with rectal temperatures obtained with recently calibrated glass mercury thermometers. With fever defined as at least 38° C (100.4° F) per rectum the noncontact tympanic thermometer in the rectal-equivalent mode had a sensitivity of 75% and a specificity of 96%. In the actual-ear mode the sensitivity dropped to just over 50% while the specificity was 100%.[6] These data show that fever in one fourth or more of young children could be missed if only the noncontact tympanic thermometer was used, but if the instrument indicated "fever," it would rarely be wrong. Studies using tympanic thermometers in adult patients have shown significant variations in readings from one ear to the other, as well as among commercial brands.[7,8] At present, tympanic thermometers do not appear to be reliable.

Without measuring their temperatures, can parents accurately determine whether young children are febrile? This was assessed in the emergency room study described in the previous paragraph. Parental sensitivity was 82% and parental specificity 77%. The sensitivity of parents' assessment of fever in their children is a bit better than that of the noncontact tympanic thermometer but is considerably less specific; parental opinions should be taken seriously.[6]

Benefits of Fever

Is fever beneficial? Should it be treated? The febrile response to infection is only part of an "acute phase response" involving the activation of numerous cytokines that cause symptoms such as somnolence and anorexia, as well as inducing a wide variety of metabolic and immunological changes that could in theory be beneficial. With few exceptions mammals, reptiles, amphibians, and fish respond to infections with fever, which suggests that such reactions have evolutionary value. One study in humans reported that rhinovirus infections treated with antipyretics were more severe and lasted longer than those not so treated, and another found that treatment of rhinovirus infections with aspirin increased viral shedding. Circumstantial evidence suggests that fever may be beneficial in some cases, but no useful data are available as to whether treatment with antipyretics causes more harm than good.[9]

Treating Fever

See discussion of fever in children.

Fever of Unknown Origin

In 10% to 30% of patients who are examined for fever of unknown origin, no diagnosis is ever made. The long-term outcome of such patients is good, and in one study the 5-year mortality rate was only 3.2%. Nonsteroidal anti-inflammatory drugs (NSAIDs) can be used for symptomatic relief if necessary.[10]

◣ REFERENCES ◥

1. Rabinowitz RP, Cookson ST, Wasserman SS, et al: Effects of anatomic site, oral stimulation, and body position on estimates of body temperature, *Arch Intern Med* 156:777-780, 1996.
2. Mackowiak PA, Wasserman SS, Levine MM: A critical appraisal of 98.6 degrees F, the upper limit of the normal body temperature, and other legacies of Carl Reinhold August Wunderlich, *JAMA* 268:1578-1580, 1992.
3. Shann F, Mackenzie A: Comparison of rectal, axillary and forehead temperatures, *Arch Pediatr Adolesc Med* 150:74-78, 1996.
4. Keeley D: Taking infants' temperatures (editorial), *BMJ* 304:931-932, 1992.
5. Zengeya ST, Blumenthal I: Modern electronic and chemical thermometers used in the axilla are inaccurate, *Eur J Pediatr* 155:1005-1008, 1996.
6. Hooker EA, Smith SW, Miles T, et al: Subjective assessment of fever by parents—comparison with measurement by noncontact tympanic thermometer and calibrated rectal glass mercury thermometer, *Ann Emerg Med* 28:313-317, 1996.

7. Manian FA, Griesenauer S: Lack of agreement between tympanic and oral temperature measurements in adult hospitalized patients, *Am J Infect Control* 26:428-430, 1998.

8. Modell JG, Katholi CR, Kumaramangalam SM, et al: Unreliability of the infrared tympanic thermometer in clinical practice: a comparative study with oral mercury and oral electronic thermometers, *South Med J* 91:649-655, 1998.

9. Mackowiak PA: Concepts of fever, *Arch Intern Med* 158:1870-1881, 1998.

10. Knockaert DC, Dujardin KS, Bobbaers HJ: Long-term follow-up of patients with undiagnosed fever of unknown origin, *Arch Intern Med* 156:618-620, 1996.

HEAT-RELATED ILLNESSES

Heat stroke is defined as a core body temperature of at least 40.5° C (105° F). Acute neurological symptoms and signs are associated with heat stroke. Hypotension is the rule, and mortality is at least 10%.[1] Even if patients with heat stroke do not die in the hospital, many survivors suffer a permanent loss of independence.[2] In contrast, heat exhaustion is due to volume depletion brought about by heat. Symptoms include sweating, dizziness, headache, nausea, vomiting, and muscle weakness. The body temperature does not have to be elevated. Many patients with heat exhaustion can be adequately treated with oral fluids and cool sponging.[1] The elderly are at increased risk for both conditions because they are less likely to be aware of excessive heat, are less likely to be aware of thirst in the early stages of dehydration, and have a prolonged latency before starting to sweat.[1,3] Children under 5 years of age are also at increased risk of heat stroke and heat exhaustion.[4]

Drugs may interfere with thermoregulation in a variety of ways. Some act by increasing muscle activity and heat production (amphetamines and cocaine), and some by blocking the parasympathetic system and thus inhibiting sweating (tricyclic antidepressants and phenothiazines). Others decrease blood flow to the skin by decreasing cardiac output (e.g., beta-blockers), by causing vasoconstriction (vasoconstrictors in decongestants), or by inducing volume depletion (diuretics, alcohol).[1]

Heat-related mortality can be decreased by increasing fluid intake (8 oz per hour regardless of thirst), decreasing physical exertion, exercising only during cool times of the day, spending more time in air-conditioned environments, and taking cool water baths.[3,4] Fans are not protective at temperatures above 32.3° C (90° F) with a relative humidity greater than 35%.[4]

In a study of excess deaths in the 1995 Chicago heat wave, increased risk was observed for persons who were confined to bed for known medical problems, who did not have air conditioners, or who were socially isolated.[5]

──────────── ◢ **REFERENCES** ◣ ────────────

1. Bross MH, Nash BT, Carlton FB Jr: Heat emergencies, *Am Fam Physician* 50:389-396, 1994.

2. Dematte JE, O'Mara K, Buescher J, et al: Near-fatal heat stroke during the 1995 heat wave in Chicago, *Ann Intern Med* 129:173-181, 1998.

3. Blum LN, Bresolin LB, Williams MA (Council on Scientific Affairs of the AMA): Heat-related illness during extreme weather emergencies, *JAMA* 279:1514, 1998.

4. Centers for Disease Control and Prevention: Heat-related illnesses and deaths—Missouri, 1998, and United States, 1979-1996, *JAMA* 282:227-228, 1999.

5. Semenza JC, Rubin CH, Falter KH, et al: Heat-related deaths during the July 1995 heat wave in Chicago, *N Engl J Med* 335:84-90, 1996.

HEMOCHROMATOSIS
(See also screening)

Major symptoms of hemochromatosis that lead to medical consultation are abdominal pain, joint pains, and weakness. Eight percent of males with this disease are impotent. Evidence of liver disease (hepatomegaly or abnormal liver enzymes) is found in 84% of cases.[1] Since diabetes is found in 20% to 50% of patients with hemochromatosis, investigating diabetic patients for the disorder might be beneficial.[2] Among patients of northern European ancestry who have hereditary hemochromatosis, 85% to 90% are homozygous for the C282Y mutation on chromosome 6. On the other hand, iron overload develops in only about three fourths of persons homozygous for the C282Y mutation on chromosome 6.[3] The homozygous C282Y mutation is present in 4 to 5:1000 persons of northern European ancestry.[4]

Whether screening for hemochromatosis should be undertaken is controversial for a number of reasons, a main one of which is that many people with chemical or genetic evidence of hemochromatosis will never have clinical symptoms.[4] If screening is to be undertaken, the single best current test appears to be serum transferrin saturation, with a cut-off point of 45% or higher. Other tests include serum ferritin levels of 300 μg/L (300 ng/mL) or higher and direct assessment of C282Y mutations using polymerase chain reaction techniques. In one Australian trial of 3011 white adults of northern European ancestry all three tests were used. Sixteen individuals (0.5%) were found to be homozygous, but of these only eight (0.26%) met the clinical criteria for hemochromatosis. Of the 16 homozygous individuals, 15 were detected by serum transferrin saturation, which had a sensitivity and a specificity of 94% but a positive predictive value of only 6%. One fourth of those who were homozygous had no elevation of ferritin levels.[3]

Adams[5] suggests that anyone in whom hemochromatosis is suspected on the basis of family history, clinical symptoms, abnormal serum transferrin saturation, or elevated serum ferritin level be tested for the genetic mutation. If the test is positive, genetic counseling and testing of family members are indicated. The role of liver biopsy to measure iron load is somewhat controversial because many types of advanced liver disease can be associated with abnormal accumulations of iron.[5]

REFERENCES

1. Desforges JF: Screening for hemochromatosis, *N Engl J Med* 328:1616-1620, 1993.
2. Conte D, Manachino D, Colli A, et al: Prevalence of genetic hemochromatosis in a cohort of Italian patients with diabetes mellitus, *Ann Intern Med* 128:370-373, 1998.
3. Olynyk JK, Cullen DJ, Aquilia S, et al: A population-based study of the clinical expression of the hemochromatosis gene, *N Engl J Med* 341:718-724, 1999.
4. Haddow JE, Bradley LA: Hereditary haemochromatosis: to screen or not: conditions for screening are not yet fulfilled (editorial), *BMJ* 319:531-532, 1999.
5. Adams PC: Hemochromatosis: clinical implications of genetic testing, *Can Med Assoc J* 159:156-158, 1998.

HIGH-ALTITUDE MEDICINE

In susceptible individuals the hypoxia associated with high altitudes can induce a variety of symptoms. The most common and least serious, which affects one sixth to one third of recreational skiers in Colorado, is acute mountain sickness. Presenting complaints are headache plus at least one of the following: fatigue or weakness, gastrointestinal complaints, lightheadedness or dizziness, and sleep disturbances.[1] Symptoms usually begin after 12 to 24 hours and peak on the second or third day.[2] More serious are high-altitude pulmonary edema and high-altitude cerebral edema. These disorders usually occur in individuals ascending to or above 2500 m (8202 ft). Symptoms of high-altitude pulmonary edema usually occur at night and include dyspnea, cough, weakness, and chest tightness. Signs include central cyanosis, rales, or wheezes (often over the right middle lobe), tachypnea, and tachycardia. High-altitude cerebral edema is manifested as mental changes and in many cases ataxia. Optimal treatment of all these conditions is descent to lower altitudes, which is mandatory for patients with pulmonary or cerebral edema. Acetazolamide (Diamox) 125-250 mg bid has been used before ascent is begun to prevent acute mountain sickness.[1] Aspirin 325 mg taken 1 hour before ascent and repeated at 4 and 8 hours has been shown to prevent the headaches of acute mountain sickness.[3]

REFERENCES

1. Harris MK, Terrio J, Miser WF, et al: High-altitude medicine, *Am Fam Physician* 57:1907-1914, 1998.
2. Peacock AJ: Oxygen at high altitude, *BMJ* 317:1063-1066, 1998.
3. Burtscher M, Likar R, Nachbauer W, et al: Aspirin for prophylaxis against headache at high altitudes: randomised, double blind, placebo controlled trial, *BMJ* 316:1057-1058, 1998.

INFORMED CONSENT

(See also attitudes, physician; cardiac arrest; investigations; maternal serum screening; oncology; patient education; prevention; prostate cancer; screening; statistics; uncertainty)

Informed consent implies that the patient has a right to consent to or refuse a medical intervention. Consent may be implicit or explicit. Explicit consent, which can be oral or written, should be obtained for any intervention that involves risk or more than mild discomfort. A recognized exception is a medical emergency in which the patient is not able to give consent.[1]

Consent has three important components[1]:

1. Disclosure. This is the provision by the physician, in a comprehensible fashion, of the essential information required for the patient to make a decision.
2. Capacity. This is the ability of the patient to understand the information given and to appreciate the consequences of his or her decision.
3. Voluntariness. This means the patient is allowed to make a decision free of coercion or manipulation.

A number of myths have arisen about informed consent.[2] One is that physicians are obliged to present alternatives in an unbiased fashion without ever stating their own opinions. This is false. Physicians should indeed present the alternatives but are free to volunteer their own opinions or to give them if requested. Informed consent is an ongoing dialogue between physician and patient. A second myth is that patients must be given complete information about any proposed interventions. This too is false. Patients should be given *reasonable* amounts of information. A third myth is that patients cannot give informed consent because the data are too complex for them to comprehend. It does not follow that because patients are unable to recall the data after the physician-patient interview, they were unable to make a rational decision at the time. A fourth myth is that physicians are compelled to inform patients of relevant medical data even if they specifically ask not to be given such information. Respect for patient autonomy in this situation (not telling them) is legally acceptable and is termed a waiver.[2]

The essential processes involved in informed consent are that patients be offered important relevant information and be allowed to ask questions about it, mull over the options, and make their decisions either on their own or on the advice of their physicians.[2]

Informed Consent for Screening Procedures

Why should patients be required to give informed consent for screening tests? The answer in brief is that the benefits are not always great,[3,4] that significant adverse consequences may be produced,[5,6] that many screening programs are experimental (if they were not, there would be no controversy),[7] and, most important, that patients, not physicians, should be the ones to determine the interventions to which they will be subjected.[7,8]

When a screening test is abnormal, further diagnostic tests, often invasive, are indicated, as are therapeutic interventions with their attendant risks (screening cascade).[5] All patients with positive tests are immediately subjected to these risks, while the benefits, which accrue to only a few, will be realized only in the future.[4] Even when benefits are conclusively proved, individual patients may not be healthy enough or live long enough to enjoy them. When presented with all the facts of a screening program, some patients may not wish to risk the immediate risks of morbidity or mortality even if the overall statistics favor a particular intervention.[7]

Because benefits are limited and harm is potentially serious, a patient should never be subjected to a case finding or screening procedure without giving informed consent.[7,8] Unfortunately, this is almost impossible to implement in daily practice for several reasons, such as lack of time and knowledge on the part of the physician and lack of understanding of complex data on the part of the patient.[6-9] Skrabanek[10] suggests another reason that physicians may be reluctant to mention the harm of screening: if they did, patients might not participate in the programs.

Despite the difficulties, informed consent for cancer screening can make a difference. This has been documented by Wolf and associates,[11] who randomly divided a group of men of predominantly lower socioeconomic status to receive either a scripted informational intervention about prostate specific antigen (PSA) screening or a single sentence about PSA. Those who received the informational intervention were much less likely to want PSA screening.

In practice, physicians often resolve the dilemma of obtaining informed consent for preventive programs by following their own inclinations without fully discussing the issues with the patients. In some cases this is because they are overconfident about their medical recommendations even though no such certainty exists in the medical literature. Such "micro-certainty" in the face of "macro-uncertainty" may adversely affect the ability of patients to participate actively in decision making and to give truly informed consent.[12]

Patient Preconceptions and Informed Consent

Physicians are often astounded to learn the error of some patients' preconceptions that may influence their decisions in giving informed consent. For example, most elderly patients grossly overestimate the success rate of cardiopulmonary resuscitation and may opt for it under the illusion that they would have an 80% or better chance of surviving to discharge when the actual figure is between zero and 15%.[13] Similar findings have been reported in younger individuals. In one study women between the ages of 40 and 50 were found to overestimate their risk of dying of breast cancer 20 fold and to overestimate the benefit of screening 6 fold.[14]

Patient Preferences and Informed Consent

Consideration of patient preferences is essential before any medical action is taken. Patients' viewpoints may surprise or even dismay their physicians. For example, a patient who has had a transient ischemic attack and has significant carotid artery stenosis may be unwilling to accept a small risk of a catastrophic adverse effect from surgical intervention (such as a stroke or death) even if the intervention has been conclusively shown to benefit many more people than it harms.[15] Another example involves deciding whether to accept chemotherapy for metastatic non–small cell cancer of the lung. Such chemotherapy improves median survival by 1.5 to 3 months and is often recommended as standard treatment in the United States. When patients who had undergone such treatments were interviewed, only 22% would have chosen this intervention had they been fully aware of both the toxicity and the limited benefits.[16]

An important concern for some physicians may be whether patients can adequately understand medical concepts and weigh cost-benefit issues rationally (as judged by physicians). This hypothesis was tested on a group of parents of young children who were asked hypothetical questions about their choices for managing fever of undetermined origin in very young children. The parents were given the kind of background data that physicians require to make these choices; they made rational, logical choices, which in the majority of cases were for minimal investigation and careful follow-up.[17]

Language and Informed Consent

The language used in obtaining informed consent may play a pivotal role in determining what option the patient chooses (see discussion of statistics).[18,19] For example, patients with known coronary artery disease and elevated cholesterol levels who met the criteria for inclusion in the Scandinavian Simvastatin Survival Study (4S) (see discussion of lipids) could be informed in several different ways about the benefits of taking HMG-CoA reductase inhibitors. The most common method would be to use the relative reduction figures and on this basis tell the patients that the medications would reduce their risk of dying by 30%. A second way would be to use the absolute reduction rates and on this basis inform them that their risk of dying would be reduced by 3.3%. A third approach would be to present the numbers necessary to treat without using emotion-laden words such as "chance" and "risk." Patients could be told that if 100 persons in their situation were not to take cholesterol-lowering medications, 92 would be alive and 8 dead after 5 years, and there is no way of knowing if they would be one of the 8 or one of the 92. They would also be told that if 100 persons in their situation were to take the medications, 95 would be alive and 5 dead after 5 years and, again, there is no way of knowing if they would be one of the 5 or one of the 95.[18] To fully understand the benefits of treatment or screening, patients must be given data in terms of numbers needed to treat or to screen.[19]

A less subtle issue is whether information is given in a fashion the patient can understand. As Surbone[20] aptly put it, if information is given in abstruse or technical terms that patients cannot comprehend, they do not have the knowledge, or the autonomy that goes with such knowledge, to make informed decisions.

Patient Decision Aids and Informed Consent

One way of facilitating communication between physicians and patients is the use of patient decision aids that give information about the benefits and risks of the proposed intervention in a detailed and accurate but comprehensible fashion.[21,22] One such system used a 29-page booklet and a 20-minute audiotape to help patients with atrial fibrillation decide whether they wanted to be treated with warfarin or aspirin. Included in the booklet were charts containing 100 icons ("happy faces" and "sad faces") that pictorially represented the risk of major and minor strokes and severe bleeding for each therapeutic option. Patients selected at random to receive this decision aid improved their understanding of the disease and the therapeutic options and were helped in decision making.[22] Such aids have some obvious problems: they are time consuming to prepare, expensive, rapidly outdated, and possibly not comprehensible to those with low literacy levels (see discussion of patient education).

Cultural Values and Informed Consent

Should all patients be told the truth about their medical conditions? In the North American context the answer is clearly yes in most instances: patients must be given autonomy and have a "right to know," medical decisions cannot be made by a patient who is ignorant of his or her diagnosis, a conspiracy of silence by the physician and the patient's family may lead the patient to die in lonely isolation, and ignorance may prevent the patient from completing "unfinished business."[23] In a number of other cultures, however, the answer is no. For example, Mediterranean countries such as Italy, Greece, and Morocco have a strong tradition that family members and not the patient should be informed of bad news.[20,23] The rationale is that the sick patient would be overwhelmed by frightening and complicated information and unable to make decisions on the basis of what he or she heard, and therefore that telling the patient would do more harm than good.[20] Similar attitudes are found in many Koreans and Mexican Americans, and it has been recommended that patients in these groups be asked whether they prefer to receive information and make their own medical decisions or to have their families handle the matter.[24] Among traditional Navajo peoples, receiving negative information, as is often necessary when issues of informed consent arise, conflicts with the concept of hózhó, which in oversimplified terms is a belief in beauty, harmony, and a positive outlook on life.[25]

What are North American physicians to do when faced with families who do not want the patient informed of his or her condition? They could of course ignore the family and inform the patient anyway, but a more humane alternative is to ask the patient what he or she wants to know. Freedman[23] calls this "offering truth." Patients are asked a series of questions that allow the physician to determine whether the patients want to know everything, a little bit, or nothing at all. Patients have every right to choose to be uninformed, and such a waiver has been supported in law.[26,27] However, if the correct course of action remains uncertain, physicians may decide to ask for a formal ethical review.[28]

❧ REFERENCES ❧

1. Etchells E, Sharpe G, Walsh P, et al: Bioethics for clinicians. 1. Consent, *Can Med Assoc J* 155:177-180, 1996.
2. Meisel A, Kuczewski M: Legal and ethical myths about informed consent, *Arch Intern Med* 156:2521-2526, 1996.
3. Marshall KG: Prevention. How much harm? How much benefit? 1. Influence of reporting methods on perception of benefits, *Can Med Assoc J* 154:1493-1499, 1996.
4. Marshall KG: Prevention. How much harm? How much benefit? 2. Ten potential pitfalls in determining the clinical significance of benefits, *Can Med Assoc J* 154:1837-1843, 1996.
5. Marshall KG: Prevention. How much harm? How much benefit? 3. Physical, psychological and social harm, *Can Med Assoc J* 155:169-176, 1996.
6. Marshall KG: Screening for prostate cancer: how can patients give informed consent? *Can Fam Physician* 39:2385-2390, 1993.
7. Marshall KG: Prevention. How much harm? How much benefit? 4. The ethics of informed consent for preventive screening programs, *Can Med Assoc J* 155:377-383, 1996.
8. Lee JM: Screening and informed consent, *N Engl J Med* 328:438-440, 1993.
9. Hofman KJ, Tambor ES, Chase GA, et al: Physicians' knowledge of genetics and genetic tests, *Acad Med* 68:625-631, 1993.
10. Skrabanek P: The physician's responsibility to the patient, *Lancet* 1:1155-1157, 1988.
11. Wolf A, Nasser JF, Wolf AM, et al: The impact of informed consent on patient interest in prostate-specific antigen screening, *Arch Intern Med* 156:1333-1336, 1996.
12. Baumann AO, Deber RB, Thompson GG: Overconfidence among physicians and nurses: the "micro-certainty, macro-uncertainty" phenomenon, *Soc Sci Med* 32:167-174, 1991.
13. Murphy DJ, Burrows D, Santilli S, et al: The influence of the probability of survival on patients' preferences regarding cardiopulmonary resuscitation, *N Engl J Med* 330:545-549, 1994.
14. Black WC, Nease RF, Tosteson A: Perceptions of breast cancer risk and screening effectiveness in women under 50, *J Natl Cancer Inst* 87:720-731, 1995.
15. Kassirer JP: Incorporating patients' preferences into medical decisions (editorial), *N Engl J Med* 330:1895-1896, 1994.
16. Silvestri G, Pritchard R, Welch HG: Preferences for chemotherapy in patients with advanced non–small cell lung cancer: descriptive study based on scripted interviews, *BMJ* 317:771-775, 1998.
17. Oppenheim PI, Sotiropoulos G, Baraff LJ: Incorporating patient preferences into practice guidelines: management of children with fever without source, *Ann Emerg Med* 24:836-841, 1994.
18. Skolbekken J-A: Communicating the risk reduction achieved by cholesterol reducing drugs, *BMJ* 316:1956-1958, 1998.
19. Steiner JF: Talking about treatment: the language of populations and the language of individuals, *Ann Intern Med* 130:618-622, 1999.
20. Surbone A: Letter from Italy: truth telling to the patient, *JAMA* 268:1661-1662, 1992.
21. O'Connor AM, Rostom A, Fiset V, et al: Decision aids for patients facing health treatment or screening decisions: systematic review, *BMJ* 319:731-734, 1999.

22. Man-Son-Hing M, Laupacis A, O'Connor AM, et al: A patient decision aid regarding antithrombotic therapy for stroke prevention in atrial fibrillation: a randomized controlled trial, *JAMA* 282:737-743, 1999.

23. Freedman B: Offering truth: one ethical approach to the uninformed cancer patient, *Arch Intern Med* 153:572-576, 1993.

24. Blackhall LJ, Murphy ST, Frank G, et al: Ethnicity and attitudes toward patient autonomy, *JAMA* 274:820-825, 1995.

25. Carrese J, Rhodes LA: Western bioethics on the Navajo reservation: benefit or harm? *JAMA* 274:826-829, 1995.

26. Hébert PC: Truth-telling in clinical practice, *Can Fam Physician* 40:2105-2113, 1994.

27. Greenlaw J: Talk about not talking (editorial), *Arch Intern Med* 153:557-558, 1993.

28. Gostin LO: Informed consent, cultural sensitivity, and respect for persons (editorial), *JAMA* 274:844-845, 1995.

INVESTIGATIONS

(See also attitudes, physician; informed consent; oncology [follow-up]; periodic health examination; statistics; uncertainty)

Multiple Tests

Multiple tests compound the problem of false-positive results. Because of the norms of the bell-shaped curve, the odds that a single test will be abnormal by chance alone are 5%. This increases to 26% for six tests, 46% for 12 tests, and 64% for 20 tests, assuming that each test is independent of the others.[1]

"Routine" Laboratory Tests

Are routine laboratory investigations a helpful form of case finding in well person care? A prospective study from the Mayo Clinic analyzed the yield of selected case-finding blood and urine tests among patients with a mean age of 63. Overall, 36% of the tests were positive (see discussion of multiple tests above), but in only 4.8% were new diagnoses (diagnostic yield) made and in only 4% was a therapeutic intervention started (therapeutic yield) as a result of the testing. The majority of therapeutic yields came from the lipid profiles (16.5%).[2] Almost identical results were previously reported in a study from Basel, Switzerland.[3]

Detrimental Effects of Investigation

Both false-positive and false-negative results of tests may have adverse consequences. False-negative results may erroneously reassure both the patient and the physician and unnecessarily delay treatment. False-positive results not only cause considerable mental distress, but also lead to a cascade of further investigations and interventions, some of which, such as angiograms, colonoscopies, and breast biopsies, involve significant morbidity and in rare instances death.[4] Although true-negative results often reassure patients, this is not always the case (see discussion of screening).[5]

Even a true-positive test may have more detrimental than beneficial effects. The individual concerned has now been labeled as an ill person,[6] and this is particularly harmful if the abnormality detected is untreatable or there is no reliable evidence that treatment does any good. In the United States the rate of testing has increased sharply in the past few years, and since a clear relationship exists between number of tests ordered and number of therapeutic interventions undertaken, the latter have also increased at a striking rate.[7-9] Examples are cardiac catheterization and cardiac revascularization,[7-9] mammography and breast surgery, imaging of the spine and back surgery, prostate biopsy and prostatectomy,[7,8] and oral glucose challenge test in pregnancy and Cesarean section.[10] Although it is possible that the increased testing and treatment are a result of increased disease and therefore clinically justified, it is more probable that many patients will not benefit from treatment of the disorders being detected. In other words, testing drives therapy. If this is so, patient care would be improved (and costs decreased) by programs directed at decreasing testing rather than decreasing therapeutic interventions, since physicians have more difficulty withholding therapy once a precise diagnosis has been made.[7]

Excessive Investigations

Feldman[11] and Woolf and Kamerow[12] have concluded that lack of awareness of the significance of sensitivity, specificity, and, particularly, positive predictive value is one cause of excessive testing (see later discussion). Other causes include pressure from peers and supervisors, demands of patients or families, and fear of litigation.[13] Woolf and Kamerow[12] suggest that physicians' attitudes are an even more important cause of excessive testing than is lack of statistical knowledge. They point out that much of medical school training is done in tertiary care hospitals where students learn that errors of omission are more serious than errors of commission. In other words, failure to detect a disease is worse than any adverse effects that might result from the testing procedure itself or the consequences of false-positive or false-negative results.

Discomfort with uncertainty is often the driving force behind testing.[12,13] As Kassirer[13] points out, such discomfort is often illogical, since high diagnostic certainty is necessary only for diseases in which treatment is not very effective and morbidity is significant. If a disease is easily treated with a therapy that has few adverse effects, treatment can reasonably be initiated even if the diagnosis is not absolutely certain.

Positive Predictive Value and Disease Prevalence

The positive predictive value of a test is the percentage of positive results that are true positives, and this varies directly with the prevalence of the disease in the community. Family physicians must understand the concept of positive predictive value if they want to avoid harming their patients through screening procedures. If the prevalence of a disease is low, the vast majority of patients with "positive" results have false-positive tests and do not have the disease[12]; these unfortunate patients go through agony until or even beyond the time that the diagnosis is clarified.[14-16]

Once the relationship between disease prevalence and positive predictive value is understood, it can be seen that the positive predictive values of tests performed on "sick" hospitalized patients are likely to be much higher than the positive predictive values of tests performed on ambulatory patients in the office setting. This is yet another reason that physicians trained primarily in hospitals are enthusiastic about tests.

REFERENCES

1. Cebul RD, Beck JR: Biochemical profiles: applications in ambulatory screening and preadmission testing of adults, *Ann Intern Med* 106:403-413, 1987.
2. Boland BJ, Wollan PC, Silverstein MD: Yield of laboratory tests for case-finding in the ambulatory general medical examination, *Am J Med* 101:142-152, 1996.
3. Ruttimann S, Dreifuss M, Clemençon D, et al: Multiple biochemical blood testing as a case-finding tool in ambulatory medical patients, *Am J Med* 94:141-148, 1993.
4. Marshall KG: Prevention. How much harm? How much benefit? 3. Physical, psychological and social harm, *Can Med Assoc J* 155:169-176, 1996.
5. McDonald IG, Jelinek VM, Panetta F, et al: Opening Pandora's box: the unpredictability of reassurance by a normal test result, *BMJ* 313:329-332, 1996.
6. Meador CK: The last well person, *N Engl J Med* 330:440-441, 1994.
7. Verrilli D, Welch G: The impact of diagnostic testing on therapeutic interventions, *JAMA* 275:1189-1191, 1996.
8. Epstein AM: Use of diagnostic tests and therapeutic procedures in a changing health care environment (editorial), *JAMA* 275:1197-1198, 1996.
9. Wennberg DE, Kellett MA, Dickens JD Jr, et al: The association between local diagnostic testing intensity and invasive cardiac procedures, *JAMA* 275:1161-1164, 1996.
10. Naylor CD, Sermer M, Chen E, et al (Toronto Trihospital Gestational Diabetes Investigators): Cesarean delivery in relation to birth weight and gestational glucose tolerance: pathophysiology or practice style? *JAMA* 275:1165-1170, 1996.
11. Feldman W: On ordering tests (editorial), *Ann RCPSC* 26:269-270, 1993.
12. Woolf SH, Kamerow DB: Testing for uncommon conditions: the heroic search for positive test results, *Arch Intern Med* 150:2451-2458, 1990.
13. Kassirer JP: Our stubborn quest for diagnostic certainty: a cause of excessive testing, *N Engl J Med* 320:1489-1491, 1989.
14. Lerman C, Trock B, Rimer BK, et al: Psychological and behavioral implications of abnormal mammograms, *Ann Intern Med* 114:657-661, 1991.
15. Lerman C, Rimer BK, Engstrom PF: Cancer risk notification: psychosocial and ethical implications, *J Clin Oncol* 9:1275-1282, 1991.
16. Wardle J, Pope R: The psychological costs of screening for cancer, *J Psychosom Res* 36:609-624, 1992.

LEG CRAMPS

Although a number of studies have concluded that quinine is no more effective than a placebo for controlling nocturnal leg cramps,[1-3] others have shown some benefit. In one such trial quinine reduced by 50% the frequency of cramps experienced by the patients, although it did not reduce their severity.[4] Another small, nonblinded evaluation from England found quinine to be more effective than going to bed with three corks tied in a sock (an interesting control group).[5] A metaanalysis of six randomized controlled crossover studies of elderly patients taking 200, 300, or 500 mg of quinine at bedtime concluded that the drug decreased the number of nights with cramps by 27% but not the intensity or duration of the cramps. The effect of quinine is cumulative, so a 4-week trial should be given before deciding whether the drug is beneficial.[6] The usual dose is 200 to 300 mg qhs.

Several nonpharmacological treatments of leg cramps have been recommended. Daniell[7] reported successful prevention of cramps within a week in 44 patients who performed stretching exercises three times a day. While barefoot, patients stood 2 to 3 feet from a wall and faced it. They placed their hands on the wall and, keeping their heels on the ground, leaned forward to the point that they felt the stretch in their calf muscles. This position was maintained for 10 seconds, and the maneuver was then repeated once after a 5-second rest. Another recommendation is to place a pillow at the bottom of the bed to keep the feet dorsiflexed; if cramps still occur, the patient should passively dorsiflex the ankle and massage the calf.[8]

REFERENCES

1. Lim SH: Randomised double-blind trial of quinine sulphate for nocturnal leg cramp, *Br J Clin Pharmacol* 11:462, 1986.
2. Smith C, Jee R, O'Neill C, Dobbs SM: Double-blind, placebo-controlled cross-over study of maintenance treatment with quinine bisulphate for night cramps, *Br J Clin Pharmacol* 21:108, 1986.
3. Warburton A, Royston JP, O'Neill CJ, et al: A quinine a day keeps the leg cramps away? *Br J Clin Pharmacol* 23:459-465, 1987.
4. Connolly PS, Shirley EA, Wasson JH, et al: Treatment of nocturnal leg cramps: a crossover trial of quinine vs. vitamin E, *Arch Intern Med* 152:1877-1880, 1992.
5. Maule B: Nocturnal cramp: quinine versus folklore, *Practitioner* 234:420-421, 1990.
6. Man-Son-Hing M, Wells G: Meta-analysis of efficacy of quinine for treatment of nocturnal leg cramps in elderly people, *BMJ* 310:13-17, 1995.
7. Daniell HW: Simple cure for nocturnal leg cramps (letter), *N Engl J Med* 301:216, 1979.
8. Weiner IH, Weiner HL: Nocturnal leg muscle cramps, *JAMA* 244:2332-2333, 1980.

MEDICAL EDUCATION

(See also investigations; skepticism; uncertainty)

Career Choice

Given the choice, physicians commonly change careers. An 11-year prospective study in Great Britain found that 30% of physicians changed careers once and 39% two or more times.[1] In Saskatchewan 60% of physicians were not following the career path they had planned, or would have planned, in their third year of medicine and 40% had made career changes after starting internship or residency.[2] A 7-year follow-up of the 1722 medical students who graduated from Canada's 16 medical schools in 1989 found that 17.5% of them had already changed career paths after starting postgraduate training.[3] As of 1994, career changes of this nature in Canada became almost impossible because of government-mandated restrictions of residency positions.[3] Likely consequences of this are that some physicians will find themselves stuck in fields they dislike, which may have negative consequences for their patients as well as themselves, training programs will probably have more unsuitable residents, undergraduates will use electives to try and make career choices rather than to broaden their education, and the absence of practice-experienced physicians in residency programs will narrow the scope of the training experience.[4] Another possible adverse consequence is that a number of specialties such as anesthesia, community medicine, neurology, psychiatry, radiation oncology, laboratory medicine, and physical medicine and rehabilitation, which have benefited from physician career changes in the past, may be unable to acquire and train adequate numbers of residents to meet the population needs.[3]

Undergraduate Medical Education

By the mid-1990s women constituted 40% of the U.S. undergraduate student body in medicine. This contrasts with a less than 10% representation two decades earlier.[5]

Women in Academic Medicine

In the United States women physicians on medical school faculties are promoted more slowly than men, even taking into account productivity and differential attrition rates from academic medicine.[6] At Johns Hopkins, institutional reforms within the department of medicine without any changes in promotion criteria resulted in a marked increase in promotion and retention of female academic staff.[7]

One reason women may not advance as rapidly is that those who have children at home tend to spend fewer hours in professional activities and far more hours in domestic activities than do male physicians. A Canadian study found that women family physicians with children at home spent a mean of 90.5 hours a week in combined professional and domestic work, whereas male family physicians with children at home spent a mean of 68.6 hours.[8]

⚓ REFERENCES ⚓

1. Parkhouse J, Ellin DJ: Reasons for doctors' career choice and change of choice, *BMJ* 296:1651-1653, 1988.
2. Shaw S, Goplen G, Houston DS: Career changes among Saskatchewan physicians, *Can Med Assoc J* 154:1035-1038, 1996.
3. Ryten E, Thurber D, Buske L: The class of 1989 and post-MD training, *Can Med Assoc J* 158:731-777, 1998.
4. Houston S: Postgraduate training: unfair to students and recent graduates (editorial), *Ann RCPSC* 29:136-137, 1996.
5. Women in Medical Services Office: *Leading change, women in medicine,* Chicago, 1995, American Medical Association.
6. Tesch BJ, Wood HM, Helwig AL, et al: Promotion of women physicians in academic medicine: glass ceiling or sticky floor? *JAMA* 273:1022-1025, 1995.
7. Fried LP, Francomano CA, MacDonald SM, et al: Career development for women in academic medicine: multiple interventions in a department of medicine, *JAMA* 276:898-905, 1996.
8. Woodward CA, Williams AP, Ferrier B, et al: Time spent on professional activities and unwaged domestic work: is it different for male and female primary care physicians who have children at home? *Can Fam Physician* 42:1928-1935, 1996.

MULTIPLE CHEMICAL SENSITIVITIES
(See also alternative medicine; breast implants; chronic fatigue syndrome; fibromyalgia; functional somatic syndromes)

Multiple chemical sensitivities, chronic fatigue syndrome, and fibromyalgia are three conditions whose existence is controversial. Believers search ever more intensely for organic causes, while unbelievers attribute the symptoms to psychiatric disorders such as depression or personality disorders. The symptoms and epidemiology of the three conditions overlap.[1] Synonyms for multiple chemical sensitivities include environmental illness, 20th-century disease, total allergy syndrome, sick building syndrome, and immune dysregulation. Between 85% and 90% of patients are women, usually between the ages of 30 and 50.[2] Other "syndromes" with nonspecific symptoms such as headache, fatigue, and trouble concentrating that appear to overlap with multiple chemical sensitivities, chronic fatigue syndrome, and fibromyalgia include some cases of irritable bowel syndrome, atypical connective tissue disease after silicone breast implants, hypoglycemia, and Gulf War illness.[3] Barsky[4] considers multiple chemical sensitivities to be a functional somatic syndrome (see discussion of functional somatic syndromes).

Since there is no agreement as to the existence of multiple chemical sensitivities, it is not surprising that there is no consensus as to its clinical presentation. Multiple symptoms are the rule, and they cover the spectrum of human misery. Some of the more common ones are fatigue, depression, sleep disturbances, poor concentration, memory loss, dizziness, weakness, joint pains, headaches, and heat intolerance. The patients are convinced their symptoms are caused by chemicals in concentrations below those considered to be toxic. The putative offending environmental agents are protean, and in an attempt to avoid them many patients stop working or seeing friends and isolate themselves in their homes.[2]

A common investigation used by "clinical ecologists" (a term that health professionals who focus on this disorder tend to give themselves) is a "challenge" test that involves inhalation of low concentrations of possible offending chemicals to determine if symptoms are produced. This procedure cannot be standardized, and the American Academy of Allergy and Immunology rejects the technique as unproven.[2] A high-technology investigative tool that some have claimed can confirm the diagnosis is single photon emission computed tomography (SPECT) scanning. However, the studies purporting this are flawed.[5] Claims that abnormalities of porphyrin metabolism cause the disorder are not supported by scientific evidence.[6] Staudenmayer[7] thoroughly investigated reports of patients suffering from multiple chemical sensitivities and found no scientific evidence supporting the belief that excessive sensitivity to minute levels of environmental chemicals causes multiple chemical sensitivities.

At least half of patients with multiple chemical sensitivities have recognized psychiatric conditions, most frequently depressive, anxiety, and somatoform disorders.[2] There are suggestions that the condition has some of the attributes of a hysterical epidemic.[5]

Multiple chemical sensitivities has become a focal point for numerous advocacy groups and litigation cases.[5] Although no scientific evidence has shown multiple chemical sensitivities to be a specific disease, it could become one as a result of court decisions,[5] political decisions,[8] and public belief.[8]

What are skeptical physicians to do when faced with patients claiming to have multiple chemical sensitivities? After sighing, they must take careful histories and perform punctilious physical examinations to rule out recognized specific physical and mental illnesses. At that point, in my opinion, they should politely but unequivocally give the patients their opinions about "multiple chemical sensitivities," outline the ways in which they may be able to help the patients, and specify the limits to what they are willing to undertake.

❧ REFERENCES ❧

1. Buchwald D, Garrity D: Comparison of patients with chronic fatigue syndrome, fibromyalgia, and multiple chemical sensitivities, *Arch Intern Med* 154:2049-2053, 1994.
2. Magill MK, Suruda A: Multiple chemical sensitivity syndrome, *Am Fam Physician* 58:721-728, 1998.
3. Kipen HM, Fiedler N: Invited commentary: sensitivities to chemicals—context and implications (editorial), *Am J Epidemiol* 150:13-16, 1999.
4. Barsky AJ, Borus JF: Functional somatic syndromes, *Ann Intern Med* 130:910-921, 1999.
5. Dehart RL: Multiple chemical sensitivity (editorial), *Am Fam Physician* 58:652-654, 1998.
6. Hahn M, Bonkovsky HL: Multiple chemical sensitivity syndrome and porphyria: a note of caution and concern, *Arch Intern Med* 157:281-285, 1997.
7. Staudenmayer H: *Environmental illness: myth and reality,* Boca Raton, Fla, 1999, Lewis.
8. Kreutzer R, Neutra RR, Lashuay N: Prevalence of people reporting sensitivities to chemicals in a population-based survey, *Am J Epidemiol* 150:1-12, 1999.

PATIENT EDUCATION
(See also informed consent; prevention)

According to one survey the average reading level of adults in the United States is grade 8 or 9 and 47% of the American population has deficient literacy skills.[1] This has enormous implications for patient care because patients with inadequate reading ability are less compliant with medical regimens. Suggested solutions are to combine written and oral instructions, present illustrations in the latter, use simple language in both, and give only essential information.[2]

❧ REFERENCES ❧

1. *Adult literacy in America: a first look at the results of the National Adult Literacy Survey,* ed 2, Washington, DC, 1993, Office of Educational Research and Improvement, Department of Education.
2. Mayeaux EJ Jr, Murphy PW, Arnold C, et al: Improving patient education for patients with low literacy skills, *Am Fam Physician* 53:205-211, 1996.

PETS
(See also animal bites; cat scratch disease; rabies; toxoplasmosis)

Specially trained dogs (service dogs) can perform a multitude of tasks to help physically disabled persons who have ambulatory difficulties. Among other things they can turn on switches, open and close doors, pull a person up from a sitting or lying position, pick up objects, pull on clothing, help a person get into or out of the bath, and pull a wheelchair. Their efficacy for patients with spinal cord injuries, muscular dystrophy, multiple sclerosis, and traumatic brain injury is sufficient to decrease the need for other helping resources and thus the overall cost of the disability. Having a service dog increases the self-esteem of the owner.[1]

Salmonellosis is associated with pet turtles and may also be transmitted by other reptiles such as iguanas and snakes. Ninety percent of asymptomatic reptiles carry *Salmonella* species in their stools. Transmission to humans may occur by direct contact with the animals or through cleaning their cages or aquariums. Children under 5, pregnant women, and immunocompromised individuals are at high risk for severe complications of *Salmonella* infections such as septicemia and meningitis.[2] The CDC recommends that no reptiles be kept in child care centers or in residences housing immunocompromised individuals or children under the age of 5.[3]

Psittacosis is caused by *Chlamydia psittaci* and can be transmitted by any bird via feces, beak secretions, or feather dust. Healthy birds may harbor the organisms, but the numbers increase significantly if the animal is sick. Humans usually have an abrupt onset of fever, sweats, and headache, followed in a few days by symptoms and signs of pneumonia and often diarrhea and vomiting. The diagnosis is a clinical one because the organisms are difficult to isolate. The treatment of choice is tetracyclines.[4]

Some pet tarantulas have urticarious hairs that if accidentally rubbed on the cornea (by hands or fingers that had previously been handling the spider) can penetrate it and seriously compromise visual acuity.[5]

◥ REFERENCES ◤

1. Allen K, Blascovich J: The value of service dogs for people with severe ambulatory disabilities, *JAMA* 275:1001-1006, 1996.
2. Centers for Disease Control and Prevention: Reptile-associated salmonellosis-selected states, 1994-95, *JAMA* 273:1898-1899, 1995.
3. Centers for Disease Control and Prevention: Reptile-associated salmonellosis—selected states, 1996-1998, *JAMA* 282:2293-2294, 1999.
4. Sax PE: Case records of the Massachusetts General Hospital Case 16-1998, *N Engl J Med* 338:1527-1535, 1998.
5. Blaikie AJ, Ellis J, Sanders R, et al: Eye disease associated with handling pet tarantulas: three case reports, *BMJ* 314:1524-1525, 1997.

PHARMACEUTICALS

(See also prescribing habits; wellness)

Adverse Drug Reactions

Adverse drug reactions are one of the leading causes of death in the United States. About half of all Food and Drug Administration (FDA)-approved drugs have serious adverse effects not detected before approval. Recent examples that have led to the withdrawal of the drugs are fenfluramine (Pondimin, Ponderal), which was associated with cardiac valvular disease, and terfenadine (Seldane), which was associated with serious cardiac arrhythmias.[1]

Drug Expiration Dates

Dry formulation drugs (e.g., tablets and capsules) stored in unopened containers generally maintain 70% to 80% of their potency for up to 10 years. Even drugs in opened containers maintain 70% to 80% of their potency for up to 2 years, especially if stored in locations that are not excessively humid. With the possible exception of tetracycline, outdated drugs are unlikely to be harmful.[2] Liquid formulations of drugs are less stable and should not be used after the expiration dates. Epinephrine is particularly unstable and must be stored in the dark. It is oxidized when exposed to air.[3]

Pharmaceutical Representatives

There is about 1 pharmaceutical representative for every 15 to 30 physicians in the United States, and estimates are that the industry spent more than $13,000 per physician on advertising in 1993.[4] Most physicians find the information given by the representatives useful.[5] Evidence indicates that pharmaceutical representatives influence the prescribing habits of physicians.[6,7] Attending continuing medical education conferences sponsored by drug companies and accepting meals and lodging paid for by the pharmaceutical industry is associated with increased prescriptions of the sponsor's medications.[7] In one study a third of residents and a quarter of faculty said that they changed their prescribing habits as a result of information gleaned from the representatives.[8] About half of U.S. residency training programs permit representatives to give presentations, and the majority allow them to provide food for conferences. In one survey 11% of the statements made by the representatives about drugs were considered inaccurate by an assessing team, but few physicians in the audience recognized these errors.[5] It should be noted that there were no controls to determine how often physicians' statements about drugs were considered inaccurate.

Effect of Pharmaceutical Industry Financial Support of Research

Does financial support from pharmaceutical manufacturers influence the opinions of researchers? The answer is unknown, but the possibility exists. In a survey of the published literature on the safety of calcium channel blockers, a strong association was found between those favoring this class of drugs and financial support of the authors by the manufacturers of calcium channel antagonists.[9]

Direct Consumer Advertising

The budget for direct-to-consumer advertising in the United States increased from $123.1 million in 1989 to over $900 million in 1997; the latter figure is more than double the price of pharmaceutical advertisements in medical journals.[10] One senior representative of the American Pharmaceutical Manufacturers proudly pointed out that in 1998 direct-to-consumer ads led 21 million consumers to seek medical advice about a condition they never considered worthy of asking about until they had seen the ad.[11] The effects of direct consumer advertising on the health of the population are unknown. Since studies of physicians have shown that the more they depend on information obtained from the pharmaceutical industry, the less appropriate are their prescribing practices, it is reasonable to assume that inappropriate expectations raised by drug advertising will be even greater in the general population.[12] These expectations will pressure some physicians into writing unwarranted prescriptions.[10,12,13]

◥ REFERENCES ◤

1. Moore TJ, Psaty BM, Furberg CD: Time to act on drug safety (editorial), *JAMA* 279:1571-1573, 1998.
2. Drugs past their expiration date, *Med Lett* 38:65-66, 1996.
3. Stability of drugs in solution, *Med Lett* 38:90, 1996.
4. Drake D, Uhlman M: *Making medicine, making money,* Kansas City, Mo, 1993, Andrews & McMeel.
5. Ziegler MG, Lew P, Singer BC: The accuracy of drug information from pharmaceutical sales representatives, *JAMA* 273:1296-1298, 1995.
6. Lexchin J: Interactions between physicians and the pharmaceutical industry: what does the literature say? *Can Med Assoc J* 149:1401-1407, 1993.

7. Wazana A: Physicians and the pharmaceutical industry: is a gift ever just a gift? *JAMA* 283:373-380, 2000.

8. Lurie N, Rich EC, Simpson DE, et al: Pharmaceutical representatives in academic medical centers: interaction with faculty and house staff, *J Gen Intern Med* 5:240-243, 1990.

9. Stelfox HT, Chua G, O'Rourke K, et al: Conflict of interest in the debate over calcium-channel antagonists, *N Engl J Med* 338:101-106, 1998.

10. Holen MF: Direct-to-consumer marketing of prescription drugs: creating consumer demand, *JAMA* 281:382-384, 1999.

11. Holmer AF: Direct-to-consumer prescription drug advertising builds bridges between patients and physicians, *JAMA* 281:380-382, 1999.

12. Lexchin J: Consequences of direct-to-consumer advertising of prescription drugs (editorial), *Can Fam Physician* 43:594-596, 1997.

13. Hoffman JR, Wilkes M: Direct to consumer advertising of prescription drugs (editorial), *BMJ* 318:1301-1302, 1999.

PHYSICIAN-PATIENT COMMUNICATIONS
(See also appeal of alternative medicine)

A review of 21 randomized controlled studies of physician-patient communication showed that effective communication correlated with improved patient outcomes. In order of frequency the reported improvements were in emotional health, symptom resolution, function, blood pressure control, blood sugar levels, and pain control.[1]

In the United States the quality of physician-patient interviews correlates with the likelihood that physicians will be sued. In an audiotape analysis comparing interviewing styles between primary care physicians who had been subject to malpractice claims and those who had not, physicians who had never been sued seemed to have a warmer relationship with patients as expressed by humor and laughter. They also used more orienting comments, such as "First I'll examine you, and then we will talk," and more facilitative comments, such as "Go on, tell me more about that." The actual content of the interview in terms of biopsychosocial balance or the provision of information was the same for both groups.[2]

REFERENCES

1. Stewart MA: Effective physician-patient communication and health outcomes: a review, *Can Med Assoc J* 152:1423-1433, 1995.

2. Levinson W, Roter DL, Mullooly JP, et al: Physician-patient communication: the relationship with malpractice claims among primary care physicians and surgeons, *JAMA* 277:553-559, 1997.

PRESCRIBING HABITS
(See also geriatrics; pharmaceuticals)

Prescription and over-the-counter drugs are the fastest growing health care expenditure in Canada. In 1993 they accounted for 15% of money spent on health care, and the annual rate of increase is 8.2%.[1] Probably many of the drugs are prescribed inappropriately, often because physicians bow to patients' real or perceived wishes for medications.

This may lead to a vicious circle in which those who received prescriptions for self-limiting illnesses in the past expect to receive them the next time they experience similar symptoms.[2] On the other hand, there is evidence that drugs are underused for some important conditions, including hypertension, myocardial infarction, and depression.[3] Properly used drugs can actually save the system money.[4]

Poor prescribing habits are of particular concern for the elderly, as discussed under "Prescribing Habits and the Elderly" in the section on geriatrics. The role of the pharmaceutical industry in influencing prescribing habits is discussed above under "Pharmaceuticals."

An occasional problem with drug prescriptions is the substitution of one drug for another with a similar name. For example, after two patients who were prescribed Losec (the original trade name of omeprazole in the United States) were given Lasix,[5] Merck Sharp & Dohme changed the name in the United States to Prilosec.[6] You just can't win; a patient for whom Prilosec was prescribed was given Prozac.[7] Another example is the case of a hospitalized women with pneumonia and pleurisy who was prescribed a Z-Pak (a blister card of six capsules of azithromycin [Zithromax]) and who instead received regular applications of an ice pack to her chest wall.[8] The recommendation of Lawyer and Despot[8] always to include generic drug names when writing prescriptions seems eminently sensible.

REFERENCES

1. *National health expenditures in Canada, 1975-1993*, Ottawa, 1994, Health Canada, pp 3-4.

2. Greenhalgh T, Gill P: Pressure to prescribe: involves a complex interplay of factors, *BMJ* 315:1482-1483, 1997.

3. MacLeod SM: Improving physician prescribing practices: bridge over troubled waters (editorial), *Can Med Assoc J* 154:675-677, 1996.

4. McIsaac W, Naylor CD, Anderson GM, et al: Reflections on a month in the life of the Ontario Drug Benefit Plan (editorial), *Can Med Assoc J* 150:473-477, 1994.

5. Fine SN, Isdorfer RM, Miskovitz PF, et al: Losec or Lasix (letter)? *N Engl J Med* 322:1674, 1990.

6. Hoffman JP: More on "Losec or Lasix?" (letter), *N Engl J Med* 323:1428, 1990.

7. Costable JM Jr, McKinley MJ: Prozac or Prilosec for gastric ulcer? (letter), *N Engl J Med* 335:600, 1996.

8. Lawyer C, Despot J: 'Z-Pak' vs Ice Pack: need for clarity and continuous quality assurance (letter), *JAMA* 278:1405, 1997.

RELIGION

Numerous studies have found a positive correlation between a variety of religious activities and decreased morbidity and mortality. For example, clerics of certain denominations have lower mortality rates than nonclerics, and church attenders have lower mortality rates than nonattenders. The problem with such studies is that they rarely account fully for confounding variables; clerics by and large have healthier life-styles than nonclerics and some people do not go to church because they are too ill or feeble. At present there is only tenuous evidence that religion or spirituality leads to better physical health.[1]

Although future well-controlled trials may show that certain religious or spiritual practices are indeed beneficial, the ethical implications this might have for physicians are difficult to know. It is taken for granted that health professionals will always respect an individual's religious beliefs, but if faith in God were shown to be therapeutically beneficial, would it be ethical for physicians to try to convert unbelievers? According to Sloan, Bagiella, and Powell[1] it would not, any more than it is ethical to advise the unmarried to marry because married people have better health. These authors also point out that linking religious beliefs to health outcomes may cause harm if patients interpret failure to get better as indicative of moral failure.[1]

◣ REFERENCES ◢

1. Sloan RP, Bagiella E, Powell T: Religion, spirituality, and medicine, *Lancet* 353:664-667, 1999.

RISK ANALYSIS
(See also attitudes, physician; investigations; positive predictive value; risk assessment in pregnancy; screening; uncertainty)

Risk and uncertainty are inextricably linked. In medicine one way of attempting to diminish the degree of uncertainty is to develop systems for placing patients in different risk categories. For example, scoring systems may be applied to pregnant women to categorize their pregnancies as "high risk" or "low risk." Various terms used to encompass risk-categorizing systems include risk approach, risk analysis, risk scoring, risk screening systems, and risk management.[1]

Three important assumptions underlie risk analysis:
1. Risk factors that will allow an accurate determination of which cohort of patients is at high risk are well established.
2. One or more interventions are available to improve the outcome of patients identified as being at high risk.
3. Above all else the physician must look for, identify, and manage the worst case scenario. This is an attitudinal issue and reflects the "maximalist" approach of "If in doubt, do something" (see discussion of physician attitudes).

Risk analysis tends to ameliorate a physician's anxiety in an ambiguous situation by reformulating the problem in a numerical fashion. High numbers equal high risk and the need to do something, whereas low numbers equal low risk about which the physician need not worry. Numbers give magical and often false reassurance because they appear to represent certainty.[2]

Developing a risk analysis protocol is extremely complex[3] and is seldom well done. Even a carefully prepared analysis in which cohorts at high risk are clearly distinguished from cohorts at low risk often does little to help the individual patient. This is because in situations in which the

prevalence rate of adverse outcomes is low, the positive predictive value of any screening system is low. As a result, many persons who will not have adverse outcomes are labeled as at "high risk" and may suffer both the psychological adverse effects of being so labeled (see discussion of labeling) and the physical adverse effects of unwarranted investigations or interventions.[4] For example, when risk evaluation is performed in pregnancy, the "high-risk" label is applied to 16% to 55% of pregnant women.[5] Unfortunately, a large percentage of adverse outcomes occur in persons who have no identifiable risk factors and so are categorized as being at "low risk." Half of all perinatal morbidity and mortality occurs in "low-risk" pregnancies.[5,6]

One thoughtful analyst of risk analysis has concluded that pregnancy risk scoring has not been proved to cause more benefit than harm.[1] This view is echoed in an editorial by Klein,[7] who points out that labeling pregnant women as at high risk may itself lead to consultations and unnecessary interventions.

◣ REFERENCES ◢

1. Hall PF: Rethinking risk (editorial), *Can Fam Physician* 40:1239-1244, 1994.
2. Postman N: *Technopoly: the surrender of culture to technology,* Mississauga, Ontario, 1992, Vintage Books.
3. Morgan MG: Risk analysis and management, *Sci Am* 269:32-41, 1993.
4. Woolf SH, Kameron DB: Testing for uncommon conditions—the heroic search for positive test results, *Arch Intern Med* 150:2451-2458, 1990.
5. Wall EM: Assessing obstetric risk: a review of obstetric risk-scoring systems, *J Fam Pract* 27:153-163, 1988.
6. Hall PF: Obstetric risk scoring: a Trojan horse, *Manitoba Med* 63:43-45, 1993.
7. Klein M: Family physician maternity care: outcomes when family physicians provide most community-based care (editorial), *Can Fam Physician* 41:546-548, 1995.

SLEEP
(See also motor vehicle accidents; sudden infant death syndrome)

Insomnia
(See also anxiety disorders; Creutzfeldt-Jakob disease; hip fractures; hormone replacement therapy; jet lag; narcolepsy; prescribing habits; restless legs syndrome; seasonal affective disorder; sleep apnea; sleep walking; snoring)

Etiology
Depression, anxiety disorders, and sleep apnea are common causes of insomnia, and it is important to rule them out (snoring is a clue for sleep apnea).[1-4] Other important causes are the intake of various chemical agents such as alcohol, nicotine, caffeine, or a variety of prescription or nonprescription drugs.[1,2,4] Even one or two glasses of wine in the evening can cause awakening around 2 or 3 AM as the seda-

tive effect wears off. The half-life of coffee is 3 to 7 hours, so some people should avoid drinking it in the afternoon or evening if they want to sleep.[1,2] Physical illnesses, particularly cardiopulmonary diseases, musculoskeletal pain, and prostate problems leading to frequent nocturnal micturitions, are independent causes of insomnia.[3] Restless legs syndrome[2,4] and sometimes periodic leg movement disorder[4] may cause insomnia, as may menopausal hot flashes.[4]

Epidemiology

Complaints of insomnia are more common in women than men, in the divorced, widowed, or separated, in lower socioeconomic groups, and in the elderly.[1] Polygraph studies show sleep in the elderly to be shallower, shorter, and more fragmented. However, older people do not have a decline in the subjective need for sleep. For some the poor quality of nighttime sleep leads to daytime somnolence.[2,4]

Nonpharmacological management

Aside from elimination of precipitating causes of insomnia such as those listed above, the following behavioral approach may be helpful[1,2,4,5]:

1. Go to bed only when sleepy.
2. Do not read, eat, or watch television in bed. Bed is for sleeping and sex.
3. If you are in bed and can't sleep, get up, go to another room, and stay up until you are really sleepy and then go back to bed. Do not watch television because the brightness of its light has an arousing effect; instead read with as dim a light as possible. If after returning to bed you still can't sleep, get up again and repeat the cycle.
4. Set the alarm for the same time every morning, and get up when it rings regardless of how little sleep you have had.
5. Never sleep during the day.

An additional approach is to document the number of hours the patient sleeps and to make bedtime that number of hours (or that number of hours plus 30 minutes) before the fixed morning wakeup time. If, for example, an insomniac sleeps only 5 hours and the morning wakeup time is to be 7 AM, bedtime should be 1:30 or 2 AM. This will probably cause the patient to accumulate a sleep deficit and fall asleep more easily. After a week the bedtime can be made earlier by 15 minutes, and further 15-minute weekly increments of time spent in bed can be added provided that at least 85% of the time in bed is spent sleeping.[1]

In a study from Virginia, elderly patients (mean age 65 years) with primary insomnia were selected at random to participate in one of three therapeutic regimens: an 8-week program of weekly small group sessions for cognitive behavioral therapy, pharmacotherapy with temazepam (Restoril), and a combination of cognitive behavioral therapy and either temazepam or placebo. The behavioral approach was essentially that described above, and the cognitive compo-

nent included rectifying unrealistic expectations about the hours of sleep required (less than 8 hours is OK), clarifying that daytime distress is not entirely the result of insomnia, and correcting fallacious beliefs about how to improve sleep. After 2 years of follow-up, excellent results were obtained with cognitive behavioral therapy, whereas the short-term benefits of temazepam had entirely dissipated. Some of the patients in the combined cognitive behavioral and temazepam arm of the study maintained improved sleep patterns, whereas others did not.[6] This study indicates that although cognitive behavioral therapy leads to excellent results, benzodiazepines have no long-term benefits in treating insomnia in the elderly.

A 16-week randomized trial of moderate-intensity aerobic exercises for elderly patients with sleep disturbances showed a significant improvement in self-rated sleep quality. Each subject performed low-impact aerobics, brisk walking, or stationary cycling four times a week for 30 to 40 minutes before the evening meal.[7]

Hypnotics

Serious side effects from taking hypnotic drugs are common, especially in the elderly, whose elimination of many of these drugs is greatly delayed.[1] Benzodiazepines are addictive, suppress memories, adversely affect cognition in patients with early dementia, and increase the risk of injury from falls and other accidents (see discussion of hip fractures).[8] According to Kupfer and Reynolds[1] no data from randomized trials have shown that taking hypnotic drugs for more than 35 days provides sustained benefits.

The following are basic principles of the pharmacotherapy of insomnia[1]:

1. Use the lowest dose possible.
2. Prescribe for a limited period (no more than 4 weeks on a regular basis).
3. Prescribe intermittent doses (two to four times a week).
4. Discontinue hypnotics gradually.

Available hypnotics are the benzodiazepines (intermediate- or short-acting compounds preferred), zolpidem (Ambien), zaleplon (Sonata), and chloral hydrate (Noctec). Zolpidem is not a benzodiazepine but has a similar therapeutic profile. How habituating it is has not been determined.[1] Although neither zolpidem or zaleplon is a benzodiazepine, both bind to benzodiazepine receptors.[9] Zopiclone (Imovane) is also a nonbenzodiazepine and has been touted as being nonaddictive in short-term use; case reports of addiction after long-term use are appearing.[10] Amnestic reactions with triazolam (Halcion) are common, and like other benzodiazepines, it is addictive.[11] I never prescribe it.

Antidepressants, especially those that are serotonin specific, have been widely used as hypnotics. No systematic studies of the efficacy of these agents for this purpose have been published. The tricyclic drugs such as amitriptyline

(Elavil) or doxepin (Sinequan) have significant anticholinergic side effects. More promising are trazodone (Desyrel), nefazodone (Serzone), and paroxetine (Paxil).[1] Trazodone 100 mg hs has been used successfully as a hypnotic in depressed patients who had persistent, exacerbated, or new-onset insomnia when being treated with fluoxetine or bupropion.[12]

Alcohol is not a good sedative because the initial central nervous system depression is followed by rebound excitation that disturbs sleep.[1,4,11]

The value of melatonin for insomnia is unknown because few adequate trials have been published and the purity of some products is questionable.[13] In a 1999 Israeli study elderly patients who had been taking benzodiazepines daily for at least 6 months were assigned at random to receive a placebo or 2 mg of a sustained release formulation of melatonin taken 2 hours before bedtime. All patients were asked to gradually decrease and then discontinue their benzodiazepines. After 6 weeks 78% of the melatonin group were no longer taking benzodiazepines compared with 25% of the placebo group.[14]

Table 48 lists a few of the drugs that are approved or used as hypnotics. In prescribing them the physician should remember that except with the antidepressants, efficacy usually dissipates in a few weeks and dependency is a major risk.[1,11]

Table 48   Hypnotics

Drugs	Usual doses
Aldehydes and Derivatives	
Chloral hydrate	500-1000 mg qhs
Benzodiazepine Derivatives	
Short acting	
Triazolam (Halcion)	0.125 mg qhs
Intermediate acting	
Oxazepam (Serax)	15-30 mg qhs
Lorazepam (Ativan)	0.5-2 mg qhs
Temazepam (Restoril)	5-30 mg qhs
Long acting	
Diazepam (Valium)	2-10 mg qhs
Flurazepam (Dalmane)	15-30 mg qhs
Cyclopyrrolones	
Zopiclone (Imovane)	3.75-14 mg qhs
Imidazopyridines	
Zolpidem (Ambien)	5-10 mg qhs
Pyrazolopyrimidines	
Zaleplon (Sonata)	10 mg qhs
Tricyclics	
Amitriptyline (Elavil)	10-75 mg qhs
Doxepin (Sinequan)	10-75 mg qhs
Modified Cyclic Derivatives	
Trazodone (Desyrel)	150-300 mg qhs
Phenylpiperazine Compounds	
Nefazodone (Serzone)	100-250 mg hs
Selective Serotonin Reuptake Inhibitors	
Paroxetine (Paxil)	20 mg qhs

◄ REFERENCES ►

1. Kupfer DJ, Reynolds CF III: Management of insomnia, *N Engl J Med* 336:341-346, 1997.
2. Mendelson W: A 96-year-old woman with insomnia, *JAMA* 277:990-996, 1997.
3. Katz DA, McHorney CA: Clinical correlates of insomnia in patients with chronic illness, *Arch Intern Med* 158:1099-1107, 1998.
4. Rajput V, Bromley SM: Chronic insomnia: a practical review, *Am Fam Physician* 60:1431-1442, 1999.
5. Bootzin RR, Perlis ML: Nonpharmacologic treatments of insomnia, *J Clin Psychiatry* 53(suppl 6):37-41, 1992.
6. Morin CM, Colecchi C, Stone J, et al: Behavioral and pharmacological therapies for late-life insomnia: a randomized controlled trial, *JAMA* 281:991-999, 1999.
7. King AC, Oman RF, Brassington GS, et al: Moderate-intensity exercise and self-rated quality of sleep in older adults: a randomized controlled trial, *JAMA* 277:32-37, 1997.
8. Bursztajn HJ: Melatonin therapy: from benzodiazepine-dependent insomnia to authenticity and autonomy (editorial), *Arch Intern Med* 159:2393-2395, 1999.
9. Zaleplon for insomnia, *Med Lett* 41:93-94, 1999.
10. Jones IR, Sullivan G: Physical dependence on zopiclone: case reports, *BMJ* 316:117, 1998.
11. Hypnotic drugs, *Med Lett* 38:59-61, 1996.
12. Nierenberg AA, Adler LA, Peselow E, et al: Trazodone for antidepressant-associated insomnia, *Am J Psychiatry* 151:1069-1072, 1994.
13. Epstein FH: Melatonin in humans, *N Engl J Med* 336:186-195, 1997.
14. Garfinkel D, Zisapel N, Wainstein J, et al: Facilitation of benzodiazepine discontinuation by melatonin: a new clinical approach, *Arch Intern Med* 159:2456-2460, 1999.

Narcolepsy

The usual sequence of symptom development in narcolepsy is as follows:
1. Hypersomnia
2. Cataplexy
3. Sleep paralysis
4. Hypnagogic/hypnopompic hallucinations

Pharmacological treatment is with methylphenidate (Ritalin). The usual dosage for adults is 10 to 30 mg/day in two or three divided doses. The maximum dose is 60 mg/day.

Sleep Apnea

(See also motor vehicle accidents; snoring)

The estimated prevalence of sleep apnea or sleep-disordered breathing in middle-aged adults is 2% to 4%. The condition is most common in middle-aged obese men. Symptoms include loud snoring, gasping, snorting, and apnea during sleep and fatigue during the day. Patients with obstructive sleep apnea are said to have an increased incidence of hypertension, ischemic heart disease, cerebrovascular disease, and motor vehicle accidents.[1,2] A systematic review of the literature was unable to confirm an association between sleep apnea and any of these outcomes except possibly motor vehicle accidents. This may be because many of the reputed adverse affects are explained by confounding variables such as obesity and smoking.[2] Other adverse effects of sleep apnea are decreased quality of social and emotional life among those affected[3] and decreased sleep quality among bed partners.[4]

Avoidance of alcohol and sedative drugs is an important initial step in the management of sleep apnea. Weight loss if it can be achieved and maintained is helpful, and for some people sleeping in the lateral position gives some relief. In some mild cases protriptyline (Triptil) or fluoxetine (Prozac) or oral appliances are helpful,[1,2] but the prime medical therapeutic modality is continuous positive airway pressure (CPAP).[1-3,5,6] Surgical procedures include palatal surgery and tracheostomy.[1] The efficacy of positive airway pressure has been questioned based on a systematic review of the evidence; possibly patients with severe symptoms benefit, but this is unproved.[2] Since then a number of prospective studies have reported excellent results with CPAP even in patients with mild or moderate sleep apnea.[3,5,6]

REFERENCES

1. Strollo PJ Jr, Rogers RM: Obstructive sleep apnea, *N Engl J Med* 334:99-104, 1996.
2. Wright J, Johns R, Watt I, et al: Health effects of obstructive sleep apnoea and the effectiveness of continuous positive airways pressure: a systematic review of the research evidence, *BMJ* 314:851-860, 1997.
3. D'Ambrosio C, Bowman T, Mohsenin V: Quality of life in patients with obstructive sleep apnea: effect of nasal continuous positive airway pressure—a prospective study, *Chest* 115:123-129, 1999.
4. Beninati W, Harris CD, Herold DL, et al: The effect of snoring and obstructive sleep apnea on the sleep quality of bed partners, *Mayo Clin Proc* 74:955-958, 1999.
5. Redline S, Adams N, Strauss ME, et al: Improvement of mild sleep-disordered breathing with CPAP compared with conservative therapy, *Am J Respir Crit Care* Med 157:858-865, 1998.
6. Polo O: Continuous positive airway pressure for treatment of sleep apnoea (editorial), *Lancet* 353:2086-2087, 1999.

Sleep Walking

About 10% to 15% of children between the ages of 5 and 12 have at least one episode of sleep walking. Between one fourth and one third of children who are sleep walkers have enuresis, and a fair number also have night terrors. The incidence is increased in patients with Tourette's syndrome. Somnambulism generally occurs in the first 3 to 4 hours of sleep during stages 3 and 4 of non-rapid-eye-movement (NREM) sleep. Injuries during the episodes are common, especially in adults. In children the condition is generally self-limited.[1]

REFERENCES

1. Masand P, Popli AP, Weilburg JB: Sleepwalking, *Am Fam Physician* 649-653, 1995.

Snoring
(See also sleep apnea)

A prospective study of Swedish men found that the incidence of habitual snoring increases until ages 50 to 60 and then declines. The single most significant risk factor in all age groups was increased weight; smoking was a significant risk factor in younger middle-aged men.[1]

A study of snoring overweight men found that sleeping on one side or using nasal decongestants had little effect. However, weight loss was effective. Men who lost 3 kg or more cut their hourly snoring rates in half, and three subjects who lost an average of 7.6 kg stopped snoring entirely.[2]

Protriptyline 5 to 20 mg qhs is reputed to reduce snoring.

REFERENCES

1. Lindberg E, Taube A, Janson C, et al: A 10-year follow-up of snoring in men, *Chest* 114:1048-1055, 1998.
2. Braver HM, Block AJ, Perri MG: Treatment for snoring—combined weight loss, sleeping on side, and nasal spray, *Chest* 107:1283-1288, 1995.

SPORTS MEDICINE
(See also acute exertional rhabdomyolysis; concussion; exercise; exercise in pregnancy; hematuria; seizures; urinalysis-blood)

Bicycle Seats

An infrequent complication of bicycle riding is pudendal neuropathy characterized by numbness of the scrotum and penile shaft. This is thought to be caused by compression of the dorsal branch of the pudendal nerve between the bicycle seat and the symphysis pubis; in many cases it results from an upward tilting of the bicycle seat. In a few case reports temporary impotence has been associated with biking, but whether a causal relationship exists is uncertain.[1]

REFERENCES

1. Weiss BD: Clinical syndromes associated with bicycle seats, *Clin Sports Med* 13:175-186, 1994.

Diarrhea, Hematochezia, and Other Gastrointestinal Symptoms in Competitive Athletes
(See also exercise-induced hematuria)

Gastrointestinal (GI) symptoms are almost the norm for competitive runners, cyclists, and triathletes. One survey divided symptoms into upper GI (nausea, belching, heartburn, chest pain, and vomiting) and lower GI (cramps, bloating, diarrhea, flatulence, urge to defecate, defecation, diarrhea, and side ache). Of runners, 71% had lower and 36% had upper GI symptoms. Of cyclists, 67% had upper and 64% lower GI symptoms.[1]

Diarrhea occurs in 20% to 25% of marathon runners.[2,3] Symptoms vary from loose stools to frank diarrhea and are associated with increased mileage or a particularly strenuous effort. Diarrhea may occur during or right after the training. About half the patients have fecal urgency and often have to stop the workout to go to the bathroom.[3]

Hematochezia may also occur in runners. Occult blood in the stool has been found in 20% of runners immediately after a marathon, and 6% had frank rectal bleeding.[4]

─────────── ◤ **REFERENCES** ◥ ───────────

1. Peters HP, Seebregts L, Akkermans LM, et al: Gastrointestinal symptoms in long-distance runners, cyclists, and triathletes: prevalence, medication, and etiology, *Am J Gastroenterol* 94:1570-1581, 1999.
2. Butcher JD: Runner's diarrhea and other intestinal problems of athletes, *Am Fam Physician* 48:623-627, 1993.
3. Keeffe EB, Lowe DK, Goss JR, Wayne R: Gastrointestinal symptoms of marathon runners, *West J Med* 141:481-484, 1984.
4. McCabe ME 3d, Peura DA, Kadakia SC, et al: Gastrointestinal blood loss associated with running a marathon, *Dig Dis Sci* 31:1229-1232, 1986.

Diving

Breath hold diving

Untrained individuals can usually hold their breath for about half a minute before the strong stimulus from carbon dioxide accumulation leads them to surface and breathe. Hyperventilation before diving blows off carbon dioxide and allows individuals to stay underwater for as long as 5 minutes. This is a dangerous practice because during ascent at the end of the dive the partial pressure of the little oxygen that remains in the lungs decreases rapidly and dramatically, which may lead to inadequate cerebral oxygen pressure, unconsciousness, and drowning.[1]

Scuba diving

A number of medical problems result from scuba diving. One of the most serious is decompression sickness, which usually manifests itself within 8 hours of the dive but may not become obvious until up to 24 hours. This disorder is usually seen in divers who have exceeded the time limits set out in standard "dive tables" for the depth attained. The most common symptom is joint pain, especially in the shoulders or elbows. Skin rash, skin marbling (cutis marmorata), and pruritus are also common. Central nervous symptoms often involve the spinal cord and cause numbness, paresthesias, and weakness. Altered mentation may be seen. Pulmonary symptoms are relatively rare and consist of substernal pain, dyspnea, and coughing ("the chokes"), which usually occur immediately after surfacing. If inert gas bubbles form in the inner ear, the patient experiences vertigo, tinnitus, and sensorineural hearing loss (inner ear decompression syndrome). Treatment of decompression sickness is recompression; this may be beneficial for patients with neurological symptoms even after the passage of several days.[2]

Other serious or even fatal consequences of scuba diving are pulmonary barotrauma and arterial gas embolism. If a diver fails to exhale while ascending (which is most likely to occur in an uncontrolled ascent), the expanding air may rupture the alveoli. Subcutaneous emphysema is a common result, pneumothorax may occur, and if air bubbles enter the pulmonary vasculature and from there the arterial circulation, cerebrovascular accident or myocardial infarction may ensue. Symptoms of arterial gas embolism usually come on immediately after the ascent, whereas those of decompression sickness develop gradually.[2] Hyperbaric oxygen is the treatment of choice for arterial gas embolism, as well as for decompression sickness.[3]

The most common form of barotrauma from scuba diving is barotitis media or "middle ear squeeze." It is caused by a failure of the eustachian tube to open, often because of an upper respiratory infection. In severe cases hemotympanum or even perforation may occur. In some cases barotrauma can also affect the inner ear (inner ear barotrauma). If the diver is unable to clear the ears because of a blocked eustachian tube, the high intracranial pressure associated with the attempt to clear them may be transmitted through the internal auditory canal to the inner ear and cause a round window tear or a rupture of the membranous labyrinth. In either case there will be sudden onset of vertigo, tinnitus, and hearing loss. As stated previously, similar symptoms may occur in decompression sickness involving the inner ear, but in that case symptoms usually develop later and more gradually.[2]

─────────── ◤ **REFERENCES** ◥ ───────────

1. Wilmshurst P: ABC of oxygen: diving and oxygen, *BMJ* 317:996-999, 1998.
2. Clenney TL, Lassen LF: Recreational scuba diving injuries, *Am Fam Physician* 53:1761-1766, 1996.
3. Tibbles PM, Edelsberg JS: Hyperbaric-oxygen therapy, *N Engl J Med* 334:1642-1648, 1996.

Drugs and Sports

Banned substances

A large number of drugs are banned for Olympic competitors. Even if prescription or nonprescription drugs are not banned, competitors must declare their use before Olympic meets. Banned substances include the following[1,2]:

1. Stimulants (epinephrine, amphetamines, cocaine, and decongestants such as pseudoephedrine, phenylephrine, and phenylpropanolamine). Many cold remedies contain decongestants.
2. Narcotics (except codeine)
3. Beta-blockers for specific sports such as archery, diving, or shooting
4. Diuretics
5. Probenecid (because it affects urine samples)
6. Anabolic steroids
7. Peptide hormones and analogues (growth hormone, adrenocorticotropic hormone, human chorionic gonadotropin, erythropoietin)
8. Tetracaine (because of the cocaine)

9. Corticosteroids by the IV, intramuscular, or oral route. Intraarticular and inhaled corticosteroids are allowed but must be reported.

10. Autologous blood transfusions ("blood doping")

Natural and herbal remedies should be avoided because some contain unlabeled banned substances. Although many banned agents can be detected by toxicological analysis, others, such as the peptide analogues, are difficult or impossible to identify.

Anabolic steroids. Illicit use of anabolic steroids is common. One U.S. survey found that 7% of male high school students had taken these drugs.[3]

Anabolic steroids increase muscle mass and strength but not aerobic capacity. There is no convincing evidence that they increase performance. A variety of anabolic steroids are used, often concomitantly and in doses up to 100 times those required for replacement therapy. Common adverse effects are acne, decreased testicular volume, and azoospermia. Other documented complications are cholestasis, peliosis hepatis (liver cysts), and hepatocellular adenomas and carcinomas. The high-density lipoprotein level is lowered and the low-density lipoprotein level elevated, the erythrocyte count is increased, and platelet numbers and platelet aggregation are augmented. Increased or decreased libido, increased aggression, psychosis, and withdrawal symptoms have been reported.[4]

Androstenedione is available in health food stores as a "dietary supplement." Claims have been made that it can increase muscle mass and strength, presumably by increasing testosterone levels.[5,6] A randomized placebo-controlled trial of oral androstenedione in young men undergoing resistance training found no evidence that androstenedione elevated testosterone levels or increased the size or strength of muscles to a greater extent than was observed in the placebo group.[6] Whether it increases athletic performance is unknown. The long-term safety of the drug has not been determined; potential side effects are those of other anabolic steroids.[5]

Creatine. Creatine is also available as a "dietary supplement." In laboratory studies it has been reported to increase performance moderately, but the majority of studies have shown no benefit in field trials. It appears to be safe and is not banned by the International Olympic Committee.[5]

REFERENCES

1. Olson R: Drugs, athletes, and family physicians: when to withhold medications and when to document prescriptions, *Can Fam Physician* 42:1953-1960, 1996.
2. MacAuley D: Drugs in sport, *BMJ* 313:211-215, 1996.
3. Buckley WE, Yesalis CE III, Friedl KE, et al: Estimated prevalence of anabolic steroid use among male high school seniors, *JAMA* 260:3441-3445, 1988.
4. Bagateli CJ, Bremner WJ: Androgens in men—uses and abuses, *N Engl J Med* 334:707-714, 1996.
5. Creatine and androstenedione—two "dietary supplements," *Med Lett* 40:105-106, 1998.
6. King DS, Sharp RL, Vukovich MD, et al: Effect of oral androstenedione on serum testosterone and adaptations to resistance training in young men: a randomized controlled trial, *JAMA* 281:2020-2028, 1999.

Female Athletes

(See also amenorrhea; eating disorders; osteoporosis; risks of exercise)

A serious problem for some female athletes is the combination of an eating disorder, amenorrhea, and osteoporosis. The incidence of this so-called female athlete triad in top women athletes has been reported to be between 15% and 62%.[1] In amenorrheic athletes bone density has been shown to be decreased not only in the spine and proximal femur, but in many other sites, including cortical weight-bearing bone.[2]

In a small retrospective study of amenorrheic runners, hormone replacement therapy with either conjugated estrogen (Premarin) 0.625 mg/day or an estradiol transdermal patch of 50 µg/day plus medroxyprogesterone acetate 10 mg/day for 14 days a month resulted in greater bone density in the treated than in the untreated cohort.[3] Birth control pills may also be effective (see discussion of amenorrhea).

REFERENCES

1. Tofler IR, Stryer BK, Micheli LJ, et al: Physical and emotional problems of elite female gymnasts, *N Engl J Med* 335:281-283, 1996.
2. Rencken ML, Chesnut CH III, Drinkwater BL: Bone density at multiple skeletal sites in amenorrheic athletes, *JAMA* 276:238-240, 1996.
3. Cumming DC: Exercise-associated amenorrhea, low bone density, and estrogen replacement therapy, *Arch Intern Med* 156:2193-2195, 1996.

Preparticipation Medical Examinations

(See also cardiac arrest; exercise)

Between one third[1] and one half[2] of cardiac deaths in young athletes in the United States are due to hypertrophic cardiomyopathy. In contrast, an Italian investigation found that hypertrophic cardiomyopathy was the cause in only 2% of cases.[3] Other causes of death in young athletes are coronary atherosclerosis, anomalous origin of the coronary arteries, and arrhythmogenic right ventricular cardiomyopathy.[3]

Can preparticipation medical examinations identify cardiac disorders? This is unlikely because the incidence of sudden cardiac death in high school athletes is very low[4,5] and because the symptoms and signs of most of the cardiac conditions leading to sudden death in young athletes are absent or minimal.[1,4,5] Over a 12-year period only three cardiac deaths were reported in Minnesota high school athletes for an annual rate of approximately 1 in 200,000 per year.[4] A review of cardiac deaths in athletes found that only 3% were identified during preparticipation examinations as having possible cardiovascular disease.[1] Although increasing the sensitivity of preparticipation examinations by improving protocols is theoretically possible,[5] large numbers of cases would still be missed and false-positive findings would increase dramatically.[6] By one estimate, if tools available to screen for sudden cardiac death had both sensitivities and specificities of 99%, the positive predictive value would be 0.5%—only 1 of 200 positives would be a true positive.[7]

Corrado and associates[3] are a little more optimistic about the benefits of preparticipation screening. They postulate that the reason only 2% of the cardiac deaths in their study of Italian athletes were due to hypertrophic cardiomyopathy was that preparticipation 12-lead electrocardiography (ECG) followed in abnormal cases (9%) by echocardiography detected most individuals with hypertrophic cardiomyopathy, who were then banned from competitive sports.[3] Screening by echocardiography is impractical. A review of five studies involving a total of 5458 students found that not a single case was detected.[8] In spite of the report by Corrado and co-workers, little evidence supports routine ECGs as part of the preparticipation examination. The U.S. Preventive Services Task Force gives preparticipation ECGs a "D" recommendation.[9]

Preparticipation medical examinations as a way of preventing sudden death also seem to have little value for marathon runners, since in a tabulation of 215,413 runners in a variety of marathons only four sudden cardiac deaths occurred for a prevalence rate of 0.002%.[10] Exercise testing is not indicated for prospective marathon runners because it is neither sensitive nor specific.[8]

At present there is no proof that preparticipation examinations can prevent death in athletes. Nevertheless, both the American Heart Association[11] and the American Academy of Family Physicians[12] recommend that preparticipation cardiovascular screening be undertaken for high school and college athletes.

Preparticipation examinations are commonly said to lead to the detection and treatment of a number of noncardiac conditions. Examination of close to 3000 athletes by members of the Mayo Clinic staff resulted in 2% being disqualified from participation (almost half because of musculoskeletal problems) and 12% being allowed to participate on condition that they receive medical follow-up, mainly for visual and musculoskeletal problems. In the vast majority of cases medical problems were identified on the basis of the history.[13]

--- ⚐ **REFERENCES** ⚐ ---

1. Maron BJ, Shirani J, Poliac LC, et al: Sudden death in young competitive athletes: clinical, demographic, and pathological profiles, *JAMA* 276:199-204, 1996.
2. Van Camp SP, Bloor CM, Mueller FO, et al: Nontraumatic sports death in high school and college athletes, *Med Sci Sports Exerc* 27:641-647, 1995.
3. Corrado D, Basso C, Schiavon M, et al: Screening for hypertrophic cardiomyopathy in young athletes, *N Engl J Med* 339:364-369, 1998.
4. Maron BJ, Gohman TE, Aeppli D: Prevalence of sudden cardiac death during competitive sports activities in Minnesota high school athletes, *J Am Coll Cardiol* 32:1881-1884, 1998.
5. Glover DW, Maron BJ: Profile of preparticipation cardiovascular screening for high school athletes, *JAMA* 279:1817-1819, 1998.
6. Matheson GO: Preparticipation screening of athletes (editorial), *JAMA* 279:1829-1830, 1998.
7. O'Connor FG, Kugler JP, Oriscello RG: Sudden death in young athletes: screening for the needle in a haystack, *Am Fam Physician* 57:2763-2770, 1998.
8. Thompson PD: The cardiovascular complications of vigorous physical activity, *Arch Intern Med* 156:2297-2302, 1996.
9. US Preventive Services Task Force: *Guide to clinical preventive services,* ed 2, Baltimore, 1996, Williams & Wilkins, pp 3-14.
10. Maron BJ, Poliac LC, Roberts WO: Risk for sudden cardiac death associated with marathon running, *J Am Coll Cardiol* 28:428-431, 1996.
11. Maron BJ, Thompson PD, Puffer JC, et al: Cardiovascular preparticipation screening of competitive athletes: a statement for health professionals from the Sudden Death Committee (clinical cardiology) and Congenital Cardiac Defects Committee (cardiovascular disease in the young), American Heart Association, *Circulation* 94:850-856, 1996.
12. American Academy of Family Practice, American Academy of Pediatrics, American Medical Society for Sports Medicine, American Orthopedic Society for Sports Medicine, American Osteopathic Academy of Sports Medicine: *Preparticipation physical evaluation,* ed 2, Minneapolis, 1997, Physician Sportsmed.
13. Smith J, Laskowski ER: The preparticipation physical examination: Mayo Clinic experience with 2,739 examinations, *Mayo Clin Proc* 73:419-429, 1998.

Pyschological Morbidity Among Olympic-Level Athletes
(See also abuse)

An assessment of Olympic-level gymnastic training programs found that training often begins between the ages of 5 and 7 years and that some children leave home by the age of 12 to obtain specialized instruction. At this point in their development they may be training for 30 to 45 hours a week and become socially isolated.[1] Tofler and associates[1] suggest that one of the driving forces behind this phenomenon is pressure from parents and coaches motivated by their need for vicarious achievement. This could be considered a form of child abuse.[1] Allowing Kerri Strug to perform a second vault during the 1996 Olympics after she had sustained a major injury to her ankle is an example of this phenomenon.[2]

--- ⚐ **REFERENCES** ⚐ ---

1. Tofler IR, Stryer BK, Micheli LJ, et al: Physical and emotional problems of elite female gymnasts, *N Engl J Med* 335:281-283, 1996.
2. O'Connor PJ, Lewis RD: Physical and emotional problems of elite female gymnasts (letter), *N Engl J Med* 336:140-141, 1997.

SURGERY

Many references to surgery are made throughout the text and may be found by searching the index for specific topics such as coronary artery bypass grafting, prostate cancer, lung cancer, breast cancer, and bites. This section deals with only a few selected areas.

Anesthesia

(See also coronary artery bypass grafting and angioplasty; pharmacological treatment of type 2 diabetes)

Routine preoperative laboratory tests and chest x-ray examination are not required for most asymptomatic low-risk surgical patients.[1] Although the guidelines of the American College of Cardiology and the American Heart Association recommend preoperative electrocardiograms (ECGs) for all patients undergoing noncardiac surgery,[2] the utility of providing this in patients under age 60 without evidence of cardiac disease is questionable.[3] Noninvasive cardiac testing is recommend only for selected patients, as determined by rather complex algorithms—in general it is reserved for patients who will be having surgery known to be associated with a significant risk of cardiac events and who have low exercise capacity or other predictors of risk such as cardiovascular disease or diabetes.[1]

It used to be taught that elective surgery should be delayed until 6 months after a myocardial infarction. Current evidence suggests that patients who have no significant abnormalities on an exercise stress test 4 to 6 weeks after infarction may be able to undergo elective surgery without undue risk.[1]

Beta-blockers prevent myocardial infarction and cardiac deaths in high-risk cardiac patients undergoing surgery. Poldermans and associates[4] suggest starting beta-blockers 1 to 2 weeks before surgery and continuing them for 2 weeks afterward. The heart rate should be reduced to 70 beats per minute preoperatively.

Diminished cognitive functioning is reported to occur in about 3% of patients subjected to coronary artery bypass grafting. Whether this is related to anesthesia or other aspects of the surgery is uncertain.[5] The results of a 1998 multicenter prospective trial indicate that anesthesia or major orthopedic, abdominal, or thoracic surgery (excluding cardiac surgery) leads to both short- and long-term cognitive deficits in elderly patients and that this phenomenon is unrelated to hypoxemia or hypotensive episodes. In this study, which compared preoperative neuropsychological tests with those taken after surgery, cognitive defects were present in 25% of patients after 1 week and 10% after 3 months.[6]

Children exposed to environmental tobacco smoke in the home have a much higher rate of respiratory complications after anesthesia than children not so exposed.[7]

Self-reported exercise tolerance is one way of assessing the risk of serious postoperative complications in adults. Patients unable to walk more than four blocks or climb two flights of stairs are at significantly increased risk.[8]

❧ REFERENCES ❧

1. Wiklund RA: Anesthesiology (first of two parts), *N Engl J Med* 337:1132-1141, 1997.
2. ACC/AHA guidelines for perioperative cardiovascular evaluation for noncardiac surgery, *Circulation* 93:1280-1317, 1996.
3. Gold BS, Young ML, Kinman JL, et al: The utility of preoperative electrocardiograms in the ambulatory surgical patient, *Arch Intern Med* 152:301-305, 1992.
4. Poldermans D, Boersma E, Bax JJ, et al: The effect of bisoprolol on perioperative mortality and myocardial infarction in high-risk patients undergoing vascular surgery, *N Engl J Med* 341:1789-1794, 1999.
5. Roach GW, Kanchuger M, Mangano M, et al: Adverse cerebral outcomes after coronary bypass surgery, *N Engl J Med* 335:1857-1863, 1996.
6. Moller JT, Cluitmans P, Rasmussen LS, et al: Long-term postoperative cognitive dysfunction in the elderly: ISPOCD1 study, *Lancet* 351:851-861, 1998.
7. Skolnick ET, Vomvolakis MA, Buck KA, et al: Exposure to environmental tobacco smoke and the risk of adverse respiratory events in children receiving general anesthesia, *Anesthesiology* 88:1144-1153, 1998.
8. Reilly DF, McNeely MJ, Doerner D, et al: Self-reported exercise tolerance and the risk of serious perioperative complications, *Arch Intern Med* 159:2185-2192, 1999.

Appendicitis

The clinical diagnosis of appendicitis may be difficult. In about 20% of cases the diagnosis is missed, and 15% to 40% of patients who have a laparotomy for appendicitis do not have the disease.[1] In most situations the most effective way of diagnosing appendicitis remains the history and physical examination. Important points in the history favoring the diagnosis are migration of the pain from the periumbilical region to the right lower quadrant and presence of pain before vomiting. Previous episodes of similar pain argue against the diagnosis. Most patients with appendicitis have right lower quadrant tenderness, guarding, or rigidity.[2]

Although ultrasound is reasonably effective in detecting a distended appendix, no studies have shown it to be superior to clinical examination in making the diagnosis of appendicitis. Plain x-ray views of the abdomen are neither sensitive nor specific.[2] Diagnostic laparoscopy has been shown to decrease the number of unnecessary appendectomies,[3] and computed tomographic (CT) scanning is an accurate diagnostic tool.[1,4] Focused helical computed tomography (helical CT) of the appendix is reported to have a sensitivity of close to 100% and a specificity of 95%. It can also establish other diagnoses when the appendix is normal.[4] A study of children with symptoms suggestive of appendicitis found that limited CT scanning with rectal contrast performed only on those who had both equivocal clinical findings and equivocal or negative ultrasound results led to the correct diagnosis in the vast majority of cases.[5]

An historical cohort study from Sweden found no evidence that infertility resulted from perforated appendices in female children or young adults.[6]

◥ REFERENCES ◤

1. Rao PM, Rhea JT, Novelline RA, et al: Effect of computed tomography of the appendix on treatment of patients and use of hospital resources, *N Engl J Med* 338:141-146, 1998.
2. Wagner JM, McKinney WP, Carpenter JL: Does this patient have appendicitis? *JAMA* 276:1589-1594, 1996.
3. Olsen JB, Myren CJ, Haahr PE: Randomized study of the value of laparoscopy before appendicectomy, *Br J Surg* 80:922-923, 1993.
4. Siegel MJ, Evens RG: Advances in the use of computed tomography, *JAMA* 281:1252-1254, 1999.
5. Garcia Pena BM, Mandl KD, Kraus SJ, et al: Ultrasonography and limited computed tomography in the diagnosis and management of appendicitis in children, *JAMA* 282:1041-1046, 1999.
6. Andersson R, Lambe M, Bergström R: Fertility patterns after appendicectomy: historical cohort study, *BMJ* 318:963-967, 1999.

Burns

Burns are classified according to the depth of the burn and the percentage of body surface covered (rule of nines).

Depth of burn

Depth of burns is determined clinically according to the following criteria.[1]

First-degree burns. First-degree burns involve only the epidermis. They are erythematous and blanch with pressure. Sensation is intact, and they are mildly painful.

Second-degree burns. Superficial second-degree burns involve the epidermis and superficial dermis, but the epithelial appendages are intact. These occur as blanching erythema with superficial blisters. Sensation is intact, and they are mildly painful. Deep second-degree burns involve the epidermis, most of the dermis, and most of the skin appendages. They appear dry, waxy, and whitish with red elements. The skin does not blanch with pressure. Sensation is present but diminished, and the burn is only slightly painful. Scarring usually occurs.

Third-degree burns. Third-degree burns involve the epidermis, all of the dermis, and all of the skin appendages. They appear white, red, tan, or charred. The skin is dry and leathery and does not blanch with pressure. It is anesthetic, and the burn is not painful. Scarring occurs.

Fourth-degree burns. Fourth-degree burns involve the same structures as third-degree burns but also underlying structures such as tendons, muscle, or bone. Their appearance is the same as that of third-degree burns. They are anesthetic.

Rule of nines

The extent of burns according to the rule of nines is as follows[1]:

Head and neck	9%
Each upper limb	9%
Each lower limb	18%
Back and buttocks	18%
Chest and abdomen	18%

Major risk factors for mortality from burns are age over 60, burn size more than 40% of body surface area, and concomitant inhalation injury.[2]

◥ REFERENCES ◤

1. Waitzman AA, Neligan PC: How to manage burns in primary care, *Can Fam Physician* 39:2394-2400, 1993.
2. Ryan CM, Schoenfeld DA, Thorpe WP, et al: Objective estimates of the probability of death from burn injuries, *N Engl J Med* 338:362-366, 1998.

Cosmetic Surgery

In many instances, liposuction can be performed under local anesthesia. By use of endoscopic techniques, procedures such as plication of the abdominal recti, lifting of sagging eyebrows, and elimination of forehead creases can be performed through minimal incisions.

◥ REFERENCES ◤

1. Heoyberghs JL: Cosmetic surgery, *BMJ* 318:512-516, 1999.

Hernias

The prevalence of groin hernias is 3% to 4%. The incidence and the risk of strangulation increase with age. Once a groin hernia develops, it never spontaneously resolves and over the years it gradually enlarges. The risk of strangulation is highest for femoral hernias but still significant for inguinal hernias with rates of 2.8% within 3 months of discovery and 4.5% within 2 years. The risk of strangulation is greatest in the 3 months after onset.[1]

There is a strong familial predisposition for groin hernias. Physical activities such as weight lifting do not cause hernias but may aggravate a hernia that has already developed.[1]

If not strangulated, most groin hernias can be repaired in outpatient (day) surgery using a local anesthetic; if a laparoscopic technique is used, regional or general anesthesia is required.[1,2] The classic way of repairing hernias is to close the defect with sutures (Shouldice hernioplasty). Tension-free hernioplasties are now generally preferred, and these require the placement of a prosthesis over the defect. Adverse effects, including postoperative pain, are minimal. Normal activities of daily living may commence immediately; jogging, golf, and similar activities within 10 to 14 days; and heavy lifting as soon as it can be done without pain. Recurrence rates are usually less than 1%.[1]

Tension-free hernioplasties can also be performed with the laparoscope with excellent results,[2,3] and in general patients have less pain and return to normal activities sooner than with open repair.[3] However, the learning curve for performing laparoscopic herniorrhaphies is long, and in some series recurrence of hernias and serious complications such as bowel perforation or vascular injury (although rare) are more common with the laparoscopic than with the open procedure.[3] If undergoing a laparoscopic repair, pick an experienced surgeon.

REFERENCES

1. Wantz GE: A 65-year-old man with an inguinal hernia, *JAMA* 277:663-669, 1997.
2. Bax T, Sheppard BC, Crass R: Surgical options in the management of groin hernias, *Am Fam Physician* 59:893-906, 1999.
3. O'Dwyer PJ, Macintyre I, Grant A, et al (MRC Laparoscopic Groin Hernia Trial Group): Laparoscopic versus open repair of groin hernia: a randomised comparison, *Lancet* 354:1185-1190, 1999.

Ingrown Toenails

A conservative way of managing ingrown toenails is to have the patient soak the affected foot for 20 to 30 minutes daily and then clean the "gutter" between the nail and the skin with a swab or a blunt object such as a butter knife.[1]

REFERENCES

1. Scherger JE: Successful technique for treating ingrown toenails (letter), *Am Fam Physician* 53:499, 1996.

Skin Excisions

One of the goals of skin excision is to avoid unsightly scars. Among the ways of achieving this are avoidance of elective excisions during the prepubertal growth spurt and early teens, since at this time the chance of hypertrophic scar formation is greater, and avoidance of incisions in the presternal area, deltoid region, or back, since poor scar formation is common in these regions. The patient should be told that complete healing takes about 1 year and that scars are often most noticeable 2 to 3 months after the initial wound.[1]

REFERENCES

1. Wilkes GH: Office excision and suture techniques for the family physician, *Can J CME* 6:49-53, 1994.

Lacerations
(See also bites)

Lacerations of the face may be sutured up to 24 hours after injury provided aggressive irrigation and debridement are used. In most cases the patient can remove the outer dressing of the wound and take a shower after a day or so. Swimming and tub baths should be avoided until healing is complete. Nonabsorbable sutures should be removed from the face in 4 to 5 days, the trunk and extremities in 7 to 10 days, and the palms and soles in 12 to 15 days. If traumatic tattooing is found, the area should be scrubbed with a brush before closure. The flap of flap-type lacerations of the anterior tibia in the elderly should be debrided of subcutaneous tissues with sharp curved scissors before being sutured. A pressure dressing should be applied.[1]

Tissue adhesives

A new cyanoacrylate tissue adhesive, octylcyanoacrylate (Dermabond), has been developed that is stronger and less brittle than previous products. It can be used on long or short facial lacerations and selected lacerations elsewhere. It should not be used on the hands or feet, over joints, in wounds crossing mucocutaneous junctions, in bite wounds, or in heavily soiled or crushed wounds. In one randomized trial the cosmetic results equaled those of sutures.[2]

Octylcyanoacrylate is used as a topical closure. The skin edges are carefully juxtaposed, and the agent is painted over the apposed edges, which are held together for another 30 seconds to allow complete polymerization to take place. The adhesive should not be permitted to seep into the wound edges because this would inhibit healing. Patients may take showers but should not soak or scrub the area. The adhesive sloughs off in 1 to 2 weeks.[2]

Infected wounds

Mupirocin (Bactroban) cream (in contrast to mupirocin ointment) became available in the United States and Canada in 1999. A comparative study of infected lacerations or abrasions found that the application of mupirocin cream three times a day was as effective as oral cephalexin (Keflex) in controlling the infections.[3]

REFERENCES

1. Martin S: Triage and care of wounds, *Can J CME* 7:29-47, 1995.
2. Quinn J, Wells G, Sutcliffe T, et al: A randomized trial comparing octylcyanoacrylate tissue adhesive and sutures in the management of lacerations, *JAMA* 277:1527-1530, 1997.
3. Kraus SJ, Eron LJ, Bottenfield GW, et al: Mupirocin cream is as effective as oral cephalexin in the treatment of secondarily infected wounds, *J Fam Pract* 47:429-433, 1998.

Puncture Wounds

Puncture wounds of the foot are usually caused by nails, and the most common serious complications are deep tissue infections. These are especially likely to occur if a foreign body is retained, a common situation when a penetrating nail has passed through sneakers and socks. Deep penetrating wounds of the feet usually have to be enlarged to allow the search for and removal of foreign bodies, as well as copious irrigation. Anesthesia may be obtained with local infiltration or a posterior tibial nerve block (posterior to the medial malleolus). A circular core of tissue 4 mm in diameter around the puncture site should be excised with a scalpel or a 4-mm punch biopsy.[1]

_____ **✏ REFERENCES ✏** _____

1. Warren D: Be prepared for summertime foot punctures, *Patient Care Can* 6:22-38, 1995.

TOXICOLOGY

(See also lead poisoning; screening)

Pharmacological agents that are particularly dangerous for children are iron supplements, tricyclic antidepressants, calcium channel blockers, beta-blockers, hypoglycemic agents, and chloroquine.[1]

The usefulness of home administration of ipecac is being questioned. Although ipecac decreases the absorption of some drugs, its use has not been proved to decrease morbidity or mortality.[1,2] A disadvantage of ipecac is that the induced nausea and vomiting may prevent the subsequent administration of activated charcoal.[2]

A single dose of activated charcoal (50 g for adults and 1 g/kg for children up to 12 years of age) is the treatment of choice for most poisonings that are likely to cause moderate or severe toxicity. Ideally, activated charcoal should be administered within 1 hour of toxin ingestion.[2] Growing evidence supports the administration of activated charcoal at home; formulations of superactivated charcoal are being developed that would facilitate administration because smaller volumes of fluid would be required. Substances not readily absorbed by activated charcoal include ferrous salts, lithium, potassium salts, ethanol, methanol, and ethylene glycol.[1]

If ipecac is to be administered, the following guidelines should be used. Ipecac is contraindicated in patients who are less than 6 months of age, who are already vomiting, who have altered mental status, or who have ingested hydrocarbons, corrosives, or sharp objects. The usual dose is 10 ml for children aged 6 to 12 months, 15 ml for children aged 1 to 12 years, and 30 ml for older adolescents. The dose of ipecac should be immediately followed with water: 5 to 15 ml/kg for infants under 1 year, a half to 1 glass for children ages 1 to 12, and 1 to 2 glasses for those over 12.[3]

For children with serious poisoning, sophisticated support systems are the cornerstone of therapy. Whole-bowel irrigation with polyethylene glycol solutions (GoLYTELY, Colyte) is frequently used.[1,2] Specific antidotes are available for digoxin, colchicine, tricyclic antidepressants, acetaminophen, beta-blockers, calcium channel blockers, benzodiazepines, and ethylene glycol. Octreotide has been shown to prevent hypoglycemia produced by sulfonylurea ingestion.[1]

Acetaminophen is probably the single most frequent cause of poisoning. The specific antidote is *N*-acetylcysteine, which is usually administered on the basis of levels of plasma acetaminophen. Patients who are taking anticonvulsants or are anorectic are at increased risk of toxicity and should be given *N*-acetylcysteine at lower plasma acetaminophen levels.[2]

Patients found to have swallowed packets of illicit drugs may be treated by watchful waiting, but if the drugs are potentially lethal, they should be removed by endoscopy from the stomach and by surgery from the small bowel.[2]

_____ **✏ REFERENCES ✏** _____

1. Liebelt EL, DeAngelis CD: Evolving trends and treatment advances in pediatric poisoning, *JAMA* 282:1113-1115, 1999.
2. Jones AL, Volans G: Management of self poisoning, *BMJ* 319:1414-1417, 1999.
3. Larsen LC, Cummings DM: Oral poisonings: guidelines for initial evaluation and treatment, *Am Fam Physician* 57:85-92, 1998.

TROPICAL MEDICINE

(See also adoption; aviation medicine; cyclosporiasis; diarrhea; diarrhea and dehydration in infants; hepatitis A; hepatitis B; immunizations; refractive errors)

Information for Travelers

General information about traveling in tropical regions, including a directory of physicians who speak English, immunization requirements, and maps showing areas of risk for malaria and yellow fever, is available from the International Association for Medical Assistance to Travelers (IAMAT), 40 Regal Road, Guelph, Ontario, Canada N1K 1B5; 417 Center Street, Lewiston, NY 14092, USA; or 57 Voirets, 2112 Grand-Lancy-Geneva, Switzerland. Updated information from the Centers for Disease Control and Prevention (CDC) is available on the Internet at http://www.cdc.gov. or by phone at (888) 232-3228. The CDC malaria hot line for physicians is (770) 488-7788.

Immunizations for Travelers

Pregnant women and immunocompromised individuals should generally not receive live virus vaccines such as oral polio, yellow fever, and measles vaccines.[1]

All travelers to tropical or developing countries should have up-to-date vaccinations against tetanus and diphtheria, and those born after 1956 need up-to-date measles vaccinations. Travelers to developing or tropical countries outside the Western Hemisphere also need to be protected against polio. Those who have never had a primary vaccination series should receive it, and those who have had such a series but never had a booster should receive a booster. Typhoid vaccination is advised for anyone going beyond the usual tourist routes in countries where typhoid is endemic. Hepatitis A vaccination should be given to those going anywhere other than Canada, the United States, Western Europe, Japan, Australia, or New Zealand. Hepatitis B vaccine should be given to individuals planning to spend long periods in endemic areas such as Africa, China, Korea, Southeast Asia, the Amazon region, Haiti, or the Dominican Republic, as well as to persons traveling to these areas for shorter periods who will possibly need dental or medical care, may have sexual contact with local inhabitants, or are going to work in a medical facility. Japanese encephalitis vaccine is advised for those visiting rice-growing rural areas in Southeast Asia; the attack rate in short-term travelers to urban areas is extremely low. Meningococcal vaccination is recommended only for those visiting areas where epidemics are in progress (often sub-Saharan Africa). Yellow fever vaccine is indicated for persons traveling to tropical areas of South America and Africa. Rabies vaccine is advised for those with occupational risk, those who will be hiking in rural areas, or those staying in endemic areas for prolonged periods. Tourists are at low risk of acquiring cholera; the parenteral cholera vaccines are not very effective, and immunization is not recommended.[1]

Dengue

Dengue is a mosquito-borne virus infection that is prevalent in Asia, Africa, the Pacific islands, and tropical and subtropical regions of the Americas. The incubation period is 5 to 8 days, and in most cases the disease is self-limited. Dengue is characterized by the sudden onset of fever and headache, often accompanied by retroorbital pain, photophobia, severe backache, muscle aches, joint pains ("break bone fever"), and sometimes lymphadenopathy and a rash that may be petechial. The fever commonly lasts 5 to 6 days. Recovery is usually rapid, but in some cases it may be prolonged.[2]

Malaria

The four species of *Plasmodium* that infect humans are *vivax, ovale, malariae,* and *falciparum. P. falciparum* is the most lethal species. All the types are spread by bite of the female *Anopheles* mosquito. Although the disease is found worldwide, the risk for travelers is greatest in sub-Saharan Africa, the Solomon islands, Papua New Guinea, and Vanuatu. The risk is low in most of Latin America and Southeast Asia and is intermediate in the Indian subcontinent and Haiti.[3]

Protection against mosquito bites is a key element in malaria prophylaxis. This involves avoiding evening or nighttime strolls because the *Anopheles* mosquito is a nocturnal feeder, wearing clothing that covers most of the body, using screens, and applying insect repellents containing up to 35% diethyltoluamide (DEET).[4] DEET (HourGuard, Skedaddle, Repel, Cutter, OFF) is currently the most effective insecticide available. Extended release products include Hour-Guard and Skedaddle. Concentrations of over 30% should not be used because they offer little additional protection but have a higher risk of neurotoxicity; 10% is the maximum concentration that should be used for children. If DEET and a sunscreen are both applied, the sun protection factor of the sunscreen is decreased by about one third. In addition to coverage of exposed skin with DEET, clothes

should be impregnated with permethrin, which is an insecticide, not a repellent.[5] A mosquito-proof netting, preferably impregnated with permethrin, that covers the bed at night is also advisable[3]; portable types with frames are available through IAMAT (see above).

Chloroquine (Aralen) is the drug of choice for the few areas of the world where non-chloroquine-resistant malaria is still extant: Central America west of the Panama Canal Zone, Mexico, Haiti, the Dominican Republic, and most of the Middle East. Cases of chloroquine-resistant malaria have been reported in Iran, Oman, Yemen, and Saudi Arabia.[1] The map of chloroquine-resistant malaria is ever changing, and travelers must consult up-to-date sources of information.[1,3]

The usual dose of chloroquine for malaria prophylaxis is 2 tablets or 500 mg (300 mg of base) weekly starting 2 weeks before departure and continuing until 8 weeks after return. For infants and children the prophylactic dose is 5 mg/kg of the base. Chloroquine may be taken during pregnancy.[3] If there is insufficient time to start prophylaxis 2 weeks before departure, a loading dose may be given. Adults should take 500 mg (300 mg base) as soon as possible and a second dose of 500 mg in 6 hours; for children the loading dose is chloroquine base 5 mg/kg as soon as possible with a second dose of 5 mg/kg in 6 hours.

When chloroquine is used to treat malaria in adults, 4 tablets (1 g) are given as a loading dose followed in 6 to 8 hours by 2 tablets (500 mg), followed by a single dose of 2 tablets (500 mg) on each of the next 2 consecutive days. The dose intervals for children with malaria are the same, but the first dose is calculated on the basis of 10 mg/kg of base (maximum 600 mg of base) and the subsequent three doses on the basis of 5 mg/kg of base.

The drug of choice for malaria prophylaxis in areas with chloroquine-resistant malaria is mefloquine (Lariam) except in regions where mefloquine-resistant malaria is present, such as the Thai-Cambodian and Thai-Burmese borders. In these places doxycycline 100 mg/day is recommended.[1,3] The usual dose of mefloquine for malaria prophylaxis is 250 mg weekly starting 1 week before departure and continuing for 4 weeks after return. The prophylactic dose for children weighing 15 to 19 kg is ¼ tablet (62.5 mg) weekly, for those weighing 20 to 30 kg is ½ tablet (125 mg) weekly, and for those weighing 31 to 45 kg is ¾ tablet (187.5 mg) weekly. Mefloquine should be taken with food, and adults should drink at least 240 ml (1 glass) of water with it. Although caution has been recommended in prescribing mefloquine to patients with cardiac conduction defects or taking medications such as quinine, chloroquine, beta-blockers, or calcium channel blockers, there is no good evidence supporting these concerns. Mefloquine appears to be safe in pregnancy.[3] A number of observational studies have suggested that mefloquine is associated with a relatively high incidence of neuropsychiatric side effects, including sleep disturbances, which may lead to noncompliance.[6] However, the data are inconclusive and the significance of these reports is uncertain.

Patients taking mefloquine prophylactically are often advised to carry a therapeutic dose of sulfadoxine-pyrimethamine (Fansidar) so they can treat themselves if high fever develops and they cannot obtain medical care.[4] The usual adult dosage of Fansidar for treatment of malaria is 3 tablets as a single dose. For children over 2 months of age the dosage is 1 tablet as a single dose for those weighing 11 to 29 kg and 2 tablets as a single dose for those weighing 30 to 45 kg. Fansidar is contraindicated in patients allergic to sulfonamides.

Although the the CDC recommends mefloquine for travelers going to the Indian subcontinent, the Philippines, and part of Indonesia, the World Health Organization advises the use of a combination of chloroquine base 300 mg weekly plus proguanil (Paludrine) 200 mg/day for travelers to these areas.[3] There is concern that the efficacy of the chloroquine-proguanil regimen is suboptimal. An alternative prophylaxis for falciparum malaria is a combination of atovaquone (Mepron) 250 mg plus proguanil 100 mg (combined by Glaxo Wellcome into one tablet called Malarone) taken once daily, which has been reported to be effective over a 10-week trial period in adults.[7]

In about 90% of travelers who acquire malaria the disease develops after they return home. The standard treatment of severe falciparum malaria, including cerebral malaria, is IV quinidine or, if that is not available, intramuscular quinine. Unfortunately, many hospital pharmacies in North America do not stock either of these drugs, and this has resulted in some deaths.[8] A new treatment that is as effective as quinine is intramuscular artemether, a drug derived from the Chinese quinghao plant.[9]

Travelers' Diarrhea

A Jamaican study found that during a 1-week stay about one fourth of tourists had diarrhea. The mean time of onset was day 4 , and adolescents and young adults were at higher risk than older adults staying at the same hotels. Tourists from Britain and other northern countries were at greater risk than those from Latin America, Southern Europe, and Japan; individuals who had traveled to subtropical countries in the recent past were at decreased risk. Almost none of the tourists surveyed followed standard dietary precautions such as avoiding salads, cold buffets, and local tap water.[10] Whether these precautions would actually have made a difference is uncertain,[10] since only one prospective study (published in 1985) has documented any benefit from such a regimen.[11] The overall incidence of diarrhea was greater in the summer than the winter. Most tourists took all their meals at the hotel where they stayed. The rate of diarrhea varied from one hotel to another, with a high of 30% and a low of 14%. Pathogens were isolated from stool cultures in only 32% of cases. The most frequently detected organisms were entero-

toxigenic *Escherichia coli,* rotaviruses, *Salmonella* species, and *Campylobacter jejuni.* Relatively rare isolates were enteric adenoviruses, *Shigella* species, *Entamoeba histolytica, Giardia lamblia,* and *Cryptosporidium.*[10]

Travelers' diarrhea lasts longer than 1 week in 10% of cases and longer than 1 month in 2% of cases.[4]

Prophylaxis of travelers' diarrhea is generally not recommended.[1,12] There are several reasons for this. From the public health perspective, widespread use of antibiotics is likely to foster antibiotic resistance. Complications of antibiotic prophylaxis include allergic reactions, photosensitivity reactions, and antibiotic-associated vaginal candidiasis and diarrhea. Since only a small percentage of people acquire travelers' diarrhea, a large number of individuals would be treated unnecessarily. Finally, the treatment of the disorder is simple and efficacious, so prophylaxis is rarely needed. However, even though antibiotic prophylaxis for travelers' diarrhea has not been proved necessary for medical conditions such as achlorhydria or AIDS, it may be recommended in the following circumstances[12]:

1. A necessary brief trip during which illness is not acceptable
2. AIDS or other immunodeficiency states
3. Active inflammatory bowel disease
4. Insulin-dependent diabetes
5. Heart disease in elderly patients
6. Chronic renal failure
7. Achlorhydria, gastrectomy, or omeprazole (Prilosec, Losec) use

If prophylaxis is to be given, the *Medical Letter* recommends one of the fluoroquinolones or, as a somewhat less effective second choice, bismuth subsalicylate (Table 49).[1]

The mainstay of treatment of travelers' diarrhea is adequate fluid replacement,[4,12] which can be supplied with commercial or homemade oral replacement solutions. Commercial oral replacement fluids are available in either a liquid form (Pedialyte, Lytren) or a powder form that has to be reconstituted with water (Gastrolyte and many other brands). For travelers the powder form is most convenient. One inexpensive alternative to commercial electrolyte solutions is the World Health Organization rehydration solution, in which 1 teaspoon (5 mg) of salt and 4 level tablespoons (40 ml) of sugar are added to 1 L of water.[13] Another, devel-

Table 49   Prophylaxis of Travelers' Diarrhea

Drugs	Usual doses
Ciprofloxacin (Cipro)	500 mg/day
Levofloxacin (Levaquin)	500 mg/day
Norfloxacin (Noroxin)	400 mg/day
Ofloxacin (Floxin)	300 mg/day
Bismuth subsalicylate (Pepto-Bismol)	2 262-mg tablets qid with meals and hs

oped at St. Justine's Children's Hospital in Montreal, is 360 ml (12 oz or 1½ cups) of orange juice without added sugar, 600 ml (20 oz or 2½ cups) of boiled water, and 2 ml (a little less than half a teaspoon) of salt.[14]

Pharmacotherapy for travelers' diarrhea may be symptomatic, antibacterial, or a combination of the two.[1] Loperamide (Imodium) or diphenoxylate-atropine (Lomotil) may be used for symptomatic treatment. However, only loperamide should be used if concomitant antibacterial treatment is to be given because the combination of antibacterials and diphenoxylate-atropine has been associated with the development of toxic megacolon.[13]

For most cases of travelers' diarrhea in adults the *Medical Letter* recommends loperamide plus a single dose of ciprofloxacin (750 mg), levofloxacin 500 mg, or ofloxacin 400 mg. With this protocol, resolution of symptoms usually occurs within 24 hours. For more severe diarrhea or diarrhea associated with fever or blood in the stools, a 3-day course of antibiotics is recommended (Table 50). The usual drug for young children is trimethoprim-sulfamethoxazole, even though many strains of *E. coli* are resistant to it.[1] Erythromycin or azithromycin (Zithromax) may be added to trimethoprim-sulfamethoxazole in areas such as Mexico where the incidence of *Campylobacter* is

Table 50   Pharmacological Management of Travelers' Diarrhea

Drugs	Usual doses
Symptomatic Control	
Loperamide (Imodium)	4 mg stat, then 2 mg after each loose stool; maximum 16 mg/day
Diphenoxylate 2.5 mg, atropine 0.025 mg (Lomotil)	2 tablets stat, then 1 tablet after each loose stool; maximum 8 tablets daily
Antibacterial	
Ciprofloxacin (Cipro)	750 mg once only or 500 bid for 3 days*
Levofloxacin (Levaquin)	500 mg once only or once daily for 3 days*
Norfloxacin (Noroxin)	400 bid for 3 days*
Ofloxacin (Floxin)	400 mg once only or 300 bid for 3 days*
Bismuth subsalicylate (Pepto-Bismol)	30 ml or 2 262-mg tablets q30min for 5 doses; regimen may be repeated on day 2
Trimethoprim-sulfamethoxazole (TMP-SMX) (Bactrim, Septra)	1 DS tablet as single dose or 1 DS tablet bid for 3 days. For children, 6 mg/kg/day of trimethoprim and 30 mg/kg/day of sulfamethoxazole in 2 divided doses

*For mild cases, a single dose of one of the quinolones may be effective. For severe cases treat for 3 days.

relatively high, and children aged 12 years or older may take fluoroquinolone if other medications are not available or effective.[15]

────────────── **❧ REFERENCES ❧** ──────────────

1. Advice for travelers, *Med Lett* 41:39-42, 1999.
2. Jelinek T, Dobler G, Hölscher M, et al: Relevance of infection with dengue virus among international travelers, *Arch Intern Med* 157:2367-2370, 1997.
3. Lobel HO, Kozarsky PE: Update on prevention of malaria for travelers, *JAMA* 278:1767-1771, 1997.
4. Advice for travelers, *Med Lett* 38:17-20, 1996.
5. Fradin MS: Mosquitoes and mosquito repellents: a clinician's guide, *Ann Intern Med* 128:931-940, 1998.
6. Croft A, Garner P: Mefloquine to prevent malaria: a systematic review of trials, *BMJ* 315:1412-1416, 1997.
7. Shanks GD, Gordon DM, Klotz FW, et al: Efficacy and safety of atovaquone/proguanil as suppressive prophylaxis for *Plasmodium falciparum* malaria, *Clin Infect Dis* 27:494-499, 1998.
8. Humar A, Sharma S, Zoutman D, et al: Fatal falciparum malaria in Canadian travellers, *Can Med Assoc J* 156:1165-1167, 1997.
9. Pittler MH, Ernst E: Artemether for severe malaria: a meta-analysis of randomized clinical trials, *Clin Infect Dis* 28:597-601, 1999.
10. Steffen R, Collard F, Tornieporth N, et al: Epidemiology, etiology, and impact of traveler's diarrhea in Jamaica, *JAMA* 281:811-817, 1999.
11. Kozicki M, Steffen R, Schär M: Boil it, cook it, peel it, or forget it, *Int J Epidemiol* 14:169-172, 1985.
12. Canadian communicable disease report, statement on travellers' diarrhea, *Can Med Assoc J* 152:205-208, 1995.
13. Hoge CW, Shlim DR, Echeverria P, et al: Epidemiology of diarrhea among expatriate residents living in a highly endemic environment, *JAMA* 275:533-538, 1996.
14. Deschênes M, Nazair P: La gastro-entérite: déshydratation, réhydratation, *Med Quebec,* March, 27-101, 1994.
15. Fischer PR: Travel with infants and children, *Infect Dis Clin North Am* 12:355-368, 1998.

UNCERTAINTY

(See also attitudes, physician; informed consent; investigations; positive predictive value; risk analysis; risk assessment in pregnancy; screening)

Some of the causes of uncertainty in physicians are their lack of knowledge of the scientific literature, limitations of scientific knowledge itself, and their unsureness as to which of these two situations applies in any particular case. If physicians are unaware of or unwilling to acknowledge their limitations, patient care will suffer because they will fail to get help when it is needed.[1] On the other hand, physicians must not become paralyzed by uncertainty. In many cases treatment should be based on probability rather than certainty. Only harm can come from a never-ending series of additional consultations and investigations (see discussion of investigations).[1,2] According to Gianakos,[1] the best physicians accept their limitations and openly acknowledge these to their peers, students, and patients.

A detrimental way for health professionals to deal with uncertainty is to deny it. For example, breast surgeons may be quite certain that the treatment they recommend is correct even though no consensus exists in the literature. Baumann and associates[3] label this the "micro-certainty, macro-uncertainty" phenomenon.

Over a decade ago Biehn[4] from the University of Western Ontario wrote about some of the methods of dealing with uncertainty in family medicine. He pointed out that family physicians probably see more patients with undifferentiated diseases than do any other groups of physicians and that this necessarily leads to uncertainty (see discussion of physician attitudes). He suggested that one of the first ways of dealing with this issue is to ensure that the presenting complaint is the patient's real reason for coming to the office and not just a ticket of admission for a hidden agenda. If the patient has a hidden agenda and the physician brings it out and deals with it, the anxiety of both the patient and the physician will drop dramatically and the vague presenting complaint is likely to resolve spontaneously.

Patients probably have even more difficulty living with uncertainty than physicians.[5,6] As Wardle and Pope[5] point out, shades of gray and risk spectrum are not part of most people's conception of illness. Angell[6] makes the same point and adds that many people believe it is possible to avoid all health risks.

⚐ REFERENCES ⚐

1. Gianakos D: Accepting limits (editorial), *Arch Intern Med* 158:1059-1061, 1998.
2. Kassirer JP: Our stubborn quest for diagnostic certainty: a cause of excessive testing, *N Engl J Med* 320:1489-1491, 1989.
3. Baumann AO, Deber RB, Thompson GG: Overconfidence among physicians and nurses: the "micro-certainty, macro-uncertainty" phenomenon, *Soc Sci Med* 32:167-174, 1991.
4. Biehn J: Managing uncertainty in family practice, *Can Med Assoc J* 126:915-917, 1982.
5. Wardle J, Pope R: The psychological costs of screening for cancer, *J Psychosom Res* 36:609-624, 1992.
6. Angell M: Shattuck Lecture—evaluating the health risks of breast implants: the interplay of medical science, the law, and public opinion, *N Engl J Med* 334:1513-1518, 1996.

NEPHROLOGY

Topics covered in this section

Chronic Renal Failure
Glomerulonephritis
Microalbuminuria
Postural Proteinuria
Urinalysis

CHRONIC RENAL FAILURE

(See also diabetic microalbuminuria; diabetic nephropathy; hypertension; microalbuminuria; nonsteroidal antiinflammatory drugs; restless legs syndrome)

Chronic renal insufficiency is caused by diabetes in 37% of cases, by hypertension in 30%, and by chronic glomerulonephritis in 12%. Other important causes include cystic kidney disease, obstructive nephropathy, drug-induced nephropathy, and ischemic renal disease.[1] End-stage renal failure is more common in black than in white men, and this correlates with an increased incidence of hypertension and lower socioeconomic status.[2]

When presented with an elevated creatinine level, physicians must try to determine the etiology of the renal disease and in particular rule out reversible conditions such as urinary obstruction. In addition to creatinine measurements, the basic workup of renal failure includes ultrasonography of the urinary tract; urinalysis; 24-hour urine collection for protein and creatinine clearance; a complete blood count; measurement of electrolytes, urea, calcium, phosphorus, glucose, total protein, and albumin; and serum protein electrophoresis. Rapidly progressive renal failure (a condition that requires emergency consultation) should be ruled out by measurement of creatinine levels at reasonably short intervals.[3]

Elective nephrology consultation is probably indicated for any patient with creatinine levels of 120 to 150 μmol/L (1.4 to 1.7 mg/dl) or higher, levels that represent a more than 50% loss of glomerular filtration function. Studies have shown that patient outcomes are better with early than with late nephrology consultations, not only because they may lead to better management of underlying diseases, but because more time is made available for the lengthy period of preparation that usually must precede long-term dialysis or renal transplantation.[3]

One of the most important therapeutic interventions for decreasing the progression of chronic renal insufficiency is adequate blood pressure control. Target levels should be 130/80 to 130/85 mm Hg or, for those with proteinuria of greater than 1 g/day, 125/75 mm Hg.[1] Angiotensin-converting enzyme (ACE) inhibitors are the agents of first choice because they clearly decrease the rate of progression to chronic renal failure in both hypertensive and normotensive patients with nondiabetic nephropathies.[4] If renal function is compromised, ACE inhibitors must be administered carefully with monitoring of renal function and serum potassium levels,[1] but some nephrologists categorically reject the notion that severe renal failure is an absolute contraindication to these agents.[4] Tight diabetic control is important for patients with diabetic nephropathy,[1] and a metaanalysis of low-protein diets in both diabetic and nondiabetic renal disease found that such diets slowed the progression of the disease.[5]

Phenacetin has long been known to cause chronic tubulointerstitial nephritis (analgesic nephropathy) and ultimately chronic renal failure. Strong circumstantial evidence has shown that other analgesics, particularly those containing acetaminophen, can also cause this disorder. Whether acetaminophen or nonsteroidal antiinflammatory drugs (NSAIDs) alone can induce this condition is uncertain. The major adverse effect of NSAIDs on the kidneys is an acute reversible renal insufficiency.[6]

Aside from dialysis or transplantation, therapeutic interventions commonly necessary for end-stage renal disease are erythropoietin to combat anemia and oral calcium carbonate or calcium acetate to bind with intestinal phosphate and thus help control elevated serum phosphate levels. The most common cause of death in patients with end-stage renal disease, regardless of whether they have had kidney transplants, is cardiac disease.[7]

Renal Transplantation

The 3-year survival rate for transplanted cadaveric kidneys in the United States is 70%. The survival rate is higher among living unrelated donors: for wife-to-husband grafts it is 87%, and for husband-to-wife grafts it is the same provided the wife has never been pregnant. If she has been pregnant, the survival rate is 76%. Good survival in spite of relatively poor histocompatibility is attributed to healthier kidneys.[8] In the United States 27% of transplanted kidneys come from living related donors, whereas in France the figure is only 4%.[9]

The long-term survival rate of recipients of renal transplants is greater than that of patients on long-term dialysis who are suitable candidates for transplants but have not received them.[10]

──────────── ⚞ **REFERENCES** ⚟ ────────────

1. Rahman M, Smith MC: Chronic renal insufficiency: a diagnostic and therapeutic approach, *Arch Intern Med* 158:1743-1752, 1998.
2. Klag MJ, Whelton PK, Randall BL, et al: End-stage renal disease in African-American and white men, *JAMA* 277:1293-1298, 1997.
3. Meddlesome DC, Barrett JB, Brownscombe LM, et al: Elevated levels of serum creatinine: recommendations for management and referral, *Can Med Assoc J* 161:413-417, 1999.
4. Ruggenenti P, Perna A, Gherardi G, et al: Renoprotective properties of ACE-inhibition in non-diabetic nephropathies with non-nephrotic proteinuria, *Lancet* 354:359-364, 1999.
5. Pedrini MT, Levey AS, Lau J, et al: The effect of dietary protein restriction on the progression of diabetic and nondiabetic renal diseases—a meta-analysis, *Ann Intern Med* 124:627-632, 1996.
6. De Broe ME, Elseviers MM: Analgesic nephropathy, *N Engl J Med* 338:446-452, 1998.
7. Walker R: General management of end stage renal disease, *BMJ* 315:1429-1432, 1997.
8. Terasaki PI, Cecka JM, Gjertson DW, et al: High survival rates of kidney transplants from spousal and living unrelated donors, *N Engl J Med* 333:333-336, 1995.
9. Soulillou J-P: Kidney transplantation from spousal donors (editorial), *N Engl J Med* 333:379-380, 1995.
10. Wolfe RA, Ashby VB, Milford EL, et al: Comparison of mortality in all patients on dialysis, patients on dialysis awaiting transplantation, and recipients of a first cadaveric transplant, *N Engl J Med* 341:1725-1730, 1999.

GLOMERULONEPHRITIS

(See also hematuria; streptococcal infections; urinalysis)

IgA Nephropathy

Worldwide, IgA nephropathy is the most common form of glomerulonephritis. For many patients the disease is innocuous, but end-stage renal disease develops in 20% to 40% of patients within 5 to 25 years of the diagnosis.[1] Males are more often affected. In over half the cases gross hematuria is the presenting condition, often in association with concurrent respiratory or gastrointestinal infections, while a third are detected incidentally because of an investigation of microscopic hematuria.[1] An important clinical clue in the latter instance is the presence of red blood cell casts.[2]

Although no specific treatment for IgA nephropathy is known, an important therapeutic intervention is rigorous control of blood pressure, preferably by use of ACE inhibitors.[1] A Mayo Clinic study of patients with IgA nephropathy and marked proteinuria showed that daily administration over 2 years of 12 g of fish oil containing 1.9 g of eicosapentaenoic acid and 1.4 g of docosahexanoic acid retarded the rate of deterioration of renal function and reduced the number of cases of end-stage renal failure.[2] A subsequent analysis of the same group of patients after a mean follow-up of 6.4 years found persistent benefit from fish oil treatment.[3]

Poststreptococcal Glomerulonephritis

Acute glomerulonephritis may follow a number of viral, bacterial, or protozoal infectious diseases. The best known is poststreptococcal glomerulonephritis, which usually affects children between the ages of 2 and 10 years. The disorder is usually manifested as gross hematuria and edema 1 to 2 weeks after a streptococcal infection. Edema usually resolves spontaneously within 2 weeks, and serum creatinine concentrations return to normal within a month. Hematuria resolves within a month, but mild proteinuria may persist for several years. Complete recovery is the norm, but hypertension or renal failure may eventuate in a few patients.[1]

──────────── ⚞ **REFERENCES** ⚟ ────────────

1. Hricik DE, Chung-Park M, Sedor JR: Glomerulonephritis, *N Engl J Med* 339:888-899, 1998.
2. Donadio JV Jr, Bergstralh EJ, Offord KP, et al (Mayo Nephrology Collaborative Group): A controlled trial of fish oil in IgA nephropathy, *N Engl J Med* 331:1194-1199, 1994.
3. Donadio JV Jr, Grande JP, Bergstralh EJ, et al: The long-term outcome of patients with IgA nephropathy treated with fish oil in a controlled trial, *J Am Soc Nephrol* 10:1772-1777, 1999.

MICROALBUMINURIA

(See also diabetes mellitus and hypertension; diabetic nephropathy)

Microalbuminuria is a urinary albumin excretion of 30 to 300 mg/24 hr. The gold standard is a 24-hour urine measurement, but because this may be difficult to achieve, a dipstick specific for microalbuminuria may be used instead. If the dipstick is used on a first morning specimen and the patient does not have a febrile illness, it is reasonably accurate. A second dipstick reading should be performed within a few months to verify the results. Microalbuminuria is an important abnormality in a number of renal conditions, but particularly diabetic nephropathy. The detection of microalbuminuria and the subsequent treatment of the patient with ACE inhibitors slow the progression of diabetic nephropathy (see discussion of diabetic nephropathy).[1]

⚑ REFERENCES ⚑

1. Cattran DC: Microalbuminuria urine dip tests: recognize limits, *Patient Care Can* 7:8-9, 1996.

POSTURAL PROTEINURIA

Patients with postural proteinuria have proteinuria only in the erect position. The diagnosis can be easily made by collecting urine samples immediately on arising in the morning and after being erect for a few hours. In some patients with postural proteinuria, protein excretion is present whenever the patient is erect, and in others it is intermittent.[1,2]

⚑ REFERENCES ⚑

1. Trempe D: L'analyse d'urine: bandelettes réactives ou sédiment urinaire? *Med Quebec* 29:25-31, 1994.
2. Rapoport A, Richardson RMA: How to tell it's proteinuria, *Patient Care Can* 5:13-18, 1994.

URINALYSIS

(See also acute bacteriuria and pyuria in the elderly; bladder cancer; diabetic nephropathy; exercise-induced hematuria; exertional rhabdomyolysis; fever without source; hematuria; IgA nephropathy)

Little is gained by a microscopic examination of urine that is dipstick negative provided the dipstick is capable of detecting leukocytes.[1] Some important features of the urinalysis are described in the following paragraphs.

Specific Gravity

The usual specific gravity of an early morning urine sample is 1014 to 1028. Heavy proteinuria or glucosuria can elevate the specific gravity.

Glucose

False-negative glucose readings may occur if the patient has taken large quantities of aspirin or vitamin C.

Blood

Dipsticks can detect as few as 2 or 3 red blood cells (RBCs) per high-power field.[1] If the dipstick is positive for blood but RBCs are not seen on microscopic examination, the explanation might be myoglobinuria or hemolysis of RBCs. False-negative readings may result if the patient has ingested large quantities of vitamin C or sometimes as a result of captopril (Capoten) therapy. Healthy people have up to 3 RBCs per high-power field in a centrifuged specimen.[2]

If the dipstick reading is positive for blood, microscopy to look for RBC casts is important. If such casts are found, the origin of the hematuria is the kidney and in the majority of cases there is underlying glomerular disease. RBC casts lyse quickly, so the urine should be examined by an experienced observer within 2 hours. The casts are better preserved in acid urine.[2]

Intermittent microscopic or even gross hematuria may be a result of vigorous exercise. In asymptomatic persons under the age of 40 with microscopic hematuria, the diagnosis can be safely made if microscopy shows RBCs but no RBC casts and if the hematuria clears within 72 hours of the precipitating physical activity.[3] If after vigorous exercise the urine is positive for blood, no RBCs are found with microscopy, and the patient is complaining of muscle pain or swelling, acute exercise-induced rhabdomyolysis should be considered. If the patient has this condition, the creatine kinase level is very high.[4]

Whether the incidental finding of microscopic hematuria in asymptomatic individuals merits a complete urological and nephrological workup is controversial. A fairly high incidence of significant disease has been reported from referral clinics where most of the patients were over 40 years of age,[2] but in a population survey the incidence of serious disease was only 2.3%.[5]

Both the Canadian Task Force on Preventive Health Care[6] and the U.S. Preventive Services Task Force[7] give a "D" recommendation for dipstick assessment of urine as a screening tool for bladder cancer in the general population.

Leukocytes

The dipstick detects neutrophils by reacting to some of the esterases these cells possess. This reaction takes place even if the white cells have lysed and are therefore not visible on microscopy.[1,2] The test is sensitive and can detect as few as 3 to 5 white blood cells (WBCs) per high-power field.[1]

Pyuria is usually defined as 5 or more WBCs per high-power field in a centrifuged specimen.[2] The presence of WBC casts suggests pyelonephritis or an autoimmune disease such as lupus.[1]

Asymptomatic pyuria and asymptomatic bacteriuria are common in elderly women and usually resolve spontaneously.[8]

Nitrites

The presence of nitrites in the urine occurs when certain bacteria convert nitrates to nitrites. This requires time, so a first voided morning specimen is the ideal specimen for testing. Ascorbic acid may cause false-negative readings.[2]

Protein

The comments that follow should not be construed as advocating routine urinalysis of asymptomatic persons. The Canadian Task Force on Preventive Health Care recommends against routine protein dipstick analysis of the adult population as a screen for chronic renal disease ("D" recommendation).[6] The reason behind this is that no effective treatment is known for the majority of serious conditions that may cause proteinuria. An exception is diabetic nephropathy in persons with insulin-dependent diabetes. For this group of patients the Canadian Task Force Preventive Health Care recommends screening for microalbuminuria ("A" recommendation).[6]

The Ames dipstick is sensitive primarily for albumin and can detect as little as15 to 20 mg/dl of protein. Results are classified as negative, trace (10 to 20 mg/dl), 1+ (30 mg/dl), 2+ (100 mg/dl), 3+ (300 mg/dl), and 4+ (1000 mg/dl).[9] Healthy persons may excrete a trace of protein, particularly if the urine is concentrated. False-positive tests may be seen with highly alkaline urine (pH 7.5 to 8.0), with very concentrated urine, and in patients with gross hematuria.[2,9] False-negative findings occur with dilute urine.[2,9,10] Further investigations are probably unnecessary in a clinically healthy person whose only abnormality on more than one urinalysis is proteinuria of 30 mg/dl or less. Anyone with 100 mg/dl or more has significant proteinuria and needs further tests.[2,10] The dipstick will not detect Bence Jones protein or microalbuminuria.[10] Detection of the latter is important in follow-up of diabetic patients and is discussed under "Diabetic Nephropathy."

Aside from tests for blood urea nitrogen and creatinine and a complete blood count, an important investigation for a patient with proteinuria is a 24-hour urine protein excretion. Creatinine excretion should be measured at the same time to ensure adequacy of the sample. Normal values of 24-hour urine creatinine excretion are 1.3 to 2.2 mmol/kg (15 to 25 mg/kg) for men and 0.9 to 1.9 mmol/kg (10 to 22 mg/kg) for women. The average excretion of protein in the urine is 40 to 80 mg/day, and the upper limit of normal is 150 mg/day or 8 to 10 mg/dl (0.08 to 0.10 g/L). Proteinuria of 3 g/day or more is always the result of glomerular disease, and patients with this test result often have the nephrotic syndrome. (Patients with the nephrotic syndrome usually excrete more than 3.5 g of protein in the urine per day.) Patients with lesser degrees of proteinuria may have glomerular or tubular disease. If urinary protein is less than 1 g/day

in an otherwise healthy person and urinalysis shows no other abnormalities, serious disease is unlikely and the patient simply requires follow-up at intervals of 3 to 6 months.[2,10]

Whether the proteinuria is persistent or intermittent is an important determination. Intermittent or transient proteinuria is generally benign and may be induced by fever, exercise, emotional stress, or posture. Postural proteinuria may be diagnosed if a voiding first thing in the morning is negative for protein whereas voidings in the erect position later in the day are positive.[10]

Screening Urinalysis

Screening urinalysis of healthy adults and children is of little value. The positive predictive value of abnormal dipstick results on screening urinalysis is approximately 12% to 16%. Considerable psychological and physical harm ensues to the many individuals who require further investigations to prove that they are normal.[11] Both the Canadian Task Force on Preventive Health Care[6] and the U.S. Preventive Services Task Force[7] give "D" or "E" recommendations for routine urinalysis during the pediatric years, as well as for such screening of the general adult population and the elderly. For pregnant women a urine culture between 12 and 16 weeks of pregnancy is recommended, and dipstick urinalysis is not an adequate substitute.[6,7]

─────────────── ◣ **REFERENCES** ◢ ───────────────

1. Kiel DP, Moskowitz MA: The urinalysis: a critical appraisal, *Med Clin North Am* 71:607-624, 1987.
2. Misdraji J, Nguyen PL: Urinalysis: when—and when not—to order, *Postgrad Med* 100:173-192, 1996.
3. Gambrell RC, Blount BW: Exercise-induced hematuria, *Am Fam Physician* 53:905-911, 1996.
4. Line RL, Rust GS: Acute exertional rhabdomyolysis, *Am Fam Physician* 52:502-506, 1995.
5. Mohr DN, Offord KP, Owen RA, et al: Asymptomatic microhematuria and urologic disease: a population-based study, *JAMA* 256:224-229, 1986.
6. Canadian Task Force on the Periodic Health Examination: *Canadian guide to clinical preventive health care,* Ottawa, 1994, Canada Communication Group—Publishing, pp 826-836.
7. US Preventive Services Task Force: *Guide to clinical preventive services,* ed 2, Baltimore, 1996, Williams & Wilkins, pp 181-186.
8. Monane M, Gurwitz JH, Lipsitz LA, et al: Epidemiologic and diagnostic aspects of bacteriuria: a longitudinal study in older women, *J Am Geriatr Soc* 43:618-622, 1995.
9. Larson TS: Evaluation of proteinuria, *Mayo Clin Proc* 69:1154-1158, 1994.
10. Rapaport A, Richardson RM: How to tell it's proteinuria, *Patient Care Can* 5:13-18, 1994.
11. Kaplan RE, Springate JE, Feld LG: Screening dipstick urinalysis: a time to change, *Pediatrics* 100:919-921, 1997.

NUTRITION

(See also alternative medicine; food poisoning; formulas. Nutrition is discussed under specific disease entities in many sections of this text.)

Topics covered in this section

Fruits, Vegetables, and Cereals
Minerals
Obesity
Vegetarians
Vitamins

FRUITS, VEGETABLES, AND CEREALS

(See also oncology)

Although the recommended daily intake of fruits and vegetables for both adults and children is a minimum of two fruits and three vegetables ("5-A-Day"), few children or adults follow these guidelines.[1] The Iowa Women's Health Study found that women who ate at least one serving of whole grain food per day had lower total, cancer, and cardiovascular mortality rates,[2] and a review of the epidemiological literature on tomato intake concluded that a high intake correlated with lower rates of numerous cancers, particularly of the prostate, lung, and stomach.[3]

⊿ REFERENCES ⊿

1. Dennison BA, Rockwell HL, Baker SL: Fruit and vegetable intake in young children, *J Am Coll Nutr* 17:371-378, 1998.
2. Jacobs DR, Meyer KA, Kushi LH, et al: Is whole grain intake associated with reduced total and cause-specific death rates in older women? The Iowa Women's Health Study, *Am J Public Health* 89:322-329, 1999.
3. Giovannucci E: Tomatoes, tomato-based products, lycopene, and cancer: review of the epidemiologic literature, *J Natl Cancer Inst* 91:317-331, 1999.

MINERALS
Zinc

Adequate intake of zinc is important for child health in developing countries. In these areas zinc supplementation of 10 to 20 mg/day decreases the incidence of diarrheal disease, improves the immune response, increases growth, and appears to enhance neuropsychological development. Claims have been made that zinc lozenges are effective treatment for the common cold, but this is controversial (see discussion of the common cold).[1]

⊿ REFERENCES ⊿

1. Gadomski A: A cure for the common cold? Zinc again (editorial), *JAMA* 279:1999-2000, 1998.

OBESITY

The inclusion of obesity under the general heading "Nutrition" is questionable, since it might better be placed under "Exercise" or given its own heading. It is placed here mainly because that is the convention.

Definition

Various definitions of "overweight" and "obesity" are used. A recent U.S. expert panel defined "overweight" as a body mass index (BMI) of 25 to 29.9 and "obese" as a BMI greater than 30. Both overweight and obese persons have increased morbidity rates from a variety of diseases (see "Adverse Consequences of Obesity").[1] In Canada, obesity is defined as a BMI greater than 27.[2]

The waist/hip ratio is another clinically significant parameter of obesity. According to Lean and associates,[3] health risks are significant if the values are above 0.95 for men and 0.80 for women. The Nurses' Health Study found that women with a waist/hip ratio greater than 0 .75 had over twice the risk for coronary artery disease as those with a lower ratio.[4]

A simple measurement of abdominal girth also seems a good index of the health risks of obesity.[3-6] Values of 102 cm (50 inches) or more for men and 88 cm (35 inches) or more for women are considered dangerous and indications for weight loss, and values of 94 to 102 cm (38 to 41 inches) in men and 80 to 88 cm (32 to 35 inches) in women are warnings not to gain weight.[3] The Nurses' Health Study reported that women with waist circumferences of 76.2 cm (30 inches) or greater had over twice the risk for coronary artery disease compared with thinner women.[4] An expert panel of the National Institutes of Health considers a waist circumference of 102 cm or 40 inches in men and 88 cm or 35 inches in women to indicate a high risk for the medical complications of obesity.[6]

⊿ REFERENCES ⊿

1. Expert Panel on the Identification, Evaluation, and Treatment of Overweight and Obesity in Adults: Executive summary of the clinical guidelines on the identification, evaluation, and treatment of overweight and obesity in adults, *Arch Intern Med* 158:1855-1867, 1998.
2. Douketis JD, Feightner JW, Attia J, et al: Periodic health examination, 1999 update. 1. Detection, prevention and treatment of obesity, *Can Med Assoc J* 160:513-525, 1999.
3. Lean MEJ, Han TS, Morrison CE: Waist circumference as a measure for indicating need for weight management, *BMJ* 311:158-161, 1995.
4. Rexrode KM, Carey VJ, Hennekens CH, et al: Abdominal adiposity and coronary heart disease in women, *JAMA* 280:1843-1848, 1998.
5. Lean ME, Han TS, Seidell JC: Impairment of health and quality of life in people with large waist circumference, *Lancet* 351:853-856, 1998.
6. Clinical guidelines on the identification, evaluation, and treatment of overweight and obesity in adults—the evidence report, *Obesity Res* 6(suppl 2):51S-209S, 1998.

Epidemiology of Obesity

The prevalence of obesity (BMI 30 or greater) in the United States has increased from 12% in 1991 to 18% in 1998. Increases have occurred in both sexes, all age groups, all races, and all educational levels, but the greatest degree of increase has been among Hispanics, persons with some college education, men and women in their twenties, and residents of the Atlantic Coast states in the South.[1] When rates of "overweight" and "obesity" are combined, the estimated prevalence among U.S. adults is 55%.[2] A Canadian population survey of individuals over the age of 12 (aboriginal people excluded) published in 1999 found that one fourth of all women and one third of all men were obese (BMI 27 or greater).[3]

A postulated explanation for the obesity epidemic is an increasingly sedentary life-style.[4-7] Pima Indians living in remote areas of Mexico where life is physically arduous are lean, whereas Pima Indians in Arizona where amenities of civilization are freely available are obese.[5] A comparison of female monozygotic twin pairs found that the more physically active twin was thinner,[6] and in women body mass index is positively correlated with number of hours spent watching television.[7] The importance of caloric intake is suggested by the positive correlation between weight and number of fast food meals consumed.[7]

Foreyt and Goodrick[8] from Baylor College of Medicine in Houston calculated that if the U.S. population continues to increase in weight at the same rate as at present, the entire adult population will meet the criterion of obesity by the year 2230. They also point out that Americans spend $33 billion a year on weight control without any benefit at a population level.

Childhood obesity is a risk factor for adult obesity (see discussion of obesity in childhood).

➷ REFERENCES ➷

1. Mokdad AH, Serdula MK, Dietz WH, et al: The spread of the obesity epidemic in the United States, 1991-1998, *JAMA* 282:1519-1522, 1999.
2. Expert Panel on the Identification, Evaluation, and Treatment of Overweight and Obesity in Adults: Executive summary of the clinical guidelines on the identification, evaluation, and treatment of overweight and obesity in adults, *Arch Intern Med* 158:1855-1867, 1998.
3. Trakas K, Lawrence K, Shear NH: Utilization of health care resources by obese Canadians, *Can Med Assoc J* 160:1457-1462, 1999.
4. Williamson DF: Descriptive epidemiology of body weight and weight change in U.S. adults, *Ann Intern Med* 119(7 pt 2):646-649, 1993.
5. Fox CS, Esparza J, Nicolson M, et al: Is a low leptin concentration, a low resting metabolic rate, or both the expression of the "thrifty genotype"? Results from Mexican Pima Indians, *Am J Clin Nutr* 68:1053-1057, 1998.
6. Samaras K, Kelly PJ, Chiano MN, et al: Genetic and environmental influences on total-body and central abdominal fat: the effect of physical activity in female twins, *Ann Intern Med* 130:873-882, 1999.
7. Jeffery RW, French SA: Epidemic obesity in the United States: are fast foods and television viewing contributing? *Am J Public Health* 88:277-280, 1998.
8. Foreyt J, Goodrick K: The ultimate triumph of obesity (editorial), *Lancet* 346:134-135, 1995.

Pathophysiology of Obesity
(See also exercise)

Obesity results from an imbalance between energy input and energy expenditure.[1] Energy is expended in a variety of ways: basal metabolic rate, postprandial thermogenesis (the excess energy required to digest and absorb food), and physical activity thermogenesis. Physical activity thermogenesis may in turn be subdivided into volitional exercise and nonexercise activity thermogenesis (NEAT), which according to Levine and associates[2] includes activities of daily living, maintenance of posture, spontaneous muscle contraction, and fidgeting (see below).[2] Specific activities of daily living were not defined in the *Science* article in which the acronym "NEAT" first appeared, but when interviewed by a Toronto reporter, Dr. Levine gave as examples of such activities walking to and from work, shoveling snow, gardening, going up and down stairs at home, and washing dishes. Basically, NEAT includes all physical activity except planned exercise programs.[3]

Most people gradually gain weight with age; a very small imbalance between intake and energy expenditure that persists over many years can result in significant weight changes. Bennett[1] points out that if a 70-kg man gains 10 kg over 20 years, the excess energy intake is equivalent to about 1 carrot stick a day.

Overeating is commonly believed to be the major cause of obesity, but evidence supporting this hypothesis is not definitive. Decreased physical activity is a more likely explanation.[1,4,5] Surveys show that although Americans have become fatter, they have been eating fewer calories and less fat. They may be participating in more leisure-time exercise programs, but they have reduced their household and occupational physical activity to such a degree that their total energy expenditure is decreased.[5]

In many individuals the body adjusts its energy output as weight changes. Those who have purposely lost weight have a decreased resting energy output, whereas those who have purposely gained weight have an increased resting energy output.[6] The mechanism by which the "set point" for body fat is modulated has not been clearly established, but leptin has been suggested as the mediating factor. Plasma leptin levels decrease with weight loss or starvation, and low levels of leptin are associated with factors fostering weight gain such as low daily energy expenditures, low sympathetic nervous system activity, and possibly hyperphagia.[7]

The set point for body fat is a powerful mechanism of homeostasis and undoubtedly explains why dieting so often fails. The only good news about the set point is that its level may gradually change as a result of the type of food ingested or the amount of energy expended on a regular basis. In the long run, both a sedentary life-style (decreased physical activity) and the sustained consumption of a high-fat diet may shift the set point to promote fat retention. Conversely, regular exercise and a persistent decrease in the fat content of the diet may shift it to promote a leaner body structure.[1]

Levine, Eberhardt, and Jensen[2] from the Mayo Clinic performed a rigorous experiment on 16 nonobese volunteers who were fed 1000 excess kcal/day for 8 weeks and whose volitional exercise was strictly controlled. Weight gain ranged from 1.4 to 7.2 kg, and there was a 10-fold variation in fat storage. Basal metabolic rate and postprandial thermogenesis increased by a small amount in all subjects, but there was little interindividual variation. However, wide variations in NEAT (see above) were observed, and this accounted for the striking differences in fat accumulation. Whether this finding can be translated into an effective therapeutic intervention is unknown but intriguing.

The optimal foraging theory offers an evolutionary explanation for our current epidemic of obesity. Animals are programmed to expend a minimum amount of energy to take in a maximum amount of high-energy food. This is beneficial when food is scarce but is harmful when no activity is required to obtain meals.[4,8] Populations with a particularly strong propensity for obesity are often referred to as having a "thrifty genotype." Whether hypoleptinemia is the mechanism by which the "thrifty genotype" is expressed is uncertain; one study of Pima Indians failed to support the hypothesis.[7]

Does a high fat intake in itself predispose to obesity? Evidence suggests that it does so by overriding the normal sensation of satiety. Obese persons tend to have a higher fat content in their diets than do normal weight individuals (see discussion of dietary advice for overweight patients).[9]

───────────── ◣ REFERENCES ◪ ─────────────

1. Bennett WI: Beyond overeating (editorial), *N Engl J Med* 332:673-674, 1995.
2. Levine JA, Eberhardt NL, Jensen MD: Role of nonexercise activity thermogenesis in resistance to fat gain in humans, *Science* 283:212-214, 1999.
3. Strauss S: Fidgeting fights flab? Fat chance, *Toronto Globe and Mail,* March 20, 1999, p D5.
4. Weinsier RL: Genes and obesity: is there reason to change our behaviors? (editorial), *Ann Intern Med* 130:938-939, 1999.
5. Heini AF, Weinsier RL: Divergent trends in obesity and fat intake patterns: the American paradox, *Am J Med* 102:259-264, 1997.
6. Leibel RL, Rosenbaum M, Hirsch J: Changes in energy expenditure resulting from altered body weight, *N Engl J Med* 332:621-628, 1995.
7. Fox CS, Esparza J, Nicolson M, et al: Is a low leptin concentration, a low resting metabolic rate, or both the expression of the "thrifty genotype"? Results from Mexican Pima Indians, *Am J Clin Nutr* 68:1053-1057, 1998.
8. Foreyt J, Goodrick K: The ultimate triumph of obesity (editorial), *Lancet* 346:134-135, 1995.
9. Toubro S, Astrup A: Randomised comparison of diets for maintaining obese subjects' weight after major weight loss: ad lib, low fat, high carbohydrate diet v fixed energy intake, *BMJ* 314:29-34, 1997.

Adverse Medical Consequences of Obesity
(See also exercise; poverty)

A number of medical conditions are associated with obesity. These include the following:
1. Hypertension[1]
2. Coronary heart disease[1-4]
3. Type 2 diabetes mellitus[1,4]
4. Gallbladder disease[1]
5. Sleep apnea[1]
6. Respiratory problems such as cough and wheezing[1,5]
7. Cancers of the endometrium,[1] breast,[1] prostate,[1] colon,[1,6] and pancreas[7]
8. Osteoarthritis[1]
9. Low back pain[5]
10. Increased total mortality[1,4,8,9]
11. Complications of pregnancy[10,11]

A progressive relationship was found between increasing BMI and coronary artery disease (CAD) in the Nurses' Health Study. The relative risk was lowest for women with a BMI less than 21 and was 3.5 for women whose BMI was greater than 29. Weight gain after the age of 18 was also a risk factor, even if the weight remained well within the "normal" limits.[3] A progressive increase in CAD risk with a BMI over 20 has also been demonstrated in British men.[4] Obesity is now thought to pose as great a risk for coronary heart disease as smoking, a sedentary life-style, and elevated blood cholesterol.[2] Obese individuals who lose 5% to 10% of their body weight may decrease their blood pressure and cholesterol levels and improve their glucose tolerance,[2] but whether this will translate into a reduced risk of cardiovascular disease is unknown.[12]

Total cohort mortality was increased sharply in the Nurses' Health Study among women with a BMI over 27; it was also increased among women who gained more than 10 kg after the age of 18. Although cardiovascular disease accounted for most of the excess mortality, cancers were also contributing factors.[8] Among British men total cohort mortality was increased when the BMI was 30 or more.[4]

Perinatal mortality[11] and the incidence of neural tube defects[10] are both elevated among the offspring of obese women.

REFERENCES

1. Expert Panel on the Identification, Evaluation, and Treatment of Overweight and Obesity in Adults: Executive summary of the clinical guidelines on the identification, evaluation, and treatment of overweight and obesity in adults, *Arch Intern Med* 158:1855-1867, 1998.
2. Eckel RH, Krauss RM (AHA Nutrition Committee): American Heart Association call to action: obesity as a major risk factor for coronary heart disease, *Circulation* 97:2099-2100, 1998.
3. Willett WC, Manson JE, Stampfer MJ, et al: Weight, weight change, and coronary heart disease in women: risk within the "normal" weight range, *JAMA* 273:461-465, 1995.
4. Shaper AG, Wannamethee G, Walker M: Body weight: implications for the prevention of coronary heart disease, stroke, and diabetes mellitus in a cohort study of middle aged men, *BMJ* 314:1311-1317, 1997.
5. Lean ME, Han TS, Seidell JC: Impairment of health and quality of life in people with large waist circumference, *Lancet* 351:853-856, 1998.
6. Ford ES: Body mass index and colon cancer in a national sample of adult US men and women, *Am J Epidemiol* 150:390-398, 1999.
7. Silverman DT, Swanson CA, Gridley G, et al: Dietary and nutritional factors and pancreatic cancer: a case-control study based on direct interviews, *J Natl Cancer Inst* 90:1710-1719, 1998.
8. Manson JE, Willett WC, Stampfer MJ, et al: Body weight and mortality among women, *N Engl J Med* 333:677-685, 1995.
9. Calle EE, Thun MJ, Petrelli JM, et al: Body-mass index and mortality in a prospective cohort of U.S. adults, *N Engl J Med* 341:1097-1105, 1999.
10. Goldenberg RL, Tamura T: Prepregnancy weight and pregnancy outcome (editorial), *JAMA* 275:1127-1128, 1996.
11. Cnattingius S, Bergström R, Lipworth L, et al: Prepregnancy weight and the risk of adverse pregnancy outcomes, *N Engl J Med* 338:147-152, 1998.
12. Kassirer JP, Angell M: Losing weight—an ill-fated New Year's resolution (editorial), *N Engl J Med* 338:52-54, 1998.

Dietary Advice for Overweight Patients
(See also pathophysiology of obesity)

Dieting rarely leads to long-term weight loss (see below). However, since other weight loss programs are equally ineffective or, in the case of pharmacological interventions, possibly dangerous, many patients seek dietary advice. Traditional suggestions are that patients eat three reasonably sized meals a day, try to avoid snacking, and decrease fat intake.

High-fat versus high-carbohydrate diets

Since a high fat intake may contribute to obesity (see discussion of pathophysiology of obesity), low-fat, high-carbohydrate diets may be beneficial. This was tested in a two-stage Danish study of the management of obesity in women. In the initial stage one group was treated with an extremely low-calorie diet in the form of a prepared liquid formulation (2 MJ/day) for 8 weeks while the other was treated with a standard, ordinary food, low-calorie diet (5 MJ/day) for 17 weeks. Both cohorts were also treated with an ephedrine-caffeine anorexiant. Both groups had lost an average of 12.6 kg (28 lb) at the completion of the initial diet. At this point anorexiant therapy was discontinued for all patients, who were then randomly assigned to either a fixed energy intake diet or an ad lib, low-fat, high-carbohydrate diet. At the end of 1 year those on the fixed energy diet had regained 11.3 kg, whereas those on the ad lib high-carbohydrate diet had regained only 5.4 kg. Weight gain in the maintenance phase did not correlate with the form of the initial diet (low calorie versus extremely low calorie).[1]

Quantity of food

Patients should be made aware of the size of average servings. They should know the difference between a 4-oz steak and a 16-oz steak. They should know that milk with a meal means one glass, not four glasses, and that thirst is quenched with water and not glass after glass of juice or soft drinks. It is quite amazing how people can fool themselves. I had one diabetic patient who was so careful of his diet that he made carrot sandwich snacks without butter, margarine, mayonnaise, or other condiments. The only problem was that he would eat 10 such sandwiches at a sitting. As he told me later, "I finally figured out that even rabbits get fat on carrots."

Calorie content of food types

Patients who are serious about weight loss should learn the caloric content of various food classes:

Proteins	4 kcal/g
Carbohydrates	4 kcal/g
Fats	9 kcal/g
Alcohol	7 kcal/g

Once patients understand the principles of caloric content, they can recognize and try to avoid or cut down on alcohol and high-calorie foods with a high fat content. Fat intake can be lowered by cutting off (and not eating) all visible fat from meat, avoiding high-calorie fast foods and most fried foods, and avoiding or minimizing margarine, butter, oils such as salad dressings, delicatessen salads drenched in oil, nuts, mayonnaise, sauces, and rich desserts such as pies, cakes, cookies, Danish pastries, and ice cream. Complex carbohydrates should make up a significant proportion of the diet.

Most vegetables are low in calories and can be eaten in large quantities. Exceptions that have moderate numbers of calories (approximating the numbers in fruit) are potatoes, lima beans, sweet corn, and green peas.

Fruit should be eaten in moderation. Fruit juices, especially apple juice, have more calories than the whole fruit. Raisins are dehydrated and so have a relatively high caloric content.

Family physicians can help patients with diet by having them keep a diary in which they record everything they eat or drink for 3 days. The physician can go over the diary with the patient at a subsequent visit.

⚟ REFERENCES ⚞

1. Toubro S, Astrup A: Randomised comparison of diets for maintaining obese subjects' weight after major weight loss: ad lib, low fat, high carbohydrate diet v fixed energy intake, *BMJ* 314:29-34, 1997.

Efficacy and Harm of Dieting

Dieting is a national U.S. (and Canadian) pastime. U.S. studies have shown that at any one time 40% of women and 20% of men are dieting.[1,2] Since only a minuscule number of people maintain weight loss after dieting,[3] very low-calorie dieting seems a largely futile and perhaps even dangerous activity. In most studies one third to two thirds of any initial weight loss is regained within a year and almost all of it within 5 years.[4] For those who initially lose weight the best predictor of the maintenance of weight loss is the frequency of exercise after the completion of dieting, and a good predictor for regaining weight is the amount of television watched.[5]

Patients who have lost weight, whether through dieting, exercise, drugs, or a combination of these modalities, must realize that because of a change in their set point their caloric requirements for maintaining this "normal" weight will be about 15% less than the calories required by someone of the same weight who was never obese (see discussion of pathophysiology of obesity).[6]

Although obesity is associated with significant morbidity, no randomized controlled trials of the effect of voluntary weight loss on total mortality have been conducted.[7] In observational studies mortality is often increased among those who lose weight, probably because the weight loss is an involuntary sequel of underlying disease.[7,8]

Dieting may lead to increased morbidity and mortality.[1,9] Dieting has been associated with decreased psychosocial functioning, binge eating, and even bulimia. Wooley and Garner[9] concluded that the detrimental effects of dieting outweigh the advantages and recommended that physicians stop prescribing a treatment that is risky and ineffective.

In the past an association between weight cycling or yo-yo dieting and increased mortality has been reported. More recent studies have found no such correlation.[10] However, weight cycling, which has been reported in over 50% of adult women, is associated with an increased risk of cholecystectomy.[11]

⚟ REFERENCES ⚞

1. Serdula M, Collins ME, Williamson DF, et al: Weight control practices of US adolescents and adults: Youth Risk Behavior Survey and Behavioral Risk Factor Surveillance System, *Ann Intern Med* 119:667-671, 1993.
2. Horm J, Anderson K: Who in America is trying to lose weight? *Ann Intern Med* 119:672-676, 1993.
3. Douketis JD, Feightner JW, Attia J, et al: Periodic health examination, 1999 update. 1. Detection, prevention and treatment of obesity, *Can Med Assoc J* 160:513-525, 1999.
4. NIH Technology Assessment Conference Panel: Methods for voluntary weight loss and control, *Ann Intern Med* 119(7 pt 2):764-770, 1993.
5. Grodstein F, Levine R, Troy L, et al: Three-year follow-up of participants in a commercial weight loss program, *Arch Intern Med* 156:1302-1306, 1996.
6. Rosenbaum M, Leibel RL, Hirsch J: Obesity, *N Engl J Med* 337:396-407, 1997.
7. Williamson DF, Pamuk E, Thun M, et al: Prospective study of intentional weight loss and mortality in overweight white men aged 40-64 years, *Am J Epidemiol* 149:491-503, 1999.
8. French SA, Folsom AR, Jeffery RW, et al: Prospective study of intentionality of weight loss and mortality in older women: the Iowa Women's Health Study, *Am J Epidemiol* 149:504-514, 1999.
9. Wooley SC, Garner DM: Dietary treatments for obesity are ineffective, *BMJ* 309:655-656, 1994.
10. Jeffery R. Does weight cycling present a health risk? *Am J Clin Nutr* 63(suppl):452S-455S, 1996.
11. Syngal S, Coakley EH, Willett WC, et al: Long-term weight patterns and risk for cholecystectomy in women, *Ann Intern Med* 130:471-477, 1999.

Exercise as a Means of Weight Control

Individuals who exercise have lower body mass indices than those who do not.[1,2] Exercise is a logical technique for inducing weight loss in the obese, since overweight persons generally do not take in more calories than lean persons but usually expend fewer calories (see discussion of pathophysiology of obesity). Weight loss induced by exercise is almost all from body fat, particularly central abdominal fat, whereas much of the weight lost in dieting is from lean body mass. Exercise alone does not lead to as much initial weight loss as dieting, but when dieting and exercise are combined, the total initial weight loss is greater. Continued exercise helps maintain weight loss.[2] Unfortunately, only one fifth of the millions of Americans who at any time are trying to lose weight both ingest fewer calories and exercise.[3]

Traditional exercise programs for weight loss involve structured programs and classes. A life-style program emphasizing increased physical activity such as walking to the corner store rather than driving or taking stairs rather then the escalator is as effective, at least over a 1-year period.[4] One study of women with a mean BMI of 32.8 found that daily brisk walking (or other equivalent aerobic exercises) increased weight loss and helped maintain the loss. Women who exercised for 30 minutes a day or more (either as a single long bout or as several short bouts) achieved greater weight loss than those who exercised for 20 minutes a day. The presence of a home treadmill increased compliance with repeated short bouts of exercise.[5]

Perhaps the most important reason to make exercise part of a weight control program is that active obese individuals have lower morbidity rates than do the sedentary obese.[6]

────────── **❧ REFERENCES ❧** ──────────

1. Thune I, Njølstad I, Løchen M-L, et al: Physical activity improves the metabolic risk profiles in men and women: the Tromsø Study, *Arch Intern Med* 158:1633-1640, 1998.
2. Grodstein F, Levine R, Troy L, et al: Three-year follow-up of participants in a commercial weight loss program, *Arch Intern Med* 156:1302-1306, 1996.
3. Serdula MK, Mokdad AH, Williamson DF, et al: Prevalence of attempting weight loss and strategies for controlling weight, *JAMA* 282:1353-1358, 1999.
4. Andersen RE, Wadden TA, Bartlett SJ, et al: Effects of lifestyle activity vs structured aerobic exercise in obese women: a randomized trial, *JAMA* 281:335-340, 1999.
5. Jakicic JM, Winters C, Lang W, et al: Effects of intermittent exercise and use of home exercise equipment on adherence, weight loss, and fitness in overweight women: a randomized trial, *JAMA* 282:1554-1560, 1999.
6. Blair SN: Evidence for success of exercise in weight loss and control, *Ann Intern Med* 119(7 pt 2):702-706, 1993.

Drug Treatment of Obesity

(See also exercise; informed consent; prevention; type 2 diabetes)

A 1996 in-depth analysis of the literature on the pharmacotherapy of obesity noted that few studies have had follow-up periods longer than 6 months and that many that have been done have not been blinded, randomized, or placebo controlled. According to this article, follow-up reports have been published on fewer than 200 patients taking anorexiant drugs of any sort for a duration of 2 or more years.[1]

When reading reports of the efficacy of anorexiants, the physician should remember that almost all studies are short term and that behavioral treatment alone has been reported to lead to an average weight loss of 8.5 kg (19 lb) by 21 weeks and 5.6 kg (12 lb) by 1 year.[1] The benefits of drugs must be measured against behaviorally obtained weight loss, not baseline weight.

The benefits of the serotonin uptake inhibitors fenfluramine (Pondimin, Ponderal) and dexfenfluramine (Redux) when used alone in the treatment of obesity are uncertain. Although initial weight loss is common, it is usually regained rapidly after cessation of the drugs.[1,2] Adverse effects of these drugs include rare but well-documented cases of primary pulmonary hypertension and a theoretical concern about neurotoxicity.[3]

The combination of fenfluramine and phentermine (e.g., Ionamin, Phentrol), which is known as "Fen/Phen," turned out to be a particularly popular product, although studies supporting its efficacy were limited and involved small numbers of patients.[1] In the mid-1990s an advertising blitz for anorexiants was mounted in North America, and this was reflected in an astonishing increase in the sale of drugs such as phentermine and fenfluramine. Many physicians in the United States set up Fen/Phen treatment programs for obesity, and some commercial weight loss chains began hiring medical consultants to prescribe anorexiants.[4] By July 1997 the U.S. Food and Drug Administration (FDA) had received 33 reports of significant valvular insufficiency (usually involving multiple valves) that was apparently related to these drugs,[5] and in late August 1997 two articles on this treatment appeared in the *New England Journal of Medicine,* one reporting valvular insufficiencies in 24 women after taking fenfluramine-phentermine therapy[6] and the other describing a case of fatal pulmonary hypertension in a woman who had taken fenfluramine-phentermine for only 23 days.[7] In September 1997 fenfluramine and dexfenfluramine were voluntarily withdrawn from the market.

What medical interventions are recommended for the large numbers of obese patients who have taken fenfluramine or dexfenfluramine in the past? According to one editorial writer, all should be given a careful clinical examination and those with a murmur or those who took the drugs for more than 3 months should have echocardiograms. Those with murmurs or significant regurgitation should receive standard prophylaxis for endocarditis.[8]

A new centrally acting prescription anorexiant is the serotonin and noradrenaline reuptake inhibitor sibutramine (Meridia). Of the few published trials of efficacy or adverse effects, most have been short term. The usual dosage is 10 to 15 mg once a day.[9]

Orlistat (Xenical) is a new product that is not an anorexiant. The drug is taken by mouth in doses of 100 to 400 mg tid and acts by inhibiting gastrointestinal lipases, especially pancreatic lipase. Two 2-year placebo-controlled trials, one in Europe[10] and one in the United States,[11] reported greater weight loss in those treated with orlistat in the first-year, weight loss phase and less weight gain in the treated group in the second-year, maintenance phase. In the U.S. study the group taking orlistat 120 mg tid lost an extra 3.5 kg during the first year compared with those taking placebo and regained 2.25 kg less during the second year compared with those taking placebo. Half the patients in both the placebo and orlistat arms of the study dropped out, and no attempt was made to assess the weight of those patients.[12] The longest published trial of orlistat has been 2 years. Gastrointestinal side effects of the drug are common, and an increase in breast cancer has been reported.[13] Although failure to absorb fat may account for some of the weight loss in patients taking orlistat, avoidance of dietary fat because of symptoms of induced steatorrhea probably accounts for most of it.[14]

Short-term experimental trials in which recombinant leptin was injected daily into obese subjects have been undertaken. Some patients respond with weight loss, but the long-term efficacy and safety of the drug are unknown.[15]

Over-the-counter products marketed as weight control agents include an ephedrine-like alkaloid, phenylpropanolamine (Acutrim, Control, Dex-A-Diet, Dexatrim Pre-Meal, Prolamine, Phenyldrine, Phenoxine). Serious adverse effects, including stroke and seizures, have been reported with the use of these agents.[16]

◣ REFERENCES ◢

1. National Task Force on the Prevention and Treatment of Obesity: Long-term pharmacotherapy in the management of obesity, *JAMA* 276:1907-1915, 1996.
2. O'Connor HT, Richman RM, Steinbeck KS, et al: Dexfenfluramine treatment of obesity: a double blind trial with post trial follow-up, *Int J Obesity* 19:181-189, 1995.
3. McCann UD, Seiden LS, Rubin LJ, et al: Brain serotonin neurotoxicity and primary pulmonary hypertension from fenfluramine and dexfenfluramine, *JAMA* 278:666-672, 1997.
4. Kushner R: The treatment of obesity: a call for prudence and professionalism (editorial), *Arch Intern Med* 157:602-604, 1997.
5. Food and Drug Administration: Health advisory on concomitant fenfluramine and phentermine use, *JAMA* 278:379, 1997.
6. Connolly HM, Crary JL, McGoon MD, et al: Valvular heart disease associated with fenfluramine-phentermine, *N Engl J Med* 337:581-588, 1997.
7. Mark EJ, Chang HT, Evans RJ, et al: Fatal pulmonary hypertension associated with short-term use of fenfluramine and phentermine, *N Engl J Med* 337:602-606, 1997.
8. Devereux RB: Appetite suppressants and valvular heart disease (editorial), *N Engl J Med* 339:765-766, 1998.
9. Sibutramine for obesity, *Med Lett* 40:32, 1998.
10. Sjöström L, Rissanen A, Andersen T, et al: Randomised placebo-controlled trial of orlistat for weight loss and prevention of weight regain in obese patients, *Lancet* 352:167-173, 1998.
11. Davidson MH, Hauptman J, DiGirolamo M, et al: Weight control and risk factor reduction in obese subjects treated for 2 years with orlistat: a randomized controlled trial, *JAMA* 281:235-242, 1999.
12. Williamson DF: Pharmacotherapy for obesity (editorial), *JAMA* 281:278-280, 1999.
13. Prescrire: orlistat; no hurry . . ., *Can Fam Physician* 45:2330-2338, 1999.
14. Garrow J: Flushing away the fat: weight loss during trials of orlistat was significant, but over half was due to diet (editorial), *BMJ* 317:830-831, 1998.
15. Heymsfield SB, Greenberg AS, Fujioka K, et al: Recombinant leptin for weight loss in obese and lean adults: a randomized, controlled, dose-escalation trial, *JAMA* 282:1568-1575, 1999.
16. Centers for Disease Control and Prevention: Adverse events associated with ephedrine-containing products—Texas, December 1993–September 1995, *JAMA* 276:1711-1712, 1996.

Surgical Treatment of Obesity

Standard surgical techniques for treating intractable morbid obesity (BMI of 40 or more or BMI of 35 or more if comorbid conditions are present) are vertical banded gastroplasty, in which a synthetic band is stapled on the stomach to decrease the gastric outlet, or a Roux-en-Y gastric bypass, in which the distal stomach is resected and the proximal pouch is anastomosed to the jejunum.[1]

◣ REFERENCES ◢

1. Semchenko A, Seim HC, Pi-Sunyer FX: Management of obesity, *Am Fam Physician Monogr* No 2, 1999.

Olestra

Olestra (Olean), a nonabsorbable fat substitute, was approved for use in certain snack foods by the FDA in 1996.[1] Olestra has been reported to cause abdominal cramps and diarrhea, particularly if large quantities are taken, and it absorbs fat-soluble vitamins. To prevent vitamin deficiencies, the manufacturer, Procter & Gamble, has added vitamins A, D, E, and K to snack foods containing olestra. According to one author no long-term clinical trials of the product have been conducted, so the full spectrum of possible adverse effects is unknown.[1] A 6-week randomized double-blind placebo-controlled trial of ad libitum eating of ordinary potato chips or olestra-containing potato chips did not reveal any differences in gastrointestinal complaints. Those who ate the most olestra chips had slightly more frequent and looser bowel movements, but this did not interfere with their activities of daily living. No oil or fecal leakage occurred. The lead author is a consultant to Procter & Gamble, and the study was funded by that company.[2] Consumer groups in the United States have claimed that olestra is a health hazard, but in 1998 an FDA advisory panel declared that olestra did not cause gastrointestinal symptoms and that it was safe.[3]

◣ REFERENCES ◢

1. Blackburn H: Olestra and the FDA, *N Engl J Med* 334:984-986, 1996.
2. Sandler RS, Zorich NL, Filloon TG, et al: Gastrointestinal symptoms in 3181 volunteers ingesting snack foods containing olestra or triglycerides: a 6-week randomized, placebo-controlled trial, *Ann Intern Med* 130:253-261, 1999.
3. Josefson D: Fat substitute declared safe, *BMJ* 316:1926, 1998.

Obesity Screening
(See also screening)

The Canadian Task Force on Preventive Health Care gives a "C" recommendation to calculating the BMI as part of the periodic health examination. It also gives a "C" recommendation for weight reduction therapy of obese adults without obesity-related diseases (e.g., diabetes or hypertension) but gives a "B" recommendation for such therapy if obese individuals have obesity-related diseases.[1] The U.S. Preventive Services Task Force gives a "B" recommendation for the periodic measurement of height and weight.[2] A National Institutes of Health expert panel recommends calculating the BMI, measuring waist circumference (upper limits of normal 102 cm or 40 inches for men and 88 cm or 35 inches for women), and treating obese individuals with two or more obesity-related diseases or risk factors.[3]

REFERENCES

1. Douketis JD, Feightner JW, Attia J, et al: Periodic health examination, 1999 update. 1. Detection, prevention and treatment of obesity, *Can Med Assoc J* 160:513-525, 1999.
2. US Preventive Services Task Force: *Guide to clinical preventive services,* ed 2, Baltimore, 1996, Williams & Wilkins, pp 219-229.
3. Clinical guidelines on the identification, evaluation, and treatment of overweight and obesity in adults—the evidence report, *Obesity Res* 6(suppl 2):51S-209S, 1998.

Obesity in Childhood

(See also cholesterol lowering studies in children; epidemiology of obesity)

In the United States obesity in children has been increasing just as it has in adults.[1] Children under age 3 who are obese but whose parents are not obese have a very low risk of becoming obese adults. Obesity in the teenage years, particularly if marked, is a risk factor for adult obesity. The risk is even greater if one or both parents are obese.[2] A twin study of children confirmed the powerful influence of genetics in determining the percentage of body fat,[3] and a cross-sectional study of German children aged 5 to 6 years found that the prevalence of obesity was less in those who had been breast fed than in those who had not.[4]

A prospective study of a small number of boys and girls followed from ages 5 to 11 found that girls but not boys decreased their energy expenditures significantly during the prepubertal period, probably in part because the social desirability of physical activity for girls decreases at that age.[5]

One fourth of U.S. children watch 4 or more hours of television daily, and two thirds watch at least 2 hours a day. These figures are exclusive of time spent playing video games, watching videos, or working or playing on the computer. Excessive TV watching correlates with increased BMI, and it is hypothesized that children are less physically active and ingest extra calories while watching TV.[6] However, whether the excessive weight in these individuals is caused by prolonged TV watching or whether overweight kids tend to watch more TV is unknown.[7] One small prospective randomized trial of third- and fourth-grade students found a slight decrease in BMI in those who had had limits set on their television, videotape, and video game time.[8]

Is there any point instituting preventive interventions for children at high risk? As far as I know, no good data are available with which to answer that question. Common sense dictates that all children, not just obese ones, be encouraged to be physically active (with strict limitation of TV time) and to eat a balanced diet.

The U.S. Preventive Services Task Force gives a "B" recommendation for the periodic measurement of height and weight of children and adults.[9] The Canadian Task Force on Preventive Health Care gives these strategies a "C" recommendation.[10] The Canadian Task Force also gives a "C" recommendation to exercise and to family-based nutrition and exercise counseling as a means of controlling obesity in children, and it gives a "D" to very low-calorie diets in preadolescents.[10]

REFERENCES

1. Troiano RP, Flegal KM, Kuczmarski RJ, et al: Overweight prevalence and trends for children and adolescents: the National Health and Nutrition Examination Surveys, 1963-91, *Arch Pediatr Adolesc Med* 149:1085-1091, 1995.
2. Whitaker RC, Wright JA, Pepe MS, et al: Predicting obesity in young adulthood from childhood and parental obesity, *N Engl J Med* 337:869-873, 1997.
3. Faith MS, Pietrobelli A, Nunez C, et al: Evidence for independent genetic influences on fat mass and body mass index in a pediatric twin sample, *Pediatrics* 104:61-67, 1999.
4. von Kries R, Koletzko B, Sauerwald T, et al: Breast feeding and obesity: cross sectional study, *BMJ* 319:147-150, 1999.
5. Goran MI, Gower BA, Nagy TR, et al: Developmental changes in energy expenditure and physical activity in children: evidence for a decline in physical activity in girls before puberty, *Pediatrics* 101:887-891, 1998.
6. Andersen RE, Crespo CJ, Bartlett SJ, et al: Relationship of physical activity and television watching with body weight and level of fatness among children: results from the Third National Health and Nutrition Examination Survey, *JAMA* 279:938-942, 1998.
7. Robinson TN: Does television cause childhood obesity? (editorial), *JAMA* 279:959-960, 1998.
8. Robinson TN: Reducing children's television viewing to prevent obesity: a randomized controlled trial, *JAMA* 282:1561-1567, 1999.
9. US Preventive Services Task Force: *Guide to clinical preventive services,* ed 2, Baltimore, 1996, Williams & Wilkins, pp 219-229.
10. Canadian Task Force on the Periodic Health Examination: Periodic health examination, 1994 update. I. Obesity in childhood, *Can Med Assoc J* 150:871-879, 1994.

VEGETARIANS

(See also antioxidants)

Vegetarians can be classified as follows:

Vegans	Eat no animal food except possibly honey
Lactovegetarians	Eat dairy products
Lacto-ovo-vegetarians	Eat dairy products and eggs

VITAMINS

(See also alternative medicine; congenital heart disease; homocysteine; neural tube defects; osteoporosis; risk factors for coronary artery disease)

Vitamin B_6 and folates may protect against coronary artery disease, possibly by lowering homocysteine levels. This is discussed in the section on risk factors for coronary artery disease.

In the past the daily requirement of a nutritional element such as a vitamin was called the "recommended daily allowance (RDA)." The current terminology (or jargon) is "recommended nutrient intake (RNI)."

Antioxidants
(See also vitamin A; vitamin C; vitamin E)

Vitamins A, C, and E have antioxidant properties, as do a variety of other compounds, including the lipid-lowering drug probucol (Lorelco). This characteristic has been claimed to protect against coronary artery disease, some cancers, and age-related macular degeneration. Many epidemiological studies have shown a lower rate of cardiovascular disease and cancer in individuals who eat a diet containing large amounts of fruits and vegetables, which are rich in antioxidant vitamins such as A and E.[1] Many believe that the antioxidant vitamins account for the decreased risk of cardiovascular disease and cancer.[1] However, Gaziano[2] points out that persons who eat more fruits and vegetables are those who lead healthy life-styles and thus a conclusion that fruits and vegetables account for their better health cannot be justified. Support for skepticism about the ability of antioxidants to protect against coronary artery disease comes from a comparative review of prospective epidemiological studies versus randomized trials of antioxidant vitamins; benefits were found in the epidemiological studies but not the randomized trials.[3] A 1997 study found that the rate of restenosis after angioplasty was significantly reduced in patients treated with the powerful antioxidant probucol but not in those treated with a combination of beta-carotene, vitamin C, and vitamin E. The weak cholesterol-lowering properties of probucol were insufficient to explain the results.[4]

If antioxidants do decrease the risk of cardiovascular disease, what is their mechanism of action? One of the more important hypotheses is that antioxidants inhibit oxidation of low-density lipoprotein and this in turn inhibits foam cell development and the generation of atherosclerotic plaques. In addition, there is evidence that antioxidants are beneficial even in the presence of established atherosclerotic plaques by enhancing plaque stability, inhibiting platelet activation, and protecting the vascular endothelium.[5]

Antioxidant vitamin supplementation may be harmful. The Finnish Alpha-Tocopherol/Beta-Carotene study showed a non–statistically significant trend toward an increased incidence of cardiovascular disease in the beta-carotene arm of the study, as well as an increased incidence of lung cancer in smokers taking supplemental beta-carotene.[6] Similar deleterious effects have been reported from an American multicenter trial of beta-carotene plus vitamin A (CARET).[7]

Toxic effects of antioxidant vitamins are rare. A few cases of vitamin A toxicity, generally from ingesting more than 100,000 units per day, are reported annually in the United States. Ascorbic acid seems to be nontoxic in doses under 4 g/day as is vitamin E in doses under 3200 mg/day.[8]

At present the best advice family physicians can give their patients on the subject of vitamins is to eat plenty of fruits and vegetables.[2,9] Supplemental antioxidant vitamins probably have little value.[9,10] (For further discussion see the sections on vitamins A and E below.)

◢ REFERENCES ◣

1. Greenberg ER, Sporn MB: Antioxidant vitamins, cancer, and cardiovascular disease (editorial), N Engl J Med 334:1189-1190, 1996.
2. Gaziano JM: Antioxidant vitamins and coronary artery disease risk, Am J Med 97(suppl 3A):18S-21S, 1994.
3. Jha P, Flather M, Lonn E, et al: The antioxidant vitamins and cardiovascular disease: a critical review of epidemiologic and clinical trial data, Ann Intern Med 123:860-872, 1995.
4. Tardif J-C, Coté G, Lespérance J, et al (Multivitamins and Probucol Study Group): Probucol and multivitamins in the prevention of restenosis after coronary angioplasty, N Engl J Med 337:365-372, 1997.
5. Diaz MN, Frei B, Vita JA, et al: Antioxidants and atherosclerotic heart disease, N Engl J Med 337:408-416, 1997.
6. Alpha-Tocopherol, Beta Carotene Cancer Prevention Study Group: The effect of vitamin E and beta carotene on the incidence of lung cancer and other cancers in male smokers, N Engl J Med 330:1029-1035, 1994.
7. Omenn GS, Goodman GE, Thornquist MD, et al: Effects of a combination of beta carotene and vitamin A on lung cancer and cardiovascular disease, N Engl J Med 334:1150-1155, 1996.
8. Meyers DG, Maloley PA, Weeks D: Safety of antioxidant vitamins, Arch Intern Med 156:925-935, 1996.
9. Tribble DL: Antioxidant consumption and risk of coronary heart disease: emphasis on vitamin C, vitamin E, and ß-carotene; a statement for healthcare professionals from the American Heart Association, Circulation 99:591-595, 1999.
10. Lonn EM, Yusuf S: Emerging approaches in preventing cardiovascular disease, BMJ 318:1337-1341, 1999.

Vitamin A
(See also antioxidants; macular degeneration; osteoporosis; vitamin A supplements in pregnancy; vitamin E)

Good dietary sources of preformed vitamin A (retinol) are milk, milk products, liver, and kidney. Beta-carotenes found in green and yellow vegetables, cantaloupe, and apricots act as a substrate that can be synthesized by the body into retinol. However, a rate-limiting factor to this process prevents excess beta-carotene ingestion from causing vitamin A toxicity.

Antioxidants, including carotenoids, have been claimed to protect against coronary artery disease. A follow-up study of the Lipid Research Clinics Primary Prevention Trial showed an inverse relationship between serum carotenoid levels and coronary heart disease.[1] Another investigation found that patients whose initial beta-carotene concentrations were in the highest quartile had about half the total and cardiovascular mortality of those whose initial beta-carotene concentrations were in the lowest quartile.[2] However, other studies have failed to confirm any protective effect[3] or have even suggested an increased incidence of cardiovascular disease.[4,5]

Antioxidants are also claimed to protect against cancer. Recent evaluations have found either no benefit[3] or in the case of beta-carotene an increased incidence of lung cancer.[4,5] For example, a Finnish study of smokers taking beta-carotene 20 mg/day for 5 to 8 years found that they had a higher incidence of lung cancer than did control subjects taking placebo,[4] and similar results were reported by the American Beta-Carotene and Retinol Efficacy Trial (CARET), in which smokers, former smokers, and persons exposed to asbestos were treated with a combination of 30 mg of beta-carotene plus 25,000 IU of retinol (vitamin A) daily.[5] A study from Dartmouth failed to demonstrate any benefit of antioxidants in preventing the recurrence of colonic polyps.[6]

A high intake of carotenoids has been shown to be inversely correlated with the incidence of age-related macular degeneration. Beta-carotene derived from vitamin A is only one of many carotenoids. In this study the specific foods associated with the reduction of age-associated macular degeneration were dark green leafy vegetables, especially spinach and collard greens. The specific carotenoids that were thought to be beneficial were lutein and zeaxanthin. Preformed vitamin A was not beneficial, nor were supplements of vitamin C or vitamin E.[7]

Supplements of vitamin A in excess of 10,000 IU have long been recognized to be teratogenic (see discussion of vitamin A supplements in pregnancy).[8] Recent studies from Scandinavia, an area of the world that has a high rate of hip fractures, have shown a positive correlation between the ingestion of preformed vitamin A (but not beta-carotenes) and osteoporosis. The high levels of vitamin A in Scandinavia are thought to result in part from a long tradition of swilling large quantities of cod liver oil and from the fortification of low-fat milk products in Sweden with vitamins D and A.[9]

⬛ REFERENCES ⬛

1. Morris DL, Kritchevsky SB, Davis CE: Serum carotenoids and coronary heart disease: the Lipid Research Clinics Coronary Prevention Trial and follow-up study, *JAMA* 272:1439-1441, 1994.
2. Greenberg ER, Baron JA, Karagas MR, et al: Mortality associated with low plasma concentration of beta carotene and the effect of oral supplementation, *JAMA* 275:699-703, 1996.
3. Nennekens CH, Buring JE, Manson JE, et al: Lack of effect of long-term supplementation with beta carotene on the incidence of malignant neoplasms and cardiovascular disease, *N Engl J Med* 334:1145-1149, 1996.
4. Alpha-Tocopherol, Beta Carotene Cancer Prevention Study Group: The effect of vitamin E and beta carotene on the incidence of lung cancer and other cancers in male smokers, *N Engl J Med* 330:1029-1035, 1994.
5. Omenn GS, Goodman GE, Thornquist MD, et al: Effects of a combination of beta carotene and vitamin A on lung cancer and cardiovascular disease, *N Engl J Med* 334:1150-1155, 1996.
6. Greenberg ER, Baron JA, Tosteson TD, et al: A clinical trial of antioxidant vitamins to prevent colorectal adenoma, *N Engl J Med* 330:1029-1035, 1994.
7. Seddon JM, Ajani UA, Sperduto RD, et al: Dietary carotenoids, vitamins A, C, and E, and advanced age-related macular degeneration, *JAMA* 272:1413-1420, 1994.

8. Rothman KJ, Moore LL, Singer MR, et al: Teratogenicity of high vitamin A intake, *N Engl J Med* 333:1369-1373, 1995.
9. Melhus H, Michaëlsson K, Kindmark A, et al: Excessive dietary intake of vitamin A is associated with reduced bone mineral density and increased risk for hip fracture, *Ann Intern Med* 129:770-778, 1998.

Vitamin C

In 1844 the British parliament required that seamen be issued lime or lemon juice on a regular basis, hence the term "Limey."

The recommended nutrient intake (RNI) of vitamin C is 35 mg for infants, 45 to 50 mg for children, and 45 to 60 mg for adults.

Ascorbic acid is essential for collagen formation; it catalyzes the hydroxylation of proline and lysine. In the absence of hydroxylation the collagen is unstable, and this is particularly manifest in blood vessel walls. Clinical manifestations of scurvy are perifollicular hemorrhages, corkscrew hairs, large ecchymoses, and hemorrhagic gingivitis. Those at risk of scurvy in North America are alcoholics, persons following fad diets, institutionalized individuals, and the isolated elderly.[1]

⬛ REFERENCES ⬛

1. Offinger KC: Scurvy: more than historical relevance, *Am Fam Physician* 48:609-613, 1993.

Vitamin D

The usual daily requirement of vitamin D for the population at large is 400 IU. Those with osteoporosis should probably have 800 IU/day. Almost all multivitamins contain 400 IU of vitamin D.

A study of elderly homebound (sunlight-deprived) patients found that many had inadequate intake and low serum levels of vitamin D.[1]

⬛ REFERENCES ⬛

1. Gloth FM III, Gundberg CM, Hollis BW, et al: Vitamin D deficiency in homebound elderly persons, *JAMA* 274:1683-1686, 1995.

Vitamin E

(See also antioxidants; coronary artery disease; tardive dyskinesia; vitamin A)

Recommended nutrient intake

The RNI of vitamin E (alpha-tocopherol) is 8 to 15 IU/day. Vitamin E is found mainly in fats. Foods high in vitamin E include vegetable oils, margarine, mayonnaise, sunflower seeds, nuts, avocados, and mangos.

Safety

The long-term safety of vitamin E supplements of 100 IU or more per day has not been studied, but toxicity appears to be low. There are reports that vitamin E can aggravate the coagulation defects of vitamin K deficiency.[1]

Cardiovascular disease

Studies have shown a decreased incidence of coronary artery disease in women and men taking vitamin E supplements at doses of 100 IU/day. There was no greater effect with higher doses, and no benefit with lower doses.[2,3] A 1998 study from Finland found that male smokers taking alpha-tocopherol 50 mg/day over a median period of 6 years had a nonsignificant 8% decrease in relative risk of dying from coronary artery disease compared with control subjects receiving placebo.[4] The Iowa Women's Health Study showed that postmenopausal women who had a high intake of foods rich in vitamin E, such as dark green leafy vegetables, seeds, nuts, vegetable oils, mayonnaise, and margarine, had a lower risk of death from coronary artery disease than did those with a low intake from dietary sources; no protective effect was noted from vitamin E supplements.[5] A randomized controlled trial in which 400 to 800 mg of vitamin E daily was given to patients with angiographically proven coronary artery disease found that this regimen decreased the incidence of nonfatal myocardial infarctions compared with the placebo-treated control subjects,[6] whereas no benefit was observed in a trial of post–myocardial infarction patients given 300 mg of vitamin E daily.[7] A large multicenter trial of patients with known coronary artery disease or at high risk of coronary artery disease found no benefit from the ingestion of 400 IU of vitamin E daily.[8] Although a diet rich in fruit, vegetables, and whole grains is a reasonable recommendation, evidence is insufficient to advise vitamin E supplementation for the primary prevention of coronary artery disease.[9]

Lung cancer

A study of the effect of vitamin E on the incidence of lung cancer in male smokers given alpha-tocopherol 50 mg/day over 5 to 7 years showed no decrease in incidence.[10]

Tardive dyskinesia

A number of studies, many of them double blind, have shown an amelioration of tardive dyskinesia with vitamin E treatment. The usual doses were 1200 to 1600 mg/day.[11-14]

◣ REFERENCES ◢

1. Kappus H, Diplock AT: Tolerance and safety of vitamin E: a toxicological position report, *Free Radical Biol Med* 13:55-74, 1992.
2. Stampfer MJ, Hennekens CH, Manson JE, et al: Vitamin E consumption and the risk of coronary disease in women, *N Engl J Med* 328:1444-1449, 1993.
3. Rimm EB, Stampfer MJ, Ascherio A, et al: Vitamin E consumption and the risk of coronary heart disease in men, *N Engl J Med* 328:1450-1456, 1993.
4. Virtamo J, Rapola JM, Ripatti S, et al: Effect of vitamin E and beta carotene on the incidence of primary nonfatal myocardial infarction and fatal coronary heart disease, *Arch Intern Med* 158:668-675, 1998.
5. Kushi LH, Folsom AR, Prineas RJ, et al: Dietary antioxidant vitamins and death from coronary heart disease in postmenopausal women, *N Engl J Med* 334:1156-1162, 1996.
6. Stephens NG, Parsons A, Schofield PM, et al: Randomised controlled trial of vitamin E in patients with coronary disease: Cambridge Heart Antioxidant Study (CHAOS), *Lancet* 347:781-786, 1996.
7. Marchioli R, Bomba E, Chieffo C, et al (GISSI-Prevenzione Investigators): Dietary supplementation with n-3 polyunsaturated fatty acids and vitamin E after myocardial infarction: results of the GISSI-Prevenzione trial, *Lancet* 354:447-455, 1999.
8. Heart Outcomes Prevention Evaluation Study Investigators: Vitamin E supplementation and cardiovascular events in high-risk patients, *N Engl J Med* 342:154-160, 2000.
9. Tribble DL: Antioxidant consumption and risk of coronary heart disease: emphasis on vitamin C, vitamin E, and ß-carotene; a statement for healthcare professionals from the American Heart Association, *Circulation* 99:591-595, 1999.
10. Alpha-Tocopherol, Beta Carotene Cancer Prevention Study Group: The effect of vitamin E and beta carotene on the incidence of lung cancer and other cancers in male smokers, *N Engl J Med* 330:1029-1035, 1994.
11. Dabiri LM, Pasta D, Darby JK, et al: Effectiveness of vitamin E for treatment of long-term tardive dyskinesia, *Am J Psychiatry* 151:925-926, 1994.
12. Adler LA, Peselow E, Rotrosen J, et al: Vitamin E treatment of tardive dyskinesia, *Am J Psychiatry* 150:1405-1407, 1993.
13. Laugharne J, Rangarajan N, Reynolds GP: Tardive dyskinesia, lipid peroxidation, and sustained amelioration with vitamin E treatment, *Int Clin Psychopharmacol* 8:151-153, 1993.
14. Egan MF, Hyde TM, Albers GW, et al: Treatment of tardive dyskinesia with vitamin E, *Am J Psychiatry* 149:773-777, 1992.

OBSTETRICS

(See also adverse medical consequences of obesity; diabetic retinopathy; postpartum depression; prematurity)

Topics covered in this section

EPIDEMIOLOGY

Since the 1960s fetal deaths have declined 70% in all maternal age groups in the United States. However, the risk of fetal death is about twice as high among women over 35 as it is among younger women.[1]

───────────────── ◥ **REFERENCES** ◤ ─────────────────

1. Frettis RC, Schmittdiel J, McLean FH, et al: Increased maternal age and the risk of fetal death, *N Engl J Med* 333:953-957, 1995.

ANTENATAL CARE FOR PHYSICIANS WHO DO NOT PRACTICE OBSTETRICS

(See also anemia; bed rest complications; risk assessment in pregnancy)

Even physicians who do not practice obstetrics have patients who are pregnant or who want to become pregnant, and the physician should be able to give them some basic counseling. For example, every woman who could become pregnant should be taking at least 0.4 mg of folate daily before conception (see discussion of neural tube defects). The following paragraphs outline some aspects of a typical antenatal protocol.[1]

Frequency of Visits

The schedule of visits should be as follows:

Initial visit	8 weeks
Weeks 8-28	Every 4 weeks
Weeks 28-36	Every 2 weeks
Week 36–term	Every week

Nutrition and Weight Gain

Recommended weight gain in pregnancy for women of normal weight is 11 to 16 kg (25 to 35 lb). Underweight women should gain about 16 to 18 kg (35 to 40 lb) and obese women about 7 to 11 kg (15 to 25 kg). For normal weight women the rate of gain should be about 1.3 to 2.3 kg (3 to 5 lb) per month in the first trimester and 0.5 to 1.0 kg (1 to 2 lb) during the second and third trimesters.[2] Failure of the mother to gain adequate weight has long been believed to put the baby at risk of intrauterine growth retardation (IUGR).[3] IUGR has many causes, including preeclampsia, diabetes, maternal smoking, a variety of infections, and some congenital anomalies,[3] but the concept that failure of maternal weight gain is an etiological factor is being challenged. Although babies born to women who gain relatively little weight during pregnancy may be small, there is no increased risk of premature deliveries with their multiple adverse outcomes. Small term babies generally do well during infancy and childhood (although some data have suggested that they are at higher risk of coronary artery disease in later life).[4] Feig and Naylor[5] advise a minimal weight gain of 6.8 kg (15 lb), but for women with a normal body mass index a maximum weight gain of 11.4 kg (25 lb).[5] Further support for the marginal importance of nutrition during pregnancy in industrialized countries comes from a British prospective study. Placental and fetal weight did not correlate with the amount of any macronutrient ingested, and among micronutrients vitamin C, for the women taking higher levels, was associated with a very small increase in placental and fetal weight.[6]

Exercise

No relationship has been found between low or moderate exercise and gestational duration. However, heavy exercise reduces the risk of preterm delivery.[7]

Uterine Growth in Pregnancy

The uterus has the features below at various stages of pregnancy:

Weeks	Uterine Size
6	Normal
8	Globular; slightly enlarged
12	Symphysis
20	Just below umbilicus
20-38	Ht/cm = weeks of pregnancy

Quickening

Quickening takes place at 16 weeks for multiparas and at 20 weeks for primiparas.

Vaginal Bleeding

About one fifth of pregnant women have vaginal bleeding during the first 20 weeks of pregnancy, and about half of these go on to spontaneous abortion. In one study women who had a spontaneous abortion were not at an increased risk of abortion in subsequent pregnancies.[8]

Initial Visit

The initial visit comprises a complete history, including experience with babies and availability of social supports, an obstetrical risk assessment (controversial; see below), a physical examination including pelvic examination, laboratory investigations, counseling, and a prescription for folic acid and iron. The usual laboratory examinations are a complete blood count, Venereal Disease Research Laboratories (VDRL) test, rubella titer, hepatitis B surface antigen (HBsAg), ABO-Rh typing, a Papanicolaou (Pap) smear, and cervical cultures for gonorrhea and *Chlamydia*. Urine cultures in asymptomatic pregnant women should be obtained between 12 and 16 weeks. If asymptomatic bacteriuria is not detected and treated, symptomatic disease will develop in 25% to 30% of those affected. Urine dipsticks that detect nitrites and leukocyte esterases are relatively insensitive and will miss 25% of cases of asymptomatic bacteriuria in pregnant women.[9]

Important points to cover in counseling include the pros and cons of HIV screening, avoidance of smoking and secondhand smoke, abstention from alcohol (an occasional single drink is probably not harmful), and eating a balanced diet. This type of counseling is best given before the patient becomes pregnant, and advice at the first prenatal visit should function as a reinforcement of what has already been said. All women who are pregnant should receive supplements containing 0.4 to 0.8 mg of folic acid.[10,11] This is most easily done by prescribing a daily multivitamin containing adequate quantities of folic acid. Whether routine iron supplementation is indicated is uncertain, and both the Canadian Task Force on Preventive Health Care[12] and the U.S. Preventive Services Task Force[13] give this a "C" recommendation. Patients should be referred to prenatal classes.

Bed Rest

In the United States, prescription of bed rest is almost the norm for a variety of complications of pregnancy, such as hypertension, incompetent cervix, premature labor, premature rupture of the membranes, placenta previa, and even twin pregnancies. No randomized controlled trials supporting this intervention have been published. Since bed rest is known to be associated with physical deconditioning and a variety of detrimental psychosocial effects, bed rest for these conditions may do more harm than good (see discussion of bed rest complications).[14]

❧ REFERENCES ❧

1. Williams T, Zaltz A: Deliver effective prenatal care, *Patient Care Can* 5:39-51, 1994.
2. Kolasa K, Weismiller DG: Nutrition during pregnancy, *Am Fam Physician* 56:205-212, 1997.
3. Vandenbosche RC, Kirchner JT: Intrauterine growth retardation, *Am Fam Physician* 58:1384-1390, 1998.
4. Kramer MS: Maternal nutrition, pregnancy outcome and public health policy, *Can Med Assoc J* 159:663-665, 1998.
5. Feig D, Naylor D: Eating for two: are guidelines for weight gain during pregnancy too liberal? *Lancet* 351:1054-1055, 1998.
6. Mathews F, Yudkin P, Neil A: Influence of maternal nutrition on outcome of pregnancy: prospective cohort study, *BMJ* 319:339-343, 1999.
7. Hatch M, Levin B, Shu X-O, et al: Maternal leisure-time exercise and timely delivery, *Am J Public Health* 88:1528-1533, 1998.
8. Everett C: Incidence and outcome of bleeding before the 20th week of pregnancy: prospective study from general practice, *BMJ* 315:32-34, 1997.
9. Tincello DG, Richmond DH: Evaluation or bleeding before the 20th week of pregnancy: prospective study from general practice, *BMJ* 316:435-437, 1997.
10. Canadian Task Force on the Periodic Health Examination: *Canadian guide to clinical preventive health care,* Ottawa, 1994, Canada Communication Group— Publishing, pp 74-81.
11. US Preventive Services Task Force: *Guide to clinical preventive services,* ed 2, Baltimore, 1996, Williams & Wilkins, pp 467-483.
12. Canadian Task Force on the Periodic Health Examination: *Canadian guide to clinical preventive health care,* Ottawa, 1994, Canada Communication Group— Publishing, pp 64-72.
13. US Preventive Services Task Force: *Guide to clinical preventive services,* ed 2, Baltimore, 1996, Williams & Wilkins, pp 231-246.
14. Maloni JA, Cohen AW, Kane JH: Prescription of activity restriction to treat high-risk pregnancies, *J Women's Health* 7:351-358, 1998.

CONGENITAL ANOMALIES

(See also drugs and chemicals in pregnancy; informed consent; positive predictive value; prevention; screening; ultrasound in pregnancy)

Risk Factors

A mother who has an infant with a congenital anomaly has a 2.5 times increased relative risk of having a second infant with a congenital anomaly. The increase is due primarily to a 7.6 times increased risk of having a child with the same anomaly. In one study the risk decreased significantly if the woman moved to another community before having the second child, which suggests an environmental cause for anomalies.[1] An analysis of the Medical Birth Registry of Norway concluded that women who themselves had birth defects had a 4% chance of bearing children with birth defects, whereas the risk for the population as a whole was 1.4%. The increased risk was confined to the specific defects carried by the mothers.[2]

A number of genetic diseases have a particularly high prevalence in certain population groups, and for many of these diseases carrier states can be identified by genetic testing. If one or both parents are noncarriers, the chances that they will have an affected child are remote; if both parents are carriers, the parents may opt for prenatal diagnosis if they go ahead with a pregnancy. Examples of these disorders are beta-thalassemia among those whose families originated around the Mediterranean or in the Middle East, Far East, Indian subcontinent, or to a lesser extent Africa[3] and Tay-Sachs disease, Gaucher disease, and cystic fibrosis among Ashkenazi Jews.[4]

When the incidence of the carrier state is high (one in eight Ashkenazi Jews tested are carriers of one of the three autosomal recessive diseases Tay-Sachs, Gaucher, or cystic fibrosis), screening couples is more desirable than screening individuals because the chance of both members of a couple being carriers is 1 in 67.[4] Screening is best done before conception. If pregnancy has already occurred, both the mother and father should be screened, and if both are positive, an amniocentesis can determined whether the fetus is affected.

Other autosomal recessive diseases that are relatively common among Ashkenazi Jews and for which screening techniques are either established or being developed are Canavan disease, Fanconi anemia type C, Bloom syndrome, and Niemann-Pick disease type A.[5]

Folic Acid

Folic acid supplements taken before conception and during pregnancy decrease the incidence of neural tube defects, as discussed in more detail below in the section on neural tube defects. Folic acid supplementation also decreases the incidence of congenital heart disease, especially conotruncal malformations, hypertrophic pyloric stenosis, urinary tract abnormalities, and congenital limb deficiencies.[6]

Amniocentesis

Indications for amniocentesis are numerous and include all women who will have reached their thirty-fifth birthday at the time of delivery, women with a past history of having an infant with chromosomal abnormalities, or women who are at high risk of having a fetus with such conditions as Tay-Sachs disease, sickle cell anemia, and thalassemia. Amniocentesis is generally performed between 15 and 20 weeks of gestation, and the estimated pregnancy loss is 0.5% to 1%. If the procedure is performed before 15 weeks, the pregnancy loss is two to three times greater.[7]

Chorionic Villus Sampling

Chorionic villus sampling is best performed between 10 and 12 weeks of gestation. The approach may be transcervical or transabdominal. When this procedure is compared with midtrimester amniocentesis, an excess of pregnancy loss between 0.5% and 4.5% is reported. However, fetal loss with chorionic villus sampling is less than that with early (before 15 weeks) amniocentesis. The indications for chorionic villus sampling are similar to those for amniocentesis except that a few conditions such as osteogenesis imperfecta are better assessed by chorionic villus sampling.[7]

Maternal Serum Screening

The traditional triple maternal serum screening (MSS) test is performed in the second trimester and consists of measurements of maternal alpha-fetoprotein (AFP), unconjugated estriol (uE_3), and human chorionic gonadotropin (hCG). The quadruple test consists of these three tests plus an assessment of inhibin A.[8] An elevated maternal AFP level at 16 to 18 weeks suggests an elevated relative risk of a neural tube defect. A low AFP level in conjunction with a low uE_3 and an elevated hCG level suggests an elevated relative risk of Down syndrome (see below).

Maternal serum screening of all pregnancies would detect an estimated 60% to 70% of infants with Down syndrome and 80% of those with open neural tube defects. However, the positive predictive value (percentage of patients with positive tests who actually have the disorder) is very low. About 8% of women undergoing maternal serum screening would have an initial positive test (6% for Down syndrome, 1.6% for neural tube defect, and the remainder for other rare fetal anomalies), but only 1% to 2% of this 8% would actually have an abnormal baby; a negative test would not guarantee the absence of the anomalies being sought.[9]

The principal reason that parents seek prenatal diagnosis is to obtain reassurance that the baby is normal. In view of the very low positive predictive value of maternal serum screening, these wishes can be only partially met at the cost of many false-positive results. MSS tests should be ordered only if the patient is aware of the implications of positive and negative tests and has given informed consent. In most situations maternal serum screening would probably do more harm than good if the patient would not consider having an abortion should defects be detected.[10]

Down Syndrome

Eighty percent of children with Down syndrome (trisomy 21) are born to women younger than 35 years of age.[11] Maternal serum screening for Down syndrome is discussed previously.

The Canadian Task Force on Preventive Health Care estimates that if all women were screened for Down syndrome with the MSS test, 58% of cases would be detected. Of women screened, 0.1% (1:1000) would have true-positive results and 3.7% would have false-positive results.[9] Put another way, the positive predictive value would be a little less than 3%. Positive predictive values are higher when screening is limited to older women. In a study of maternal serum screening in women 35 years of age or older, 89% of Down syndrome cases were detected (11% false-negative rate), but the false-positive rate was 25%.[12]

Both the Canadian Task Force on Preventive Health Care[9] and the U.S. Preventive Services Task Force[13] give a "B" recommendation to maternal serum screening of women under the age of 35, within the context of a comprehensive program, and they also give a "B" recommendation for chorionic villus sampling or amniocentesis in pregnant women over the age of 35. An alternative to amniocentesis or chorionic villus sampling for women over 35 could be maternal serum screening.[9,13]

A new technique of screening for trisomy 21 is the assessment of nuchal translucency thickness (a reflection of nuchal edema) by ultrasonography between weeks 10 and 14. This procedure is reported to detect not only trisomy 21, but also a number of other chromosomal defects. In one report of such a screening intervention using specially trained ultrasonographers, 80% of trisomy 21 pregnancies were identified, but because the positive predictive value of the test is low, 30 invasive tests (amniocentesis or chorionic villus sampling) were required to detect one affected infant. This is similar to the number of invasive tests required to detect one affected infant when maternal serum screening is used to find the disorder.[14] Sensitivity for detecting Down syndrome in the first trimester is improved by combining ultrasound assessment of nuchal translucency with measurements of serum pregnancy-associated plasma protein A and the free beta subunit of human chorionic gonadotropin. In Down syndrome, serum levels of pregnancy-associated plasma protein A tend to be low and levels of the free beta subunit of human chorionic gonadotropin high. However, even with this combination, the false-positive rate remains high.[8] Improved specificity (fewer false positives) could be achieved by combining first- and second-trimester screening results (integrated test).[8] Whether integrated testing would be acceptable to patients is uncertain, since many women would either have to live for several weeks with abnormal results from first-trimester testing while awaiting second-trimester results or not be told first-trimester results until the second-trimester tests were also done.[11]

Neural Tube Defects

The incidence of neural tube defects varies from a low of 5 per 10,000 live births in Switzerland to a high of 57 in Northern China. The rate is 9 in the United States and 33 in Mexico.[15]

Between 90% and 95% of neural tube defects occur in families with no history of the disorder. However, the risk is much higher if there is a family history of neural tube defects. If a woman has had one affected infant, the chance of having a second affected infant is increased 10 fold for an absolute rate of 2% to 3%.[16]

Daily administration of folic acid for the month before conception and for the first trimester reduces the incidence of neural tube defects by at least 50%. Although this is well known, only about one third of U.S. women of childbearing age take folic acid supplements.[17]

Secondary prevention of neural tube defects is based on screening maternal serum for AFP. If the AFP level is elevated, a confirmatory repeat examination is performed followed by high-resolution ultrasonography and, if the latter is not definitive, amniocentesis with assessment of amniotic fluid AFP. In low-risk women, ultrasonography alone may be an adequate screening technique.[16,18]

Both the U.S. Preventive Services Task Force[18] and the Canadian Task Force on Preventive Health Care[16] give an "A" recommendation for prescribing folic acid 4 mg/day to women with a family or personal history of having an infant with a neural tube defect and for prescribing 0.4 mg/day[16] or 0.4 to 0.8 mg/day[18] to all women capable of becoming pregnant. (Most multivitamins contain at least 0.4 mg of folic acid, but a few contain less. Patients should be instructed to check the label carefully before purchasing a particular brand.) MSS for AFP at 16 to 18 weeks gets a "B" recommendation from both task forces provided it is part of a quality-controlled program.[16,18]

The Canadian Task Force states that ultrasonography may be adequate for low-risk women if performed between 16 and 18 weeks ("B" recommendation),[16] whereas the U.S. Preventive Services Task Force gives midtrimester ultrasound screening for this purpose a "C" recommendation.[18]

Congenital Heart Disease

A case-control study found that women who took multivitamins around the time of conception had a 43% lower risk of having babies with conotruncal defects of the heart. The major defects involved were tetralogy of Fallot, transposition of the great vessels, and truncus arteriosus.[19]

Increased nuchal translucency detected by ultrasound between 10 and 14 weeks of gestation is present in most fetuses that have major cardiac malformations (the translucency is caused by edema).[20] Whether such screening with subsequent assessment by specialist fetal echocardiography causes more harm than good is uncertain. Screening would find a fetus with increased nuchal translucency in 5% of all pregnant women, but the positive predictive value of the test is low—123 women would have to undergo fetal echocardiography to detect one viable infant with major cardiac anomalies.

─────────────── ❧ **REFERENCES** ❧ ───────────────

1. Lie RT, Wilcox AJ, Skærven R: A population-based study of the risk of recurrence of birth defects, *N Engl J Med* 331:1-4, 1994.
2. Skjaerven R, Wilcox AJ, Lie RT: A population-based study of survival and childbearing among female subjects with birth defects and the risk of recurrence in their children, *N Engl J Med* 340:1057-1062, 1999.
3. Cao A, Saba L, Galanello R, et al: Molecular diagnosis and carrier screening for β thalassemia, *JAMA* 278:1273-1277, 1997.
4. Eng CM, Schechter C, Robinwitz J, et al: Prenatal genetic carrier testing using triple disease screening, *JAMA* 278:1268-1272, 1997.
5. Kronn D, Jansen V, Ostrer H: Carrier screening for cystic fibrosis, Gaucher disease and Tay-Sachs disease in the Ashkenazi Jewish population, *Arch Intern Med* 158:777-781, 1998.
6. Czeizel AE: Nutritional supplementation and prevention of congenital abnormalities, *Curr Opin Obstet Gynecol* 7:88-94, 1995.
7. Kuller JA, Laifer SA: Contemporary approaches to prenatal diagnosis, *Am Fam Physician* 52:2277-2281, 1995.
8. Wald NJ, Watt HC, Hackshaw AK: Integrated screening for Down's syndrome based on tests performed during the first and second trimesters, *N Engl J Med* 341:461-467, 1999.
9. Dick PT (Canadian Task Force on the Periodic Health Examination): Periodic health examination, 1996 update. I. Prenatal screening for and diagnosis of Down syndrome, *Can Med Assoc J* 154:465-479, 1996.
10. Zamorski MA: Prenatal diagnosis: more than meets the eye (editorial), *Am Fam Physician* 52:2173-2177, 1995.
11. Copel JA, Bahado-Singh RO: Prenatal screening for Down's syndrome — a search for the family's values (editorial), *N Engl J Med* 341:521-522, 1999.

12. Haddow JE, Palomaki GE, Knight GJ, et al: Reducing the need for amniocentesis in women 35 years of age or older with serum markers for screening, *N Engl J Med* 330:1114-1118, 1994.

13. US Preventive Services Task Force: *Guide to clinical preventive services,* ed 2, Baltimore, 1996, Williams & Wilkins, pp 449-465.

14. Snijders RJ, Noble P, Sebire N, et al: UK multicentre project on assessment of risk of trisomy 21 by maternal age and fetal nuchal-translucency thickness at 10-14 weeks of gestation, *Lancet* 352:343-346, 1998.

15. Botto LD, Moore CA, Khoury MJ, et al: Neural-tube defects, *N Engl J Med* 341:1509-1519, 1999.

16. Canadian Task Force on the Periodic Health Examination: Periodic health examination, 1994 update. III. Primary and secondary prevention of neural tube defects, *Can Med Assoc J* 151:159-166, 1994.

17. From the Centers for Disease Control and Prevention: Use of folic acid–containing supplements among women of childbearing age—United States, 1997, *JAMA* 279:1430, 1998.

18. US Preventive Services Task Force: *Guide to clinical preventive services,* ed 2, Baltimore, 1996, Williams & Wilkins, pp 467-483.

19. Botto LD, Khoury MJ, Mulinare J, et al: Periconceptional multivitamin use and the occurrence of conotruncal heart defects—results from a population-based, case-control study, *Pediatrics* 98:911-917, 1996.

20. Hyett J, Perdu M, Sharland G, et al: Using fetal nuchal translucency to screen for major congenital cardiac defects at 10-14 weeks of gestation: population based cohort study, *BMJ* 318:81-85, 1999.

21. Mol BW: Down's syndrome, cardiac anomalies, and nuchal translucency: fetal heart failure might link nuchal translucency and Down's syndrome (editorial), *BMJ* 318:70-71, 1999.

DRUGS AND CHEMICALS IN PREGNANCY

(See also alopecia; breast feeding; hypertensive disorders of pregnancy; nausea and vomiting in pregnancy)

Acid-Suppressing Drugs

H_2 blockers do not appear to be teratogenic. The best studied is ranitidine (Zantac). Few studies have been done with proton pump inhibitors, but so far no evidence has been found that omeprazole (Prilosec, Losec) is associated with an increased risk of malformations.[1] Misoprostol (Cytotec and one of the drugs in Arthrotec) should not be used because of an increased risk of Möbius' syndrome (congenital facial paralysis).[2,3]

⊿ REFERENCES ⊾

1. Lalkin A, Magee L, Addis A, et al: Motherrisk update: acid-suppressing drugs during pregnancy, *Can Fam Physician* 43:1923-1924, 1997.

2. Koren G, Pastuszak A, Ito S: Drugs in pregnancy, *N Engl J Med* 338:1128-1137, 1998.

3. Pastusazak AL, Schüler L, Speck-Martins CE, et al: Use of misoprostol during pregnancy and Möbius' syndrome in infants, *N Engl J Med* 338:1881-1885, 1998.

Alcohol

(See also attention deficit disorder; conduct disorder)

Epidemiological evidence suggests that the incidence of the fetal alcohol syndrome is 10% in pregnant women who drink fewer than eight drinks a week and up to 30% to 40% in women who drink more than that. It also seems likely that binge drinking is particularly likely to cause the syndrome. Many women who have had a few social drinks before they were aware they were pregnant become panic stricken at the thought they may have harmed their infant, but no reliable evidence has shown that mild social drinking in pregnancy is detrimental.[1]

Characteristics of the fetal alcohol syndrome are prenatal and postnatal growth retardation, microcephaly, hypotonia, mental retardation, microphthalmia, short palpebral fissures (distance from inner to outer canthi), thin upper lip, and poorly developed philtrum (groove on upper lip). Some of the facial abnormalities are difficult to discern in the newborn but become more obvious as the child develops. In recent years it has become apparent that full-blown fetal alcohol syndrome did not always develop in children born to women who drank excessively during pregnancy. Instead many children manifested selective cognitive disabilities, behavioral dysfunction such as poor ability to socialize, and in later life delinquency, substance abuse, and inappropriate sexual activity. This modified syndrome is called fetal alcohol effects.[2]

⊿ REFERENCES ⊾

1. Koren G: Alcohol consumption in early pregnancy: how much will harm a fetus? *Can Fam Physician* 42:2141-2143, 1996.

2. Koren G, Loebstein R, Nulman I: Fetal alcohol syndrome: role of the family physician, *Can Fam Physician* 44:38-39, 1998.

Analgesics and Nonsteroidal Antiinflammatory Drugs

The analgesic drugs of choice in pregnancy are acetaminophen and codeine. Nonsteroidal antiinflammatory drugs and aspirin may be used in the first trimester but should not be used in the latter half of pregnancy, particularly the third trimester, because of an increased risk of constriction or closure of the fetal ductus arteriosus.[1]

⊿ REFERENCES ⊾

1. Koren G, Pastuszak A, Ito S: Drugs in pregnancy, *N Engl J Med* 338:1128-1137, 1998.

Antibacterials and Antiviral Agents

Acyclovir

Acyclovir (Zovirax) is not approved for use in pregnant women, but no evidence has shown that it is teratogenic.[1]

Clindamycin

Vaginal clindamycin is probably safe in pregnancy.[1]

Erythromycin estolate

Erythromycin estolate is contraindicated in pregnancy.[1]

Metronidazole

Oral metronidazole (Flagyl) is usually considered to be contraindicated in the first trimester, but vaginal metronidazole is probably safe.[1] Six prospective studies and one retrospective study of oral metronidazole use during the first trimester of pregnancy, as well as a metaanalysis of all seven of these studies, showed no increased incidence of teratogenesis.[2]

Quinolones

Quinolones such as norfloxacin (Noroxin), ofloxacin (Floxin), and ciprofloxacin (Cipro) are contraindicated in children because they have been shown to cause arthropathy in the weight-bearing joints of immature animals. However, they have not been shown to cause birth defects in experimental animals or in the limited studies that have been done in humans.[3] According to the *Medical Letter,* fluoroquinolones are contraindicated in pregnancy.[1]

Sulfonamides

Sulfonamides may be given in the first two trimesters of pregnancy.

Tetracyclines

Tetracyclines are contraindicated in pregnancy.[1]

REFERENCES

1. Drugs for sexually transmitted diseases, *Med Lett* 37:117-122, 1995.
2. Burtin P, Taddio A, Ariburnu O, et al: Safety of metronidazole in pregnancy: a meta-analysis, *Am J Obstet Gynecol* 172:525-529, 1995.
3. Koren G: Use of the new quinolones during pregnancy, *Can Fam Physician* 42:1097-1099, 1996.

Anticonvulsants in Pregnancy

(See also seizures)

Pregnant patients with seizure disorders who are not taking medications have an approximate risk of having an infant with congenital anomalies of 3% compared with a rate of 2% in the general population; if they are taking one antiepileptic medication, the rate is also 3%, but it increases to 5% with two, 10% with three, and 20% with four.[1] Benzodiazepines in combination with other antiepileptic drugs are also associated with an increased incidence of congenital anomalies.[2]

A common syndrome resulting from a variety of antiepileptic drugs is facial dimorphism, cleft lip, cleft palate, cardiac defects, hypoplasia of the digits, and nail dysplasia. Originally described as a complication of phenytoin (Dilantin), this syndrome is now known to be associated with other antiepileptic drugs, including carbamazepine (Tegretol) and valproate (Depakene, Depakote).[1] Phenytoin (Dilantin) is

associated with an increased risk of low intelligent quotients.[3,4] This effect is not seen with carbamazepine (Tegretol), which therefore is the anticonvulsant of choice in pregnancy.[4] Patients taking carbamazepine[1,3] or valproate[1,5] have an increased risk of neural tube defects. These patients should be given 4 or 5 mg of folate daily before and after conception, even though no studies evaluating the efficacy of such a protocol have been published.[1,5]

REFERENCES

1. Brodie MJ, Dichter MA: Antiepileptic drugs, *N Engl J Med* 334:168-175, 1996.
2. Samrén EB, van Duijn CM, Christiaens GC, et al: Antiepileptic drug regimens and major congenital abnormalities in the offspring, *Ann Neurol* 46:739-746, 1999.
3. Koren G: In utero exposure to phenytoin or carbamazepine, *Can Fam Physician* 41:1862-1863, 1995.
4. Scolnik D, Nulman I, Rovet J, et al: Neurodevelopment of children exposed in utero to phenytoin and carbamazepine monotherapy, *JAMA* 271:767-770, 1994.
5. Koren G: Safe use of valproic acid during pregnancy, *Can Fam Physician* 45:1451-1453, 1999.

Antihistamines

(See also antihistamines)

Tripelennamine (Pyribenzamine), chlorpheniramine (Chlor-Trimeton, Chlor-Tripolon), dexchlorpheniramine (Polaramine), dimenhydrinate (Dramamine, Gravol), and loratadine (Claritin) are all classified by the U.S. Food and Drug Administration as being in Category B, which means probably safe with no toxicity demonstrated in animal studies or controlled trials in women.[1] A 1997 metaanalysis of over 200,000 women who were exposed to a variety of antihistamines in the first trimester of pregnancy not only found no increase in the risk of congenital anomalies, but documented a slight decrease in risk. Possibly the use of antihistamines to control nausea and vomiting in pregnancy actually improves fetal outcomes.[2]

REFERENCES

1. Peggs JF, Shimp SA, Opdycke RAC: Antihistamines: the old and the new, *Am Fam Physician* 52:593-600, 1995.
2. Koren G: Antihistamines are safe during the first trimester, *Can Fam Physician* 43:33-34, 1997.

Antihypertensives

Antihypertensives are discussed in the section on hypertensive disorders of pregnancy.

Asthma Medications

None of the common asthma medications, including beta$_2$-adrenergic agonists, inhaled and oral steroids, cromolyn, and theophylline, have been shown to be teratogenic.[1,2] In one study asthmatic patients taking oral steroids had a slightly increased incidence of preeclampsia,[2] but since severe asthma is associated with maternal and fetal mortality, the benefits outweigh the risks.[1,2] Unfortunately, pregnant women with acute asthma exacerbations are less likely than nonpregnant women to receive oral corticosteroids during emergency room visits and are more likely to have continuing exacerbations. Pregnancy is an indication, not a contraindication, for prescribing oral corticosteroids during an asthmatic exacerbation.[3]

―――――――――― ◣ **REFERENCES** ◥ ―――――――――

1. Bailey B, Addis A: Motherrisk update: asthma during pregnancy, *Can Fam Physician* 43:1717-1718, 1997.
2. Schatz M, Zeiger RS, Harden K, et al: The safety of asthma and allergy medications during pregnancy, *J Allergy Clin Immunol* 100:301-306, 1997.
3. Cydulka RK, Emerman CL, Schreiber D, et al: Acute asthma among pregnant women presenting to the emergency department, *Am J Respir Crit Care Med* 160:887-892, 1999.

Caffeine

A case-control study found that the offspring of pregnant women drinking more than four cups of coffee a day had an increased risk of dying of sudden infant death syndrome.[1]

―――――――――― ◣ **REFERENCES** ◥ ―――――――――

1. Ford RP, Schluter PJ, Mitchell EA, et al: Heavy caffeine intake in pregnancy and sudden infant death syndrome, *Arch Dis Childhood* 78:9-13, 1998.

Chemicals

Aspartame,[1] cosmetics,[2] and hair care products[3] have not been reported to cause adverse effects in pregnancy. Pregnant women should not be exposed to mercury. Occupational exposure to mercury is increased in the amalgamation and paint production industries and in dentistry. The main dietary source is contaminated fish and seafood.[4] Organic solvents are teratogenic in experimental animals. A meta-analysis of five studies concluded that exposure to organic solvents during pregnancy increased the risk of major malformation (odds ratio 1.64),[5] but according to one prospective study the increase was seen predominantly in women who reported symptoms from their exposure to solvents.[6]

―――――――――― ◣ **REFERENCES** ◥ ―――――――――

1. Zuber C, Librizzi RJ, Bolognese RJ: Do aspartame and video display terminals pose pregnancy risks? *Postgrad Obstet Gynecol* 9:1-5, 1989.
2. Zuber C, Hom M, Vought L, et al: Common chemical exposures in pregnancy: cosmetics, paint fumes, and cold medications, *Postgrad Obstet Gynecol* 12:1-6, 1992.
3. Koren G: Hair care during pregnancy, *Can Fam Physician* 42:625-626, 1996.
4. Moienafshari R, Bar-Oz B, Koren G: Occupational exposure to mercury: what is a safe level? *Can Fam Physician* 45:43-45, 1999.
5. McMartin KI, Koren G: Exposure to organic solvents: does it adversely affect pregnancy? *Can Fam Physician* 45:1671-1673, 1999.
6. Khattak S, K-Moghtader G, McMartin K, et al: Pregnancy outcome following gestational exposure to organic solvents: a prospective controlled study, *JAMA* 281:1106-1109, 1999.

Dermatological Medications

Isotretinoin (Accutane) is teratogenic and strictly contraindicated in pregnancy,[1] and tazarotene (Tazorac) may be teratogenic.[2] A small series found no adverse effects to the fetus when women used topical tretinoin during pregnancy.[3]

―――――――――― ◣ **REFERENCES** ◥ ―――――――――

1. Atanackovic G, Koren G: Young women taking isotretinoin still conceive: role of physicians in preventing disaster, *Can Fam Physician* 45:289-292, 1999.
2. Federman DG, Froelich CW, Kirsner RS: Topical psoriasis therapy, *Am Fam Physician* 59:957-962, 1999.
3. Shapiro L, Pastuszak A, Curto G, et al: Is topical tretinoin safe during the first trimester? *Can Fam Physician* 44:495-498, 1998.

Dextromethorphan

Dextromethorphan is not teratogenic.[1]

―――――――――― ◣ **REFERENCES** ◥ ―――――――――

1. Einarson A, Koren G: Dextromethorphan, *Can Fam Physician* 45:2309-2310, 1999.

Psychiatric Medications

Antidepressants

A follow-up study of children exposed to tricyclic antidepressants or fluoxetine (Prozac) in the first trimester of pregnancy showed no abnormalities of cognitive, language, or behavioral development.[1,2] Several cohort studies have failed to document any risk of teratogenesis from taking fluoxetine in pregnancy,[3] and a prospective controlled study of women taking one of the selective serotonin reuptake inhibitors fluoxetine (Prozac), paroxetine (Paxil), and sertraline (Zoloft) during pregnancy also failed to find any evidence of adverse effects on the fetus.[4] No evidence of teratogenicity has been found in the few published studies of tricyclic antidepressants taken during the first trimester.[5]

Antipsychotics

The psychotic state itself may adversely affect fetal outcome, and neuroleptics may result in a very slight increase in congenital anomalies. Patients taking phenothiazines have a rate of 2.4% compared with a background rate of 2%.[5]

Benzodiazepines

There have been conflicting reports as to whether benzodiazepines increase the risk of cleft palate or cleft lip when taken during pregnancy. Since many women become pregnant while taking these drugs, anxiety and even some pregnancy terminations have resulted from concern about this eventuality. A recent analysis of the literature found that pooled data from cohort studies showed no relationship between first-trimester benzodiazepine use and facial clefts, whereas pooled data from case-control studies found a small but significant increase in both facial clefts and other major malformations. If facial clefts are present in a fetus, they may be detected by fetal ultrasound level 2 ultrasonography.[6]

Lithium

The incidence of Ebstein's anomaly is increased in patients taking lithium in the first trimester. Although the relative risk is increased 10 to 20 fold, the condition is rare; the absolute risk is about 1 : 1000 or 0.1%.[5] Ebstein's anomaly is distal displacement of the tricuspid valve into the right ventricle, which usually results in inadequate right ventricular outflow, tricuspid regurgitation, and sometimes cyanotic heart disease from a right-to-left atrial shunt.

≥ REFERENCES ≤

1. Koren G: First-trimester exposure to fluoxetine (Prozac): does it affect pregnancy outcome? *Can Fam Physician* 42:43-44, 1996.
2. Nulman I, Rovet J, Stewart DE, et al: Neurodevelopement of children exposed in utero to antidepressant drugs, *N Engl J Med* 336:258-262, 1997.
3. Robert E: Treating depression in pregnancy (editorial), *N Engl J Med* 335:1056-1059, 1996.
4. Kulin NA, Pastuszak A, Sage SR, et al: Pregnancy outcome following maternal use of the new selective serotonin reuptake inhibitors: a prospective controlled multicenter study, *JAMA* 279:609-610, 1998.
5. Altshuler LL, Cohen L, Szuba MP, et al: Pharmacologic management of psychiatric illness during pregnancy; dilemmas and guidelines, *Am J Psychiatry* 153:592-606, 1996.
6. Dolovich LR, Addis A, Vaillancourt JM, et al: Benzodiazepine use in pregnancy and major malformations or oral cleft: meta-analysis of cohort and case-control studies, *BMJ* 317:839-843, 1998.

Vitamin A Supplements in Pregnancy
(See also vitamin A)

In one study the odds ratio of having a child with a congenital anomaly was 4.8 for women taking vitamin A supplements of 10,000 IU or more compared with those taking 5000 IU or less. Among women taking more than 10,000 units, about 1 in 57 had a baby with congenital malformation attributable to the vitamin. These data do not apply to beta-carotene.

≥ REFERENCES ≤

1. Rothman KJ, Moore LL, Singer MR, et al: Teratogenicity of high vitamin A intake, *N Engl J Med* 333:1369-1373, 1995.

EPISIOTOMY

Midline episiotomies are almost routine procedures for the delivery of primiparous women in many North American obstetrical practices. Episiotomies have been thought to reduce the mechanical and metabolic morbidity of the infant, prevent perineal relaxation, and decrease the incidence of perineal pain, urinary incontinence, and sexual dysfunction.[1,2] As documented in a randomized controlled trial by Klein and associates,[2,3] there is no substance to these hypotheses. Patients who had episiotomies not only had more pain and sexual dysfunction, but also had a much higher incidence of third- and fourth-degree tears.[3] Labrecque and co-workers[4] in a retrospective cohort study involving over 4000 women also found a much higher rate of third- and fourth-degree tears in patients who had episiotomies. Family physicians who refer their patients for obstetrical care should determine whether their consultants are believers or nonbelievers in episiotomy because believers have great difficulty staying the knife even when they have agreed ahead of time to try to do so.[5]

≥ REFERENCES ≤

1. Helewa ME: Episiotomy and severe perineal trauma: of science and fiction (editorial), *Can Med Assoc J* 156:811-813, 1997.
2. Klein M, Gauthier R, Robbins JM, et al: Relation of episiotomy to perineal trauma and morbidity, sexual dysfunction, and pelvic floor relaxation, *Am J Obstet Gynecol* 171:591-598, 1994.
3. Klein MC, Gauthier RC, Jorgensen SH, et al: Does episiotomy prevent perineal trauma and pelvic floor relaxation? *Online J Curr Clin Trials* [serial online], Jul 1, 2 (Doc No 10), 1992.
4. Labrecque M, Baillargeon L, Dallaire M, et al: Association between median episiotomy and severe perineal lacerations in primiparous women, *Can Med Assoc J* 156:797-802, 1997.
5. Klein MC, Kaczorowski J, Robbins JM, et al: Physicians' beliefs and behaviour during a randomized controlled trial of episiotomy: consequences for women in their care, *Can Med Assoc J* 153:769-779, 1995.

EXERCISE IN PREGNANCY

Pregnancy is not a contraindication to exercises. A meta-analysis of moderate exercise in pregnancy (three to six times a week) found no adverse effects from a variety of exercise programs, including weight lifting, jogging, swimming, and biking.[1] Theoretical concerns about exercise and pregnancy are discussed in the ensuing paragraphs.

Hyperthermia

Exercise can increase body temperature to 39° to 40° C, and in experimental animals elevated temperature in the first trimester is associated with an increase in neural tube defects. No prospective studies have shown an increase in congenital malformations in humans as a result of increased body temperature brought about by exercise.[2]

Redistribution of Splanchnic Blood Flow

Splanchnic blood flow decreases significantly with exercise. No studies have shown that this has significant adverse effects.[2]

Fetal Distress

In most cases the fetal heart rate responds to maternal exercise by an increase of about 10 beats/min; in a few cases transient bradycardia occurs. No human studies have demonstrated an increased incidence of fetal distress as a result of exercise.[2]

Abortion

Few studies have considered the relationship between exercise around the time of conception or in the first trimester and the rate of spontaneous abortion. Available data show no increase in the rate of abortion among those who exercise,[2] but a decrease in the loss of fetuses with normal karyotypes.[3]

Labor

Exercise is not associated with premature rupture of the membranes or premature labor.[2]

Injury

Even though ligaments are lax in pregnancy, maternal injury rates are not reported to be increased in exercising pregnant women.[2]

Maternal Weight Gain

Normal maternal weight gain is not altered by exercise.[2]

Contraindications to Exercise in Pregnancy

Although the evidence clearly supports moderate exercise in normal pregnancies, this does not necessarily apply to women with a past history of obstetrical problems or current medical or obstetrical conditions that could be adversely affected by exercise. Obstetrical problems that are considered to be relative or absolute contraindications to exercise are two or more previous spontaneous abortions, an incompetent cervix, vaginal bleeding or placenta previa, ruptured membranes or premature labor, preeclampsia or toxemia, multiple pregnancies, and fetal growth retardation. General medical conditions that are relative or absolute contraindications to exercise are eating disorders, very low body fat, some forms of heart disease, anemia, and a number of other serious systemic diseases.[4]

───────────── ◣ **REFERENCES** ◪ ─────────────

1. Lokey EA, Tran ZV, Wells CL, et al: Effects of physical exercise on pregnancy outcomes: a meta-analytic review, *Med Sci Sports Exerc* 23:1234-1239, 1991.
2. Stevenson L: Exercise in pregnancy. I. Update on pathophysiology, *Can Fam Physician* 43:97-104, 1997.
3. Latka M, Kline J, Hatch M: Exercise and spontaneous abortion of known karyotype, *Epidemiology* 10:73-75, 1999.
4. Stevenson L: Exercise in pregnancy. II. Recommendations for individuals, *Can Fam Physician* 43:107-111, 1997.

GESTATIONAL DIABETES MELLITUS

(See also attitudes, physician; screening; surrogate outcomes)

Risk Factors

Gestational diabetes is said to affect 3% to 4% of pregnancies.[1] The following are classic risk factors[2]:
1. First-degree relative with diabetes
2. Older age
3. Obesity
4. Previous pregnancy with gestational diabetes
5. Previous macrosomatic infant
6. Previous unexplained near-term fetal death

Up to 50% of women with gestational diabetes have none of these risk factors.[2]

Pros and Cons of Screening

Patients with gestational diabetes mellitus have an increased incidence of macrosomatic infants, a higher rate of preeclampsia, and more Cesarean sections. Over the long term, one third of them will develop type 2 diabetes.[1] Identifying and treating patients with this condition have been assumed to decrease the morbidity of both infants and mothers, as well as infant mortality. In practice, even though treatment decreases the incidence of macrosomia,[3] this has not decreased the Cesarean section rate or altered maternal or neonatal morbidity.[1,2] Why the Cesarean section rate has not decreased is uncertain, but it may be because of the practice style of the attending obstetricians, which in this case is a propensity to perform Cesarean sections on patients with gestational diabetes even in the absence of specific clinical indications.[3] Both the U.S. Preventive Services Task Force[4] and the Canadian Task Force on Preventive Health Care[5] have concluded that the evidence is insufficient to recommend universal screening, and they give this procedure a "C" recommendation. At present the vast majority of North American women are screened for gestational diabetes.[1]

An alternative to universal screening is selective screening of high-risk women, an approach endorsed by the American College of Obstetricians and Gynecologists,[6] the American Diabetes Association,[7] and the Canadian Diabetes Association.[8] In practice, almost all pregnant women would be screened because the only ones considered to be at low risk are thin white women under the age of 25 who have not had large babies and who have no family history of diabetes.[8] As the Canadian guidelines point out, these recommendations are based on expert opinion, not evidence.[8]

Method of Screening for Gestational Diabetes

Screening is usually performed between 24 and 28 weeks of gestation by measuring plasma glucose level 1 hour after a

50-g oral glucose load that can be given at any time of day regardless of when meals are taken. If the level is 7.8 mmol/L (140 mg/dl) or higher, a glucose tolerance test is indicated; if the level is 10.3 mmol/L (185 mg/dl) or higher, gestational diabetes mellitus can be diagnosed.[8]

The optimal glucose tolerance test involves measuring a fasting plasma glucose level followed by plasma glucose levels 1 and 2 hours after the oral ingestion of 75 mg of glucose. The upper limits of normal are 5.3 mmol/L (95 mg/dl) for the fasting specimen, 10.6 mmol/L (190 mg/dl) for the 1-hour specimen, and 8.9 mmol/L (160 mg/dl) for the 2-hour specimen. If any two readings exceed these limits, gestational diabetes is diagnosed; if only one is exceeded, the diagnosis is "impaired glucose tolerance of pregnancy."[8]

Management

Initial management of gestational diabetes is diet, exercise, and careful home glucose monitoring. Optimal glucose levels are no higher than 5.3 mmol/L (95 mg/dl) fasting, no higher than 7.8 mmol/L (140 mg/dl) 1 hour postprandial, and no higher than 6.7 mmol/L (120 mg/dl) 2 hours postprandial. If optimal glucose levels cannot be maintained by diet and exercise, insulin therapy should be started.[8] Although most protocols for insulin treatment of gestational diabetes involve twice daily doses of mixtures of regular and intermediate-acting insulins, an Israeli study found better control of mothers' diabetes and less hyperbilirubinemia and fewer hypoglycemic reactions in infants if a four-dose insulin regimen was used—three doses of regular insulin before meals and a dose of intermediate-acting insulin at bedtime.[9]

◤ REFERENCES ◢

1. Naylor CD, Sermer M, Chen E, et al: Selective screening for gestational diabetes mellitus, *N Engl J Med* 337:1591-1596, 1997.
2. Greene MF: Screening for gestational diabetes mellitus (editorial), *N Engl J Med* 337:1625-1626, 1997.
3. Naylor CD, Sermer M, Chen E, et al (Toronto Trihospital Gestational Diabetes Investigators): Cesarean delivery in relation to birth weight and gestational glucose tolerance: pathophysiology or practice style? *JAMA* 275:1165-1170, 1996.
4. US Preventive Services Task Force: *Guide to clinical preventive services,* ed 2, Baltimore, 1996, Williams & Wilkins, pp 193-208.
5. Canadian Task Force on the Periodic Health Examination: *Clinical preventive health care,* Ottawa, 1994, Canadian Communication Group—Publishing, pp 16-23.
6. *Diabetes and pregnancy,* ACOG technical bulletin 200, Washington, DC, 1994, American College of Obstetricians and Gynecologists.
7. Expert Committee on the Diagnosis and Classification of Diabetes Mellitus: Report of the Expert Committee on the Diagnosis and Classification of Diabetes Mellitus, *Diabetes Care* 20:1183-1197, 1997.
8. Meltzer S, Leither L, Daneman D, et al: 1998 Clinical practice guidelines for the management of diabetes in Canada, *Can Med Assoc J* 159(suppl 8):SI-S29, 1998.
9. Nachum Z, Ben-Shlomo I, Shalev E: Twice daily versus four times daily insulin dose regimens for diabetes in pregnancy: randomised controlled trial, *BMJ* 319:1223-1227, 1999.

GROUP B STREPTOCOCCAL DISEASE
(See also clinical practice guidelines; prevention; screening)

Group B *Streptococcus (Streptococcus agalactiae)* is an important cause of neonatal infections, and in high-risk circumstances, which are outlined below, the administration of intrapartum antibiotics decreases the incidence of neonatal infection.[1,2] Early prenatal screening of women for group B *Streptococcus* does not predict whether colonization will exist at the time of delivery,[1] and treatment of women carrying group B *Streptococcus* before delivery does not decrease the incidence of neonatal sepsis.[1,3,4] The efficacy of detecting *Streptococcus* B by cultures increases if swabs are taken from both the lower third of the vagina and the anorectal canal and if the microbiology laboratory uses selective rather than nonselective growth medium.[1,5]

An estimated 15% to 40% of pregnant women will have a positive vaginal or rectal culture for group B *Streptococcus,* and vertical transmission of the organism to the neonate occurs in 40% to 73% of women who carry the organism. However, infection develops in only 1% to 2% of infants who are colonized.[2] Risk factors during labor for neonatal infection with group B *Streptococcus* include preterm labor, premature rupture of membranes, prolonged rupture of membranes, and fever.[2,3]

Guidelines for the detection and management of group B *Streptococcus* in pregnancy have been issued by the Centers for Disease Control and Prevention and are supported by the American College of Obstetricians and Gynecologists and the American Academy of Pediatrics. They are as follows[6]:

1. Screening of all women between weeks 35 and 37 and treatment during labor of all women who are carriers whether or not they have risk factors. If culture results are not available at the time of delivery, treatment should be instituted only if risk factors are present (see below).[6] Cultures should be taken from both the lower vagina and the anorectum using one or two swabs.[6] One major problem with implementing this approach in regions where antenatal care takes place in private offices is ensuring that the antenatal culture results are available in the hospital at the time of delivery.[4] Other problems identified by surveys of obstetricians in the United States are that cultures are often taken from the vagina only and not the vagina and rectum[1,3] and, more important, that the vast majority of clinicians treat detected carriers as soon as the culture reports are received (during the antepartum period) even though the literature clearly states that this is an unacceptable practice.[1-4]

2. No screening for *Streptococcus* B is performed, but treatment is given to all women who have risk factors: gestation less than 37 weeks, rupture of membranes greater than 18 hours, and temperature of 38° C (100.4° F) or higher.[6] In one study only 15% of surveyed obstetricians actually used antibiotics when these conditions were met.[1]

3. Special categories.[6]

   a. Women who have previously delivered a child in whom group B streptococcal disease developed do not need to be screened for the organism because all of them should be treated during the intrapartum period anyway.

   b. Women who are found to have symptomatic or asymptomatic group B streptococcal bacteriuria should be treated both at the time of diagnosis and during the intrapartum period; vaginal and rectal screening is unnecessary because they should be treated anyway.

------------------------ ◤ REFERENCES ◣ ------------------------

1. Jafari HS, Schuchat A, Hilsdon R, et al: Barriers to prevention of perinatal group B streptococcal disease, *Pediatr Infect Dis J* 14:662-667, 1995.

2. Gigante J, Hickson GB, Entman SS, et al: Universal screening for group B *Streptococcus:* recommendations and obstetricians' practice decisions, *Obstet Gynecol* 85:440-443, 1995.

3. Mercer BM, Ramsey RD, Sibai BM: Prenatal screening for group B *Streptococcus.* I. Impact of antepartum screening on antenatal prophylaxis and intrapartum care, *Am J Obstet Gynecol* 173:837-841, 1995.

4. Larsen JW, Dooley SL: Group B streptococcal infections: an obstetrical viewpoint, *Pediatrics* 91:148-149, 1993.

5. Mercer BM, Briggs R: Group B *Streptococcus* and pregnancy, *Pediatr Ann* 25:206-214, 1996.

6. American Academy of Pediatrics Committee on Infectious Diseases and Committee on Fetus and Newborn: Revised guidelines for prevention of early-onset group B streptococcal (GBS) infection, *Pediatrics* 99:489-496, 1997.

HYPERTENSIVE DISORDERS OF PREGNANCY

(See also hypertension)

Classification

The hypertensive disorders of pregnancy may be divided into four main categories. The terminology used for these disorders is confusing. In the list below, traditional terms are followed in parentheses by terms recommended by the Canadian Hypertension Society[1,2]:

1. Chronic hypertension (preexisting hypertension)

2. Gestational hypertension (gestational hypertension without proteinuria)

3. Preeclampsia (gestational hypertension with proteinuria)

4. Chronic hypertension with superimposed preeclampsia (preexisting hypertension plus superimposed gestational hypertension with proteinuria)

Definition

Hypertension in pregnancy has been traditionally defined as any reading over 140/90 mm Hg.[1,2] In addition, several guidelines have recommended that the diagnosis be made if there is an increase of the systolic level by 30 mm Hg or of the diastolic level by 15 mm Hg compared with average readings before 20 weeks' gestation.[3,4] The Canadian Hypertension Society rejects changing blood pressure levels during pregnancy as a criterion for hypertension because rises above these levels occur commonly and do not result in the detection of more true cases of hypertension than are found by using absolute figures alone.[2,5]

Prevention

A 1996 metaanalysis concluded that calcium supplements were effective in preventing preeclampsia,[6] whereas a large randomized trial found no benefit.[7] A further evaluation of these two studies concluded that calcium supplementation has no value for low-risk women but may be of value for high-risk women and that more studies are necessary.[8]

Laboratory Investigations

Standard investigations for patients with hypertensive disorders of pregnancy include a complete blood count and platelet count, urinalysis, and measurements of serum uric acid, serum creatinine, and liver enzymes.[2]

Nonpharmacological Management

Nonpharmacological interventions may be used for the management of patients with systolic readings of 140 to 150 mm Hg or diastolic readings of 90/100 mm Hg provided there are no complicating maternal or fetal conditions requiring pharmacological interventions. At present this consists primarily of watchful waiting; the traditional therapeutic modalities of strict bed rest and salt restriction have no value.[5]

Pharmacological Management

Medications are required for all women with systolic pressures above 169 mm Hg or diastolic pressures above 109 mm Hg.[1,9] Decisions about pharmacotherapy have to take into account the gestational age, the presence or absence of proteinuria, and perhaps evidence of end organ damage such as cardiac hypertrophy.[9]

Many antihypertensive drugs are either contraindicated in pregnancy or inadequately studied. Methyldopa (Aldomet) is the drug of first choice for outpatient pharmacotherapy in nonsevere hypertension. Second-line drugs for nonsevere hypertension in pregnancy include labetalol (Trandate), pindolol (Visken), oxprenolol (Trasicor), and nifedipine (Adalat, Procardia). For severe hypertension of pregnancy the first-line drug is hydralazine (Apresoline) and second-line drugs are labetalol and nifedipine. ACE inhibitors and angiotensin II receptor antagonists are contraindicated in pregnancy.[1,9]

Chronic Hypertension (Preexisting Hypertension)

The diagnosis of chronic hypertension is made when patients have a history of hypertension before pregnancy or when the blood pressure is 140/90 mm Hg or higher before 20 weeks of gestation. Use of the latter criterion results in many missed cases because blood pressure normally drops during the second trimester. In the majority of trials of antihypertensive drug treatment for mildly hypertensive women no beneficial effects for mother or fetus have been noted in the treatment groups compared with the placebo or the no medication groups. Most women with chronic hypertension who have systolic levels below 170 or diastolic levels below 110 mm Hg do not require pharmacotherapy.[1]

Gestational Hypertension (Gestational Hypertension Without Proteinuria)

Gestational hypertension is the new onset of hypertension after 20 weeks' gestation without associated symptoms or signs of preeclampsia. In general, drug treatment is not required and pregnancy outcome is good.[1]

Preeclampsia (Gestational Hypertension with Proteinuria)

A working clinical definition of preeclampsia is hypertension plus hyperuricemia or proteinuria. (Proteinuria is defined as 1+ on dipstick on two or more occasions, or 300 mg [0.3 g] or higher in a 24-hour urine collection.) The severity of preeclampsia is measured by the degree of hypertension and proteinuria. Edema is common but is not necessary for the diagnosis.[1,3] The problem with this or any other clinical definition is that patients may have the disorder without hypertension or proteinuria. For example, 20% of women in whom seizures (eclampsia) later develop have diastolic blood pressure readings below 90 mm Hg or no proteinuria.[1]

A probable explanation for the lack of hypertension or proteinuria in some women who later have serious disease is that one of the basic pathophysiological abnormalities is reduced vascular perfusion, which is often localized. If decreased perfusion does not involve the glomeruli, proteinuria will not occur. Another basic abnormality in preeclampsia is endothelial cell dysfunction, which can cause increased vascular permeability with edema, thromboses, and low platelet counts.[1,3]

Risk factors for preeclampsia include first pregnancy, family history of preeclampsia, previous personal history of preeclampsia, older age, preexisting hypertension, diabetes, multiple pregnancies, hydatidiform mole, and hydrops fetalis.[3] Women with preeclampsia are at greater risk for seizures, cerebral hemorrhage, liver and renal failure, disseminated intravascular coagulation, abruptio placentae, and fetal growth retardation.[1] Although a number of reports have suggested that low-dose aspirin might prevent preeclampsia, this has not been substantiated by subsequent randomized controlled trials.[10,11]

Management of mild preeclampsia is controversial. Whether bed rest, hospitalization, antihypertensive therapy,

or prophylactic anticonvulsants are beneficial is unknown, but it is generally agreed that if the woman is at 34 weeks or more and the cervix is favorable for induction, immediate delivery should be undertaken. In all cases close monitoring (weight, fetal status, blood pressure, proteinuria, and platelet count) is needed because the preeclampsia may progress rapidly.[1]

Women with severe preeclampsia who are at 34 or more weeks of gestation require immediate delivery, as do many who are at an earlier stage. For those with a diastolic pressure of 110 mm Hg or more, the usual medical treatment is IV hydralazine (Apresoline) or, if it is contraindicated, IV labetalol or oral nifedipine.[1,9]

Prophylactic anticonvulsants are often given to patients with severe preeclampsia even though no good evidence supports such an intervention. In North America magnesium sulfate is the drug most frequently used, whereas in Europe the more common practice has been antihypertensive therapy with or without phenytoin (Dilantin).[1] One trial comparing the prophylactic use of magnesium sulfate with phenytoin in women with preeclampsia demonstrated a small benefit for the magnesium sulfate–treated group.[12] Magnesium sulfate is the anticonvulsant of choice for women with eclampsia.[13] It is the drug recommended by the Canadian Hypertension Society.[9]

HELLP Syndrome

The acronym HELLP stands for *h*emolysis, *e*levated *l*iver enzymes, and *l*ow *p*latelet counts. It most frequently occurs as a complication of severe preeclampsia, but it can develop in pregnant women who are normotensive and have no proteinuria and even in postpartum women. Ninety percent of patients with the HELLP syndrome have right upper quadrant pain secondary to focal hepatic necrosis. At the slightest suspicion of this condition a complete blood count and blood smear should be obtained. The blood smear may reveal the presence of fragmented red cells (schistocytes), which are usually seen in microangiopathic conditions such as this.[14]

_____ ◥ **REFERENCES** ◤ _____

1. Sibai BM: Treatment of hypertension in pregnant women, *N Engl J Med* 335:257-265, 1996.
2. Helewa ME, Burrows RF, Smith J, et al: Report of the Canadian Hypertension Society Consensus Conference. 1. Definitions, evaluation and classification of hypertensive disorders in pregnancy, *Can Med Assoc J* 157:715-725, 1997.
3. Zamorski MA, Green LA: Preeclampsia and hypertensive disorders of pregnancy, *Am Fam Physician* 53:1595-1604, 1996.
4. National High Blood Pressure Education Program Working Group report on high blood pressure in pregnancy, *Am J Obstet Gynecol* 163(5 Pt 1):1691-1712, 1990.
5. Moutquin J-M, Garner PR, Burrows RF: Report of the Canadian Hypertension Society Consensus Conference. 2. Nonpharmacologic management and prevention of hypertensive disorders in pregnancy, *Can Med Assoc J* 157:907-919, 1997.

6. Bucher HC, Guyatt GH, Cook RJ, et al: Effect of calcium supplementation on pregnancy-induced hypertension and preeclampsia: a meta-analysis of randomized controlled trials, *JAMA* 275:1113-1117, 1996.

7. Levine RJ, Hauth JC, Curet LB, et al: Trial of calcium to prevent preeclampsia, *N Engl J Med* 337:69-76, 1997.

8. DerSimonian R, Levine RJ: Resolving discrepancies between a meta-analysis and a subsequent large controlled trial, *JAMA* 282:664-670, 1999.

9. Rey É, LeLorier J, Burgess E, et al: Report of the Canadian Hypertension Society Consensus Conference. 3. Pharmacologic treatment of hypertensive disorders in pregnancy, *Can Med Assoc J* 157:1245-1254, 1997.

10. Cartis S, Sibai V, Hauth J, et al: Low-dose aspirin to prevent preeclampsia in women at high risk, *N Engl J Med* 338:701-705, 1998.

11. Duley L: Aspirin for preventing and treating pre-eclampsia: large trials continue to show no benefit (editorial), *BMJ* 318:751-752, 1999.

12. Lucas MJ, Leveno KJ, Cunningham FG: A comparison of magnesium sulfate with phenytoin for the prevention of preeclampsia, *N Engl J Med* 333:201-205, 1995.

13. Eclampsia Trial Collaborative Group: Which anticonvulsant for women with eclampsia? Evidence from the Collaborative Eclampsia Trial, *Lancet* 242:1455-1463, 1995.

14. Stone JH: HELLP syndrome: hemolysis, elevated liver enzymes, and low platelets, *JAMA* 280:559-562, 1998.

INFECTIOUS DISEASES IN PREGNANCY

(See also erythema infectiosum; HIV and AIDS)

Erythema Infectiosum

Erythema infectiosum is caused by parvovirus B19 and usually affects children between the ages of 5 and 14 years. It is contagious for 5 to 10 days before the onset of the rash, but not once the rash has appeared. Fifty percent of adults have acquired immunity. Among infants carried by women who became infected with parvovirus B19 during the first 20 weeks of pregnancy, 20% develop a nonimmune form of hydrops fetalis because of transient red blood cell aplasia. Although a few cases of fetal loss result from this infection, spontaneous recovery without sequelae is the usual outcome.[1]

Pregnant women who have been exposed to erythema infectiosum should be tested for specific IgG and IgM antibodies. If IgG antibody is present, the patient is immune, and if neither antibody is present, she is not infected but remains at risk. If IgM antibodies develop, the woman should be carefully monitored with serial ultrasounds to detect the presence of hydrops. In a very few cases fetal blood transfusions are indicated, but in most instances the condition resolves spontaneously.[1]

Herpes Simplex

The risk of transmitting herpes simplex virus (HSV) to the neonate is up to 50% in cases of primary herpes, whereas for women with recurrent episodes it is only 2% to 3%

with vaginal birth even in the presence of lesions. The lesser risk with recurrent herpes is due in part to a lesser quantity of virus and in part to the presence of protective IgG in the baby. Serial cultures of HSV during the last weeks of pregnancy are no longer advised. The current recommendation of both the Society of Obstetricians and Gynecologists of Canada and the American College of Obstetricians and Gynecologists is to examine the vulva, buttocks, and thighs for lesions and offer Cesarean section if they are present.[2]

HIV and AIDS

The risks of vertical transmission of HIV and methods of management of the infection in pregnant women are discussed in the section on HIV and AIDS.

Mumps

Mumps is very rare in pregnancy. It is not known to be teratogenic. Women who have the disease in the first trimester have a higher incidence of spontaneous abortions.[3]

Rubella

Rubella is contagious from a few days before the appearance of the rash until 5 to 7 days after its development. About half of those who acquire the disease are asymptomatic. In North America lack of immunity is most common in recent immigrants and refugees.[4]

Major features of the congenital rubella syndrome are cataracts, sensorineural hearing loss, and congenital heart disease, especially patent ductus arteriosus and pulmonary stenosis. Other features that may be seen are microphthalmia, retinopathy, and intrauterine growth retardation. The congenital rubella syndrome occurs only when the mother is infected with rubella in the first 20 weeks of gestation, and the earlier the infection occurs, the greater the risk. Between one fifth and one third of infants born to mothers infected during the first 20 weeks of pregnancy are affected. Although rubella vaccine is contraindicated in pregnancy, no cases of congenital rubella syndrome have been reported in women who accidentally received such vaccinations in early pregnancy.[4]

If a woman whose immune status to rubella is unknown is exposed to the disease, she should be tested for rubella IgG within 7 days. If the test is positive, the patient is immune, but if it is negative, she should be tested for rubella IgG and IgM after 3 weeks. Recent infection is indicated by either the new development of IgM or a four-fold or greater increase in IgG. If serological tests are positive, infection of the fetus can be diagnosed prenatally by testing fetal blood for rubella-specific IgM or by chorionic villus biopsy and polymerase chain reaction assessment.[4]

Rubeola

Rubeola is very rare in pregnancy. No evidence of teratogenesis or spontaneous abortion in infected women has been reported. The risk of premature labor, spontaneous abortion, and neonatal mortality is slightly increased.[5]

Toxoplasmosis

Toxoplasmosis acquired by the mother during pregnancy, even if asymptomatic, may infect the fetus and cause a variety of disorders such as chorioretinitis, developmental delay, and hearing loss.[6] The risk of vertical transmission is much greater in late pregnancy than in early pregnancy, but the risk of clinical disease in the infant is much greater when maternal infection is acquired early in pregnancy.[7]

About two thirds of women in Canada have no protective immunity. Measures for preventing infection include avoiding undercooked meat and unpasteurized milk; carefully washing raw foods, utensils, counters, and hands during the preparation of food; wearing gloves while gardening; and washing hands after contact with soil or sand. Cats, particularly kittens, can transmit the infection through their feces. Cats should not be fed undercooked meat, and kitty litter should be changed daily because the toxoplasmosis oocysts take 2 to 3 days to become infectious. If possible the litter change should be done by a nonpregnant person. However, it can safely be done by the pregnant woman if she wears gloves, washes her hands afterward, and disinfects the litter box with boiling water (see also discussion of HIV and AIDS).[6]

Screening pregnant women for toxoplasmosis is a routine practice in some European countries such as Austria and France. A systematic literature review concluded that the value of screening pregnant women for toxoplasmosis or treating those who are infected is uncertain.[8]

Varicella

The risk of acquiring varicella in pregnancy is low, 1 to 7 per 10,000 pregnancies. The disease is infectious from 2 days before the onset of the eruption until all the vesicles have crusted, which usually takes about 5 days.[9] The most feared complication of varicella in pregnancy is congenital varicella embryopathy (limb hypoplasia, skin scarring, eye defects, and neurological abnormalities). When mothers are infected in the first 20 weeks of pregnancy, 2.2% of infants are affected by the syndrome.[10] Treatment of the mother with antiviral medications does not alter that risk.[9]

Varicella in pregnancy puts the mother at increased risk because the mortality of varicella pneumonia during pregnancy is high. Should maternal varicella develop during the peripartum period, the infant is at high risk for varicella and should receive varicella zoster immune globulin (VZIG).[9]

If a pregnant women with no history of chickenpox is exposed to an infected person, her antibody status should be determined (over 85% of women who do not know if they have had chickenpox are found to be immune). If she is antibody negative, or if serological results are unavailable within 96 hours of exposure, she should be given passive immunization with VZIG[9]; the usual dose is 4 vials each containing 125 units. If given within 96 hours of exposure, VZIG is likely to abort the disease; if given later, it may modify the disease.[9]

◣ REFERENCES ◤

1. Mankuta D, Bar-Oz B, Koren G: Erythema infectiosum (fifth disease) and pregnancy, *Can Fam Physician* 45:603-605, 1999.
2. Sanderson F: Perinatal viral infections: 5 scenarios to manage, *Patient Care Can* 7(1):43-60, 1996.
3. Boucher M: Les maladies virales de l'enfance et de la grossesse: petit guide pratico-pratique, *Clin Mar* 10:55-70, 1995.
4. Bar-Oz B, Ford-Jones L, Koren G: Congenital rubella syndrome, *Can Fam Physician* 45:1865-1867, 1999.
5. Stein SJ, Greenspoon JS: Rubeola during pregnancy, *Obstet Gynecol* 78:925-929, 1991.
6. Phillips E: Toxoplasmosis, *Can Fam Physician* 44:1823-1825, 1998.
7. Dunn D, Wallon M, Peyron F, et al: Mother-to child transmission of toxoplasmosis: risk estimates for clinical counselling, *Lancet* 353:1829-1833, 1999.
8. Wallon M, Liou C, Garner P, et al: Congenital toxoplasmosis: systematic review of evidence of efficacy of treatment in pregnancy, *BMJ* 318:1511-1514, 1999.
9. Hudson SP: Selected viral infections in pregnancy, *J SOGC* 16:1245-1251, 1994.
10. Inocencion G, Loebstein R, Lalkin A, et al: Managing exposure to chickenpox during pregnancy, *Can Fam Physician* 44:745-747, 1998.

NAUSEA AND VOMITING IN PREGNANCY

(See also nausea and vomiting)

Diet

Meals should be frequent and small with increased carbohydrate and decreased fat. Suggested nutrients for severe nausea are crackers, unbuttered toast, broth, pretzels, and nondiet ginger ale.[1] Iron may have to be omitted until symptoms are better.

Medications

Doxylamine succinate 10 mg in combination with pyridoxine HCl 10 mg is marketed in Canada under the trade name Diclectin. It is an effective and safe antiemetic during pregnancy and was approved for use in pregnancy by the Health Protection Branch of Health and Welfare Canada in 1990. Many studies have shown that it is not teratogenic.[2-4] A similar formulation in the United States called Bendectin was voluntarily withdrawn by the manufacturer in 1983 because of a profusion of legal suits stemming largely from the claims of an Australian obstetrician and gynecologist that his studies had indicated that the drug was teratogenic. Subsequent investigations proved these claims to be fraudulent—no evidence was ever found verifying that such studies had been undertaken. In 1989 the Medical Tribunal of New South Wales in Australia revoked this physician's license to practice. Unfortunately, U.S. patients are still deprived of the medication.[4] Pyridoxine is used in this formulation not only to prevent vitamin B_6 deficiency in pregnancy, but also because it has some independent antinauseant effect.[5]

Although doxylamine combined with pyridoxine is not available in the United States, doxylamine alone as 25-mg tablets may be obtained for insomnia under the trade name Unisom Nighttime Sleep-Aid.

An alternative drug for nausea and vomiting of pregnancy is dimenhydrinate (Dramamine, Gravol). The usual dose is 50 to 100 mg qid prn.

❧ REFERENCES ❧

1. Kolasa K, Weismiller DG: Nutrition during pregnancy, *Am Fam Physician* 56:205-212, 1997.
2. Jewell MD: Debendox (Bendectin) for nausea in pregnancy. In Enkin MW, Keirse MJN, Renfrew MJ, Neilson JP, eds: *Pregnancy and childbirth module,* Cochrane Database of Systematic Reviews, Review No 07703, April 30, 1993, Oxford, Eng, Update Software.
3. Caddick R, Colliton IE, Dushinski B, et al: Guidelines for the management of nausea and vomiting in pregnancy, *SOGC Clin Pract Guidelines* No 12, November 1995.
4. Fortin CA, Lalonde AB: The Bendectin Affair (of legal and general interest), *J SOGC* 17:61-63, 1995.
5. Vutyavanich T, Supreeya W, Ruangsri R: Pyridoxine for nausea and vomiting of pregnancy—a randomized double-blind, placebo-controlled trial, *Am J Obstet Gynecol* 173:881-884, 1995.

RISK ASSESSMENT IN PREGNANCY

(See also attitudes, physician; prevention; risk analysis)

Many pregnancy risk assessment protocols have been developed. On the basis of these, 16% to 55% of pregnancies are labeled high risk, yet half of perinatal mortality and morbidity occurs in "low-risk" pregnancies.[1-3] One thoughtful analyst of this subject concluded that pregnancy risk scoring has not been proved to do more good than harm.[1] Klein[4] speculated that categorizing women as being at high risk is in itself a factor leading to increased consultations and interventions and asked whether risk scoring may not actually make women sick.

❧ REFERENCES ❧

1. Hall PF: Rethinking risk (editorial), *Can Fam Physician* 40:1239-1244, 1994.
2. Wall EM: Assessing obstetric risk: a review of obstetric risk-scoring systems, *J Fam Pract* 27:153-163, 1988.
3. Hall PF: Obstetric risk scoring: a Trojan horse, *Manitoba Med* 63:43-45, 1993.
4. Klein M: Family physician maternity care: outcomes when family physicians provide most community-based care (editorial), *Can Fam Physician* 41:546-548, 1995.

SMOKING IN PREGNANCY

(See also poverty)

Known detrimental effects of smoking in pregnancy include increased risks of the following[1]:
1. Intrauterine growth retardation
2. Low-birth-weight babies
3. Preterm birth
4. Spontaneous abortion
5. Placenta previa
6. Abruptio placentae

Correlations have been observed between smoking in pregnancy and behavioral problems in the offspring, such as conduct disorder in childhood[2,3] and criminal behavior in adulthood[4] among males and substance abuse in adolescence among females.[3]

Because the adverse effects of smoking are well known, between 40% and 60% of pregnant women smokers quit on their own before the first prenatal visit. Women who continue to smoke during pregnancy are usually heavier smokers, and thus far attempts to help them give up cigarettes have been largely unsuccessful.[5]

❧ REFERENCES ❧

1. Brosky G: Why do pregnant women smoke and can we help them quit? (editorial), *Can Med Assoc J* 152:163-166, 1995.
2. Fergusson DM, Woodward LJ, Horwood J: Maternal smoking during pregnancy and psychiatric adjustment in late adolescence, *Arch Gen Psychiatry* 55:721-727, 1998.
3. Weissman MM, Warner V, Wickramaratne PJ, et al: Maternal smoking during pregnancy and psychopathology in offspring followed to adulthood, *J Am Acad Child Adolesc Psychiatry* 38:892-899, 1999.
4. Brennan PA, Grekin ER, Mednick SA: Maternal smoking during pregnancy and adult male criminal outcomes, *Arch Gen Psychiatry* 56:215-219, 1999.
5. Ershoff DH, Quinn VP, Boyd NR, et al: The Kaiser Permanente Prenatal Smoking-Cessation Trial: when more isn't better, what is enough? *Am J Prevent Med* 17:161-168, 1999.

ULTRASOUND IN PREGNANCY

(See also congenital anomalies; Down syndrome; informed consent)

Routine ultrasound is usually scheduled at 18 weeks, and a number of fetal abnormalities may be detected at this stage of gestation.[1-5] However, the sensitivity is low (17%[1] to 40%[2]), as is the positive predictive value.[5] Gestational age can be assessed and multiple pregnancies detected,[3,4] and in many cases fetal sex can be determined.[1] Studies comparing patients undergoing routine antenatal ultrasound with those having selective ultrasound (when clinically indicated) have shown that those in the routine ultrasound group had twin pregnancies accurately diagnosed in all cases, a lower frequency of induction for apparent postterm pregnancy, fewer low-weight babies, and more induced abortions for fetal abnormalities.[3,4]

Whether a single routine ultrasound screening during the second trimester of pregnancy actually improves perinatal morbidity and mortality is another question. Probably it does not, but this is still an area of heated controversy. Evidence-based reviews of numerous trials addressing this issue[4,6,7] have concluded that except in one study, the Helsinki Ultrasound Trial,[2] no decreased perinatal morbidity or mortality has been documented. The Helsinki study,[2] which has been updated since these reviews were published,[8] reported a decrease in perinatal mortality in the screened group. The explanation was that more children with severe congenital malformation were being born and dying in the control group, and the difference disappeared if the induced abortions for congenital anomalies in the screened group were categorized as deaths.[7] A South African trial that was reported in 1996 found no differences in perinatal outcome between the ultrasound-screened and the control groups.[9]

The U.S. Preventive Services Task Force[6] gives a single routine midtrimester ultrasound screening a "C" recommendation, while the Canadian Task Force on Preventive Health Care[7] gives it a "B."

New developments in ultrasound technology have made it possible to detect many congenital anomalies in the first trimester.[10,11] However, the positive predictive value is low, so many women have to undergo amniocentesis or chorionic villus sampling to detect one abnormality (see congenital anomalies).[10] Two other problems occur with first-trimester ultrasound.[11] Many pregnancies complicated by fetal abnormalities terminate in spontaneous abortion, and diagnosing these abnormalities by ultrasound forces the parents to make decisions about induced termination that might otherwise be unnecessary.[11] In many cases true informed consent is not obtained for the ultrasound. Women may believe the only purpose of the procedure is to determine gestational age, and some would not agree to it if they were aware of its potential to raise suspicions of congenital malformations.[11,12]

REFERENCES

1. Ewigman BG, Crane JP, Frigoletto FD, et al (RADIUS Study Group): Effect of prenatal ultrasound screening on perinatal outcome, *N Engl J Med* 329:821-827, 1993.
2. Saari-Kemppainen A, Karjalainen O, Ylostalo P, et al: Ultrasound screening and perinatal mortality: controlled trial of systematic one-stage screening in pregnancy; the Helsinki Ultrasound Trial, *Lancet* 336:387-391, 1990.
3. Enkin M, Keirse MJ, Renfrew M, et al, eds: *A guide to effective care in pregnancy and childbirth,* ed 2, Oxford, Eng, 1995, Oxford University Press, pp 41-42.
4. Neilson JP: Routine ultrasound in early pregnancy. In Enkin MW, Keirse MJNC, Renfrew MJ, Neilson JP, eds: *Pregnancy and childbirth module,* Cochrane Database of Systematic Reviews, Review No 03872, June 9, 1993, Oxford, Eng, 1994, Update Software.
5. Buskens E, Grobbee DE, Frohn-Mulder IM, et al: Efficacy of routine fetal ultrasound screening for congenital heart disease in normal pregnancy, *Circulation* 94:67-72, 1996.
6. US Preventive Services Task Force: *Guide to clinical preventive services,* ed 2, Baltimore, 1996, Williams & Wilkins, pp 407-417.
7. Canadian Task Force on the Periodic Health Examination: *Canadian guide to clinical preventive health care,* Ottawa, 1994, Canada Communication Group—Publishing, pp 4-14.
8. Leivo T, Tuominen R, Saarikemppainen A, et al: Cost-effectiveness of one-stage ultrasound screening in pregnancy—a report from the Helsinki Ultrasound Trial, *Ultrasound Obstet Gynecol* 7:309-314, 1996.
9. Geerts LT, Brand EJ, Theron GB: Routine obstetric ultrasound examinations in South Africa—cost and effect on perinatal outcome—a prospective randomised controlled trial, *Br J Obstet Gynaecol* 103:501-507, 1996.
10. Snijders RJ, Noble P, Sebire N, et al: UK multicentre project on assessment of risk of trisomy 21 by maternal age and fetal nuchal-translucency thickness at 10-14 weeks of gestation, *Lancet* 352:343-346, 1998.
11. McFadyen A, Gledhill J, Whitlow B, et al: First trimester ultrasound screening: carries ethical and psychological implications (editorial), *BMJ* 317:694-695, 1998.
12. Price BE: Scanning during pregnancy is often for doctors' benefit rather than parents' (letter), *BMJ* 318:1489, 1999.

VIDEO DISPLAY TERMINALS

There is no good evidence that video display terminals lead to adverse effects in pregnancy.[1]

REFERENCES

1. Zuber C, Librizzi RJ, Bolognese RJ: Do aspartame and video display terminals pose pregnancy risks? *Postgrad Obstet Gynecol* 9:1-5, 1989.

ONCOLOGY, PAIN, PALLIATIVE CARE, NAUSEA AND VOMITING

Topics covered in this section

Nausea and Vomiting
Oncology
Pain, Chronic
Palliative Care

NAUSEA AND VOMITING

(See also cachexia; motion sickness; nausea and vomiting in pregnancy; oncology; palliative care)

Pathophysiology

The causes of nausea and vomiting include the following:

1. Direct irritation of visceral afferents from the gut (vagal), often from distention of portions of gut that are not usually distended such as the antrum of the stomach
2. Stimulation of the chemoreceptor trigger zone in the medulla by toxins, drugs, or metabolic disorders.

3. Stimulation of the medullary vomiting center via the vestibular system as occurs in motion sickness and labyrinthitis
4. Stimulation of the medullary vomiting center via cortical input such as fear and pain

Neuroreceptors Mediating Vomiting

Neuroreceptors mediating vomiting include dopaminic (D_2), HT_3 (serotonin), histaminic (H_1), and muscarinic cholinergic. Few of us will remember this esoterica of neuropharmacology, but I include it because it is the basis of the theory that the prescriber should try to choose a drug specific for the neurotransmitters that have been activated in the particular situation. All-purpose antiemetics are the phenothiazines, which act on dopaminic, histaminic, and muscarinic receptors, but none is as potent as the more selective drugs (see later discussion).

Specific Disorders and the Choice of Antiemetic Drugs

Table 51 lists some of the common indications for antiemetics, the choice of drugs, and in most cases the usual adult doses. One of the better drugs for nausea and vomiting in pregnancy is the combination of doxylamine succinate and pyridoxine HCl. This drug is available in Canada but is no longer marketed in the United States. The reasons for this are discussed in more detail in the section on nausea and vomiting in pregnancy. Two other drugs that are available in Canada but not in the United States are betahistine (Serc) and nabilone (Cesamet). Betahistine, an H_1 agonist, is used for Ménière's disease. It acts by inhibiting neuronal impulses in the lateral vestibular nucleus. Nabilone is a synthetic cannabinoid that is sometimes used for chemotherapy-induced nausea and vomiting. The use of antiemetics for chemotherapy is discussed in the following paragraphs.

Antiemetics for Chemotherapy

Although in urban areas chemotherapy is usually administered by oncologists, family physicians still have to discuss the pros and cons of this treatment with their patients and help them deal with medication-induced side effects. In rural areas family physicians do everything.

Two types of nausea and vomiting may occur with chemotherapy: immediate, which takes place within the first 24 hours, and delayed, which develops from days 2 to 5. Drugs that are effective for ameliorating immediate nausea and vomiting may be different from drugs effective for the delayed form. For this reason combination therapies are often used. To complicate matters, vomiting is commonly better controlled than nausea.[1]

Emetic Potential of Chemotherapeutic Drugs

The degree of nausea and vomiting induced by a chemotherapeutic agent is called its emetogenic potential. The choice of an antiemetic in chemotherapy is determined in

Table 51   Antiemetics

Indications and drugs	Usual doses
Pregnancy	
Doxylamine succinate 10 mg–pyridoxine HCl 10 mg (Diclectin)	2 tablets hs and 1 tablet qam prn
Dimenhydrinate (Dramamine, Gravol)	50-100 mg qid
Motion Sickness	
Dimenhydrinate (Dramamine, Gravol)	50-100 mg qid
Scopolamine (Transderm-Scop, Transderm V)	Apply patch to postauricular area 12 hours before onset of motion; change every 72 hours prn
Ménière's Disease	
Betahistine (Serc)	4-8 mg q8h
Dimenhydrinate (Gravol, Dramamine)	50-100 mg qid
Diphenhydramine (Benadryl)	25-50 mg tid-qid
Narcotic Induced	
Prochlorperazine (Compazine, Stemetil)	5-10 mg po or rectally tid or qid
Haloperidol (Haldol)	1-2 mg daily or bid
Pseudoobstruction	
Metoclopramide (Maxeran)	5-10 mg tid-qid
Domperidone (Motilium)	10 mg qid
Cisapride (Prepulsid)	5-10 mg tid-qid
Chemotherapy	
Dexamethasone (Decadron)	See text for doses
Prochlorperazine (Compazine, Stemetil)	See text for doses
Haloperidol (Haldol)	See text for doses
Domperidone (Motilium)	See text for doses
Nabilone (Cesamet)	See text for doses
Dolasetron (Anzemet)	See text for doses
Granisetron (Kytril)	See text for doses
Odansetron (Zofran)	See text for doses
Metoclopramide (Maxeran)	See text for doses

part by the emetogenic potential of the chemotherapeutic agents being used.[2-4] This correlation is shown in Table 52. The emetogenic potential of some commonly used chemotherapeutic agents is given in Table 53.[2-4]

Single Versus Combination Antiemetic Drugs for Chemotherapy

Single antiemetic drugs are generally used for mild or moderately emetogenic chemotherapy, and combination drugs for moderate or highly emetogenic chemotherapy. Examples of initial single-dose or multiple-dose regimens are given in Tables 54 and 55. The literature on the use of antiemetics for patients undergoing chemotherapy is vast, and only selected examples are given here. Some of the combined regimens can be very effective. In an Italian study using dexamethasone and granisetron (initial doses shown in Example 3 in Table 55), a combination of dexamethasone (Decadron) and granisetron controlled both immediate and delayed nausea and vomiting in 93% of patients receiving moderately eme-

Table 52 Choice of Antiemetics Based on Emetogenic Potential of Chemotherapeutic Agents

Drug	Emetogenic potential
Steroids	
Dexamethasone (Decadron)	Mild, moderate, marked
Phenothiazines	
Prochlorperazine (Compazine, Stemetil)	Mild, moderate
Butyrophenones	
Haloperidol (Haldol)	Mild, moderate
Domperidone (Motilium)	Mild, moderate
Cannabinoids	
Nabilone (Cesamet)	Mild, moderate
5-HT$_3$ Receptor Antagonists	
Granisetron (Kytril)	Mild, moderate, marked
Odansetron (Zofran)	Mild, moderate, marked
Substituted Benzamides	
Metoclopramide (Maxeran)	Mild, moderate, marked

Table 53 Emetic Potential of Chemotherapeutic Drugs

Mild	Moderate	High
Fluorouracil	Cyclophosphamide	Cisplatin
Methotrexate	Doxorubicin	Mechlorethamine HCl
Etoposide	Carboplatin	(nitrogen mustard)
Vincristine	Mitomycin	Streptozocin
Bleomycin	Asparaginase	Dacarbazine
	Azacitidine	Carmustine
		Dactinomycin

Table 54 Initial Doses of Antiemetic Drugs in Selected Single-Dose Regimens

Drug	Initial dose
Example 1	
Prochlorperazine (Compazine, Stemetil)	5-10 mg po or IV or a 25-mg rectal suppository
Example 2	
Dexamethasone (Decadron)	10-20 mg IV
Example 3	
Ondansetron (Zofran)	8 mg po or 10 mg IV
Example 4	
Nabilone (Cesamet)	1-2 mg the night before chemotherapy and 1-2 mg 1-3 hours before chemotherapy

Table 55 Initial Doses of Antiemetic Drugs in Selected Combined Regimens

Drug	Initial dose
Example 1	
Dexamethasone (Decadron)	20 mg IV plus
Metoclopramide (Maxeran)	3 mg/kg IV q2h × 2
Diphenhydramine (Benadryl)	25-50 mg IV q2h × 2
Lorazepam (Ativan)	1-2 mg IV
Example 2	
Dexamethasone (Decadron)	20 mg IV
Ondansetron (Zofran)	8-10 mg IV
Example 3	
Dexamethasone (Decadron)	8 mg IV
Granisetron (Kytril)	3 mg IV

❧ REFERENCES ❧

1. Italian Group for Antiemetic Research: Dexamethasone, granisetron, or both for the prevention of nausea and vomiting during chemotherapy for cancer, *N Engl J Med* 332:1-5, 1995.
2. Grunberg SM, Hesketh PJ: Control of chemotherapy-induced emesis, *N Engl J Med* 329:1790-1796, 1993.
3. *Le traitement des nausées et vomissements causés par la radiothérapie et la chimiothérapie,* Québec, 1993, Le Lorier J Redacteur, Gouvernement du Québec.
4. Drugs for vomiting caused by cancer chemotherapy, *Med Lett* 35:14-26, 1993.

ONCOLOGY

(See also informed consent; nausea and vomiting; pain; palliative care)

Most oncology topics are covered in the discussions of specific neoplasms, palliative care, pain, and nausea and vomiting.

Epidemiology and Primary Prevention

(See also Mediterranean diet; oncology)

Ecological, cohort, and case-control studies have found that a high intake of fruits and vegetables and a low intake of fat and protein are associated with a decreased risk of many common neoplasms.[1] A high intake of tomatoes (which are rich in lycopene) correlates with a decreased risk of numerous cancers, especially of the prostate, stomach, and lung.[2] Preliminary data suggest that the Mediterranean diet, which is so valuable for the prevention of coronary artery disease, is also associated with a lower incidence of a number of neoplasms.[1,3]

In animal studies overfeeding is associated with an increased risk of cancer and calorie restriction with a decreased risk. Cohorts of women who suffered food deprivation during wartime had lower rates of breast cancer. Perhaps related to childhood caloric intake is the observation that tall men are at greater risk than short men for non-smoking-related cancers.[4]

togenic chemotherapy. This two-drug combination gave better results for immediate nausea and vomiting than either drug alone, whereas dexamethasone alone was as effective as the two-drug combination in controlling delayed nausea and vomiting.[1] Granisetron is closely related to other 5-HT$_3$ receptor antagonists such as odansetron (Zofran) and dolasetron (Anzemet).[1]

REFERENCES

1. Hakim I: Mediterranean diets and cancer prevention, *Arch Intern Med* 158:1169-1170, 1998.
2. Giovannucci E: Tomatoes, tomato-based products, lycopene, and cancer: review of the epidemiologic literature, *J Natl Cancer Inst* 91:317-331, 1999.
3. de Lorgeril M, Salen P, Martin J-L, et al: Mediterranean dietary pattern in a randomized trial: prolonged survival and possible reduced cancer rate, *Arch Intern Med* 158:1181-1187, 1998.
4. Albanes D: Height, early energy intake, and cancer (editorial), *BMJ* 317:1331-1332, 1998.

Clinical Trials

Evidence to date suggests that cancer patients participating in clinical trials have a longer survival than patients treated outside of such trials.[1-4]

REFERENCES

1. Stiller CA: Survival of patients with cancer: those included in clinical trials do better, *BMJ* 99:1058-1059, 1989.
2. Stiller CA, Draper GJ: Treatment centre size, entry to trials, and survival in acute lymphoblastic leukemia, *Arch Dis Child* 64:657-661, 1989.
3. Karjalainen S, Palva I: Do treatment protocols improve end results: a study of survival of patients with multiple myeloma in Finland, *BMJ* 299:1069-1072, 1989.
4. Weijer C: The breast cancer research scandal: addressing the issues (editorial), *Can Med Assoc J* 152:1195-1197, 1995.

Chemotherapy

(See also nausea and vomiting)

A relatively new chemotherapeutic agent is paclitaxel (Taxol), which is derived from the bark of the Pacific yew tree. This drug has been effective in a number of patients who no longer responded to conventional chemotherapy. It is commonly used for tumors of the ovaries, lung, breast, and head and neck.[1] Further discussion of chemotherapy can be found in sections on specific neoplasms throughout the text.

REFERENCES

1. Rowinsky EK, Donehower RC: Paclitaxel (Taxol), *N Engl J Med* 332:1004-1014, 1995.

Radiation Therapy

Radiation therapy is associated with fatigue in about half of all patients who are subjected to it.[1]

REFERENCES

1. Smets EM, Willems-Groot AF, Garssen B, et al: Fatigue and radiotherapy: (A) experience in patients undergoing treatment, *Br J Cancer* 78:899-906, 1998.

Follow-Up of Patients with Cancer Who Have Had Curative Treatments

(See also informed consent; investigations)

Traditional medical practice involves extensive follow-up investigations of patients who have had curative surgery for cancer. The usual argument for this policy is to detect and treat recurrences at an early stage. Evaluation of such protocols for patients with breast cancer,[1,2] melanoma,[3] colon cancer,[4-6] endometrial carcinoma,[7] small cell lung cancer,[8] and squamous cell carcinoma of the head and neck[9] have shown little or no survival advantage from their use. Among patients with Hodgkin's disease, only 11% of relapses were detected by physical examination or routine investigation whereas 89% were found through the investigation of newly developed symptoms.[10]

A recent update from the Canadian Task Force on Preventive Health Care gives an "E" recommendation to blood work and diagnostic imaging such as bone scans as part of follow-up management of patients with breast cancer; mammography and breast examination by health professionals is given a "C."[11] According to the American Society of Clinical Oncology, evidence fails to support bone scans, chest x-ray examination, liver ultrasound, liver computed tomography, hematological blood counts, or tumor markers as routine follow-up procedures after treatment of breast cancer. The society does recommend monthly breast self-examination; annual mammography; and a careful history and physical examination every 3 to 6 months for 3 years, then every 6 to 12 months for 2 years, and annually thereafter.[12] Current guidelines for surveillance of patients with colon cancer also advise against many traditional investigations such as complete blood counts, liver function tests, fecal occult blood tests, chest x-ray examination, computed tomography, and pelvic imaging (see "Management of Colorectal Cancer").[13]

Aside from cost, the disadvantage of intensive follow-up investigations is a possible impairment of the patient's quality of life. In a study of patients with breast cancer, twice as many preferred reducing rather than increasing the frequency of follow-up visits.[14] Tests are time consuming and sometimes uncomfortable. False-positive tests may take weeks to be clarified, and true positives that detect incurable disease in otherwise asymptomatic patients do not seem to be beneficial.[15] At present few patients are given these data, so they do not have the opportunity to exercise informed consent concerning the intensity of follow-up they would prefer.

REFERENCES

1. GIVIO Investigators: Impact of follow-up testing on survival and health-related quality of life in breast cancer patients: a multicenter randomized controlled trial, *JAMA* 271:1587-1592, 1994.
2. Del Turco MR, Palli D, Cariddi A, et al: Intensive diagnostic follow-up after treatment of primary breast cancer: a randomized trial; National Research Council Project on Breast Cancer Follow-up, *JAMA* 271:1593-1997, 1994.

3. Weiss M, Loprinzi CL, Creagan ET, et al: Utility of follow-up tests for detecting disease recurrence of surgically resected primary malignant melanoma. In *Proceedings of the Annual Meeting of the American Society of Clinical Oncology,* March 1995, Los Angeles, Abstract 893.

4. Kjeldsen BJ, Kronborg O, Fenger C, et al: A prospective randomized study of follow-up after radical surgery for colorectal cancer, *Br J Surg* 84:666-669, 1997.

5. Makela JT, Laitinen SO, Kairaluoma MI: Five-year follow-up after radical surgery for colorectal cancer—results of a prospective-randomized trial, *Arch Surg* 130:1062-1067, 1995.

6. Schoemaker D, Black R, Giles L, et al: Yearly colonoscopy, liver CT, and chest radiography do not influence 5-year survival of colorectal cancer patients, *Gastroenterology* 114:7-14, 1998.

7. Agboola OO, Grunfeld E, Coyle D, et al: Costs and benefits of routine follow-up after curative treatment for endometrial cancer, *Can Med Assoc J* 157:879-886, 1997.

8. Perez EA, Loprinzi CL, Sloan JA, et al: Utility of screening procedures for detecting recurrence of disease after complete response in patients with small cell lung carcinoma, *Cancer* 80:676-680, 1997.

9. Cooney TR, Poulsen MG: Is routine follow-up useful after combined-modality therapy for advanced head and neck cancer? *Arch Otolaryngol Head Neck Surg* 125:379-382, 1999.

10. Radford JA, Eardley A, Woodman C, et al: Follow up policy after treatment for Hodgkin's disease: too many clinic visits and routine tests? A review of hospital records, *BMJ* 314:343-346, 1997.

11. Temple LK, Wang EE, McLeod RS, et al (Canadian Task Force on Preventive Health Care): Preventive health care, 1999 update. 3. Follow-up after breast cancer, *Can Med Assoc J* 161:1001-1008, 1999.

12. Smith TJ, Davidson NE, Schapira DV, et al: American Society of Clinical Oncology 1998 update of recommended breast cancer surveillance guidelines, *J Clin Oncol* 17:1080-1082, 1999.

13. Desch CE, Benson AB III, Smith TJ, et al: Recommended colorectal cancer surveillance guidelines by the American Society of Clinical Oncology, *J Clin Oncol* 17:1312-1321, 1999.

14. Gulliford T, Opomu M, Wilson E, et al: Popularity of less frequent follow up for breast cancer in randomised study—initial findings from the Hotline Study, *BMJ* 314:174-177, 1997.

15. Loprinzi CL: Follow-up testing for curatively treated cancer survivors: what to do? (editorial), *JAMA* 273:1877-1878, 1995.

Paraneoplastic Syndromes

Some of the paraneoplastic syndromes are listed in Table 56.

PAIN, CHRONIC

(See also constipation; metastatic breast cancer; multiple myeloma; nausea and vomiting; palliative care)

Pain and Cancer

Between 65% and 85% of patients with advanced cancer suffer from pain, but this can be effectively controlled in 85% to 95% of cases.[1] Health care workers often underestimate the severity of chronic pain.[2]

Table 56   Paraneoplastic Syndromes

Hypercalcemia (hormonally mediated)
Cushing's syndrome (ectopic production of adrenocorticotropic hormone)
Hyponatremia (ectopic production of antidiuretic hormone)
Clubbing
Hypertrophic osteoarthropathy
Peripheral neuropathies
Cerebellar degeneration
Myasthenia gravis
Lambert-Eaton myasthenic syndrome (more severe in lower limbs and proximal muscles and improves temporarily with exercise)
Polymyositis
Dermatomyositis
Sudden appearance of seborrheic keratoses (Leser-Trélat sign)
Acanthosis nigricans
Paraneoplastic pemphigus
Migratory thrombophlebitis (Trousseau's syndrome)

Categories of Pain Control Drugs

Classes of pain control drugs include the following[1,2]:

Nonopioids	Acetaminophen, acetylsalicylic acid (ASA), nonsteroidal antiinflammatory drugs (NSAIDs), tramadol
Weak opioids	Codeine
Strong opioids	Morphine, hydromorphone, oxycodone, fentanyl
Adjuvants	Corticosteroids, psychotropic drugs, anticonvulsants

Analgesic Ladder

The World Health Organization stepwise protocol for chronic pain control (analgesic ladder) is to start with non-opioids, add a mild opioid such as orally administered codeine to a maximum of 120 mg q4h, and end up replacing the mild opioid with a potent opioid such as oral morphine. Adjuvants should be used at each step if indicated.[1,2]

Nonopioids

Standard nonopioids that may be used alone for the treatment of mild cancer pain are acetaminophen, aspirin, NSAIDs, and perhaps tramadol (Ultram). Doses should be titrated upward to their maximal levels, and if one agent in this class is ineffective, another may be tried. However, if pain is moderate or severe, narcotics should be started immediately.[1,2] The maximum analgesic effect of aspirin or acetaminophen is obtained with doses of 650 to 1300 mg. Other NSAIDs have potency equal to or greater than acetaminophen and aspirin. For example, ibuprofen 400 mg is equivalent to acetaminophen-codeine combinations, and ketorolac (Toradol) 120 mg intramuscularly or IV is equivalent to 12 mg of morphine intramuscularly. If one NSAID does not give adequate pain relief, another should be tried because patients respond in variable fashion to different drugs within this class. Although aspirin causes irreversible inhibition of platelet aggregation, other NSAIDs cause a reversible inhibition of aggregation that disappears as the drug blood levels fall.[3]

Tramadol is a relatively new nonopioid analgesic. The usual dose is 50 to 100 mg q4-6h. Tramadol 50 mg is equivalent to codeine 60 mg, and tramadol 100 mg is equivalent to aspirin 650 mg plus codeine 60 mg.[3] The role of tramadol in the management of chronic cancer pain is uncertain, but it may be useful for patients who have mild to moderate chronic pain that is not relieved by acetaminophen and who cannot tolerate NSAIDs.[1]

Weak Opioids

The standard "weak" opioid used for chronic pain is codeine. The equivalency of oral codeine to oral morphine is approximately 10:1. That is, 60 mg of codeine phosphate po is roughly equivalent to 6 mg of morphine sulfate po.[3]

Codeine comes in three basic forms: short-acting codeine phosphate, long-acting codeine preparations (Codeine Contin), and short-acting codeine phosphate in combination with another analgesic such as acetaminophen or ASA plus or minus caffeine (Tylenol 3 or 4, Empirin 30 or 60, Empracet 30 or 60). A major limitation of dosage in the combination forms is the adjuvant drugs (acetaminophen, ASA, caffeine). The numbers 8, 15, and 30 following a trade name (e.g., Empirin 30) refer to the milligrams of codeine in the product. In the case of Tylenol the numbers 1, 2, 3, and 4 refer to 8, 15, 30, and 60 mg of codeine, respectively.

Sorting out the available preparations becomes even more difficult when products with the same names in Canada and the United States are compared. In the United States Tylenol 2 and Tylenol 3 contain acetaminophen 300 mg plus codeine 15 and 30 mg, respectively. In Canada the same ingredients are present but with the addition of 15 mg of caffeine. Tylenol 1 is available only in Canada and contains 300 mg of acetaminophen, 8 mg of codeine, and 15 mg of caffeine. In both countries Tylenol 4 contains 300 mg of acetaminophen and 60 mg of codeine.

Since these various combinations have many brand names, physicians must check the specific ingredients carefully before prescribing them. One way to avoid mistakes is to write out the generic names of the combinations desired such as "acetaminophen 325 mg plus codeine 30 mg."

A long-acting formulation of codeine, Codeine Contin, is available in Canada. It is supplied as scored 100-, 150-, and 200-mg tablets. The total daily dosage is about 25% less than the total daily dosage of codeine phosphate, and it is given in two equal doses q12h.

Strong Opioids

Strong opioids include morphine, hydromorphone (Dilaudid), oxycodone (Roxicodone, Percodan, Percocet), and fentanyl (Duragesic).

Morphine

The usual strong opioid that is given for chronic pain is morphine. A significant first-pass effect occurs with oral morphine. When it is given as a single dose at the initiation of treatment, the potency ratio of oral to subcutaneous or IV morphine is 1:6 or 1:8. With repeated oral doses the ratio becomes 1:2 or 1:3. That is, the parenteral dose is only two to three times as potent as the oral dose.

For control of chronic pain, medications are given by the oral route if possible because this results in more even blood levels. The next best alternative is the rectal route, and the least desirable is the parenteral route. Initially, short-acting preparations such as solutions or tablets of morphine sulfate should be used. Dosage intervals should be close enough to prevent recurrence of pain (q3-4h for morphine sulfate). If pain does recur, the next dose should be increased by 25% to 50%. Half of the regular dose should be kept available to be given as needed (q1-2h for morphine) in case of breakthrough pain. Initially the patient should be awakened at regular intervals during the night to receive the analgesic doses, but when the patient's condition becomes stable, this can be avoided by giving 1.5 to 2 times the usual dose at bedtime. Once pain is controlled by short-acting oral or rectal opioids, patients may be switched to longer acting oral preparations (e.g., Kadian, MS Contin, Oramorph SR, M-Eslon). In the case of morphine the total daily dose of the long-acting preparations is equal to the total daily dose of short-acting morphine but is given in 2 divided doses at 12-hour intervals. Short-acting formulations of the long-acting narcotics should be made available to the patient in case of breakthrough pain.[1,2]

Hydromorphone

Hydromorphone (Dilaudid) may be taken orally, rectally, or by injection. Oral formulations are available as solutions, short-acting tablets, and in Canada slow release tablets (Hydromorph Contin). Hydromorphone is four to five times as potent as morphine, and it is also more soluble than morphine. The increased solubility means that if high-dose parenteral injections are required, the volume required for equipotent doses is less for hydromorphone than for morphine.

Oxycodone

Although their names sound similar, oxycodone is a narcotic that is 10 times more potent than codeine. Its analgesic effect is comparable to that of morphine. In one study of cancer patients with chronic pain controlled by oral oxycodone, it was possible to change to the same dosage of oral morphine with no loss of pain control.[4]

In Canada the only formulations of short-acting oxycodone available for oral use are in combination with acetaminophen (Percocet) or ASA (Percodan), which limit the dosage. In the United States short-acting oxycodone is available alone (Roxicodone) or, as in Canada, in combination with acetaminophen (Percocet, Roxicet) or ASA (Percodan, Roxiprin). A controlled release formulation of oxycodone (OxyContin) has recently become available; in one study of cancer pain control it was found to be as effective as controlled release hydromorphone.[5]

Although oxycodone may be a useful drug for patients with chronic cancer pain, it is a popular drug of abuse.[6] Physicians should therefore not prescribe oxycodone for short-duration musculoskeletal pain.

Fentanyl

Fentanyl (Duragesic) is available as transdermal patches that come in various strengths and are applied to the arms or torso for 72 hours. (Some patients, especially smokers, may metabolize the drug more rapidly and have to change the patches every 48 hours.) The patches do not become fully effective until they have been in place for at least 12 hours. In general, chronic pain should first be controlled by oral narcotics and then the patient can be switched to fentanyl using the conversion figures on the package insert.[7]

Switching Opioids

Patients with chronic pain may require a change of narcotic medications. Sometimes this is done because pain relief is inadequate and an equivalent dose of another narcotic is more effective and sometimes because the original narcotic has adverse effects. The dose of the new narcotic is usually determined by reference to equivalency tables. Quoted equivalencies are only rough approximations, and individual patients may require higher or lower doses than those listed.[8]

Supplementary Drugs

All patients taking narcotics should be given laxatives preventively (see discussion of constipation), antiemetics as necessary (see section on nausea and vomiting), and in most cases, adjuvant drugs.[1,2]

Psychomotor Function

Long-term use of narcotics does not appear to impair psychomotor functions such as those required to drive a car.[9]

Opioids to Avoid in the Treatment of Chronic Pain

Physicians should avoid prescribing meperidine (Demerol) for chronic pain. Meperidine has a short duration of action (1 to 3 hours) and poor oral absorption (oral/parenteral ratio is 4:1), and repeated doses may lead to central nervous system toxicity.

Pentazocine (Talwin) has poor bioavailability by the oral route, a short duration of action, and many neuropsychiatric side effects. It is an opioid agonist-antagonist and may induce withdrawal symptoms in opioid-dependent patients.

Propoxyphene (Darvon) is an opioid with the potency of about 600 mg of aspirin.[1,2] Its value for relief of chronic pain is questionable.[2]

Adjuvant Analgesic Drugs

The main classes of adjuvant analgesic drugs for the management of chronic pain are NSAIDs, tricyclic antidepressants, anticonvulsants, corticosteroids, and bisphosphonates.

Nonsteroidal antiinflammatory drugs

NSAIDs are particularly useful as adjunct treatment for bony metastases. A metaanalysis of NSAIDs in the treatment of cancer pain came to the conclusion that the analgesic effect of this class of drugs in standard doses was roughly equivalent to 5 to 10 mg of intramuscular morphine. Increasing the dosage of the NSAID or adding a weak opioid such as codeine did not augment the analgesic effect but did result in more adverse reactions.[10]

Tricyclic antidepressants and anticonvulsants

Tricyclic antidepressants are highly valuable for neuropathic pain.[3] Serotonergic reuptake inhibitors such as imipramine (Tofranil) and amitriptyline (Elavil) are more effective in controlling pain that are norepinephrine reuptake inhibitors such as desipramine (Norpramin, Pertofrane) and doxepin (Sinequan). However, both groups are usually effective, and desipramine often causes fewer side effects. Usual analgesic doses are 75 to 100 mg/day.

The common symptoms of neuropathic pain are hyperalgesia and constant burning pain. Severe pain is experienced from even slight pressure such as clothes, and paresthesias are often present. Some authors have stressed the importance of distinguishing neuropathic pain from the lancinating pain of neuralgia such as tic douloureux because neuralgia does not usually respond to tricyclics or to steroids but is often helped by anticonvulsants such as carbamazepine (Tegretol).[11] However, evidence is accumulating that anticonvulsants such as carbamazepine, phenytoin (Dilantin), and gabapentin (Neurontin) can be effective for any type of pain caused by peripheral nerve dysfunction.[3]

Corticosteroids

Corticosteroids are extremely useful adjuvant drugs. They have antiinflammatory and antiemetic activity, stimulate the appetite, and often elevate the mood. Some of the indications for their use in control of chronic pain are as follows:

1. Increased intracranial pressure
2. Spinal cord compression
3. Nerve compression
4. Visceral distention
5. Lymphedema
6. Osseous metastases unresponsive to NSAIDs
7. Soft tissue infiltration
8. Intractable pain not responsive to opioids

In critical situations treatment should start with large IV doses followed by oral doses of a drug such as dexamethasone (Decadron) in the ranges listed below:

Increased intracranial pressure	4-12 mg tid-qid
Nerve compression	4-8 mg bid-tid
Intractable pain	4-8 mg tid-qid
Soft tissue infiltration	2-4 mg bid

Bisphosphonates

The bisphosphonate pamidronate (Aredia) given IV may lead to significant pain relief in some cases of metastatic bone disease[11,12] or in multiple myeloma[13] (see sections on metastatic breast cancer and multiple myeloma).

Opioids for Chronic Nonmalignant Pain

Narcotics often relieve chronic nonmalignant pain associated with such conditions as osteoarthritis, low back disorders, chronic soft tissue disorders, postherpetic neuralgia,[14] and phantom limb sensation.[15] Physical dependence may develop, but most patients can be successfully withdrawn from opioids through a tapering process.[14,15] However, since family physicians often face patients with drug-seeking behavior, they must try to distinguish legitimate from illegitimate demands for narcotics. Clues to addictive behavior include a personal or family history of substance abuse, repeated reports of lost or stolen prescriptions, claims that nonopioids give no relief, dosage requests out of proportion to the degree of pain, claims that controlled-release opioids are ineffective, and refusal to try tapering opioids. Narcotics should be prescribed only when it is clear that other agents do not work, and in most cases controlled-release rather than short-acting agents should be chosen. In some instances a check for double-doctoring or the use of multiple pharmacies is advisable.[14]

◢ REFERENCES ◣

1. Levy MH: Pharmacologic treatment of cancer pain, *N Engl J Med* 335:1124-1132, 1996.
2. Montauk SL, Martin J: Treating chronic pain, *Am Fam Physician* 55:1151-1160, 1997.
3. Drugs for pain, *Med Lett* 40:79-84, 1998.
4. Glare PA, Walsh TD: Dose-ranging study of oxycodone for chronic pain in advanced cancer, *J Clin Oncol* 11:973-978, 1993.
5. Hagen NA, Babul N: Comparative clinical efficacy and safety of a novel controlled-release oxycodone formulation and controlled-release hydromorphone in the treatment of cancer pain, *Cancer* 79:1428-1437, 1997.
6. Hess, H: Police probe ring selling popular painkillers: computers used to produce forged prescriptions in narcotics for growing black market, *Toronto Globe and Mail,* Jan 14, 1997, p A6.
7. Woodroffe MA, Hays H: Fentanyl transdermal system: pain management at home, *Can Fam Physician* 43:268-272, 1997.
8. Moulin DE: Relative potency estimates of analgesics—are they perceived or real? *Pain Res Manage* 1:195-196, 1996.
9. Vainio A, Ollila J, Matikainen E, et al: Driving ability in cancer patients receiving long-term morphine analgesia, *Lancet* 346:667-670, 1995.
10. Eisenberg E, Berdey CS, Carr DB, et al: Efficacy and safety of nonsteroidal antiinflammatory drugs for cancer pain: a meta-analysis, *J Clin Oncol* 12:2756-2765, 1994.
11. Davis CL, Hardy JR: Palliative care, *BMJ* 308:1359-1362, 1994.
12. Hortobagyl GN, Theriault RL, Porter L, et al: Efficacy of pamidronate in reducing skeletal complications in patients with breast cancer and lytic bone metastases, *N Engl J Med* 335:1785-1791, 1996.
13. Berenson JR, Lichtenstein A, Porter L, et al (Myeloma Aredia Study Group): Efficacy of pamidronate in reducing skeletal events in patients with advanced multiple myeloma, *N Engl J Med* 334:529-530, 1996.
14. Drake AC, Stewart JH: Efficacy and abuse potential of opioid analgesics and the treatment of chronic noncancer pain, *Pain Res Manage* 4:104-109, 1999.
15. Fuchs PN, Gamsa A. Chronic use of opioids for nonmalignant pain: a prospective study, *Pain Res Manage* 2:101-107, 1997.

PALLIATIVE CARE

(See also nausea and vomiting; pain)

Cachexia

(See also nausea and vomiting)

Cancer cachexia is due to tumor-induced metabolic abnormalities that lead to lipolysis and loss of muscle and skeletal protein. Corticosteroids have been shown to increase appetite, food intake, and well-being, but not weight gain. The beneficial effects dissipate after about 1 month. Megestrol acetate (Megace) increases appetite, food intake, sense of well-being, and weight gain. The usual therapeutic dose is between 480 and 800 mg/day.[1]

◢ REFERENCES ◣

1. Bruera E, Neumann CM: Management of specific symptom complexes in patients receiving palliative care, *Can Med Assoc J* 158:1717-1726, 1998.

Dehydration and Fluid Replacement

Patients dying in hospices rarely receive parenteral fluids and do not appear to suffer as a result. Patients dying in hospitals often receive parenteral fluids until the time of death. Does dehydration decrease the quality of life in the terminally ill? There are no definitive data indicating whether at the end of life parenteral fluids decrease thirst, dry mouth sensation, or nausea, increase cognitive functioning, or prolong survival. By the same token there are no reliable data substantiating serious adverse effects of parenteral fluid administration, such as pain from venipunctures, fluid overload and congestive failure, or increased nausea and vomiting in the presence of intestinal obstruction.[1] However, a growing body of literature suggests that dying or seriously ill patients do not suffer from the withdrawal of parenteral nutrition, tube feedings, or IV fluids. In these circumstances thirst is rare, and the discomfort of a dry mouth can be controlled by avoiding drugs that aggravate the condition and by using glycerine swabs, ice chips, and sips of water.[2]

◢ REFERENCES ◣

1. Burge FI: Dehydration and provision of fluids in palliative care: what is the evidence? *Can Fam Physician* 42:2383-2388, 1996.

2. Brody H, Campbell ML, Faber-Langendoen K, et al: Withdrawing intensive life-sustaining treatment—recommendations for compassionate clinical management, *N Engl J Med* 336:652-657, 1997.

Dyspnea

Dyspnea is a subjective symptom that often correlates poorly with objective measurements of pulmonary function. In some cases it is caused by coexistent diseases such as chronic obstructive pulmonary disease or pneumonia and is relieved by treatment with bronchodilators or antibiotics. When the cause is not obvious, a trial of oxygen should given.[1] Systemic opioids have proved effective for many patients with cancer-related dyspnea.[1] Although some reports have claimed that nebulized opioids are also effective, at least two randomized controlled trials failed to find any benefit from the nebulized administration of these drugs.[2,3] If a patient already taking regular doses of morphine for pain control becomes dyspneic, relief may often be achieved by increasing the every 4 hours dose equivalent of morphine by 25%.[4] Benzodiazepines are frequently used but probably have value only if the dyspnea is related to panic disorder or severe anxiety. Corticosteroids are thought to be useful for patients with carcinomatous lymphangitis or the superior vena cava syndrome.[1]

≥ REFERENCES ≤

1. Bruera E, Neumann CM: Management of specific symptom complexes in patients receiving palliative care, *Can Med Assoc J* 158:1717-1726, 1998.
2. Davis C: The role of nebulised drugs in palliating respiratory symptoms of malignant disease, *Eur J Palliative Care* 2:9-15, 1995.
3. Noseda A, Carpiaux J-P, Markstein C, et al: Disabling dyspnea in patients with advanced disease: lack of effect of nebulized morphine, *Eur Respir J* 10:1079-1083, 1997.
4. Allard P, Lamontagne C, Bernard P, et al: How effective are supplementary doses of opioids for dyspnea in terminally ill cancer patients? A randomized continuous sequential clinical trial, *J Pain Symptom Manage* 17:256-265, 1999.

Intestinal Obstruction

(See also antiemetics for pseudoobstruction)

Bowel obstruction occurs in close to one half of patients with advanced ovarian cancer and in about one fourth of patients with advanced colorectal cancers.[1]

No randomized controlled trials deal with the medical management of bowel obstruction in terminally ill patients. A number of studies have shown effective palliation lasting several months by the use of a variety of drugs, usually in combination.[1]

Colicky pain can be controlled with scopolamine (also called hyoscine), atropine, or loperamide (Imodium). Scopolamine may be given subcutaneously, often in large doses, or as two skin patches (Transderm-Scop, Transderm-V) that should be changed every 3 days. Patches take 12 to 24 hours to become effective.[2] The more continuous pain of distended bowel, tumor masses, or hepatic distention is managed with narcotics. Nausea and vomiting are often controlled with a phenothiazine such as chlorpromazine (Thorazine, Largactil), with prochlorperazine (Compazine, Stemetil), or with butyrophenones such as haloperidol (Haldol). In a few cases obstruction can be alleviated by giving corticosteroids such as dexamethasone (Decadron). If the obstruction is partial, metoclopramide (Maxeran) may be beneficial.[1,2]

≥ REFERENCES ≤

1. Frank C: Medical management of intestinal obstruction in terminal care, *Can Fam Physician* 43:259-265, 1997.
2. Miron S: Occlusion intestinale traitement palliatif, *Méd Québec,* Feb 1994, pp 89-94.

Patient Perspectives

In a qualitative study, patients receiving palliative care gave the following as their five most important issues[1]:

1. Obtaining adequate control of pain and other symptoms
2. Avoiding measures that inappropriately prolong dying
3. Achieving and maintaining control of their own lives as long as they are capable of doing so, and being sure that if they become incapable, the wishes of their chosen proxy will be respected
4. Relieving to the greatest extent possible the burden their deaths would impose on loved ones
5. Achieving full and intimate involvement with loved ones

≥ REFERENCES ≤

1. Singer PA, Martin DK, Kelner M: Quality end-of-life care: patients' perspectives, *JAMA* 281:163-168, 1999.

Prognosis of Terminally Ill Patients

A Canadian study found that physicians tend to overestimate life expectancy in patients with advanced cancer. As a result a number of patients may be deprived of hospice or other palliative care treatment programs.[1]

≥ REFERENCES ≤

1. Vigano A, Dorgan M, Bruera E, et al: The relative accuracy of the clinical estimation of the duration of life for patients with end of life cancer, *Cancer* 86:170-176, 1999.

Spinal cord compression

Malignant spinal cord compression is a medical emergency that occurs in 1% to 2% of patients with cancer, usually those who have breast or prostate cancer with bone metastases or who have myeloma. Permanent loss of motor power or bowel or bladder function is likely unless the patient is referred for treatment within 24 hours of the onset of symptoms.[1]

REFERENCES

1. Husband DF: Malignant spinal cord compression: prospective study of delays in referral and treatment, *BMJ* 317:18-21, 1998.

Superior Vena Cava Syndrome

Lung cancer (usually small cell) and non-Hodgkin's lymphoma are the most common causes of the superior vena cava syndrome. Dyspnea, cough, a sensation of fullness in the head, and facial or arm swelling are common early complaints. Neck or chest wall venous distention is usually found on examination. The treatment of choice is chemotherapy, often combined with radiation therapy; corticosteroids may give temporary relief.[1]

REFERENCES

1. Chow E, Danjoux C, Andersson L: Superior vena cava syndrome, *Patient Care Can* 10:57-62, 1999.

OPHTHALMOLOGY

Topics covered in this section

Cataracts
Central Serous Chorioretinopathy
Congenital Lacrimal Obstruction
Corneal Lesions
Corneal Transplants
Glaucoma, Acute Angle Closure
Glaucoma, Open Angle
Macular Degeneration
Refractive Errors
Topical Ophthalmic Medications

CATARACTS

(See also macular degeneration)

Epidemiology

Cataracts are more common in black than white populations,[1] and diabetes is a well-recognized risk factor.[1,2] Both oral and inhaled corticosteroids are risk factors in adults,[3,4] but most other commonly used drugs are not associated with cataract development.[5] Aspirin is not protective against cataracts.[5] An association has been reported between excessive exposure to ultraviolet B (UV-B) light and cataracts.[4] Effective protection against UV-B may be obtained by wearing sunglasses. A wide-brimmed hat cuts the exposure by 30% to 50%.[6] Other probable risk factors for cataracts are hypertension,[1] central obesity,[1] and smoking.[2]

Symptoms and Signs

Several symptoms suggest cataracts as the cause of visual changes. One of the early ones is "second sight." The presence of an early cataract may change the refractive index of the lens so that the patient can begin to read without glasses. However, vision dims progressively, which is particularly noticeable at night; the patient needs very bright lights to read or to perform fine work. Another suggestive symptom is the presence of haloes around street lights or the headlights of approaching cars. This and the associated glare make many patients spontaneously stop driving at night. Monocular diplopia is also a symptom of cataracts.[7,8]

Most cataracts can be detected with direct ophthalmoscopy. The examiner should set the lens wheel to 4+ diopters and examine the red reflex with the ophthalmoscope 15 to 20 cm from the patient's eye. Cataracts are usually seen as dark specks or a haze against the red reflex.[4]

Both cataracts and age-related macular degeneration are common causes of visual loss in the elderly. Clues that the cause is macular degeneration rather than cataracts are loss of color discrimination and spontaneous use of a magnifying glass by the patient.[7]

Treatment

Before cataract surgery it is important to try to predict the degree of visual recovery that can be expected. Such surgery is pointless if macular degeneration will prevent visual acuity from being improved by the procedure. Ophthalmologists use two techniques for assessment: potential acuity measurement (PAM) and laser interferometry. Both procedures are painless and test macular function through small "windows" in the cataracts.[7]

Cataracts can be removed at any stage of their development; it is a myth that surgery must wait until the cataract is "ripe."[7,8] In fact, even if visual acuity is nearly normal, cataract removal is indicated if glare results in significant disability.[8]

Current techniques of cataract removal by extraction or phacoemulsification use an extracapsular approach. This means that the cataract is extracted from within the lens capsule, leaving the capsule behind to support the implant. In about one third of patients the capsule becomes cloudy in the first few weeks or months after surgery. Clear vision is instantly reestablished by use of a laser beam (yttrium aluminum garnet [YAG]) to cut a hole in the capsule.[7,8]

REFERENCES

1. Leske MC, Wu S-Y, Hennis A, et al: Diabetes, hypertension, and central obesity as cataract risk factors in a black population: the Barbados Eye Study, *Ophthalmology* 106:35-41, 1999.
2. West S: Does smoke get in your eyes? (editorial), *JAMA* 268:1025-1026, 1992.
3. Garbe E, Suissa S, LeLorier J: Association of inhaled corticosteroid use with cataract extraction in elderly patients, *JAMA* 280:539-543, 1998.
4. Chylack LT Jr: Cataracts and inhaled corticosteroids (editorial), *N Engl J Med* 337:46-48, 1997.

5. Cumming RG, Mitchell P: Medications and cataract: the Blue Mountains Eye Study, *Ophthalmology* 105:1751-1758, 1998.
6. West SK, Duncan DD, Munoz B, et al: Sunlight exposure and risk of lens opacities in a population-based study: the Salisbury Eye Evaluation Project, *JAMA* 280:714-718, 1998.
7. Fowler JH: Investigating cataracts—unveiling vision loss, *Can J Diagn* 11:64-77, 1994.
8. Obstbaum SA: An 82-year-old woman with cataracts, *JAMA* 275:1675-1680, 1996.

CENTRAL SEROUS CHORIORETINOPATHY

Central serous retinopathy is a disorder of the eye that usually involves young or middle-aged men. The clinical presentation is painless decreased or distorted vision in one eye. The underlying mechanism is accumulation of serous fluid between the retina and the choroid. The etiology is unknown, but the condition seems to affect individuals with type A personality and to be related to psychological stress. The vast majority of patients spontaneously regain normal visual acuity over a period of weeks or months.[1]

◣ REFERENCES ◢

1. Sharma S: Ophthaproblem: central serous chorioretinopathy, *Can Fam Physician* 44:1827, 1833-1834, 1998.

CONGENITAL LACRIMAL OBSTRUCTION

Congenital lacrimal duct obstruction is common and results in symptoms in 6% to 20% of neonates. In 80% of cases the obstruction is unilateral. In 90% of cases the obstruction spontaneously resolves within a year, and spontaneous resolution is usually seen in the remaining children during the second year of life. Symptoms are watering of the eye and crusting of the lids so that they are stuck together in the morning. Except in the case of a secondary infection, the globe remains white. Treatment is reassurance and explanation to the parents, cleaning of the lids on a regular basis, and topical antibiotics for obvious secondary conjunctivitis (red eye and increased exudate) if it arises. Probing of the lacrimal system during the first year is unnecessary in most instances and may cause strictures. One study has shown that massaging the lacrimal sac while occluding the canaliculi opens the canal in a number of cases.[1]

◣ REFERENCES ◢

1. Young JD, MacEwen CJ: Managing congenital lacrimal obstruction in general practice, *BMJ* 315:293-296, 1997.

CORNEAL LESIONS

(See also contact lenses; topical ophthalmic medications)

Care should be taken not to misdiagnose a corneal herpetic infection as a corneal abrasion. Herpetic lesions have a typical dendritic appearance, and because of decreased corneal sensitivity in the region of the lesion the corneal reflex is diminished.

Antibiotic ointment is not necessary in the routine treatment of corneal abrasions, and there is no published evidence supporting its use. A topical mydriatic such as homatropine or cyclopentolate (Cyclogyl) may be used for pain relief (see discussion of topical ophthalmic medications), and the eye may be patched if desired (see next paragraph).[1]

Simple corneal abrasions may be treated without eye patches. Abrasions 1 cm in diameter or smaller heal faster and with less pain when no patch is used.[2] Cold compresses and oral nonsteroidal antiinflammatory drugs (NSAIDs) may give adequate pain relief,[3] but a good alternative is topical ophthalmic NSAID drops such as ketorolac tromethamine (Acular) 0.5% qid.[4]

The wearing of contact lenses may be associated with corneal lesions that appear to be simple abrasions (see discussion of contact lenses). Such lesions should never be patched because the condition may in fact be infectious keratitis, which is usually caused by *Pseudomonas aeruginosa* or a protozoan of the *Acanthamoeba* species. This type of keratitis is more common in persons wearing overnight contact lenses or extended-wear contact lenses. Immediate ophthalmological consultation is highly desirable.[5] Patching is contraindicated in patients with infectious keratitis. *Pseudomonas* infection is treated by the frequent instillation of antibiotics such as an aminoglycoside (gentamicin [Garamycin Ophthalmic] or tobramycin [Tobrex]) or a quinolone (ciprofloxacin [Ciloxan], norfloxacin [Chibroxin], or ofloxacin [Ocuflox]) and follow-up within 24 hours (see section on topical ophthalmic medications). Steroid drops should never be used.[6]

◣ REFERENCES ◢

1. King JW, Brison RJ: Do topical antibiotics help corneal epithelial trauma? *Can Fam Physician* 39:2349-2352, 1993.
2. Kaiser PK (Corneal Abrasion Patching Study Group): A comparison of pressure patching versus no patching for corneal abrasions due to trauma or foreign body removal, *Ophthalmology* 102:1936-1942, 1995.
3. Mindlin AM: Treatment of corneal abrasions (letter), *JAMA* 275:837, 1996.
4. Kaiser PK, Pineda R II: A study of topical nonsteroidal antiinflammatory drops and no pressure patching in the treatment of corneal abrasions, *Ophthalmology* 104:1353-1359, 1997.
5. Sharma S: Ophthaproblem: contact lens (*Acanthamoeba*) keratitis, *Can Fam Physician* 44:1605, 1615, 1998.
6. Jampel HD: Patching for corneal abrasions, *JAMA* 274:1504, 1995.

CORNEAL TRANSPLANTS

The most common indication for corneal transplantation is corneal edema developing as a complication of cataract surgery. Human lymphocyte antigen tissue typing is unnecessary. Success, as measured by a clear cornea, is greater than 90%, but many patients are left with significant astigmatism requiring thick lenses for correction. Risk of graft rejection is lifelong but greatest in the first year; it is controlled primarily by prophylactic or therapeutic topical steroids.[1]

◀ REFERENCES ▶

1. Weston BC, White GL Jr: Corneal transplantation, *Am Fam Physician* 54:1945-1948, 1996.

GLAUCOMA, ACUTE ANGLE CLOSURE
(See also glaucoma, open angle)

Epidemiology

Acute angle closure glaucoma has its peak incidence in the sixth and seventh decades. It occurs more frequently in hypermetropic eyes (long-sighted eyes) because the globe in such an eye is smaller than normal and therefore more crowded internally. It is possible to tell whether someone is hypermetropic by checking their glasses; the lenses are positive and act like magnifying glasses.[1]

Prodromal Symptoms

Patients with acute angle closure glaucoma usually have had prodromal symptoms resulting from temporary increases in intraocular pressure. Such preliminary symptoms include slight blurring of vision, mild headaches, and occasionally seeing haloes around objects. Precipitating factors are those causing pupillary dilation such as the dim light of a movie theater, the adrenergic response to anger or anxiety, and anticholinergic medications such as tricyclic antidepressants.[1]

Sometimes a narrow angle can be detected in patients at risk of angle closure glaucoma by shining a penlight on the temporal side of the iris while checking to see whether the nasal side of the iris remains in shadow because of forward tenting of the iris.

Symptoms and Signs

A patient with fully developed angle closure glaucoma complains of agonizing eye pain, blurred vision, and often headache. Nausea and vomiting are common, and sometimes the patient has abdominal and chest pain. The eye is red with a ciliary flush, the cornea is steamy, and the pupil is dilated, fixed, and usually vertically oval. Ballottement of the globe often reveals a stony hard consistency, although failure to detect this sign does not rule out acute glaucoma. Visual acuity is markedly diminished.[1]

Management

Immediate management of acute angle closure glaucoma is directed toward lowering the intraocular pressure with medication. One three-stage protocol is as follows[1]:

1. Instill 2 drops of a topical beta-blocker such as timolol (Timoptic 0.5%) plus 2 drops of pilocarpine 2%.
2. If the attack has not stopped in 15 minutes, give acetazolamide (Diamox) 200 to 500 mg plus an osmotic diuretic, such as glycerol solution in orange juice, 1.5 to 2

g/kg, or mannitol 1 g/kg IV over a 20-minute period. This step may be repeated twice at 2-hour intervals.
3. Perform surgery, usually in the form of laser iridotomy.

◀ REFERENCES ▶

1. Balazsi AG: Looking into the signs of glaucoma, *Can J Diagn* 10:65-85, 1993.

GLAUCOMA, OPEN ANGLE
(See also asthma; glaucoma, acute angle closure; screening; surrogate endpoint)

Terminology

Ocular hypertension and glaucoma are not synonymous. Glaucoma is characterized by damage to the optic nerve that is manifested as visual field defects. Although most patients with glaucoma have elevated intraocular pressures (greater than 21 mm Hg), at least 15% of patients have normal pressures—"normal-tension glaucoma." However, many individuals have elevated intraocular pressures but no evidence of glaucoma ("ocular hypertension").[1] Although ocular hypertension is considered a risk factor for glaucoma, over 70% of patients with pressures that are consistently between 21 and 35 mm Hg do not have glaucomatous changes.[2]

Risk Factors

Recognized risk factors for open angle glaucoma include the following:

1. Age over 65
2. Family history of glaucoma
3. Black race
4. Severe myopia
5. Diabetes
6. Elevated intraocular pressure
7. Previous eye trauma
8. Previous eye surgery
9. Oral corticosteroid use[3]
10. Long-term use of ocular adrenocorticosteroids
11. High-dose continuous inhaled corticosteroid use (see discussion of asthma)[4]

Screening

Standard screening techniques are tonometry and funduscopy, but they are neither sensitive nor specific. Perimetry is too complex to be a practical screening tool.[2] Both the Canadian Task Force on Preventive Health Care[5] and the U.S. Preventive Services Task Force[6] give a "C" recommendation to screening maneuvers for glaucoma. An alternative strategy is to limit screening to those at high risk. At particularly high risk are individuals over the age of 65 (especially those over the age of 75), persons with a sibling who has glaucoma, and blacks.[7] The efficacy of screening high-risk persons is unknown.

Clinical Signs

As noted in the section on screening, the sensitivity and specificity of the various signs of open angle glaucoma are low. These signs include the following[8]:

1. Afferent pupillary defect (Marcus Gunn pupil)
2. Elevated intraocular pressure measured with Schiötz or applanation tonometry
3. Cup/disc ratio greater than 0.7
4. Difference of more than 0.2 in the cup/disc ratio between the two eyes
5. Oval cup with the vertical diameter greater than the horizontal diameter
6. Notching of the cup
7. Occasionally splinter hemorrhages at the disc margins
8. Visual field defects, especially in the nasal quadrants

Treatment

The principle underlying both medical and surgical treatment of glaucoma is that lowering intraocular pressure will arrest the progression of the disease. Unfortunately, there are no conclusive data confirming this hypothesis. All standard modalities of treatment can lower intraocular pressure by varying degrees (a surrogate endpoint), but no reliable randomized placebo-controlled trials have shown that treatment arrests the deterioration of visual fields (a clinically important endpoint).[9]

A wide variety of topical drugs are available for lowering intraocular pressure (Table 57).[1,10] Beta-blockers are the drugs of first choice, but respiratory and cardiovascular adverse effects are common. Because these topical drugs are absorbed directly into the systemic circulation through the nasolacrimal duct and nasal mucosa, no first-pass liver metabolism occurs; 1 drop of 0.5% timolol solution in each eye is equivalent to a 10-mg oral dose. Specific adverse effects include diminished pulmonary function in about one fourth of patients and a significantly increased incidence of falls, which can be devastating in the elderly.[11] A simple technique for decreasing systemic absorption while at the same time increasing ophthalmic absorption is to occlude the nasolacrimal duct with pressure from a finger or simply by closing the eyes firmly for 5 minutes after applying the drops.[10]

The cholinergic agonist pilocarpine, the traditional alternative to beta-blockers, must be taken four times a day, has local side effects, and can cause confusion.[11] Other effective alternatives include alpha$_2$-adrenergic agonists, topical carbonic anhydrase inhibitors, and prostaglandin analogues (Table 57). If one drug does not work, another may be tried or a combination of topical drugs can be used.[10]

While oral carbonic anhydrase inhibitors are usually prescribed for acute angle closure glaucoma, they are occasionally used for patients with chronic open angle glaucoma. Caution is needed because they can cause metabolic acidosis, paresthesias, altered taste, and, rarely, aplastic anemia and other blood dyscrasias.[10] The two most frequently used drugs in this class are acetazolamide (Diamox) 250 mg to 1 g daily in divided doses and methazolamide (Neptazane) 50 to 100 mg bid or tid.

If medical therapy fails or the adverse effects are unacceptable, the next option is either laser trabeculoplasty, which has about a 50% 5-year success rate in the elderly, or surgical trabeculectomy.[12] In laser trabeculoplasty a low-power argon laser beam is focused on the trabecular meshwork. This usually increases the outflow of aqueous humor with a resultant decrease in the intraocular pressure of about 30%.[2] In Great Britain many centers are now opting for surgery as first-line therapy.[1]

Table 57   Topical Medications for Chronic Open Angle Glaucoma

Drugs	Usual dose
Topical Nonselective Beta-Blockers	
Carteolol (Ocupress) 1%	1 drop bid
Levobunolol (AK Beta, Betagan) 0.25% and 0.5%	1 drop bid
Metipranolol (Optipranolol) 0.3%	1 drop bid
Timolol (Betimol, Timoptic) 0.25% and 0.5%	1 drop bid except for Timoptic-XE, which is 1 drop daily
Topical Cardioselective Beta-Blockers	
Betaxolol (Betoptic) 0.25% and 0.5%	1 drop bid
Topical Alpha$_2$-Adrenergic Receptor Agonists	
Apraclonidine (Iopidine) 0.5%	1 drop tid
Brimonidine tartrate (Alphagan) 0.2%	1 drop tid
Topical Cholinergic Myopics	
Pilocarpine 1%, 2%, 4% and 6%	1-2 drops qid
Topical Carbonic Anhydrase Inhibitors	
Brinzolamide (Azopt) 1%	1 drop tid
Dorzolamide (Trusopt) 2%	1 drop tid
Topical Prostaglandin Analogues	
Latanoprost (Xalatan) 0.005% (50 μg/ml)	1 drop qhs

⬆ REFERENCES ⬆

1. Lewis PR, Phillips TG, Sassani JW: Topical therapies for glaucoma: what family physicians need to know, *Am Fam Physician* 59:1871-1879, 1999.
2. Tucker JB: Screening for open-angle glaucoma, *Am Fam Physician* 148:75-80, 1993.
3. Garbe E, Lelorier J, Boivin J-F, et al: Risk of ocular hypertension or open-angle glaucoma in elderly patients on oral glucocorticoids, *Lancet* 350:979-982, 1997.
4. Garbe E, LeLorier J, Boivin J-F, Suissa S: Inhaled and nasal glucocorticoids and the risks of ocular hypertension or open-angle glaucoma, *JAMA* 277:722-727, 1997.
5. Canadian Task Force on the Periodic Health Examination: Periodic health examination, 1995 update. 3. Screening for visual problems among elderly patients, *Can Med Assoc J* 152:1211-1222, 1995.
6. US Preventive Services Task Force: *Guide to clinical preventive services,* ed 2, Baltimore, 1996, Williams & Wilkins, pp 383-391.

7. Rosenberg LF: Glaucoma: early detection and therapy for prevention of vision loss, *Am Fam Physician* 52:2289-2298, 1995.

8. Balazsi AG: Looking into the signs of glaucoma, *Can J Diagn* 10:65-85, 1993.

9. Rossetti L, Marchetti I, Orzalesi N, et al: Randomized clinical trials on medical treatment of glaucoma: are they an appropriate guide to clinical practice? *Arch Ophthalmol* 111:96-103, 1993.

10. Alward WL: Medical management of glaucoma, *N Engl J Med* 339:1298-1307, 1998.

11. Brimonidine—an alpha-2-agonist for glaucoma, *Med Lett* 39:54-55, 1997.

12. Diggory P, Franks W: Medical treatment of glaucoma—reappraisal of the risks, *Br J Ophthalmol* 80:85-89, 1996.

MACULAR DEGENERATION
(See also cataracts; vitamin A)

Both age-related macular degeneration and cataracts are common causes of visual loss in the elderly. Clues that the cause is macular degeneration rather than cataracts are loss of color discrimination and spontaneous use of a magnifying glass by the patient.[1]

Age-related macular degeneration is the most common cause of irreversible blindness among persons over the age of 65. It accounts for 40% to 50% of new cases of blindness in Canada. Its incidence is about 1% in 55-year-olds and rises to 15% by age 80.[2] With funduscopy, drusen and pigment stippling may be seen in the macular area. Smoking is a risk factor for the development of macular degeneration in both men[3] and women,[4] and prolonged exposure to sunlight might also increase risk of the disease.[5]

The U.S. Preventive Services Task Force[6] and the Canadian Task Force on Preventive Health Care[2] give a "C" recommendation to funduscopy for the detection of age-related macular degeneration. Both these organizations give a "B" recommendation to visual acuity testing in the elderly.[2,6]

Some studies have suggested that certain carotenoids, especially lutein and zeaxanthin, which are found in dark green leafy vegetables such as spinach and collard greens, have a protective effect against age-related macular degeneration. Vitamin A, beta-carotene, and supplements of vitamins C and E have not been found to be protective.[7]

A preliminary 1-year trial found that IV injection of verteporfin (a drug activated by light) followed by exposure of the affected macula to a laser beam prevented further visual loss in some patients with macular edema.[8]

--- ⚑ **REFERENCES** ⚑ ---

1. Fowler JH: Investigating cataracts—unveiling vision loss, *Can J Diagn* 11:64-77, 1994.

2. Canadian Task Force on the Periodic Health Examination: Periodic health examination, 1995 update. III. Screening for visual problems among elderly patients, *Can Med Assoc J* 152:1211-1222, 1995.

3. Christen WG, Glynn RJ, Manson JE, et al: A prospective study of cigarette smoking and risk of age-related macular degeneration in men, *JAMA* 276:1147-1151, 1996.

4. Seddon JM, Willett WC, Speizer FE, et al: A prospective study of cigarette smoking and age-related macular degeneration in women, *JAMA* 276:1141-1146, 1996.

5. Cruickshanks KJ, Klein R, Klein BE: Sunlight and age-related macular degeneration: the Beaver Dam Eye Study, *Arch Ophthalmol* 111:514-518, 1993.

6. US Preventive Services Task Force: *Guide to clinical preventive services,* ed 2, Baltimore, 1996, Williams & Wilkins, pp 373-391.

7. Seddon JM, Ajani UA, Sperduto RD, et al: Dietary carotenoids, vitamins A, C, and E, and advanced age-related macular degeneration, *JAMA* 272:1413-1420, 1994.

8. Treatment of Age-related Macular Degeneration with Photodynamic Therapy (TAP) Study Group: Photodynamic therapy of subfoveal choroidal neovascularization in age-related macular degeneration with verteporfin, *Arch Ophthalmol* 117:1329-1345, 1999.

REFRACTIVE ERRORS
Contact Lenses

A rare but serious complication of contact lens use that may lead to blindness is microbial keratitis or corneal ulceration, which is usually caused by *Pseudomonas* or *Serratia* species. A study from the Netherlands found the annual incidence among daily-wear soft contact lens wearers was 3.5 per 10,000 users.[1] Microbial keratitis can occur with daily-wear lenses or disposable lenses even when they are used correctly and taken out at night,[1,2] but the risk is much greater if the lenses are worn overnight.[1] Pain and visual loss are the usual presenting symptoms. Urgent treatment with hourly instillation of topical antibiotics is required (systemic antibiotics are not effective). Patients traveling to remote areas may be advised to include topical ophthalmic antibiotics in an emergency medical kit.[2]

Surgical Correction

The two surgical techniques that are most frequently used to correct refractive errors are photorefractive keratectomy (PRK) and laser-assisted in situ keratomileusis (LASIK). Both are performed with an excimer laser that emits ultraviolet light, which has the ability to decompose (photoablate) the superficial tissue layers at which it is directed without causing significant thermal damage to surrounding tissues. In PRK the laser is applied to the intact eye and ablates both the covering epithelium and the underlying stroma. The patient is left with a large iatrogenic corneal abrasion that takes several days to heal; topical NSAIDs are commonly prescribed during the healing phase. In LASIK a microtome is used to cut a very thin corneal flap, which is folded back so that the laser can be applied directly to the corneal stroma. The flap is then replaced, and because the epithelium is still intact, healing and full visual recovery are rapid. LASIK is a relatively new procedure; complications are related to preparing the flap in most cases and are more common with inexperienced operators.[3]

Myopia (short sightedness), hyperopia (long sightedness), and astigmatism can be corrected surgically. The cornea (which contributes about two thirds of the refractive power of the eye) is sculpted with laser so that the curvature is altered. In the case of myopia the globe is too large and the image is focused anterior to the retina; correction is achieved by flattening (ablating) the central portion of the cornea to decrease curvature and thus move the focal point posteriorly. In the case of hyperopia the globe is too small and the image is focused posterior to the retina; correction is achieved by leaving the central area intact while ablating a peripheral ring around the margin of the cornea to increase curvature and thus move the focal point anteriorly. Astigmatism is corrected by sculpting selected meridians of the cornea.[3]

Nearly normal visual acuity is achieved in most patients, but in some, especially those with marked refractive errors, a degree of "regression" develops over 6 months so that the patient remains slightly hyperopic or myopic. Some patients experience glare or haloes postoperatively, especially at night, but these diminish slowly with time.[3]

PRK and LASIK are outpatient procedures that take only a few minutes to perform. They are generally contraindicated in persons under the age of 18.[3]

─────────────── **◣ REFERENCES ◢** ───────────────

1. Cheng KH, Leung SL, Hoekman HW, et al: Incidence of contact-lens-associated microbial keratitis and its related morbidity, *Lancet* 354:181-185, 1999.
2. Donzis PB: Corneal ulcers from contact lenses during travel to remote areas (letter), *N Engl J Med* 338:1629-1630, 1998.
3. Yu EY, Jackson WB: Recent advances in refractive surgery, *Can Med Assoc J* 160:1329-1337, 1999.

TOPICAL OPHTHALMIC MEDICATIONS

(See also allergic rhinitis; glaucoma)

Eyedrop Instillation in Children

Instilling eyedrops in recalcitrant children is difficult. Confrontation may be avoided by having the child lie supine with eyes closed while the drops are applied to the lids near the medical canthus. When the eyes are opened, most of the drops flow onto the conjunctiva. A British ophthalmologist evaluated this technique using pilocarpine. When the degree of pupillary dilatation was measured, it was calculated that 66% of the drug entered the eye.[1]

Anesthetics

A frequently used topical anesthetic is proparacaine (Alcaine, Ophthaine, Ophthetic). The usual dose for removing corneal foreign bodies and other procedures is 1 or 2 drops of a 0.5% solution.

Antibacterials

A variety of topical antibiotics are available, and a number of them are listed in Table 58. These are all available in the

Table 58   Topical Ophthalmic Antibacterials

Generic names	Trade names
Aminoglycosides	
Gentamicin	Garamycin
Tobramycin	Tobrex, AKTob
Fluoroquinolones	
Ciprofloxacin	Ciloxan
Norfloxacin	Chibroxin
Ofloxacin	Ocuflox
Sulfonamides	
Sulfacetamide sodium	Sodium Sulamyd
Other	
Chloramphenicol	Chloroptic

form of ophthalmic drops and ointments. Dosages vary slightly among products, but as a general rule for severe conjunctivitis, 1 or 2 drops is instilled every 1 to 2 hours while the patient is awake for the first 1 to 2 days and the dose is then reduced to q4-6h for the next few days. If the infection is mild, drops are applied q4-6h. Ointments may be applied at bedtime. Sulfacetamide sodium (Sodium Sulamyd) comes as a 10% and a 30% solution; most family physicians use the 10% solution. Tobramycin ophthalmic products are safe for children of all ages. The safety of fluoroquinolone ophthalmic preparations for children under 1 year of age has not been established. Although the odds are slim that chloramphenicol eye drops would cause aplastic anemia,[2,3] 23 cases of serious hematological toxicity have been reported in a U.S. national register.[4] Since other antibiotic drops are available, prudence dictates reservation in the use of chloramphenicol.[5]

Antihistamines, Vasoconstrictors, and Mast Cell Stabilizers

Topical antihistamines or antihistamines combined with vasoconstrictors may give relief to some patients with allergic conjunctivitis. Emedastine difumarate (Emadine) 1 to 2 drops in each eye qid, Levocabastine (Livostin) 1 drop in each eye daily, olopatadine (Patanol) 1 to 2 drops in each eye bid, and ketotifen (Zaditor) 1 drop in each eye q8h to q12h are examples of ophthalmic antihistamines.

Many antihistamine-vasoconstrictor combinations are available over the counter. The use of these agents has been associated with induction of both acute and chronic conjunctivitis.[6] Examples of these combination drugs are naphazoline plus pheniramine (Naphcon-A) and naphazoline plus antazoline (Vasocon-A). The usual dose is 1 or 2 drops in each eye every 3 to 4 hours.

Topical vasoconstrictors alone decrease redness of the eyes in patients with allergic conjunctivitis, and many of these are available over the counter. Examples are phenylephrine (Neo-Synephrine), tetrahydrozoline (Visine), and naphazoline (Clear Eyes, Naphcon).

Two mast cell stabilizers that may relieve symptoms of allergic conjunctivitis are cromolyn sodium (Crolom, Opticrom) and lodoxamide (Alomide). The usual dose for each is 1 or 2 drops qid.

Ketorolac (Acular), a topical ophthalmic NSAID, has been used for treatment of allergic conjunctivitis.

Cycloplegic Mydriatics

Drugs that paralyze the ciliary muscle and thus inhibit accommodation are cycloplegics, and of course those that dilate the pupils are mydriatics. Many agents do both. Short-acting cycloplegic mydriatics such as tropicamide (Mydriacyl) 0.5% or 1% are generally used by family physicians for dilating the pupil to facilitate funduscopy. Longer acting drugs such as cyclopentolate (Cyclogyl) 1% or 2% or homatropine 2% or 5% may be used to relieve ciliary spasm (and pain) from corneal abrasions or for the treatment of iritis or uveitis.

Glaucoma Medications

Glaucoma medications are discussed in the earlier section on glaucoma.

Nonsteroidal Antiinflammatory Drugs

Ophthalmic NSAIDs relieve the pain of corneal abrasion. Some of the available agents are flurbiprofen (Ocufen), diclofenac (Voltaren), and ketorolac (Acular).

Tears and Lubricants

A large number of artificial tear preparations are available without prescription for symptomatic treatment of dry eyes. The usual dose is 1 to 2 drops q1-4h. Examples are hydroxypropyl methylcellulose (Isopto Tears, Lacril, Tears Naturale), polyvinyl alcohol (Hypotears, Liquifilm, Tears Plus), and polysorbate (Teardrops). Lubricating ointments containing white petrolatum and mineral oil may be applied to dry eyes at bedtime. They are often used in cases of Bell's palsy to prevent the cornea from drying. Examples are DuraTears and Lacri-Lube.

────────────── ◢ **REFERENCES** ◣ ──────────────

1. Smith SE: Eyedrop instillation for reluctant children, *Br J Ophthalmol* 75:480-481, 1991.
2. Wiholm B-E, Kelly JP, Kaufman D, et al: Relation of aplastic anaemia to use of chloramphenicol eye drops in two international case-control studies, *BMJ* 316:666, 1998.
3. Lancaster T, Swart AM, Jick H: Risk of serious haematological toxicity with use of chloramphenicol eye drops in a British general practice database, *BMJ* 316:667, 1998.
4. Doona M, Walsh JB: Use of chloramphenicol as topical eye medication: time to cry halt? *BMJ* 310:1217-1218, 1995.
5. Doona M, Walsh JB: Topical chloramphenicol is an outmoded treatment (letter), *BMJ* 316:1903, 1998.
6. Soparkar CN, Wilhelmus KR, Koch DD, et al: Acute and chronic conjunctivitis due to over-the-counter ophthalmic decongestants, *Arch Ophthalmol* 115:34-48, 1997.

OTOLARYNGOLOGY

(See also dysphagia)

Topics covered in this section

Ear
Motion Sickness
Mouth
Nose
Pharynx
Sinuses
Vertigo

EAR
External Ear

Foreign bodies

Many foreign bodies may be removed from the external auditory canal by syringing. This method should not be used for organic materials (e.g., peas, beans) because they may absorb the water and swell. It should not be used for disk batteries such as those in watches and hearing aids because when exposed to water they may leak and cause severe tissue damage. Small children often require a general anesthetic before removal of foreign bodies.[1]

Instilling mineral oil or 2% lidocaine into the canal will kill live insects. The remains may then be gently syringed out.[1]

Otitis externa

Seborrheic dermatitis and other skin conditions can affect the ear canal and cause otitis externa. A common treatment for these conditions is steroid drops alone such as betamethasone (Betnesol Otic) or steroid drops combined with other ingredients such as hydrocortisone plus acetic acid and propylene glycol (VoSol HC Otic).

A variety of bacterial organisms, especially *Staphylococcus aureus* and *Pseudomonas aeruginosa,* have been associated with otitis externa, but in many cases an infectious etiology cannot be ascertained. The most consistently observed predisposing factor is frequent water exposure,[2,3] and one reported method of preventing the condition is to instill 2 to 4 drops of an equal mixture of vinegar (5% acetic acid) and rubbing alcohol (70% isopropyl alcohol) into the ear canals immediately after coming out of the water.[3] Swimming in freshwater lakes has led to outbreaks of *P. aeruginosa* otitis externa.[4] Fungal infections, whether caused by *Candida* or *Aspergillus niger,* are rare in North America.

Medications for bacterial otitis externa often include aminoglycosides (gentamicin, neomycin, or framycetin). Ototoxicity from the use of gentamicin (Garasone Otic) drops has been reported in patients with perforated drums. In patients with perforations topical drugs containing aminoglycosides should not be used or should be used for as short a time as possible, applied to an ear wick (gauze strip) rather than directly into the canal, and discontinued immediately if tinnitus, hearing loss, vertigo, or imbalance develops.[5]

Most of the topical antibiotics used for otitis externa are combinations of antibiotics and steroids; the corticosteroids are used to diminish inflammation and prevent obstruction of the canal. Combinations of hydrocortisone, neomycin, and polymyxin B (e.g., Cortisporin Otic) and hydrocortisone and ciprofloxacin (Cipro HC Otic) are available in both the United States and Canada. In Canada combinations of betamethasone and gentamicin (Garasone Otic) or of dexamethasone, framycetin, and gramicidin (Sofracort) are also on the market, and chloramphenicol drops without steroids (Chloromycetin Otic) and ofloxacin (Floxin Otic) drops without steroids may be obtained in the United States.

Indications for systemic antibiotics in the treatment of external otitis are few. According to one U.S. survey, however, 40% of patients with external otitis received both topical and systemic medications, and in most cases the systemic antibiotics were not active against *S. aureus* or *P. aeruginosa*.[6]

Wax

An effective ceruminolytic is a liquid formulation of docusate (Colace, Regulex). Between 8 and 10 drops should be instilled into the canal and left for 10 minutes, followed by instrumental or lavage removal of the cerumen.[7]

❧ REFERENCES ❧

1. Ansley JF, Cunningham MJ: Treatment of aural foreign bodies in children, *Pediatrics* 101:638-641, 1998.
2. Russell JD, Donnelly M, McShane DP, et al: What causes acute otitis externa? *J Laryngol Otol* 107:898-901, 1993.
3. Larimore WL, Hartman JR, Shupe TB, et al: Diary from a week in practice, *Am Fam Physician* 55:2651, 1997.
4. van Asperen IA, de Rover CM, Schijven JF, et al: Risk of otitis externa after swimming in recreational fresh water lakes containing *Pseudomonas aeruginosa*, *BMJ* 311:1407-1410, 1995.
5. Canadian Adverse Drug Reaction Newsletter: Aminoglycoside ear drops and ototoxicity, *Can Med Assoc J* 156:1056, 1997.
6. Halpern MT, Palmer CS, Seidlin M: Treatment patterns for otitis externa, *J Am Board Fam Pract* 12:1-7, 1999.
7. Chen DA, Caparosa RJ: A nonprescription cerumenolytic, *Am J Otol* 12:475-476, 1991.

Middle Ear

(See also aviation medicine; scuba diving)

Otitis media

(See also middle ear effusion; tonsillectomy)

Acute otitis media. Based on tympanocentesis as the gold standard, at least 40% of patients in whom acute otitis media is diagnosed on the basis of clinical findings do not have the disease. Pneumatic otoscopy may increase the specificity of diagnosis but is not commonly used in practice.[1]

Symptoms of upper respiratory tract infection such as cough or rhinorrhea are seen in 94% of children with acute otitis media. In the absence of such symptoms the diagnosis of otitis media is unlikely.[2] In one study the positive predictive value of ear pain as a symptom of acute otitis media in children with upper respiratory tract symptoms was 83%; however, 40% of children with otitis media did not have pain.[3]

Viruses alone or in combination with bacteria are the major causes of otitis media.[4,5] The most common viruses are respiratory syncytial viruses and parainfluenza and influenza viruses.[4] The most common bacterial pathogens are *Streptococcus pneumoniae, Haemophilus influenzae,* and *Branhamella (Moraxella) catarrhalis.*[4,5]

About 30% to 40% of *Haemophilus* and 50% to 90% of *Branhamella* organisms produce beta-lactamase and are resistant to amoxicillin in vitro. In some areas 40% of pneumococci are resistant to trimethoprim-sulfamethoxazole, and a few are resistant to penicillin. However, this in vitro resistance does not usually translate into clinical ineffectiveness. Should antibiotics be used for otitis media (see below), most authorities recommend amoxicillin as the first choice or trimethoprim-sulfamethoxazole (Septra, Bactrim) as the least expensive alternative.[5] Although the standard dose of amoxicillin is 40 to 45 mg/kg/day, an expert committee convened by the Centers for Disease Control and Prevention recommended that 80 to 90 mg/kg/day be used when drug-resistant *S. pneumoniae* was suspected to be present in the community.[6] Suggested indications for using beta-lactamase-stable drugs, such as amoxicillin–clavulanic acid (Augmentin, Clavulin), erythromycin-sulfisoxazole (Pediazole), or a second- or third-generation cephalosporin, are persistent symptoms for more than 48 to 72 hours while the patient is taking the initial antibiotic, development of otitis media while the patient is taking amoxicillin, or an episode of otitis media within the previous 2 months that did not respond to amoxicillin.[7]

No solid guidelines for optimal duration of treatment with antibiotics have been established. Good results have been reported with 2, 3, 5, and 10 days.[9] One metaanalysis concluded that for uncomplicated acute otitis media in children a 5-day course was as effective as a 10-day course. The power of the study was insufficient to determine whether this was true for children under 2 years of age or those with perforated drums,[9] and therefore 10 days should probably be used in these circumstances.[1]

Reputed advantages of routinely using antibiotics for acute otitis media are that these drugs decrease the duration of symptoms and the rate of complications. Careful review of the literature does not substantiate this. Some studies found no improvement in outcomes with antibiotics,[8] and others reported only a slight advantage.[10] One metaanalysis found that after 24 hours 60% of children were pain free regardless of whether they received antibiotics and that between days 2 and 7 only 14% of the control patients had persistent pain. This analysis also found a decreased incidence of contralateral otitis media in the antibiotic-treated group.[10]

Persistent ear pain in children with otitis media is not necessarily due to persistent bacterial infection. One study of children treated with antibiotics found that 62% had persistent symptoms even when bacteriological cure was shown by tympanostomy cultures.[11] Viral infection is probably a major cause of this phenomenon.[12]

A cogent reason for avoiding antibiotic use for otitis media is a rising incidence of antibiotic resistance that correlates with increasing use of these drugs in ambulatory children.[8,13] Is it safe not to use antibiotics? In most of the developed world they are prescribed routinely, but a notable exception is the Netherlands. In that country guidelines recommend no initial use of antibiotics. For children 2 years and over, reevaluation is suggested after 3 days if symptoms persist, and at that time antibiotics may be prescribed. For children 6 months to 2 years, antibiotics are also withheld initially, but reassessment by visit or phone after 24 hours is required. No controlled trials of this approach have been published, but persistence of symptoms for more than 3 to 4 days has been noted in only 3% of children and serious complications have been extremely rare.[8]

Recurrent otitis media. The first-line management of recurrent otitis media is to make sure that environmental risk factors are eliminated. Important ones are eliminating exposure to tobacco smoke, using small rather than large day care facilities,[14] and if feasible, taking pacifiers away from the children (a Finnish prospective study of children under 3 years attending day care found that those who used pacifiers had 25% more episodes of acute otitis media than those who did not[15]).

According to some experts three episodes of otitis media occurring within a 6-month period are an indication for prophylactic antibiotics.[14] These are usually given daily for several months, especially during the winter. Some physicians give antibiotics only at the onset of an upper respiratory tract infection, but this does not seem to be as effective. Prophylactic regimens include amoxicillin 20 mg/kg/day as a single dose or in 2 divided doses or sulfisoxazole 75 mg/kg/day as a single dose or in 2 divided doses. Prophylactic antibiotics are at least as effective as ventilation tubes in preventing further infections.[16]

How strong is the evidence supporting the prophylactic administration of antibiotics for otitis media? A 1993 meta-analysis of a number of trials found a small benefit,[17] whereas a more recent randomized placebo-controlled trial found none.[18] Furthermore, the natural history of recurrent otitis media tends to make one think twice about the need for antibiotic prophylaxis. A study in northern Finland followed 222 children with recurrent otitis media, defined as three episodes within 6 months or four episodes within 1 year. None of the children received prophylactic antibiotics or had ventilation tubes. During the first 6 months after recurrent otitis media was diagnosed, 38% had no subsequent ear infections, 28% had one further episode, 18% two further episodes, and 12% three or more further episodes. In only 4% did chronic

otitis media with effusion develop. The major risk factor for recurrent infections was age under 16 months.[19]

Among children with recurrent otitis media, adenoidectomy or adenotonsillectomy leads to a slight short-term decrease in recurrence rates, but in view of the surgical morbidity, few indications exist for such interventions.[20]

➤ REFERENCES ➤

1. Pichichero ME: Changing the treatment paradigm for acute otitis media in children (editorial), *JAMA* 279:1748-1750, 1998.
2. Ruuskanen O, Heikkinen T: Otitis media: etiology and diagnosis, *Postgrad Med* 13(suppl 1):S23-S26, 1994.
3. Heikkinen T, Ruuskanen O: Signs and symptoms predicting acute otitis media, *Arch Pediatr Adolesc Med* 149:26-29, 1995.
4. Heikkinen T, Thint M, Chonmaitree T: Prevalence of various respiratory viruses in the middle ear during acute otitis media, *N Engl J Med* 340:260-264, 1999.
5. Drugs for treatment of acute otitis media in children, *Med Lett* 36:19-21, 1994.
6. Dowell SF, Butler JC, Giebink GS, et al: Acute otitis media: management and surveillance in an era of pneumococcal resistance—a report from the Drug-Resistant Streptococcus Pneumoniae Therapeutic Working Group, *Pediatr Infect Dis J* 18:1-9, 1999.
7. Paradise JL: Treatment guidelines for otitis media: the need for breadth and flexibility, *Postgrad Med* 14:429-435, 1995.
8. Froom J, Culpepper L, Jacobs M, et al: Antimicrobials for acute otitis media? A review from the International Primary Care Network, *BMJ* 315:98-102, 1997.
9. Kozyrsky J AL, Hildes-Ripstein E, Longstaffe A, et al: Treatment of acute otitis media with a shortened course of antibiotics: a meta-analysis, *JAMA* 279:1736-1742, 1998.
10. Del Mar C, Glasziou P, Hayem M: Are antibiotics indicated as initial treatment for children with acute otitis media? A meta-analysis, *BMJ* 314:1526-1529, 1997.
11. Marchant CD, Carlin SA, Johnson CE, et al: Measuring the comparative efficacy of antibacterial agents for acute otitis media: the "Polyanna phenomenon," *J Pediatr* 120:72-77, 1992.
12. Arola M, Ziegler T, Ruuskanen O: Respiratory virus infection as a cause of prolonged symptoms in acute otitis media, *J Pediatr* 116:697-701, 1990.
13. Aronoff SC: Antimicrobials in children and the problem of drug resistance (editorial), *Am Fam Physician* 54:44-56, 1996.
14. Giebink GS: Preventing otitis media, *Ann Otol Rhinol Laryngol* 163(suppl):20-23, 1994.
15. Niemela M, Uhari M, Mottonen M: A pacifier increases the risk of recurrent acute otitis media in children in day care centers, *Pediatrics* 96:884-888, 1995.
16. Berman S: Otitis media in children, *N Engl J Med* 332:1560-1565, 1995.
17. Williams R, Chalmers T, Stange KC, et al: Use of antibiotics in preventing recurrent acute otitis media and in treating otitis media with effusion, *JAMA* 270:1344-1351, 1993.
18. Roark R, Berman S: Continuous twice daily or once daily amoxicillin prophylaxis compared with placebo for children with recurrent acute otitis media, *Pediatr Infect Dis J* 16:376-381, 1997.

19. Alho OP, Laara E, Oja H: What is the natural history of recurrent acute otitis media in infancy, *J Fam Pract* 43:258-264, 1996.
20. Paradise JL, Bluestone CD, Colborn DK: Adenoidectomy and adenotonsillectomy for recurrent acute otitis media, *JAMA* 282:945-953, 1999.

Middle ear effusion

(See also otitis media)

The management of otitis media with effusion has traditionally involved the insertion of ventilation tubes. This is the second most common surgical procedure in U.S. children, superseded only by circumcision.[1]

Risk factors for otitis media with effusions include bottle feeding, exposure to passive smoke, and attendance at day care or other group infant facilities.[2]

Longitudinal studies of young children with middle ear effusions have shown that by 3 months 50% of effusions have resolved spontaneously and that resolution continues thereafter at a constant rate so that by 1 year few children still have an effusion.[2]

Suggested initial treatment is observation and probably antibiotics. Antibiotics have been shown to increase the resolution rate by 14%.[2] However, expectant watching of these children for 4 to 6 months is quite safe if they do not have significant hearing loss or other symptoms.[3] A cogent reason for avoiding antibiotics whenever possible in the treatment of serous otitis media is to slow the development of antibiotic-resistant organisms.[4]

The rationale for myringotomy with tube insertion is primarily to improve hearing and prevent difficulties in language development. However, no conclusive evidence has been presented to support or reject this hypothesis. The Otitis Media Panel recommends that myringotomy with tube insertion be considered for a child who has had bilateral effusions for a total of 3 months and who has a hearing deficit of at least 20 dB in the better hearing ear.[2] In a study in the United Kingdom, children who met these criteria were selected at random either to receive immediate placement of ventilation tubes or to be observed for a further 9 months with placement of tubes at that time if hearing deficits persisted. Eighty-five percent of children in the watchful waiting arm of the study required tubes (15% were spared surgery). Expressive language scores were slightly lower in the watchful waiting group at 9 months, but by 18 months no differences between the groups were detectable.[5]

Treatments that are not recommended include antihistamines, decongestants, corticosteroids, and tonsillectomy.[2]

Adenoidectomy is a controversial issue. Some experts, as represented by the Otitis Media Panel,[2] believe there is almost no indication for adenoidectomy in the treatment of serous otitis media, others that it has a role in primary treatment with or without ventilation tubes,[6,7] and still others that it is indicated if treatment with ventilation tubes is unsuccessful.[8]

A historical note: During World War II a number of flyers and submariners in the U.S. military were subjected to nasopharyngeal irradiation to shrink nasopharyngeal lymphoid tissue and thus prevent barotrauma to the ear.[9]

⤳ REFERENCES ⤳

1. Berman S: Otitis media in children, *N Engl J Med* 332:1560-1565, 1995.
2. Otitis Media Guideline Panel: Managing otitis media with effusion in young children, *Am Fam Physician* 50:1003-1010, 1994.
3. Aronoff SC: Antimicrobials in children and the problem of drug resistance (editorial), *Am Fam Physician* 54:44-56, 1996.
4. Paradise JL: Managing otitis media: a time for change (editorial), *Pediatrics* 96:712-715, 1995.
5. Maw R, Wilks J, Harvey I, et al: Early surgery compared with watchful waiting for glue ear and effect on language development in preschool children: a randomised trial, *Lancet* 353:960-963, 1999.
6. Bicknell PG: Role of adenotonsillectomy in the management of pediatric ear, nose and throat infections, *Postgrad Med* 13:S75-S78, 1994.
7. Maw AR: Tonsils and adenoids: their relation to secretory otitis media, *Acta Otorhinolaryngol* 40:81-88, 1988.
8. Paradise JL, Bluestone CD, Rogers KD, et al: Efficacy of adenoidectomy for recurrent otitis media in children previously treated with tympanostomy-tube placement: results of parallel randomized and nonrandomized trials, *JAMA* 263:2066-2073, 1990.
9. Skolnick AA: Discovery of 50-year-old naval logbook may aid follow-up study of radium-exposed veterans, *JAMA* 276:1628-1630, 1996.

Inner Ear

(See also vertigo)

Benign positional vertigo, Ménière's disease, and vestibular neuronitis are discussed in the section on vertigo.

Hearing impairment

Audiological assessment of children. Conventional audiometry can rarely be performed on children under 4 years of age, but a variety of other techniques can assess hearing capabilities even in infants. Two important tests are otoacoustic emissions and auditory brainstem responses. In response to environmental sounds the cochlea generates very soft sounds of its own. These otoacoustic emissions can be detected by a small probe placed in the ear canal (with young infants this is best done when they are asleep). The otoacoustic emissions test cannot determine the threshold of hearing loss, but such threshold can be determined by the auditory brainstem response. When auditory brainstem responses are assessed, scalp electrodes detect changes in brain activity in response to sound. Older children are asked to lie quietly during the procedure, and younger children are assessed during natural or hypnotic-induced sleep or even during general anesthesia.[1]

Cochlear implants. Modern cochlear implants use multi-electrode arrays that provide several channels of stimulation. The electrodes are implanted into the cochlea near the auditory nerve. At present 2 years is the lower age limit for implants. Most cochlear implants may be damaged by magnetic resonance imaging.[2] The value of cochlear implants is controversial.[3] It is claimed that both adults and children with profound sensorineural hearing loss receive significant benefit, including improved speech and reading ability because of supplemental information from the implant.[2] On the other hand, many deaf people function well in society and do not consider themselves to have a disability requiring medical therapy (see discussion of cultural aspects of deafness below).[3,4]

Hearing aids. Digital hearing aids not only amplify specific frequencies, but also distinguish speech from background noise and suppress the background noise. As a result, amplified sounds are less distorted than with many earlier devices.[5] Traditional hearing aids are behind-the-ear models, but improved technology has allowed the development of in-the-ear, in-the-canal, and completely-in-the-canal models. Behind-the-ear aids are generally used for children because changes in the canal with growth would require up to four changes a year for in-canal types.[1]

Screening for hearing loss in the elderly. A Dutch study found that the sensitivity and specificity of the whispered voice test were excellent compared with formal audiograms for detecting hearing losses greater than 30 dB (a level of loss causing social disability). Screening audiograms and auriscopes with built-in audiometric devices had high sensitivities for losses greater than 40 dB, but specificities were low. The whispered voice test is much less expensive.[6]

The Canadian Task Force on Preventive Health Care[7] and the U.S. Preventive Services Task Force[8] both give "B" recommendations to screening elderly people for hearing impairment.

Smoking. Both active smoking and passive smoking are associated with an increased risk of hearing loss.[9]

Cultural aspects of deafness. Many deaf people, particularly those who were born deaf, identify with the "Deaf" community. Members of the "Deaf" community use American sign language and tend not to use vocal speech or to lip read. They form a cultural minority that is often not well understood by the dominant hearing community. For example, to attract someone's attention, members of the "Deaf" community tend to touch the other person, which is acceptable in their culture but often deemed intrusive and offensive in the dominant culture. Because most severely hearing-impaired children have parents with normal hearing, the "Deaf" culture is imparted to them by residential schools and peers rather than by parents.

A critically important issue for members of "Deaf World Culture" is cochlear implants (see earlier discussion). The issue is not only that members of the culture do not consider hearing loss a disability, but that if cochlear implants became the norm and they proved to be effective (still a matter of controversy), the "Deaf "culture would become extinct.[4]

───────────── **REFERENCES** ─────────────

1. Papaioannou V: Audiological assessment and (re)habilitation in children, *Patient Care Can* 10(1):32-41, 1999.
2. NIH Consensus Conference: Cochlear implants in adults and children: NIH Consensus Development Panel on Cochlear Implants in Adults and Children, *JAMA* 274:1955-1961, 1995.
3. Swanson L: Cochlear implants: the head-on collision between medical technology and the right to be deaf, *Can Med Assoc J* 157:929-932, 1997.
4. Lane H, Bahan B: Ethics of cochlear implantation in young children: a review and reply from a deaf-world perspective, *Otol Head Neck Surg* 119:297-313, 1998.
5. Werner J, Gottschlich S: Recent advances: otorhinolaryngology, *BMJ* 315:354-357, 1997.
6. Eekhof JA, de Bock GH, de Laat JA, et al: The whispered voice: the best test for screening for hearing impairment in general practice? *Br J Gen Pract* 46:473-474, 1996.
7. Canadian Task Force on the Periodic Health Examination: *Canadian guide to clinical preventive health care,* Ottawa, 1994, Canada Communication Group—Publishing, pp 954-963.
8. US Preventive Services Task Force: *Guide to clinical preventive services,* ed 2, Baltimore, 1996, Williams & Wilkins, pp 393-405.
9. Cruickshanks KJ, Klein R, Klein BE, et al: Cigarette smoking and hearing loss: the Epidemiology of Hearing Loss Study, *JAMA* 279:1715-1719, 1998.
10. Barnett S: Clinical and cultural issues in caring for deaf people, *Fam Med* 31:17-22, 1999.

Tinnitus

Healthy individuals frequently experience intermittent tinnitus lasting a few minutes. Although tinnitus lasting weeks, months, or years may occur in individuals with normal hearing, it is usually associated with hearing loss. The most frequent causes of such hearing loss are sensorineural loss as occurs in presbycusis, noise-induced hearing loss, and Ménière's disease. Tinnitus may also be induced by middle ear disease such as otitis media, serous otitis media, and otosclerosis, external ear disease such as an occluding wax plug, and certain drugs such as aspirin. With time most people become less bothered by their tinnitus. The most important therapeutic intervention is reassurance. For some patients with hearing impairment as well as tinnitus, hearing aids ameliorate both symptoms. A few patients benefit from tinnitus-masking devices that can be worn in or behind the ear.[1]

───────────── **REFERENCES** ─────────────

1. Vesterager V: Tinnitus—investigation and management, *BMJ* 314:728-732, 1997.

MOTION SICKNESS

The traditional medications for motion sickness are H_1 receptor antagonists such as dimenhydrinate (Dramamine,

Gravol) 50 to 100 mg qid, preferably given 1 to 2 hours before onset of motion, and scopolamine patches (Transderm-Scop, <u>Transderm-V</u>) applied to the postauricular area 12 hours before onset of motion and changed every 72 hours.[1]

REFERENCES

1. Nicholson AN, Pascoe PA, Spencer MB, et al: Jet lag and motion sickness, *Br Med Bull* 49:285-304, 1993.

MOUTH
Aphthous Ulcers
(See also treatment of specific AIDS-related disorders)

About 4% of patients with recurrent oral ulcers have a gluten enteropathy. The ulcers respond to a gluten-free diet.[1]

A number of studies have suggested that thalidomide (Synovir) in doses of 50 to 200 mg/day is effective in treating and preventing aphthous ulcers in both HIV-negative and HIV-positive patients.[2]

A blinded study from Israel found that the application of a solution of sucralfate (Sulcrate) to aphthous ulcers four times a day using an applicator stick not only decreased the duration of pain and the time until healing, but also increased the duration of remissions.[3]

Amlexanox (Aphthasol), an inhibitor of inflammatory mediators, is marketed as a 5% oral paste to be applied to the ulcers four times a day. Controlled trials have shown it to be effective.[4]

REFERENCES

1. Srinivasan U, Weir DG, Feighery C, et al: Emergence of classic enteropathy after longstanding gluten sensitive oral ulceration, *BMJ* 316:206-207, 1998.
2. New uses of thalidomide, *Med Lett* 38:15-16, 1996.
3. Rattan J, Schneider M, Arber N, et al: Sucralfate suspension as a treatment of recurrent aphthous stomatitis, *J Intern Med* 236:341-343, 1994.
4. Khandwala A, Vaninwegen RG, Alfano MC: 5-Percent amlexanox oral paste, a new treatment for recurrent minor aphthous ulcers. 1. Clinical demonstration of acceleration of healing and resolution of pain, *Oral Surg Oral Med Oral Pathol* 83:222-230, 1997.

NOSE

Allergic and vasomotor rhinitis are discussed in the immunology section.

PHARYNX
Pharyngitis
(See also streptococcal infections)

Symptomatic relief of the symptoms of pharyngitis may be obtained by gargling with 15 ml (1 tbsp) of benzydamine (<u>Tantum</u>) every 1½ to 3 hours and especially before meals.

Tonsillectomy
(See also otitis media; streptococcal infections)

Absolute indications for tonsillectomy are obstructive tonsils causing sleep apnea or obstructive tonsils unresponsive to antibiotics, which cause failure to thrive or progressive weight loss.[1-3] Elective indications are recurrent acute tonsillitis (with each episode seen and documented by a physician) defined as more than five episodes in 1 year, seven in 2 years, and nine in 3 years; peritonsillar abscess (one episode only is a controversial indication); obstructive tonsils without sleep apnea or cor pulmonale; and chronic bad breath from retention of debris in tonsillar crypts.[1-3]

Recurrent otitis media and glue ear are not recognized indications for tonsillectomy (see discussion of otitis media).

REFERENCES

1. Bluestone CD: Current indications for tonsillectomy adenoidectomy, *Ann Otol Rhinol Laryngol* 101:58-64, 1992.
2. Benjamin B: Guidelines on tonsillectomy and adenoidectomy, *J Paediatr Child Health* 28:136-140, 1992.
3. Fabian MC, Smitheringale A: Tonsillitis—making the right decisions, *Can J Diagn* 11:53-63, 1994.

SINUSES
Sinusitis

Acute sinusitis lasts 1 to 3 weeks. Chronic sinusitis is defined as disease lasting more than 3 months, as three or more recurrent infections annually, or as repeated failures of medical therapy to cure the condition.[1]

Making a clinical diagnosis of acute bacterial sinusitis is difficult. Symptoms and signs of particular value are "double sickening," in which a patient with a cold begins to improve and then finds that symptoms worsen[2]; facial pain, particularly if unilateral; maxillary toothache; purulent nasal secretions; poor response to decongestants[1,2]; and abnormal transillumination.[1] This last sign is of value only if transillumination is performed by an experienced operator in a completely dark room.[1] If on a clinical basis a patient has either a high or low probability of having sinusitis, x-ray examination adds little.[1,2] In inconclusive cases or when the patient has frontal pain leading to a concern about frontal sinusitis (which can be complicated by a brain abscess), x-ray studies might be helpful.[1] Before the age of 6 years only the maxillary and ethmoid sinuses are sufficiently developed to be seen consistently on radiographs.

In both adults and children, *Haemophilus influenzae* and *Streptococcus pneumoniae* account for about 70% of cases of bacterial sinusitis. In children most of the remaining cases are due to *Branhamella (Moraxella) catarrhalis*.[1,2] In adults other etiological agents include *Staphylococcus aureus, Streptococcus pyogenes, B. catarrhalis,* anaerobes, and gram-negative organisms.[1]

Antibiotics are considered standard treatment for sinusitis but may not always be necessary. A randomized placebo-controlled trial of amoxicillin for radiologically proven maxillary sinusitis in patients of general practitioners found no benefit from the antibiotic in terms of rapidity of symptom resolution, complications, or recurrences.[3]

Although one trial of children with sinusitis has shown that a 3-day course of trimethoprim-sulfamethoxazole (Septra, Bactrim) was as effective as a 10-day course,[4] the standard duration of therapy for this disease remains 10 days. Beta-lactamase agents do not offer any significant advantage as first-line therapy for acute bacterial sinusitis. The antibiotics of first choice are amoxicillin 500 mg q8h (40 mg/kg/day in 3 divided doses for children) or trimethoprim-sulfamethoxazole 160/800 mg q12h (8/40 mg/kg/day in 2 divided doses for children). Second-line drugs include cefuroxime axetil (Ceftin), Cefaclor (Ceclor), cefixime (Suprax), clarithromycin (Biaxin), erythromycin-sulfisoxazole (Pediazole), and amoxicillin-clavulanate (Augmentin, Clavulin).[1,2]

Although no placebo-controlled trials have substantiated it, use of a topical nasal decongestant spray such as oxymetazoline (Dristan Long Lasting Nasal) or xylometazoline (Otrivin) two or three times a day or phenylephrine (Neo-Synephrine) three or four times a day for 3 to 4 days may be helpful.[1]

The organisms causing chronic sinusitis are similar to those causing acute sinusitis except that anaerobes are much more common. An effective regimen for this condition is cefuroxime axetil (Ceftin) 500 mg q12h plus metronidazole (Flagyl) 500 mg q6-8h. An alternative is clindamycin.[5]

REFERENCES

1. Low DE, Desrosiers M, McSherry J, et al: A practical guide for the diagnosis and treatment of acute sinusitis, *Can Med Assoc J* 156(suppl 6):S1-S14, 1997.
2. Fagnan LJ: Acute sinusitis: a cost-effective approach to diagnosis and treatment, *Am Fam Physician* 58:1795-1802, 1998.
3. Van Buchem FL, Knottnerus JA, Schrijnemaekers VJ, et al: Primary-care-based randomised placebo-controlled trial of antibiotic treatment in acute maxillary sinusitis, *Lancet* 349:683-687, 1997.
4. Williams JW Jr, Holleman DR Jr, Samsa GP, et al: Randomized controlled trial of 3 vs 10 days of trimethoprim/sulfamethoxazole for acute maxillary sinusitis, *JAMA* 273:1015-1021, 1995.
5. Brook I, Yocum P: Antimicrobial management of chronic sinusitis in children, *J Laryngol Otol* 109:1159-1162, 1995.

VERTIGO
(See also motion sickness)

Vertigo can be caused by ear disease (peripheral vertigo) or central nervous system disease (central vertigo). Clues that vertigo is central include the presence of other central nervous symptoms or signs, spontaneous nystagmus that changes direction (in peripheral disease the direction of nystagmus is constant), and inability to walk (patients with peripheral vertigo do not like to walk, but they can). However, the symptoms and signs of inferior cerebellar infarction may be identical to those of peripheral disease.[1]

REFERENCES

1. Baloh RW: Vertigo, *Lancet* 352:1841-1846, 1998.

Benign Positional Vertigo

Benign positional vertigo is caused by the accumulation of particles (probably otoconia) in the endolymph of the posterior semicircular canal. These appear to interfere with the free flow of endolymph and cause vertigo with head movements. The mean age of patients with benign positional vertigo is 54; about 20% of cases are a result of head trauma, and 10% are a sequel of acute vestibular neuronitis. The natural history of benign positional vertigo is one of gradual resolution over weeks or even years, with many people having remissions and exacerbations.[1]

The diagnosis of benign positional vertigo is confirmed by performing the Dix-Hallpike (Hallpike) maneuver. The examiner helps the patient, who is seated on the examining table, to lie rapidly back so that his or her head, which is rotated to one side by about 45 degrees, hangs down over the upper edge of the examining table by about 45 degrees. Characteristic findings in patients with benign positional vertigo are latency, adaptability, and fatigability, as well as rotary (torsional) nystagmus toward the dependent ear and the subjective sensation of vertigo. Latency refers to the fact that the patient does not experience vertigo or demonstrate nystagmus immediately after lying back on the table, but only after a latent period of a few seconds. Adaptability means that after the patient experiences 20 to 60 seconds of vertigo and nystagmus while lying back on the table, both stop spontaneously. Fatigability means that if the Hallpike maneuver is repeated one or more times, both vertigo and nystagmus diminish in intensity or disappear.[1] Patients with a central nervous system cause of vertigo usually do not exhibit latency, adaptability, or fatigability.

Epley's canalith repositioning procedure

In recent years head maneuvers have been described as a means of permanently controlling the symptoms of benign positional vertigo.[1,2] The theory is that the particles lodged in the posterior semicircular canal can be made to fall into the utricle, where they will do no further harm. The method described below is that of Epley,[2] who reported a 77% success rate after only one treatment session. The recurrence rate is about 15% per year.[1]

The Epley canalith repositioning procedure is performed as follows.[1,2] The affected ear is first determined by the Hallpike maneuver. It is the ear that is dependent when symptoms are produced. Each movement in the particle repositioning maneuver (Epley's maneuver) is performed rapidly and then maintained for at least 30 seconds[2] or until symptoms have subsided.[1] The initial maneuver is identical to the Hallpike maneuver. The seated patient is assisted in lying back on the examining table so that the head hangs over the edge of the table with the neck extended about 45 degrees and rotated 45 degrees toward the affected side. The physician supports the patient's head in this position while giving reassurance that the vertigo will subside. Next the head is rapidly rotated through 90 degrees to the opposite side. After remaining in this position for a short period, the patient is assisted in rolling over onto his or her side, the direction of the roll being in the direction the face was pointing in the last maneuver. The head rotation of 45 degrees is maintained throughout this maneuver so that at its completion the patient, although lying on his or her side, is looking toward the floor. After a short delay the patient is helped to a sitting position while continuing to keep the head rotated. The final maneuver is to rotate the head back to the straight-ahead position and flex the neck by about 20 degrees.

In cases of treatment failure the procedure may be repeated immediately. In some patients both ears are affected; in those cases only one side is treated at a time.[2]

The original studies recommended that patients try to keep the head in the vertical position for 48 hours (sleeping on the back with two or three pillows). However, a 1996 study found no benefit from this type of posttreatment protocol.[3]

Modified Epley's procedure

Radtke and associates have developed a modified Epley's procedure that patients perform three times daily at home until symptoms have resolved. The patient sits on a bed with a pillow placed so that when the patient lies down it will rest under the shoulders. The seated patient turns the head 45 degrees toward the affected side and rapidly lies down—the shoulders rest on the pillow, and the occiput on the bed. After 30 seconds the head is rapidly turned 90 degrees to the opposite side, and after another 30 seconds the patient rolls onto one side in the direction the head is pointing while maintaining the head rotation. Thus the patient ends up lying on one side with the face facing the bed. After 30 seconds the patient sits up and turns, ending up seated on the edge of the bed with the feet on the floor.[4]

Habituation exercises of Brandt and Daroff

An older home treatment for benign positional vertigo is the positional or habituation exercises of Brandt and Daroff.[1,4,5] The patient begins by sitting on the side of the bed with feet on the floor and the head turned 45 degrees to one side. The patient rapidly lies down on one side in the direction opposite to which he or she is looking so that the portion of the occiput behind the ear touches the mattress. The patient then sits up, turns the head so it points 45 degrees in the opposite direction, and lies down quickly on the opposite side. Every position is maintained for at least 30 seconds.[5]

◥ REFERENCES ◤

1. Furman JM, Cass SP: Benign paroxysmal positional vertigo, *N Engl J Med* 341:1590-1596, 1999.
2. Epley JM: The canalith repositioning procedure for treatment of benign paroxysmal positional vertigo, *Otolaryngol Head Neck Surg* 107:399-404, 1992.
3. Massoud EA, Ireland DF: Post-treatment instructions in the nonsurgical management of benign paroxysmal positional vertigo, *J Otolaryngol* 25:121-125, 1996.
4. Radtke A, Neuhauser H, von Brevern M, et al: A modified Epley's procedure for self-treatment of benign positional vertigo, *Neurology* 53:1358-1360, 1999.
5. Lempert T, Gresty MA, Bronstein AM: Benign positional vertigo: recognition and treatment, *BMJ* 311:489-491, 1995.

Ménière's Disease
(See also nausea and vomiting)

The four characteristic symptoms of Ménière's disease are episodic vertigo, fluctuating sensorineural hearing loss, tinnitus, and sense of fullness in the ear. Rarely are all these symptoms present at the onset of the disease; only in later episodes will the diagnosis become evident. Two of the major conditions to consider in the differential diagnosis are benign positional vertigo and vestibular neuronitis.[1]

Ménière's disease is characterized by remissions and exacerbations, and over the long term 70% of patients experience a long-term remission.[2] This fact, along with the lack of a significant number of controlled trials on treatment of the disease, has led to a huge variety of unproven management protocols. Medical regimens include limitations on the intake of salt, caffeine, alcohol, and tobacco, as well as the prescription of many classes of drugs, including diuretics, vasodilators, benzodiazepines, tricyclic antidepressants, antihistamines, and neuroleptics. The antihistamines, which include meclizine (Antivert, Bonine, Bonamine), promethazine (Phenergan), and dimenhydrinate (Dramamine, Gravol), and neuroleptics, such as prochlorperazine (Compazine, Stemetil), are used as antinauseants during the acute attack, whereas the other agents are used for long-term prophylaxis.[1,2]

Canadian physicians should be aware that in Canada Antivert contains both meclizine and niacin, whereas in the United States Antivert contains no niacin. As far as I can determine, the vasodilator niacin has no beneficial effects on Ménière's disease.

One drug that has been assessed positively in controlled trials of Ménière's disease is betahistine (Serc), which is usually prescribed as 4 to 8 mg q8h.[2-4] Its mode of action is thought to be an inhibition of neuronal impulses to the lateral vestibular nucleus.[4] Betahistine is currently the favored form of medical treatment for Ménière's disease in Canada and Europe.[2]

The value of surgical treatments that decompress the labyrinth or shunt endolymph is controversial. Patients with no serviceable hearing may obtain complete relief of symptoms at the cost of total hearing loss through a complete labyrinthectomy.[1,2]

REFERENCES

1. Knox GW, McPherson A: Meniere's disease: differential diagnosis and treatment, *Am Fam Physician* 55:1185-1190, 1997.
2. Saeed SR: Diagnosis and treatment of Ménière's disease, *BMJ* 316:368-372, 1998.
3. Fraysse B, Bebear JP, Dubreuil C, et al: Betahistine dihydrochloride versus flunarizine: a double-blind study on recurrent vertigo with or without cochlear syndrome typical of Meniere's disease, *Acta Otolaryngol* 490(suppl):1-10, 1991.
4. Aantaa E: Treatment of acute vestibular vertigo, *Acta Otolaryngol* 479(suppl):44-47, 1991.

Vestibular Neuritis

Vestibular neuritis or vestibular neuronitis is presumed to be secondary to a viral infection. Presenting symptoms of severe vertigo, nausea, vomiting, and postural instability develop rapidly and begin to improve within a few days. Severe vertigo resolves within a week, but complete resolution of symptoms may take several weeks or even a few months.[1]

The differential diagnosis of acute onset vertigo includes many disorders. Patients with benign positional vertigo have brief symptoms brought on by positional changes and do not have vertigo when they are not moving. Patients with acoustic neuromas rarely have severe vertigo, and patients with Ménière's disease usually give a typical history (see previous discussion). The most important disorders to rule out in a patient with acute vertigo are brainstem or inferior cerebellar infarcts. Most patients with brainstem infarcts have other central nervous symptoms and signs, but these may be absent or subtle in cases of inferior cerebellar infarction.[1]

Three clues that help differentiate central nervous system (central) from vestibular (peripheral) lesions are the direction of nystagmus, the ability to inhibit nystagmus by fixation, and the ability of the patient to walk. With central lesions the quick component of nystagmus may change direction when the patient looks in different directions, whereas the direction of the quick component always remains the same in peripheral lesions. In peripheral lesions nystagmus is usually inhibited by fixation, whereas in central lesions it is not; this can be assessed by observing the optic disc of one eye with an ophthalmoscope while the patient alternately covers and uncovers the other eye. If pressed, patients with peripheral disease can walk, although they are unsteady and nauseated; patients with inferior cerebellar infarcts are rarely able to walk.[1]

Vertigo in young patients who do not have risk factors for cerebrovascular accident is almost always due to peripheral lesions. Older patients with risk factors for stroke who do not have obvious localizing neurological signs may have an inferior cerebellar infarct, especially if they are unable to walk. Such patients require further evaluation.[1]

REFERENCES

1. Hotson JR, Baloh RW: Acute vestibular syndrome, *N Engl J Med* 339:680-685, 1998.

PEDIATRICS

ACCIDENTS

(See also child abuse; guns; motor vehicle accidents; substance abuse)

Trampoline injuries are particularly common in children, and the number has escalated in the past decade. Most are caused by backyard trampolines. The majority of injuries are soft tissue injuries and fracture or dislocation of the limbs. However, after football, trampoline is the sport most commonly causing permanent paralysis from neck injuries. Attempted flips are the most common cause of severe neurological injury.[1,2] The American Academy of Pediatrics recommends the abolition of trampolines from homes and the banning of trampolines from regular physical education classes in schools.[2]

Power lawn mowers are an important cause of injury to children, especially those under the age of 6. In most cases the injury is from direct contact with the blades, but in a few instances penetrating injuries occur from objects propelled by the rotating blades.[3]

According to some reports a correlation exists between childhood injuries and the numbers of hours that children watch television. A possible explanation is that television distorts reality and encourages children to participate in excessive risk-taking activities.[4]

◤ REFERENCES ◢

1. Smith GA: Injuries to children in the United States related to trampolines, 1990-95: a national epidemic, *Pediatrics* 101:406-412, 1998.
2. American Academy of Pediatrics Committee on Injury and Poison Prevention and Committee on Sports Medicine and Fitness: Trampolines at home, school, and recreational centers, *Pediatrics* 103:1053-1056, 1999.
3. Munoz-Juárez M, Drugas GT, Hallett JW, et al: Vena caval implement: an unusual lawn mower injury in a child, *Mayo Clin Proc* 73:537-540, 1998.
4. Uberos DJ, Gómez A, Munoz A, et al: Television and childhood injuries: is there a connection? (letter), *Arch Pediatr Adolesc Med* 152:712-713, 1998.

ADOPTION
International Adoption

International adoptees should be screened for human immunodeficiency virus (HIV), hepatitis B and C, congenital syphilis, lead poisoning, tuberculosis (by Mantoux testing), and parasites. HIV and hepatitis B and C screening should be repeated after 6 months. Vision and hearing should be assessed, growth and development should be carefully monitored, and according to some experts, anemia, thyroid dysfunction, and renal dysfunction should be ruled out. Even if children have records of immunization from their native countries, their immunity may be inadequate; they should either be assessed for antibody levels or have repeat immunizations.[1]

◤ REFERENCES ◢

1. Miller LC: Caring for internationally adopted children, *N Engl J Med* 341:1539-1540, 1999.

ASTHMA IN CHILDREN
(See also allergic rhinitis—environmental control; asthma)

About half of all children have one or more episodes of wheezing before the age of 3 years, usually in association with respiratory infections, but only one fourth still have wheezing episodes at the age of 6. A history of maternal asthma is associated with an increased risk of the child's continuing to wheeze at the age of 6, maternal smoking with an increased incidence of wheezing before the age of 3,[1] and exposure to passive smoke with a delayed resolution of acute asthmatic attacks.[2] The morbidity rate from asthma among poor inner city children is particularly high, almost certainly because of sensitivity to cockroaches and continued exposure to them.[3]

Between 30% and 70% of children with asthma have marked improvement or resolution of symptoms by the time they become adults. Such resolution is seen more often in patients with milder forms of the disease.[4]

Inhaled medications are the ideal way of controlling asthma in both children and adults. For children who cannot use that method the first choice of an oral agent is usually a beta$_2$-adrenergic agonist such as metaproterenol (Alupent), which has the generic name orciprenaline in Canada. The usual dose of this product is 10 mg tid prn for children aged 4 to 12 years and 20 mg tid prn for children over 12. In some instances a theophylline derivative such as oxtriphylline (Choledyl) is still used. For children under 5 the dosage is 24 to 36 mg/kg/day divided into 3 equal doses given at 8-hour intervals. The usual dose for children over the age of 5 is 22 mg/kg/day divided into 4 equal doses. Both metaproterenol and oxtriphylline can cause hyperactivity, nausea, and vomiting.

As in adults, inhaled corticosteroids are indicated for most children with moderate or severe asthma. The bulk of evidence based on short- and intermediate-duration studies is that standard pediatric doses of inhaled glucocorticoids do not affect a child's growth.[5,6] It may be that a subset of children with severe asthma taking more than 400 µg of inhaled steroids daily have some decrease in growth.[7] Wheezing in association with upper respiratory infections is probably a separate entity from atopic asthma, and in this situation inhaled corticosteroids may be ineffective.[8]

A number of authors have claimed that persistent cough may be the only symptom of asthma in children (cough variant asthma). According to others, the existence of such a syndrome is questionable. The pathways for cough and bronchoconstriction are different, and a common trigger such as an upper respiratory tract infection may affect both. In some asthmatic children coughing overshadows wheezing, which may be missed, but most children with cough but no associated wheezing or dyspnea do not have asthma. Labeling cough alone as asthma is one reason that the reported incidence of asthma has been increasing.[9] A randomized placebo-controlled trial of albuterol (salbutamol) or inhaled corticosteroids for children only with cough failed to show any benefit.[10] The authors questioned whether cough without other evidence of airway obstruction is ever due to asthma.[9] When the diagnosis of asthma is unclear, a short trial of asthma medications may be indicated in some children but no evidence supports a prolonged course of inhaled corticosteroids.[9]

Asthma is discussed in detail under "Respirology."

───────────── ◥ **REFERENCES** ◤ ─────────────

1. Martinez FD, Wright AL, Taussig LM, et al: Asthma and wheezing in the first six years of life, *N Engl J Med* 332:133-138, 1995.
2. Abulhosn RS, Morray BH, Llewellyn CE, et al: Passive smoke exposure impairs recovery after hospitalization for acute asthma, *Arch Pediatr Adolesc Med* 151:135-139, 1997.
3. Rosenstreich D, Kattan M, Baker D, et al: The role of cockroach allergy and exposure to cockroach allergen in causing morbidity among inner-city children with asthma, *N Engl J Med* 336:1356-1363, 1997.
4. O'Connor GT, Weiss ST, Speizer FE: The epidemiology of asthma. In Gershwin ME, ed: *Bronchial asthma,* ed 2, Orlando, Fla, 1986, Grune & Stratton.
5. Wolthers OD: Long-, intermediate- and short-term growth studies in asthmatic children treated with inhaled glucocorticosteroids, *Eur Respir J* 9:821-827, 1996.
6. Allen DB, Bronsky EA, LaForce CF, et al: Growth in asthmatic children treated with fluticasone propionate, *J Pediatr* 132:472-477, 1998.
7. McCown C, Neville RG, Thomas GE, et al: Effect of asthma and its treatment on growth: four year follow up of cohort of children from general practices in Tayside, Scotland, *BMJ* 316:668-672, 1998.
8. Doull IJ, Lampe FC, Smith S, et al: Effect of inhaled corticosteroids on episodes of wheezing associated with viral infection in school age children: randomised double blind placebo controlled trial, *BMJ* 315:858-862, 1997.
9. Chang AB: Isolated cough: probably not asthma, *Arch Dis Child* 80:211-213, 1999.
10. Chang AB, Phelan PD, Carlin JB, et al: A randomised, placebo controlled trial of inhaled salbutamol and beclomethasone for recurrent cough, *Arch Dis Child* 79:6-11, 1998.

ATTENTION DEFICIT/HYPERACTIVITY DISORDER

(See also antisocial personality disorder; conduct disorder; fetal alcohol effects; Tourette's syndrome)

Between 3% and 5% of children in North America are diagnosed as having attention deficit/hyperactivity disorder (ADHD), and boys are more often affected than girls. The actual number of affected girls is probably higher than is generally reported because fewer girls than boys with ADHD have oppositional or conduct disorder and therefore fewer are brought to medical attention. Even when girls are seen by physicians, the diagnosis of ADHD may be missed because it is often overshadowed by comorbid conditions such as anxiety disorders, mood disorders, or substance abuse.[1]

A family history of ADHD is common; 30% of first-degree relatives of children with ADHD also have the condition. The increased risk for siblings is fivefold for boys and threefold for girls.[2] A family history of conversion disorder, sociopathy, and alcoholism may also be elicited.[3]

Common comorbid conditions of ADHD are learning disabilities (25% to 35% of children)[3,4]; oppositional disorder and conduct disorders in boys[3,4]; and anxiety disorders, mood disorders, and substance abuse in girls.[1] Children

with ADHD are at increased risk for antisocial personality disorder or drug abuse disorder when they reach adulthood. This risk is particularly marked if the child meets the criteria for both ADHD and conduct disorder.[5]

The diagnosis of ADHD is based on the history.[3,4] The fourth edition of the *Diagnostic and Statistical Manual of Mental Disorders (DSM IV)* divides the symptoms into the two major categories of inattention and hyperactivity/impulsivity. Each category contains nine sets of symptoms, and the diagnosis is made if the child has six of the listed symptoms in either category, has had symptoms before the age of 7 years, has symptoms in two or more settings (such as school and home), and suffers impairment in social, academic, or occupational functioning because of the symptoms. The following are examples of symptoms associated with inattention[2]:

1. Fails to pay attention to detail at school and makes careless mistakes
2. Has difficulty sustaining attention when playing or performing tasks
3. May not seem to listen when spoken to directly
4. Is often distracted

These are examples of symptoms of hyperactivity/impulsivity[3]:

1. Often squirms in chair or fidgets with hands or feet
2. Often runs or climbs excessively
3. Often talks excessively
4. May have difficulty waiting his or her turn
5. Often blurts out an answer before a question is completed

Children with ADHD may not display any symptoms when in a physician's office, so short periods of observation are not sufficient to rule out the diagnosis.[1,2] Usually the practitioner must question a number of observers from different settings to obtain a diagnostic history. Questionnaires such as the Connors Parent Rating Scales and the Connors Teacher Rating Scales are useful.[2] Although ADHD may be diagnosed in preschool children, the validity of making the diagnoses in this age group is uncertain.[4] The conditions most commonly misdiagnosed as ADHD are depression and anxiety disorders. In general, ADHD begins at an earlier age and has an unremitting course, whereas mood and anxiety disorders tend to present at a somewhat older age and have episodic courses.[4]

Not all children "outgrow" ADHD; about half continue to benefit from medications during adulthood.[1] Recognizing the disorder may be particularly difficult in adults if it was not identified in childhood. Presenting problems in adults usually involve difficulties in work or school performance, inattention, or hyperactivity. The diagnosis cannot be made unless the history shows that the problems started by age 7 and were persistently present thereafter.[6]

A 1995 metaanalysis found no correlation between sugar intake and childhood hyperactivity or cognitive functioning.[7]

A well-designed comparison of behavioral therapy, medication therapy, and combined medication and behavioral therapy for children with ADHD found that after 14 months medication therapy gave the best results and that combined medication and behavioral therapy offered little added advantage.[8]

The medication of first choice for ADHD is methylphenidate (Ritalin). The usual dosage is 0.3 to 0.7 mg/kg/dose given two or three times daily. Most children under 8 years take 5 mg bid, and most of those 8 years and older take 10 mg bid.[1] The duration of action of methylphenidate tablets is only 3 to 4 hours, so frequent doses are often necessary. For schoolchildren this often means a morning and noon dose with a third dose in the late afternoon or at suppertime. If giving a noon dose at school is difficult, slow release tablets (20 mg), which have a duration of action of 6 to 8 hours, may be tried.[1] Unfortunately, the slow release tablets are not always effective because blood levels rise slowly and peak levels are low.[6,9]

Dextroamphetamine (Dexedrine, Dextrostat) is as effective as methylphenidate. Some children respond only to methylphenidate, and others only to dextroamphetamine.[10]

Other drugs that have been used for the treatment of ADHD are pemoline (Cylert), tricyclic antidepressants, and clonidine (Catapres). Pemoline can cause toxic hepatitis, and deaths have been reported from the use of tricyclic antidepressants and clonidine in children.[10]

Management of ADHD in adults has not been well studied.[11] Although methylphenidate 10 mg bid may be sufficient,[1] more typical regimens involve up to 30 mg tid or qid.[11]

──────────── ◣ REFERENCES ◢ ────────────

1. Biederman J, Faraone SV, Mick E, et al: Clinical correlates of ADHD in females: findings from a large group of girls ascertained from pediatric and psychiatric referral sources, *J Am Acad Child Adolesc Psychiatry* 38:966-975, 1999.
2. Taylor ME: Evaluation and management of attention-deficit hyperactivity disorder, *Am Fam Physician* 55:887-901, 1997.
3. American Psychiatric Association: *Diagnostic and statistical manual of mental disorders,* ed 4, Washington, DC, 1994, The Association, pp 78-85.
4. Zametkin AJ: Attention-deficit disorder: born to be hyperactive? *JAMA* 273:1871-1874, 1995.
5. Lynam DR: Early identification of chronic offenders: who is the fledgling psychopath? *Psychol Bull* 120:209-234, 1996.
6. Biederman J: A 55-year-old man with attention-deficit/hyperactivity disorder, *JAMA* 280:1086-1092, 1998.
7. Wolraich ML, Wilson DB, White W: The effect of sugar on behavior or cognition in children: a meta-analysis, *JAMA* 274:1617-1621, 1995.
8. MTA Cooperative Group: A 14-month randomized clinical trial of treatment strategies for attention-deficit/hyperactivity disorder, *Arch Gen Psychiatry* 56:1073-1086, 1999.
9. Lawrence JD, Carson DS: Optimizing ADHD therapy with sustained-release methylphenidate, *Am Fam Physician* 55: 1705-1709, 1997.
10. Elia J, Ambrosini PJ, Rapoport JL: Treatment of attention-deficit-hyperactivity disorder, *N Engl J Med* 340:780-788, 1999.
11. Wilens TE, Biederman J, Spencer TJ: Pharmacotherapy of adult attention deficit/hyperactivity disorder, *Psychiatr Clin North Am* 5:1-16, 1998.

AUTISM

Autism, Asperger's syndrome, childhood disintegrative disorder, and Rett's syndrome are all conditions that fit into the category of pervasive developmental disorders. Affected children have deficits in one or more areas, including reciprocal social interaction, verbal and nonverbal communication, and imaginative play. Their interests and activities are usually markedly restricted.[1]

Autism is four times more frequent in boys than in girls. The classic image of an autistic child sitting alone compulsively rocking represents only a small percentage of affected individuals. Autistic children have difficulty with social interactions, and inadequate eye contact is an important clinical sign. Some autistic children display acceptable initial eye contact but tend not to maintain it. Autistic children rarely have close friends, since their interests are limited and often considered "odd" or "weird" by others. Although some affected children are mute, others have excellent vocabularies. However, they tend to indulge in monologues about whatever interests them and have great difficulty sustaining a give-and-take conversation.[1]

The prognosis for autistic children has not been fully defined. Intensive behavioral treatment has been said to improve outcome. Unfortunately, desperate parents often latch onto questionable regimens.[1] A single IV injection of secretin is of no value.[2]

Many consider Asperger's syndrome to represent the highest functioning level of autism. Patients have normal cognition and language but tend to talk pedantically about their own esoteric interests. Patients with childhood disintegrative disorder develop normally until the age of 2 and then regress to acquire the characteristics of autistic children.

Rett's syndrome affects only girls. They display severe neurodevelopmental delay and pathognomonic hand-wringing. Deceleration of head growth is part of the syndrome.[1]

──────────── ◣ REFERENCES ◢ ────────────

1. Gara L, Goldfarb C: The autistic child: what can you do? *Can J Diagn* 16(2):147-155, 1999.
2. Sandler AD, Sutton KA, DeWeese J, et al: Lack of benefit of a single dose of synthetic human secretin in the treatment of autism and pervasive developmental disorder, *N Engl J Med* 341:1801-1806, 1999.

BREAST FEEDING

(See also breast implants; diarrhea and dehydration in infants; formulas; neonatal jaundice; obesity in childhood)

These are signs of successful breast feeding in the neonate[1]:

1. Eight to ten feedings a day
2. Audible swallowing
3. Six to eight wet diapers a day
4. Three to five bowel movements a day
5. Birth weight regained by 2 weeks

It is difficult to say with certainty that a nursing mother may safely take a given drug, but a large number of drugs are usually compatible with breast feeding. Drugs such as ergot derivatives, bromocriptine, and oral contraceptives are generally contraindicated because they can inhibit lactation. Other contraindicated drugs include all drugs of abuse, alcohol, nicotine, antineoplastic drugs, iodine-containing substances, gold, and radioactive substances. Lithium is often considered a contraindication to nursing, but this is uncertain. Antidepressants, antipsychotics, and short-acting benzodiazepines are probably safe.[2] Silicone breast implants are not a contraindication to nursing.[3]

A critical review of the literature found no adverse effects on the infants of nursing mothers who were taking amitriptyline (Elavil), nortriptyline (Aventyl), desipramine (Norpramin, Pertofrane), clomipramine (Anafranil), dothiepin (Prothiaden), or sertraline (Zoloft). Among healthy full-term infants none of these drugs or their metabolites were detectable in the infants' serum. Some adverse effects were reported when the mother was taking doxepin (Sinequan) or fluoxetine (Prozac) while breast feeding, and these two drugs have been detected in infant serum. The authors suggest that if a nursing mother requires antidepressants and continues to breast feed, serum levels of the drug be measured in infants under 10 weeks of age once a maternal therapeutic dose of the drug has been reached. Measurement of serum levels in infants over 10 weeks is needed only if they display symptoms.[4]

In the first 6 months of life breast-fed babies have lower rates of cough, wheeze, diarrhea, and otitis media and fewer sick baby visits than do non-breast-fed or only occasionally breast-fed infants.[5] Exclusive breast feeding for the first 4 months of life has also been associated with a decreased incidence of asthma at 6 years of age.[6] Physicians should encourage both parents to accept this form of infant feeding.[7] The American Academy of Pediatrics recommends exclusive breast feeding as the ideal nutrition during the first 6 months of life and states that no other solids or liquids are required during this period. Breast feeding should continue for at least a year, but iron-enriched solids should be added in the second 6 months of life.[8] In some cases breast feeding simply does not work, and the mother should not be made to feel guilty about this.[9]

✑ REFERENCES ✑

1. Spencer JP: Practical nutrition for the healthy term infant, *Am Fam Physician* 54:138-144, 1996.
2. Bailey B, Ito S: Breast-feeding and maternal drug use, *Pediatr Clin North Am* 44:41-54, 1997.
3. Koren G, Ito S: Do silicone breast implants affect breastfeeding? *Can Fam Physician* 44:2641-2642, 1998.
4. Wisner KL, Perel JM, Findling RL: Antidepressant treatment during breast-feeding, *Am J Psychiatry* 153:1132-1137, 1996.
5. Raisler J, Alexander C, O'Campo P: Breast-feeding and infant illness: a dose-response relationship? *Am J Public Health* 89: 25-30, 1999.
6. Oddy WH, Holt PG, Sly PD, et al: Association between breast feeding and asthma in 6 year old children: findings of a prospective birth cohort study, *BMJ* 319:815-819, 1999.
7. Sharma M, Petosa R: Impact of expectant fathers in breast-feeding decisions, *J Am Diet Assoc* 97:1311-1313, 1997.
8. American Academy of Pediatrics Work Group on Breastfeeding: Breastfeeding and the use of human milk, *Pediatrics* 100: 1035-1039, 1997.
9. Bennison J: Breast feeding does not always work, *BMJ* 315: 754, 1997.

BRONCHIOLITIS

Bronchiolitis is a common disease of infants that is usually caused by the respiratory syncytial virus. The peak age is 2 to 6 months, although the condition occurs in children up to 2 years of age. It is more common in premature infants and those from lower socioeconomic environments. After a 3-day incubation period, upper respiratory tract symptoms, including rhinorrhea and cough, occur. Between 2 and 3 days after the onset of symptoms, respiratory distress and appetite loss develop. Physical findings are tachycardia, tachypnea, cyanosis, an increase in the anteroposterior diameter of the chest, intercostal and subcostal retractions, hyperresonance, prolonged expiration, wheezes, and fine crackles. Because the diaphragm is depressed by hyperinflation, the liver and spleen are easily palpable. When the diagnosis is suspected, investigation, including chest x-ray examination, is indicated. In many cases the child requires admission to the hospital.[1]

✑ REFERENCES ✑

1. Jeng M-J, Lemen R: Respiratory syncytial virus bronchiolitis, *Am Fam Physician* 55:1139-1146, 1997.

BULLYING

Bullying in schools is common, and both bullies and those who are bullied have increased rates of psychological and psychosomatic symptoms. Children who are bullied have been reported to be at greater risk for bed wetting, insomnia, school phobias, depression, suicidal ideation, and psychosomatic symptoms such as abdominal pain and headaches.[1,2] Bullies also commonly have psychosomatic symptoms[1] and, like those they bully, are at increased risk of depression and suicide.[2]

❧ REFERENCES ❧

1. Forero R, McLellan L, Rissel C, et al: Bullying behaviour and psychosocial health among school students in New South Wales, Australia: cross sectional survey, *BMJ* 319:344-348, 1999.
2. Kaltiala-Heino R, Rimpelä M, Marttunen M, et al: Bullying, depression, and suicidal ideation in Finnish adolescents: school survey, *BMJ* 319:348-351, 1999.

CIRCUMCISION AND DISORDERS OF THE FORESKIN
(See also circumcision, female; urinary tract infections in children)

The prevalence of circumcision varies widely in the developed world. In the United States 80% of boys are circumcised, in Canada and Australia 40%, and in the United Kingdom 6%.[1] Purported medical reasons for circumcision include a decreased risk of urinary tract infections, phimosis, paraphimosis, balanitis, sexually transmitted diseases, and penile cancer.

Although urinary tract infections in the first year of life have been reported to be 20 times more common in uncircumcised than in circumcised boys, more recent data suggest that the increased risk in the uncircumcised is more like fourfold or tenfold and that the absolute risk for a urinary tract infection of an uncircumcised boy is about 1%.[2] To and associates[3] calculated that 195 circumcisions would have to be performed to prevent one hospital admission for urinary tract infection in the first year of life.

Circumcision prevents phimosis and paraphimosis, but since these conditions are neither frequent nor serious, they hardly merit preventive surgical intervention. "Pathological" or "cicatrizing" phimosis must be distinguished from "developmental" or "physiological" phimosis.[1,4] Pathological phimosis consists of fibrous adhesions between the foreskin and the glans and, according to one study, is secondary to balanitis xerotica obliterans (lichen sclerosus et atrophicus) in 84% of cases. Pathological phimosis is an absolute indication for circumcision but is rare, with an estimated incidence of only 4:10,000 boys per year.[4] In contrast, physiological phimosis, which results from the normal embryological fusion of the foreskin to the glans, is present in over 95% of newborn boys. Over the years the foreskin gradually separates from the glans, allowing the prepuce to be retracted in 20% of males by 6 months, 50% by 1 year, 90% by 3 years, and 99% by 17 years.[5]

Pathological phimosis can be distinguished from physiological phimosis by a gentle attempt to retract the foreskin. If pathological phimosis is present, the tip of the penis will adopt the shape of a cone; if physiological phimosis is present, the tip of the foreskin will pucker and spread out slightly so that the penis resembles a small sea anemone.[1] For most cases of physiological phimosis the only intervention required of physicians is parental reassurance. Forceful retraction of the foreskin is contraindicated, but once retraction can be accomplished with ease, the foreskin should be pulled back when bathing so the glans can be washed. Ballooning of the foreskin while urinating is common in children with physiological phimosis; the urine is partially diverted under the foreskin but drains freely, and the condition is inconsequential.[6] Pharmacological treatment of physiological phimosis consists of unrolling the foreskin once a day for a total of 4 to 6 weeks so that 0.05% betamethasone can be applied topically to the portions of the foreskin and glans that have been exposed. Topical corticosteroids speed the separation of the foreskin from the glans and thus "cure" physiological phimosis.[1]

Paraphimosis is a fixed retraction of the foreskin; treatment is manual reduction, often under anesthesia. Because paraphimosis rarely recurs, a single episode is not an indication for circumcision.[6]

Most cases of mild balanitis respond to topical cleansing, although more advanced cases may require oral antibiotics. Recurrent balanitis is one indication for using topical steroids to hasten the resolution of physiological phimosis.[6]

Some studies have reported a higher incidence of syphilis[1] and HIV[1,7] infections in uncircumcised men, but others have failed to find any relationship between circumcision and sexually transmitted diseases.[8] Although the risk of penile cancer is less in the circumcised than the uncircumcised, cancer of the penis is so rare that the association has little clinical import.[1]

Circumcision has been claimed to lead to a decrease in sexual satisfaction in adult life; data on this topic are sparse, but one observational study failed to confirm the hypothesis.[8]

Neonatal circumcision without anesthesia is painful.[2,9,10] Three modalities of anesthesia are in common use: a 5% eutectic mixture of the local anesthetics lidocaine and prilocaine (EMLA cream) applied to the penis under an occlusive dressing 60 to 90 minutes before the procedure, a dorsal penile nerve block, and a subcutaneous circumferential ring block at the midshaft of the penis.[2] A comparison of 30% topical lidocaine, 5% lidocaine/prilocaine (EMLA cream), and placebo found both topical anesthetics to be superior to placebo and found EMLA cream to be superior to lidocaine cream.[9] On the other hand, a comparative evaluation of EMLA cream, dorsal penile nerve block, and penile ring block found ring block to be the most effective procedure and topical EMLA cream the least.[10]

The complication rates of neonatal circumcision are usually considered to be on the order of 0.2% to 0.6%. Most are minor episodes of bleeding or local infection.[11] Persad and associates[12] reported an 8% rate of meatal stenosis.[12]

Should routine circumcision be recommended? The position of both the American Academy of Pediatrics[2] and the Canadian Pediatric Society[13] is that it should not.

◥ REFERENCES ◣

1. Dewan PA, Tieu HC, Chieng BS: Phimosis: is circumcision necessary? *J Paediatr Child Health* 32:285-289, 1996.
2. American Academy of Pediatrics Task Force on Circumcision: Circumcision policy statement, *Pediatrics* 103:686-693, 1999.
3. To T, Agha M, Kick PT, et al: Cohort study on circumcision of newborn boys and subsequent risk of urinary-tract infection, *Lancet* 352:1813-1816, 1998.
4. Shankar KR, Rickwood AM: The incidence of phimosis in boys, *BJU Int* 84:101-102, 1999.
5. Øster J: Further fate of the foreskin: incidence of preputial adhesions, phimosis and smegma among Danish schoolboys, *Arch Dis Child* 43:200-203, 1968.
6. Simpson ET, Barraclough P: The management of the paediatric foreskin, *Aust Fam Physician* 27:381-383, 1998.
7. Halperin DT, Bailey RC: Male circumcision and HIV infection: 10 years and counting, *Lancet* 354:1813-1815, 1999.
8. Laumann EO, Masi CM, Zuckerman EW: Circumcision in the United States: prevalence, prophylactic effects, and sexual practice, *JAMA* 277:1052-1057, 1997.
9. Woodman PJ: Topical lidocaine-prilocaine versus lidocaine for neonatal circumcision: a randomized controlled trial, *Obstet Gynecol* 93:775-779, 1999.
10. Lander J, Brady-Fryer B, Metcalfe JB, et al: Comparison of ring block, dorsal penile nerve block, and topical anesthesia for neonatal circumcision: a randomized controlled trial, *JAMA* 278:2157-2162, 1997.
11. Tran PT, Giacomantonio M: Routine neonatal circumcision? *Can Fam Physician* 42:2201-2204, 1996.
12. Persad R, Sharma S, McTavish J, et al: Clinical presentation and pathophysiology of meatal stenosis following circumcision, *Br J Urol* 75:91-93, 1995.
13. Fetus and Newborn Committee, Canadian Paediatric Society: Neonatal circumcision revisited, *Can Med Assoc J* 154:769-780, 1996.

COLIC

(See also formulas)

The classic definition of colic is excessive crying that occurs in the first 3 months of an otherwise healthy infant's life, lasts longer than 3 hours a day, takes place on more than 3 days a week, and is longer than 3 weeks in duration. A more practical definition is excessive crying in a healthy, thriving infant. Colic occurs as frequently in breastfed as in bottle-fed babies and almost always resolves by 4 months.[1]

Symptoms

Crying in colicky babies varies a great deal from day to day, is typically paroxysmal, and, older literature to the contrary, occurs at any time of day. During these episodes the babies are almost impossible to soothe, but in the intervals they are settled and normal.[2]

How much do normal infants cry? In 1962 Brazelton[3] reported on 80 normal infants. The median daily crying time was 1¾ hours in the second week of life, 2¾ hours at 6 weeks, and less than 1 hour by the 12th week.

Etiology

The etiology of colic is unknown. Some of the major hypotheses are that it results from a gastrointestinal disturbance, that it reflects suboptimal parent-child interactions, that it is a variant of normal, and that it consists of a variety of different conditions that at present cannot be distinguished.[1]

Management

A 1998 systematic review of infantile colic assessed behavioral, dietary, and pharmacological interventions.[1]

Behavior

Overresponse to and overstimulation of crying infants probably does more harm than good. The physician should inform the parents that colic is a self-limited condition and nothing they have done or are doing causes it. When infants cry, they should be checked for hunger or for wet or dirty diapers. If neither of these is the cause of crying, parents should avoid exhausting themselves with prolonged carrying or holding of the infant and should try to find someone else to share in the caring. No reliable evidence supports use of infant carriers, vibration devices, or recordings of car sounds.[1]

Diet

For over 40 years a debate has raged over the value of eliminating cow's milk from the diet of children with colic and substituting lactose-free, soy or protein hydrolysate formulas. A systematic review concluded that substituting a protein hydrolysate formula is often beneficial but that no substantial evidence supports soy, lactose-free, or fiber-enriched formulas. Since intact cow's milk protein may be found in human breast milk, nursing mothers with colicky infants might try eliminating milk products from their diet.[1]

Medications

Dicyclomine (Bentyl, Bentylol) has been proved effective but is not recommended because of rare but potentially serious adverse effects. There is no evidence that simethicone has value.[1]

◥ REFERENCES ◣

1. Lucassen PL, Assendelft WJ, van Eijk JT, et al: Effectiveness of treatments for infantile colic: systematic review, *BMJ* 316:1563-1569, 1998.
2. Wolke D, Meyer R: Excessive infant crying: a controlled study of mothers helping mothers, *Pediatrics* 94:322-332, 1994.
3. Brazelton TB: Crying in infancy, *Pediatrics* 29:579, 1962.

CONDUCT DISORDER

(See also antisocial personality disorder; attention deficit/hyperactivity disorder; fetal alcohol effects)

Conduct disorder is the most common psychiatric disorder of childhood,[1] with somewhere between 8% and 12% of 15-year-olds meeting the criteria for the condition.[2] The ratio of boys to girls has usually been quoted as 3:1,[1] but the true ratio may be closer to unity.[2] About 40% of 6- to 8-year-olds in whom conduct disorder is diagnosed become adolescent delinquents, and as adults they are at high risk for antisocial personality disorder, substance abuse, and participation in criminal activities.[1] The risk for girls appears to be as high as for boys.[2] The prognosis is particularly poor if the child has both conduct disorder and attention deficit disorder.[3] Children with conduct disorders often have dyslexia.[1]

Although genetics is a significant component of conduct disorder, childrearing practices play an important role. Parenting deficits associated with poor prognosis are inadequate supervision, harsh and erratic discipline, rejection of the child, little or no involvement with the child, and parental conflict. Parental training programs are a very important part of the treatment program.[1]

Maternal smoking during pregnancy appears to be an additional risk factor.[4]

◤ REFERENCES ◥

1. Scott S: Aggressive behaviour in childhood, *BMJ* 316:202-206, 1998.
2. Pajer KA: What happens to "bad" girls? A review of the adult outcomes of antisocial adolescent girls, *Am J Psychiatry* 155:862-870, 1998.
3. Taylor E, Chadwick O, Heptinstall E, et al: Hyperactivity and conduct problems as risk factors for adolescent development, *J Am Acad Child Adolesc Psychiatry* 35:1213-1226, 1996.
4. Fergusson DM, Woodward LJ, Horwood J: Maternal smoking during pregnancy and psychiatric adjustment in late adolescence, *Arch Gen Psychiatry* 55:721-727, 1998.

CROUP

Croup is characterized by a barking cough, a hoarse voice, and stridor and is usually caused by a virus. Traditional treatment is exposure to humidified air (mist tents or a running shower in a closed bathroom), but no good studies have documented the efficacy of these approaches.[1] It is now evident that intramuscular,[2,3] oral,[2,4,5] or inhaled[2,4] corticosteroids or a combination of inhaled and oral corticosteroids[6] is effective for therapy. Symptomatic improvement is evident as early as 6 hours.[2] In most trials the dose of oral or intramuscular dexamethasone has been 0.6 mg/kg, but 0.15 mg/kg by the oral route appears to be equally effective.[1] Inhaled steroid may be given as 4 ml of a budesonide (Pulmicort) solution (2 mg) in an updraft nebulizer with continuous flow oxygen at 5 to 6 L/min.[6]

◤ REFERENCES ◥

1. Jaffe DM: The treatment of croup with glucocorticoids (editorial), *N Engl J Med* 339:553-555, 1998.
2. Ausejo M, Saenz A, Pham B, et al: The effectiveness of glucocorticoids in treating croup: meta-analysis, *BMJ* 319:595-600, 1999.
3. Johnson DW, Jacobson S, Edney PC, et al: A comparison of nebulized budesonide, intramuscular dexamethasone, and placebo for moderately severe croup, *N Engl J Med* 339:498-503, 1998.
4. Geelhoed GC, Macdonald WB: Oral and inhaled steroids in croup: a randomized, placebo-controlled trial, *Pediatr Pulmonol* 20:355-361, 1995.
5. Geelhoed GC, Macdonald WB: Oral dexamethasone in the treatment of croup: 0.13 mg/kg versus 0.3 mg/kg versus 0.6 mg/kg, *Pediatr Pulmonol* 20:362-368, 1995.
6. Klassen TP, Watters LK, Feldman ME, et al: Efficacy of nebulized budesonide in dexamethasone-treated outpatients with croup, *Pediatrics* 97:463-466, 1996.

DEVELOPMENTAL COORDINATION DELAY
(See also well-baby care)

Developmental coordination delay is a failure of motor coordination development to such a degree that it adversely affects the child's activities of daily living or academic performance. The condition can be diagnosed only if other causative medical conditions have been ruled out. Boys are affected more often than girls, and the prevalence rate is probably about 6%. Manifestations may include delays in early milestones such as crawling and walking and difficulty cutting with scissors, tying shoelaces, doing up buttons, riding a bike, or being proficient at sports. These children are often labeled clumsy. The physical deficits tend to persist, and many children do not "grow out of them." Adolescent psychosocial problems are common, possibly because of low self-esteem.[1,2] Treatment results are uncertain, but explanations and organized teaching of specific activities with the assistance of occupational therapists are probably helpful.[2]

◤ REFERENCES ◥

1. American Psychiatric Association: *Diagnostic and statistical manual of mental disorders,* ed 4, Washington, DC, 1994, American Psychiatric Association, pp 53-55.
2. Fox AM, Lent B: Clumsy children: primer on developmental coordination disorder, *Can Fam Physician* 42:1965-1971, 1996.

DIAPER RASH

Diaper rash or diaper dermatitis is a descriptive term for dermatitis occurring in the diaper area. The two most common causes are irritant diaper dermatitis and *Candida* dermatitis. These two conditions can be distinguished by physical examination. Irritant diaper dermatitis tends to spare the creases and is accentuated on convex surfaces such as the lower abdomen, buttocks, thighs, and genitalia. *Candida* dermatitis almost always involves the inguinal creases, and usually the infant has red plaques with white scales and satellite lesions.[1,2] The cause of irritant diaper dermatitis is primarily contact with moisture from urine. Contributing factors are fecal enzymes and irritant chemicals.[1,2]

Treatment and prevention of both irritant and *Candida* diaper dermatitis consist of measures to keep the diaper area dry. This can involve exposure to air for as long as possible, as well as the use of highly absorbent (superabsorbent) disposable diapers and frequent changes of diapers.[1,2] Superabsorbent disposable diapers have been shown to be more effective than cloth diapers in the prevention and treatment of diaper dermatitis.[1] Pharmacological agents of choice are barrier creams such as A & D ointment or Desitin. Topical antifungal agents such as nystatin (Mycostatin), clotrimazole (Canesten), or miconazole (Monistat Derm Cream) should be gently rubbed into the area several times a day, and treatment should be continued for at least 7 days after the rash has cleared.[1] A low-potency corticosteroid such as 1% hydrocortisone applied four times a day may help alleviate symptoms in more severe cases[1,2] but is not a necessary component of treatment.[1] Parents should be instructed to apply antifungal and corticosteroid creams before applying barrier creams.[1]

⚓ REFERENCES ⚓

1. Ipp M: Pediatric dermatology: recognizing, treating what's serious, *Patient Care Can* 7:20-32, 1996.
2. Sires UI, Mallory SB: Diaper dermatitis: how to treat and prevent, *Postgrad Med* 98:79-84, 1995.

DIARRHEA AND DEHYDRATION IN INFANTS
(See also breast feeding; formulas; tropical medicine)

In the United States about half of all cases of diarrhea in infants are caused by rotavirus. Breast feeding does not prevent rotavirus infection but does diminish the severity of the disease.[1]

In 1996 the American Academy of Pediatrics published guidelines for the management of gastroenteritis in children between the ages of 1 month and 5 years. These were some of the principal recommendations[2]:

1. Children with mild diarrhea and no dehydration do not require glucose-electrolyte solutions and may be given a regular diet including milk.
2. Oral rehydration therapy is the initial treatment of choice for children with mild or moderate dehydration.
3. Any one of a variety of glucose-electrolyte solutions may be used for oral rehydration therapy. Examples of commercial products are Naturalyte, Pediatric electrolyte, Pedialyte, Infalyte, Rehydralyte, Gastrolyte, and WHO/UNICEF oral rehydration salts.
4. Chicken broth, soft drinks, apple juice, and sports beverages (such as Gatorade) should not be used. Chicken broth has too much salt and no glucose, and the rest have too much glucose and inadequate salt.
5. The replacement volume of glucose-electrolyte replacement fluid for mild diarrhea is 50 ml/kg over a 4-hour period plus replacement of continuing losses. An additional 10 ml/kg should be given after each stool.
6. The replacement volume of glucose-electrolyte replacement fluid for moderate diarrhea is 100 ml/kg over a 4-hour period plus replacement of continuing losses. An additional 10 ml/kg should be given after each stool.
7. The secret of successful oral rehydration therapy in children who are vomiting is to give small amounts at frequent intervals. Every 1 to 2 minutes the child should be given 5 ml (1 tsp) of solution; as rehydration occurs and vomiting diminishes, larger amounts may be given at less frequent intervals.
8. Once rehydration is achieved, other fluids, including milk, and, if age appropriate, solid foods should be added.
9. Early refeeding does not worsen diarrhea and may even improve it. The majority of children tolerate full-strength milk and have no need for lactose-free formulations.
10. Any food may be used after a bout of diarrhea, but the best tolerated seem to be complex carbohydrates such as bread, potatoes, and rice, lean meats, yogurt, fruits, and vegetables. Fatty foods and high-sucrose foods (dessert-type foods and soft drinks) are less well accepted.
11. IV fluids are indicated for severe dehydration, shock or near shock, or moderate dehydration if the child cannot retain orally administered fluids because of persistent vomiting.
12. Antidiarrheal drugs should not be used.

These guidelines differ from the traditional approach in two important ways. They recommend the rapid reintroduction of whole milk rather than switching to a soy-based or other lactose-free formula for 1 to 2 weeks before going back to milk, and they recommend the rapid introduction of food with only minor concern about which types. A 1994 metaanalysis found that except for infants with severe dehydration, there was no benefit in switching to a lactose-free formula or in diluting the formula.[3] Analysis of the literature has shown no adverse effects from the early introduction of solids[4] and no advantage to using the BRAT diet of bananas, rice, applesauce, and tea.[5]

An inexpensive alternative to commercial electrolyte solutions that was developed at St. Justine's Children's Hospital in Montreal is 360 ml (12 oz or 1½ cups) of orange juice without added sugar, 600 ml (20 oz or 2½ cups) of boiled water, and 2 ml (a little less than ½ tsp) of salt.[6]

Evidence increasingly shows that cereal-based solutions containing complex rather than simple carbohydrates are effective. None is commercially available in North America at present, but one can be made up with ½ cup of dry precooked baby rice cereal, 2 cups of water, and ¼ tsp of salt. (Care should be taken to measure the salt accurately; if the solution tastes salty, too much has been added.[7])

⚓ REFERENCES ⚓

1. Newburg DS, Peterson JA, Ruiz-Palacios GM, et al: Role of human-milk lactadherin in protection against symptomatic rotavirus infection, *Lancet* 351:1160-1164, 1998.

2. Nazarian LF, Berman JH, Brown G, et al: Practice parameter: the management of acute gastroenteritis in young children, *Pediatrics* 97:424-435, 1996.

3. Brown KH, Peerson JM, Fontaine O: Use of nonhuman milks in the dietary management of young children with acute diarrhea: a meta-analysis of clinical trials, *Pediatrics* 93:17-27, 1994.

4. Brown KH: Dietary management of acute childhood diarrhea: optimal timing of feeding and appropriate use of milks and mixed diets, *J Pediatr* 118:S92-S98, 1991.

5. Meyers A: Modern management of acute diarrhea and dehydration in children, *Am Fam Physician* 51:1103-1115, 1995.

6. Deschênes M, Nazair P: La gastro-entérite: déshydratation, réhydratation, *Med Québec*, March 1994, pp 27-101.

7. Meyers A: Modern management of acute diarrhea and dehydration in children, *Am Fam Physician* 51:1103-1115, 1995.

ENURESIS

Enuresis is failure to achieve bladder control by age 5.[1,2] Enuresis is primary (no period of continence) in 90% of cases and secondary (reversion to incontinence after an extended period of dryness) in 10%. Secondary incontinence is often associated with psychological stress. Daytime incontinence is rare and needs a more thorough investigation than nocturnal enuresis.[2]

The overall incidence of primary nocturnal enuresis is about 15% to 20% among 5-year-olds, 5% to 7% among 10-year-olds, and 2% to 4% among 12- to 14-year-olds. The spontaneous remission rate is 15% per year.[2] Boys are affected twice as often as girls. Enuresis may be familial; if one parent was affected, the incidence among the offspring is 40%, and if both parents were affected, the incidence is 70%.[1,2]

If by history and physical examination (including a careful neurological examination) no abnormalities are detected other than nocturnal enuresis, the only investigation required is a urinalysis, which should include specific gravity as a screen for diabetes insipidus. Urine culture is necessary only if symptoms suggest a urinary tract infection.[1]

The usual initial intervention is motivational therapy. Parents and the child are informed about the nature of the condition and are told that neither parents nor child is responsible for its development but that with concerted effort improvement may occur. Charts of dry and wet nights are set up, and rewards are given for each night the child is dry. Within a year about 25% of children achieve complete resolution, which is somewhat better than the spontaneous resolution rate of 15%. Another 70% of children improve. If after 6 months motivational therapy is unsuccessful, behavioral conditioning is usually attempted with use of an alarm system, which may be a sound device or a vibratory device.[1] Alarm systems are triggered by sensor pads that detect moisture. Older systems use a pad on which the child sleeps, whereas newer ones use a small Velcro pad that is attached to the child's undergarments.[3] Cendron[1] recommends using alarm systems only for children 7 years old or older. Alarm

systems should be continued until the child has been consistently dry for a 3-week period. The reported success rate is 70%, but the relapse rate is 20 to 30%.[1]

Two drugs commonly used for enuresis are imipramine (Tofranil) and desmopressin (DDAVP). Imipramine is usually first given as 25 mg 1 hour before bedtime. This may be increased to 50 mg for children aged 7 to 12 and 75 mg for older children. Treatment is usually continued for 3 to 6 months, after which time the child is gradually weaned from the drug. The long-term cure rate is about 25%. The usual initial dose of desmopressin (DDAVP) is 20 µg (1 spray in each nostril) at bedtime. After 2 weeks the dose can be increased to 40 µg or, for children over the age of 12, to 60 µg. When used for long-term control, treatment should be continued for 3 to 6 months and then reduced by 10-µg increments per month. DDAVP may also be used intermittently for special occasions such as sleepovers or camping trips.[1]

◼ REFERENCES ◣

1. Cendron M: Primary nocturnal enuresis, *Am Fam Physician* 59: 1205-1214, 1999.

2. Ullom-Minnich MR: Diagnosis and management of nocturnal enuresis, *Am Fam Physician* 54:2259-2266, 1996.

3. Tietjen DN, Husmann DA: Nocturnal enuresis: a guide to evaluation and treatment, *Mayo Clin Proc* 71:857-862, 1996.

ERYTHEMA INFECTIOSUM
(See also infectious diseases in pregnancy)

Erythema infectiosum is also called fifth disease or "slapped-cheek" disease. It is caused by human parvovirus B19. Clinical manifestations begin with nonspecific symptoms, including headache, mild fever, and gastrointestinal symptoms. After a few days the typical pruritic rash appears on the cheeks ("slapped-cheek" appearance). Between 1 and 4 days later a lacy maculopapular rash may develop on the trunk and extremities; this rash tends to wax and wane and lasts 1 to 3 weeks. Infection is thought to be spread by respiratory secretions, but by the time the rash has appeared, the child can no longer spread infection. Most individuals who are positive serologically for parvovirus B19 have no recollection of having had symptomatic disease.[1]

Infection of pregnant women with parvovirus B19 infection may cause a nonimmune form of hydrops fetalis (see discussion of infectious diseases in pregnancy). In some cases, particularly in adult women, infection causes arthralgias or arthritis. In most instances joint symptoms resolve spontaneously in 1 to 3 weeks, but in about one fifth of cases symptoms persist for months or even years.[1]

◼ REFERENCES ◣

1. Sabella C, Goldfarb J: Parvovirus B19 infections, *Am Fam Physician* 60:1455-1460, 1999.

FEBRILE SEIZURES
(See also fever in children; seizures)

Are children without evident neurological disorders who have febrile seizures at greater risk for epilepsy than other children? Population studies in both the United States and the United Kingdom show that in most cases the risk increase is very small.[1-4] For example, the background risk for epilepsy in the general population of children is 1.4%, and among children with simple febrile seizures it is about 2.4%. However, the relatively small subgroup of children with "complex" febrile seizures (defined as focal, lasting more than 15 minutes, or recurring during the same febrile illness) are at higher risk for seizure disorders.[1,2] In one study the rate was 6% to 8% among children with only one "complex" feature, 17% to 22% among those with two, and 49% among those with three.[1]

At 10 years of age, children who had had either simple or "complex" febrile seizures in the early years of life demonstrated intellectual functioning, academic progress, and behavior that were as good as in children who never had febrile seizures.[5]

In one study children with a history of febrile seizures were assigned at random to be treated during any subsequent febrile episodes with acetaminophen, diazepam, acetaminophen plus diazepam, or placebo. The rate of febrile seizures was identical in all groups.[6]

⚐ REFERENCES ⚑

1. Annegars JF, Hauser WA, Shirts SB, et al: Factors prognostic of unprovoked seizures after febrile convulsions, *N Engl J Med* 316:493-498, 1987.
2. Verity CM, Golding J: Risk of epilepsy after febrile convulsions: a national cohort study, *BMJ* 303:1373-1376, 1991.
3. Robinson RJ: Febrile convulsions: further reassuring news about prognosis (editorial), *BMJ* 303:1345-1346, 1991.
4. Shinnar S, Berg AT, Moshe SL, et al: The risk of seizure recurrence after a first unprovoked afebrile seizure in childhood—an extended follow-up, *Pediatrics* 98:216-225, 1996.
5. Verity CM, Greenwood R, Golding J: Long-term intellectual and behavioral outcomes of children with febrile convulsions, *N Engl J Med* 338:1723-1728, 1998.
6. Uhari M: Effect of acetaminophen and of low intermittent doses of diazepam on prevention of recurrences of febrile seizures, *J Pediatr* 126:991-995, 1995.

FEVER IN CHILDREN
(See also febrile seizures; fever; urinalysis)

Various types of thermometers and the ability of parents to determine whether their children are febrile are discussed under "Fever."

Antipyretics

The standard symptomatic treatment of fever in children has been acetaminophen (Tempra), approximately 50/mg/kg/day in 4 divided doses or 15 mg/kg/dose q4-6h. A double-blind study of febrile children under 12 years of age compared ibuprofen (Advil, Motrin) 20 mg/kg/day with acetaminophen (Tempra, Tylenol) 50 mg/kg/day. No difference in efficacy or adverse effects was observed.[1]

When acetaminophen is prescribed for children, it is important to remember that drops are more concentrated than syrups and that various strengths of both chewable and regular tablets are available.

Sponging

Sponging is rarely if ever indicated except when temperatures exceed 40° to 41° C. If this technique is used, a single oral dose of an antipyretic should be given first and the sponging fluid should be lukewarm (neutral to the touch). Cold water or alcohol should never be used. Cold water causes shivering and raises body temperature, and alcohol may be inhaled and cause hypoglycemia and coma.[2]

Fever Without Source

The common practice for fever without source in children under 3 months of age has been to do a complete workup for sepsis and to treat them with antibiotics pending culture results. In some cases this may not be necessary.[3-6] The main reason for an aggressive approach to this problem was that before mass immunization for *Haemophilus influenzae*, meningitis developed in 5% to 10% of children who had fever without source. At present *Streptococcus pneumoniae* is the causative organism in the majority of cases that are found to be bacteremic. This bacterium rarely causes meningitis in young infants, and most cases resolve without treatment.[3,4]

Baraff and associates[3] suggest the following management protocols for children with rectal temperatures of 38° C (100.4° F) or higher and no clinically evident focus of infection.

Infants under 28 days

All infants under 28 days of age, with or without a toxic appearance, should be admitted to the hospital and have a complete workup for sepsis, including blood, urine, and cerebrospinal fluid cultures. Most cases are treated with parenteral antibiotics pending culture results. For selected "low-risk" (criteria listed below) infants who do not appear toxic, acceptable management would be the same sepsis workup with careful observation but no antibiotic therapy pending culture results.

Infants 28 to 90 days

A variety of approaches may be taken for infants between the ages of 28 and 90 days. If they appear toxic, they should be admitted to the hospital, have a complete sepsis workup, including blood, urine, and cerebrospinal fluid cultures, and be treated with parenteral antibiotics pending culture results.

Two options exist for the management of fever in "low-risk" infants in this age range. (Low risk is defined as previously healthy, nontoxic, no evidence of focal infection [excluding otitis media], white blood cell count of 5000 to 15,000/mm^3 [5 to 15 × 10^9/L], fewer than 1500 band cells/mm^3 [1.5 × 10^9/L], normal urinalysis findings, and if diarrhea is present, fewer than 5 white blood cells per high-power field in stool.) Both approaches may be accomplished on an outpatient basis provided the parents are reliable and close follow-up can be ensured. Protocol 1 is a sepsis workup, including blood, urine, and cerebrospinal fluid cultures. Ceftriaxone 50 mg/kg (maximum 1 g) intramuscularly is given stat, and follow-up takes place within 24 hours. At follow-up a second dose of ceftriaxone may be given. Protocol 2 involves no sepsis workup other than a urine culture, no antibiotics (unless needed to treat otitis media), careful observation by parents, and physician follow-up within 24 hours.

Children aged 3 to 36 months

Toxic-appearing children should be admitted to the hospital, have a complete sepsis workup, including blood, urine, and cerebrospinal fluid cultures, and be treated with parenteral antibiotics pending culture results.

The management of previously healthy, non-toxic-appearing children aged 3 to 36 months depends on the rectal temperature. If it is below 39° C (102.2° F), no diagnostic tests or antibiotics are needed. The child should be treated as an outpatient with acetaminophen 15 mg/kg/dose q4h and should be reassessed if the fever persists for more than 48 hours or if the clinical condition deteriorates. If the temperature is 39° C (102° F) or higher, management may in most cases be on an outpatient basis after the following workup:

1. Urine culture for boys under 6 months of age and girls under 2 years of age or for any child who has a positive urine dipstick test for leukocyte esterase or nitrites. Urine dipsticks may be negative in up to 20% of young children with urinary tract infections, which is why culture is recommended for all young children regardless of the dipstick results.
2. Stool cultures if stool contains blood and mucus or more than 5 white blood cells per high-power field
3. Chest x-ray examination if respiratory symptoms are present
4. Blood cultures for all children in this category or for those with a white blood cell count of 15,000/mm^3 (15 × 10^9/L) or higher
5. Antibiotics either for all children in this category or for those with a white blood cell count of 15,000/mm^3 (15 × 10^9/L) or higher
6. Acetaminophen 15 mg/kg per dose q4h
7. Follow-up in 24 to 48 hours

Although chest x-ray examination in febrile children under 2 years of age who do not have physical signs of pulmonary infection has generally not proved valuable, a 1999 paper reported the presence of occult pneumonia (as interpreted by radiologists) in 19% of children aged 5 years or less who had temperatures of 39° C (102° F) or higher, white blood cell counts of 20,000/mm^3 or higher, and no abnormal lung findings on examination.[7] Whether detection of these cases has clinical significance is uncertain because most would probably have resolved without treatment and the few that did not could be identified and treated with a close follow-up protocol.[8]

❧ REFERENCES ❧

1. McIntyre J, Hull D: Comparing efficacy and tolerability of ibuprofen and paracetamol in fever, *Arch Dis Child* 74:164-167, 1996.
2. Impicciatore P, Pandolfini C, Casella N, et al: Reliability of health information for the public on the World Wide Web: systematic survey of advice on managing fever in children at home, *BMJ* 314:1875-1881, 1997.
3. Baraff LJ, Bass JW, Fleisher GR, et al: Practice guideline for the management of infants and children 0-36 months of age with fever without source, *Pediatrics* 92:1-12, 1993.
4. Long SS: Antibiotic therapy in febrile children: "best-laid schemes . . .," *J Pediatr* 124:585-588, 1994.
5. Daaleman TP: Fever without source in infants and young children, *Am Fam Physician* 54:2503-2512, 1996.
6. Jaskiewicz JA, McCarthy CA, Richardson AC, et al: Febrile infants at low risk for serious bacterial infection—an appraisal of the Rochester criteria and implications for management, *Pediatrics* 94:390-396, 1994.
7. Bachur R, Perry H, Harper MB: Occult pneumonias: empiric chest radiographs in febrile children with leukocytosis, *Ann Emerg Med* 33:166-173, 1999.
8. Green SM, Rothrock SG: Evaluation styles for well-appearing febrile children: are you a "risk-minimizer" or a "test-minimizer"? (editorial), *Ann Emerg Med* 33:211-214, 1999.

FORMULAS

(See also breast feeding; colic; diarrhea and dehydration in infants)

Infant formulas have as their bases cow's milk, soy, or protein hydrolysates (Table 59). The last named are the most expensive. Almost all formulas come with or without iron fortification, and almost all are available as ready-to-feed (the most expensive), as liquid concentrates that require dilution, and as powders that require reconstitution (the least expensive).[1] Bottle-fed infants should probably receive iron-fortified formulas from birth because otherwise they are at risk for iron deficiency anemia.[1,2] (The iron is not required to prevent iron deficiency until 4 to 6 months, but because parents rarely change the formulas begun in the neonatal period, iron-fortified formulas should be used from the beginning of bottle feeding.) Although iron deficiency anemia has been claimed to be associated with developmental disadvantage, iron supplementation of bottle-fed infants in developed countries does not appear to improve developmental status.[3] The Canadian Task Force on Preventive Health Care gives iron-fortified formulas a "B" rating,[2] and the U.S. Preventive Services Task Force gives them a "C."[4]

Table 59 Selected Examples of Infant Formulas

Formula	Manufacturer and comments
Milk-Based Formulas	
Bonamil	Wyeth, casein dominant
Carnation Goodstart	Carnation, partial protein hydrolysate
Enfamil, Enfalac	Mead Johnson, whey-dominant protein
Lactofree, Enfalac Lactose Free	Mead Johnson, lactose free
SMA	Wyeth, whey dominant
Similac	Ross
Similac LF	Ross, lactose free
Soy-Based Formulas	
Enfalac Soy	Mead Johnson, contains sucrose
Prosobee	Mead Johnson, does not contain sucrose
Gerber Soy Formula	Gerber
Isomil	Ross
Nursoy	Wyeth
Soyalac	Nutricia–Loma Linda
Protein Hydrolysates	
Alimentum	Ross
Nutramigen	Mead Johnson

Most cow's milk–based formulas contain lactose (some are produced as lactose free), whereas soy-based formulas and protein hydrolysates do not. Traditionally infants with diarrhea were switched to non-lactose-containing formulas or to formulas diluted with water. A 1994 metaanalysis of 29 randomized trials found that if infants with severe dehydration were excluded, no benefit was achieved by switching to soy-based formulas or protein hydrolysates or by diluting formulas with water (see discussion of diarrhea and dehydration in infants).[5]

Whether infantile colic responds to protein hydrolysates is controversial (see discussion of colic). The Committee on Nutrition of the American Academy of Pediatrics claims that no evidence supports the use of protein hydrolysates for colic,[6] but papers with contrary views keep appearing.[7]

REFERENCES

1. Spencer JP: Practical nutrition for the healthy term infant, *Am Fam Physician* 54:138-144, 1996.
2. Canadian Task Force on the Periodic Health Examination: *Clinical preventive health care,* Ottawa, 1994, Canadian Communication Group—Publishing, pp 244-255.
3. Morley R, Abbott R, Fairweather-Tait S, et al: Iron fortified follow on formula from 9 to 18 months improves iron status but not development or growth: a randomised trial, *Arch Dis Child* 81:247-252, 1999.
4. US Preventive Services Task Force: *Guide to clinical preventive services,* ed 2, Baltimore, 1996, Williams & Wilkins, pp 231-246.
5. Brown KH, Peerson JM, Fontaine O: Use of nonhuman milks in the dietary management of young children with acute diarrhea: a meta-analysis of clinical trials, *Pediatrics* 93:17-27, 1994.
6. American Academy of Pediatrics, Committee on Nutrition: Hypoallergenic infant formulas, *Pediatrics* 83:1068-1069, 1989.
7. Hill DJ, Hudson IL, Sheffield LJ, et al: A low allergen diet is a significant intervention in infantile colic: results of a community-based study, *J Allergy Clin Immunol* 96:886-892, 1995.

FRAGILE X SYNDROME

The fragile X syndrome is a sex-linked disorder, and its full expression is seen only in males. Males who are affected usually have great difficulty at school and are unable to live independently as adults. Female carriers may have minor learning disabilities. Screening programs have been recommended so that women who are carriers can decide whether to have prenatal testing if they become pregnant.[1]

REFERENCES

1. Turner G, Robinson H, Wake S, et al: Case finding for the fragile X syndrome and its consequences, *BMJ* 315:1223-1236, 1997.

GROWTH HORMONE

Studies evaluating the efficacy of growth hormone for short normal children give conflicting results. Most claim little benefit,[1,2] but one long-term U.S. multicenter study reported an increased adult height of about 9 cm in boys and 6 cm in girls compared with the heights achieved by untreated children in other studies.[3] Children who are treated with growth hormone require three to seven injections a week for many years.[3]

REFERENCES

1. Coste J, Letrait M, Carel JC, et al: Long term results of growth hormone treatment in France in children of short stature: population, register based study, *BMJ* 315:708-713, 1997.
2. Hindmarsh PC, Brook CG: Final height of short normal children treated with growth hormone, *Lancet* 348:13-16, 1996.
3. Hintz R, Attie K, Baptista J, et al: Effect of growth hormone treatment on adult height of children with idiopathic short stature, *N Engl J Med* 340:502-507, 1999.

INTUSSUSCEPTION

Intussusception occurs most frequently between the ages of 5 and 9 months. Males are affected twice as often as females. The classic triad of vomiting, abdominal pain, and bloody diarrhea is seen in only one third of patients. The most common symptoms are colicky abdominal pain, irritability, and vomiting. Fever, lethargy, and diarrhea may also be presenting symptoms.[1]

REFERENCES

1. Winslow BT, Westfall JM, Nicholas RA: Intussusception, *Am Fam Physician* 54:213-217, 1996.

LABIAL FUSION

Labial fusion is usually seen in girls between the age of 3 months and 4 years. It results from denudation of the squamous epithelium of the labia minora, which is usually caused by a chemical or infectious vulvitis. Fusion begins at the posterior fourchette and progresses anteriorly toward the clitoris; in more advanced cases some degree of urinary obstruction may predispose the child to urinary tract infection. Treatment consists of the daily or twice-daily application of small amounts of estrogen cream (Premarin) to the fused area. Applications are continued until the adhesions lyse, which usually occurs within 3 to 4 weeks. Once the labia have separated, an ointment such as Vaseline should be applied to them for at least a month to prevent readhesion.[1]

❧ REFERENCES ❧

1. Leung AK, Robson WL, Wong B: Labial fusion, *Paediatr Child Health* 1:216-218, 1996.

LEAD POISONING

In October 1991 the U.S. Centers for Disease Control and Prevention (CDC) redefined lead poisoning by lowering acceptable blood lead levels to 10 μg/dl (0.48 μmol/L). Both the CDC and the American Academy of Pediatrics had recommended universal lead level screening for children younger than 6 years, but these guidelines have now been revised. Current recommendations are that children known to live in communities where 27% or more of the housing was built before 1950, or in communities where more than 12% of children have been documented to have blood lead levels of 10 μg/dl or higher, still require blood test screening, as do children living in communities where this type of data is unavailable. All other children should be screened by risk questionnaires, which include determining whether the child lives in or regularly visits a house or child care facility built before 1950; lives in or regularly visits a house or child care facility built before 1978 that has been renovated within the last 6 months; or has a sibling or playmate who has or has had lead poisoning. If the answer to any question is positive or if the answer is unknown, blood levels should be determined.[1]

Questions should also be asked about the presence of vinyl miniblinds, which are a newly discovered source of lead poisoning. Until recently lead was used as a stabilizing agent in the manufacturing process, and as the blinds aged, lead dust formed on the surface of the blinds.[2]

If families with small children are not able to move out of homes contaminated with lead, a partially effective alternative is regular intensive cleaning of the house, concentrating on wet mopping of floors, damp sponging of walls and other surfaces, and high-efficiency particle-accumulating vacuuming.[3]

Published evidence has suggested that lead levels even lower than 10 μg/dl (0.48 μmol/L) may lead to lower IQ levels.[4] An association has also been reported between elevated lead levels and an increased incidence of dental caries.[5]

❧ REFERENCES ❧

1. American Academy of Pediatrics Committee on Environmental Health: Screening for elevated blood lead levels, *Pediatrics* 101:1072-1078, 1998.
2. Norman EH, Hertz-Picciotto I, Salmen DA, et al: Childhood lead poisoning and vinyl miniblind exposure, *Arch Pediatr Adolesc Med* 151:1033-1037, 1997.
3. Rhoads GG, Ettinger AS, Weisel CP, et al: The effect of dust lead control on blood lead in toddlers: a randomized trial, *Pediatrics* 103:551-555, 1999.
4. Matte TD: Reducing blood lead levels: benefits and strategies (editorial), *JAMA* 281:2340-2342, 1999.
5. Moss ME, Lanphear BP, Auinger P: Association of dental caries and blood lead levels, *JAMA* 281:2294-2298, 1999.

NEONATAL JAUNDICE
(See also breast feeding)

Unconjugated hyperbilirubinemia or physiological jaundice of the newborn is extremely common. It is more frequent and more severe in premature, Asian, and breast-fed infants. The unconjugated bilirubin tends to peak about the fourth day of life and then gradually declines over several weeks. The difference between normal full-term breast-fed and bottle-fed babies is that in most studies both the peaks and the duration of jaundice tend to be higher in the breast-fed babies.[1,2]

Gartner[2] has marshaled considerable evidence that the initial hyperbilirubinemia of the breast-fed infant is a form of starvation jaundice and that when feeding is started early and given frequently, the bilirubin peaks of breast-fed infants are not higher than those of bottle-fed babies. He has suggested that although bottle-fed babies may thrive on six feedings a day, breast-fed infants probably require 10 in the early days and weeks of life. According to him, breast-fed babies should not be given glucose and water supplementation because this decreases their milk intake.

The differential diagnosis of physiological jaundice must consider a wide variety of conditions, including extrahepatic and intrahepatic biliary obstructions, liver disease, various metabolic abnormalities, hemolytic disorders, large hematomas, sepsis, hypothyroidism, and bowel obstruction.[1]

Not all jaundiced babies need extensive investigation. The Canadian Paediatric Society recommends that all babies who are being considered for phototherapy have a complete blood cell count and smear, measurement of conjugated and unconjugated bilirubin, blood grouping with antibody testing, and further tests such as measurement of glucose-6-phosphate dehydrogenase for those whose ethnicity (Asian, African, or Mediterranean descent) puts them at risk of glucose-6-phosphate deficiency.[3]

No national or international consensus has defined a threshold level of bilirubin that would mandate phototherapy for term infants without additional risk factors.[3] The 1994 recommendations of the American Academy of Pediatrics are that phototherapy be instituted in term infants aged 25 to 48 hours when the bilirubin is 15 mg/dl (260 μmol/L) or higher, in those aged 49 to 72 hours when it is 18 mg/dl (310 μmol/L) or higher, and in those over the age of 72 hours when it is 20 mg/dl (340 μmol/L) or higher.[4] The Canadian Paediatric Society takes a more cautious approach and advises starting phototherapy in infants aged 24 hours if the bilirubin is 10 mg/dl (170 μmol/L) or higher, in infants aged 48 hours if it is 15 mg/dl (260 μmol/L) or higher, and in those aged 72 hours if it is 18 mg/dl (310 μmol/L) or higher.[3] Infants at increased risk for kernicterus (gestational age under 37 weeks and birth weight less than 2500 g, hemolysis, jaundice at less than 24 hours of age, sepsis, and need for resuscitation at birth) should receive phototherapy at lower levels of bilirubin than are indicated for healthy term infants.[3]

Even though breast feeding is associated with higher bilirubin levels than bottle feeding, breast feeding is not contraindicated during phototherapy. However, the babies should be well hydrated because dehydration may raise bilirubin levels and phototherapy itself may aggravate dehydration.[3]

--------------------- ⚡ **REFERENCES** ⚡ ---------------------

1. Lasker MR, Holzman IR: Neonatal jaundice: when to treat, when to watch and wait, *Postgrad Med* 99:187-193, 197-198, 1996.
2. Gartner LM: On the question of the relationship between breastfeeding and jaundice in the first 5 days of life, *Semin Perinatol* 18:502-509, 1994.
3. Fetus and Newborn Committee of the Canadian Paediatric Society: Approach to the management of hyperbilirubinemia in term newborn infants: a joint statement with the College of Family Physicians of Canada, *Paediatr Child Health* 4:161-164, 1999.
4. Provisional Committee for Quality Improvement and Subcommittee on Hyperbilirubinemia: Practice parameter: management of hyperbilirubinemia in the healthy term newborn, *Pediatrics* 94:558-565, 1994.

PNEUMONIA IN CHILDREN
(See also pneumonia)

The incidence of pneumonia in North American children is highest before age 5 and then decreases. Risk factors include prematurity, low socioeconomic status, exposure to passive smoke, and attendance at day care.[1]

Clinical signs of pneumonia in young children can be deceptive. Most studies consider tachypnea to be an important sign.[1,2] Normal respiratory rates in awake babies during the first week of life are about 50 per minute, and these decrease to around 40 per minute at 6 months.[2] One set of guidelines states that tachypnea is present if the rate is greater than 60 per minute in infants under 2 months of age, greater than 50 per minute if aged 2 to 12 months, and greater than 40 per minute for young children over 1 year of age.[1,2]

Ideally, respiratory rate should be measured for 1 minute or for two 30-second periods when the child is awake and not crying. Intercostal, subcostal, or suprasternal notch retraction suggests more severe disease. Other suggestive signs are nasal flaring and grunting. Depending on respiratory rates alone will lead to a failure of diagnosis in a number of cases and overdiagnosis in considerably more (sensitivity and specificity are not ideal). However, pneumonia can be excluded with confidence if the child lacks all the following signs: respiratory distress, tachypnea, crackles, and decreased breath sounds.[1,2]

The causative organisms of pneumonia in children are determined largely by age. Under the age of 2 years, viruses are predominant, but *Chlamydia trachomatis, Mycoplasma pneumoniae, Streptococcus pneumoniae, Haemophilus influenzae* type b, and nontypable *H. influenzae* cause some infections. Among children aged 2 or older, *S. pneumoniae, M. pneumoniae,* and *C. trachomatis* become the predominant pathogens, although the organisms primarily responsible for infections in infants and toddlers still account for a number of infections in this age group. *Staphylococcus aureus* is a cause of severe pneumonia necessitating admission to an intensive care unit in all age groups.[1]

Management varies with age and severity of infection. In general, children under the age of 3 months are admitted, as are those who are toxic, in severe respiratory distress, vomiting, or dehydrated or have not responded to oral antibiotics as outpatients. The recommended antibiotics for outpatient treatment of pneumonia in children, as outlined by a Canadian Consensus Panel of Pediatric Infectious Disease specialists and a microbiologist, are[1]:

1. For children 3 months to 5 years: amoxicillin 40 mg/kg/day in 3 divided doses, or erythromycin 40 mg/kg/day in 4 divided doses, or clarithromycin (Biaxin) 15 mg/kg/day in 2 divided doses. Treatment duration for all regimens is 7 to 10 days.
2. For children 5 to 18 years: erythromycin 40 mg/kg/day in 4 divided doses or clarithromycin (Biaxin) 15 mg/kg/day in 2 divided doses. Treatment duration for both regimens is 7 days.

--------------------- ⚡ **REFERENCES** ⚡ ---------------------

1. Jadavji T, Law B, Lebel MG, et al: A practical guide for the diagnosis and treatment of pediatric pneumonia, *Can Med Assoc J* 156(suppl):S703-S711, 1997.
2. Margolis P, Gadomski A: Does this infant have pneumonia? *JAMA* 279:308-313, 1998.

PRETERM INFANTS

A follow-up study of surviving premature infants weighing less than 750 g at birth found that these children were at high risk for neurobehavioral dysfunction and poor school performance.[1] The rate of mental retardation (intelligence quotient below 70) was 21% versus 2% in the control group of full-term children, the rate of cerebral palsy was 9% versus none, and the rate of severe visual disability was 25.5% versus 2%. Children weighing between 750 and 1499 g at birth also had higher disability rates in all categories but to a lesser degree than the children under 750 g at birth.[1]

A prospective evaluation of premature births in northern England found that one fourth of those born at less than 26 weeks of gestation and surviving past 1 year had severe disabilities. Ten percent were incapable of meaningful communication or independent mobility.[2]

An increased incidence of neurocognitive and behavioral dysfunction in adolescents who had been born preterm has been documented. In a British study 20% required extra educational provisions, reading age was generally lower than that of control subjects, and over half had abnormal magnetic resonance imaging brain scans.[3] A Canadian study of adolescents who had been extremely low-birth-weight infants (less than 1000 g) found that these children had significantly more limitations in the areas of cognition, sensation, and self-care and experienced more pain than was the case with control subjects. Despite this the majority viewed their health-related quality of life as quite satisfactory.[4]

Being the mother of a very low-birth-weight child increases psychological stress as measured at 1 month regardless of whether the child is labeled as having a high risk of neurodevelopmental impairment. At 2 years mothers of very low-birth-weight children at high risk of impairment had an increased incidence of depression, but by 3 years psychological distress was no greater in these mothers than in mothers of term babies.[5]

⚓ REFERENCES ⚓

1. Hack M, Taylor G, Klein N, et al: School-age outcomes in children with birth weights under 750g, *N Engl J Med* 331:753-759, 1994.
2. Tin W, Wariyar U, Hey E (Northern Neonatal Network): Changing prognosis for babies of less than 28 weeks' gestation in the north of England between 1983 and 1994, *BMJ* 314:107-111, 1997.
3. Stewart AL, Rifkin L, Amess PN, et al: Brain structure and neurocognitive and behavioural function in adolescents who were born very preterm, *Lancet* 353:1653-1657, 1999.
4. Saigal S, Feeny D, Rosenbaum P, et al: Self-perceived health status and health-related quality of life of extremely low-birth-weight-infants at adolescence, *JAMA* 276:453-459, 1996.
5. Singer LT, Salvator A, Guo S, et al: Paternal psychological distress and parenting stress after the birth of a very low-birth-weight infant, *JAMA* 281:799-805, 1999.

PUBERTY

Normal puberty begins in girls between the ages of 8 and 13 and in boys between the ages of 9 and 14. In 85% of girls the initial manifestation of puberty is breast development or thelarche, whereas in 15% it is the growth of pubic hair. Acceleration in growth occurs at this stage. Pubic hair growth or pubarche usually begins 6 months after thelarche, and axillary hair appears 2 years after the development of pubic hair. Menarche follows thelarche by about 2 years.[1] Growth velocity peaks at about 12.5 years (8 cm or 3.2 inches per year), and growth ceases around 16 years.[2] For boys the initial manifestation of puberty is almost always testicular enlargement, which is followed in about 6 months by the development of pubic hair. The penis enlarges 12 to 18 months after testicular enlargement, and facial and axillary hair appears 2 years after the development of pubic hair.[1] Growth velocity peaks at about 14 years (10 cm or 4 inches per year), and growth ceases at around 17 years.[2]

Precocious puberty is defined as the development of secondary sexual characteristics before the age of 8 years in girls and before the age of 9.5 years in boys. The most important differential diagnoses are isolated premature thelarche and isolated premature pubarche, since neither of these conditions has clinical significance and neither requires treatment.[1,3] The diagnosis of true precocious puberty is important because a few cases are caused by virilizing tumors and because in other cases premature closure of the epiphyses may lead to abnormally short adult stature.[1,3]

⚓ REFERENCES ⚓

1. Lee PA: Advances in the management of precocious puberty, *Clin Pediatr* 33:54-61, 1994.
2. Blondell RD, Foster MB, Dave K: Disorders of puberty, *Am Fam Physician* 60:209-218, 1999.
3. Merke DP, Cutler GB Jr: Evaluation and management of precocious puberty, *Arch Dis Child* 75:269-271, 1996.

PYLORIC STENOSIS

Hypertrophic pyloric stenosis usually presents as projectile, nonbilious vomiting in infants under 3 months of age. Three times as many boys as girls are affected, and the condition is more common in first-born children than in subsequent siblings.[1]

Classic clinical signs are visible gastric peristalsis and a palpable "olive." The sensitivity of these signs has decreased in recent years, probably because of earlier referral and therefore less fully developed lesions. In one recent study clinical diagnosis was possible in only about half the cases. If an olive is palpable, imaging studies are not necessary.[1]

Aspiration of gastric contents with a no. 8 feeding tube after a fast of 90 minutes may be used as an initial investigative technique when no olive is palpable. Over 90% of infants with pyloric stenosis will have an aspirate volume equal to or greater than 5 ml.[1]

Ultrasound and upper gastrointestinal x-ray series are the standard imaging techniques for diagnosing pyloric stenosis. If an initial ultrasound fails to demonstrate pyloric stenosis, an upper gastrointestinal series is needed.[1]

⚓ REFERENCES ⚓

1. Mandell GA, Wolfson PJ, Adkins S, et al: Cost-effective imaging approach to the nonbilious vomiting infant, *Pediatrics* 103:1198-1202, 1999.

REYE'S SYNDROME

Reye's syndrome was first described in Australia in 1963. The major abnormalities are a fatty liver and encephalopathy. The condition usually develops within 3 weeks after the onset of a viral illness (often varicella, upper respiratory tract infection, or gastroenteritis), and the major clinical manifestations are progressive vomiting, mental status changes, and eventually coma. Laboratory tests usually show elevations of alanine aminotransferase (ALT), aspartate aminotransferase (AST), and ammonia levels. Although the median age for Reye's syndrome is 6 years, the disease has been reported in infants under 1 year of age and in adolescents as old as 17 years.[1]

A clear association between Reye's syndrome and aspirin use was established by 1980. A major public health campaign warning parents about the dangers of aspirin in children was mounted, and as a result the incidence of Reye's syndrome dropped dramatically. Because Reye's syndrome is now rare, children with encephalopathy and evidence of liver dysfunction should be investigated for inborn metabolic disorders because some of these can mimic Reye's syndrome.[1]

◿ REFERENCES ◣

1. Belay ED, Bresee JS, Holman RC, et al: Reye's syndrome in the United States from 1981 through 1997, *N Engl J Med* 340:1377-1382, 1999.

ROSEOLA INFANTUM

Roseola infantum is thought to be caused by human herpesvirus type 6 (HHV-6). The incubation period is 7 to 17 days with a mean of 10 days. Most cases occur between 6 and 18 months of age, and the disorder is rare over the age of 3.

SINGLE-PARENT FAMILIES

(See also abuse; antisocial personality disorder; poverty)

Approximately 24% of American children live with only one parent and another 15% live in melded families. About half of American children have or will have lived with one parent. Of single-parent families, 86% are headed by the mother and 63% are white. Most single parents are in their twenties and thirties, and the situation is usually a result of separation or divorce.[1]

Births to unwed women increased in the United States from 18% in 1980 to 31% in 1995.[2] Part of this increase may be explained by a decrease in the birth rate among married women, and it must also be realized that 25% of single mothers are living in a common-law relationship. Although the out-of-wedlock birth rate has increased in teenagers, it has increased more sharply in women aged 20 to 29. The illegitimacy rate among blacks is about 2.5 times that among whites, but over the last decade there has been a decrease among blacks and an increase among whites. The most striking correlates of out-of-wedlock births are failure to graduate from high school and poverty.[2] Children, especially boys, who are subject to high-conflict divorce have a two to four times greater frequency of emotional and behavioral problems than is the norm in the community. Girls are particularly prone to respond poorly to court-ordered joint custody or frequent visitations.[3]

There is little evidence that welfare fosters single motherhood; a more likely explanation for the high rate of single parenthood among the poor is that disadvantaged young men and women do not see marriage as a realistic possibility.[2] While pregnancy and birth rates among single teenagers have been increasing in the United States so that they are now among the highest in the developed world,[4] they have been decreasing in Sweden. This may be related to a much higher level of contraceptive use and sex education in Sweden.[1]

In the absence of intensive follow-up, one third of pregnant adolescents will become pregnant again within a year and nearly one half within 2 years.[5] Unfortunately, interventions to alter this pattern of behavior, such as peer support groups, are often failures.[6]

Children from single-parent families are at double the risk for behavioral problems, dropping out of high school, failing a grade, being out of work, and in the case of girls becoming teenage mothers. This applies across all economic levels, but the rates are halved in the better off.[1]

◿ REFERENCES ◣

1. McLanahan S, Sandefur G: *Growing up with a single parent: what hurts, what helps,* Cambridge, Mass, 1994, Harvard University Press.
2. Usdansky ML: Single motherhood: stereotypes vs. statistics, *New York Times,* February 11, 1996, Sect 4, p 4.
3. Meurer JR, Meurer LN, Holloway RL: Clinical problems and counseling for single-parent families, *Am Fam Physician* 54: 864-870, 1996.
4. Spitz AM, Velebil P, Koonin LM, et al: Pregnancy, abortion, and birth rates among US adolescents—1980, 1985, and 1990, *JAMA* 275:989-994, 1996.
5. Stevens-Simon C, White M: Adolescent pregnancy, *Pediatr Ann* 20:322-331, 1991.
6. Stevens-Simon C, Dolgan JI, Kelly L, et al: The effect of monetary incentives and peer support groups on repeat adolescent pregnancies: a randomized trial of the Dollar-a-Day program, *JAMA* 277:977-982, 1997.

STUTTERING

Stuttering occurs in 3% to 5% of preschool-age children and is three to four times more common in boys than girls. In about 80% of cases stuttering resolves spontaneously by age 16. Consultation with a speech therapist is indicated if the child is over 4 years of age, has had consistent stuttering for at least 3 months, and manifests struggling behavior while stuttering. Some of the important therapeutic techniques are to avoid criticizing the child and to encourage slow speaking. Parents can model this by speaking or reading slowly to their children.[1]

REFERENCES

1. Lawrence M, Barclay DM III: Stuttering: a brief review, *Am Fam Physician* 57:2175-2178, 1998.

SUDDEN INFANT DEATH SYNDROME
(See also cardiac arrest)

Important risk factors for sudden infant death syndrome (SIDS) include the following:

1. Sleeping in the prone position[1]
2. Sleeping on one side[1]
3. Sleeping in the mother's bed all night, especially if she smokes[1]
4. Maternal smoking during pregnancy and postnatally[3]
5. Passive exposure to smoke[1-3]
6. Poverty[1]
7. Young maternal age[1]
8. Heavy caffeine intake during pregnancy[4]

Important preventive measures against SIDS are to avoid sleeping in the prone position (the back is the preferred position)[1,2] and to ban cigarettes from the environment both antenatally[3] and postnatally.[1-3]

REFERENCES

1. Brooke H, Gibson A, Tappin D, et al: Case-control study of sudden infant death syndrome in Scotland, 1992-95, *BMJ* 314:1516-1520, 1997.
2. Mitchell E: Cot death—the story so far, *BMJ* 319:1461-1462, 1999.
3. Klonoff-Cohen HS, Edelstein SL, Lefkowitz ES, et al: The effect of passive smoking and tobacco exposure through breast milk on sudden infant death syndrome, *JAMA* 273:795-798, 1995.
4. Ford RP, Schluter PJ, Mitchell EA, et al: Heavy caffeine intake in pregnancy and sudden infant death syndrome, *Arch Dis Child* 78:9-13, 1998.

URINARY TRACT INFECTIONS IN CHILDREN
(See also circumcision, male; labial fusion; urinary tract infections)

Before the age of 3 months, urinary tract infections (UTIs) are more common in males than females, but after that time females are more likely to be affected. About 8% of girls and 2% of boys have a UTI during childhood, and in 5% to 15% of these cases renal scarring develops. Renal scarring is associated with an increased incidence of recurrent pyelonephritis in adulthood, poor renal growth, hypertension, and end-stage renal failure.[1] Renal scarring as a complication of UTI is most common before 1 year of age and is rare in children over the age of 5. Whether vesicoureteral reflux causes renal scarring is uncertain.[2]

Urine culture is necessary to make a diagnosis of UTIs in children. Dipstick results for nitrites and leukocyte esterases are insufficiently sensitive, with a false-negative rate of up to 20%.[3] Urinary tract infection is defined as a pure bacterial growth of more than 10^5 colony-forming units per milliliter in voided or clean-catch urine or the presence of any pathogens in suprapubic aspirates. Counts lower than 10^5 are clinically significant in boys and in catheter-obtained specimens. Acute infections should be treated for 7 to 10 days; some retrospective studies have concluded that immediate empirical treatment results in less renal scarring than does delayed treatment.[1]

Diagnostic imaging procedures commonly used to detect vesicoureteral reflux or obstructive lesions in children with UTIs are ultrasonography, renal scintigraphy, and voiding cystourethrography. No consensus exists as to which children should be investigated, mainly because no published randomized trials deal with the issue. Three suggested options are as follows:

1. Investigate all children.[1]
2. Investigate all males regardless of age and all females under the age of 5 years. Females over the age of 5 years require imaging only if they have systemic symptoms or (perhaps) recurrent UTIs.[2]
3. Investigate any child with a UTI acquired before toilet training has begun. For children over this age with reliable parents who will ensure adequate follow-up, omit imaging for a first infection but provide it if the child has a recurrence.[3]

Delays in performance of imaging can be safely addressed by providing interim prophylactic antibiotic coverage.

Degrees of vesicoureteral reflux are categorized from I (mild) to V (severe). For lesser degrees of reflux the outcome is as good with medical therapy as with surgery.[1] First-line treatment for most cases of reflux is antibiotic prophylaxis, usually with nitrofurantoin 1 to 2 mg/kg once daily or trimethoprim/sulfamethoxazole (trimethoprim 2 to 4 mg/kg) once daily. Annual cystograms are obtained, and antibiotics are usually discontinued when the reflux has resolved. If breakthrough UTIs occur, surgical correction of the reflux may be indicated.[3]

REFERENCES

1. Larcombe J: Urinary tract infection in children, *BMJ* 319:1173-1175, 1999.
2. Ahmed SM, Swedlund SK: Evaluation and treatment of urinary tract infections in children, *Am Fam Physician* 57:1573-1580, 1998.
3. Ross JH, Kay R: Pediatric urinary tract infection and reflux, *Am Fam Physician* 59:1472-1478, 1999.

VARICELLA IN CHILDREN
(See also varicella; varicella vaccines)

Treatment of varicella in otherwise healthy children with acyclovir (Zovirax) is of questionable value. Defervescence may occur 1 to 2 days earlier than in untreated patients, and there may be fewer skin lesions. However, treatment does not appear to decrease the rate of transmission of the infection, reduce complications, or cause less scarring.[1] Immunization against varicella is discussed in the section on varicella vaccines.

――――――――― ◣ REFERENCES ◢ ―――――――――

1. Balfour HH JR, Kelly JM, Suarez CS, et al: Acyclovir treatment of varicella in otherwise healthy children, *J Pediatr* 116:633-639, 1990.

WELL-BABY CARE
(See also developmental coordination delay)

Numerous protocols for well-baby care have been published. One that is well organized, relevant, easy to use, and evidence based is the *Rourke Baby Record: Evidence-Based Infant/Child Health Maintenance Guide*.[1,2]

――――――――― ◣ REFERENCES ◢ ―――――――――

1. Panagiotou L, Rourke LL, Rourke JT, et al: Evidence-based well-baby care. 1. Overview of the next generation of the Rourke Baby Record, *Can Fam Physician* 44:558-567, 1998.
2. Panagiotou L, Rourke LL, Rourke JT, et al: Evidence-based will-baby care. 2. Education and advice section of the next generation of the Rourke Baby Record, *Can Fam Physician* 44: 568-572, 1998.

PSYCHIATRY

(See also alcohol; attention deficit/hyperactivity disorder; conduct disorder; female athlete triad; single-parent families)

Topics covered in this section

Abuse
Aggression
Anxiety Disorders
Creativity
Eating Disorders
False Memories
Functional Somatic Syndrome
Mood Disorders
Personality Disorders
Psychoses
Psychotherapy
Substance Abuse and Gambling

ABUSE
(See also aggression; false memories; guns; single-parent families; sports medicine)

Childhood Abuse

Although adults who have been abused as children have both an increased risk of developing personality disorders[1] and an increased number of risk factors for poor physical health,[2] children are resilient and the majority of those who are abused do not have psychopathological problems as adults.[3]

An important clue to abuse is bruising. In one study of normal children (no suspicion of abuse), bruising was present in only 0.6% of those under 6 months of age and 1.7% of those under 9 months of age. Once children started to cruise, bruising became common, especially over the knees and anterior tibiae and on the forehead. In this study none of the children manifested bruising on the hands or buttocks and almost none had bruising of the face (nose and cheeks).[4]

A specific form of childhood abuse is the shaken baby syndrome. The victims are usually male infants, and most are under 6 months of age. The perpetrators are men in 90% of cases, most often the biological father and next most frequently the mother's boyfriend. When a woman is responsible, she is usually a caretaker, not the mother. A wide variety of injuries may occur,[5] but the most serious is head trauma ("abusive head trauma").[6] The shaken baby syndrome accounts for more than half of all nonaccidental pediatric deaths, and the psychomotor and social development of survivors is often impaired.[5]

Many cases of abusive head trauma are missed either because the examining physician fails to suspect the condition or because of errors in the interpretation of cranial computed tomographic (CT) scans. Many infants with intracranial hemorrhage have no systemic symptoms,[7] and when symptoms are present, they are often nonspecific (e.g., vomiting, fever, and irritability).[6] Intracranial hemorrhage is most frequently missed if the child appears well and if the physician interprets the family structure as nonsuspect (usually white with the parents living together).[6] A critically important sign is the presence of scalp hematomas.[6,7] The authors of a Harvard study concluded that if a child over the age of 3 months is asymptomatic and does not have a scalp hematoma, radiographic imagining of the brain is unnecessary.[7]

A classic sign of abusive head trauma causing subdural hematomas is the presence of retinal hemorrhages, which tend to be concentrated in the region of the maculae. Injuries may result from shaking alone, from striking the head against a hard object, or from other forms of trauma.[5] One investigative protocol for suspected child abuse includes retinal examination by an ophthalmologist, a complete blood cell count, coagulation studies, CT or magnetic resonance imaging of the head, skeletal survey, and a multidisciplinary social assessment.[8] If a spinal tap has been performed, the fluid should be assessed for xanthochromia and, according to some authors, a pediatric radiologist should be asked to review the CT images.[6]

Domestic Violence

The lifetime prevalence of intimate partner abuse or domestic violence is extraordinarily high. In a survey of women treated in the emergency rooms of 11 community hospitals, 37% reported a lifetime prevalence of emotional or physical abuse and 14% had suffered physical or sexual abuse in the past year.[9] In another emergency room study a single question asking patients whether anyone had punched, kicked, hit, or hurt them in some other way in the past year detected over two thirds of abused patients as established by a standardized 19-item questionnaire.[10] In 90% of cases the abuser is male.[11] The risk of physical abuse is greatly increased if the male partner is abusing drugs or alcohol.[12,13]

Domestic abuse takes many forms. One classification breaks abuse down into these categories[14]:

1. Emotional abuse
2. Environmental abuse (e.g., made to feel afraid of being in own home or car)
3. Social abuse (e.g., control over friends; public scenes)
4. Financial abuse
5. Religious abuse (e.g., use of religion to control; mocking of religious beliefs)
6. Physical abuse
7. Sexual abuse
8. Ritual abuse (e.g., forced participation in rituals; mutilations)

Another form of abuse is interfering with adequate medical treatment for chronic diseases, for example, by hiding insulin syringes.[11]

The value of screening for domestic abuse has not been determined, largely because the efficacy of therapeutic interventions is unknown.[15] Because the adverse effects of abuse are so serious, a logical case can be made for screening pending the results of controlled trials. In one suggested protocol for screening, the health professional introduces the topic by saying that because domestic abuse is a serious health problem, patients are now routinely asked about it. Two suggested questions are, "Do you ever feel unsafe at home?" and "Has anyone at home hit you or tried to injure you in any way?"[11]

In surveys of women who have been abused, most have said they would welcome being asked about it and would be willing to discuss it.[11]

Current guidelines advise against marital counseling in the management of domestic abuse because such an intervention could increase the risk of further abuse. Even bringing up the issue of abuse on a one-to-one basis with the male partner (with the female partner's consent) might lead to escalation of violence.[16] Immediate management is to ensure the safety of the abused partner, using when possible a team approach involving nurses, social workers, and other community resources. One option is to move the abused woman and her children to a shelter and obtain a restraining order against the abusive partner. For women who are unwilling to accept this, outside emergency contacts and support services can be set up and advice given about techniques for improving safety at home (e.g., hiding weapons, ensuring that money and documents are easily accessible, and establishing a method of quickly accessing a phone).[11]

Elderly Abuse

Elderly abuse has been divided into the following categories[17]:

1. Physical violence
2. Psychological or emotional abuse
3. Material or financial exploitation
4. Neglect (intentional or unintentional)

Two thirds of abuse cases are perpetrated by spouses and one third by adult offspring. Specific risk factors that have been identified among caregivers are a history of mental illness or substance abuse, a history of violent or antisocial behavior, and significant financial dependence on the elderly person.[17]

Although elderly abuse is obviously a serious issue, the value of physician screening for this problem is uncertain. Both the U.S. Preventive Services Task Force[18] and the Canadian Task Force on Preventive Health Care[19] give case finding for elderly abuse a "C" rating.

Sexual Abuse

An anonymous survey of adolescent schoolchildren in a Midwestern state found a 10% prevalence of sexual abuse. The female/male ratio was 4:1, and the rate was twice as high among blacks and Native Americans as among whites.[20] In a Swiss study perpetrators were known to the children in two thirds of the cases and family members were responsible for 20.5% of events against girls and 6.3% of events against boys. A little less than half the events were experienced before the age of 12.[21]

Girls who have been sexually abused as children are six times more likely to report later sexual victimization than are nonabused girls, and boys who have been sexually abused are twice as likely to report sexual aggression as are nonabused boys. Persistent exposure to family violence may an important factor in determining whether sexually abused boys later become sexual abusers.[22] One study found that boys at highest risk of sexual abuse were under 13, socioeconomically deprived, and not living with their fathers. Most perpetrators were known to the victim but not related to him and were self-declared heterosexuals. Boys who had been sexually abused rarely informed their primary care physicians of these events. Sequelae included an increased incidence of high-risk sexual behaviors, substance abuse, anxiety disorders, mood disorders, poor school performance, and legal troubles.[23]

Genital examination of girls who had been subject to penetration was normal in 44% of cases; an intact hymen did not rule out penetration.[24]

◥ REFERENCES ◤

1. Johnson JG, Cohen P, Brown J, et al: Childhood maltreatment increases risk for personality disorders during early adulthood, *Arch Gen Psychiatry* 56:600-606, 1999.

2. Felitti VJ, Anda RF, Nordenberg D, et al: Relationship of childhood abuse and household dysfunction to many of the leading causes of death in adults: the Adverse Childhood Experiences (ACE) Study, *Am J Prev Med* 14:245-258, 1998.

3. Paris J: Does childhood trauma cause personality disorders in adults? *Can J Psychiatry* 43:148-153, 1998.

4. Sugar NF, Taylor JA, Feldman KW, et al: Bruises in infants and toddlers: those who don't cruise rarely bruise, *Arch Pediatr Adolesc Med* 153:399-403, 1999.

5. Lancon JA, Haines D, Parent A: Anatomy of the shaken baby syndrome, *Anat Rec (New Anat)* 253:13-18, 1998.

6. Jenny C, Hymel KP, Ritzen A, et al: Analysis of missed cases of abusive head trauma, *JAMA* 281:621-626, 1999.

7. Greenes DS, Schutzman SA: Clinical indicators of intracranial injury in head-injured infants, *Pediatrics* 104:861-867, 1999.

8. Jayawant S, Rawlinson A, Gibbon F, et al: Subdural haemorrhages in infants: population based study, *BMJ* 317:1558-1561, 1998.

9. Dearwater SR, Coben JH, Campbell JC, et al: Prevalence of intimate partner abuse in women treated at community hospital emergency departments, *JAMA* 280:433-438, 1998.

10. Feldhaus KM, Koziol-Mclain J, Amsbury HL, et al: Accuracy of 3 brief screening questions for detecting partner violence in the emergency department, *JAMA* 277:1357-1361, 1997.

11. Eisnstat SA, Bancroft L: Domestic violence, *N Engl J Med* 341:886-892, 1999.

12. Kyriacou DN, Anglin D, Taliaferro E, et al: Risk factors for injury to women from domestic violence, *N Engl J Med* 341:1892-1898, 1999.

13. Grisso JA, Schwarz DF, Hirschinger N, et al: Violent injuries among women in an urban area,. *N Engl J Med* 341:1899-1905, 1999.

14. Martin F, Younger-Lewis C: More than meets the eye: recognizing and responding to spousal abuse, *Can Med Assoc J* 157:1555-1558, 1997.

15. Rodriguez MA, Bauer HM, McLoughlin E, et al: Screening and intervention for intimate partner abuse: practices and attitudes of primary care physicians, *JAMA* 282:468-474, 1999.

16. Ferris LE, Norton P, Dunn EV, et al: Clinical factors affecting physicians' management decisions in cases of female partner abuse, *Fam Med* 31:415-425, 1999.

17. Lachs MS, Pillemer K: Abuse and neglect of elderly persons, *N Engl J Med* 332:437-443, 1995.

18. US Preventive Services Task Force: *Guide to clinical preventive services,* ed 2, Baltimore, 1996, Williams & Wilkins, pp 555-565.

19. Canadian Task Force on the Periodic Health Examination: *Canadian guide to clinical preventive health care,* Ottawa, 1994, Canada Communication Group—Publishing, pp 921-929.

20. Lodico MA, Gruber E, Diclemente RJ: Childhood sexual abuse and coercive sex among school-based adolescents in a Midwestern state, *J Adolesc Health* 18:211-217, 1996.

21. Halpérin DS, Bouvier P, Jaffé PD, et al: Prevalence of child sexual abuse among adolescents in Geneva: results of a cross sectional survey, *BMJ* 312:1326-1329, 1996.

22. Skuse D, Bentovim A, Hodges J, et al: Risk factors for development of sexually abusive behaviour in sexually victimised adolescent boys: cross sectional study, *BMJ* 317:175-179, 1998.

23. Holmes WC, Slap GB: Sexual abuse of boys: definition, prevalence, correlates, sequelae, and management, *JAMA* 280:1855-1862, 1998.

24. Adams JA, Knudson S: Genital findings in adolescent girls referred for suspected sexual abuse, *Arch Pediatr Adolesc Med* 150:850-857, 1996

AGGRESSION

(See also abuse; conduct disorder; guns; personality disorders; suicide)

On the basis of a literature search, the optimal drugs for short-term management of aggression seem to be high-potency antipsychotics or short-acting benzodiazepines. A variety of drugs have been used to treat chronic aggressive behavior. For adults without other psychiatric disorders lithium and propranolol (Inderal) are probably the first-line drugs.[1] Relatively high doses of propranolol also appear to be effective for pathological aggression in children.[2] Selective serotonin reuptake inhibitors (SSRIs)[3] and possibly divalproex sodium[4] help control aggression in patients with personality disorders.

◣ REFERENCES ◢

1. Pabis DJ, Stanislav SW: Pharmacotherapy of aggressive behavior, *Ann Pharmacother* 30:278-287, 1996.

2. Simeon JG: Propranolol in aggressive children and adolescents, *Child Adolesc Psychopharmacol News* 2:11-12, 1997.

3. Kavoussi R, Coccaro E: Psychopharmacologic treatment of hostility and aggressive disorders, *Psychiatr Clin North Am* 5:53-67, 1998.

4. Kavoussi RJ, Coccaro EF: Divalproex sodium for impulsive aggressive behavior in patients with personality disorder, *J Clin Psychiatry* 59:676-680, 1998.

ANXIETY DISORDERS

(See also alcohol; chest pain; depression; fibromyalgia; insomnia; motor vehicle accidents; palpitations; serotonin syndrome, Tourette's syndrome)

Classification

The following conditions are included under the rubric of anxiety disorders:

1. Generalized anxiety disorder
2. Panic disorder
3. Phobias (simple, social, agoraphobia)
4. Obsessive-compulsive disorder
5. Posttraumatic stress disorder

Nonpharmacological Therapy

Discontinuing or at least decreasing central nervous system stimulants and depressants such as caffeine, alcohol, and hypnotic drugs is an essential initial step in treatment of anxiety disorders.[1] For some, a regular aerobic exercise program is beneficial.[2] Psychotherapy, alone or in combination with pharmacotherapy, is an essential therapeutic strategy for all of the anxiety disorders.[3]

Medications

Benzodiazepines should not be used to treat anxiety disorders because they are addictive. The drugs of choice are antidepressants (tricyclics, selective serotonin reuptake inhibitors [SSRIs], and monoamine oxidase [MAO] inhibitors) and perhaps buspirone (Table 60). All are at least as effective as benzodiazepines.[1,3-7]

Imipramine (Tofranil) and other tricyclic antidepressants, including clomipramine (Anafranil), have been shown to be effective in panic disorders. Because initiation of treatment with this class of drugs is often associated with increased anxiety, the physician should start with low doses such as imipramine 10 mg/day and gradually increase the dose until

symptoms are controlled. For some patients a low dose is sufficient, whereas others may require the full therapeutic dose as used for depression. Clomipramine is the tricyclic of choice for obsessive-compulsive disorder. The dosage should not exceed 250 mg/day because of the risk for seizures.[3]

SSRIs are the pharmacological agents of choice for panic attacks, phobic disorders, obsessive-compulsive disorder, and posttraumatic stress disorder. In general, doses are low for phobic disorders and panic attacks and high for obsessive-compulsive disorder.[3] A metaanalysis of the pharmacotherapy of panic disorder found that not only were SSRIs more effective than placebo, but also they were more effective than imipramine (Tofranil) or alprazolam (Xanax).[4]

Although rarely used now, the MAO inhibitors phenelzine (Nardil) and tranylcypromine (Parnate) are effective in panic disorders and phobic disorders.[3]

Buspirone (Buspar) is a member of a class of antianxiety agents that is not sedative, has little potential for abuse, and is not associated with withdrawal symptoms. Its primary use is for generalized anxiety disorder.[3,6]

Beta-blockers are often useful for limited or focused social phobias (performance anxiety) such as may occur before making a speech, performing on a musical instrument, or taking an examination.[3,8,9] Positive results have been reported with single doses of atenolol (Tenormin) 100 mg, nadolol (Corgard) 40 mg, oxprenolol (Trasicor) 40 mg, and propranolol (Inderal) 40 mg.[8] Patients should take a test dose before any important performance to ensure that no unexpected adverse effects occur.[9]

Obsessive-Compulsive Disorder

The lifetime prevalence of obsessive-compulsive disorder is 2% to 3%. It is the fourth most common psychiatric disorder after substance abuse, phobias, and affective disorders. It has a higher prevalence rate than panic disorders or schizophrenia. Obsessive-compulsive disorder often begins in childhood, and onset over the age of 40 is rare. Slightly more females than males are affected.[10] The natural history of the untreated disorder is improvement in over 80% of cases. Even after several decades, however, only 20% of patients have made a complete recovery and 28% have "recovered" but continue to have symptoms that do not cause distress or interfere with daily activities.[11]

Cognitive-behavioral therapy is almost always an essential component of the treatment of obsessive-compulsive disorder, but medications also play an important role. Patients with obsessive-compulsive disorder are often slow to respond to medications and may require larger doses of antidepressants than are necessary for depression. Once they respond, they will probably require long-term or indefinite therapy because of the high relapse rate after discontinuation of medications.[3,10]

The tricyclic antidepressant clomipramine (Anafranil) has long been known to be effective in the treatment of

Table 60   Pharmacotherapy of Anxiety Disorders

Drugs	Usual doses and comments
Benzodiazepines	Addictive; lead to rebound anxiety as blood levels drop; antidepressants preferable
Alprazolam (Xanax)	0.125-0.25 mg tid or qid
Clonazepam (Rivotril)	0.5 mg bid or tid
Diazepam (Valium)	2-10 mg bid-qid
Lorazepam (Ativan)	2-3 mg/day in 3 divided doses
Azapirones	
Buspirone (Buspar)	20-30 mg/day in 2 or 3 divided doses
Tricyclics	
Imipramine (Tofranil)	Panic and phobic disorder (low doses)
Desipramine (Norpramin, Pertofrane)	Panic and phobic disorder (low doses)
Nortriptyline (Aventyl)	Panic and phobic disorder (low doses)
Clomipramine (Anafranil)	Obsessive-compulsive disorder (high doses)
Selective Serotonin Reuptake Inhibitors	Panic and phobic disorder (low doses); obsessive-compulsive disorder (high doses)
Citalopram (Celexa)	
Fluoxetine (Prozac)	
Fluvoxamine (Luvox)	
Paroxetine (Paxil)	
Sertraline (Zoloft)	
MAO Inhibitors	Panic and phobic disorders
Phenelzine (Nardil)	30 mg qam and 15-30 mg at noon
Tranylcypromine (Parnate)	20 mg qam and 10 mg in the afternoon
Azapirones	Generalized anxiety disorder
Buspirone (Buspar)	20-30 mg/day in two or three divided doses
Beta-Blockers	Focused social phobias (performance anxiety)
Atenolol (Tenormin)	Single dose; start low and increase prn
Nadolol (Corgard)	Single dose; start low and increase prn
Oxprenolol (Trasicor)	Single dose; start low and increase prn
Propranolol (Inderal)	Single dose; start low and increase prn

obsessive-compulsive disorder, but SSRIs are equally effective and generally better tolerated. High doses and prolonged treatment are usually required; initial response to the drug may not be evident for up to 3 months. If a patient fails to respond to one SSRI, another should be tried.[3] Clomipramine,[12] fluoxetine,[12] and sertraline[13] have been shown to be effective in children and adolescents with obsessive-compulsive disorder. The dosage range for fluoxetine in obsessive-compulsive disorder is 20 to 80 mg/day, for fluvoxamine is 100 to 300 mg/day, and for sertraline is 50 to 200 mg/day. It is advisable to start with a low dose and, for nonresponders, increase to the maximum dose over 6 to 8 weeks.[3]

Social Phobias

Social phobias are overwhelming irrational fears of being scrutinized or ridiculed by others.[7] Social phobias may be generalized or limited to specific events such as public speaking. Generalized social phobias are incapacitating because affected individuals fear being observed or evaluated by others in a wide range of circumstances. Phobic persons may avoid going to restaurants, have difficulty communicating with others at work or at school, withdraw from most social activities, and in more advanced cases drop out of school or the workforce.[7,14]

Social phobia is the third most common psychiatric condition in the United States, exceeded only by major depression and substance abuse.[7,14] The point prevalence of the disorder is 4.5%, but few of those affected are identified by primary care physicians.[14] Patients with generalized phobias do not voluntarily express their fears. To uncover the disease, the physician must ask specific questions about whether embarrassment or "fear of looking stupid" prevents socializing or other activities.[7] Social phobias almost always begin in adolescence, and onset after age 25 is rare. Comorbid psychiatric disorders such as major depression, dysthymia, panic disorder, obsessive-compulsive disorder, and alcohol and other substance abuse are extremely common.[7,14] Some phobic patients use alcohol or other drugs to alleviate their anxieties; 16% are alcoholics.[7]

Cognitive-behavioral therapy and medications control social phobias. Effective drugs are MAO inhibitors and SSRIs.[7,14] Paroxetine (Paxil)[14] and fluvoxamine (Luvox)[15] have been shown to be beneficial in multicenter randomized placebo-controlled trials. One small study found that when symptoms were controlled with daily fluoxetine (Prozac), remission could be maintained by once weekly doses because of the long-half life of the drug.[16] Tricyclics are not useful,[7] and benzodiazepines should not be used because of the high risk of addiction.[3,7,14]

Panic Disorder

Although benzodiazepines initially relieve symptoms, they are associated with a high incidence of withdrawal symptoms and relapse when discontinued. The drugs of choice for panic disorder are the SSRIs. If benzodiazepines have any role, it is only as very short-term bridge therapy until treatment with antidepressants is begun. Alternatives to the SSRIs are tricyclic antidepressants, MAO inhibitors, or in some cases valproate.[3]

Posttraumatic Stress Disorder

The widespread belief that the intensity and duration of trauma correlate with the frequency of subsequent posttraumatic stress disorder (PTSD) may be incorrect. Major stresses are common, and posttraumatic stress disorder is rare. More important, a dose-response curve cannot be shown. In many cases the trauma experienced by patients with posttraumatic stress disorder is much less severe than that faced by others who did not have psychiatric sequelae. The risk for posttraumatic stress disorder is determined predominantly by preexisting personality traits, especially the tendency to respond to events with negative emotions.[17]

Survivors of the terrorist bombing that destroyed the Alfred P. Murrah Federal Building in Oklahoma City in April 1995 almost all had at least some symptoms characteristic of posttraumatic stress disorder, most commonly difficulty concentrating, exaggerated startle response, intrusive memories, and insomnia. These symptoms alone do not fulfill the diagnostic criteria for posttraumatic stress disorder and were rarely associated with functional impairment or other psychiatric disorders. Such symptoms are probably best considered a normal reaction to extreme stress and can be managed by education, general support, and reassurance. One third of the victims of the Oklahoma City bombing were found to have posttraumatic stress disorder; major risk factors were previous psychiatric disorders, severity of injuries, loss of loved ones, female sex, and preexisting psychopathological conditions. The symptoms of posttraumatic stress disorder came on within hours of the bombing, and in two thirds of those affected other psychiatric disorders, usually depression, developed.[18] These findings are consistent with previous studies, which have found that most patients with posttraumatic stress disorder suffer from other Axis I psychiatric disorders, most often depression, another anxiety disorder, or substance abuse.[19]

Teams of professionals are frequently mobilized to rush to disaster scenes and debrief surviving victims and their families with the hope that this will prevent posttraumatic stress disorder. No well-designed controlled studies evaluating the efficacy of such an approach have been published.[17]

The natural history of posttraumatic stress disorder is one of spontaneous improvement in most instances, and this makes therapeutic interventions difficult to evaluate unless adequate control subjects are available. Psychotherapy in which patients relive their experiences is not helpful and in some studies has been found to be harmful. Behavioral therapy may be beneficial, but the most valuable type of therapy deals with predisposing negative character traits.[17] Few randomized trials of pharmacotherapy have been published. Results of open label trials (in which both patients and physicians are aware of the specific medications that are being taken) suggest that SSRIs, particularly fluvoxamine, decrease core symptoms such as numbing, avoidance, and hyperarousal, and some evidence suggests that clonidine (Catapres) ameliorates intrusive recollections, nightmares, hypervigilance, and outbursts of anger. Benzodiazepines decrease anxiety but have no beneficial effect on the core symptoms of posttraumatic stress disorder. Because comorbid substance abuse is common, they should rarely be prescribed.[19]

◣ REFERENCES ◢

1. Antony MM, Swinson RP: *Anxiety disorders and their treatment: a critical review of the evidence-based literature,* Ottawa, 1996, Publications Health Canada, pp 1-101.
2. Petruzello SJ, Landers DM, Hatfield BD, et al: A meta-analysis on the anxiety-reducing effects of acute and chronic exercise, *Sports Med* 11:143-182, 1991.
3. Layton ME, Dager SR: Treatment of anxiety disorders, *Psychiatr Clin North Am* 5:183-209, 1998.
4. Boyer W: Serotonin uptake inhibitors are superior to imipramine and alprazolam in alleviating panic attacks: a meta-analysis, *Int Clin Psychopharmacol* 10:45-49, 1995.
5. Piccinelli M, Pini S, Bellantuono C, et al: Efficacy of drug treatment in obsessive-compulsive disorder: a meta-analytic review, *Br J Psychol* 166:424-443, 1995.
6. Cadieux RJ: Azapirones: an alternative to benzodiazepines for anxiety, *Am Fam Physician* 53:2349-2353, 1996.
7. Bruce TJ, Saeed SA: Social anxiety disorder: a common, underrecognized mental disorder, *Am Fam Physician* 60:2311-2322, 1999.
8. Jefferson JW: Social phobia: everyone's disorder? *J Clin Psychiatry* 57(suppl 6):28-32, 1996.
9. Jefferson JW: Social phobia: a pharmacologic treatment overview, *J Clin Psychiatry* 56(suppl 5):18-24, 1995.
10. Warneke L: Anxiety disorders: focus on obsessive-compulsive disorder, *Can Fam Physician* 39:1612-1621, 1993.
11. Skoog G, Skoog I: A 40-year follow-up of patients with obsessive-compulsive disorder, *Arch Gen Psychiatry* 56:121-127, 1999.
12. Heyman I: Children with obsessive compulsive disorder should have access to specific psychopharmacological and behavioral treatments (editorial), *BMJ* 315:444, 1997.
13. March JS, Biederman J, Wolkow R: Sertraline in children and adolescents with obsessive-compulsive disorder: a multicenter randomized controlled trial, *JAMA* 280:1752-1756, 1998.
14. Stein MB, Liebowitz MR, Lydiard B, et al: Paroxetine treatment of generalized social phobia (social anxiety disorder): a randomized controlled trial, *JAMA* 280:708-713, 1998.
15. Stein MB, Fyer AJ, Davidson JR, et al: Fluvoxamine treatment of social phobia (social anxiety disorder): a double-blind, placebo-controlled study, *Am J Psychiatry* 156:756-760, 1999.
16. Emmanuel NP, Ware MR, Brawman-Mintzer O, et al: Once-weekly dosing of fluoxetine in the maintenance of remission in panic disorder, *J Clin Psychiatry* 60:299-301, 1999.
17. Bowman ML: Individual differences in posttraumatic distress: problems with the DSM-IV model, *Can J Psychiatry* 44:21-33, 1999.
18. North CS, Nixon SJ, Shariat S, et al: Psychiatric disorders among survivors of the Oklahoma City bombing, *JAMA* 282:755-762, 1999.
19. Friedman MJ: Current and future drug treatment for posttraumatic stress disorder patients, *Psychiatr Ann* 28:461-468, 1998.

CREATIVITY

Creative artists are popularly believed to be prone to psychopathology. To elucidate this issue, Post[1] read 350 biographies of world-famous creative people in an attempt to discern the presence or absence of psychiatric disorders. He found that personality deviations were increased among visual artists and writers. Alcoholism was common among writers, artists, and composers, and depression was frequent among writers. Scientists were, as a group, mentally stable. (And boring?)

◣ REFERENCES ◢

1. Post F: Creativity and psychopathology: a study of 291 world-famous men, *Br J Psychiatry* 165:22-34, 1994.

EATING DISORDERS
(See also diabetic retinopathy)

An Australian cohort study found that 8% of 15-year-old girls dieted at a "severe level" and 60% at a "moderate level." The risk for an eating disorder was increased 18-fold in severe-level dieters and 5-fold in moderate-level dieters compared with nondieters. An additional risk factor for eating disorders was a high level of psychiatric morbidity. The authors recommend exercise rather than dieting as the optimal strategy for weight control in adolescents.[1]

A school survey of thousands of Minnesota adolescents found that those with unhealthy weight loss behaviors as manifested by induced vomiting or the use of diet pills, laxatives, or diuretics had a higher incidence of other maladjusted behavior patterns such as suicide attempts, alcohol, tobacco, and drug use, unprotected sexual intercourse, and multiple sex partners.[2]

Women with type 1 diabetes have an increased incidence of bulimia and anorexia. Some women skip or reduce insulin doses in an attempt to lose weight.[3] Patients with type 1 diabetes who have eating disorders are at increased risk of retinopathy (see discussion of diabetic retinopathy).

◣ REFERENCES ◢

1. Patton GC, Selzer R, Carlin JB, et al: Onset of adolescent eating disorders: population based cohort study over 3 years, *BMJ* 318:765-768, 1999.
2. Neumark-Sztainer D, Story M, French SA: Covariations of unhealthy weight loss behaviors and other high-risk behaviors among adolescents, *Arch Pediatr Adolesc Med* 150:304-308, 1996.
3. Jacobson AM: The psychological care of patients with insulin-dependent diabetes mellitus, *N Engl J Med* 334:1249-1253, 1996.

Anorexia Nervosa

(See also Addison's disease; amenorrhea; bulimia; euthyroid sick syndrome; female athletes)

Four major criteria must be met to make the diagnosis of anorexia nervosa: weight loss, intense fear of gaining weight, disturbance in body image, and amenorrhea.[1,2]

Epidemiology

Anorexia nervosa can be fatal. Crude mortality rates as high as 18% after 30 years have been reported.[1] Suicide accounts for a high proportion of the excess mortality.[2] The ratio of women to men with anorexia nervosa is 10:1 to 20:1. Anorexia is rare in prepubertal children, particularly in boys. Tumors affecting the hypothalamus or brainstem may be the cause of an anorexia-like symptom complex, and sometimes repeated neuroradiological examinations are necessary to detect them.[3]

Negative self-evaluation and perfectionism are character traits predisposing to anorexia nervosa, but unlike patients with bulimia nervosa, those with anorexia are not more likely to have been exposed to dieting by other family members or to have heard negative comments about their eating habits.[4] Patients with eating disorders have an increased incidence of mood, anxiety, and personality disorders.[2]

Physical findings

Physical findings in advanced anorexia are those of starvation: emaciation, bradycardia, hypotension, hypothermia, atrophy of breasts, dry skin, yellow palms and soles from hypercarotenemia, and lanugo hair.[2]

Investigations

Routine laboratory investigations for patients with anorexia nervosa should include a complete blood cell count (increased incidence of anemia, leukopenia, and thrombocytopenia) and measurements of electrolytes (hyponatremia is common, but in the absence of vomiting, laxative, or diuretic abuse hypokalemia is rare), fasting glucose level (hypoglycemia is common but usually asymptomatic), and bone density (50% of patients have a bone density that is more than 2 standard deviations below normal). Patients with anorexia nervosa may manifest the euthyroid sick syndrome, and a prolonged QT interval is often seen on the electrocardiogram.[2] "Routine" tests performed in an emergency room may produce entirely normal results even though the patient is in imminent danger of death from a cardiac arrhythmia.

Management

Hospitalization and controlled refeeding are essential for critically ill patients.[1,2] Most individuals whose weight is 75% or less of expected body weight fit in this category.[2] The major therapeutic modality for long-term management is cognitive-behavioral psychotherapy.[1] A randomized trial found that both behavioral family system therapy and ego-oriented individual therapy (plus collateral sessions with the parents) were effective but that more rapid improvement occurred with the behavioral family therapy.[5] Many patients have symptoms of depression, but this is often a direct result of starvation and symptoms usually resolve as weight returns toward normal.[1] Although antidepressants are ineffective for anorexia, they may be useful for associated depression or anxiety disorders or perhaps for preventing relapses, but only when the weight has increased to about 75% of normal.[1,2]

The prevention of osteoporosis is another important goal of therapy—amenorrheic women must regain sufficient weight to permit functioning of the hypothalamic-pituitary-ovarian axis. In one study menses returned within 6 months in most women whose body weight had returned to at least 90% of "standard body weight" charts. The actual weight for return of menses was 2 kg (4.4 lb) more than the weight at which menses ceased. Rise of serum estradiol to levels of 110 pmol/L (30 pg/mL) showed a good correlation with return of menses. Other indicators of improvement are an increase in ovarian size or the presence of a dominant ovarian follicle on ultrasonography.[6] Estrogen replacement therapy has been prescribed to ameliorate bone loss in anorectic women, but its efficacy for this purpose has not been established. Whether bisphosphonates have value is unknown. Expert opinion is that all patients should receive daily calcium supplements of 1000 to 1500 mg plus a multivitamin containing 400 IU of vitamin D.[2]

Prognosis

Predictors of a poor outcome for anorexia nervosa are age at onset over 18 years, vomiting, laxative abuse, alcohol or substance abuse, and numerous hospitalizations. After 10 years about one fourth of patients have recovered, one fourth are bulimic, one third are functioning reasonably well, and one tenth are still anorectic.[1]

─────────────── ◥ REFERENCES ◢ ───────────────

1. Halmi KA: A 24-year-old woman with anorexia nervosa, *JAMA* 279:1992-1998, 1998.
2. Becker AE, Grinspoon SK, Klibanski A, et al: Eating disorders, *N Engl J Med* 340:1092-1098, 1999.
3. DeVile CJ, Sufraz R, Lask BD, et al: Occult intracranial tumours masquerading as early onset anorexia nervosa, *BMJ* 311:1359-1360, 1995.
4. Fairburn CG, Cooper Z, Doll HA, et al: Risk factors for anorexia nervosa: three integrated case-control comparisons, *Arch Gen Psychiatry* 56:468-476, 1999.
5. Robin AL, Siegel PT, Moye AW, et al: A controlled comparison of family versus individual therapy for adolescents with anorexia nervosa, *J Am Acad Child Adolesc Psychiatry* 38:1482-1489, 1999.
6. Golden NH, Jacobson MS, Schebendach J, et al: Resumption of menses in anorexia nervosa, *Arch Pediatr Adolesc Med* 151:16-21, 1997.

Bulimia
(See also anorexia nervosa)

Bulimia nervosa affects between 1% and 3% of adolescent and young adult females. The course is chronic with remissions and exacerbations. Patients commonly have comorbid psychiatric conditions, particularly affective disorders, personality disorders, and substance abuse.[1] Bulimic individuals are more likely than nonbulimic women and children to have had mothers who were obese during their childhood, to have been exposed to family members who were dieting, and to have been the object of negative remarks about their eating habits, appearance, or weight.[2]

Characteristic physical findings in bulimia include the following[1]:

1. Parotid swelling ("chipmunk cheeks") seen in about 25% of patients
2. Calluses or red marks on the backs of the hands as a result of trauma from teeth during induced vomiting
3. Damaged teeth from acid erosion of enamel; this usually involves the occlusal surfaces of the molars and the lingual surfaces of the other teeth

A number of laboratory tests may be abnormal in patients with bulimia. About 50% have an elevated amylase level. Other common abnormalities reflect a hypokalemic hypochloremic alkalosis induced by vomiting: a urine pH greater than 8 (25% of cases), decreased potassium and chloride levels, and an increased bicarbonate level. The sodium concentration is usually normal. Electrolyte abnormalities may persist for 2 to 7 days after the last binge.

The natural history of bulimia has not been well defined. According to one review of 88 studies in which follow-up took place, about half of bulimic women had fully recovered by 5 to 10 years, 20% still met the criteria for bulimia, and the remainder experienced relapses. Relapses were most common in the first 4 years after diagnosis.[3] Women with substance abuse problems have a lower rate of recovery.[4]

If a bulimic patient also has a substance disorder, the substance disorder has to be treated before bulimia can be effectively managed. Proven options for the treatment of bulimia are antidepressants, cognitive-behavioral therapy, or a combination of the two. Antidepressants that have been shown to be more effective than placebos include the tricyclics (desipramine [Norpramin, Pertofrane] 150 to 300 mg/day, imipramine [Tofranil] 175 to 300 mg/day), the MAO inhibitor phenelzine (Nardil) 60 to 80 mg/day, and fluoxetine (Prozac) 20 to 60 mg/day. In studies of fluoxetine the best results were reported with 60 mg/day. Cognitive-behavioral therapy alone seems to be better than medications alone, but best results are obtained with a combination of cognitive-behavioral therapy and medications.[1]

─────────────── ❧ **REFERENCES** ❧ ───────────────

1. McGilley BM, Pryor TL: Assessment and treatment of bulimia nervosa, *Am Fam Physician* 57:2743-2750, 1998.

2. Fairburn CG, Cooper Z, Doll HA, et al: Risk factors for anorexia nervosa: three integrated case-control comparisons, *Arch Gen Psychiatry* 56:468-476, 1999.

3. Keel PK, Mitchell JE: Outcome in bulimia nervosa, *Am J Psychiatry* 154:313-321, 1997.

4. Keel PK, Mitchell JE, Miller KB, et al: Long-term outcome of bulimia nervosa, *Arch Gen Psychiatry* 56:63-69, 1999.

FALSE MEMORIES
(See also abuse)

Whether repressed memories of childhood sexual abuse exist and can be recovered through psychotherapy is an emotionally heated issue. Supporting the existence of repressed memories is a study by Williams[1] of 129 women with previously documented histories of sexual abuse in childhood; 38% did not recall the abuse that had occurred more than 17 years previously. The younger they were at the time of abuse, the less likely they were to remember. This and other studies of a similar nature have been criticized by Pope[2] on the grounds that the patients were not directly asked about the alleged events and therefore may have chosen not to disclose them. He and his associates found that in all studies where patients were directly asked about the traumatic incidents, they reported remembering them. Penfold[3] concluded that both true and fabricated memories may be recovered. Frankel[4] found little evidence supporting the validity of recovered memories of abuse but did not rule them out in all cases. The British Royal College of Psychiatrists strongly opposes techniques that use suggestion or persuasion to unearth hidden memories and encourages therapists to express any doubts they may have about the historical accuracy of reputed recovered memories.[5] A more radical view is that of Ofshe and Watters,[6] who consider the recovery of false memories to be pseudoscience that causes a great deal of harm to patients and their families.

Closely related to the issue of recovered memories and childhood sexual abuse is the question of multiple personality disorders, which is called dissociative identity disorder in *DSM IV*. This is because those who believe in multiple personalities think that childhood sexual abuse is a common basis for them. According to Merskey,[7] the number of diagnosed cases has increased remarkably in recent years and this is because a few psychiatrists are making large numbers of such diagnoses. In his view a large number of cases probably are iatrogenically produced.[8]

─────────────── ❧ **REFERENCES** ❧ ───────────────

1. Williams SM: Recall of childhood trauma: a prospective study of women's memories of child sexual abuse, *J Consult Clin Psychol* 62:1167-1176, 1994.

2. Pope HG Jr: Recovered memories of childhood sexual abuse (editorial), *BMJ* 316:488-489, 1998.

3. Penfold PS: The repressed memory controversy: is there middle ground? *Can Med Assoc J* 155:647-653, 1996.

4. Frankel FH: Discovering new memories in psychotherapy—childhood revisited, fantasy, or both? *N Engl J Med* 333:591-594, 1995.

5. Royal College of Psychiatrists: Reported recovered memories of child sexual abuse: recommendations for good practice and implications for training, continuing professional development and research, *Psychiatr Bull* 21:663-665, 1997.

6. Ofshe R, Watters E: *Making monsters: false memories, psychotherapy, and sexual hysteria,* New York, 1994, Scribner's.

7. Merskey H: Multiple personality disorder and false memory syndrome, *Br J Psychiatry* 166:281-283, 1995.

8. Merskey H: The manufacture of personalities: the production of multiple personality disorder, *Br J Psychiatry* 160:327-340, 1992.

FUNCTIONAL SOMATIC SYNDROMES

(See also chronic fatigue syndrome; fibromyalgia; hypoglycemia; irritable bowel syndrome; Lyme disease; multiple chemical sensitivities; silicone breast implants; whiplash)

Barsky[1] has lumped together a group of syndromes that are characterized by symptoms of suffering and disability but that do not fit into the categories of specific psychiatric or organic diseases:

1. Chronic fatigue syndrome
2. Fibromyalgia
3. Multiple chemical sensitivities
4. Irritable bowel syndrome
5. Hypoglycemia
6. Candidiasis hypersensitivity
7. Gulf War syndrome
8. Sick building syndrome
9. Systemic reactions to silicone breast implants
10. Repetition stress injury
11. Chronic whiplash
12. Chronic Lyme disease
13. Certain food allergies

Symptoms of all these disorders tend to be diffuse and nonspecific, and overlap of symptoms among the disorders is common. Identical symptoms are prevalent in healthy populations, but they are often not brought to medical attention, or if they are, they are rapidly resolved with reassurance.[1]

Typical symptoms of functional somatic syndromes are fatigue, insomnia, weakness, headaches, muscle aches, joint pains, nausea and other gastrointestinal complaints, palpitations, shortness of breath, dizziness or lightheadedness, sore throat, dry mouth, decreased concentration, poor memory, irritability, depression, and anxiety. With such a rich choice of complaints many physicians concentrate on those with which they are most familiar; if patients consult a rheumatologist, the diagnosis is likely to be fibromyalgia, whereas if they consult a gastroenterologist, it is likely to be irritable bowel syndrome.[1]

Specific psychiatric diagnoses, particularly depression, anxiety disorders, and somatoform disorder, are more common in patients with functional somatic syndromes than in the general population.[1]

A striking characteristic of functional somatic syndromes is the patients' lack of response to reassurance from negative medical examinations and from explanations of the role of stress in producing body discomfort. Possible explanations are a decreasing trust in science in general and physicians in particular, sensational and alarmist reports in the mass media, litigation and disability issues, and the growing presence of advocacy groups together with clinics and physicians "specializing" in these disorders.[1]

Barsky[1] suggests that functional somatic syndromes originate from the many somatic complaints that are normal experiences of healthy people. A process of amplification perpetuates and aggravates the symptoms in some persons, leading to the development of a "disorder." Prospective patients learn by word of mouth or from the media about a "disease" that would fit their symptoms. They find out about its other manifestations and realize that they are suffering from them as well: "The suspicion of disease heightens bodily awareness, symptom perception, and distress, and these in turn, reinforce the belief that the sufferer is sick."[1]

Management is difficult. The following steps are suggested[1]:

1. Assessment to rule out organic disease (without over-investigation)
2. Assessment for specific psychiatric disorders
3. Establishment of a therapeutic alliance with patient
4. Establishment of restoration of function as the goal of treatment
5. Limited reassurance
6. Referral for cognitive-behavioral therapy if the first five steps are unsuccessful

Comorbid psychiatric conditions such as depression may require antidepressants.[1]

——————— ⚑ REFERENCES ⚑ ———————

1. Barsky AJ, Borus JF: Functional somatic syndromes, *Ann Intern Med* 130:910-921, 1999.

MOOD DISORDERS
Bipolar Affective Disorder

(See also depression; hypothyroidism; seizures; serotonin syndrome; subclinical hypothyroidism)

About half of all patients with bipolar disorder have a parent with an affective disorder. About one fourth of the children who have one parent with a bipolar disorder have an affective disorder.[1]

First symptoms of bipolar disorder usually occur between the ages of 15 and 19, but a 3- to 10-year lag time between the onset of symptoms and treatment is common.[2] Inadequately treated patients may have more than 10 episodes of biphasic mood dysregulation during their lifetime, and episodes can become more frequent as the patient ages.[3]

A diagnosis of bipolar I disorder requires the patient to have had at least one full-blown manic episode; there may or may not have been a depressive episode. The diagnosis of bipolar II disorder can be made if the patient has had one or more major depressions, as well as one or more hypomanic episodes, provided that no true manic attacks have occurred.[4] The diagnosis of hypomania is difficult and in many cases is made only in retrospect.[5]

Management

Recent evidence suggests that either lithium or valproate may be the drug of first choice for classic mania or hypomania with euphoric mood, that lithium, valproate, or carbamazepine may be used for mixed episodes or dysphoric mood, and that for mania with rapid cycling, either valproate or carbamazepine is the drug of first choice.[6] Patients with bipolar depression should receive antidepressants only if they are already taking lithium, valproate, or carbamazepine.[7]

Few studies have examined the efficacy of psychosocial interventions in bipolar disorder, and the information available is mostly narrative or suffers from variable methodological quality. Only psychoeducation, cognitive therapy, and brief inpatient family therapy interventions have been supported by small randomized control trials. These interventions have been helpful in the depressed phase of illness, not the manic phase.[8] Given the nature of bipolar illness, basic psychoeducation for the patient and family provides significant opportunity to both manage and reduce stigmatization of persons with this chronic disease.

Prodromal symptoms of relapse. Relapse rates of 50% at 1 year and 70% at 5 years after an initial manic episode have been reported. A randomized controlled trial found that bipolar patients who were instructed to identify the specific life situations and prodromal symptoms that preceded their manic or depressive relapses were able to seek earlier treatment than control subjects who received the usual care. Early treatment resulted in fewer manic episodes but had no effect on frequency of depressive episodes.[9]

Lithium. Lithium is classically used for bipolar disorders. It is effective in controlling acute mania, but a delay of 1 to 2 weeks is usual before any amelioration of symptoms and substantial improvement is commonly not evident for 3 to 4 weeks. In practice, neuroleptics or benzodiazepines are usually added to the lithium to control the agitation and excessive activity of acute mania. The usual dosage of lithium is 1200 to 1800 mg/day in acute mania and 900 to 1500 mg/day for maintenance therapy. In the beginning lithium is given twice or three times a day to minimize the adverse effects of nausea and tremor, but as soon as possible only a single daily dose should be given at bedtime. Aside from convenience, a single dose is thought to decrease the risk of renal damage. Lithium is useful in cyclothymic disorder and as a potentiating agent for tricyclic or SSRI antidepressants in cases of refractory depression.[10]

The most common adverse effect of lithium is hand tremor, which occurs in one fourth to one half of patients.[10]

This can be minimized by lowering the dose or by adding a beta-blocker.[7] Other side effects are leukocytosis, hypothyroidism, subclinical hypothyroidism, acne, and polyuria because of reduced urinary concentrating ability.[7,10] An estimated one fourth to one half of patients taking lithium for bipolar disease discontinue the drug, usually because of adverse effects.[11] Patients taking lithium should be warned to drink plenty of fluids in hot weather.[10] Diuretics should be avoided. Concomitant use of nonsteroidal antiinflammatory agents may lead to lithium toxicity.[12]

Before lithium therapy commences, recommended laboratory investigations are a complete blood cell count, urinalysis, electrocardiography if the patient is over age 50, and measurement of TSH, BUN, creatinine, and electrolytes.[10]

During the initiation of therapy, lithium levels should be assessed every 5 to 7 days, as well as 5 to 7 days after any change in dosage. During maintenance therapy lithium levels should be checked every 1 to 2 months in the early period and every 6 to 12 months once the patient's condition is stable while receiving the drug. Lithium levels should be measured 10 to 12 hours after the last lithium dose. The therapeutic range for maintenance therapy is 0.6 to 1 mmol/L (0.6 to 1 mEq/L), whereas for acute mania the aim is 0.8 to 1.4 mmol/L (0.8 to 1.4 mEq/L). Toxic levels are 1.2 mmol/L (1.2 mEq/L) or greater. TSH and creatinine levels should be checked annually.[10]

Anticonvulsants. Carbamazepine (Tegretol) and valproic acid (Depakene) or divalproex (Depakote, Epival) are effective for mania.[1,7,11] Adverse effects include nausea, weight gain, diarrhea, and tremor; the last can be treated with beta-blockers.[7] Carbamazepine and lithium seem to be less useful for rapid cycling, whereas divalproex is more effective for this clinical scenario. Patients treated with any of these drugs should have regular monitoring of serum levels, which should be maintained at the same level as for seizure control (see discussion of seizures). Lamotrigine (Lamictal) in doses of 200 mg/day has been shown to be effective monotherapy for the depressive phase of bipolar 1 disorders, and it did not increase the risk of rapid cycling or mania.[13] Topiramate (Topamax) 100 to 400 mg/day in 2 divided doses is also beginning to show promise and has the added advantage of weight loss as a side effect.

Atypical antipsychotics. Atypical antipsychotic agents (e.g., olanzapine, risperidone, quetiapine, clozapine) may be effective treatments for bipolar disorder, especially as adjunctive treatments for acute mania. However, currently available research studies have had mainly open label (both patients and physicians are aware of the specific medications that are being taken), uncontrolled designs, and further research is necessary before the definitive efficacy of these agents in bipolar disorder is established.[14]

Electroconvulsive therapy. Patients whose disorder is refractory to standard therapy and those who are rapidly cycling often respond to ECT.[15]

◢ REFERENCES ◣

1. Werder SF: An update on the diagnosis and treatment of mania in bipolar disorder, *Am Fam Physician* 51:1126-1136, 1995.

2. Yatham LN, Kusumakar V, Parikh SV, et al: Bipolar depression: treatment options, *Can J Psychiatry* 42(suppl 2):87S-91S, 1997.

3. Goldberg JF, Harrow M, Grossman LS: Recurrent affective syndromes in bipolar and unipolar mood disorders at follow-up, *Br J Psychiatry* 166:382-385, 1995.

4. American Psychiatric Association: *Diagnostic and statistical manual of mental disorders,* ed 4, Washington, DC, 1994, American Psychiatric Association, pp 350-358.

5. Cassano GB, Dell'Osso L, Frank E, et al: The bipolar spectrum: a clinical reality in search of diagnostic criteria and an assessment methodology, *J Affect Disord* 54:319-328, 1999.

6. Francis A, Docherty JP, Kahn DA: The expert consensus guideline series: treatment of bipolar disorder, *J Clin Psychiatry* 57(suppl 12A):1-89, 1996.

7. Drugs for psychiatric disorders, *Med Lett* 39:33-40, 1997.

8. Parikh SV, Kusumakar V, Haslam RS, et al: Psychosocial intervention as an adjunct to pharmacotherapy in bipolar disorder, *Can J Psychiatry* 42(suppl 2):74S-78S, 1997.

9. Perry A, Tarrier N, Morriss R, et al: Randomised controlled trial of efficacy of teaching patients with bipolar disorder to identify early symptoms of relapse and obtain treatment, *BMJ* 318:149-153, 1999.

10. Price LH, Heninger GR: Lithium in the treatment of mood disorders, *N Engl J Med* 331:591-598, 1994.

11. Joffe RT: Valproate in bipolar disorder: the Canadian perspective, *Can J Psychiatry* 38(3 suppl 2):S46-S50, 1993.

12. Ragheb M: The clinical significance of lithium–nonsteroidal antiinflammatory drug interactions, *J Clin Psychopharmacol* 10:350-354, 1990.

13. Calabrese JR, Bowden CL, Sachs GS, et al: A double-blind placebo-controlled study of lamotrigine monotherapy in outpatients with bipolar I depression, *J Clin Psychiatry* 60:79-88, 1999.

14. Ghaemi SN, Goodwin FK: Use of atypical antipsychotic agents in bipolar and schizoaffective disorders: review of the empirical literature, *J Clin Psychopharmacol* 19:354-361, 1999.

15. Mukerjee S, Sacheim HA, Schnur DB: Electroconvulsive therapy of acute manic episodes: a review of 50 years experience, *Am J Psychiatry* 151:169-176, 1994.

Depression

(See also alternative medicine; anxiety disorders; bipolar affective disorder; chest pain; cocaine; fibromyalgia; guns; insomnia; premenstrual dysphoric disorder; serotonin syndrome; sexual abuse; sexual dysfunction)

Epidemiology

A community survey of depression in several different countries using *DSM III* criteria found striking variations in prevalence rates. The highest incidence was in Beirut and Paris and the lowest in Taiwan and Korea. Common to most countries were an association with substance abuse and anxiety disorders, a higher rate in females than in males, and higher rates in divorced or separated individuals compared with married individuals. This survey found little variation in the prevalence of bipolar disorder.[1]

The incidence of smoking is much higher among individuals who have ever been depressed compared with those who have not, and the success rate in quitting among smokers who have ever been depressed is much lower than among those who have never been depressed.[2]

A prospective case-control study from New York found that two thirds of adolescents in whom a major depression had been diagnosed had at least one recurrent episode of depression within the next 10 to 15 years, compared with one third of nondepressed adolescents.[3]

Unexplained medical symptoms and frequent medical visits

Primary care physicians commonly see depression manifested as physical symptoms, especially when anxiety is also present. One recent trial in a health maintenance organization in the United States screened 7203 patients who heavily used medical care for depression; 20% were found to have a current major depression or major depression in partial remission. In a year these depressed patients had significantly higher numbers of office visits and days in the hospital than did patients without depression.[4] An international study has also confirmed the relationship between somatic symptoms and depression.[5]

A challenge for family physicians is to convert patients to the idea that physical symptoms may have a mental source. One useful practice pearl is to tell patients at the beginning of a medical workup that up to one third of problems seen in family medicine are caused by mental health disorders (a good example is a tension headache or "butterflies") but that the physician will begin by ruling out important physical causes. This gets the possibility of a mental health issue on the table early rather than backing into it. Another approach is to devote one clinical visit to a walk-through diagnostic aid (e.g., the Hamilton Depression Rating Scale). Having an objective score may make the diagnosis more meaningful to patients, as well as further delineate their condition.

Suicide

Although the highest suicide rate is found among men over the age of 69,[6] the incidence of suicide among the young has been increasing in the Western world. This is particularly marked among aboriginal peoples.[7] The availability of guns appears to increase the risk of suicide (see discussion of guns). Over 90% of people who commit suicide have a diagnosable psychiatric illness; depression and alcoholism head the list, but bipolar affective disorder and schizophrenia are also common.[6] Systematic reviews have not found evidence that suicide prevention interventions for ambulatory patients are effective.[8] However, a recent comprehensive program mounted by the U.S. Air Force, involving multiple agencies (mental health, family support centers, child and youth development, health and wellness centers, chaplains, and family advocacy) and a wide spectrum of military personnel, including military leaders, supervisors, attorneys, and health professionals, dramatically decreased the suicide rate of air force personnel.[9]

Psychotherapy

A 1997 metaanalysis concluded that interpersonal psychotherapy (therapy dealing with the relationships between the patient and significant others) or cognitive-behavioral psychotherapy is as effective as antidepressants for the treatment of mild depression. This was not the case for more severe recurrent depressions, in which a combination of psychotherapy and antidepressants was more effective than psychotherapy alone.[10] However, a 1999 metaanalysis using original data (megaanalysis) from four studies comparing medications against cognitive-behavioral therapy for severely depressed outpatients found that cognitive-behavioral therapy was as effective as medications.[11] This is an exciting and provocative study, but family physicians should be aware that in most of the trials cognitive-behavioral therapy was given by skilled and highly trained therapists and therefore questions remain about replicability of this approach in the family medicine setting.

Cognitive-behavioral therapy is aimed at changing the way a person thinks and behaves, especially changing self-defeating thinking styles and behavior patterns. It usually involves a fixed number of sessions and in this respect is appropriate for the family medicine setting. "Cognitive" refers to negative thinking and associated feelings, which take place at an automatic level (e.g., "I'm worthless"; "I'm fat"; "I can't do this"). "Behavior" is self-explanatory and is based on the negative beliefs. Unlike traditional psychoanalysis, cognitive-behavioral therapy is "here and now" therapy in which past issues are reviewed only to clarify a patient's present observations and attitudes. Although standard practice for treating recurrent depression involves long-term antidepressant therapy (see below), a preliminary study suggests that cognitive-behavioral therapy dealing not only with residual symptoms such as anxiety and irritability, but also with maladaptive life-styles (interpersonal friction, excessive work, inadequate sleep) and a sense of inadequate well-being, may be an effective alternative to medications in reducing the risk of relapses.[12] Interpersonal psychotherapy has also proved effective for depression.[13]

Antidepressants

At present most physicians choose SSRIs as first-line antidepressants. This is not because they are more effective than tricyclics (they are not), but because they have fewer adverse effects and therefore patient compliance should be better. Furthermore, they are less toxic when taken as an overdose.[14,15]

A major problem with antidepressants is that beneficial effects are rarely seen before 2 to 4 weeks has elapsed, a situation that is aggravated by some of the SSRIs that cause stimulation and insomnia. Because of this some clinicians add a long-acting benzodiazepine to SSRIs during the first few weeks of treatment, especially if anxiety is a major component of the depression. A double-blind randomized trial of patients with moderate to severe depression found that those treated with fluoxetine (Prozac) 20 to 40 mg/day plus clonazepam (Rivotril) 0.5 to 1 mg at bedtime had marked improvement in the Hamilton Depression Rating Scale during the first 3 weeks of treatment compared with those who received fluoxetine plus placebo. The clonazepam was tapered and discontinued between the third and fourth weeks, and this was associated with a temporary worsening of symptoms.[16] Although benzodiazepines are helpful for many patients at the initiation of SSRIs, prescribing them for anyone with a current or past history of alcohol or other substance abuse would be foolish. Perhaps the most important way to improve compliance is to tell patients that they might feel worse before they feel better. This prepares them for the reality that they may have the side effects but obtain little relief for the first 2 to 4 weeks. An effort should be made to customize therapy for the patient, as by scheduling sedative medications at bedtime, having the patient take nausea-inducing medications with meals, and starting at a lower dose if anxiety is a prominent symptom.

Early discontinuation of antidepressants has been shown to increase the risk of relapse.[17] Three major factors predicting length of therapy are recurrence (number of episodes), severity, and duration. First episodes of depression have a 50% risk of recurrence, second episodes a 70% risk, and third episodes a 90% risk.[18] For a mild first episode of short duration, 6 months of antidepressants is generally recommended. For a longer or more severe first episode, medications should be continued for at least 12 months. For patients with recurrent depression antidepressants should be continued for many years or for life. Current evidence suggests that full therapeutic doses should be used for maintenance therapy.[14]

Drug interactions with antidepressants, particularly those that involve inhibition of one or more of the 30 or so isoenzymes of the cytochrome P450 system, are a major concern. Many antipsychotics and antidepressants, including most of the SSRIs, have this effect, which could result in toxic elevations of the blood levels of concurrently taken medications. The combination of some of the SSRIs with tricyclics (resulting in toxic levels of tricyclics) is particularly notable, but this situation also occurs when certain SSRIs are combined with certain antipsychotics or benzodiazepines, carbamazepine (Tegretol), theophylline, terfenadine (Seldane), and astemizole (Hismanal), among other medications.[19]

Withdrawal or discontinuation reactions are common when antidepressants are stopped. A variety of symptoms have been described, including nausea, diarrhea and abdominal pain, dizziness, paresthesias, sleep disturbances, and mood changes. These symptoms should not be assumed to reflect recurrence of the original psychiatric disorder. Discontinuation reactions occur within days of discontinuing the drug and resolve rapidly, whereas recurrence of depression is usually seen only after a few weeks has elapsed. When antidepressants are discontinued, slow tapering over 4 weeks has been recommended; this may not be necessary when switching from one SSRI to another.[20]

Tricyclics and related antidepressants. In most cases tricyclics are no longer the first therapeutic choice for depression (see discussion of antidepressants). Exceptions are made if the patient has previously been successfully treated with a drug from this class and did not suffer significant adverse reactions or if cost is an important consideration. Patients suffering from neuropathic pain as well as depression often benefit from tricyclic agents.[21] For the elderly, low-dose desipramine (Norpramin, Pertofrane) or nortriptyline (Aventyl) is a good choice[22] because they have fewer anticholinergic effects and are less sedating than most other tricyclics.[15] Some of the more frequently used tricyclics are listed in Table 61.

If tricyclics are used for young or middle-aged adult outpatients, the starting dose is usually 25 or 50 mg/day. It is increased by 25 mg every 3 to 5 days until a therapeutic level of 150 mg is reached. The exceptions are protriptyline (Triptil), which has a therapeutic dose range of 30 to 60 mg/day (it is three times as potent as amitriptyline), and nortriptyline (Aventyl), for which the usual therapeutic dose is 75 to 100 mg/day (it is twice as potent as amitriptyline). Tricyclic antidepressants can usually be given as a single daily dose, most commonly at bedtime. If side effects are distressing, divided doses can be tried. Some patients find that

desipramine and protriptyline cause insomnia if given at bedtime. Doses are usually much lower for elderly patients.

Important adverse effects include urinary retention and, rarely, fatal arrhythmias. Because of the latter, use of the tricyclics should be avoided for patients with heart disease.[15] In children and adolescents tricyclics should be avoided or used with caution because they have caused sudden cardiac death in this age group. Weight gain is a common adverse effect; the worst offender is amitriptyline (Elavil), whereas the drug least likely to induce this effect is desipramine.[22] Like the SSRIs, tricyclics are associated with a fairly high incidence of sexual dysfunction, usually in the form of anorgasmia or ejaculatory delay.[23]

Amoxapine (Asendin) has both antipsychotic and antidepressant properties and may be useful in cases of psychotic depression.[24] Drugs closely related to the tricyclics are maprotiline (Ludiomil) and mirtazapine (Remeron), which are tetracyclics, and trazodone (Desyrel), which is a modified cyclic. Trazodone is sedative and has been used successfully in doses of 100 mg at bedtime as a hypnotic in depressed patients who had persistent, exacerbated, or new-onset insomnia when being treated with fluoxetine or bupropion.[25] Priapism is a rare complication of trazodone therapy.

Tricyclics have been used for a number of conditions other than depression, including insomnia, chronic pain, enuresis, urinary incontinence, panic disorder, phobic disorder, obsessive-compulsive disorder, premature ejaculation, and snoring. These issues are discussed elsewhere in the text.

Specific serotonin reuptake inhibitors. At present SSRIs are probably the drugs of first choice for treatment of depression (Table 62). They have fewer reported adverse effects than tricyclics, and patients are more likely to continue taking SSRIs or to reach full therapeutic levels than are those taking tricyclics. However, when outcomes were measured at 6 months, no difference was found between patients taking fluoxetine (Prozac) and those taking either desipramine (Norpramin, Pertofrane) or imipramine (Tofranil). Although SSRIs have been shown to be effective in the elderly, some studies have found tricyclics to be slightly superior.[26]

In addition to their use in depression, SSRIs are effective for anxiety disorders, including panic disorder, phobic disorder, and obsessive-compulsive disorder, and in bulimia. Nausea is an important adverse effect that can be mitigated by giving the drug with meals.

Table 61   Tricyclics and Related Antidepressants

Drugs	Usual doses
Tricyclics	
Amitriptyline (Elavil)	150 mg qhs
Amoxapine (Asendin)	150 mg qhs; has antipsychotic properties
Clomipramine (Anafranil)	50-250 mg/day
Desipramine (Norpramin, Pertofrane)	150 mg qhs; half of this for elderly
Doxepin (Sinequan)	150 mg qhs
Imipramine (Tofranil)	150 mg qhs
Nortriptyline (Aventyl)	75-100 mg/day; half of this for elderly
Protriptyline (Triptil)	15-30 mg/day
Trimipramine (Surmontil)	150 mg qhs
Tetracyclic Derivatives	
Maprotiline (Ludiomil)	150 mg qhs
Mirtazapine (Remeron)	15-45 mg qhs
Modified Cyclic Derivatives	
Trazodone (Desyrel)	150-300 mg qhs

Table 62   Selective Serotonin Reuptake Inhibitors for Depression

Drugs	Usual doses
Citalopram (Celexa)	20-40 mg/day qam or qpm
Fluoxetine (Prozac)	20-60 mg/day qam
Fluvoxamine (Luvox)	50-150 mg/day qhs
Paroxetine (Paxil)	20 mg/day qam
Sertraline (Zoloft)	50-200 mg/day with evening meal

Sexual dysfunction is an adverse effect with all the SSRIs. It is often underreported because patients were not directly asked about this issue. Sexual dysfunction may manifest itself as decreased libido, difficulty with arousal, or delayed or absent orgasm (anorgasmia). Anorgasmia occurs in about one fifth of men taking SSRIs, and this is independent of ejaculation.[23] Management of sexual dysfunction in patients taking SSRIs is controversial, and recommendations are often based on case reports. Suggested protocols include reducing the dosage of the SSRI, maintaining the dose and hoping that tolerance and return of orgasms will come with time, waiting until the SSRI can be discontinued, or switching to another class of antidepressants that is not reputed to cause this problem as frequently, such as nefazodone (Serzone) or bupropion (Wellbutrin).[27,28] One study of 30 outpatients taking fluoxetine (Prozac), paroxetine (Paxil), or sertraline (Zoloft) assessed the value of discontinuing the drug after the Thursday morning dose and restarting it on Sunday at noon. Improved sexual functioning during the weekend was noted by those taking paroxetine and sertraline but not by those taking fluoxetine (presumably because of the long half-life of the latter).[27] In another study 39 women with anorgasmia when taking fluoxetine (Prozac) were switched to bupropion (Wellbutrin), and 90% had complete or partial resolution of the problem.[28]

Other pharmacological interventions that have been tried include adding another drug such as yohimbine (Yocon), bethanechol (Urecholine), buspirone (Buspar), amantadine (Symmetrel), dexamphetamine (Dexedrine), pemoline (Cylert), and cyproheptadine (Periactin).[23,27] That so many drugs have been tried suggests that none works well.

Guidelines for switching antidepressants. When a patient is switched from an SSRI to another antidepressant, no washout period (time interval to allow blood levels of original antidepressant to diminish) is required except in the following situations[18]:

1. Switching to moclobemide (Manerix) necessitates a 1-week washout
2. Switching to a monoamine oxidase inhibitor necessitates a 1-week washout
3. Switching from fluoxetine to any other antidepressant necessitates a 5-week washout

Switching from moclobemide to any other antidepressant necessitates a 3-day washout, and switching from a monoamine oxidase inhibitor to another antidepressant necessitates a 2-week washout.[18]

Other newer antidepressants. An increasing number of new classes of antidepressants have been developed, and several of these are listed in Table 63. Venlafaxine (Effexor), which is chemically unrelated to the SSRIs, inhibits both serotonin and norepinephrine reuptake. In higher doses it may cause diastolic hypertension.[15]

Nefazodone (Serzone) acts through the blockade of serotonin type 2 (5-HT$_2$) receptors, as well as the inhibition of serotonin reuptake. Drug interactions have been reported with astemizole (Hismanal), terfenadine (Seldane), cisapride (Propulsid), and MAO inhibitors. Although nefazodone is chemically related to trazodone, it does not appear to cause priapism.[22,29] One of its advantages is that it is not associated with an increased incidence of sexual dysfunction.[22]

Bupropion (Wellbutrin) is not chemically related to other antidepressants, and its mechanism of action is unknown. Early use of bupropion increases the risk of seizures in those already at risk (e.g., patients with anorexia). Other adverse effects include agitation and insomnia. Bupropion does not appear to cause sexual dysfunction.[15,22,28] Some clinicians are using bupropion in combination with other antidepressants in nonresponsive patients, but as yet there is little data on the value of this strategy. Bupropion is the base molecule for both Wellbutrin and Zyban, the smoking cessation drug. Wellbutrin and Zyban should not be prescribed together.

Monoamine oxidase inhibitors. First-generation MAO inhibitors include phenelzine (Nardil) and tranylcypromine (Parnate) (Table 64). They are effective in the treatment of depression and panic disorder, but because of adverse effects they are rarely used at present. If these drugs are prescribed, the initial doses should be low and built up gradually at weekly intervals. Patients must be warned stringently to avoid all sympathomimetic drugs (cold remedies containing ephedrine or related drugs) and meperidine (Demerol). Foods to be avoided while taking these drugs include "natural" or "herbal" food supplements (because they may contain ephedrine),[30] aged cheeses, pickled herring, chicken livers, yeast extracts, meat extracts such as Bovril or Oxo, broad bean pods, red wines, beer, and ripe bananas. A newer selective MAO-A inhibitor (reversible inhibitor of mono-

Table 63   Other Newer Antidepressants

Drugs	Usual doses
Phenethylamine	
Venlafaxine (Effexor XR)	75-375 mg/day
Phenylpiperazine	
Nefazodone (Serzone)	100-250 mg bid
Aminoketone	
Bupropion (Wellbutrin SR)	100 mg tid

Table 64   MAO Inhibitors

Drugs	Usual doses
Nonselective MAO Inhibitors	
Phenelzine (Nardil)	30 mg qam and 15-30 mg at noon
Tranylcypromine sulfate (Parnate)	20 mg qam and 10 mg in the afternoon
Selective MAO-A Inhibitors	
Moclobemide (Manerix)	150 mg bid or 100 mg tid

MAO, Monoamine oxidase.

amine oxidase A [RIMA]) is moclobemide (Manerix). The drug can be started at its full therapeutic dose of 100 mg tid or 150 mg bid, and dietary restrictions are not required.[31]

Bipolar disease and antidepressants. When seeing a depressed patient, the physician should check carefully for a personal or family history of bipolar disorders. Antidepressants should not be prescribed for someone with a bipolar disorder unless the patient is already taking lithium or unless mania may be precipitated. A patient who is depressed but has a family history of bipolar disorder should be watched closely for mania if antidepressants are prescribed. A patient with bipolar disorder may become manic from the rapid withdrawal of antidepressants.

Relapses after treatment with antidepressants. Relapses after successful pharmacotherapy for depression are common. In one study of patients with diagnoses of depression alone, dysthymia alone, or dysthymia plus depression (double depression) who had responded to desipramine (Norpramin, Pertofrane), continuation of the drug over a 2-year period resulted in a relapse rate of 11% compared with those assigned at random to receive placebo, whose relapse rate was 52%. Most of the relapses occurred in the 6 months after stopping the active drug. The relapse rate was highest in patients with pure dysthymia or dysthymia plus depression.[32]

Electroconvulsive therapy

Electroconvulsive therapy (ECT) is most commonly prescribed for severely depressed patients who do not respond to antidepressants. The usual course of therapy is three times a week for 6 to 12 treatments. ECT is also effective in mania. However, if a patient who responds to ECT is not put on maintenance therapy with antidepressants or lithium, the relapse rate is high. An occasional patient needs maintenance ECT at weekly or monthly intervals.[33] ECT may be administered bilaterally or unilaterally. Amnesia for some events in the weeks following treatment is an important adverse consequence, although in most cases full cognitive function returns within a few weeks. Unilateral ECT causes fewer cognitive disturbances, but 20% of patients do not respond to this form of treatment.[34]

Herbal products

A popular folk remedy for depression is St. John's wort (*Hypericum perforatum*). A systematic review and meta-analysis of 23 randomized trials of this agent found it to be more effective than placebo and as effective as standard antidepressants for the treatment of mild or moderately severe depression.[35] However, as an accompanying editorial,[36] the *Medical Letter*,[37] and others[38] point out, the methodology in many of these trials was poor: variable populations, short-duration trials, and subtherapeutic doses of control tricyclic antidepressants. A recent Cochrane review found evidence that St. John's wort was better than placebo for mild to moderate depression but that more work is needed to assess the comparative value of other antidepressants and the long-

term outcomes.[39] Trials sponsored by the new U.S. Office for Alternative Medicine are examining the efficacy and side effect profile of St. John's wort compared with SSRIs for major depression. A specific concern in North America is that herbal products are not regulated, so patients cannot be assured of receiving what is stated on the bottle label (see discussion of alternative medicine).

━━━━━━━━━━　❧ **REFERENCES** ❧　━━━━━━━━━━

1. Weissman MM, Bland RC, Canino GJ, et al: Cross-national epidemiology of major depression and bipolar disorder, *JAMA* 276:293-299, 1996.
2. Glassman AH: Cigarette smoking: implications for psychiatric illness, *Am J Psychiatry* 150:546-553, 1993.
3. Weissman MM, Wolk S, Goldstein RB, et al: Depressed adolescents grown up, *JAMA* 281:1707-1713, 1999.
4. Pearson SD, Katzelnick DJ, Simon GE, et al: Depression among high utilizers of medical care, *J Gen Intern Med* 14:461-468, 1999.
5. Simon GE, VonKorff M, Piccinelli M, et al: An international study of the relation between somatic symptoms and depression, *N Engl J Med* 341:1329-1335, 1999.
6. Hirschfeld RM, Russell JM: Assessment and treatment of suicidal patients, *N Engl J Med* 337:910-915, 1997.
7. Malchy B, Enns MW, Young TK, et al: Suicide among Manitoba's aboriginal people, 1988-94, *Can Med Assoc J* 156:1133-1138, 1997.
8. Geddes J: Suicide and homicide by people with mental illness: We still don't know how to prevent most of these deaths (editorial), *BMJ* 318:1225-1226, 1999.
9. Suicide prevention among active duty air force personnel—United States, 1990-1999, *MMWR* 48:1053-1057, 1999.
10. Thase ME, Greenhouse JB, Frank E, et al: Treatment of major depression with psychotherapy or psychotherapy-pharmacotherapy combinations, *Arch Gen Psychiatry* 54:1009-1015, 1997.
11. DeRubeis RJ, Gelfand LA, Tang TZ, et al: Medications versus cognitive behavior therapy for severely depressed outpatients: mega-analysis of four randomized comparisons, *Am J Psychiatry* 156:1007-1013, 1999.
12. Fava GA, Rafanelli C, Grandi S, et al: Prevention of recurrent depression with cognitive-behavioral therapy: preliminary findings, *Arch Gen Psychiatry* 55:816-820, 1998.
13. Reynolds CF 3rd, Frank E, Perel JM, et al: Nortriptyline and interpersonal psychotherapy as maintenance therapies for recurrent major depression: a randomized controlled trial in patients older than 59 years, *JAMA* 281:39-45, 1999.
14. Hirschfeld RM: Long-term drug treatment of unipolar depression, *Int Clin Psychopharmacol* 11:211-217, 1996.
15. Drugs for depression and anxiety, *Med Lett* 41:33-38, 1999.
16. Smith WT, Londborg PD, Glaudin V, et al: Short-term augmentation of fluoxetine with clonazepam in the treatment of depression: a double-blind study, *Am J Psychiatry* 155:1339-1345, 1998.
17. Reimherr FW, Amsterdam JD, Quitkin FM, et al: Optimal length of continuation therapy in depression: a prospective assessment during long-term fluoxetine treatment, *Am J Psychiatry* 155:1247-1253, 1998.

18. Kennedy SH, Bakish D, Evans M, et al: *CANMAT guidelines for the diagnosis and pharmacologic treatment of depression,* Toronto, 1999, Ontario Ministry of Health.

19. Nemeroff CB, DeVane Cl, Pollock BG: Newer antidepressants and the cytochrome P450 system, *Am J Psychiatry* 153:311-320, 1996.

20. Haddad P, Lejoyeux M, Young A: Antidepressant discontinuation reactions: are preventable and simple to treat (editorial), *BMJ* 316:1105-1106, 1998.

21. McQuay HJ, Tramer M, Nye BA, et al: A systematic review of antidepressants in neuropathic pain, *Pain* 68:217-227, 1996.

22. Andrews JM, Nemeroff CB: Contemporary management of depression, *Am J Med* 97:24S-32S, 1994.

23. Segraves RT: Antidepressant-induced orgasm disorder, *J Sex Marital Ther* 21:192-201, 1995.

24. Anton RF Jr, Burch EA Jr: Amoxapine versus amitriptyline combined with perphenazine in the treatment of psychotic depression, *Am J Psychiatry* 147:1203-1208, 1990.

25. Nierenberg AA, Adler LA, Peselow E, et al: Trazodone for antidepressant-associated insomnia, *Am J Psychiatry* 151: 1069-1072, 1994.

26. Lebowitz BD, Pearson JL, Schneider LS, et al: Diagnosis and treatment of depression in late life: consensus statement update, *JAMA* 278:1186-1190, 1997.

27. Rothschild AJ: Selective serotonin reuptake inhibitor–induced sexual dysfunction: efficacy of a drug holiday, *Am J Psychiatry* 152:1514-1516, 1995.

28. Walker PW, Cole JO, Gardner EA, et al: Improvement in fluoxetine-associated sex dysfunction in patients switched to bupropion, *J Clin Psychiatry* 54:459-465, 1993.

29. Robinson DS, Roberts DL, Smith JM, et al: The safety profile of nefazodone, *J Clin Psychiatry* 57(suppl 2):31-38, 1996.

30. Centers for Disease Control and Prevention: Adverse events associated with ephedrine-containing products—Texas, December 1993–September 1995, *JAMA* 276:1711-1712, 1996.

31. Freeman H: Moclobemide, *Lancet* 342:1528-1532, 1993.

32. Kocsis JH, Friedman RA, Markowitz JC, et al: Maintenance therapy for chronic depression—a controlled clinical trial of desipramine, *Arch Gen Psychiatry* 53:769-774, 1996.

33. Banazak DA: Electroconvulsive therapy: a guide for family physicians, *Am Fam Physician* 53:273-278, 1996.

34. Kraus RP, Chandarana P: "Say, are you psychiatrists still using ECT?" *Can Med Assoc J* 157:1375-1377, 1997.

35. Linde K, Ramirez G, Mulrow CD, et al: St John's wort for depression—an overview and meta-analysis of randomised clinical trials, *BMJ* 313:253-258, 1996.

36. de Smet PA, Nolen WA: St John's wort as an antidepressant (editorial), *BMJ* 313:253-258, 1996.

37. St. John's wort, *Med Lett* 39:107-108, 1997.

38. Evans MF, Morgenstern K: St. John's wort: an herbal remedy for depression? *Can Fam Physician* 43:1735-1736, 1997.

39. Linde K, Mulrow CD: *St. John's wort for depression,* Cochrane Library, Issue 4, Oxford, 1999, Update Software.

Treatment-resistant depression

In general, 60% to 70% of depressed patients respond to the initial antidepressant used and a further 10% to 15% to a second antidepressant or ECT.[1]

When faced with a depressed patient who fails to respond to treatment, the physician must first reassess the diagnosis and management to date. Is an underlying disease such as hypothyroidism or an interfering comorbidity such as substance abuse or an anxiety disorder present?[2] According to Joffe[2] and Berber[3] the following are the main options for dealing with truly refractory depression. (These can be remembered with the mnemonic "OSCAR."[3])

1. Optimization. The first step is always optimization, that is, to ensure that an adequate dose of the initial antidepressant has been prescribed, that the patient has been compliant in taking it, and that it has been given for a sufficient duration, which is usually 6 weeks. In the case of tricyclic antidepressants, measuring blood levels may be helpful.[2] If a patient is a partial responder, an increase in the dose (if tolerated) may be effective.

2. Substitution. If a patient has no response, a different antidepressant should be considered. The literature suggests that the response rate after switching classes is about 50% to 60% as opposed to 20% to 30% when switching within the same class. However, preliminary evidence based on open trials indicates that this may not be the case with the SSRIs; the response rate from substituting a second SSRI has been reported to be 50% to 60%.[2,4,5]

3. Combination. Combination refers to combining two antidepressants from two different classes, for example, an SSRI and a tricyclic.[2] This is a new and promising area of research.

4. Augmentation. Augmentation is the addition to an antidepressant of another drug that on its own is not known to have antidepressant effects. Examples are lithium, triiodothyronine or liothyronine (Cytomel), buspirone (Buspar), and psychostimulants such as dextroamphetamine (Dexedrine) or methylphenidate (Ritalin). Most of the studies to date have involved lithium and triiodothyronine.[2]

5. Review. This is a general but important concept that reminds physicians to reassess management to date, including mobilization of local resources and psychotherapeutic interventions.[3]

Which strategies should be used? Few controlled trials have been conducted in this area, so the data on which recommendations are based come mostly from open trials. Optimization is obviously the first step for all patients. The traditional second step has been substitution, which can be very effective; the main disadvantage is the time taken to discontinue the first antidepressant and build up the second one to a full therapeutic level. Augmentation has the advantage that time is not lost from stopping one drug and starting another and that if a response is to occur, it sometimes does so within days and usually within 2 to 3 weeks. Combinations of antidepressants can also be effective, and time is not lost; care must be taken that toxicity is not induced through one agent's interference with the metabolism of the other (see discussion of antidepressants).[6]

The preceding discussion has been limited to drug therapy for treatment-resistant depression. ECT is an alternative that perhaps should be used at an earlier stage in the therapeutic regimen than is currently the practice.[7]

REFERENCES

1. Warneke L: Management of resistant depression, *Can Fam Physician* 42:1973-1980, 1996.
2. Joffe RT, Levitt AJ, Sokolov ST: Augmentation strategies—focus on anxiolytics, *J Clin Psychiatry* 57(suppl 7):25-33, 1996.
3. Berber MJ: Pharmacological treatment of depression: consulting with Dr. Oscar, *Can Fam Physician* 45:2663-2668, 1999.
4. Joffe RT, Levitt AJ, Sokolov ST, et al: Response to an open trial of a second SSRI in major depression, *J Clin Psychiatry* 57:114-115, 1996.
5. Thase ME, Blomgern SL, Birkett MA, et al: Fluoxetine treatment of patients with major depressive disorder who failed initial treatment with sertraline, *J Clin Psychiatry* 58:16-21, 1997.
6. Joffe RT, Levitt AJ: Antidepressant failure: augmentation or substitution? (editorial), *J Psychiatry Neurosci* 20:7-9, 1995.
7. Joffe RT, Kellner CH: The role of ECT in refractory depression (editorial), *Convuls Ther* 11:77-79, 1995.

Dysthymic disorder

For dysthymic disorder to be diagnosed, the patient must experience a depressed mood almost continuously for 2 years (1 year for a child), as well as have two or more of the symptoms usually associated with depression such as changes in eating or sleeping patterns, poor concentration, fatigue, and low self-esteem or feelings of hopelessness.[1]

The diagnosis of dysthymic disorder cannot be made if during the initial 2 years (1 year for a child) the patient has had major depression. However, if a major depression occurs before or after this period, the patient is given both diagnoses (dysthymic disorder and major depressive disorder) or is referred to as having "double depression." Other conditions that exclude the diagnosis of dysthymic disorder are a diagnosis of mania, hypomania, a mixed episode, or cyclothymia.[1]

Antidepressants are effective not only for controlling the depressive symptoms of dysthymic disorder,[2-4] but also for improving psychosocial functioning.[3] Both tricyclics and SSRIs are effective, but SSRIs are currently the preferred class of drugs.[2-4] Preliminary studies suggest that venlafaxine (Effexor) built up to a maximum dose of 225 mg/day is also effective.[5] According to one author, treatment should start with small doses and increase slowly. Response may take many weeks, and the best that may be achieved for some patients, especially those with comorbid personality disorders, is a 25% to 30% improvement.[2]

In a placebo-controlled study, dysthymic patients who responded to desipramine were selected at random to continue the desipramine (Norpramin, Pertofrane) or to take a placebo for a 2-year period. The relapse rate was much higher

in the placebo group, and most such events occurred during the first 6 months after stopping the drug.[6]

REFERENCES

1. American Psychiatric Association: *Diagnostic and statistical manual of mental disorders,* ed 4, Washington, DC, 1994, American Psychiatric Association, pp 345-349.
2. Sansone RA, Sansone LA: Dysthymic disorder: the chronic depression, *Am Fam Physician* 53:2588-2596, 1996.
3. Kocsis JH, Zisook S, Davidson J, et al: Double-blind comparison of sertraline, imipramine, and placebo in the treatment of dysthymia: psychosocial outcomes, *Am J Psychiatry* 154:390-395, 1997.
4. Thase ME, Fava M, Halbreich U, et al: A placebo-controlled, randomized clinical trial comparing sertraline and imipramine for the treatment of dysthymia, *Arch Gen Psychiatry* 53:777-784, 1996.
5. Dunner DL, Hendrickson HE, Bea C, et al: Venlafaxine in dysthymic disorder, *J Clin Psychiatry* 58:528-531, 1997.
6. Kocsis JH, Friedman RA, Markowitz JC, et al: Maintenance therapy for chronic depression—a controlled clinical trial of desipramine, *Arch Gen Psychiatry* 53:769-774, 1996.

Postpartum depression

Postpartum depression occurs within 6 to 12 weeks of delivery in about 10% of pregnancies. It should be distinguished from postnatal blues, which are experienced by 50% to 80% of women and are mild and self-limited, and postpartum or puerperal psychosis, which affects about 0.2% of pregnant women. The "blues" appear 2 to 7 days after delivery and usually resolve within 2 weeks. Treatment is reassurance and support.[2]

The duration of untreated postpartum depression is usually 2 to 6 months, which is similar to depression occurring at any other time. Women whose initial manifestation of an affective disorder is postpartum depression are at increased risk for subsequent postpartum depressions. Women with postpartum depression who have had a past history of depressions unrelated to pregnancy are not at increased risk for subsequent postpartum depression.[3] A previous stillbirth is also a risk factor for postpartum depression, particularly if the subsequent pregnancy occurs within 12 months of that event.[4]

Children of women with postpartum depression have been found to have some degree of cognitive impairment and emotional and behavioral problems when evaluated at ages 18 months and 4 to 5 years. Whether treatment of postpartum depression alters this outcome is uncertain, but preliminary studies are encouraging.[3] One explanation for this finding is that associative learning in young infants is related to the quality of the "child-directed speech" to which they are exposed. Among other characteristics, child-directed speech is distinguished by exaggerated modulation of tone, increased amplitude, longer pauses, and more repetitions. Depressed mothers are less capable of generating child-directed speech than are nondepressed mothers.[5]

Therefore detection and treatment of postpartum depression are priorities because treatment improves the quality of life of both mother and infant.

Although a number of studies have shown counseling and psychotherapy to be beneficial,[3] most workers advocate pharmacotherapy (even for nursing mothers) because withholding drugs has serious consequences for mother, baby, and other family members. First-choice drugs are SSRIs.[6] Tricyclics are also effective, and ECT leads to rapid improvement in refractory cases.[1]

An open clinical trial in a small group of women with a past history of postpartum depression compared the effects of antidepressants given immediately after delivery against clinical monitoring only. The rate of recurrent postpartum depression was much higher in the group not receiving antidepressants.[7]

REFERENCES

1. Murray D: Oestrogen and postnatal depression (editorial), *Lancet* 347:918-919, 1996.
2. Epperson CN: Postpartum major depression: detection and treatment, *Am Fam Physician* 59:2247-2254, 1999.
3. Cooper PJ, Murray L: Postnatal depression, *BMJ* 316:1884-1886, 1998.
4. Hughes PM, Turton P, Evans CD: Stillbirth as risk factor for depression and anxiety in the subsequent pregnancy: cohort study, *BMJ* 318:1721-1724, 1999.
5. Kaplan PS, Bachorowski J-A, Zarlengo-Strouse P: Child-directed speech produced by mothers with symptoms of depression fails to promote associative learning in 4-month-old infants, *Child Dev* 70:560-570, 1999.
6. Kulinn NA, Pastuszak A, Sage SR, et al: Pregnancy outcome following maternal use of the new selective serotonin reuptake inhibitors: a prospective controlled multicenter study, *JAMA* 279:609-610, 1998.
7. Wisner KL, Wheeler S: Prevention of recurrent postpartum major depression, *Hosp Commun Psychiatry* 45:1191-1196, 1994.

Seasonal Affective Disorder

Between 10% and 15% of patients with mood disorders are said to suffer from seasonal affective disorder (SAD). Patients with SAD usually have "atypical" symptoms of depression: overeating, carbohydrate craving, weight gain, and oversleeping. They show a marked lack of energy. Symptoms usually begin in October or November and are worst in January and February. Spontaneous recovery occurs in April or May. SAD is usually unipolar, but 20% have a type II bipolar disorder.[1]

The usual protocol for light therapy involves exposure to a fluorescent light box rated at 10,000 lux for 30 to 45 minutes a day between 6 and 8 AM. Response is usually seen in 1 to 3 weeks but may occur earlier.[2] Patients can read while in front of the lights; ultraviolet light (less than 400 nm) should be filtered out.[1] One study comparing 1.5 hours of light therapy of approximately 6000 lux against sham negative ion generator placebos found light therapy to be effective, but benefits were not generally noted until 3 weeks had elapsed.[3] Light therapy works best if it is used in the morning.[4]

Few studies have considered the efficacy of medications for SAD; fluoxetine (Prozac)[1,5,6] and moclobemide[6] are probably beneficial.

REFERENCES

1. Tam EM, Lam RW, Levitt AJ: Treatment of seasonal affective disorder—a review, *Can J Psychiatry* 40:457-466, 1995.
2. Levitt AJ, Wesson VA, Joffe RT, et al: A controlled comparison of light box and head-mounted units in the treatment of seasonal depression, *J Clin Psychiatry* 57:105-110, 1996.
3. Eastman CI, Young MA, Fogg LF, et al: Bright light treatment of winter depression: a placebo-controlled trial, *Arch Gen Psychiatry* 55:883-889, 1998.
4. Lewy AJ, Bauer VK, Cutler NL, et al: Morning vs evening light treatment of patients with winter depression, *Arch Gen Psychiatry* 55:890-896, 1998.
5. Lam RW, Gorman CP, Michalon M, et al: Multicenter, placebo-controlled study of fluoxetine in seasonal affective disorder, *Am J Psychiatry* 152:1765-1770, 1995.
6. Kennedy SH, Bakish D, Evans M, et al: *CANMAT guidelines for the diagnosis and pharmacologic treatment of depression,* Toronto, 1999, Ontario Ministry of Health.

Serotonin Syndrome
(See also neuroleptic malignant syndrome)

The serotonin syndrome is characterized by an excess of serotonin in the brainstem, which in most cases is precipitated by giving two or more serotonergic drugs concurrently. The diagnosis is often missed because symptoms are nonspecific; they involve cognition and behavior, the autonomic nervous system, and the neuromuscular system. The following are some of the symptoms[1,2]:

1. Cognition-behavior—confusion, disorientation, agitation, irritability, anxiety
2. Autonomic—hyperthermia, diaphoresis, flushing, sinus tachycardia, hypertension, dilated pupils, lacrimation, nausea, diarrhea
3. Neuromuscular—restlessness, myoclonus, muscle rigidity, trismus, teeth chattering, tremor, opisthotonos

Symptoms develop within 24 hours of taking the offending drug and are commonly apparent within 1 to 2 hours. Responsible drugs are most often those used to treat affective disorders, obsessive-compulsive disorders, and Parkinson's disease. Meperidine and dextromethorphan can also precipitate this syndrome. The disorder usually follows the addition of a second drug, for example, an SSRI given to a patient with Parkinson's disease being treated with selegiline (Eldepryl) or levodopa. Among the more frequently responsible drugs are SSRIs, MAO inhibitors, antiparkinsonian drugs (selegiline [Eldepryl], amantadine [Symmetrel], levodopa [Sinemet, Prolopa], bromocriptine [Parlodel]), dextromethorphan, meperidine (Demerol), cocaine, and amphetamines. Some other drugs that have been reported to cause the syndrome are tricyclics, especially clomipramine (Anafranil) and imipramine (Tofranil), lithium, fenfluramine (Pondimin, Ponderal), and bupropion (Wellbutrin).[1]

Treatment is discontinuation of the offending drug and supportive therapy. A variety of therapeutic agents have been mentioned in case reports, but no specific agent has been shown to be beneficial.[2]

―――――――――― ❧ **REFERENCES** ❧ ――――――――――

1. Mills KC: Serotonin syndrome, *Am Fam Physician* 52:1475-1482, 1995.
2. Martin TG: Serotonin syndrome, *Ann Emerg Med* 28:520-526, 1996.

PERSONALITY DISORDERS

(See also abuse; aggression; attention deficit/hyperactivity disorder; conduct disorder)

Classification

The major personality disorders or Axis II disorders are borderline personality disorder, antisocial personality disorder, narcissistic personality disorder, histrionic personality disorder, dependent personality disorder, avoidant personality disorder, schizotypal personality disorder, schizoid personality disorder, paranoid personality disorder, and obsessive-compulsive personality disorder.[1]

Etiology

Childhood neglect and abuse increase the risk for personality disorders (see discussion of abuse).

Aggressive Behavior

The management of aggression in patients with personality disorders is discussed in the section on aggression.

Antisocial Personality Disorder

A diagnosis of antisocial personality disorder can be made only in individuals over the age of 18. Criteria for the diagnosis are a consistent disregard for the rights of others and violation of those rights from the age of 15, as well as a history of conduct disorder starting before the age of 15.[1] A significant risk factor for the development of antisocial personality disorder is antecedent attention deficit/hyperactivity disorder.[2]

The overall reported prevalence rate of antisocial personality disorder in the Western world is between 2% and 4%, and males outnumber females by a ratio of between 5:1 and 7:1. Persons with this disorder are often fearless and may be heroes in combat situations. In most cases criminal behavior dies out by middle age but difficulties in interpersonal relationships persist.[3]

Antisocial personality disorder is rare in East Asian countries such as Taiwan and Japan, possibly because of the cohesiveness of traditional families in these environments. Support for this explanation comes from the observation that in Europe and North America important risk factors for the development of antisocial personality disorder are antisocial behavior in the father, parental alcoholism, childhood physical abuse, and separation from or loss of a parent. The common denominator is lack of parental supervision and discipline. Current evidence suggests that to acquire an antisocial personality disorder, a person must have the genetic potential and then be exposed to an environment conducive to its development.[3]

The definition of antisocial personality disorder in *DSM IV* is based largely on behavior[1] and does not fully embrace the concept of psychopathy that Frick and co-workers[4] point out is characterized by superficial charm and the absence of enduring relationships, empathy, guilt, and anxiety. The distinction is important because persons who meet the criteria of antisocial personality disorder often have low intelligence and adverse family backgrounds, whereas those defined by psychopathic traits are notable for their narcissism and striking lack of anxiety.

Borderline Personality Disorder

Axis I comorbid conditions are the norm for patients with borderline personality. In one study mood disorders were found in 96%, anxiety disorders in 88% (posttraumatic stress disorder in 56%, panic disorder in 48%, and social phobias in 46%), substance use disorders in 64%, and eating disorders in 53%.[5]

Patients with borderline personality disorder are the bane of physicians because none of the reasonable suggestions made by physicians work or are implemented by the patient. Borderline patients obtain a sense of control if they can sabotage the interventions recommended by their physicians.[6]

According to Dawson,[6] an essential aspect of the management of borderline patients is for the physician to refuse to play the role of an ever more powerful paternal figure looking after an increasingly regressing child. The physician should make it clear that the patient is a competent adult who is capable of taking responsibility for his or her own life and health; the physician is a helper but is of secondary importance and cannot take responsibility for the patient's self-destructive behavior. This process of establishing and maintaining a different type of social contract with the patient is called relationship management. Dawson describes a variety of interviewing techniques that may be helpful in establishing and maintaining this contract. A key element is for the physician to refrain from jumping in with empathetic words or gestures when the patient begins to complain about the miseries of life.

Other useful suggestions in the management of borderline patients in primary care are the following[7]:

1. Set and observe limits. A verbal contract is often useful in spelling out such items as fixed but limited appointments, necessity of coming on time and not canceling, limited number of telephone calls, and contingency plans for overwhelming suicidal ideation.

2. Follow a behavioral approach to psychotherapy that focuses on helping the patients understand how to get on with their lives.

3. Recognize and treat concomitant Axis I disorders.

4. Arrange for judicious psychiatric consultations (not referrals).

5. If all the above are unsuccessful, inform the patient that you will not be able to continue being his or her physician.

▰ REFERENCES ▰

1. American Psychiatric Association: *Diagnostic and statistical manual of mental disorders,* ed 4, Washington, DC, 1994, The Association, pp 629-673.

2. Mannuzza S, Klein RG, Bessler A, et al: Adult outcome of hyperactive boys: educational achievement, occupational rank, and psychiatric status, *Arch Gen Psychiatry* 50:565-576, 1993.

3. Paris J: Antisocial personality disorder: a biopsychosocial model, *Can J Psychiatry* 41:75-80, 1996.

4. Frick PJ, O'Brien BS, Wootton JM, et al: Psychopathy and conduct problems in children, *J Abnorm Psychol* 103:700-707, 1994.

5. Zanarini MC, Frankenburg FR, Dubo ED, et al: Axis I comorbidity of borderline personality disorder, *Am J Psychiatry* 155: 1733-1739, 1998.

6. Dawson DF: Relationship management and the borderline patient, *Can Fam Physician* 39:833-839, 1993.

7. Paré M, Linehan MM, Oldham JM, et al: Dx: personality disorder . . . now what? *Patient Care Can* 7:63-85, 1996.

PSYCHOSES

(See also nausea and vomiting; serotonin syndrome; vitamin E)

Schizophrenia

The natural course of schizophrenia is deterioration, which is usually greatest in the first few years after diagnosis. However, rate of progression varies markedly from one individual to another. Prognosis is better for women than men, for those who have a later onset of disease, for those who respond well to an initial course of medication, and for those who live in a relatively serene family environment. Prognosis is considerably worse if negative symptoms are prominent, if the patient also has a substance abuse disorder, and if social and cognitive functioning were poor before the onset of illness. The longer the duration of untreated psychosis, the worse the prognosis.[1]

Early treatment of schizophrenia is recommended in the hope that this will improve prognosis. Aside from medications, treatment should include social skills training, family psychoeducational training, and a protected employment environment. Atypical neuroleptics are probably the drugs of choice, but proof of this is not yet available.[1]

Substance abuse is common among schizophrenics; 75% smoke,[2] and the current rate of other forms of substance abuse (alcohol, cannabis, amphetamines, antihistamines, and analgesics) is 20%. The lifetime rate for these forms of substance abuse is 80%.[3]

A combination of cognitive and behavioral characteristics may presage the development of schizophrenia. An Israeli study compared the results of compulsory draft board psychological tests of adolescent males who later became schizophrenic with the results of male adolescents who did not develop schizophrenia. None of the subjects included in the study manifested clinical evidence of mental illness or mental retardation at the time of testing. Those who later became schizophrenic had significantly lower scores in all domains but particularly in social functioning, organizational ability, and cognitive functioning.[4]

Neuroleptics

The classification and usual dosages of selected neuroleptics are recorded in Table 65.

Risperidone (Risperdal), olanzapine (Zyprexa), clozapine (Clozaril), and quetiapine (Seroquel) are new "atypical" or "second-generation" antipsychotics.[1,3,5] As a group they appear to improve negative symptoms such as apathy, lack of initiative, disorganization, depression, and hostility, and they may improve cognitive functioning.[1,3,5] Atypical neuroleptics also appear to have fewer extrapyramidal side effects than "typical" or "first-generation" antipsychotics (in

Table 65 Neuroleptics

Drugs	Usual doses
Typical (First-Generation) Antipsychotics	
Butyrophenone derivatives	
Haloperidol (Haldol)	5-20 mg/day
Phenothiazines, aliphatic	
Chlorpromazine (Thorazine, Largactil)	25-400 mg/day
Methotrimeprazine (Nozinan)	6-75 mg/day
Phenothiazines, piperazine	
Trifluoperazine (Stelazine)	6-20 mg/day
Prochlorperazine (Compazine, Stemetil)	5-10 mg tid or qid; usually used for nausea and vomiting
Fluphenazine enanthate (Prolixin Enanthate, Moditen)	25 mg (12.5-100 mg) IM q2 weeks
Fluphenazine decanoate (Prolixin Decanoate, Modecate)	25 mg (12.5-50 mg) IM q3 weeks
Phenothiazines, piperidine	
Thioridazine (Mellaril)	25-400 mg/day
Tricyclic dibenzoxazepine derivatives	
Loxapine (Loxapac)	60-100 mg/day
Atypical (Second-Generation) Antipsychotics	
Clozapine (Clozaril)	300-600 mg/day
Olanzapine (Zyprexa)	10-20 mg/day
Risperidone (Risperdal)	2-6 mg/day
Sertindole (Serlect)	16-20 mg/day
Quetiapine (Seroquel)	100 mg tid–200 mg bid

the case of risperidone this is true only if the dose is no more than 8 mg/day[5]). One trial comparing low-dose haloperidol (mean dose 3.7 mg/day) to low-dose risperidone (mean dose 3.2 mg per day) in patients who had not received neuroleptics found no difference between the groups in the incidence of dystonia, parkinsonism, akathisia, or dyskinesia.[6] Second-generation drugs are chemically diverse, so failure of response to one does not mean that another will not be effective.[3]

A major adverse effect of many second-generation neuroleptics is weight gain. In a comparative U.S. study of four second-generation agents (clozapine, olanzapine, risperidone, and sertindole [Serlect]) and the first-generation neuroleptic haloperidol, the most weight gain was associated with clozapine and olanzapine, and the least weight gain with haloperidol and sertindole.[7]

Clozapine has been particularly valuable in treating patients who have failed to respond to first-generation neuroleptics.[1,3,5] Agranulocytosis has been reported in 1% to 2% of patients, so weekly monitoring of white blood cell counts is necessary. Clozapine lowers the seizure threshold.[5]

Typical or "first-generation" antipsychotic drugs have often been divided into two groups: low potency and high potency. The low-potency group, which includes drugs such as chlorpromazine (Thorazine, Largactil), tends to cause sedation and hypotension but to have relatively few extrapyramidal effects. High-potency drugs such as haloperidol (Haldol) are less sedating and cause less hypotension but are associated with greater extrapyramidal effects.[8]

The cumulative relapse rate 5 years after a first episode of schizophrenia is 82%; the rate is approximately five times greater in patients who discontinue neuroleptics than in those who continue to take their medications. Robinson and associates[9] advise that after a first psychotic episode neuroleptics be taken continuously for at least 2 years. Kane[8] recommends neuroleptic treatment for 1 to 2 years after a first episode of schizophrenia and for 5 years or even indefinitely for anyone who has had two or more episodes. The relapse rate while taking medications is 15% to 20% per year.

In outpatient settings the dosage of neuroleptics should be relatively low initially and should be increased gradually. Maximum control of psychotic thought processes may take weeks or even months,[7] whereas agitation may be rapidly controlled because of the sedative effects of neuroleptics or supplementally administered benzodiazepines. Follow-up every 2 weeks is adequate to monitor psychotic thought processes, whereas daily assessments may be necessary to evaluate agitation.

In the past, very large doses of neuroleptics were used for some patients. The current view is that doses greater than 10 to 20 mg of haloperidol or its equivalent add little if any additional therapeutic benefit.[8] Some workers suggest that if 2 to 5 mg of haloperidol or the equivalent is not effective, one of the atypical antipsychotics such as olanzapine or risperidone should be substituted,[10] while others recommend the

preferential use of atypical antipsychotics as first-line therapy.[1,3] However, if the patient's disorder is well controlled with first-generation agents, switching to second-generation drugs is not recommended.[3]

Much or all of the neuroleptic dose can be given at bedtime if nocturnal sedation is required. If daytime agitation is a problem, the total daily dose may be divided so that a portion of it is given during the day.

The following are some of the more important adverse effects of neuroleptics:

1. Seizures. In general the neuroleptics lower the seizure threshold. The incidence of seizures is particularly high with clozapine (Clozaril).
2. Interaction with tricyclics. The neuroleptics inhibit the metabolism of tricyclics and so raise their blood levels.
3. Hypotension. All of the phenothiazines may cause a marked hypotensive effect through alpha-adrenergic blockade. Phenothiazines should be used with extreme caution in the elderly.
4. Anticholinergic effects. The anticholinergic effects of neuroleptics are most marked in the aliphatic phenothiazines (chlorpromazine [Thorazine, Largactil], methotrimeprazine [Nozinan]).
5. Sedation. All of the neuroleptics are sedative, but of those commonly used, the most sedative seem to be methotrimeprazine (Nozinan), chlorpromazine (Thorazine, Largactil), and thioridazine (Mellaril).
6. Prolactin elevation. Neuroleptics raise prolactin levels and may cause galactorrhea.
7. Tardive dyskinesia. The risk of tardive dyskinesia is generally related to dose, treatment duration, and age. Tardive dyskinesia is three to five times more common in elderly than in young patients treated with conventional antipsychotics, and after 3 years of treatment the rate of tardive dyskinesia surpasses 50%.[11] The most effective treatment is to decrease or withdraw the offending neuroleptic, but evidence suggests that vitamin E in doses of 800 to 1600 mg daily can ameliorate symptoms.[3] Occasional spontaneous remissions have been reported.[12] Tardive dyskinesia appears to be less common with second-generation than with first-generation neuroleptics.[1]
8. Neuroleptic malignant syndrome. The cardinal features of the neuroleptic malignant syndrome are hyperpyrexia, muscle rigidity, altered mental status, and autonomic instability (variations in pulse and blood pressure). Patients may have elevated creatinine kinase levels, myoglobinuria from rhabdomyolysis, and acute renal failure. The mortality rate of untreated persons is 20%. The disorder usually occurs within the first few weeks of starting a neuroleptic or of increasing the dose. Treatment is discontinuation of the neuroleptic, fluids, and administration of dantrolene (Dantrium), bromocriptine (Parlodel), or per-

golide (Permax).[8] (See also the discussion of serotonin syndrome.)

9. Extrapyramidal effects. The extrapyramidal effects of neuroleptics include dystonias, opisthotonos, oculogyric crises, Parkinson-like symptoms, and akathisia. Among first-generation neuroleptics, those commonly causing this type of adverse effect are the butyrophenone derivatives (haloperidol [Haldol]). Extrapyramidal effects are rare with the aliphatic phenothiazine derivatives (chlorpromazine [Thorazine, Largactil], methotrimeprazine [Nozinan]) and are relatively uncommon with the usual oral doses of the piperidine phenothiazine derivatives (thioridazine [Mellaril]). The incidence of extrapyramidal side effects with the piperazine phenothiazine derivatives depends on the dosage. These effects are uncommon with the usual outpatient doses of trifluoperazine (Stelazine) but very common with the long-acting intramuscular forms (fluphenazine enanthate [Prolixin Enanthate, Moditen] and fluphenazine decanoate [Prolixin Decanoate, Modecate]). Extrapyramidal reactions are relatively rare with the newer atypical antipsychotics. Acute dystonic reactions can be controlled by a single injection of diphenhydramine (Benadryl) 50 mg. Other extrapyramidal effects are controlled by benztropine (Cogentin) or procyclidine (Kemadrin). At usual outpatient doses, one rarely needs antiparkinsonian drugs with chlorpromazine, methotrimeprazine, trifluoperazine, or thioridazine. Most patients taking haloperidol require them on a regular basis, and patients taking the long-acting intramuscular formulations of fluphenazine enanthate or fluphenazine decanoate require them only during the first week or two after the injections. The usual dosage of benztropine is 1 to 4 mg/day as a single dose or in 2 divided doses, whereas that of procyclidine (Kemadrin) is 7.5 to 20 mg/day in 3 divided doses.

10. Akathisia. Akathisia is an extrapyramidal effect that causes the patient to feel extremely restless. The main modality of treatment is to lower the dose of the neuroleptic, but some patients may respond to antiparkinsonian agents, beta-blockers, or benzodiazepines.[3] In view of the high risk of substance abuse in schizophrenic patients, benzodiazepines should be prescribed with caution.

11. Weight gain. Weight gain may occur with both first- and second-generation neuroleptics but is most marked with many of the second-generation agents (see above).[7]

◣ REFERENCES ◤

1. Malla AK, Norman RM, Voruganti LP: Improving outcome in schizophrenia: the case for early intervention, *Can Med Assoc J* 160:843-846, 1999.

2. Glassman AH: Cigarette smoking: implications for psychiatric illness, *Am J Psychiatry* 150:546-553, 1993.

3. Working Group for the Canadian Psychiatric Association and the Canadian Alliance for Research on Schizophrenia: Canadian clinical practice guidelines for the treatment of schizophrenia, *Can J Psychiatry* 43(suppl 2 revised):S25-S40, 1998.

4. Davidson M, Reichenberg A, Rabinowitz J, et al: Behavioral and intellectual markers for schizophrenia in apparently healthy male adolescents, *Am J Psychiatry* 156:1328-1335, 1999.

5. Csernansky JG: Psychopharmacologic treatment of schizophrenia, *Psychiatr Clin North Am* 5:161-182, 1998.

6. Rosebush PI, Mazurek MF: Neurologic side effects in neuroleptic-naïve patients treated with haloperidol or risperidone, *Neurology* 52:782-785, 1999.

7. Wirshing DA, Wirshing WC, Kysar L, et al: Novel antipsychotics: comparison of weight gain liabilities, *J Clin Psychiatry* 60:358-363, 1999.

8. Kane JM: Schizophrenia, *N Engl J Med* 334:34-41, 1996.

9. Robinson D, Woerner MG, Alvir JM, et al: Predictors of relapse following response from a first episode of schizophrenia or schizoaffective disorder, *Arch Gen Psychiatry* 56:241-247, 1999.

10. Kapur S: Receptor imaging studies in the treatment of schizophrenia, *Psychiatry Rounds* 2(1):1-5, 1998.

11. Woerner MG, Ma J, Alvir J, et al: Prospective study of tardive dyskinesia in the elderly: rates and risk factors, *Am J Psychiatry* 155:1521-1528, 1998.

12. Latimer PR: Tardive dyskinesia: a review, *Can J Psychiatry* 40(suppl 2):49S-54S, 1995.

PSYCHOTHERAPY
(See also depression)

A study of brief psychotherapy from the Jewish General Hospital in Montreal concluded that it was effective for patients with a variety of psychiatric diagnoses and that the experience of the therapists did not seem to influence the outcomes. The success rate was as good when psychotherapy was conducted by medical students, family medicine residents, and psychiatry residents under supervision as it was for staff psychiatrists.[1]

One metaanalysis concluded that interpersonal and cognitive-behavioral therapies were as effective as antidepressants for mild depression but that for severe recurrent depression a combination of antidepressants and psychotherapy was more effective than psychotherapy alone (see discussion of depression).[2]

◣ REFERENCES ◤

1. Propst A, Paris J, Rosberger Z: Do therapist experience, diagnosis and functional level predict outcome in short term psychotherapy? *Can J Psychiatry* 39:168-176, 1994.

2. Thase ME, Greenhouse JB, Frank E, et al: Treatment of major depression with psychotherapy or psychotherapy-pharmacotherapy combinations, *Arch Gen Psychiatry* 54:1009-1015, 1997.

SUBSTANCE ABUSE AND GAMBLING

(See also alcohol; breast feeding; serotonin syndrome; sports medicine)

Substance Abuse

Nihilism in the face of substance abuse is unjustified because treatment is effective in about 50% of cases. Where appropriate, family physicians should refer their addicted patients to addiction treatment centers that offer immediate and long-term care in inpatient, outpatient, or residential facilities and that use diverse programs such as pharmacotherapy, behavioral therapy, substance use monitoring, and peer support groups.[1]

An uncontrollable compulsion to seek the drug or drugs of choice is a fundamental characteristic of addiction and is at least as important as physical dependence. Treatment of drug-seeking compulsion is central to any effective therapeutic program.[1]

Two main categories of substance abusers are those (usually adolescents) who use drugs for the pleasurable or novel sensations they induce and those who use drugs as a means of dealing with life's problems. Many patients in the latter category are self-treating a mental disorder, often depression; paradoxically, the chosen drugs of abuse usually aggravate the underlying mental condition. Patients with addiction and other mental disorders should generally receive concurrent treatment for both conditions.[1]

Heredity is an important risk factor for substance abuse. First-degree relatives of abusers have an eight times higher risk of drug abuse than relatives of non–drug abusers. However, with the exception of cannabis, a familial history of drug abuse does not appear to increase the risk of alcoholism among first-degree relatives. A high percentage of the first-degree relatives of substance abusers smoke.[2]

Substance use has been increasing among adolescents in North America and the United Kingdom. A survey of high-school adolescents in the Canadian province of Nova Scotia found that approximately half of the students drank alcohol, a third smoked cigarettes, a third smoked cannabis, a fifth used all three agents, and a third used none of them. Use of all three drugs correlated with low academic achievement, older age, and a higher risk of "harm."[3]

Further evidence of the harm of adolescent drug use comes from a study of about 1800 male and female adolescents (mean age 15.7 years) in the Canadian province of Quebec. Half of those evaluated had used illegal drugs at least once, and a third had used them more than five times in their life. (Over two thirds of those who ever used illegal drugs used them more than five times.) If only one drug was used, it was almost always marijuana, whereas if two were used, they were usually marijuana and hallucinogens. Among those who had taken drugs on more than five occasions 94% of the boys and 85% of the girls reported at least one drug-related problem: used drugs in the morning; drugged or high while at school; played sports while drugged; drove a motor vehicle while drugged; had arguments with friends or parents because of drugs; got into fights because of drugs; or had trouble with the police because of drugs. Once the threshold of five uses of illicit drugs in a lifetime was surpassed, drug problems seemed to become the norm. Alcohol was used more frequently in this adolescent population but led to problems less frequently.[4]

Caffeine

Caffeine increases arousal and vigilance and decreases reaction times and fatigue.[5] Withdrawal symptoms are reported in both adults[6] and children[5] and may persist for up to a week. Symptoms of withdrawal include feelings of anxiety or depression, fatigue and headaches in adults,[6] and decreased attention span in children.[5] Whether caffeine is a "gateway" drug for children that is predictive of an increased risk of using illicit drugs is unknown.[5]

Cocaine

A New York City study found that two thirds of deaths from cocaine were due to fatal injuries caused by homicide, suicide, traffic accidents, and falls and that one third were due to drug overdose.[7] Mortality from cocaine overdoses increases dramatically during heat waves. This may be because cocaine increases core body temperature through a variety of mechanisms, including increased muscular activity, peripheral vasoconstriction, and direct action on the hypothalamus.[8] Chronic cocaine use leads to dose-related decrements in neurocognitive functioning such as attention, concentration, planning, executive functioning, and mental flexibility even after 1 month of abstinence. Such changes may be partially responsible for the difficulty many patients have in maintaining long-term abstinence.[9]

Treatment programs for cocaine abuse may be long term or short term, inpatient or outpatient. No specific pharmacological therapy for this addiction is available.[10] A variety of treatment programs have been used for cocaine addiction. Some of the major ones are individual drug counseling, group drug counseling, cognitive therapy, and supportive-expressive psychodynamic therapy. One study comparing a number of these approaches found that best results were obtained with a combination of individual drug counseling and group drug counseling. The authors postulated that a coherent focus on the importance of stopping drugs was an effective initial intervention and that once this was accomplished, other psychotherapies might be beneficial for patients with comorbid psychiatric conditions.[11]

An evaluation of outcomes from a number of United States programs found that after 1 year about one fourth of patients returned to regular cocaine use. Patients with multiple problems such as using several drugs of abuse, having an alcohol problem, participating in criminal activities, being unemployed, having few social supports, or suffering from clinically significant anxiety or depression had a worse prognosis. For patients with multiple problems, residential treatment lasting at least 3 months seemed necessary.[10]

Marijuana

Most studies of the long-term cognitive effects of heavy marijuana use have methodological flaws, and whether long-term adverse effects on the central nervous system occur is simply not known. In contrast, numerous studies clearly indicate long-term cognitive deficits from prolonged heavy drinking.[12]

Gambling

The lifetime prevalence of gambling disorders in the United States is about 5%. A survey of family practice patients in Wisconsin found the prevalence rate for gambling disorders to be 6.2%. Those at greatest risk were nonwhite unmarried males under the age of 30 with low educational achievement and low income.[13]

⬥ REFERENCES ⬥

1. Leshner AI: Science-based views of drug addiction and its treatment, *JAMA* 282:1314-1316, 1999.
2. Merikangas KR, Stolar M, Stevens DE, et al: Familial transmission of substance use disorders, *Arch Gen Psychiatry* 55:973-979, 1998.
3. Poulin C, Elliott D: Alcohol, tobacco and cannabis use among Nova Scotia adolescents: implications for prevention and harm reduction, *Can Med Assoc J* 156:1387-1393, 1997.
4. Zoccolillo M, Vitaro F, Tremblay RE: Problem drug and alcohol use in a community sample of adolescents, *J Am Acad Child Adolesc Psychiatry* 38:900-907, 1999.
5. Bernstein GA, Carroll ME, Dean NW, et al: Caffeine withdrawal in normal school-age children, *J Am Acad Child Adolesc Psychiatry* 37:858-865, 1998.
6. Silverman K, Evans SM, Strain EC, et al: Withdrawal syndrome after the double-blind cessation of caffeine consumption, *N Engl J Med* 327:1109-1114, 1992.
7. Parzuk PM, Tardiff K, Leon AC, et al: Fatal injuries after cocaine use as a leading cause of death among young adults in New York City, *N Engl J Med* 332:1753-1757, 1995.
8. Marzuk PM, Tardiff K, Leon AC, et al: Ambient temperature and mortality from unintentional cocaine overdose, *JAMA* 279:1795-1800, 1998.
9. Bolla KI, Rothman R, Cadet JL: Dose-related neurobehavioral effects of chronic cocaine use, *J Neuropsychiatry Clin Neurosci* 11:361-369, 1999.
10. Simpson DD, Joe GW, Fletcher BW, et al: A national evaluation of treatment outcomes for cocaine dependence, *Arch Gen Psychiatry* 56:507-514, 1999.
11. Crits-Christoph P, Siqueland L, Blaine J, et al: Psychosocial treatments for cocaine dependence: National Institute on Drug Abuse Collaborative Cocaine Treatment Study, *Arch Gen Psychiatry* 56:493-502, 1999.
12. Block RI: Does heavy marijuana use impair human cognition and brain function? (editorial), *JAMA* 275:560-561, 1996.
13. Pasternak AV, Fleming MF: Prevalence of gambling disorders in a primary care setting, *Arch Fam Med* 8:515-520, 1999.

RESPIROLOGY

(See also thrombophlebitis)

Topics covered in this section

ASTHMA

(See also allergic rhinitis; aspirin; asthma in children; cough)

Epidemiology, Diagnosis, and Classification

Asthma usually first manifests itself in childhood or young adulthood. Between 30% and 70% of children with asthma have marked improvement or resolution of symptoms by the time they become adults. Such resolution is seen more often in patients with milder forms of the disease.[1] In many women symptoms of asthma worsen during the premenstrual or menstrual phases of the cycle.[2]

According to the National Asthma Education and Preventive Program (NAEPP), spirometry is necessary to make a diagnosis of asthma. Peak flow meter readings are useful for following the course of asthma, but reference standards have not been established for making the diagnosis with these devices.[3]

NAEPP classifies asthma into four categories according to a number of clinical and laboratory criteria. These are the categories and some of the clinical criteria[3]:

1. Mild intermittent (symptoms twice a week or less and night symptoms twice a month or less)
2. Mild persistent (symptoms more than twice a week but less than once a day and night symptoms more than twice a month)
3. Moderate persistent (daily symptoms, daily use of short-acting beta-agonists, and nocturnal symptoms more than once a week)
4. Severe persistent (continual symptoms during the day and frequent symptoms at night)

In mild intermittent asthma the peak expiratory flow rate (PEFR) has a variability of less than 20%, in mild persistent asthma the variability is 20% to 30%, and in moderate and severe persistent asthma the variability is greater than 30%.[3]

The issue of cough variant asthma is discussed in the sections on cough and asthma in children.

────────── ◤ REFERENCES ◢ ──────────

1. O'Connor GT, Weiss ST, Speizer FE: The epidemiology of asthma. In Gershwin ME, ed: *Bronchial asthma,* ed 2, Orlando, Fla, 1986, Grune & Stratton.
2. Case AM, Reid RL: Effects of the menstrual cycle on medical disorders, *Arch Intern Med* 158:1405-1412, 1998.
3. National Asthma Education Program: *Guidelines for the diagnosis and management of asthma: expert panel report,* NIH Pub No 91-3042, Bethesda, Md, 1991, National Heart, Lung, and Blood Institute, National Institutes of Health.

Spirometry and Peak Flow Measurements

The NAEPP guidelines recommend that in the diagnosis and management of asthma physicians use objective measurements of pulmonary function such as forced expiratory volume in one second (FEV_1) before and after inhaling a short-acting bronchodilator. This is measured at the initial visit, after the asthma has been stabilized by treatment, and every 1 to 2 years thereafter.[1]

Patients with moderate to severe persistent asthma are advised by NAEPP to monitor peak flow volumes at home using peak flow meters. The argument for doing so is that some patients cannot perceive decreasing values of FEV_1 and therefore would benefit from objective measurements. This recommendation is based on expert opinion, since some studies have not shown that determining PEFR at home makes any difference.[1] For example, Malo and associates[2] found that patient self-assessment diaries (recording nocturnal symptoms, persistent morning dyspnea after bronchodilator inhalation, shorter duration of benefit after bronchodilator inhalation, and inability to go to work or school) were as accurate in detecting exacerbations as was the determination of PEFR.[2] Chan-Yeung and associates[3] reported that symptom diaries were more effective in identifying exacerbations than were twice-daily PEFR readings. On the other hand, a randomized study of patients who were selected because they required emergency room treatment for asthma found that those using a peak flow–based action plan had far fewer subsequent emergency room visits than did those assigned to a symptom-based action plan or no action plan. The authors suggest that the subset of asthmatic patients who require emergency treatment may include a disproportionate number of individuals who have poor perceptions of their deteriorating respiratory status.[4]

Different commercial brands of peak flow meters give different readings. Therefore the patient should always use the same meter. The purpose of determining PEFR at home is to be able to compare the daily results to the patient's personal best readings. The personal best is obtained by recording the best of readings taken immediately after inhaling short-acting bronchodilators during a 2- to 3-week period when the asthma is well controlled. If the daily readings are more than 80% of the personal best, control is good. If they are 50% to 80%, caution is indicated, a beta$_2$-agonist should be taken immediately, and further adjustment of medica-

tions is probably indicated. If the readings are less that 50% of personal best, a beta$_2$-agonist should be taken and immediate medical care obtained.[1]

In general, PEFR should be obtained in the morning. If the values fall below 80% of personal best, more frequent monitoring may be indicated.[1]

────────── ◤ REFERENCES ◢ ──────────

1. National Asthma Education and Prevention Program (National Heart, Lung, and Blood Institute), Second Expert Panel on the Management of Asthma: *Expert panel report 2: guidelines for the diagnosis and management of asthma,* NIH Pub No 97-4051, Bethesda, Md, 1997, National Institutes of Health.
2. Malo J-L, L'Archevêque J, Trudeau C, et al: Should we monitor peak expiratory flow rates or record symptoms with a simple diary in the management of asthma? *J Allergy Clin Immunol* 91:702-709, 1993.
3. Chan-Yeung M, Chan JH, Manfreda J, et al: Changes in peak flow, symptom score, and the use of medications during acute exacerbations of asthma, *Am J Respir Crit Care Med* 154:889-893, 1996.
4. Cowie RL, Revitt SG, Underwood MF, et al: The effect of a peak flow-based action plan in the prevention of exacerbations of asthma, *Chest* 112:1534-1538, 1997.

Delivery Systems for Inhaled Medications

Types of delivery systems

Delivery systems for inhaled medications used for outpatients are generally divided into two major categories: metered dose inhalers (MDIs) with propellants and dry powder inhalers (inspiratory flow–generated aerosols). If the patient cannot generate an adequate airflow, the latter devices are ineffective.[1]

Although traditional practice is to use nebulizers to deliver beta$_2$-agonists to hospitalized patients and young children, the supervised use of MDIs with spacer devices has proved as effective in the emergency setting as nebulizer therapy for both adults[2] and children.[3]

Metered dose inhalers

When MDIs are used, the open mouth technique is said to be more effective than the closed mouth technique. The open mouth technique is performed as follows[4]:

1. Remove the cap of the MDI.
2. Shake the MDI several times.
3. Hold the MDI vertically about 2.5 to 5 cm (1 to 2 inches) from the open mouth.
4. Tilt the head slightly backward.
5. Exhale normally (not a forced or maximum exhalation).
6. Breathe in at a moderate rate, and activate the MDI in the middle of inspiration.
7. Hold the breath for 10 seconds or more.

Whether an MDI is full or empty can be determined by placing it in a bowl of water. If it sinks, it is full, and if it floats sideways, it is empty.[4]

Not all patients are able to use MDIs correctly. In a study of elderly subjects with a mean age of 70, only about half used the devices properly 1 week after an extensive instructional session. Major determinants of failure have been shown to be cognitive impairments and weak hand strength.[5] These problems may be overcome with the use of spacers (see below).

Spacers

Spacers or aerochambers are designed to be used with MDIs. Large particles are precipitated out in the chamber, slightly higher effective doses reach the lungs, and much less drug is deposited in the oropharynx and therefore is swallowed and absorbed systemically (see the discussion of local side effects of inhaled steroids). MDIs connected to spacers require less coordination to use than MDIs alone, so they are particularly helpful for children, the aged, the disabled, and the uncoordinated. Proper use of spacers requires that the MDI be activated only once for each inhalation and that the inhalation be started as soon as possible after the activation.[6] Spacers for very young children and infants come with masks that are applied to the child's face. Many studies have demonstrated that the delivery of bronchodilators by MDIs with spacers is at least as effective for young children with acute asthma as small-volume nebulizers.[7]

Commercial spacers are expensive. Home-made spacers may be created by inserting an MDI into the bottom of a polystyrene cup (the open end is pressed against the child's face to act as a face mask) or by inserting an MDI into the bottom of a soft drink bottle (the neck is held in the mouth and the lips create a seal). A comparison of these two types of home-made devices and a commercial spacer in the treatment of acute asthma found that the commercial and soft drink bottle spacers were equally effective while only a small benefit was achieved with the cup. A 500-ml soft drink bottle was used in this study. The bottom was cut out with a hot wire molded to the exact shape of the mouthpiece of the MDI, and the MDI was immediately inserted and sealed in place with glue. Before use the bottle was primed with 15 activations of the MDI to decrease the electrostatic charge on its inner surface (rinsing with detergent is equally effective).[8]

Turbuhalers

The dose of medication from a Turbuhaler is made accessible by turning the bottom of the device. The instructions that come with the apparatus are clear, and the pharmacist is a good resource if problems occur. The basic way of using a dry powder inhaler is as follows[4]:
1. Prepare the dose.
2. Expire fully (forced or maximum expiration).
3. Close the mouth tightly around the mouthpiece.
4. Inhale fully and rapidly.

The inhalation technique with a Turbuhaler differs from that of the MDI, in which expiration is not forced and inspiration is at a moderate rate. The patient using a Turbuhaler will not feel the medication going into the airways as is usu-

ally the case with MDIs. Medications available with Turbuhalers include terbutaline (Bricanyl) and budesonide (Pulmicort). Children over the age of 8 years can easily learn to use Turbuhalers.[9]

Concentration of drugs reaching the lungs

Reports of concentrations of medications reaching the lungs from various delivery systems vary from one reference to another. All figures indicate that use of an MDI plus an aerochamber or use of a Turbuhaler leads to a greater concentration of medication deposition in the lungs than does an MDI alone. One report showed that a Turbuhaler delivers about twice as much steroid to the lungs as do standard MDIs.[10] Another study found that with a Turbuhaler a normal inhalation resulted in almost twice as much pulmonary delivery as did a slow inhalation.[11]

❧ REFERENCES ❧

1. Fong PM, Sinclair D: Inhalation devices for asthma, *Can Fam Physician* 39:2377-2382, 1993.
2. Turner MO, Patel A, Ginsburg S, et al: Bronchodilator delivery in acute airflow obstruction: a meta-analysis, *Arch Intern Med* 1736-1744, 1997.
3. Kelly HW, Murphy S: Beta-adrenergic agonists for acute, severe asthma, *Ann Pharmacother* 26:81-91, 1992.
4. Szefler SJ, Chambers CV: Diagnosis and management of asthma, *Am Fam Physician* Monogr No 2 1995, pp 1-25.
5. Gray SL, Williams DM, Pulliam CC, et al: Characteristics predicting incorrect metered-dose inhaler technique in older subjects, *Arch Intern Med* 156:948-988, 1996.
6. O'Callaghan C, Barry P: Spacer devices in the treatment of asthma: amount of drug delivered to the patient can vary greatly (editorial), *BMJ* 314:1061-1062, 1997.
7. Amirav I, Newhouse MT: Metered-dose inhaler accessory devices in acute asthma, *Arch Pediatr Adolesc Med* 151:876-882, 1997.
8. Zar HJ, Brown G, Donson H, et al: Home-made spacers for bronchodilator therapy in children with acute asthma: a randomised trial, *Lancet* 354:979-982, 1999.
9. De Boeck K, Alifier M, Warnier G: Is the correct use of a dry powder inhaler (Turbohaler) age dependent? *J Allergy Clin Immunol* 103:763-767, 1999.
10. Thorsson L, Edsbäcker S, Conradson TB: Lung deposition of budesonide from Turbuhaler is twice that from a pressurized metered-dose inhaler P-MDI, *Eur Respir J* 7:1839-1844, 1994.
11. Borgstrom L, Bondesson E, Moren F, et al: Lung deposition of budesonide inhaled via Turbuhaler: a comparison with terbutaline sulphate in normal subjects, *Eur Respir J* 7:69-73, 1994.

Principles of Asthma Pharmacotherapy
(See also drugs and chemicals in pregnancy)

Four of the major goals of the pharmacotherapy of asthma are to ameliorate symptoms, maintain near-normal pulmonary function, maintain normal activity levels, and prevent exacerbations and emergency room visits.[1]

Drugs for asthma may be divided into two main categories: long-term control medications (controllers) and quick-relief medications (relievers). Long-term control medications include corticosteroids, cromolyn sodium and nedocromil, long-acting beta$_2$-agonists, methylxanthines, and leukotriene modifiers. Quick-relief medications are short-acting beta$_2$-agonists and anticholinergics.[1,2] Specific drug regimens are discussed in the next section.

Asthma is caused by inflammation of the airways, and the most effective therapeutic drugs are antiinflammatory agents. Corticosteroids are the most potent antiinflammatories, and for most patients with stable moderate or severe asthma, twice-daily use of inhaled formulations of these agents is the cornerstone of treatment (Table 66).[1-4] Oral corticosteroids are used primarily (and liberally) for acute flare-ups of asthma,[1,3] and unless the patient is extremely ill, the oral route is just as effective as the parenteral one (see discussion of emergency treatment of asthma).[1] Inhaled steroids should be given concurrently with the oral steroids and continued after the oral steroids have been stopped.[2]

Leukotriene modifiers are a new category of oral agents that have both antiinflammatory and bronchodilator activity.[1,4,5] Included in this class are zafirlukast (Accolate), montelukast (Singulair), and zileuton (Zyflo) (Table 67).[4] Leukotriene modifiers are logical choices as add-on or second-line drugs for patients whose asthma is inadequately controlled with inhaled steroids[1,2,4] but may be used as first-line therapy in patients with mild persistent asthma.[1,5] Long-acting beta$_2$-agonists such as salmeterol (Serevent) or formoterol (Oxeze, Foradil) (Table 66) are also good second-line drugs for patients whose control is inadequate

with inhaled steroids or who require very high doses of inhaled steroids. For a few patients theophylline may be an effective add-on drug,[1,2,4] but even at low doses it is often not well tolerated (see later discussion).[3]

Cromones such as sodium cromoglycate (Intal) or nedocromil (Tilade) (Table 66) have mild antiinflammatory properties and are sometimes useful for patients with mild asthma,[1,3,4] especially for children who have an exercise or allergic component to their disease.[4]

Short-acting beta$_2$-adrenergic agonists should be used alone only for very mild asthma and for exercise-induced asthma (Table 66). If a person with mild asthma needs daily inhalations of a beta$_2$-agonist, or if the person needs increasing doses of these agents, he or she probably requires the addition of antiinflammatory medications such as inhaled corticosteroids.[1,2,4] Patients with mild asthma do as well taking beta$_2$-agonists on an as-needed basis as they do taking regularly scheduled doses.[6] Large doses of beta$_2$-agonists along with steroids are used for the emergency treatment of asthma (see later discussion).[1,2]

NAEPP advises a "step care" approach to the treatment of asthma. The physician can start treatment at the level of the patients' symptoms and augment it if necessary. Alternatively, therapy can be initiated at a higher level, and once symptoms are controlled, the number or doses of medications can be carefully decreased as tolerated (see discussion of classification of asthma). In general, patients with mild intermittent asthma do not need daily medication, those with mild persistent asthma require a daily antiinflammatory drug such as a low-dose inhaled steroid, cromolyn (Intal), or zafirlukast (Accolate), those with moderate persistent asthma need a daily medium-dose inhaled corticosteroid, and those with severe persistent asthma should have daily high-dose inhaled corticosteroids plus oral corticosteroids plus long-acting bronchodilators such as salmeterol, a leukotriene antagonist, or theophylline.[1]

Some of the key recommendations of the NAEPP for the home management of exacerbations of asthma are as follows[1]:

1. Start with up to three treatments of two to four inhalations of a beta$_2$-agonist at 20-minute intervals
2. If the response is good (resolution of symptoms and PEFR greater than 80% of predicted or personal best), take a beta$_2$-agonist q3-4h for 1 to 2 days. If taking corticosteroids, double the dose for 7 to 10 days.
3. If the response is incomplete (PEFR 50% to 80% of predicted or personal best and persistent shortness of breath and wheezing), continue taking a beta$_2$-agonist as above and add an oral steroid.
4. If the response is poor (PEFR less than 50% of predicted or personal best and marked shortness of breath and wheezing) take more beta$_2$-agonist immediately, add an oral corticosteroid, and if no response occurs within a very short time, obtain emergency medical care.

Table 66   Inhaled Medications for Asthma

Names	Delivery systems
Beta$_2$-Adrenergic Agonists, Nonselective	
Metaproterenol or orciprenaline (Alupent)	MDI
Beta$_2$-Adrenergic Agonists, Selective, Short Acting	
Albuterol or salbutamol (Proventil, Ventolin)	MDI
Fenoterol (Berotec)	MDI
Pirbuterol (Maxair)	MDI
Terbutaline (Bricanyl, Brethaire)	Turbuhaler
Beta$_2$-Adrenergic Agonists, Selective, Long Acting	
Formoterol (Oxeze, Foradil)	Dry powder capsule and inhaler device
Salmeterol (Serevent)	MDI
Anticholinergics	
Ipratropium bromide (Atrovent)	MDI
Corticosteroids	
Beclomethasone dipropionate (Beclovent, Becloforte)	MDI
Budesonide (Pulmicort)	Turbuhaler
Fluticasone propionate (Flovent)	MDI
Flunisolide (Aerobid, Bronalide)	MDI
Triamcinolone acetonide (Azmacort)	MDI
Cromones	
Cromolyn or sodium cromoglycate (Intal)	MDI
Nedocromil sodium (Tilade)	MDI

According to studies from a few centers, gastroesophageal reflux may cause asthma, probably through reflex bronchoconstriction precipitated by esophageal irritation from refluxed gastric contents.[7-10] In many of these cases GERD is asymptomatic and can be diagnosed only with tests such as 24-hour esophageal pH monitoring.[7] Harding and associates[8] state that treatment with dietary and positional modifications and proton pump inhibitors such as omeprazole (Prilosec, Losec) 20 mg bid for 3 months (shorter treatment duration may not be effective) causes improvement in most patients with proven GERD and asthma.[8] The evidence supporting these claims is tenuous. Most studies have involved small numbers of patients, few studies have been controlled or randomized, and follow-up periods have been short.[10,11]

◁ REFERENCES ▷

1. National Asthma Education and Prevention Program (National Heart, Lung, and Blood Institute) Second Expert Panel on the Management of Asthma: *Expert panel report 2: guidelines for the diagnosis and management of asthma,* NIH Pub No 97-4051, Bethesda, Md, 1997, National Institutes of Health.
2. Boulet L-P, Becker A, Bérubé D, et al: Summary of recommendations from the Canadian Asthma Consensus Report, 1999, *Can Med Assoc J* 161(suppl 11):S1-S12, 1999.
3. Drugs for asthma, *Med Lett* 37:1-4, 1995.
4. Lipworth BJ: Modern drug treatment of chronic asthma, *BMJ* 318:380-384, 1999.
5. Smith LJ: Newer asthma therapies (editorial), *Ann Intern Med* 130:531-532, 1999.
6. Drazen JM, Israel E, Boushey HA, et al: Comparison of regularly scheduled with as-needed use of albuterol in mild asthma, *N Engl J Med* 335:841-847, 1996.
7. Irwin RS, Curley FJ, French CL: Difficult-to-control asthma: contributing factors and outcome of a systematic management protocol, *Chest* 103:1662-1669, 1993.
8. Harding SM, Richter JE, Guzzo MR, et al: Asthma and gastroesophageal reflux: acid suppressive therapy improves asthma outcome, *Am J Med* 100:395-405, 1996.
9. Harding SM, Richter JE: The role of gastroesophageal reflux in chronic cough and asthma, *Chest* 111:1389-1402, 1997.
10. Vandenplas Y: Asthma and gastroesophageal reflux, *J Pediatr Gastroenterol Nutr* 24:89-99, 1997.
11. Field S, Sutherland LR: Does medical antireflux therapy improve asthma in asthmatics with gastroesophageal reflux? A critical review of the literature, *Chest* 114:275-283, 1998.

Drugs for Asthma

(See also cataracts; Churg-Strauss syndrome; glaucoma, open angle)

Beta₂-adrenergic agonists, short acting

Beta₂-adrenergic agonists such as albuterol (or as it is called in Canada, salbutamol) (Proventil, Ventolin) are potent bronchodilators. A number of the available agents that are administered by inhalation are listed in Table 66. They are used in large doses for the emergency management of asthma in conjunction with steroids (see discussion of emergency treatment of asthma), for the management of exercise- or cold-induced asthma (see discussion of exercise-induced asthma), and as adjunctive treatment for patients taking inhaled steroids for moderate or severe asthma. For a few patients with mild intermittent asthma, beta₂-adrenergic agonists may be used as sole therapy (see discussion of pharmacotherapy for asthma).[1]

Oral forms of beta₂-agonists may be used for children who cannot take the inhaled agents. Metaproterenol (or as it is called in Canada orciprenaline) (Alupent) is available not only as an MDI, but as a syrup and tablets. The usual oral dose is 10 mg tid prn for children 4 to 12 years of age and 20 mg tid prn for children over 12.

Beta₂-adrenergic agonists, long acting

An increasing body of evidence supports the use of long-acting beta₂-agonists such as salmeterol (Serevent) or formoterol (Oxeze, Foradil) as adjuncts in the treatment of patients whose moderate persistent asthma is inadequately controlled by standard doses of inhaled corticosteroids (Table 66). Improvements noted with such regimens include reduction of the daily symptoms and number of exacerbations and augmentation of measured lung function.[2]

Salmeterol appears to be especially useful for preventing nocturnal asthma attacks and exercise-induced asthma.[3] If salmeterol is used, short-acting beta₂-agonists may still be needed for acute exacerbations. Salmeterol must never be used by patients to treat an acute asthmatic attack, since this has caused fatalities.[4] Long-acting beta₂-agonists may have a role in the management of exercise-induced asthma (see discussion of exercise-induced asthma).

Inhaled corticosteroids

A number of the available inhaled steroids are listed in Table 66.

Increasing dose during exacerbations. Physicians commonly recommend that asthmatics taking regular doses of inhaled corticosteroids increase the dose at the onset of a cold or the beginning of an asthmatic exacerbation. Little evidence in the literature deals with this topic. One randomized double-blind placebo-controlled trial of such a protocol in children with mild to moderate asthma found no benefit from doubling the inhaled steroid dose for 3 days.[5]

Systemic side effects. Potential adverse effects of inhaled corticosteroids are adrenal suppression, osteoporosis, growth suppression, cataracts, and ocular hypertension. Such reactions have rarely been observed in adults if the daily dose was less than 800 µg/day or in children if it was less than 400 µg/day. If asthma is inadequately controlled with usual doses of inhaled corticosteroids, addition of a second-line drug such as a leukotriene modifier or a long-acting beta₂-agonist is usually better than increasing the dose of inhaled steroids even further.[6]

Budesonide (Pulmicort) has less systemic bioavailability than beclomethasone (Beclovent) because the rate of bio-transformation on first pass in the liver is greater with budesonide and because budesonide does not have active metabolites. The clinical significance of these findings is unclear, but choosing budesonide for patients requiring higher doses seems reasonable, since no important systemic effects have been noted with daily doses of 1600 to 2000 µg.[7] Fluticasone propionate (FloVent) produces a greater dose-related adrenal suppression than budesonide, especially at doses greater than 800 µg/day.[6]

The effect of inhaled steroids on growth in children is discussed under "Asthma" in the pediatrics section.

Local side effects. Local side effects of inhaled steroids include thrush and dysphonia or hoarseness, which is probably due to steroid myopathy of laryngeal muscles. These adverse effects, particularly dysphonia, occur less frequently when using spacers, diskhalers, or Turbuhalers.[8] In one study the incidence of dysphonia with Turbuhalers was 6% compared with 21% in patients using MDIs.[9] With the spacer or aerochamber, many large particles are precipitated out in the chamber, so fewer fall on the buccal or pharyngeal mucosa. With the diskhalers and Turbuhalers the drug is delivered by rapid active inhalation, which causes partial closure of the false cords, giving some protection to the larynx. The Turbuhaler is particularly useful, at least in theory, because the medication is not adsorbed to lactose, so there are fewer large particles to precipitate out in the mouth and pharynx. In addition to spacer devices, rinsing out the mouth and gargling with water after steroid inhalation are said to decrease the incidence of thrush.[8]

Oral corticosteroids

When oral steroids are used for asthma, a 10- to 14-day course of 0.6 mg/kg/day as a single morning dose (about 40 mg/day for most patients) can be safely given without tapering.[7] Oral steroids in doses of 40 to 60 mg/day are as effective as IV corticosteroids for acute asthmatic attacks treated in the ambulatory setting.[1]

If patients require long-term oral corticosteroid treatment, an effort should be made to prevent the development of osteoporosis through life-style modifications such as discontinuation of smoking, exercise, and calcium and vitamin D supplementation. In some cases hormone replacement therapy may be used, and in others bisphosphonates might be helpful (see also discussion of osteoporosis).[10]

Cromones

Cromolyn, which is also called sodium or disodium cromoglycate (Intal), may be useful for mild asthma in children and as a prophylactic agent for exercise and cold-induced asthma. It is supplied as an MDI, and the usual dose is 2 to 4 puffs tid or qid. Up to 6 weeks may be necessary to determine whether the drug is effective. Nedocromil sodium (Ti-lade) is also supplied as an MDI. The usual dosage for adults and children over the age of 6 is two activations qid. Both cromolyn and nedocromil are less effective than inhaled corticosteroids in moderate or severe asthma.[11]

Leukotriene modifiers

Leukotriene modifiers are a new category of oral agents used for the treatment of asthma (Table 67). They block both the proinflammatory and potent bronchoconstrictor activity of cysteinyl leukotrienes within the airways. Some such as zafirlukast (Accolate) and montelukast (Singulair) are cysteinyl leukotriene receptor antagonists, whereas others such as zileuton (Zyflo) inhibit the synthesis of cysteinyl leukotriene. Although these drugs have been reported to be as effective in controlling asthmatic symptoms in patients with mild or moderate asthma as 400 to 500 µg/day of inhaled beclomethasone (Beclovent), other data suggest that they are not quite as potent as inhaled corticosteroids. Leukotriene modifiers are particularly useful for patients with exercise- and cold-induced asthma and for those with bronchospastic reactions to aspirin and other nonsteroidal antiinflammatory reactions. They have been shown to decrease the number of nighttime awakenings, and their use in patients taking corticosteroids may lead to lower requirements for the steroids.[6,12,13] A few cases of Churg-Strauss syndrome have been reported in patients taking leukotriene modifiers (see discussion of Churg-Strauss syndrome).

Theophylline preparations

Theophylline preparations are sometimes helpful in asthma or chronic obstructive pulmonary disease. They are indicated for patients (such as toddlers) unable or unwilling to use inhaled agents and as additive therapy for patients whose disease is not well controlled with adequate doses of inhaled steroids,[14,15] particularly if nocturnal asthma is a problem.[16] In one study of patients whose asthma was poorly controlled with 800 µg of inhaled budesonide (Pulmicort) daily, the addition of a low-dose sustained release theophylline product was just as effective in improving outcomes as was doubling the daily dose of budesonide. This benefit was achieved even though the median blood theophylline level was 8.7 µg/ml, which is below accepted therapeutic levels.[15]

Aside from producing bronchodilation, theophylline products may have some antiinflammatory and bronchopro-

Table 67	Leukotriene Modifiers
Drug	**Usual doses**
Zafirlukast (Accolate)	20 mg po bid 1 hour ac or 2 hours pc for adults and children ≥12 years
Montelukast (Singulair)	10 mg po once daily in the evening for adults and children ≥15 years; 5 mg once daily in the evening for children aged 6-14
Zileuton (Zyflo)	600 mg po qid for adults

tective effects and are reputed to decrease diaphragmatic muscle fatigue.[14-16] Toxicity is an ever present hazard, especially for the elderly, and in patients taking theophylline on a long-term basis toxicity can become manifest at therapeutic blood levels.[17] Some comfort might be taken from evidence that the drug may be effective at subtherapeutic levels,[15,16] but prudence dictates extreme caution in prescribing it.

Therapeutic blood levels of theophylline are between 55 and 110 μmol/L (10 and 20 μg/ml). For monitoring of serum concentrations, levels should be assessed 4 to 8 hours after the last dose once a steady state is achieved. A steady state is reached about 3 days after the initiation of therapy or a change in dose, provided the medications are taken regularly.[14]

Two of the available sustained-release theophylline preparations are Uniphyl, which is usually started at 400 to 600 mg as a single dose in the evening with or within 1 to 2 hours of a meal, and Theo-Dur, which is usually started at 200 to 300 mg q12h. Oxtriphylline (Choledyl) is short acting and is usually prescribed as 200 mg qid for adults. The usual dosage for children under 5 years is 24 to 36 mg/kg/day divided into 3 equal doses given at 8-hour intervals. The dosage for children over the age of 5 is 22 mg/kg/day divided into 4 equal doses.

❧ REFERENCES ❧

1. National Asthma Education and Prevention Program (National Heart, Lung, and Blood Institute) Second Expert Panel on the Management of Asthma: *Expert panel report 2: guidelines for the diagnosis and management of asthma,* NIH Pub No 97-4051, Bethesda, Md, 1997, National Institutes of Health.
2. Pauwels R, Löfdahl C-G, Postma DS, et al: Effect of inhaled formoterol and budesonide on exacerbations of asthma, *N Engl J Med* 337:1405-1411, 1997.
3. Nelson HS: ß-Adrenergic bronchodilators, *N Engl J Med* 333:499-506, 1995.
4. Bone RC: Another word of caution regarding a new long-acting bronchodilator (editorial), *JAMA* 273:967-968, 1995.
5. Garrett J, Williams S, Wong C, et al: Treatment of acute asthmatic exacerbations with an increased dose of inhaled steroid, *Arch Dis Child* 79:12-17, 1998.
6. Lipworth BJ: Modern drug treatment of chronic asthma, *BMJ* 318:380-384, 1999.
7. Bai TR: Glucocorticosteroid treatment of asthma, *Can Fam Physician* 41:1921-1927, 1995.
8. Barnes PJ, Pedersen S: Efficacy and safety of inhaled corticosteroids in asthma: report of a workshop held in Eze, France, October 1992, *Am Rev Respir Dis* 148:S1-S26, 1993.
9. Selroos SO, Backman R, Forsen K-O, et al: Local side effects during four years treatment with inhaled corticosteroids—a comparison between metered dose inhalers and Turbuhalers, *Allergy* 49:888-890, 1994.
10. Cowan S, Ernst P: Bisphosphonates and glucocorticoid-induced osteoporosis: implications for patients with respiratory diseases (editorial), *Thorax* 53:331-332, 1998.
11. Drugs for asthma, *Med Lett* 37:1-4, 1995.
12. Sampson A, Holgate S: Leukotriene modifiers in the treatment of asthma: look promising across the board of asthma severity (editorial), *BMJ* 316:1257-1258, 1998.
13. Drazen J, Israel E, O'Byrne PM: Treatment of asthma with drugs modifying the leukotriene pathway, *N Engl J Med* 340:197-206, 1999.
14. Weinberger M, Hendeles L: Theophylline in asthma, *N Engl J Med* 334:1380-1388, 1996.
15. Evans DJ, Taylor DA, Zetterstrom O, et al: A comparison of low-dose inhaled budesonide plus theophylline and high-dose inhaled budesonide for moderate asthma, *N Engl J Med* 337:1412-1418, 1997.
16. D'Alonzo GE: Theophylline revisited, *Allergy Asthma Proc* 17:335-339, 1996.
17. Shannon M: Life-threatening events after theophylline overdose: a 10-year prospective analysis, *Arch Intern Med* 159:989-994, 1999.

Emergency Treatment of Asthma

Short-acting beta[2]-agonists are the drugs of choice for the initial emergency treatment of asthma (Table 66). MDIs are as effective as wet nebulization if patients are capable of using the devices.[1,2]

NAEPP recommends 4 to 8 puffs of a short-acting beta[2]-agonist every 20 minutes for up to 4 hours and then every 1 to 4 hours as needed. The addition of 4 to 8 puffs of ipratropium bromide (Atrovent) may give some benefit. Systemic corticosteroids should be given immediately. The oral route is as effective as the IV route and should be used whenever possible. The recommended dose of steroids for very ill patients is 120 to 180 mg of prednisone or the equivalent daily for the first 48 hours, reduced to 60 to 80 mg/day thereafter, for a total duration of 7 to 10 days in most instances. For less severely ill patients who can be followed at home, the recommended steroid dose is 40 to 60 mg/day (1 to 2 mg/kg/day for children). If long-term inhaled corticosteroids are planned, they should be started immediately and given concurrently with the systemic steroids.[1]

The guidelines published by the Canadian Association of Emergency Physicians, the Canadian Thoracic Society, and the Association des Médecins d'Urgence du Québec are basically similar to those of NAEPP. MDIs are considered more effective than wet nebulization for the emergency treatment of asthma and should be used whenever possible. In severe asthma a spacer is recommended, but for moderate asthma it is optional. The suggested dosage is 4 to 8 puffs every 15 to 20 minutes. In severe cases 1 puff may be given every minute up to a maximum of 20 puffs. Anticholinergic therapy (ipratropium bromide [Atrovent]) is recommended for severe asthma and may be useful in moderate asthma. Unless systemic steroids are contraindicated, they should be started as soon as possible. The oral route is as efficacious as an IV infusion. Oral steroids such as prednisone in doses of 30 to 60 mg/day should be continued for 7 to 14 days, and tapering is not required for this duration of treatment. Inhaled steroids should be prescribed on discharge and given concomitantly with the oral steroids.[2]

The combined use of oral and inhaled corticosteroids is supported by a randomized controlled trial of patients discharged from the emergency room taking oral prednisone 50 mg/day for 7 days plus either placebo or budesonide (Pulmicort) 800 μg (2 inhalations) bid for 21 days. Those receiving the budesonide had better quality of life and fewer relapses than those receiving the placebo.[3]

Evidence supporting the use of anticholinergic drugs in the emergency treatment of asthma is tenuous. In a series of 384 asthmatic adults treated in the emergency room of a New York hospital with either nebulized albuterol (salbutamol, Ventolin, Proventil) or nebulized albuterol plus ipratropium bromide (Atrovent), no differences in outcome were detectable.[4] A similar study from Cleveland also failed to show any benefit from ipratropium.[5] However, a randomized placebo-controlled trial of 427 asthmatic children treated in the emergency room at Johns Hopkins Hospital in Baltimore found that the addition of ipratropium bromide to standard albuterol therapy led to a reduction in the duration of stay and amount of treatment required before discharge.[6]

◥ REFERENCES ◤

1. National Asthma Education and Prevention Program (National Heart, Lung, and Blood Institute) Second Expert Panel on the Management of Asthma: *Expert panel report 2: guidelines for the diagnosis and management of asthma,* NIH Pub No 97-4051, Bethesda, Md, 1997, National Institutes of Health.
2. Beveridge RC, Grunfeld AF, Hodder RV, et al (CAEP/CTS Asthma Advisory Committee): Guidelines for the emergency management of asthma in adults, *Can Med Assoc J* 155:25-37, 1996.
3. Rowe BH, Bota GW, Fabris L, et al: Inhaled budesonide in addition to oral corticosteroids to prevent asthma relapse following discharge from the emergency department: a randomized controlled trial, *JAMA* 281:2119-2126, 1999.
4. Karpel JP, Schacter EN, Fanta C, et al: A comparison of ipratropium and albuterol vs albuterol alone for the treatment of acute asthma, *Chest* 611-616, 1996.
5. Mcfadden ER, Elsanadi N, Strauss L, et al: The influence of parasympatholytics on the resolution of acute attacks of asthma, *Am J Med* 102:7-13, 1997.
6. Zorc JJ, Pusic MV, Ogborn J, et al: Ipratropium bromide added to asthma treatment in the pediatric emergency department, *Pediatrics* 103:748-752, 1999.

Immunotherapy

Immunotherapy for asthma is controversial although it has been used for over 70 years.[1] One study showed minimal benefits for seasonal allergic asthma to ragweed as measured by skin test sensitivity, bronchoconstrictor response to ragweed, and peak expiratory flow and reduction of medications in the first year, but this was not sustained during the second year.[2] Few asthmatic patients are allergic to only one allergen; many are allergic to house dust mites, cat dander, molds, and cockroaches, and there is little evidence that immunotherapy with these agents has any value.[1] A double-blind, placebo-controlled trial of multiple-allergen immunotherapy in children with moderate to severe year-round asthma demonstrated no beneficial effect after at least 18 months of therapy.[3] Metaanalyses have concluded that there may be some benefit but that because of the adverse effects, the benefits may not outweigh the harm.[4,5]

◥ REFERENCES ◤

1. Barnes PJ: Is immunotherapy for asthma worthwhile? (editorial), *N Engl J Med* 334:531-532, 1996.
2. Creticos PS, Reed CE, Norman PS, et al: Ragweed immunotherapy in adult asthma, *N Engl J Med* 334:501-506, 1996.
3. Adkinson NF Jr, Eggleston PA, Eney D, et al: A controlled trial of immunotherapy for asthma in allergic children, *N Engl J Med* 336:324-331, 1997.
4. Abramson MJ, Puy RM, Weiner JM: Is allergen immunotherapy effective in asthma? A meta-analysis of randomized controlled trials, *Am J Respir Crit Care Med* 151:969-974. 1995.
5. Sigman K, Mazer B: Immunotherapy for childhood asthma: is there a rationale for its use? *Ann Allergy Asthma Immunol* 76: 299-305, 1996.

Exercise-Induced Asthma

Exercise-induced asthma is present in almost every patient who has asthma. Exercise-induced bronchoconstriction often goes unrecognized by patients or physicians, and it probably causes many adults and children to avoid vigorous sports or other activities. Factors likely to aggravate the condition are intense exercise, low temperature, and low humidity.[1] For symptoms to occur, exercise must be maintained for more than 2 minutes.[2]

In patients with exercise-induced asthma, symptoms usually develop shortly after they stop exercising. Spontaneous recovery is usually complete within half an hour to an hour.[2] A few individuals experience a late response with symptoms developing 6 to 10 hours after exercise.[3]

An interesting feature of exercise-induced asthma is that a preliminary bout of mild to moderate exercise decreases the degree of bronchoconstriction during subsequent strenuous exercise (tachyphylaxis). This protective effect lasts for about 40 minutes and can be used therapeutically by athletes if they make a point of doing moderate warm-up exercises before participating in strenuous exercise. The warm-up should last 15 to 30 minutes and be followed by a 15-minute rest before vigorous exercise.[3]

Aside from warm-up exercises, management of exercise-induced asthma usually involves taking an inhaled beta₂-adrenergic agonist such as albuterol or salbutamol (Proventil, Ventolin), cromolyn (sodium cromoglycate, Intal), or nedocromil sodium (Tilade) 10 to 15 minutes before the exercise. For many patients these regimens offer incomplete protection against asthma.[1] Alternatives that may offer significant improvements are the use of long-acting beta[2]-agonists[4,5] or a leukotriene-receptor antagonist.[6,7] In one study of adults salmeterol (Serevent) 2 puffs (42 μg) bid for 1 month was more effective than placebo. In the first few days of treatment the drug was effective for at least 9 hours, but by 30 days of treatment the duration of protection was much shorter.[4] A single 50-μg dose of salmeterol given to children aged 4 and 11 years gave good protection against exercise-induced asthma for up to 12 hours.[5] A trial of montelukast (Singulair) 10 mg once daily at bedtime in patients with exercise-induced asthma found that many experienced significant improvement and that this effect persisted for the full 3 months of the study.[6]

Patients with established asthma whose symptoms are aggravated by exercise usually note a considerable improvement in their exercise-induced symptoms when their asthma is treated with regular doses of inhaled corticosteroids.[1]

◢ REFERENCES ◣

1. Hansen-Flaschen J, Schotland H: New treatments for exercise-induced asthma (editorial), *N Engl J Med* 339:192-193, 1998.
2. McFadden ER Jr, Gilbert IA: Exercise-induced asthma, *N Engl J Med* 330:1362-1367, 1994.
3. D'Urzo AD: Exercise-induced asthma: what family physicians should do, *Can Fam Physician* 41:1900-1906, 1995.
4. Nelson J, Strauss L, Skowronski M, et al: Effect of long-term salmeterol treatment on exercise-induced asthma, *N Engl J Med* 339:141-146, 1998.
5. Blake K, Pearlman DS, Scott C, et al: Prevention of exercise-induced bronchospasm in pediatric asthma patients: a comparison of salmeterol powder and albuterol, *Ann Allergy Asthma Immunol* 82:205-211, 1999.
6. Leff JA, Busse WW, Pearlman D, et al: Montelukast, a leukotriene-receptor antagonist, for the treatment of mild asthma and exercise-induced bronchoconstrictio, *N Engl J Med* 339:147-152, 1998.
7. Drazen J, Israel E, O'Byrne PM: Treatment of asthma with drugs modifying the leukotriene pathway, *N Engl J Med* 340:197-206, 1999.

BRONCHITIS, ACUTE
(See also antibiotic resistance; asthma; cough)

Acute bronchitis may be defined as cough and sputum developing in previously healthy individuals, usually after an upper respiratory tract infection. Other diseases, especially asthma and flare-ups of COPD, should be ruled out. The vast majority of cases appear to be caused by viruses. A metaanalysis of eight randomized controlled trials of antibiotics (erythromycin, doxycycline, trimethoprim/sulfamethoxazole) found that duration of cough and sputum production was decreased by half a day in those receiving antibiotics—a statistically significant but clinically insignificant result.[1] Some studies have shown beneficial effects from the use of oral and inhaled albuterol (salbutamol, Proventil, Ventolin) and inhaled fenoterol (Berotec).[2]

◢ REFERENCES ◣

1. Bent S, Saint S, Vittinghoff E, et al: Antibiotics in acute bronchitis: a meta-analysis, *Am J Med* 107:62-67, 1999.
2. Hueston WJ, Mainous AG III: Acute bronchitis, *Am Fam Physician* 57:1270-1276, 1998.

CHRONIC BRONCHITIS AND EMPHYSEMA
(See also asthma; bronchitis, acute)

Chronic obstructive pulmonary disease (COPD) is a chronic slowly progressive disease characterized by airway obstruction that is largely fixed but may be partially reversible by bronchodilator or other therapy. COPD encompasses both chronic bronchitis and emphysema, which are now thought to be variants of the same basic disorder. It also includes some cases of chronic asthma.[1]

Spirometry is required to confirm the diagnosis of COPD; the forced expiratory volume in 1 second (FEV_1) is less than 80% of the predicted value. Measurement of PEFR is usually inadequate for making the diagnosis, but if there is more than a 20% variability in the absolute measurements of serial PEFRs, the diagnosis of asthma should be considered.[1] Patients with COPD may be said to have chronic bronchitis if they have excessive cough, productive of sputum on most days, for at least 3 months a year during at least 2 consecutive years.[2]

Epidemiology

Smoking is the major risk factor for COPD and accounts for 80% to 90% of cases, although clinically significant COPD develops in only 15% of smokers. Alpha[1]-antitrypsin deficiency accounts for less than 1% of cases.[2]

Management of Stable Chronic Obstructive Pulmonary Disease

Stopping smoking is the prime therapeutic intervention for COPD, even when the disease is advanced. Loss of pulmonary function is not restored when smoking is discontinued, but the age-related decline in FEV_1 is significantly reduced.[1]

Inhaled short-acting beta-agonists and inhaled anticholinergics give symptomatic relief, and failure of pulmonary function testing to show a bronchodilator response does not mean the patient will not respond clinically.[1,2] British guidelines advise using either a beta-agonist such as albuterol (salbutamol, Proventil, Ventolin) or ipratropium bromide (Atrovent) on an "as needed" basis for mild or moderate disease but changing to regular doses with more severe disease. If the first class of drug chosen is ineffective, the alternative class should be substituted. If that is unsuccessful, a combination of the two should be tried (an MDI containing both ipratropium bromide and albuterol/salbutamol [Combivent] is available).[1] The American Thoracic Society advises starting with both ipratropium and a selective beta-agonist aerosol in all except the mildest cases.[2] This approach is supported by studies in which a combination of ipratropium bromide and albuterol resulted in greater improvement in pulmonary function than did albuterol alone.[3,4] One study also found that patients with COPD who were taking ipratropium bromide plus albuterol or were taking ipratropium bromide alone had fewer exacerbations than did patients taking only albuterol.[4] Third-line drugs are sustained release theophyllines. Theophyllines are not very effective, and toxicity is always a danger.[1] These medications and their delivery systems are discussed in more detail in the section on asthma.

Between 10% and 20% of patients with COPD respond to corticosteroids. According to the British Thoracic Society, suitability for corticosteroid therapy is determined by spirometry when the patient's condition is stable and the patient is taking bronchodilators. Measurements taken before and after a 2-week course of prednisone or prednisolone 30 mg/day are compared, and patients are considered responsive to steroids if the FEV_1 improves; subjective improvement is not an adequate endpoint. Those who respond should be given a trial of inhaled corticosteroids with daily doses of up to 1000 μg of beclomethasone (Beclovent), 800 μg of budesonide (Pulmicort), or 500 μg of fluticasone (FloVent).[1] A recent study raises the question of whether evaluation of responses to oral steroids is always necessary. In this multicenter placebo-controlled trial of fluticasone 500 μg bid given to patients who had documented COPD but whose responses to oral steroids were not evaluated by pulmonary function studies, those receiving fluticasone had fewer moderate or severe exacerbations, a greater improvement in lung function and walking distance, and less cough and sputum production.[5]

Respiratory rehabilitation for patients with COPD is defined as an exercise training program of at least 4 weeks' duration. A metaanalysis of 14 studies of this intervention concluded that it reduced the amount of dyspnea and improved the patients' ability to cope with the disease.[6]

Home oxygen therapy has proved useful for selected patients with advanced COPD. Criteria for this therapy are that the patient be clinically stable and have a resting arterial partial pressure of oxygen (PaO_2) of 55 mm Hg or less or of 60 mm Hg or less if there is tissue hypoxia as manifested by polycythemia or cor pulmonale.[7] In properly selected patients home oxygen therapy decreases mortality, secondary polycythemia, and pulmonary hypertension and improves neuropsychological functioning. Home oxygen therapy should be continuous for at least 15 hours a day, usually with an oxygen concentrator set at a flow of 2 to 4 L/min and delivery by nasal prongs.[1]

Selected patients with emphysema benefit from bilateral lung reduction surgery, which can be accomplished through a thoracoscopic approach. Lung function and dyspnea improve immediately, and according to a 2-year follow-up study mortality is lower than in patients having unilateral lung reduction surgery.[8]

Management of Exacerbations

Chest x-ray examination is not necessary for patients who are well enough to be managed at home and who respond to treatment, but it should be part of the initial workup for patients admitted to the hospital.[1]

First-line treatment for the outpatient management of exacerbations of COPD is to add beta-agonists or anticholinergics to the usual therapeutic regimen and maximize doses. Oral corticosteroids should be used only if patients are already taking them, the response to oral corticosteroids has been previously documented, there is no response to bronchodilator therapy, or this is the first presentation of airflow obstruction.[1] Patients with COPD exacerbations who require admission are usually given oral prednisone or prednisolone 20 to 40 mg/day. The benefit of this intervention has been confirmed by a prospective randomized double-blind trial.[9]

Whether antibiotics are useful in exacerbations of COPD is controversial. Viral infections are associated with about one third of exacerbations, but the data on the role of bacteria are less clear.[7] Recent British guidelines suggest that antibiotics are useful only if the patient complains of two of the following three symptoms: increased breathlessness, increased sputum volume, and development of purulent sputum. According to these guidelines, there is little evidence that newer antibiotics are better than older ones such as tetracycline or amoxicillin.[1]

A Canadian algorithm for the use of antibiotics in cases of COPD with exacerbations categorizes patients according to risk factors as follows[7]:

1. Patients under age 65 with no or only moderate impairment of pulmonary function and fewer than four exacerbations annually. If antibiotics are used, the choices should be amoxicillin, trimethoprim-sulfamethoxazole, or tetracyclines.

2. Patients who are over the age of 65, or who have an FEV_1 less than 50%, or who have four or more exacerbations annually, or who have comorbid medical illnesses (congestive heart failure, diabetes, chronic renal failure, chronic liver disease). If antibiotics are used, the choices should be second- or third-generation cephalosporins, trimethoprim-sulfamethoxazole, or amoxicillin–clavulanic acid (Augmentin, Clavulin).

_____ ⬥ REFERENCES ⬥ _____

1. British Thoracic Society Standards of Care Committee: Guidelines for the management of chronic obstructive pulmonary disease, *Thorax* 52(suppl 5):S1-S28, 1997.

2. Celli BR, Snider GL, Heffner J, et al: Standards for the diagnosis and care of patients with chronic obstructive pulmonary disease, *Am J Respir Crit Care Med* 152:S77-S121, 1995.

3. Campbell S: For COPD a combination of ipratropium bromide and albuterol sulfate is more effective than albuterol base, *Arch Intern Med* 159:156-160, 1999.

4. Friedman M, Serby CW, Menjoge SS, et al: Pharmacoeconomic evaluation of a combination of ipratropium plus albuterol compared with ipratropium alone and albuterol alone in COPD, *Chest* 115:635-641, 1999.

5. Paggiaro PL, Dahle R, Bakran I, et al: Multicentre randomised placebo-controlled trial of inhaled fluticasone propionate in patients with chronic obstructive pulmonary disease, *Lancet* 351: 773-780, 1998.

6. Lacasse Y, Wong E, Guyatt GH, et al: Meta-analysis of respiratory rehabilitation in chronic obstructive pulmonary disease, *Lancet* 348:1115-1119, 1996.

7. Proceedings from the Canadian Bronchitis Symposium, Toronto, Ontario, Canada, February 18-19, 1994: recommendations on the management of chronic bronchitis, *Can Med Assoc J* 151(suppl):S1-S23, 1994.

8. Serna DL, Brenner M, Osann KE, et al: Survival after unilateral versus bilateral lung volume reduction surgery for emphysema, *J Thorac Cardiovasc Surg* 118:1101-1109, 1999.

9. Davies L, Angus RM, Calverley PM: Oral corticosteroids in patients admitted to hospital with exacerbations of chronic obstructive pulmonary disease: a prospective randomised controlled trial, *Lancet* 354:465-460, 1999.

COUGH

(See also angiotensin-converting enzyme inhibitors; asthma; asthma in children; bronchitis, acute; esophageal reflux; pain; pertussis; serotonin syndrome)

What are the usual causes of cough lasting more than 2 or 3 weeks? A study in the Netherlands that took place in a primary care setting evaluated patients with coughs lasting at least 2 weeks. Even though individuals with known diagnoses of asthma or COPD were excluded from the study, 50% of the patients had one or the other of these two disorders. Clinical findings pointing to these diagnoses included a history of heavy smoking, dyspnea, or symptoms precipitated by allergens and the findings on examination of wheezing or prolonged expiration.[1]

According to Mello and co-workers,[2,3] over 99% of patients in their studies who had persistent troublesome cough of longer than 3 weeks' duration (more than 5 years in the vast majority of cases), who were nonsmokers, who were not taking angiotensin-converting enzyme (ACE) inhibitors, and who had normal or stable x-ray findings had one or a combination of three diagnoses: asthma, postnasal drip, and gastroesophageal reflux disease (GERD). The character of the cough (paroxysmal, barking, dry or productive) was not helpful in making the diagnosis.[2] This is a neat categorization, but it seems to apply primarily to patients who have had persistent cough for many years, and even then the literature supporting postnasal drip and GERD as frequent causes of cough is tenuous (see below). Furthermore, the claim that 99% of patients with chronic cough have asthma, GERD, or postnasal drip is inconsistent with other studies that have found pertussis responsible for 16% of chronic coughs in adults (see discussion of pertussis).[4] Psychogenic or habit cough is yet another cause of chronic cough.[5]

Asthma

The diagnosis of asthma as a cause of chronic cough may often be verified by a trial of inhaled beta-agonist. The symptom should diminish significantly within a week of starting a dosage regimen of 2 inhalations q4h while awake (see discussion of cough variant asthma in children).[5,6]

Postnasal Drip

The evidence supporting postnasal drip as a pathogenetic factor for chronic cough is partly theoretical (afferent fibers for the cough reflex are present in the upper airways and may be sensitized by inflammation) and partly based on observations from a few referral centers that cough was resolved when selected patients with coughing that had lasted 3 weeks to several years were given a first-generation antihistamine-decongestant combination such as azatadine 1 mg plus sustained release pseudoephedrine 120 mg (Trinalin) bid.[2,5,7,8] These trials had no placebo controls,[2,7,8] disappearance of the cough often took many weeks,[8] and the diagnosis was presumptive because the signs and symptoms of postnasal drip are nonspecific and a "definitive diagnosis . . . cannot be made from history and physical examination alone."[9] Pratter[7] suggests that nonsmoking patients with prolonged cough not caused by clinically apparent asthma, ACE inhibitors, or other evident causes should be treated initially with an antihistamine-decongestant combination. If no improvement is seen within a week, empirical treatment with albuterol (salbutamol, Proventil, Ventolin) should be given, and only if that fails should workup for GERD be instituted. Subsequent papers have emphasized the importance of using first-generation H_1 blockers rather than the second-generation nonsedating formulations for treating cough thought to be caused by postnasal drip.[2,5,9]

Gastroesophageal Reflux

Whether GERD is a cause of chronic cough in a significant number of patients is controversial. The theoretical pathogenesis of GERD-associated cough is either stimulation of the afferent loop of a cough reflex through irritating reflux of gastric contents in the lower esophagus or through microaspiration; the former hypothesis is currently considered the most frequent cause.[5,10] Evidence supporting this is based on elaborate investigations of the lower esophagus in small numbers of patients with chronic cough. Some workers have found that during 24-hour pH monitoring of the esophagus in patients with chronic cough, cough was often associated with episodes of reflux.[11] Other investigators have been unable to document such an association.[12] According to the proponents of GERD as a cause of chronic cough, symptoms of reflux such as heartburn are the exception. In one study of 12 patients in whom GERD was diagnosed, nine (75%) had no symptoms other than cough[11]; the diagnosis was made on the basis of extensive esophageal investigations.

Does treatment of GERD cure chronic cough? According to Harding[10] it can, but intensive and prolonged therapy is required and resolution is usually not seen for several months. Aside from dietary modifications and elevation of the head of the bed, Harding recommends the use of proton pump inhibitors such as omeprazole (Prilosec, Losec) 20 to 40 mg/day or lansoprazole (Prevacid) 30 to 60 mg/day.

Cough Suppressants

Cough suppressants are sometimes used for patients whose lives are made miserable by spasms of coughing caused by an upper respiratory infection. The usual drug has been dextromethorphan 15 to 30 mg q4-6h or sometimes codeine (usually as a syrup containing 10 mg/5 ml) 20 to 30 mg q4-6h.[13] Although codeine and dextromethorphan have been shown to ameliorate cough in adults, no good studies documenting efficacy or safety of these drugs in children are available.[14]

Many cold remedies contain dextromethorphan but usually in combination with sympathomimetics such as pseudoephedrine and often analgesics. As a general rule physicians should prescribe nothing, or dextromethorphan or codeine alone. Each physician should find a commercial product that contains only dextromethorphan and stick to it. A rare but important adverse effect of dextromethorphan is induction of the serotonin syndrome (see discussion of serotonin syndrome). This is most likely to occur in patients already taking SSRIs, MAO inhibitors, or antiparkinsonian drugs.

A trial of albuterol (salbutamol) for "acute bronchitis" from two family medicine centers in the United States showed that albuterol therapy with an MDI was more effective than erythromycin in controlling the cough. Adding erythromycin to the albuterol regimen gave no added benefit.[15] A metaanalysis of randomized controlled trials comparing placebo to antibiotics for acute cough found no benefit from the antibiotics and an increased incidence of adverse effects in patients who took them.[16]

Oxycodone (Percocet, Percodan, Roxicodone, Roxicet, Roxiprin) should not be prescribed for cough. Although it works, it is a narcotic that is as potent as morphine and in many areas is a popular drug of abuse.

❧ REFERENCES ❧

1. Thiadens HA, de Bock GH, Dekker FW, et al: Identifying asthma and chronic obstructive pulmonary disease in patients with persistent cough presenting to general practitioners: descriptive study, *BMJ* 316:1286-1290, 1998.
2. Mello CJ, Irwin RS, Curley FJ: Predictive values of the character, timing and complications of chronic cough in diagnosing its cause, *Arch Intern Med* 156:997-1003, 1996.
3. Smyrnios NA, Irwin RS, Curley FJ, et al: From a prospective study of chronic cough: diagnostic and therapeutic aspects in older adults, *Arch Intern Med* 158:1222-1228, 1998.
4. Birkebaek NH, Kristiansen M, Seefeldt T, et al: *Bordetella pertussis* and chronic cough in adults, *Clin Infect Dis* 29:1239-1242, 1999.
5. Irwin RS, Boulet LP, Cloutier MM, et al: Managing cough as a defense mechanism and as a symptom: a consensus panel report of the American College of Chest Physicians, *Chest* 114(suppl 2):133S-181S, 1998.
6. Irwin RS, French CT, Smyrnios NA, et al: Interpretation of positive results of a methacholine inhalation challenge and 1 week of inhaled bronchodilator use in diagnosing and treating cough-variant asthma, *Arch Intern Med* 157:1981-1987, 1997.
7. Pratter MR, Bartter T, Akers S, et al: An algorithmic approach to chronic cough, *Ann Intern Med* 119:977-983, 1993.
8. Irwin RS, Curley FJ, French CL: Chronic cough: the spectrum and frequency of causes, key components of the diagnostic evaluation, and outcome of specific therapy, *Am Rev Respir Dis* 141:640-647, 1990.
9. Irwin RS, Boulet L-P, Cloutier MM, et al: Managing cough as a defense mechanism and as a symptom: a consensus panel report of the American College of Chest Physicians, *Chest* 114: 133S-135S, 1998.
10. Harding SM, Richter JE: The role of gastroesophageal reflux in chronic cough and asthma, *Chest* 111:1389-1402, 1997.
11. Irwin RS, French CL, Curley FJ, et al: Chronic cough due to gastroesophageal reflux: clinical, diagnostic, and pathogenetic aspects, *Chest* 104:1511-1517, 1993.
12. Laukka MA, Cameron AJ, Schei AJ: Gastroesophageal reflux and chronic cough: which comes first? *J Clin Gastroenterol* 19:100-104, 1994.
13. Irwin RS, Curley FJ, Bennett FM: Appropriate use of antitussives and protussives: a practical review, *Drugs* 46:80-91, 1993.
14. American Academy of Pediatrics Committee on Drugs: Use of codeine- and dextromethorphan-containing cough remedies in children, *Pediatrics* 99:918-920, 1997.
15. Hueston WJ: Albuterol delivered by metered-dose inhaler to treat acute bronchitis, *J Fam Pract* 39:437-440, 1994.
16. Fahey T, Stocks N, Thomas T: Quantitative systematic review of randomised controlled trials comparing antibiotic with placebo for acute cough in adults, *BMJ* 316:906-910, 1998.

LUNG CANCER
(See also informed consent; lead time bias; length bias; screening)

The two main categories of lung cancer are small cell lung cancer, accounting for one fourth of all cases, and non–small cell lung cancer, constituting the remainder. Non–small cell lung cancers are squamous cell carcinomas, adenocarcinomas, and large cell carcinomas.[1]

Smoking accounts for 90% of cases of lung cancer, and the disease will develop in 20% of smokers. The overall prognosis of the disease is abysmal; about 90% of patients are dead within a year of the diagnosis.[2]

Even after the data were controlled for smoking, men in the Harvard Alumni Study who regularly participated in moderate exercise such as walking or climbing stairs had a lower incidence of lung cancer than those who were sedentary. Possible explanations are that increased breathing leads to more rapid expulsion of carcinogens or that exercise enhances the immune system.[3]

A chest roentenogram showing an isolated pulmonary nodule is one method of presentation of lung cancer. About two thirds of such nodules are benign (usually granulomas or hamartomas). Malignancy is more likely if the lesion is large, spiculated, or in the upper lobe and if the patient is older, smokes, or has a past history of cancer.[4]

Surgery is considered the treatment of choice for patients with non–small cell lung cancer who can undergo an operation, but fewer than 20% of patients have operable disease and of these, fewer than 50% will survive 5 years. In a very few instances patients with localized disease may be cured by radiation therapy. Overall, the 5-year survival rate for non–small cell cancer of the lung is less than 10%.[1]

Chemotherapy can increase the median survival of patients with non–small cell lung cancer by 1.5 to 3 months but at the cost of considerable toxicity. When fully informed, few patients would choose it (see discussion of informed consent).[5]

Over half of patients with small cell lung cancer have extensive disease at the time of diagnosis. For these patients median survival without treatment is 6 to 12 weeks, whereas with treatment it is 10 to 12 months. Standard management is chemotherapy using agents such as etoposide and cisplatin plus thoracic irradiation if the disease is localized. Median survival for those with localized disease treated with chemotherapy plus thoracic irradiation is 18 months, and in some trials such patients have had 44% 2-year and 22% 5-year survival rates. Improved survival in those with localized disease has also been reported when prophylactic cranial irradiation is added to the treatment regimen.[6]

The value of chest x-ray examination or sputum cytology as a screening tool to detect lung cancer in smokers was the basis of a number of reports in the 1980s and early 1990s. Although 5-year survival rates were increased, long-term mortality was not, presumably because of lead time and length bias. The U.S. Preventive Services Task Force gives both chest x-ray and sputum cytology screening a "D" recommendation,[7] and the Canadian Task Force on Preventive Health Care gives chest x-ray screening a "D" and sputum cytology an "E."[8] Unfortunately, closure of controversial issues is rarely permanent, and studies suggesting that chest x-ray screening of smokers is efficacious continue to appear. A 1998 Finnish study reported the 5-year survival of patients with lung cancer detected by a single screening x-ray study to be 19%, compared with 10% for control subjects with lung cancer who were not screened.[9] Length bias? Lead time bias?

◥ REFERENCES ◤

1. Simmonds P: Managing patients with lung cancer (editorial), *BMJ* 319:527-528, 1999.
2. Sethi T: Lung cancer, *BMJ* 314:652-655, 1997.
3. Lee I-M, Sesso HD, Paffenbarger RS: Physical activity and risk of lung cancer, *Int J Epidemiol* 28:620-625, 1999.
4. Swensen SJ, Silverstein MC, Ilstrup DM, et al: The probability of malignancy in solitary pulmonary nodules: application to small radiologically indeterminate nodules, *Arch Intern Med* 157:849-855, 1997.
5. Silvestri G, Pritchard R, Welch HG: Preferences for chemotherapy in patients with advanced non–small cell lung cancer: descriptive study based on scripted interviews, *BMJ* 317:771-775, 1998.
6. Carney DN: Prophylactic cranial irradiation and small-cell lung cancer (editorial), *N Engl J Med* 341:524-526, 1999.
7. US Preventive Services Task Force: *Guide to clinical preventive services,* ed 2, Baltimore, 1996, Williams & Wilkins, pp 135-139.
8. Canadian Task Force on the Periodic Health Examination: *Canadian guide to clinical preventive health care,* Ottawa, 1994, Canada Communication Group—Publishing, pp 779-786.
9. Salomaa E-R, Liippo K, Taylor P, et al: Prognosis of patients with lung cancer found in a single chest radiograph screening, *Chest* 114:1514-1518, 1998.

PNEUMONIA

(See also pneumonia in children)

Diagnosis and Investigation

Symptoms of pneumonia are usually less frequent and severe in elderly patients than in younger ones.[1] Fever and audible crackles occur in 80% of patients with pneumonia. Most have a respiratory rate greater than 20 breaths/min, but only 30% have signs of consolidation.[2] Unfortunately, these and other symptoms and signs are nonspecific, and none of the findings on the history or physical examination, including the presence or absence of crackles, allows a definitive ruling in or ruling out of the disease.[3]

It is not possible to determine which of the five organisms that most commonly cause community-acquired pneumonia in adults (*Streptococcus pneumoniae, Haemophilus influenzae, Legionella* species, *Chlamydia pneumoniae,* or gram-negative rods) is responsible for the disease on the basis of history, physical examination, laboratory investigations (such as white blood cell count), or chest x-ray examination.[4] The clinical and radiological presentations seem to be more a matter of host response than the nature of the infecting organisms.[5] Sputum culture is not helpful in most cases of community-acquired pneumonia; one third of patients cannot produce sputum, one third have already been treated with antibiotics, and one fourth are infected with organisms not easily cultured.[2] False-positive results of sputum cultures are common because of colonization of organisms in the oropharynx, and the false-negative rate in pneumococcal infections approaches 50%. However, sputum cultures and Gram's stain may detect unusual organisms such as *Histoplasma, Pneumocystis carinii,* and *Mycobacterium tuberculosis.*[5] Gram's stain (but not sputum cultures) has shown value in the diagnosis of community-acquired bacteriemic pneumococcal pneumonia in patients admitted to the hospital.[6] Blood cultures are positive in no more than 25% of cases; the positivity rate is greatest if the organism is *S. pneumoniae*.[2,5] For the majority of patients with community-acquired pneumonia, treatment is empirical.[5]

Prognosis

Prognosis is an important factor in determining whether patients with pneumonia require admission. Criteria for determining prognosis have not been standardized, as is evident from the variability of admission rates for this condition from one geographical location to another.[1] Fine and associates[7] have developed a series of prediction rules that separate patients with good prognoses who can generally be treated at home from those with poor prognoses who should be admitted to the hospital. Predictors of increased risk of death based on the history and physical examination are as follows:

1. Age over 50
2. Coexisting illnesses (neoplasia, congestive heart failure, cerebrovascular disease, renal disease, and liver disease)
3. Altered mental status
4. Pulse 125 beats/min or faster
5. Respiratory rate 30 breaths/min or faster
6. Systolic blood pressure less than 90 mm Hg
7. Temperature less than 35° C or greater than 39° C

Management

Recommended treatment regimens for pneumonias treated on an outpatient basis vary from one author to another and from one country to another.[1] The pathogenic organisms tend to vary with age and with the presence of comorbid illnesses. Common to all groups are *S. pneumoniae* and *H. influenzae*. Otherwise well patients under the age of 65 tend to have a number of infections caused by *Mycoplasma pneumoniae* and *C. pneumoniae*. Individuals with comorbid illnesses or over the age of 65 are also at risk of infections caused by oral anaerobes, gram-negative rods, *Staphylococcus aureus*, and *Legionella*.[8]

The 1993 American and Canadian guidelines for the outpatient treatment of pneumonia in otherwise well patients under the age of 60 (or 65) are to use a macrolide (erythromycin, clarithromycin [Biaxin], or azithromycin [Zithromax]), with tetracycline as an acceptable alternative. For patients over the age of 60 (or 65), or for anyone with a comorbid illness, acceptable treatment options are a second-generation cephalosporin such as cefaclor (Ceclor) or cefuroxime axetil (Ceftin), trimethoprim-sulfamethoxazole (Septra, Bactrim), or a penicillin plus a beta-lactamase inhibitor (amoxicillin plus clavulanate potassium [Augmentin, Clavulin]), with the addition of a macrolide to any of these regimens if *Legionella* is suspected.[8,9] Two 1999 American nonrandomized retrospective studies of hospitalized patients with community-acquired pneumonia found

that the early addition of macrolides decreased morbidity and mortality.[10,11] An accompanying editorial questions whether selection bias may not account for these findings.[12]

The 1998 recommendations of the *Medical Letter*[13] and the Infectious Diseases Society of America[14] are somewhat different. For otherwise healthy, relatively young individuals, drugs of first choice are oral macrolides, doxycycline, or some of the newer fluoroquinolones such as levofloxacin (Levaquin), grepafloxacin (Raxar), sparfloxacin, or trovafloxacin (Trovan). These fluoroquinolones not only have good antipneumococcal activity but are also effective against *Legionella, Mycoplasma,* and *Chlamydia*.[13,14] Alternatives are amoxicillin/clavulanate or a second-generation cephalosporin such as cefuroxime, cefpodoxime (Vantin), or cefprozil (Cefzil).[14] For older patients or those with comorbid illnesses one of the listed fluoroquinolones is the preferred therapeutic agent.[13] Since these recommendation were published, trovafloxacin has been reported to cause fatal hepatic damage (see discussion of antibacterials) and grepafloxacin has been withdrawn from the market because of the risk of serious ventricular arrhythmias.

Although *L. pneumoniae* may occur in epidemics, 2% to 15% of sporadic community-acquired pneumonias are caused by this organism; patients with the disease are usually sick enough to require admission. Aside from respiratory symptoms and fever, gastrointestinal problems, especially diarrhea, are common.[15]

───────────── ◢ **REFERENCES** ◣ ─────────────

1. Bartlett JG, Mundy LM: Community-acquired pneumonia, *N Engl J Med* 333:1618-1624, 1995.
2. Marrie TJ: Community-acquired pneumonia, *Clin Infect Dis* 18:502-515, 1994.
3. Metlay JP, Kapoor WN, Fine MJ: Does this patient have community-acquired pneumonia? Diagnosing pneumonia by history and physical examination, *JAMA* 278:1440-1445, 1997.
4. Kauppinen MT, Laehde S, Syrjaelae H: Roentgenographic findings of pneumonia caused by *Chlamydia pneumoniae*: a comparison with *Streptococcus pneumoniae, Arch Intern Med* 156:1851-1856, 1996.
5. Antoniou M, Grossman RF: Etiological diagnosis of pneumonia: a goal worth pursuing? *Can J Infect Dis* 6:281-283, 1995.
6. Watanakunakorn C, Bailey TA: Adult bacteremic pneumococcal pneumonia in a community teaching hospital, 1992-1996: a detailed analysis of 108 cases, *Arch Intern Med* 157:1965-1971, 1997.
7. Fine MF, Auble TE, Yealy DM, et al: A prediction rule to identify low-risk patients with community acquired pneumonia, *N Engl J Med* 336:243-250, 1997.
8. Treatment of community acquired pneumonia in adults—conference report, *Can J Infect Dis,* Jan/Feb, vol 4, no 1, 1993.
9. Niederman MS, Bass JB Jr, Campbell GD, et al: American Thoracic Society guidelines for the initial management of adults with community-acquired pneumonia: diagnosis, assessment of severity, and initial antimicrobial therapy, *Am Rev Respir Dis* 148:1418-1426, 1993.

10. Gleason PP, Meehan TP, Fine JM, et al: Associations between initial antimicrobial therapy and medical outcomes for hospitalized elderly patients with pneumonia, *Arch Intern Med* 159:2562-2572, 1999.

11. Stahl JE, Barza M, DesJardin J, et al: Effect of macrolides as part of initial empiric therapy on length of stay in patients hospitalized with community-acquired pneumonia, *Arch Intern Med* 159:2576-2580, 1999.

12. Dowell SF: The best treatment for pneumonia: new cues, but no definitive answers (editorial), *Arch Intern Med* 159:2511-2512, 1999.

13. The choice of antibacterial drugs, *Med Lett* 40:33-42, 1998.

14. Bartlett JG, Breiman RF, Mandell LA, et al: Community-acquired pneumonia in adults: guidelines for management, *Clin Infect Dis* 26:811-838, 1998.

15. Stout JE, Yu VL: Legionellosis, *N Engl J Med* 337:682-687, 1997.

PNEUMOTHORAX

Spontaneous pneumothorax is traditionally treated by inserting a thoracostomy tube. A British study has demonstrated that simple aspiration of air with a 16- or 18-gauge needle resulted in less discomfort and a shorter hospital stay than thoracostomy tube placement. In this series aspiration technique was successful in 28 of 35 patients. In 7 patients the aspiration technique failed and tube placement was required.[1]

An emergency treatment for tension pneumothorax is to create a one-way valve with an 18-gauge needle and a portion of a latex glove. The needle is inserted into the pleural space through the second intercostal space. The tip of one finger of a latex glove is cut off and fitted over the hub of the needle, and portions of the cut edges are taped to the proximal shaft of the needle without making an airtight seal between these edges and the needle shaft. This creates a one-way valve, allowing egress but not ingress of air through the needle.[2]

◤ REFERENCES ◢

1. Harvey J, Prescott RJ: Simple aspiration versus intercostal tube drainage for spontaneous pneumothorax in patients with normal lungs, *BMJ* 309:1338-1339, 1994.

2. Earp-Jones A: Lifesaving finger, *Patient Care Can* 7:18, 1996.

SARCOID

Sarcoid is a worldwide disease affecting both sexes, all races, and all ages. It is more common and more aggressive in blacks than in whites and most frequently occurs in persons under the age of 40.[1]

A common clinical presentation of sarcoid is peripheral arthritis, often associated with erythema nodosum. Almost all patients have involvement of the ankles, and other frequently affected joints are the knees, wrists, and elbows. The arthritis is rarely monarticular, and it does not cause joint destruction. Chest x-ray examination usually shows hilar adenopathy.[1,2] Between 20% and 50% of cases of sarcoid are manifested as arthralgias, erythema nodosum, and bilateral hilar adenopathy, a constellation of findings known as Löfgren's syndrome. Löfgren's syndrome has the best prognosis of any of the variants of sarcoid.[1] In one study of this form of clinical presentation the mean duration of the arthropathy was about 4 months, recurrence of arthritis after resolution of the initial episode occurred in 4%, and chronic pulmonary sarcoidosis developed in 8% of cases. Except for cases with pulmonary involvement in which corticosteroids are indicated, the treatment of choice is nonsteroidal antiinflammatory drugs.[2]

Most cases of sarcoid are probably asymptomatic; a number of these are identified by finding hilar adenopathy on chest roentgenograms taken for other reasons. Among patients with only hilar adenopathy the disease remits spontaneously in 60% to 80% of cases. For patients with hilar adenopathy plus pulmonary infiltrates, spontaneous remission occurs in 50% to 60% of cases, whereas if there are only pulmonary infiltrates without hilar adenopathy, spontaneous remission is seen in less than 30%. The prognosis is worse in patients over 40, blacks, and those whose symptoms last longer than 6 months.[1]

No specific laboratory investigations are used for sarcoidosis. The serum level of angiotensin-converting enzyme may be elevated, but this finding has little diagnostic value because it is nonspecific; the Kveim-Siltzbach test is of historical interest only.[1]

◤ REFERENCES ◢

1. Newman LS, Rose CS, Maier LA: Sarcoidosis, *N Engl J Med* 336:1224-1234, 1997.

2. Gran JT, Bohmer E: Acute sarcoid arthritis: a favourable outcome? A retrospective survey of 49 patients with review of the literature, *Scand J Rheumatol* 25:70-73, 1996.

SMOKING

(See also detrimental effects of alcohol; smoking in pregnancy)

Topics covered in this section

Epidemiology
Beneficial Effects of Smoking
Detrimental Effects of Smoking
Quitting Smoking
Tobacco Industry

EPIDEMIOLOGY

(See also detrimental effects of alcohol; poverty)

The prevalence of smoking among Americans over the age of 17 fell from 42.4% in 1965 to 25.5% in 1990. In 1992 the prevalence was 26.5%. The increase was partly explained by a change in definition to include intermittent as well as daily smokers.[1]

The highest rates of smoking in 1992 were in the 25- to 44-year-old group (31%) and among those below the poverty line (35%). Slightly more men (29%) than women (25%) smoked, and smoking incidence declined with years of education.[1] Persons who had not started smoking during adolescence were unlikely ever to become smokers.[2] Rates of adolescent smoking have increased significantly in the 1990s. A study of U.S. college students found that the prevalence of smoking was 22.3% in 1993 and 28.5% in 1997; one fourth of these smokers began to smoke regularly after they entered college.[3] According to a 1994-1995 survey conducted by Statistics Canada, 28% of full-time Canadian workers smoked. The rate for male-dominated outdoor blue-collar occupations was 43%, whereas for white-collar workers it was 18%. Among workers who were ill or on disability the rate was 52%.[4]

Although overall smoking rates have fallen in the developed world, they have been increasing in the developing world and represent a major public health problem in these regions. For example, in Shanghai, China, 63% of males and 4% of females smoke; most smokers spend a quarter of their income on cigarettes.[5] Physicians in China are heavy smokers as well; in a 1989 survey in Beijing, 68% were found to smoke.[6] At present smoking accounts for an estimated 4 million deaths a year split evenly between rich and poor countries. If current patterns of smoking persist, by the year 2030 smoking will be responsible for 10 million deaths annually and 70% of these will be in developing countries.[7]

Alcohol abusers tend to be heavy smokers.[8,9] In fact, a history of heavy smoking may alert the clinician to unacknowledged alcohol abuse.[9]

Increases in the price of cigarettes are associated with a decreased prevalence of smoking, particularly among the young, the poor, and members of minority groups.[10]

--- ◣ **REFERENCES** ◥ ---

1. Cigarette smoking among adults—United States, 1992, and changes in the definition of current cigarette smoking, *MMWR* 43:342-346, 1994.
2. Department of Health and Human Services: *Preventing tobacco use among young people: a report of the Surgeon General,* Washington, DC, 1994, US Government Printing Office, pp 5, 58.
3. Wechsler H, Rigotti NA, Gledhill-Hoyt J, et al: Increased levels of cigarette use among college students: a cause for national concern, *JAMA* 280:1673-1678, 1998.
4. Buske L: Smoking: an occupational hazard, *Can Med Assoc J* 160:630, 1999.
5. Yang G, Fan L, Tan J, et al: Smoking in China: findings of the 1996 National Prevalence Survey, *JAMA* 282:1247-1253, 1999.
6. Skolnick AA: Answer sought for "tobacco giant" China's problem, *JAMA* 275:1220-1221, 1996.
7. Lopez AD: Counting the dead in China: measuring tobacco's impact in the developing world (editorial), *BMJ* 317:1399-1400, 1998.
8. Hurt RD, Offord KP, Croghan IT, et al: Mortality following inpatient addictions treatment: role of tobacco use in a community-based cohort, *JAMA* 275:1097-1103, 1996.
9. Valiant GE, Schnurr PP, Baron JA, et al: A prospective study of the effects of cigarette smoking and alcohol abuse on mortality, *J Gen Intern Med* 6:299-304, 1991.
10. Centers for Disease Control and Prevention: Response to increases in cigarette prices by race/ethnicity, income, and age groups—United States, 1976-1993, *JAMA* 280:1979-1980, 1998.

BENEFICIAL EFFECTS OF SMOKING

Epidemiological evidence has been presented that smoking is "good" for ulcerative colitis. The disease is more common in nonsmokers than in smokers, the initial onset of the disease often correlates with discontinuing smoking, and smoking may control the symptoms of the disease.[1] These apparently beneficial effects are not seen in Crohn's disease. In a randomized double-blind study of 72 patients with ulcerative colitis, nicotine patches improved the symptoms in the treated patients.[2] An editorial accompanying the report cautions against general use of such therapy at this time.[1] The use of nicotine patches to help maintain remission in ulcerative colitis has not proved beneficial.[3]

The incidence of Parkinson's disease has been reported to be less in smokers than in nonsmokers, and this relationship is dose dependent.[4] The reason may be that the brains of smokers have a very low level of monoamine oxidase B (MAO-B), which causes the breakdown of dopamine.[5]

In a case-controlled study the incidence of endometrial cancer was found to be lower in postmenopausal smokers than in postmenopausal nonsmokers. This is thought to occur because smoking has the ability to inactivate estrogens to some degree.[6] Some epidemiological studies have found that smokers have a lower risk of osteoarthritis than nonsmokers[7] and that women who smoke during pregnancy are at decreased risk of having infants with neural tube defects.[8]

A paradoxical benefit of smoking is that it may reduce per capita health costs. This is because far fewer smokers than nonsmokers live long enough to suffer the ravages of old age and incur the associated health care costs.[9]

--- ◣ **REFERENCES** ◥ ---

1. Hanauer SB: Nicotine for colitis—the smoke has not yet cleared (editorial), *N Engl J Med* 330:856-857, 1994.
2. Pullan RD, Rhodes J, Ganesh S, et al: Transdermal nicotine for active ulcerative colitis, *N Engl J Med* 330:811-815, 1994.
3. Thomas GAO, Mani V, Williams GT, et al: Transdermal nicotine as maintenance therapy for ulcerative colitis, *N Engl J Med* 332:988-992, 1995.
4. Gorell JM, Rybicki BA, Cole C, et al: Smoking and Parkinson's disease: a dose-response relationship, *Neurology* 52:115-119, 1999.

5. Fowler JS, Volkow ND, Wang GJ, et al: Inhibition of mono-amine oxidase B in the brains of smokers, *Nature* 379:733-736, 1996.

6. Lesko SM, Rosenberg L, Kaufman DW, et al: Cigarette smoking and the risk of endometrial cancer, *N Engl J Med* 313:593-596, 1985.

7. Cooper C, Inskip H, Croft P, et al: Individual risk factors for hip osteoarthritis: obesity, hip injury, and physical activity, *Am J Epidemiol* 147:516-522, 1998.

8. Källén K: Maternal smoking, body mass index, and neural tube defects, *Am J Epidemiol* 147:1103-1111, 1998.

9. Barendregt JJ, Bonneux L, van der Maas PF: The health care costs of smoking, *N Engl J Med* 337:1052-1057, 1997.

DETRIMENTAL EFFECTS OF SMOKING

(See also smoking in pregnancy)

Cigarette Smoking

Smoking contributes to increased mortality rates from multiple causes. McGinnis and colleagues[1] estimate that smoking accounts for 19% of U.S. deaths, which puts it ahead of all other causes of preventable deaths. Diet and activity patterns came second, accounting for 14% of deaths.[1] In a 40-year study of British physicians the excess total mortality of continuing smokers between the ages of 45 and 64 was three times that of nonsmokers, while for continuing smokers aged 65 to 84 it was twice that of nonsmokers. The authors of this study concluded that half of all regular smokers are likely to die from their habit.[2] Extrapolating from a 15-year follow-up of the British Regional Heart Study, Phillips and colleagues[3] concluded that only 42% of 20-year-old smokers who continued to smoke all their lives would still be alive by age 73 compared with 78% of 20-year-old nonsmokers who never took up the habit.

Observational studies have shown that mortality rates gradually decrease in smokers who quit and that by 20 years rates approach those of never smokers. Little if any benefit is observed in the first 5 years after quitting, probably because many smokers who stop do so when they become ill.[4]

In the United States smoking is responsible for about 30% of all cancer deaths. The overall cancer death rate in smokers is twice that of nonsmokers, and the cancer death rate for heavy smokers is four times that of nonsmokers. Cancers related to smoking include those of the lung, oral cavity, larynx, esophagus, stomach, pancreas, colon, uterine cervix, bladder, ureter and kidney, and breast. In addition, about 14% of leukemias are thought to be caused by smoking.[5]

Cardiovascular diseases associated with smoking are coronary artery disease, myocardial infarction, sudden death, strokes, subarachnoid hemorrhages, peripheral vascular disease, and aortic aneurysms. Smoking is known to decrease the oxygen-carrying power of the blood because of carbon monoxide production, to activate platelets, and to foster the development of atherosclerosis.[5]

Respiratory diseases in adults caused by smoking include lung cancer, chronic obstructive pulmonary disease, and pneumonia. Smokers have an increased death rate from influenza.[5] Smoking even as few as five cigarettes a day in adolescence diminishes the normal growth of lung function, particularly in girls.[6]

Smoking during pregnancy is associated with intrauterine growth retardation, low-birth-weight infants, preterm births, placenta previa, abruptio placentae, and a higher incidence of miscarriages of viable infants.[7] Maternal smoking may also be a risk factor for conduct disorder in male offspring and substance abuse in female offspring.[8] Smokers have been reported to have a lower fertility rate than nonsmokers,[9] and smokers are more likely to suffer from menopausal hot flashes than are nonsmokers.[10]

Smoking has been found to increase the risk of acquiring type 2 diabetes.[11] It also adversely affects thyroid function.[12,13] It is associated with an increased incidence of Graves' disease and even more so with Graves' ophthalmopathy[12] and may also be a contributing factor to the development of subclinical hypothyroidism even if it does not aggravate the clinical manifestations.[13]

Smoking is associated with numerous other maladies. The relapse rate of Crohn's disease is greater in smokers than nonsmokers.[14] The risk of age-related macular degeneration is increased in both male[15] and female[16] smokers, and it is likely that smoking is also a risk factor for cataracts.[17] Snoring[18] and hearing loss are more common in smokers than nonsmokers.[19] Sun-exposed smokers have a higher incidence of wrinkles and skin cancers than sun-exposed nonsmokers.[20] Smokers are at increased risk for periodontal disease.[21] Cigarettes are the leading cause of fire fatalities,[22] smokers are more likely than nonsmokers to develop Alzheimer's disease,[23] smokers who are involved in heavy physical work have more low back pain than nonsmokers involved in similar activities,[24] and some studies have shown an association between smoking and rheumatoid arthritis.[25]

Passive Smoking

Children exposed to passive smoke have a higher incidence of asthma, bronchitis, pneumonia, middle ear effusions, tonsillectomies, adenoidectomies, and deaths (usually from lower respiratory tract infections or fires).[26] They also have an increased rate of respiratory complications after anesthesia.[27] Infants exposed to cigarette smoke have an increased risk of sudden infant death syndrome (SIDS),[28] and exposure of pregnant women to cigarette smoke correlates with an increased risk of fetal growth retardation.[29] Nonsmokers exposed to secondhand smoke have an increased incidence of both fatal and nonfatal cardiac events,[30] strokes,[31] lung cancer,[32] breast cancer,[33] and hearing loss.[19]

Pipe and Cigar Smoking

Regular cigar smokers have a moderately increased risk of coronary artery disease, chronic obstructive lung disease, and cancers of the oropharynx, nose, larynx, esophagus, and lung.[34] Although elevated, the mortality rates for ischemic heart disease, lung cancer, and chronic obstructive lung disease are lower among pipe and cigar smokers than among cigarette smokers. In part this is because the former smoke less tobacco and in part because they tend to inhale less. Cigarette smokers who switch to cigars or pipes achieve a decreased mortality rate for these diseases, but to a lesser degree than cigar and pipe smokers who have never smoked cigarettes. This is probably because those who switch inhale more.[35]

❧ REFERENCES ❧

1. McGinnis JM, Foege WH: Actual causes of death in the United States, *JAMA* 270:2207-2211, 1993.
2. Doll R, Peto R, Wheatley K, et al: Mortality in relation to smoking: 40 years' observations on male British doctors, *BMJ* 309:901-911, 1994.
3. Phillips AN, Wannamethee SG, Walker M, et al: Life expectancy in men who have never smoked and those who have smoked continuously: 15 year follow up of large cohort of middle aged British men, *BMJ* 313:907-908, 1996.
4. Enstrom JE, Heath CW Jr: Smoking cessation and mortality trends among 118,000 Californians, 1960-1997, *Epidemiology* 10:500-512, 1999.
5. Bartecchi CE, MacKenzie TD, Schrier RW: The human costs of tobacco use (first of two parts), *N Engl J Med* 330:907-912, 1994.
6. Gold DR, Wang X, Wypij D, et al: Effects of cigarette smoking on lung function in adolescent boys and girls, *N Engl J Med* 335:931-937, 1996.
7. Brosky G: Why do pregnant women smoke and can we help them quit? (editorial), *Can Med Assoc J* 152:163-166, 1995.
8. Weissman MM, Warner V, Wickramaratne PJ, et al: Maternal smoking during pregnancy and psychopathology in offspring followed to adulthood, *J Am Acad Child Adolesc Psychiatry* 38:892-899, 1999.
9. Bolumar F, Olsen J, Boldsen J (European Study Group on Infertility and Subfecundity): Smoking reduces fecundity: a European multicenter study on infertility and subfecundity, *Am J Epidemiol* 143:578-587, 1996.
10. Staropoli CA, Flaws JA, Bush TL, et al: Predictors of menopausal hot flashes, *J Women's Health* 7:1149-1155, 1998.
11. Rimm EB, Chan J, Stampfer MJ, et al: Prospective study of cigarette smoking, alcohol use, and the risk of diabetes in men, *BMJ* 210:545-546, 1995.
12. Prummel MF, Wiersinga WM: Smoking and risk of Graves' disease, *JAMA* 269:479-482, 1993.
13. Müller B, Zulewski H, Huber P, et al: Impaired action of thyroid hormone associated with smoking in women with hypothyroidism, *N Engl J Med* 333:964-969, 1995.
14. Timmer A, Sutherland LR, Martin F (Canadian Mesalamine for Remission of Crohn's Disease Study Group): Oral contraceptive use and smoking are risk factors for relapse in Crohn's disease, *Gastroenterology* 114:1143-1150, 1998.
15. Christen WG, Glynn RJ, Manson JE, et al: A prospective study of cigarette smoking and risk of age-related macular degeneration in men, *JAMA* 276:1147-1151, 1996.
16. Seddon JM, Willett WC, Speizer FE, et al: A prospective study of cigarette smoking and age-related macular degeneration in women, *JAMA* 276:1141-1146, 1996.
17. West S: Does smoke get in your eyes? (editorial), *JAMA* 268:1025-1026, 1992.
18. Lindberg E, Taube A, Janson C, et al: A 10-year follow-up of snoring in men, *Chest* 114:1048-1055, 1998.
19. Cruickshanks KJ, Klein R, Klein BE, et al: Cigarette smoking and hearing loss: the Epidemiology of Hearing Loss Study, *JAMA* 279:1715-1719, 1998.
20. Gilchrest BA: A review of skin ageing and its medical therapy, *Br J Dermatol* 135:867-875, 1996.
21. Watts TL: Periodontitis for medical practitioners, *BMJ* 316:993-996, 1998.
22. McGuire A: Cigarettes and fire deaths, *NY State J Med* 83:1296-1298, 1983.
23. Ott A, Slooter AJ, Hofman A, et al: Smoking and risk of dementia and Alzheimer's disease in a population-based cohort study: the Rotterdam Study, *Lancet* 351:1840-1843, 1998.
24. Eriksen W, Natvig B, Bruusgaard D: Smoking, heavy physical work and low back pain: a four-year prospective study, *Occup Med* 49:155-160, 1999.
25. Karlson EW, Lee I-M, Cook NR, et al: A retrospective cohort study of cigarette smoking and risk of rheumatoid arthritis in female health professionals, *Arthritis Rheum* 42:910-917, 1999.
26. Difranza JR, Lew RA: Morbidity and mortality in children associated with the use of tobacco products by other people, *Pediatrics* 97:560-668, 1996.
27. Skolnick ET, Vomvolakis MA, Buck KA, et al: Exposure to environmental tobacco smoke and the risk of adverse respiratory events in children receiving general anesthesia, *Anesthesiology* 88:1144-1153, 1998.
28. Klonoff-Cohen HS, Edelstein SL, Lefkowitz ES, et al: The effect of passive smoking and tobacco exposure through breast milk on sudden infant death syndrome, *JAMA* 273:795-798, 1995.
29. California Environmental Protection Agency, Office of Environmental Health Hazard Assessment: *Health effects of exposure to environmental tobacco smoke,* Sacramento, 1997, California Environmental Protection Agency. (http://www.calepa.cahwnet.gov/oehha/docs/finalets.htm).
30. He J, Vupputuri S, Allen K, et al: Passive smoking and the risk of coronary heart disease—a meta-analysis of epidemiologic studies, *N Engl J Med* 340:920-926, 1999.
31. You RX, Thrift AG, McNeil JJ, et al: Ischemic stroke risk and passive exposure to spouses' cigarette smoking, *Am J Public Health* 89:572-575, 1999.
32. Hackshaw AK, Law MR, Wald NJ: The accumulated evidence on lung cancer and environmental tobacco smoke, *BMJ* 315:980-988, 1997.
33. Lash TL, Aschengrau A: Active and passive cigarette smoking and the occurrence of breast cancer, *Am J Epidemiol* 149:5-12, 1999.
34. Iribarren C, Tekawa I, Sidney S, et al: Effect of cigar smoking on the risk of cardiovascular disease, chronic obstructive pulmonary disease, and cancer in men, *N Engl J Med* 340:1773-1780, 1999.
35. Wald NJ, Watt HC: Prospective study of effect of switching from cigarettes to pipes or cigars on mortality from three smoking related diseases, *BMJ* 314:1860-1863, 1997.

QUITTING SMOKING

(See also prevention; ulcerative colitis)

Motivation

What techniques should a family physician use to help patients give up smoking? Guidelines based on an extensive literature review have been developed by the U.S. Agency for Health Care Policy and Research (AHCPR). Some of the essential points of these guidelines are that smoking status should be determined for every patient at every visit and that for smokers the desire to quit or not quit should be assessed. For smokers who do not plan to quit, an attempt should be made to motivate them to do so, and for those who want to quit, a detailed plan should be worked out.[1] Astonishingly, the majority of U.S. smokers do not believe that they are at increased risk of myocardial infarction or cancer; correction of this misconception should probably be a central issue when trying to motivate them to quit.[2]

Numerous studies have clearly demonstrated that the rate of quitting is increased by psychosocial interventions and that this base rate can be doubled by adding pharmacotherapy in the form of either nicotine replacement or antidepressants. Psychosocial therapy may be effectively given face to face or over the telephone; a number of pharmaceutical manufacturers offer such telephone services. Because the chances of stopping smoking are greatly increased by pharmacotherapy (nicotine replacement therapy or antidepressants), some experts in the field recommend that this treatment option be offered to all smokers.[3]

Patients go through several stages to make life-style changes such as quitting smoking, and it is important for the physician to deal with the stage the patient is in (see behavioral changes for prevention under "Prevention").[4]

Increased anxiety is often given as a rationale for not quitting smoking. In fact, after the first week since quitting, anxiety levels decrease.[5]

A systematic review of 188 randomized controlled trials of smoking cessation found that personal advice from a physician during a single consultation resulted in a 2% success rate measured 1 year later. Additional support such as follow-up letters or visits had a positive but variable benefit. Patients at high risk (pregnant patients and those with coronary artery disease) had a cessation rate of about 8%. Behavior modification techniques in individual or group sessions with a psychologist had a 2% success rate. No data were given for hypnosis, and acupuncture was not effective. Nicotine replacement therapy led to a 13% success rate.[6]

Two major factors that predict success in quitting are low nicotine dependence and successful abstinence during the first 2 weeks after quitting.[7] One study has even shown that success on the first day of quitting correlates with improved long-term success.[8] Another important variable is patient age; individuals over age 30 are more likely to succeed in quitting than are younger individuals.[9]

Pharmacotherapy

A 4- to 5-year follow-up study of heavy smokers (20 or more cigarettes a day) randomly assigned to 21-, 14-, or 7-mg nicotine patches or placebo patches reported continuous abstinence rates of 20%, 10%, 12%, and 7%, respectively. Regardless of initial treatment, individuals in this trial who were still abstaining at 1 year were unlikely to relapse.[9] Combinations of patches and gum[2] or of patches and nasal spray may also be used.[10] In one trial the abstinence rates among patients who used the patch for 5 months and the spray for 1 year were 27% at 1 year and 16% at 6 years, whereas the rates for the control subjects who used a patch plus placebo spray were 11% and 9%, respectively. Nicotine patches release the drug slowly, and blood levels approximate the trough levels found in smokers. Addition of nicotine nasal spray, gum, or inhalers to patches gives more rapid peaks of nicotine that are similar to those experienced by smokers.[10]

A common consequence of quitting smoking is weight gain. In one study the average excess weight gain at 10 years among persons who had quit smoking compared with control subjects who had never smoked was 4.4 kg (10 lb) for men and 5 kg (11 lb) for women.[11] Among heavy smokers who were evaluated 4 to 5 years after quitting with the help of nicotine patches or placebo, mean weight gain was 10 kg (22 lb) for men and 8 kg (18 lb) for women. Maximum weight gain was 24 kg (53 lb), but 7% of patients actually lost weight.[9] Weight gain may be less in patients taking bupropion (see below).

If all endeavors to give up smoking fail, encouraging the patient to switch to cigars or pipes might be worthwhile (see discussion of detrimental effects of smoking).[12]

One hypothesis to explain why smokers enjoy smoking is that nicotine stimulates the release of dopamine in the brain and it is this neurotransmitter than leads to "feeling good" after a cigarette. Other investigations suggest that the brains of smokers have very low levels of monoamine oxidase B (MAO-B), which normally breaks down dopamine, and this too would contribute to the "good feeling" experienced by having a smoke.[13] By extrapolation, it is logical to think that quitting might be facilitated by antidepressants. A 7-week course of sustained release bupropion (Zyban) in doses of either 150 once a day or 300 mg/day (150 mg bid) given to smokers with no history of depression resulted in abstinence rates at 1 year of 23% compared with 12% among control subjects. In this study weight gain among abstainers was greatest for those taking a placebo and least for those taking 300 mg of bupropion daily.[14] Another study compared bupropion 150 mg bid, nicotine patch alone, nicotine patch plus bupropion 150 mg bid, and placebo over a 9-week period. At the end of 1 year, abstinence rates were 30% in the bupropion only group, 36% in the bupropion plus patch group, and about 16% in the placebo and patch only groups.[15] Nortriptyline (Aventyl, Pamelor) in doses of 50 to 100 mg/day has also been shown to increase abstinence rates among smokers with[16] and without[16,17] a history of depression.

A relationship between smoking and depression is supported by the observation that smokers with a history of major depression have a high recurrence rate if they quit successfully. In a 3-month follow-up of 126 individuals who had quit smoking successfully, the incidence of major depression was 2% among those with no history of depression, 17% among those with a history of a single episode of depression, and 30% for those with a history of recurrent depressions.[18]

Formulations of Nicotine Replacement Therapy

Nicotine replacement therapy is available in the form of 2- and 4-mg nicotine-containing chewing gum (Nicorette), nicotine-containing transdermal patches with various concentrations of nicotine (Habitrol, Nicoderm, Nicotrol, and ProStep), and more recently a nicotine-containing nasal spray (Nicotrol nasal spray) and a nicotine inhaler (Nicotrol Inhaler) (Table 68).

Nicotine chewing gum (Table 68)

Nicotine chewing gum is available in 2- and 4-mg formulations. The 2-mg formulation is recommended for those who smoke fewer than 25 cigarettes a day, and the 4-mg formulation is for those who smoke more. Scheduled dosage of 1 or 2 pieces of gum per hour gives better results than ad libitum usage. The usual manufacturer's recommendations are to use the gum for 6 weeks and then taper use over another 6 weeks. However, much longer usage has not been associated with an increase in adverse effects, and even use of the drug while the patient continues to smoke has not been associated with an increase in cardiovascular disease.[2]

Nicotine polacrilex should not be chewed like ordinary gum. The gum should be chewed a few times and then held in the mouth for a minute or so before repeating the cycle. This prevents nicotine rushes. Each piece should be used for about 30 minutes.[19]

Table 68   Nicotine Replacement Therapy

Drug names	Drug concentrations
Nicotine Polacrilex Chewing Gum	
Nicorette	2 mg
Nicorette DS, Nicorette Plus	4 mg
Nicotine Transdermal Systems	
Habitrol	21, 14, 7 (mg absorbed/24 hr)
Nicoderm	21, 14, 7 (mg absorbed/24 hr)
Nicotrol	15, 10, 5 (mg absorbed/16 hr)
ProStep	22, 11 (mg absorbed/24 hr)
Nicotine Nasal Spray	
Nicotrol NS	0.5 mg per activation
Nicotine Inhaler	
Nicotrol Inhaler	2 mg absorbed from 80 deep inhalations over 20 min

Nicotine patches (Table 68)

Nicotine patches are safe for patients with known stable coronary artery disease.[20] Patients smoking more than 10 cigarettes per day should be started on the highest dose patches, while those who smoke less may be started on midrange patches.

Patches should be applied to hairless areas of the skin, and the site changed daily to prevent irritation. Habitrol, Nicoderm, and ProStep are changed every 24 hours, whereas Nicotrol is applied first thing in the morning and removed at bedtime (16 hours of use).

Nicotine nasal spray

Nicotine nasal spray results in a more rapid rise in nicotine blood levels than is obtained with patches, gum, or an inhaler.[2] The usual dose of the nicotine nasal spray (Nicotrol NS) is two activations in each nostril (a total of 4 mg) with a maximum of 5 doses an hour or 40 doses a day.

Nicotine inhaler

The nicotine inhaler looks like a cigarette. The patient inserts a 10-mg nicotine cartridge into the mouthpiece and puffs on it to obtain the nicotine. Taking 80 deep puffs over 20 minutes releases 4 mg of nicotine; of this amount, 2 mg is absorbed. The nicotine is deposited on and absorbed from the buccal mucosa (less than 5% reaches the lungs), and therefore the pharmacological effects are similar to those obtained from nicotine gum.[2]

❧ REFERENCES ❧

1. Fiore MC, Wetter DW, Bailey WC, et al (Smoking Cessation Clinical Practice Guideline Panel and Staff): The Agency for Health Care Policy and Research Smoking Cessation clinical practice guideline, *JAMA* 275:1270-1280, 1996.
2. Ayanian JZ, Cleary PD: Perceived risks of heart disease and cancer among cigarette smokers, *JAMA* 281:1019-1021, 1999.
3. Hughes JR, Goldstein MG, Hurt RD, et al: Recent advances in the pharmacotherapy of smoking, *JAMA* 281:72-76, 1999.
4. Prochaska JO: Why do we behave the way we do? *Can J Cardiol* 11(suppl A):20A-25A, 1995.
5. West R, Hajek P: What happens to anxiety levels on giving up smoking? *Am J Psychiatry* 154:1589-1592, 1997.
6. Law M, Tang JL: An analysis of the effectiveness of interventions intended to help people stop smoking, *Arch Intern Med* 155:1933-1941, 1995.
7. Kenford SL, Fiore MC, Jorenby DE, et al: Predicting smoking cessation: who will quit with and without the nicotine patch? *JAMA* 271:589-594, 1994.
8. Westman EC, Behm FM, Simel DL, et al: Smoking behavior on the first 1997 day of a quit attempt predicts long-term abstinence, *Arch Intern Med* 157:335-340, 1997.
9. Daughton DM, Fortmann SP, Glover ED, et al: The smoking cessation efficacy of varying doses of nicotine patch delivery systems 4-5 years post-quit day, *Prev Med* 28:113-118, 1999.
10. Blondal T, Gudmundsson LJ, Olafsdottir I, et al: Nicotine nasal spray with nicotine patch for smoking cessation: randomised trial with six year follow up, *BMJ* 318:285-289, 1999.

11. Flegal KM, Troiano RP, Pamuk ER, et al: The influence of smoking cessation on the prevalence of overweight in the United States, *N Engl J Med* 333:1165-1170, 1995.

12. Wald NJ, Watt HC: Prospective study of effect of switching from cigarettes to pipes or cigars on mortality from three smoking related diseases, *BMJ* 314:1860-1863, 1997.

13. Fowler JS, Volkow ND, Wang GJ, et al: Inhibition of mono-amine oxidase B in the brains of smokers, *Nature* 379:733-736, 1996.

14. Hurt RD, Sachs DP, Glover ED, et al: A comparison of sustained-release bupropion and placebo for smoking cessation, *N Engl J Med* 337:1195-1202, 1997.

15. Jorenby DE, Leischow SJ, Nides MA, et al: A controlled trial of sustained-release bupropion, a nicotine patch, or both for smoking cessation, *N Engl J Med* 340:685-691, 1999.

16. Hall SM, Reus VI, Munoz RF, et al: Nortriptyline and cognitive-behavioral therapy in the treatment of cigarette smoking, *Arch Gen Psychiatry* 55:683-690, 1998.

17. Prochazka AV, Weaver MJ, Keller RT, et al: A randomized trial of nortriptyline for smoking cessation, *Arch Intern Med* 158:2035-2039, 1998.

18. Covey LS, Glassman AH, Stetner F: Major depression following smoking cessation, *Am J Psychiatry* 154:263-265, 1997.

19. Henningfield JE: Nicotine medications for smoking cessation, *N Engl J Med* 333:1196-1203, 1995.

20. Joseph AM, Norman SM, Ferry LH, et al: The safety of trans-dermal nicotine as an aid to smoking cessation in patients with cardiac disease, *N Engl J Med* 335:1792-1798, 1996.

TOBACCO INDUSTRY

Between 1990 and 1991, U.S. cigarette manufacturers increased their advertising budgets by 16% to $4.6 billion per year.[1] There is persuasive circumstantial evidence that much of the industry's advertising has been aimed at children. In 1988 RJR Nabisco introduced a marketing campaign featuring Old Joe Camel.[2] Fischer and associates[3] found that 80% of 6-year-olds and 30% of 3-year-olds were able to associate a picture of Old Joe Camel with a pack of cigarettes. Between the introduction of the campaign in 1988 and 1990 the proportion of smokers under the age of 18 who smoked Camels increased from 0.5% to 32%.[4] A longitudinal evaluation of adolescents in California has provided more direct evidence that tobacco promotional activities are effective in encouraging the onset of smoking in this age group.[5]

The tobacco industry has long been suspected of knowing that nicotine was addictive and that smoking caused numerous serious diseases. Evidence that industry executives were fully cognizant of the detrimental effects of their products has been cumulative, but the most damning was the publication of the "Brown and Williamson Documents" (Brown and Williamson Tobacco Corporation) and the statements of a one-time tobacco lobbyist, Victor L. Crawford, in whom metastatic squamous cell carcinoma of the tongue developed, almost certainly as a result of smoking. Most of the July 19, 1995, issue of *JAMA* is devoted to this subject,[6] which has been elaborated on in the 1996 book *The Cigarette Papers*.[7] Further documentation of the duplicity of the

tobacco industry through such activities as promoting "low-tar, low-nicotine" cigarettes and manipulating the pH of cigarettes to create more free (as opposed to bound) nicotine is found in the court documents of the Minnesota Tobacco Trial.[8] A 1998 editorial from *JAMA* does not mince words: "The tobacco makers have shown themselves to be a rogue industry, unwilling to abide by ordinary ethical business rules and social standards. . . . These actions are morally reprehensible."[9]

One of the arguments put forward in support of the tobacco industry is that economic benefits derive from producing and marketing the product. On a global basis tobacco accounts for an estimated 16 million to 140 million jobs.[10] However, according to a World Bank study the net global economic effect of tobacco is a loss of $200 billion.[11] A computer simulation of the economic effects of eliminating the tobacco industry in the United States concluded that although many jobs would be lost in the Southeast, these would be offset by new jobs developed in the rest of the country because of the increased discretionary spending of all the former smokers.[12] Another economic argument propagated by the tobacco industry is that ordinances requiring restaurants and bars to be smoke free would have a devastating effect on tourism and income. No studies have found this to occur, and some even point to an improvement in tourist business.[13]

◣ REFERENCES ◢

1. Cigarette smoking among adults—United States, 1992, and changes in the definition of current cigarette smoking, *MMWR* 43:342-346, 1994.

2. MacKenzie TD, Bartecchi CE, Schrier RW: The human costs of tobacco use (second of two parts), *N Engl J Med* 330:975-980, 1994.

3. Fischer PM, Schwartz MP, Richards JW Jr, et al: Brand logo recognition by children aged 3 to 6 years: Mickey Mouse and Old Joe the Camel, *JAMA* 266:3145-3148, 1991.

4. DiFranza JR, Richards JW, Paulman PM et al: RJR Nabisco's cartoon camel promotes Camel cigarettes to children, *JAMA* 266:3149-3153, 1991.

5. Pierce JP, Choi WS, Gilpin EA, et al: Tobacco industry promotion of cigarettes and adolescent smoking, *JAMA* 279:511-515, 1998.

6. The Brown and Williamson Documents, *JAMA* 274:199-202, 219-258, 1995.

7. Glantz SA, Slade J, Bero LA, et al: *The cigarette papers,* Berkeley, 1996, University of California Press.

8. Hurt RD, Robertson CR: Prying open the door to the tobacco industry's secrets about nicotine, *JAMA* 280:1173-1181, 1998.

9. Koop CE, Kessler DC, Lundberg GD: Reinventing American tobacco policy: sounding the medical community's voice (editorial), *JAMA* 279:550-552, 1998.

10. Phillips A, deSavigny D, Law MM: As Canadians butt out, the developing world lights up (editorial), *Can Med Assoc J* 153:1111-1114, 1995.

11. Barnum H: The economic burden of the global trade in tobacco, *Tobacco Control* 3:358-361, 1994.

12. Warner KE, Fulton GA, Nicolas P, et al: Employment implications of declining tobacco product sales for the regional economies of the United States, *JAMA* 275:1241-1246, 1996.

13. Glantz SA, Charlesworth A: Tourism and hotel revenues before and after passage of smoke-free restaurant ordinances, *JAMA* 281:1911-1918, 1999.

UROLOGY

Topics covered in this section

Bladder
Hematuria
Incontinence
Infertility, Male
Penis
Prostate
Renal Cell Carcinoma
Renal Colic
Sexual Dysfunction
Testes
Urinary Tract Infections
Vasectomy
Vasovasostomy

BLADDER
Acute Urinary Retention

In most cases the cause of acute urinary retention is unknown. Elderly men are at greatest risk; the chance of suffering acute retention within 5 years is 1 in 10 for men in their seventies and 1 in 3 for men in their eighties. Acute urinary retention in younger people or women of any age requires careful investigation; medications and neurological diseases are common precipitants.

The immediate management of acute urinary retention in elderly men is catheterization. After a variable period of catheterization some men may be able to void spontaneously, although the recurrence rate of acute retention is reported to be 50% within a week and 68% within a year. Ability to void after removal of the catheter is more likely if the catheter has been left in place for a week and if the man has taken an alpha-adrenergic blocker (such as terazosin [Hytrin]) while catheterized.[1]

◣ REFERENCES ◤

1. Emberton M, Anson K: Acute urinary retention in men: an age old problem, *BMJ* 318:921-925, 1999.

Bladder Cancer
(See also hematuria; urinalysis)

Physicians sometimes order routine urinalyses as a screening technique for bladder cancer. There is no evidence that early diagnosis improves survival,[1] and because of this,

the Canadian Task Force on Preventive Health Care[2] and the U.S. Preventive Services Task Force[3] give urinalysis for the detection of bladder cancer in the general population a "D" recommendation. For similar reasons they give a "D" recommendation for urine cytology screening for bladder cancer in the general population.[2,3]

Bladder cancers are common tumors that occur more frequently in men and in smokers.[4] A prospective epidemiological study of male health professionals found that a high intake of fluids was associated with a decreased risk of bladder cancer.[5]

The usual clinical presentation is painless frank hematuria. Diagnosis is usually based on flexible cystoscopy and biopsy. In 80% of cases the tumor is confined to the mucosa (superficial tumors), while 20% are invasive. The prognosis of superficial tumors is excellent. They are usually treated with transurethral resection followed by the instillation of chemotherapeutic drugs or bacille Calmette Guerin (BCG) into the bladder. Adjuvant therapy prolongs disease-free intervals but does not prevent invasion. Invasive tumors are highly malignant and are generally treated with cystectomy, often with adjuvant chemotherapy or radiation therapy. The 5-year survival with invasive tumors is 50%.[4]

◣ REFERENCES ◤

1. Gulliford MC, Petruckevich A, Burney PGI: Survival with bladder cancer, evaluation of delay in treatment, type of surgeon, and modality of treatment, *BMJ* 303:437-440, 1991.

2. Canadian Task Force on the Periodic Health Examination: *Canadian guide to clinical preventive health care,* Ottawa, 1994, Canada Communication Group—Publishing, pp 826-836.

3. US Preventive Services Task Force: *Guide to clinical preventive services,* ed 2, Baltimore, 1996, Williams & Wilkins, pp 181-186.

4. van der Meijden AP: Bladder cancer, *BMJ* 317:1366-1369, 1998.

5. Michaud DS, Spiegelman D, Clinton SK, et al: Fluid intake and the risk of bladder cancer in men, *N Engl J Med* 340:1390-1397, 1999.

Catheters, Urethral
(See also urinalysis; bacteriuria and pyuria in the elderly; urinary tract infections)

Permanent indwelling Silastic catheters are usually changed every 3 to 12 weeks. Bacteriuria develops in virtually all patients with long-term urinary catheters,[1,2] but despite this, changing the catheter almost never leads to sepsis.[1] Complications associated with long-term indwelling catheters include obstruction by encrustations, bladder and kidney stones, pyelonephritis, renal failure, bacteremia, and bladder cancer.[2,3] Options to long-term catheterization are intermittent self-catheterization, which can be performed with a clean but nonsterile technique, and condom catheters. Intermittent self-catheterization is effective and has few adverse effects. Condom catheters have on rare occasion been responsible for penile ulceration, necrosis, and gangrene,[2] but the major concern about these devices stems from a report that the incidence of urinary tract infections (UTIs) was greater in patients using condom catheters than in those with indwelling catheters.[4] The validity of this report has been questioned in large part because the diagnosis of UTIs was based on cultures, and unless special precautions are taken, cultures of urine obtained from condom devices are likely to have a high false-positive rate because of the growth of organisms on the penile skin.[3] Earlier studies of men in nursing homes found that the incidence of clinical UTIs was 2.5 times greater in those with indwelling catheters than in control subjects using condom catheters.[5]

The Canadian Task Force on Preventive Health Care gives an "E" rating to screening and treatment of asymptomatic bacteriuria in patients with indwelling catheters.[6]

────────────── ⚐ REFERENCES ⚐ ──────────────

1. Bregenzer T, Frei R, Widmer AF, et al: Low risk of bacteremia during catheter replacement in patients with long-term urinary catheters, *Arch Intern Med* 157:521-525, 1997.
2. Stickler DJ, Zimakoff J: Complications of urinary tract infections associated with devices used for long-term bladder management, *J Hosp Infect* 28:177-194, 1994.
3. Warren JW: Urethral catheters, condom catheters, and nosocomial urinary tract infections (editorial), *Infect Control Hosp Epidemiol* 17:212-214, 1996.
4. Zimakoff J, Stickler DJ, Pontoppidan B, et al: Bladder management and urinary tract infections in Danish hospitals, nursing homes and home care: a national prevalence study, *Infect Control Hosp Epidemiol* 17:215-221, 1996.
5. Ouslander JG, Greengold B, Chen S: Complications of chronic indwelling urinary catheters among male nursing home patients: a prospective study, *J Urol* 138:1191-1195, 1987.
6. Canadian Task Force on the Periodic Health Examination: *Canadian guide to clinical preventive health care,* Ottawa, 1994, Canada Communication Group—Publishing, pp 966-967.

Interstitial Cystitis

Interstitial cystitis is a disease of unknown etiology and uncertain management. It usually affects middle-aged women and is characterized by urinary frequency (more than eight times during the day and twice at night), urgency, and perineal, suprapubic, or pelvic pain that is relieved in part by voiding. The diagnosis can be made only if other diseases such as bacterial urinary tract infection or bladder cancer are ruled out and if cystoscopy reveals multiple mucosal glomerulations or pinpoint hemorrhages. There are no specific findings on bladder biopsy.[1,2] A variety of treatments have been used; intravesical instillation of dimethyl sulfoxide (DMSO) is currently one of the favored ones.[2]

────────────── ⚐ REFERENCES ⚐ ──────────────

1. Keller MS, McCarthy DO, Neider RS: Measurement of symptoms of interstitial cystitis: a pilot study, *Urol Clin North Am* 21:67-71, 1994.
2. Thompson AC, Christmas TJ: Interstitial cystitis—an update, *Br J Urol* 78:813-820, 1996.

HEMATURIA

(See also acute exertional rhabdomyolysis; bladder cancer; diarrhea and hematochezia in runners; IgA nephropathy; urinalysis)

In a study from the Mayo Clinic, microscopic hematuria (defined as the presence of any red blood cells in a high-power field) occurred in 13% of asymptomatic men and postmenopausal women. Younger women were excluded from the study because of the high rate of contamination of the urine with menstrual flow. After a 5½-year follow-up, only 0.5% of the patients were found to have renal cell cancer or bladder cancer.[1]

In a study from a British "hematuria clinic" no diagnosis was reached in 20% of the cases. In the same clinic infections accounted for the most cases (25%), followed by benign prostatic hyperplasia (22%).[2]

Not all red urine is caused by blood. Aside from myoglobinuria and hemoglobinuria, a variety of ingested substances can give a reddish urine. These include beets, berries, food coloring, cascara-containing laxatives, ibuprofen (Motrin, Advil), phenazopyridine (Pyridium), phenytoin (Dilantin), quinine, sulfamethoxazole (Septra, Bactrim), chloroquine (Aralen), and rifampin.[3]

Exercise-Induced Hematuria

Exercise-induced hematuria is a common condition that is usually microscopic but may be macroscopic.[3,4] It affects both sexes and is associated both with contact sports such as boxing and football and with noncontact sports such as swimming, track, and rowing. There are a variety of pathophysiological explanations—ischemic damage to the nephrons from renal vessel constriction, more marked constriction of the efferent than the afferent glomerular arterioles, and repeated trauma to the bladder mucosa caused by the posterior wall slapping against the base.[4]

The differential diagnosis includes exercise-induced rhabdomyolysis and march hemoglobinuria. In neither of these cases are red blood cells found in the urine. In exercise-induced hematuria a urine dipstick test is positive for blood and the urinalysis reveals red blood cells. The diagnosis can be safely made in asymptomatic individuals under the age of 40 with microscopic hematuria if there are red blood cells, no red blood cell casts, and clearance of hematuria within 72 hours of the precipitating physical activity.[3,5] The presence of gross hematuria raises the question of urothelial neoplasm, and the presence of red blood cell casts suggests a glomerular disease. Patients with exercise-induced hematuria will not damage their kidneys if they continue participating in the activities that elicit the phenomenon.[3]

────────────── ⚐ REFERENCES ⚐ ──────────────

1. Mohr DN, Offord KP, Owen RA, et al: Asymptomatic microhematuria and urologic disease: a population-based study, *JAMA* 256:224-229, 1986.
2. Paul AB, Collie DA, Wild SR, et al: An integrated haematuria clinic, *Br J Clin Pract* 47:128-130, 1993.

3. Gambrell RC, Blount BW: Exercise-induced hematuria, *Am Fam Physician* 53:905-911, 1996.
4. Abarbanel J, Benet AE, Lask D, Kimche D: Sports hematuria, *J Urol* 143:887-890, 1990.
5. Cianflocco AJ: Renal complications of exercise, *Clin Sports Med* 11:437-451, 1992.

INCONTINENCE

(See also geriatrics)

Classification

Urinary incontinence may be classified as transient or long standing.[1] The two most common causes of persistent urinary incontinence are stress incontinence and detrusor overactivity (detrusor instability, detrusor hyperreactivity, urge incontinence).[1] Although overflow incontinence accounts for only 5% to 10% of cases of urinary incontinence, it should be ruled out in all cases.[1,2]

Transient urinary incontinence

The following are important causes of transient incontinence[1]:

1. Delirium
2. Urinary tract infections (not asymptomatic bacteriuria)
3. Atrophic urethritis and vaginitis
4. Medications, especially polypharmacy (sedatives, hypnotics, anticholinergics such as antipsychotics and tricyclic antidepressants, narcotics, alpha-adrenergic antagonists, dihydropyridine calcium channel blockers, diuretics)
5. Excess urine output
6. Restricted mobility
7. Fecal impaction

Stress incontinence

Stress incontinence is one of the major forms of incontinence in women, and its diagnosis can often be made with reasonable certainty on the basis of the history.[1] If the patient is mentally competent and denies that incontinence occurs instantaneously with a stress maneuver, the diagnosis of stress incontinence can be ruled out with 90% certainty.[1] An important aggravating factor in some cases of stress incontinence is the treatment of hypertension with alpha-adrenergic blockers such as terazosin (Hytrin), doxazosin (Cardura), labetalol (Trandate), methyldopa (Aldomet), and clonidine (Catapres). These drugs inhibit the alpha-adrenergic receptors of the internal sphincter, which stimulate its closure. If possible they should be discontinued.[2]

Specific management of stress incontinence may involve behavioral techniques, pharmacological agents, or a combination of the two. A standard behavioral technique is pelvic muscle–strengthening exercises, an approach first described by Kegel in 1948. A 1999 study of women with stress incontinence compared a group that performed pelvic muscle exercises three times a day to a nonexercising control group. Each exercise session consisted of near maximum contraction of the pelvic muscles held for 6 to 8 seconds and repeated up to 12 times with 6 seconds of rest between contractions. Marked improvement in incontinence was observed in the exercising group.[3] A report on elderly women with stress incontinence found that three fourths became continent when they followed this procedure.[4] Contracting the pelvic floor muscles beginning 1 second before coughing has been reported effective in a clinic setting.[5]

First-line pharmacological treatment for stress incontinence is probably estrogens.[2] These should be given in the usual doses for hormonal replacement therapy, and when indicated progestins should be added. Beneficial effects may be delayed for several weeks. Estrogen acts by thickening the mucosa of the urethra and trigone and also seems to increase the sensitivity and numbers of alpha-adrenergic receptors, which supply and cause contraction of the internal urethral sphincter.[2] Beneficial effects have not been found in all studies. A randomized double-blind placebo-controlled study found no improvement when a group of postmenopausal women with stress incontinence, detrusor instability, or both were treated with equine estrogens (Premarin) 0.625 mg and medroxyprogesterone (Provera) 10 mg given cyclically over 3 months.[6]

Detrusor overactivity

Detrusor overactivity or urge incontinence is characterized by the sudden onset of an intense desire to void or even a sudden gush of urine unrelated to a stress maneuver without any urge to void.[1] It is a common problem in the elderly and is caused by failure of cortical centers to inhibit detrusor activity or by spontaneous premature contractions of the detrusor muscle. Exacerbating factors are excessive caffeine intake, beta-blockers (beta-adrenergic stimulation inhibits the detrusor muscle), and sedatives.[2]

Bladder training is the usual initial therapeutic intervention for patients with detrusor overactivity.[1,7] The intervals between periods of incontinence are recorded, and the patient is instructed to void before that interval ends. For example, if incontinence occurs after 3 hours, the patient should void after 2 hours and consciously suppress any voiding urges during those first 2 hours. After this routine is established and the incontinence is controlled, the intervals between voidings are gradually lengthened.[1] An alternative that proved effective in one study was teaching patients to contract the pelvic muscles voluntarily without contracting the abdominal muscles whenever they had the urge to urinate. The program consisted of an initial session of anorectal biofeedback, three follow-up sessions with trained nurse practitioners, and a series of pelvic muscle contraction exercises done three times daily at home.[8]

Pharmacotherapy for detrusor overactivity may be tried if behavioral approaches and removal of exacerbating factors fail. Commonly used drugs are those with antimuscarinic activity that leads to relaxation of the detrusor muscle.[1,2] When these drugs are used, care should be taken not to induce urinary retention.[2] Oxybutynin (Ditropan) is one of the most commonly used drugs. Although the usual recommended dose is 5 mg bid or tid, many patients respond to 2.5 mg tid and at that dosage patients have fewer adverse effects. Maximum benefit may not be observed for several weeks.[7]

Some other antimuscarinic drugs and their usual doses are flavoxate (Urispas) 200 mg tid to qid, tolterodine (Detrol) 1 to 2 mg bid, dicyclomine (Bentyl, Bentylol) 10 to 30 mg qid, propantheline (Pro-Banthine) 15 to 30 mg qid, and imipramine (Tofranil) and desipramine (Norpramin, Pertofrane) in low doses.

Eradicating bacteriuria in incontinent nursing home residents did not improve the degree of incontinence.[9]

Overflow incontinence

Overflow incontinence may be due to obstructive lesions, to neurological disorders such as multiple sclerosis or diabetic neuropathy with denervation of the detrusor muscle, or to the secondary effects of medications such as the tricyclic antidepressants (the anticholinergic actions inhibit detrusor muscle contraction).[1] Abdominal assessment for a distended bladder is thus an essential part of the examination of a patient complaining of incontinence. The presence of a distended bladder points to overflow incontinence, although the absence of this finding does not rule it out.

Pharmacotherapy for inadequate detrusor muscle function is not very effective, but the cholinergic drug bethanechol (Urecholine) 10 to 25 mg tid or qid may be tried. Adverse effects include diarrhea and abdominal cramps, bradycardia, hypotension, and bronchospasm.[1]

─────────────── ◣ **REFERENCES** ◢ ───────────────

1. Resnick NM: An 89-year-old woman with urinary incontinence, *JAMA* 276:1832-1840, 1996.
2. Mold JW: Pharmacotherapy of urinary incontinence, *Am Fam Physician* 54:673-680, 1996.
3. Bø K, Talseth T, Holme I: Single blind, randomised controlled trial of pelvic floor exercises, electrical stimulation, vaginal cones, and no treatment in management of genuine stress incontinence in women, *BMJ* 318:487-493, 1999.
4. Norton PA, Baker JE: Postural changes can reduce leakage in women with stress urinary incontinence, *Obstet Gynecol* 84:770-774, 1994.
5. Miller JM, Ashton-Miller JA, DeLancey JO: A pelvic muscle precontraction can reduce cough-related urine loss in selected women with mild SUI, *J Am Geriatr Soc* 46:870-874, 1998.
6. Fantl JA, Bump RC, Robinson D, et al (Continence Program for Women Research Group): Efficacy of estrogen supplementation in the treatment of urinary incontinence, *Obstet Gynecol* 88:745-749, 1996.
7. Resnick NM: Improving treatment of urinary incontinence (editorial), *JAMA* 280:2034-2035, 1998.
8. Burio KL, Locher JL, Goode PS, et al: Behavioral vs drug treatment for urge urinary incontinence in older women: a randomized controlled trial, *JAMA* 280:1995-2000, 1998.
9. Ouslander JG, Schapira M, Schnelle JF, et al: Does eradicating bacteriuria affect the severity of chronic urinary incontinence in nursing home residents? *Ann Intern Med* 122:749-754, 1995.

INFERTILITY, MALE
(See also infertility, female; vasovasostomy)

An estimated 15% of couples have fertility problems. The problem rests exclusively with the male in 30% of cases and partly with the male in another 20%. Unfortunately, the causes of the male abnormalities usually remain unknown even after a thorough workup.[1]

Factors believed to adversely affect spermatogenesis include medications (cimetidine, sulfasalazine, nitrofurantoin, tetracyclines, colchicine), illicit drugs (marijuana, cocaine, anabolic steroids), cigarette smoking, and excessive heat exposure from hot tubs.[1,2]

Varicoceles are present in about one fourth of men seeking help for infertility. Whether varicoceles are etiologically related to infertility is unknown, and if treating them provides any benefit, it is minimal after the age of 30. Although infertile men should avoid soaking in a hot tub, which can raise scrotal temperatures, saunas and hot showers are not contraindicated.[2] Wearing briefs rather than boxer shorts does not alter scrotal temperatures, and there is no evidence that switching to boxer shorts increases fertility.[3]

Infection is a rare cause of male infertility even though considerable literature supports such a relationship.[1] Nevertheless, the patient should be tested for *Chlamydia trachomatis,* usually with a fresh urine sample.[2] Antisperm antibodies may be associated with male infertility, but the role of corticosteroid treatment under these circumstances is controversial.[4]

Semen analysis is the major investigation of the male in cases of infertility. The normal values given by the World Health Organization (20 million or more sperm/ml[3] and 60% progressive motility) are derived from population studies of normal and infertile men. They are not applicable to individual men, since good fertility has been documented with motile sperm counts even lower than 1 million/ml[3].[2]

When infertility is related to sperm dysfunction in the male, the intracytoplasmic injection of a single sperm or spermatid into the ovum is used in many centers (see discussion of female infertility). If the ejaculate contains no sperm, sperm may be obtained from the testes. Needle aspiration results in a retrieval rate of about 10%, whereas open testicular biopsy (which can be done with patient under local anesthesia) has a retrieval rate of around 50%.[5] Preoperative genetic screening of men with nonobstructive azoospermia may be desirable; one study in which screening was done found genetic abnormalities in 17%.[6]

Intracytoplasmic sperm injection (ICSI) was first reported in 1992, so no long-term studies of children conceived by this technique are available. One trial comparing children conceived naturally or by in vitro fertilization (IVF) with those conceived by ICSI at 1 year of age found no differences in major congenital anomalies among the groups, although a greater number of children conceived by ICSI had lower scores on a mental development index than in the other two groups.[7] A subsequent study of 17-month-old children found no clinically significant differences in mental development between ICSI-conceived children and naturally conceived control subjects.[8]

REFERENCES

1. Howards SS: Treatment of male infertility, *N Engl J Med* 332:312-317, 1995.
2. Hargreave TB, Mills JA: Investigating and managing infertility in general practice, *BMJ* 316:1438-1441, 1998.
3. Munkelwitz R, Gilbert BR: Are boxer shorts really better? A critical analysis of the role of underwear type in male subfertility, *J Urol* 160:1329-1333, 1998.
4. Haas GG Jr: Antisperm antibodies in infertile men, *JAMA* 275:885, 1996.
5. Silber SJ: The cure and proliferation of male infertility (editorial), *J Urol* 160:2072-2073, 1998.
6. Rucker GB, Mielnik A, King P, et al: Preoperative screening for genetic abnormalities in men with nonobstructive azoospermia before testicular sperm extraction, *J Urol* 160:2068-2071, 1998.
7. Bowen JR, Gibson FL, Leslie GI, et al: Medical and developmental outcome at 1 year for children conceived by intracytoplasmic sperm injection, *Lancet* 351:1529-1534, 1998.
8. Sutcliffe AG, Taylor B, Thornton S, et al: Children born after intracytoplasmic sperm injection: population control study, *BMJ* 318:704-705, 1999.

PENIS
Paraphimosis

A technique for nonoperative treatment of paraphimosis is to wrap the penis with a 4×4 gauze liberally coated with 5% lidocaine ointment. When the wrapping is applied, more pressure should be placed over the distal than the proximal penis. After 5 to 10 minutes the glans swelling should have diminished and it should be possible to pull the foreskin back over the glans.[1]

Pearly Penile Papules

Pearly penile papules are normal anatomical structures found around the corona of the penis in up to 20% of young men. They are smooth, whitish elevations and are said to be more common in blacks and in the uncircumcised. Treatment is reassurance.

Peyronie's Disease

Peyronie's disease is a disorder of unknown etiology characterized by a curvature of the penis caused by inelastic scar or plaque formation. The incidence is increased in patients with Dupuytren's contracture. Some patients cannot perform vaginal penetration because of the penile curvature or because of distal flaccidity. Pain and tenderness in the region of the plaque may be the presenting symptoms. The condition resolves spontaneously in 20% to 50% of patients. Local corticosteroid injections are sometimes helpful, but in more intractable cases surgery is necessary.[2]

REFERENCES

1. Olson C: Emergency treatment of paraphimosis, *Can Fam Physician* 44:1253, 1998.
2. Fitkin J, Ho GT: Peyronie's disease: current management, *Am Fam Physician* 60:549-554, 1999.

PROSTATE
Benign Prostatic Hyperplasia
(See also alternative medicine)

Symptoms

The major symptoms of benign prostatic hyperplasia are found in the American Urological Association questionnaire, which was developed to give a quantitative estimate of symptomatic distress.[1] The seven symptoms of significance are as follows:

1. Sensation of incomplete bladder emptying
2. Increased daytime urinary frequency (less than 2-hour intervals)
3. Increased frequency of nighttime urination
4. Urinary urgency
5. Involuntary interruptions of stream when urinating
6. Weak stream
7. Straining to begin urination

Surgical treatment

The standard surgical treatment of benign prostatic hyperplasia is transurethral resection. For patients with moderate to severe symptoms, immediate results are excellent.[2,3] However, 20% to 25% of patients do not have long-term satisfactory outcomes, and the reoperation rate in men followed for 10 or more years is 15% to 20%. Reported complications of surgery include retrograde ejaculation in about three fourths of the patients, impotence in 5% to 10%, some degree of urinary incontinence in 2% to 4%, postoperative urinary tract infections in 5% to 10%, and blood transfusions in 5% to 10%.[2] In one study of men who were sexually active both before and after transurethral prostatic resections, half reported absent or altered orgasm.[4] Because of the potential complications of surgery, and because there is now good evidence that benign prostatic hyperplasia is not always a progressive disease, watchful waiting is a reasonable therapeutic option for many patients with mild or moderate symptoms (see section on watchful waiting below).[3]

Aside from transurethral and retropubic prostatectomy, a surgical option for treating benign prostatic hyperplasia is a transurethral incision of the prostate. This is a relatively simple intervention that is effective in many instances. It is used particularly for men with small prostate glands, for those who want to avoid retrograde ejaculation, and for those who are debilitated and therefore not good candidates for more extensive procedures. Another option for some patients is a permanently indwelling prostatic stent. Procedures under development include microwave and laser therapies.[2] Transurethral microwave thermotherapy can be given using topical urethral anesthesia. In one study comparing this procedure to oral terazosin (Hytrin), greater improvement was seen in the terazosin patients at 6 weeks, but the microwave-treated patients had better outcomes at 6 and 12 months.[5]

Medical treatment

Alpha$_1$-adrenergic blocking agents relieve the symptoms of benign prostatic hyperplasia by relaxing the smooth muscles within the prostate. Four such agents that have been used for this purpose are terazosin (Hytrin), doxazosin (Cardura), prazosin (Minipress), and tamsulosin (Flomax). Most of the studies to date have involved terazosin, which improved urine flow rates and symptoms in 50% to 70% of patients.[6] The usual dosages of these agents are terazosin 5 to 10 mg qhs, doxazosin 4 to 8 mg qhs, and tamsulosin 0.4 to 0.8 mg once daily.

Finasteride (Proscar) inhibits 5-alpha-reductase, an intracellular enzyme that metabolizes testosterone into the more potent dihydrotestosterone. Use of this drug (usual dose is 5 mg daily) causes atrophy of the prostate.[7] Finasteride is more effective than placebo, but only a small number of treated patients benefit.[7,8] In one 4-year double-blind, randomized, placebo-controlled trial, 80 men had to be treated for 1 year to prevent one man from requiring surgery and 100 men had to be treated for 1 year to prevent one man from having urinary retention.[8] Side effects, which include impotence and breast tenderness, are relatively infrequent.[7]

A 1996 Veterans Administration study compared placebo to finasteride (Proscar), terazosin (Hytrin), and a combination of terazosin and finasteride. Finasteride was no more effective than placebo, terazosin resulted in significant symptom relief, and the addition of finasteride to terazosin gave no additional benefit.[6] Although finasteride was ineffective in this study, it was effective in two previous randomized controlled studies,[10,11] as well as in at least one subsequent study.[9] This may have been because the subjects had much larger prostates than was the case in the Veterans Administration trial. Relatively small prostates may respond to the muscle relaxation of an alpha$_1$-adrenergic antagonist such as terazosin, whereas larger prostates may respond only if epithelial elements are caused to atrophy through the use of a 5-alpha-reductase drug such as finasteride.[9,12]

Alternative medical treatment

A systematic review concluded that saw palmetto extracts (Permixon) were more effective in improving urinary symptoms in patients with benign prostatic hyperplasia than placebo and as effective as finasteride. Long-term benefits have not been evaluated.[13]

Watchful waiting

The simplest form of treatment is no treatment. A review of five studies on the natural history of moderately symptomatic benign prostatic hyperplasia concluded that over time, 40% of the men improve, 45% have no change in symptoms, and 15% deteriorate.[2] A recent collaborative study from nine U.S. centers compared transurethral resection with watchful waiting for 800 men with benign prostatic hypertrophy. At the end of 3 years 24% of those who were in the watchful waiting group underwent surgery.[3]

Prevention

Data from the Health Professionals Follow-up Study found that moderate exercise such as walking decreased the risk of symptoms associated with benign prostatic hyperplasia.[14]

⚓ REFERENCES ⚓

1. Barry MJ, Fowler FJ Jr, O'Leary MP, et al (Measurement Committee of the American Urological Association): The American Urological Association symptom index for benign prostatic hyperplasia, *J Urol* 148:1549-1557, 1992.
2. Oesterling JE: Benign prostatic hyperplasia: medical and minimally invasive treatment options, *N Engl J Med* 332:99-109, 1995.
3. Wasson JH, Reda DJ, Bruskewitz RC, et al: A comparison of transurethral surgery with watchful waiting for moderate symptoms of benign prostatic hyperplasia, *N Engl J Med* 332:75-79, 1995.
4. Dunsmuir WD, Emberton M, Neal DE (Steering Group of the National Prostatectomy Audit): There is significant sexual dissatisfaction following TURP, *Br J Urol* 77:161A, 1996.
5. Djavan R, Roehrborn CG, Shariat S, et al: Prospective randomized comparison of high energy transurethral microwave thermotherapy versus α-blocker treatment of patients with benign prostatic hyperplasia, *J Urol* 161:139-143, 1999.
6. Lepor H, Williford WO, Barry MJ, et al: The efficacy of terazosin, finasteride, or both in benign prostatic hyperplasia, *N Engl J Med* 335:533-539, 1996.
7. Wasson JH: Finasteride to prevent morbidity from benign prostatic hyperplasia (editorial), *N Engl J Med* 338:612-613, 1998.
8. McConnell JD, Bruskewitz R, Walsh P, et al: The effect of finasteride on the risk of acute urinary retention and the need for surgical treatment among men with benign prostatic hyperplasia, *N Engl J Med* 338:557-563, 1998.
9. Nickel JC, Fradet Y, Boake RC, et al: Efficacy and safety of finasteride therapy for benign prostatic hyperplasia: results of a 2-year randomized controlled trial (the PROSPECT Study), *Can Med Assoc J* 155:1251-1259, 1996.
10. Gormley GJ, Stoner E, Bruskewitz RC, et al: The effect of finasteride in men with benign prostatic hyperplasia, *N Engl J Med* 327:1185-1191, 1992.
11. Finasteride Study Group: Finasteride (MK-906) in the treatment of benign prostatic hyperplasia, *Prostate* 22:291-299, 1993.
12. Walsh PC: Treatment of benign prostatic hyperplasia (editorial), *N Engl J Med* 335:586-587, 1996.

13. Wilt TJ, Ishani A, Stark G, et al: Saw palmetto extracts for treatment of benign prostatic hyperplasia, *JAMA* 280:1604-1609, 1998.

14. Platz EA, Kawachi I, Rimm EB, et al: Physical activity and benign prostatic hyperplasia, *Arch Intern Med* 158:2349-2356, 1998.

Prostate Cancer

(See also detrimental effects of investigations; prevention; screening; vasectomy)

Staging and histological grading

The two main methods of staging prostate cancer are Whitmore staging and the TNM system. These are outlined in Tables 69 and 70. Two ways of grading prostate cancer by histological features are shown in Table 71.

Epidemiology

(See also BRCA1 and BRCA2 mutations; management of prostate cancer; prostate specific antigen; screening; vasectomy)

Excluding skin cancer, the most common cancer in the United States is prostate cancer. Prostate cancer is the second leading cause of cancer death in men; 20% to 25% of men with prostate cancer die of their disease. In the United States, breast cancer kills as many people as prostate cancer and lung cancer kills three times as many.[1] Other causes of

death also exceed deaths from prostate cancer; for every prostate cancer death in the United States there are 3 accidental deaths, 5 deaths from stroke, and 20 deaths from heart disease.[2]

The incidence of prostate cancer in United States has risen dramatically in the past decade, with much of the increase attributable to an epidemic of prostate specific antigen (PSA) testing.[3] A consequence of this has been a sharp increase in the rate of radical prostatectomies in North America. For example, the number of radical prostatectomies performed under Medicare in the United States increased 5.6-fold between 1987 and 1992.[4] The rate of radical prostatectomy is not evenly distributed across the United States; in the Pacific Northwest it is over twice that in New England and the Mid-Atlantic region.[5]

Prostate cancer incidence has a large geographical and racial variation. The disease is very rare in Asia and highly prevalent in Northern Europe and North America. The incidence in Asians in North America rises in later generations but not to the degree of incidence in white North Americans.[6] In North America the incidence in blacks is about 1.5 times that in whites.

Prostate cancers in black men between the ages of 50 and 59 are of higher grade, are more often locally advanced, and are more often fatal than those in white men in the same age range. Half of black men in this age range who have locally advanced disease have a PSA level lower than 4 ng/ml, and this observation has been used as an argument for screening black men in their forties and for using lower PSA cut-off points.[7] Whether such a policy would save any lives is unknown, but it would certainly subject many men to psychologically and physically traumatic interventions (see discussion of prostate specific antigen).

The relative risk of prostate cancer increases by 2- to 2.5-fold in all races if one first-degree relative has had prostate cancer. If two first-degree relatives have had the disease, the relative risk increases 4-fold for whites and Asians and up to 10-fold for blacks.[6] A Swedish study found that the risk for prostate cancer in an unaffected man if he had two or more first-degree relatives with prostate cancer was 5% by age 60, 15% by age 70, and 30% by age 80.[8]

A rare form, "hereditary prostate cancer," accounts for 43% of prostate cancers diagnosed before 55 years of age. This form appears to have a dominant mode of inheritance with high penetrance.[9] These tumors tend to be high grade and more advanced at diagnosis than nonhereditary prostate cancers.[10] Hereditary prostate cancer accounts for less than

Table 69   Whitmore Staging of Prostate Cancer

Classification	Description
A1	Single nonpalpable microscopic focus (<5% of gland)
A2	Single nonpalpable focus (>5% of gland)
B1	Palpable localized nodule limited to one lobe
B2	Palpable localized nodules involving both lobes
C	Localized disease extending beyond the capsule
D	Distant metastases

Table 70   TNM Classification of Prostate Cancer (Tumor Only)

Classification	Description
T1	Clinically inapparent; not palpable or visible on imaging
T1a	Incidental histological finding ≤5% of tissue resected
T1b	Incidental histological finding >5% of tissue resected
T1c	Identified by blind biopsy done because of elevated prostate specific antigen
T2	Palpable; confined to the prostate
T2a	Involves half a lobe or less
T2b	Involves more than half a lobe but not both lobes
T2c	Involves both lobes
T3	Extends through prostate capsule
T4	Fixed or invades structures other than seminal vesicles

Table 71   Histological Grading of Prostate Cancer

Degree of differentiation	Gleason score
Well differentiated (grade 1)	2-4
Moderately differentiated (grade 2)	5-7
Poorly differentiated (grade 3)	8-10

10% of families with a family history of prostate cancer.[8] In a few cases hereditary prostate cancer may be related to a BRCA1 or BRCA2 mutation (see discussion of BRCA1 and BRCA2 mutations in the section on breast cancer).

Whether PSA and digital rectal examination (DRE) screening will decrease mortality in men who have two or more first-degree relatives with prostate cancer or who have a first-degree relative with prostate cancer diagnosed at an early age is unknown. Because the risk is so high, most physicians working in the field recommend screening in this situation, even if many would not recommend it for the general population (see below).[8-10]

The age at which prostate cancer develops in the father is an important factor in determining the son's risk. In a Swedish study in which prostate cancer diagnoses were made without PSA testing (with PSA testing the age at diagnosis of prostate cancer is decreased by about 5 years), sons were not at increased risk if the fathers were 80 or older at the time of diagnosis, whereas if the father's cancer was diagnosed before age 70, the son's risk was increased 3 fold.[8]

A variety of life-style characteristics have been reported to increase the risk for prostate cancer, but the evidence supporting these observations is poor. Claims have been made that consumption of large amounts of dietary fat increases the risk of the disease whereas eating large amounts of tofu or tomatoes (which contain lycopene) decreases it. Some studies have reported a decreased risk in patients taking daily supplements of selenium (200 μg/day of selenomethionine). Being sedentary is considered a risk factor, while having had a vasectomy is not (see discussion of vasectomy).[6]

◣ REFERENCES ◢

1. American Cancer Society: *Cancer facts and figures, 1998,* Atlanta, 1998, The Society.
2. Woolf SH: Public health perspective: the health policy implications of screening for prostate cancer, *J Urol* 152:1685-1688, 1994.
3. Hankey BF, Feuer EJ, Clegg LX, et al: Cancer surveillance series: interpreting trends in prostate cancer. I. Evidence of the effects of screening in recent prostate cancer incidence, mortality, and survival rates, *J Natl Cancer Inst* 91:1017-1024, 1999.
4. Olsson CA, Goluboff ET: Detection and treatment of prostate cancer: perspective of the urologist, *J Urol* 152:1695-1699, 1994.
5. Lu-Yao GL, McLerran D, Wasson J, et al (Prostate Patient Outcomes Research Team): An assessment of radical prostatectomy: time trends, geographic variation, and outcomes, *JAMA* 269:2633-2636, 1993.
6. Gallagher RP, Fleshner N: Prostate cancer. 3. Individual risk factors, *Can Med Assoc J* 159:807-813, 1998.
7. Powell IJ, Banerjee M, Sakr W, et al: Should African-American men be tested for prostate carcinoma at an earlier age than white men? *Cancer* 85:472-477, 1999.
8. Grönberg H, Wiklund F, Damber J-E: Age specific risks of familial prostate carcinoma: a basis for screening recommendations in high risk populations, *Cancer* 86:477-483, 1999.
9. McLellan DL, Norman RW: Hereditary aspects of prostate cancer, *Can Med Assoc J* 153:895-900, 1995.
10. Grönberg H, Isaacs SD, Smith JR, et al: Characteristics of prostate cancer in families potentially linked to the hereditary prostate cancer 1 (HPC1) locus, *JAMA* 278:1251-1255, 1997.

Digital rectal examination

(See also informed consent; prevention; prostate specific antigen; screening)

Digital rectal examination (DRE) is the traditional method of screening for prostate cancer. DRE in unselected populations of men older than 50 will be abnormal in 7% to 15% of cases, and of these, 15% to 30% will prove to be cancer (positive predictive value). The negative predictive value of DRE is low (the normal rectal examination would miss many cancers).[1]

If lives are to be saved by DRE, the detected tumors must be confined to the prostate because any extension through the capsule makes cure virtually impossible. Half of prostate cancers detected by DRE either have extended beyond the capsule or are not surgically resectable for other reasons.[2]

An additional twist to the issue of screening for prostate cancer by DRE or by PSA screening is that about one fourth of the cancers detected by either method are found as a result of serendipity. For DRE this means that the palpable prostatic lump is benign but that blind biopsies detect tumors that are less than 1 cm^3 in volume elsewhere in the prostate. In the case of PSA screening it also means the detection by blind biopsy of tumors less than 1 cm^3 in volume because tumors that small are unlikely to raise PSA levels. Whether small tumors detected by serendipity are clinically significant is unknown. If they are, and if treatment is effective (see below), finding them by any method is useful; if they are not, detection can only result in great psychological and physical harm.[3]

Does the detection of prostate cancer by DRE save lives? There are no controlled trials assessing this issue, so the answer is unknown.[4] If DRE does save lives, the numbers are probably very small. The U.S. Preventive Services Task Force gives digital rectal examination for prostate screening a "D" recommendation,[5] and the Canadian Task Force on Preventive Health Care gives it a "C."[6] The American College of Physicians does not recommend DRE screening but rather advises physicians to discuss the pros and cons with each patient and in this manner come to a decision.[1] In contrast, the American Cancer Society advises all men over the age of 50 who have life expectancies of at least 10 years to have annual DREs and PSA tests.[7]

◣ REFERENCES ◢

1. American College of Physicians: Clinical guideline. 3. Screening for prostate cancer, *Ann Intern Med* 126:480-484, 1997.
2. Karakiewicz PI, Aprikian AG: Prostate cancer. 5. Diagnostic tools for early detection, *Can Med Assoc J* 159:1139-1146, 1998.

3. Collins MM, Ransohoff DF, Barry MJ: Early detection of prostate cancer: serendipity strikes again, *JAMA* 278:1516-1519, 1997.
4. Coley CM, Barry MJ, Fleming C, et al: Clinical guideline. 1. Early detection of prostate cancer: prior probability and effectiveness of tests, *Ann Intern Med* 126:394-406, 1997.
5. US Preventive Services Task Force: *Guide to clinical preventive services*, ed 2, Baltimore, 1996, Williams & Wilkins, pp 119-134.
6. Canadian Task Force on the Periodic Health Examination: *Canadian guide to clinical preventive health care*, Ottawa, 1994, Canada Communication Group—Publishing, pp 817-823.
7. Von Eschenbach A, Ho R, Murphy GP, et al: American Cancer Society guideline for the early detection of prostate cancer: update 1997, *CA Cancer J Clin* 47:261-264, 1997.

Prostate specific antigen

(See also digital rectal examination; informed consent; prevention; radical prostatectomy; screening; surrogate outcomes)

History. PSA testing became widely available in North America in the mid-1980s. In the United States in 1988, 1.2% of men had had PSA testing, whereas by 1994, 40% had had the test. Initial PSA testing peaked in 1992 with a rate of 19%; since then the annual rate of initial screening has declined.[1]

Causes of elevated prostate specific antigen. Causes of elevated PSA include prostate cancer, benign prostatic hyperplasia (BPH), prostatitis, urinary retention, and prostate surgery. Prostate cancer cells generate more PSA than do normal or hyperplastic prostate cells, and well-differentiated prostate cancer generates more PSA than poorly differentiated cancer. Cancers with a volume less than 1 ml are unlikely to raise the PSA level.[2] DRE does not cause a clinically significant elevation of PSA,[2] but ejaculation may result in a temporary elevation; if PSA testing is to be performed, the patient should refrain from ejaculation for 48 hours beforehand.[3]

PSA levels in men without prostate cancer increase markedly with age, almost certainly because of an increased incidence of BPH. Proposals have been made to establish age-specific reference standards, but these have not been generally accepted.[2]

A variety of methods for increasing the specificity of PSA determinations are under active investigation. These include PSA velocity, which is a measurement of the rate of change of PSA over time; PSA density, which correlates prostatic gland volume as determined by ultrasound with PSA levels; and the percentage of free serum PSA (for unknown reasons, patients with prostate cancer have relatively less free PSA than do patients with normal glands or BPH). None of these tools has been sufficiently evaluated to merit general clinical application.[2] However, many men are by default subjected to PSA velocity. These are individuals who are found to have elevated PSA levels but in whom no prostate cancer is detected even after careful transrectal ultrasound and multiple prostatic biopsies. Such patients are usually monitored with serial PSA levels taken at 6-month intervals, and since no conclusions can be drawn until at least three readings have been obtained, they remain in limbo for at least 18 months. Even then, results may be suspect because for any one individual PSA results from two or more samples taken within a short period of time may vary by as much as 24% and laboratory variability of results is reported to be between 10% and 45%. The psychological trauma of such a situation is evident.[4]

Early detection of prostate cancer with prostate specific antigen. Does PSA screening result in the detection of more localized and therefore operable prostate cancers? The answer is clearly yes, since the rate of pathologically advanced cancers detected by initial or serial PSA screening is about half that found by DRE.[5] In one series only a third of tumors detected by PSA screening were advanced; for PSAs between 4.1 and 9.9 ng/ml, a quarter of the cancers were advanced, whereas for PSAs over 10 ng/ml, over 50% of the cancers had extended beyond the capsule.[6]

If a PSA screening program is undertaken, how many men will have "positive" results requiring further investigation? The answer is many. Smith, Catalona, and their co-workers[6] reviewed numerous studies and concluded that in initial PSA screenings between 10% and 15% of men have values above 4 ng/mL, and about the same number of men have suspicious findings on DRE. Since many of these men have both an abnormal DRE and an abnormal PSA, between 15% and 25% of men participating in an initial prostate cancer screening program are advised to have further investigation such as transrectal ultrasonography and prostate biopsy.[6] These numbers are the averages for all ages. Rates of positivity for a combination of DRE and PSA screening broken down by age are 15% for men aged 50 to 59, 28% for those aged 60 to 69, and 40% for those aged 70 to 79.[1]

The number of men with "positive" PSA tests who actually have cancer (positive predictive value) is low. Figures from the literature range from 8% to 33%.[7]

The fact that a patient has a normal PSA does not mean he does not have prostate cancer. In one series of men with PSA levels of 2.6 to 4.0 ng/ml and normal prostate examinations, 22% were found to have prostate cancer when subjected to directed or undirected biopsies.[8]

Benefits and harm of prostate specific antigen screening. The fact that PSA screening results in a "stage shift" to less advanced tumors does not necessarily mean that treatment will improve mortality. Small tumors are merely surrogate endpoints for decreased mortality, and apparent short-term beneficial results of treatment may be spurious because of lead time bias and length bias (see section on prevention). Only an impeccable prospective randomized controlled trial will determine whether PSA screening actually saves lives.

In 1999 Labrie and associates from Quebec City published the results of a PSA screening trial. They obtained the names of men between the ages of 45 and 80 from voting lists and mailed letters to a randomized group inviting them to participate in a PSA screening program. The authors reported that after a mean follow-up of 8 years those screened had a 67% relative reduction in prostate cancer mortality.[9] Critics point out that this study was not a randomized controlled trial of PSA screening but rather a randomized controlled trial of inviting men to participate in screening. Only 23% of those invited accepted, and as in any preventive program that depends on voluntary participation, the volunteers were likely to be more healthy than those who did not volunteer (healthy user effect). When the study results were analyzed on an "intention-to-screen" basis, the relative reduction rate of prostate cancer mortality was only 6%; that is, approximately 30,000 men had to be screened for 1 year to save one life or 3000 had to be screened for 10 years to save one life. Other difficulties apparent with this trial were that the upper limit of normal for PSA was set at 3 ng/ml, which is lower than the usually accepted limit of 4 ng/ml, and the exact number of men in the control group who had PSA screening during the progress of the study was not established.[10] This trial does not resolve the issue of whether PSA screening saves lives.

Proponents of PSA screening and radical prostatectomy were elated by reports that between 1991 and 1995 annual prostate cancer mortality in the United States decreased by 6.7% (from 26.7 to 24.9 deaths per 100,000 men).[11-13] Attributing this reduction to PSA screening is premature, since other explanations are equally tenable. The most cogent argument against a causal relationship is that the interval between a significant rate of population screening and the decrease in mortality is too short[11]; most prostate cancers detected by screening are well differentiated and even if untreated would not be expected to affect mortality for many years. Misclassification of death certificates probably accounts for some of the apparent decrease in mortality.[12]

Ordering a PSA test has far-reaching implications because it begins an almost irreversible diagnostic and treatment cascade that can cause significant harm (see sections on prevention and screening).[14] Many patients will have a false-positive result and suffer the psychological consequences this entails. Others will be told they have inoperable cancer—an emotional catastrophe that might have been delayed by months or years had the diagnosis been made when the disease declared itself clinically. Physical harm is inevitable for a patient with a positive PSA test result because of the morbidity resulting from prostatic biopsies and, if localized cancer is found, radical prostatectomy or radiation therapy.[15] The specific adverse effects of treating prostate cancer are discussed in the later section on management of localized prostate cancer.

Informed consent for prostate specific antigen screening. Because the benefits of PSA screening have not been proved and PSA screening may cause significant harm, ethical practice demands that patients be informed of the pros and cons of PSA testing before being screened.[15-18] When they are, many will choose not to have the test.[16,17]

Clinical practice guidelines. Both the U.S. Preventive Services Task Force[19] and the Canadian Task Force on Preventive Health Care[20] give a "D" recommendation to PSA screening. The American College of Physicians does not recommend routine screening but advises its members to discuss the pros and cons with their patients and decide on an individual basis.[18]

The American Cancer Society recommends annual PSA testing and DRE for all men aged 50 or over who have a life expectancy of at least 10 years.[21] Both the American Urological Association[22] and the Canadian Urological Association initially recommended screening all men between 50 and 70 for PSA, but in 1994 the Canadian association reversed its stand.[23]

The American Urological Association guidelines recommend that PSA screening not be done for men with a life expectancy less than 10 years, since they are far more likely to die from other causes. In spite of this recommendation, screening of elderly men for PSA is widespread. A recent survey of U.S. primary care physicians found that PSA screening was ordered routinely for 65% of men aged 70 to 74, 58% of men aged 75 to 79, and 53% of men aged 80 or over.[24] It is no wonder that about one third of all radical prostatectomies are performed in men over the age of 70.[25]

Whether PSA screening is beneficial for high-risk groups such as black Americans or men with strong family histories is unknown.

⚛ REFERENCES ✍

1. Hankey BF, Feuer EJ, Clegg LX, et al: Cancer surveillance series: interpreting trends in prostate cancer. I. Evidence of the effects of screening in recent prostate cancer incidence, mortality, and survival rates, *J Natl Cancer Inst* 91:1017-1024, 1999.

2. Coley CM, Barry MJ, Fleming C, et al: Clinical guideline. 1. Early detection of prostate cancer. 1. Prior probability and effectiveness of tests, *Ann Intern Med* 126:394-406, 1997.

3. Tchetgen M-B, Song JT, Strawderman M, et al: Ejaculation increases the serum prostate-specific antigen concentration, *Urology* 47:511-516, 1996.

4. Karakiewicz PI, Aprikian AG: Prostate cancer. 5. Diagnostic tools for early detection, *Can Med Assoc J* 159:1139-1146, 1998.

5. Catalona WJ, Richie JP, Ahmann FR, et al: Comparison of digital rectal examination and serum prostate specific antigen in the early detection of prostate cancer: results of a multicenter clinical trial of 6,630 men, *J Urol* 151:1283-1290, 1994.

6. Smith DS, Catalona WJ, Herschman JD: Longitudinal screening for prostate cancer with prostate-specific antigen, *JAMA* 276:1309-1315, 1996.

7. Feightner JW: The early detection and treatment of prostate cancer: the perspective of the Canadian Task Force on the Periodic Health Examination, *J Urol* 152:1682-1684, 1994.

8. Catalona WJ, Smith DS, Wolfert RL, et al: Evaluation of percentage of free serum prostate-specific antigen to improve specificity of prostate cancer screening, *JAMA* 274:1214-1220, 1995.

9. Labrie F, Candas B, Dupont A, et al: Screening decreases prostate cancer death: first analysis of the 1988 Quebec Prospective Randomized Controlled Trial, *Prostate* 38:83-91, 1999.

10. Ruffin M: POEMS: does inviting men to screen for prostate cancer reduce disease-specific mortality? *J Fam Pract* 48:581-582, 1999.

11. Etzioni R, Legler JM, Feuer EJ, et al: Cancer surveillance series: interpreting trends in prostate cancer. III. Quantifying the link between population prostate-specific antigen testing and recent declines in prostate cancer mortality, *J Natl Cancer Inst* 91:1033-1039, 1999.

12. Feuer EJ, Merrill RM, Hankey B: Cancer surveillance series: interpreting trends in prostate cancer. II. Cause of death misclassification and the recent rise and fall in prostate cancer mortality, *J Natl Cancer Inst* 91:1025-1032, 1999.

13. Hankey BF, Feuer EJ, Clegg LX, et al: Cancer surveillance series: interpreting trends in prostate cancer. I. Evidence of the effects of screening in recent prostate cancer incidence, mortality, and survival rates, *J Natl Cancer Inst* 91:1017-1024, 1999.

14. Marshall KG: Prevention. How much harm? How much benefit? 3. Physical, psychological and social harm, *Can Med Assoc J* 155:169-176, 1996.

15. Marshall KG: Screening for prostate cancer: how can patients give informed consent? *Can Fam Physician* 39:2385-2390, 1993.

16. Wolf A, Nasser JF, Wolf AM, et al: The impact of informed consent on patient interest in prostate-specific antigen screening, *Arch Intern Med* 156:1333-1336, 1996.

17. Mazur DJ, Hickam DH: Patient preferences for management of localized prostate cancer, *West J Med* 165:26-30, 1996.

18. American College of Physicians: Clinical guideline. 3. Screening for prostate cancer, *Ann Intern Med* 126:480-484, 1997.

19. US Preventive Services Task Force: *Guide to clinical preventive services,* ed 2, Baltimore, 1996, Williams & Wilkins, pp 119-134.

20. Canadian Task Force on the Periodic Health Examination: *Canadian guide to clinical preventive health care,* Ottawa, 1994, Canada Communication Group—Publishing, pp 812-823.

21. Von Eschenbach A, Ho R, Murphy GP, et al: American Cancer Society guideline for the early detection of prostate cancer: update 1997, *CA Cancer J Clin* 47:261-264, 1997.

22. American Urological Association: Early detection of prostate cancer and use of transrectal ultrasound. In *American Urological Association 1992 policy statement book,* Baltimore, Md, 1992, The Association, vol 4, p 20.

23. Collins JP: Detection of prostate cancer (letter), *Can Med Assoc J* 152:328-329, 1995.

24. Fowler FJ, Bin L, Collins MM, et al: Prostate cancer screening and beliefs about treatment efficacy: a national survey of primary care physicians and urologists, *Am J Med* 104:526-532, 1998.

25. Murphy GP, Mettlin C, Menck H, et al: National patterns of prostate cancer treatment by radical prostatectomy: results of a survey by the American College of Surgeons Commission on Cancer, *J Urol* 152:1817-1819, 1994.

Transrectal ultrasound

Transrectal ultrasound was developed in 1986 and is the initial investigative tool used when a PSA concentration is elevated or a prostate lesion is felt on DRE. It is reported to cause pain in only 5% of patients.[1] It is not a good screening tool for prostate cancer and has received a "D" recommendation for this purpose from both the Canadian Task Force on Preventive Health Care[2] and the U.S. Preventive Services Task Force.[3]

❧ REFERENCES ❧

1. Hermansson CG, Hugosson J, Pedersen KV: Transrectal ultrasound examination of the prostate: complications and acceptance by patients, *Br J Urol* 71:457-459, 1993.

2. Canadian Task Force on the Periodic Health Examination: *Canadian guide to clinical preventive health care,* Ottawa, 1994, Canada Communication Group—Publishing, pp 812-823.

3. US Preventive Services Task Force: *Guide to clinical preventive services,* ed 2, Baltimore, 1996, Williams & Wilkins, pp 119-134.

Biopsy of prostate

The incidence of pain from needle biopsies of the prostate is variously reported as being between 8%[1] and 31%.[2] Hematuria and hemospermia combined occur in over half of patients who have had needle biopsies.[2,3] Infection rates vary from about 1% to 6% and are lower in those given prophylactic antibiotics.[1,3] In a very few cases septicemia and even death have been reported.[4] Another rare complication is acute urinary retention.[2]

❧ REFERENCES ❧

1. Hermansson CG, Hugosson J, Pedersen KV: Transrectal ultrasound examination of the prostate: complications and acceptance by patients, *Br J Urol* 71:457-459, 1993.

2. Webb JA, Shanmuganathan K, McLean A: Complications of ultrasound-guided transperineal prostate biopsy: a prospective study, *Br J Urol* 72:775-777, 1993.

3. Gustafsson O, Norming U, Nyman CR, et al: Complications following combined transrectal aspiration and core biopsy of the prostate, *Scand J Urol Nephrol* 24:249-251, 1990.

4. Brewster SF, Rooney N, Kabala J, et al: Fatal anaerobic infection following transrectal biopsy of a rare prostatic tumour, *Br J Urol* 72:977-978, 1993.

Management of Clinically Localized Prostate Cancer
(See also prostate specific antigen)

Therapeutic options. The standard treatment options for patients with clinically localized prostate cancer (no metastases and no spread beyond the capsule) are radical prostatectomy, external beam radiation therapy, brachytherapy through computer optimized transperineal implantation of radioactive material into the prostate, and watchful waiting.[1]

Radical prostatectomy. Only one prospective randomized trial comparing prostatectomy with watchful waiting has been completed. The Veterans Administration Cooperative Urological Research Group (VACURG) study enrolled relatively few men and failed to show any benefit from surgery.[2]

It has been criticized for a variety of methodological deficits. The benefits and harm of PSA screening are discussed above under "Prostate Specific Antigen."

Whether radical prostatectomy saves lives is unknown, but most experts agree that if it does, patients most likely to benefit are those whose cancers have high Gleason scores.[3] Unfortunately, cure is extremely unlikely if tumor has extended beyond the capsule of the prostate, and in two thirds of high-grade cancers this has already occurred by the time of diagnosis.[4]

"Successful" removal of the prostate is not synonymous with cure. Fowler and associates[5] found that after radical prostatectomy, recurrent prostate cancer was detected in 16% of patients by 2 years, 22% by 3 years, and 28% by 4 years. Lu-Yao and co-workers[6] reported that one fourth of men who underwent "curative" prostatectomy required additional cancer treatment by 5 years.

In most centers follow-up management after "curative" radical prostatectomy involves regular PSA assessments, DRE, and bone scans. DRE and bone scans are superfluous in men with undetectable PSA levels, since in these circumstances recurrences are almost unknown.[7]

Adverse effects from radical prostatectomy are common. An American College of Surgeons survey evaluated the outcomes of 2122 patients who underwent surgery in 484 U.S. institutions in 1990. The operative mortality rate was 0.7%, and 56.6% of men who were potent before the surgery were left impotent. Complete incontinence was reported in 3.6% of men, 4.1% required more than two pads daily, 11.2% required two or fewer pads daily, 23.1% had occasional incontinence but did not use pads, and 58% were totally continent.[8] A more recent population survey of men who had radical prostatectomies found that 18 or more months after surgery 1.6% had no urinary control, 6.8% had frequent urinary leakage, and 40.2% had occasional urinary leakage. The impotence rate among men who were potent before surgery varied from 56% for those who had bilateral nerve-sparing surgery to 65.6% for those who had non-nerve-sparing surgery.[9]

Radiation therapy. A 1998 report that compared external beam radiation therapy, radical prostatectomy, and brachytherapy for localized prostate cancer using PSA levels as a surrogate outcome for successful control of the tumor concluded that after 5 years the three modalities were equally effective for low-risk patients (low Gleason scores, relatively low PSA levels, and less advanced staging), whereas for patients at higher risk, brachytherapy was less effective than external beam radiation or radical prostatectomy.[10] Whether rising PSA levels after treatment actually correlate with increased mortality is known, so the clinical significance of this study is uncertain, although it does cast a shadow on the efficacy of brachytherapy.[1] A subsequent report of a 10-year follow-up of men who received brachytherapy for prostate cancer was more encouraging. The overall survival was 65%, and 64% of patients were clini-

cally and biochemically free of disease at 10 years; 2% of patients had died of prostate cancer, and only 6% had had metastases. The results of brachytherapy reported in this study are comparable to the published results of radical prostatectomy.[11]

About one fourth of patients undergoing external beam radiation therapy have genitourinary symptoms such as frequency, urgency, dysuria, and nocturia during the initial 2 months of therapy, and close to half have gastrointestinal symptoms such as tenesmus and diarrhea. These symptoms usually resolve within a few weeks. The most common long-term sequela is impotence, which affects about 50% of men. A dry ejaculate is common in those who remain potent. Long-term rectal or genitourinary symptoms are relatively infrequent. Brachytherapy has fewer adverse effects. The rate of impotence is low; a number of patients may have late urinary tract or gastrointestinal symptoms.[12]

Watchful waiting. Several studies of watchful waiting have been published, and almost all have shown similar results. Men with well-differentiated tumors (low Gleason scores, in the range of 2 to 5) do extremely well, and few die of prostate cancer even after follow-up periods of 10 to 15 years, whereas the majority of men who have the most undifferentiated tumors (Gleason scores of 8 to 10) die of prostate cancer. In a recent study by Albertsen and associates[13] of men followed by watchful waiting, 33% of the cancers had Gleason scores of 2 to 5, 56% had scores of 6 to 7, and only 10% had scores of 8 to 10. As one would expect, the older the patients were at the time of diagnosis, the more likely they were to die of diseases other than prostate cancer.

Because no treatment modality has been proved to be better than another,[1] patients with localized prostate cancer and their physicians must base therapeutic decisions on the data currently available. This is clearly articulated in the 1995 guidelines of the American Urological Association, which included the following points[14]:

1. Life expectancy and overall health status are more important than age in determining suitability for surgery.
2. Patients should be informed of the accepted treatment modalities, including radical prostatectomy, radiation, and watchful waiting.
3. The estimated benefits and harm of each modality should be discussed with the patient.

------------------------------   ⚞ REFERENCES ⚟   _____

1. Chodak GW: Comparing treatments for localized prostate cancer—persisting uncertainty (editorial), *JAMA* 280:1008-1010, 1998.
2. Iversen P, Madsen PW, Corle D: Radical prostatectomy versus expectant treatment for early carcinoma of the prostate: twenty-three year follow-up of a prospective randomized study, *Scand J Urol Nephrol* 172(suppl):65-72, 1995.
3. Lu-Yao GL, Yao S-L: Population-based study of long-term survival in patients with clinically localised prostate cancer, *Lancet* 349:906-910, 1997.

4. Goldenberg SL, Ramsey EW, Jewett MA: Prostate cancer. 6. Surgical treatment of localized disease, *Can Med Assoc J* 159:1265-1271, 1998.

5. Fowler FJ Jr, Barry MJ, Lu-Yao G, et al: Patient-reported complications and follow-up treatment after radical prostatectomy: the national Medicare experience, 1988-1990 (updated June 1993), *Urology* 42:622-629, 1993.

6. Lu-Yao GL, Potosky AL, Albertsen PC, et al: Follow-up cancer treatments after radical prostatectomy: a population-based study, *J Natl Cancer Inst* 88:116-173, 1996.

7. Pound CR, Christens-Barry OW, Gurganus RT, et al: Digital rectal examination and imaging studies are unnecessary in men with undetectable prostate specific antigen following radical prostatectomy, *J Urol* 162:1337-1340, 1999.

8. Murphy GP, Mettlin C, Menck H, et al: National patterns of prostate cancer treatment by radical prostatectomy: results of a survey by the American College of Surgeons Commission on Cancer, *J Urol* 152:1817-1819, 1994.

9. Stanford JL, Feng Z, Hamilton AS: Urinary and sexual function after radical prostatectomy for clinically localized prostate cancer: the Prostate Cancer Outcomes Study, *JAMA* 283:354-360, 2000.

10. D'Amico AV, Whittington R, Malkowicz B, et al: Biochemical outcome after radical prostatectomy, external beam radiation therapy, or interstitial radiation therapy for clinically localized prostate cancer, *JAMA* 280:969-974, 1998.

11. Ragde H, Elgamal A-A A, Snow PB, et al: Ten-year disease free survival after transperineal sonography-guided iodine-125 brachytherapy with or without 45-gray external beam irradiation in the treatment of patients with clinically localized, low to high Gleason grade prostate carcinoma, *Cancer* 83:989-1001, 1998.

12. Warde P, Catton C, Gospodarowicz MK: Prostate cancer. 7. Radiation therapy for localized disease, *Can Med Assoc J* 159:1381-1388, 1998.

13. Albertsen PC, Hanley JA, Gleason DF, et al: Competing risk analysis of men aged 55-74 years at diagnosis managed conservatively for clinically localized prostate cancer, *JAMA* 280:975-980, 1998.

14. Middleton RG, Thompson IM, Austenfeld MS, et al (Prostate Cancer Clinical Guidelines Panel, American Urological Association): Summary report on the management of clinically localized prostate cancer, *J Urol* 154:2144-2148, 1995.

Advanced prostate cancer

About 80% of patients with metastatic prostate cancer respond to androgen ablation, and the median disease-free survival is 2 to 3 years. With treatment PSA levels fall to normal in nearly three fourths of patients. If after 6 months of therapy PSA levels are greater than 4 ng/ml, median survival is 18 months, whereas if the levels are below 4 ng/ml, median survival is 40 months. Rising PSA levels predate clinical recurrence by 6 to 12 months.[1]

Major adverse effects of androgen ablation are loss of libido and potency, hot flashes, gynecomastia, fatigue, and after many years of use loss of muscle mass, osteoporosis, adverse lipid profiles, glucose intolerance, and perhaps depression and irritability.[1]

Current evidence supports the initiation of androgen ablation therapy as soon as the clinical diagnosis of locally advanced or metastatic disease is made.[1] Whether this applies to men who are asymptomatic but whose PSA levels begin to rise after radical prostatectomy or radiation therapy for prostate cancer is uncertain. Although early treatment with hormone therapy may delay clinical progression, clear evidence that this results in improved prostate cancer survival has not been presented[2] and the long-term adverse effects of therapy may outweigh possible benefits.[1] Support for withholding hormonal therapy for many patients whose PSA level rises after prostatectomy comes from a Johns Hopkins study in which patients with rising PSA levels after surgery were followed with watchful waiting. Five years after a rise of PSA was documented, two thirds of the men still had no clinical evidence of tumor recurrence, and among those in whom metastatic disease did develop, the median time until death from prostate cancer was 5 years. Indicators of poor prognosis were high Gleason scores, rise of PSA level in the first 2 to 5 years after surgery, and PSA doubling time of less than 10 months.[3]

Castration is as effective as any pharmacological method of androgen ablation and generally has fewer adverse physical effects. It is irreversible and for many is psychologically traumatic. The bulk of evidence has not shown that adding pharmacological androgen ablation to castration (to suppress adrenal androgens) gives additional benefit.[1]

Several classes of pharmacological agents may be used to induce androgen ablation. Luteinizing hormone–releasing hormone (LH-RH) agonists that suppress the hypothalamic release of LH-RH include goserelin (Zoladex), leuprolide (Lupron), and buserelin (Suprefact). They are given by injection at 1- to 3-month intervals. Antiandrogens compete with androgens for androgen receptors on cell membranes and are divided into two classes: nonsteroidal antiandrogens such as flutamide (Eulexin, Euflex), nilutamide (Nilandron, Anandron), and bicalutamide (Casodex), and steroidal antiandrogens such as cyproterone acetate (Androcur) and megestrol (Megace). Steroidal antiandrogens control hot flashes.[1]

LH-RH agonists cause an initial rise in LH and testosterone lasting about 2 weeks—the so-called flare phenomenon. This reaction can be blocked by giving nonsteroidal antiandrogens or cyproterone acetate.[1]

Clinical trials are evaluating the feasibility of intermittent androgen ablation. If survival is as good as that achieved with continuous treatment, quality of life may be better because adverse effects such as impotence dissipate during the months when no treatment is given.[1]

Chemotherapy is ineffective in prolonging life in patients with hormone-refractory prostate cancer. However, mitoxantrone (Novantrone) combined with prednisone gives pain relief to a number of patients. The role of bisphosphonates in controlling symptoms from bone metastases is being evaluated.

REFERENCES

1. Gleave ME, Bruchovsky N, Moore MJ, et al: Prostate cancer. 9. Treatment of advanced disease, *Can Med Assoc J* 160:225-232, 1999.
2. Scher HI: Management of prostate cancer after prostatectomy: treating the patient, not the PSA (editorial), *JAMA* 281:1642-1645, 1999.
3. Pound CR, Partin AW, Eisenberger MA, et al: Natural history of progression after PSA elevation following radical prostatectomy, *JAMA* 281:1591-1597, 1999.

Prostatitis

Uncertainty about the pathogenesis of some forms of prostatitis is reflected in competing classifications. Until recently the generally accepted classification of prostatitis has been as follows[1]:

I. Acute bacterial prostatitis
II. Chronic prostatitis
   A. Chronic bacterial prostatitis
   B. Nonbacterial prostatitis
   C. Prostatodynia

A new consensus classification developed under the aegis of the National Institutes of Health is as follows[2]:

I. Acute bacterial prostatitis
II. Chronic bacterial prostatitis
III. Chronic prostatitis/chronic pelvic pain syndrome
   A. Inflammatory
   B. Noninflammatory
IV. Asymptomatic inflammatory prostatitis

Acute bacterial prostatitis is the most straightforward form of prostatitis. It usually affects younger men and is caused by *Escherichia coli* in 80% of cases and other gram-negative rods or enterococci in most other instances. Patients are clinically ill with fever, malaise, and often low back pain or perineal pain. The prostate is enlarged, very tender, and warm. It should not be massaged. Urinalysis shows leukocytes, and urine culture is usually positive for the organism. Treatment is administration of fluoroquinolones such as ciprofloxacin, trimethoprim-sulfamethoxazole, or doxycycline for 4 to 6 weeks.[1]

Chronic bacterial prostatitis is a disease of elderly men and is usually manifested as recurring urinary tract infections, often with suprapubic, perineal, low back, or testicular pain. The prostate may or may not be tender. White blood cells and lipid-laden macrophages are found in the prostatic secretions, and cultures of prostatic secretions and voided urine after prostatic massage are positive for bacteria. Treatment is usually with a fluoroquinolone or sometimes doxycycline for 3 to 4 months.[1] Chronic bacterial prostatitis comprises a very small percentage of all cases of chronic prostatitis.[1,2]

The cause of chronic prostatitis/chronic pelvic pain syndrome is unknown.[1,2] Chronic pain in the perineum, scrotum, penis, pelvis, or lower back is often associated with urinary urgency, nocturia, weak stream, dribbling, dysuria,

and sexual dysfunction such as painful ejaculations, postejaculatory pain, and hematospermia. The prostate may or may not be tender.[1]

In the inflammatory form of chronic prostatitis/chronic pelvic pain syndrome, white blood cells and lipid-laden macrophages are found in prostatic secretions, but cultures of these secretions and urine voided after prostatic massage are negative. No treatment modality has proved to be effective. A trial of doxycycline, minocycline, or erythromycin for at least 6 weeks is often given in case *Chlamydia trachomatis* or *Ureaplasma urealyticum* is the cause of the condition.[1]

Patients with noninflammatory chronic prostatitis/chronic pelvic pain syndrome have similar symptoms and signs to those of patients with the inflammatory form, but no white blood cells or macrophages are found in prostatic secretions.[1,2] Treatments that have been tried include alpha-adrenergic blockers such as terazosin (Hytrin), nonsteroidal antiinflammatory drugs, diazepam, hot sitz baths, avoidance of spicy foods or excessive alcohol, and even transurethral microwave thermotherapy.[1] Such a smorgasbord of therapeutic recommendations is clear evidence that no treatment has been shown to be effective.

Asymptomatic inflammatory prostatitis is the classification used for asymptomatic patients who for one reason or another have a prostatic biopsy and are found on histological examination to have "prostatitis."[2]

REFERENCES

1. Roberts RO, Lieber MM, Bostwick DG, et al: A review of clinical and pathological prostatitis syndromes, *Urology* 49:809-821, 1997.
2. Krieger JN, Nyberg L Jr, Nickel JC: NIH consensus definition and classification of prostatitis (letter), *JAMA* 282:236-237, 1999.

RENAL CELL CARCINOMA

The highest incidence of renal cell carcinoma is in Scandinavia and North America. It is twice as common in men as in women and twice as common in smokers as in nonsmokers. Treatment is surgical with an overall cure rate of 58%. An occasional patient in whom a solitary metastasis develops after nephrectomy is cured by surgical removal of the metastasis. Chemotherapy has little value.[1]

REFERENCES

1. Motzer RJ, Bander NH, Nanus DM: Renal-cell carcinoma, *N Engl J Med* 335:865-875, 1996.

RENAL COLIC

(See also hyperparathyroidism)

Epidemiology

The lifetime incidence of nephrolithias in the United States is 15% for men and 7% for women. The incidence increases with age, peaking at 65. Half of all patients who have experienced a bout of renal colic will have a subsequent episode within 10 years.[1]

High-Calcium Diet

High calcium intake is not associated with an increased risk of kidney stones. In fact, the reverse may be true. As calcium intake is reduced, oxalate absorption increases, leading to hyperoxaluria and the formation of calcium oxalate stones.[1]

Diagnostic Imaging

Although excretory urography has been the gold standard for diagnosing ureteral calculi, unenhanced helical computed tomography (helical CT) is faster, safer, and more accurate. It has the additional advantage of detecting many nonurological causes of abdominal or flank pain.[1,2]

Hematuria in the Diagnosis of Renal Colic

In a study of patients proved by helical CT to have ureteral stones, 26% had no red blood cells on urine microscopy and 34% had negative results with urinary dipsticks. On the other hand, 40% of patients with symptoms of renal colic and microscopic hematuria did not have urolithiasis; non–urinary tract disorders associated with hematuria included torsion of ovarian masses, appendicitis, and diverticulitis.[2]

Investigations

Recommended investigations for patients with a first episode of nephrolithiasis are ultrasonography or CT scanning, urinalysis, stone analysis (if the stone can be recovered), and measurements of blood urea nitrogen and creatinine, electrolytes, uric acid, calcium, and phosphate. If the calcium level is elevated or in the high normal range, the parathormone level should be measured. Analyses of 24-hour urine collections are usually reserved for patients with recurrent stones.[1]

Natural History of Ureteral Calculi

Most ureteral stones pass spontaneously, especially if they are small and in the distal ureter. One prospective study found that the average time for stone passage was 8.2 days for stones 2 mm or smaller, 12.2 days for 2- to 4-mm stones, and 22.1 days for stones greater than 4 mm. Some 2- to 4-mm stones took 40 days to pass. Degree of pain was unrelated to time of passage.[3]

Urgent urological intervention (direct vision ureteroscopy or shock wave lithotripsy) is necessary if the stone is greater than 6 mm or if the patient has renal failure, a solitary kidney, urinary obstruction, or a significant urinary infection.[4] Delayed intervention is indicated when pain cannot be adequately controlled,[3,4] the patient is unwilling to wait any longer,[3] or the stone fails to pass after 2 months.[4]

Nonsteroidal Antiinflammatory Drugs in the Treatment of Renal Colic

In Europe parenteral NSAIDs are frequently used to relieve the pain of acute renal colic.[5,6] The drugs most frequently used are diclofenac (Voltaren) and indomethacin (Indocid). A metaanalysis of randomized controlled studies in which these drugs were administered parenterally showed them to have excellent analgesic effects compared with placebo and to be equal to or better than analgesics.[5] The only NSAID available for parental use in North America is ketorolac (Toradol), and in one study 90 mg of ketorolac administered intramuscularly was as effective as 100 mg of meperidine intramuscularly.[6] A British study found that a 100-mg rectal suppository of diclofenac was more effective than 100 mg of meperidine plus 12.5 mg of prochlorperazine (Compazine, Stemetil) intramuscularly.[7]

Prevention of Recurrent Nephrolithiasis

The most important way of preventing recurrent stones is a high fluid (preferably water) intake. Patients should drink 2.5 to 3 L per day (more in hot weather or if exercising) and should drink 8 to 12 oz before bedtime to counter urine concentration during sleep. For patients with recurrent stone formation pharmacotherapy is tailored to biochemical abnormalities detected by 24-hour urine collections. Thiazides are commonly used to decrease urinary calcium excretion and are often combined with potassium citrate 20 to 30 mEq bid. Potassium citrate not only counters hypokalemia, but also increases urinary citrate levels, which helps prevent the formation of both calcium and uric acid stones.[1]

◣ REFERENCES ◣

1. Goldfarb DS, Coe FL: Prevention of recurrent nephrolithiasis, *Am Fam Physician* 60:2269-2276, 1999.
2. Bove P, Kaplan D, Dalrymple N, et al: Reexamining the value of hematuria testing in patients with acute flank pain, *J Urol* 162:685-687, 1999.
3. Miller OF, Kane CJ: Time to stone passage for observed ureteral calculi: a guide for patient education, *J Urol* 162:688-691, 1999.
4. Preminger GM: Editorial comment on Miller OF, Kane CJ: Time to stone passage for observed ureteral calculi: a guide for patient education, *J Urol* 162:690-691, 1999.
5. Labrecque M, Dostaler L-P, Rousselle R, et al: Efficacy of nonsteroidal anti-inflammatory drugs in the treatment of acute renal colic, *Arch Intern Med* 154:1381-1387, 1994.
6. Oosterlinck W, Philp NH, Charig C, et al: A double-blind single dose comparison of intramuscular ketorolac tromethamine and pethidine in the treatment of renal colic, *J Clin Pharmacol* 30:336-341, 1990.
7. Thompson JF, Pike JM, Chumas PD, et al: Rectal diclofenac compared with pethidine injection in acute renal colic, *BMJ* 299:1140-1141, 1989.

SEXUAL DYSFUNCTION IN MALES
(See also benign prostatic hypertrophy; radical prostatectomy; selective serotonin reuptake inhibitors; sexual dysfunction in females; tricyclic derivatives)

Abnormalities of sexual function include problems with libido, erections, ejaculation, and orgasm. Absence or altered sensations of orgasm may occur independent of erections or ejaculation. For example, normal ejaculation but anorgasmia or altered sensation of orgasm has been reported in some patients with multiple sclerosis and Parkinson's disease and in up to half of patients subjected to transurethral prostatic resection. Although patients who have had anterolateral cordotomy for the relief of chronic pain often become anorgasmic, one third of men with complete spinal cord transection report that they have normal orgasms.[1]

An important cause of sexual dysfunction, particularly anorgasmia, is the use of antidepressants, particularly the selective serotonin reuptake inhibitors.[2]

◀ REFERENCES ▶

1. Dunsmuir WD, Emberton M: Surgery, drugs, and the male orgasm: informed consent can't be assumed unless effects on orgasm have been discussed (editorial), *BMJ* 314:319-320, 1997.
2. Segraves RT: Antidepressant-induced orgasm disorder, *J Sex Marital Ther* 21:192-201, 1995.

Erectile Dysfunction
Erectile dysfunction is the inability to achieve and maintain an erection sufficient for satisfactory sexual coitus to occur.[1]

Epidemiology
In one community study the incidence of complete impotence increased from 5% at age 40 to 15% at age 70. In this study, impotence was classified into degrees such as minimal, moderate, or complete. If all degrees of impotence are included, 40% of 40-year-olds and 67% of 70-year-olds have the disorder.[2] Unfortunately, degrees of impotence are not well defined; perhaps the normal physiological changes of aging are being categorized as the milder degrees of sexual dysfunction (see below).

Physiology of erections
Parasympathetic nerves cause dilatation of arterioles and the corpora cavernosa; as the corpora cavernosa and corpus spongiosum fill, outflow veins are compressed, augmenting the erection. Detumescence is brought about by sympathetic impulses, causing ejaculation and vasoconstriction along with diminished parasympathetic tone.[1,3]

Age-related changes in male sexual functioning
Normal changes with aging are reported to include these[1]:
1. Gradual decrease in sexual desire
2. More time and stimulation required to achieve erections. Achieving erections becomes more dependent

on direct physical stimulation than on psychic stimulation.
3. Decline in the degree of penile rigidity when erection is achieved
4. More time required to achieve orgasm
5. Decreased semen volume
6. Increased latency between erections

One of the problems of defining the normal aging changes in sexual functioning is that data are often scanty or ancient. For example, in one 1995 review of the subject,[4] the only reference given to changes in penile rigidity during erections in the elderly was the famous 1948 Kinsey Report.[5]

Etiology of impotence
An estimated 80% of erectile dysfunction is physiological, and only 20% is psychological. Diseases associated with impotence include diabetes, hypertension, occlusive vascular disease, neurological disorders, and in a few cases hormonal disorders.[3] The Massachusetts Male Aging Study found the rates of complete impotence to be 28% in diabetics, 39% in those with heart disease, and 15% in those being treated for hypertension.[2] Other important factors are alcohol abuse, a temporary failure as a result of drinking too much on a single occasion ("martini syndrome"), smoking, illicit drugs, and a variety of pharmacological agents, of which the most important are beta-blockers and diuretics, psychotropic agents, and H_2-blockers.[3]

Important psychological causes of erectile dysfunction are depression, taking up with a casual partner, and a long period of abstinence ("widower syndrome"). Sudden onset of impotence or the preservation of nocturnal erections and erections with masturbation suggests psychogenic causes.[3]

Investigations
If specific diseases are suspected as a result of the history and examination, appropriate investigations should be instituted; prolactin and free testosterone should be assessed in most cases.[1]

Oral medications
In a retrospective study from the Walter Reed Army Medical Center in Washington, D.C., 78% of impotent men with no known risk factors for erectile dysfunction had a positive response to trazodone (Desyrel). Positive responses were greatest in men who had symptoms for less than 12 months but were recorded in only 16% of those who had had symptoms for more than 5 years. Poor responses were found among smokers, men over the age of 60, and those with peripheral vascular disease.[6] A prospective study of psychogenic impotence from Milan found a positive response in 71% of the men treated with trazodone 50 mg/day plus yohimbine 15 mg/day.[7] Priapism is a rare but serious complication of trazodone and other drugs with alpha-adrenergic blocking attributes such as prazosin and several

antipsychotics. Drugs of this nature should not be given to patients with a past history of priapism or prolonged erections.[8] The usual dose of trazodone is 50 to 300 mg qhs.

Yohimbine (Yocon, Yohimex) is a presynaptic alpha$_2$-adrenergic receptor antagonist. The 1996 guidelines of the American Urological Association for the management of impotence advise against the use of yohimbine on the grounds that in controlled studies it has been no more effective than placebo.[9] However, a 1997 systematic review of randomized placebo-controlled double-blind trials of yohimbine found that it was indeed effective, with between 34% and 73% of patients responding.[10] If the drug is used, it is usually built up to a maintenance dose of 5.4 to 6 mg tid.

The most recently marketed oral medication for impotence is sildenafil (Viagra). Vascular dilatation of the penis is mediated by cyclic guanosine monophosphate (cyclic GMP). For full erection, there has to be an adequate supply of this agent. Sildenafil inhibits the enzyme phosphodiesterase-5, which breaks down cyclic GMP.[11-13] If the drug is taken when fasting, peak plasma levels are reached in about 1 hour; a fatty meal delays absorption.[12] Sildenafil does not lead to automatic erections; it facilitates them when the usual psychic or physical stimuli are encountered. The drug is said to be effective in about 90% of men with no known organic cause of impotence and in 50% of diabetic patients with documented organic erectile dysfunction.[1] Adverse effects of sildenafil include headaches, hypotension, and transient visual disturbances such as blue-green halos and decreased color discrimination.[11-13] Because of its hypotensive effect, it is contraindicated in men taking nitrates.[12,13] Drug interactions leading to increased plasma levels of sildenafil may occur with cimetidine, erythromycin, itraconazole, and ketoconazole.

Sildenafil is useful for wilting flowers; 0.5 mg in solution preserves the turgidity of cut flowers for up to a week longer than would be expected. The mechanism is the same as in humans: retardation of the breakdown of cyclic GMP.[14]

Corpora cavernosa injections

A variety of pharmacological agents can be injected into the corpora cavernosa to cause erections.[1,15] The drugs act by inhibiting sympathetic tone and thus dilating the arterioles and relaxing the smooth muscle of the corpora cavernosa. According to the guidelines of the American Urological Association, alprostadil (prostaglandin E$_1$, Caverject, Prostin VR) is the drug of choice for initial vasoactive drug injection therapy.[9]

Complications of intracavernosal injections are rare and, with the exception of priapism, usually mild. They include hematomas, temporary penile pain, prolonged erection (4 to 6 hours), priapism, fibrous nodules, and penile curvature.[15]

Alprostadil, or prostaglandin E$_1$ (Caverject), is supplied as single-dose vials of 10 or 20 μg of alprostadil powder plus 1-ml syringes (and ½-inch no. 30 needles) prefilled with diluent. The usual dose is variable but in many patients is between 5 and 20 μg. Dosage is determined empirically during initial visits to the physician. At these initial visits the goal is to achieve an erection sufficient for intercourse but lasting less than 1 hour. The initial dose is usually 2.5 μg, and this is increased by increments of 5 μg if no response occurs and 2.5 μg if there is a partial response. When a response takes place, the patient should stay in the physician's office until detumescence has occurred.

Injections are made into one (not both) of the corpora cavernosa. The manufacturer suggests a 24-hour interval between injections and a maximum of three injections a week. Erection usually takes place within 5 to 10 minutes. Injection sites should be rotated around the corpora cavernosa.

Prolonged erections or priapism requires treatment, which is usually instituted for erections lasting longer than 3 hours. A Vacutainer should be used to aspirate 40 to 60 ml of blood from one of the corpora cavernosa, and if detumescence does not occur, ice is applied for 20 minutes. If the erection still persists, 0.1 to 0.2 ml (50 to 100 μg) of a 0.05% solution of phenylephrine (Neo-Synephrine) is injected into the corpora cavernosa every 2 to 5 minutes until detumescence occurs.

Transurethral medications

Alprostadil can be given by a transurethral route. In a study of 1511 men with organic impotence, 66% were able to achieve erections in the clinic through the intraurethral application of alprostadil in doses of 125 or 250 μg. The drug was applied by a proprietary device (MUSE, Vivus, Menlo Park, Calif.) with a hollow stem 3.5 cm long that was fully inserted into the urethra. Men who achieved erections in the clinic were given home trials in which drug was compared with placebo. Among those taking the drug, about three quarters of applications resulted in intercourse or orgasm compared with only 15% among those receiving placebo.[16]

Tumescence devices

A penis ring or "cock ring" can be used for men who obtain an erection but fail to maintain it. The elastic ring has an adjustable tension and is placed over the base of the shaft of the penis once an erection is obtained. The tension is adjusted to be sufficient to prevent venous outflow and so maintain the erection, but not to be of such a degree that ejaculation is blocked because this might be painful.

Patients who are unable to obtain an erection may sometimes be assisted in doing so by applying a negative suction pump (vacuum tumescence device) over the penis that draws blood into the organ so that an erection is achieved. An elastic ring, similar to a penis ring, is then slipped over the base of the penis to maintain the erection. Pain on ejaculation has been a problem with some of these devices. One of the more recent products of this nature is the ErecAid system Esteem, manufactured by Osbon Medical Systems.

REFERENCES

1. Wagner G, de Tejada IS: Update on male erectile dysfunction, *BMJ* 316:678-682, 1998.
2. Feldman HA, Goldstein I, Hatzichristou DG, et al: Impotence and its medical and psychosocial correlates: results of the Massachusetts Male Aging Study, *J Urol* 151:54-61, 1994.
3. Dewire DM: Evaluation and treatment of erectile dysfunction, *Am Fam Physician* 53:2101-2106, 1996.
4. Schiavi R, Rehman J: Sexuality and aging, *Urol Clin North Am* 22:711-726, 1995.
5. Kinsey AC, Pomeroy WB, Martin CE: *Sexual behaviour in human male,* Philadelphia, 1948, WB Saunders.
6. Lance R, Albo M, Costabile RA, et al: Oral trazodone as empirical therapy for erectile dysfunction: a retrospective review, *Urology* 46:117-120, 1995.
7. Montorsi F, Strambi LF, Guazzoni G, et al: Effect of yohimbine-trazodone on psychogenic impotence: a randomized double-blind, placebo-controlled study, *Urology* 44:732-736, 1994.
8. Thompson JW Jr, Ware MR, Blashfield RK: Psychotropic medication and priapism: a comprehensive review, *J Clin Psychiatry* 51:430-443, 1990.
9. Guidelines for treating erectile dysfunction issued, *JAMA* 277:7-8, 1997.
10. Ernst E, Pittler MH: Yohimbine for erectile dysfunction: a systematic review and meta-analysis of randomized clinical trials, *J Urol* 159:433-436, 1998.
11. Goldstein I, Lue TF, Padma-Nathan H, et al: Oral sildenafil in the treatment of erectile dysfunction, *N Engl J Med* 338:1397-1404, 1998.
12. Sildenafil: an oral drug for impotence, *Med Lett* 40:51-52, 1998.
13. Gregoire A: Viagra: on release: evidence on the effectiveness of sildenafil is good (editorial), *BMJ* 317:759-760, 1998.
14. Siegel-Itzkovich J: Viagra makes flowers stand up straight, *BMJ* 319:274, 1999.
15. Linet OI, Ogring FG: Efficacy and safety of intracavernosal alprostadil in men with erectile dysfunction, *N Engl J Med* 334:873-877, 1996.
16. Padma-Nathan H, Hellstrom WJ, Kaiser FE, et al: Treatment of men with erectile dysfunction with transurethral alprostadil, *N Engl J Med* 336:1-7, 1997.

Premature Ejaculation

(See also selective serotonin reuptake inhibitors)

Premature ejaculation is the most common form of sexual dysfunction in men, with an estimated lifetime prevalence of 75%.[1]

The tricyclic agent clomipramine (Anafranil) and the selective serotinin reuptake inhibitors fluoxetine (Prozac), sertraline (Zoloft), and paroxetine (Paxil) have all been effective in treating premature ejaculation.[1-4] Doses of clomipramine were 25 to 50 mg/day,[2] sertraline 50 mg/day,[1] and paroxetine 20 to 40 mg/day.[3] A single-blind placebo-controlled crossover trial found that 20 mg of paroxetine taken 3 to 4 hours before intercourse effectively improved ejaculatory latency and that this benefit was even greater if preceded by 10 mg of paroxetine daily for an initial 3-week period.[4] In a study of sertraline, resolution of symptoms persisted in two thirds of the patients after staged withdrawal of the drug.[1]

REFERENCES

1. McMahon CG: Treatment of premature ejaculation with sertraline hydrochloride: a single-blind placebo controlled crossover study, *J Urol* 159:1935-1938, 1998.
2. Althof SE, Levine SB, Corty EW, et al: A double-blind crossover trial of clomipramine for rapid ejaculation in 15 couples, *J Clin Psychiatry* 56:402-407, 1995.
3. Waldinger MD, Hengeveld MW, Zwinderman AH: Paroxetine treatment of premature ejaculation: a double-blind, randomized, placebo-controlled study, *Am J Psychiatry* 151:1377-1379, 1994.
4. McMahon CG, Touma K: Treatment of premature ejaculation with paroxetine hydrochloride as needed: 2 singe-blind placebo controlled crossover studies, *J Urol* 161:1826-1830, 1999.

TESTES

Testicular Cancer

(See also clinical practice guidelines; prevention; screening)

Ninety-five percent of testicular tumors are germ cell tumors. They are more common in whites than blacks and in cryptorchid testes. The two major types of germ cell tumors are seminomas, with a peak incidence in the twenties, and nonseminomatous germ cell tumors (embryonal carcinoma, yolk cell carcinoma, teratoma, and choriocarcinoma) with a peak incidence in the thirties. A painless testicular mass is highly suggestive of testicular tumor, but in most cases men have pain and swelling or increased testicular induration.[1]

The initial investigation of a suspected testicular mass is ultrasound, and if it indicates a mass within the testes, the diagnosis is cancer until proved otherwise.[2] Both seminomas and nonseminomatous germ cell tumors may cause elevations of human chorionic gonadotropin levels, whereas only nonseminomatous germ cell tumors increase alpha-fetoprotein.[1,2]

The overall cure rate for all germ cell tumors is greater than 90%. Most cases of seminomas are treated with orchiectomy plus retroperitoneal and pelvic lymph node irradiation, whereas nonseminomatous germ cell tumors are usually treated with orchiectomy with or without pelvic lymph node resection. Recurrences or widespread disease can usually be cured by chemotherapy, although the prognosis is considerably worse if there are hepatic, cerebral, or osseous metastases.[1] A protocol for high-risk nonseminomatous germ cell tumors that appears to have excellent results is orchiectomy plus immediate administration of two courses of adjuvant chemotherapy.[3]

Widely variable recommendations have been proposed for testicular examination as a means of cancer screening. Some of these are listed in Table 72.[4]

Table 72 Recommendations for Testicular Examinations by Physicians

Authority	Recommendations
Canadian Task Force on Preventive Health Care	Only if history of cryptorchidism, infertility, atrophic testes, or ambiguous genitalia
U.S. Preventive Services Task Force	Ages 13-39 only if history of cryptorchidism, orchiopexy, or testicular atrophy
National Cancer Institute	Routine as part of periodic health examination
American Cancer Society	Every 3 years from 20-39 and thereafter annually
American Urological Association	Regularly starting at age 15
American Academy of Family Physicians	Ages 13-18 if history of cryptorchidism, orchiopexy, or testicular atrophy; as part of periodic health examination ages 19-39

REFERENCES

1. Bosl GJ, Motzer RJ: Testicular germ-cell cancer, *N Engl J Med* 337:242-259, 1997.
2. Kinkade S: Testicular cancer, *Am Fam Physician* 59:2539-2544, 1999.
3. Böhlen D, Borner M, Sonntag RW, et al: Long-term results following adjuvant chemotherapy in patients with clinical stage I testicular nonseminomatous malignant germ cell tumors with high risk factors, *J Urol* 161:1148-1152, 1999.
4. US Public Health Service: Cancer detection in adults by physical examination, *Am Fam Physician* 51:871-885, 1995.

Torsion of Testis and Testicular Appendage

Testicle

Testicular torsion is a surgical emergency. Salvage of the testis is possible in over 80% of cases provided surgery is performed within 6 hours,[1] but after 12 hours the prognosis is poor.[2] The disorder affects predominantly young men, but the middle aged are not immune. Sudden pain is the usual presenting symptom, often associated with nausea and vomiting. The testis is swollen and tender, lies higher in the scrotum than the opposite testis, and often has a transverse lie. Within a few hours the scrotum becomes erythematous and edematous and specific anatomical structures can no longer be palpated within the scrotum. Unlike in epididymitis, elevation of the scrotum usually does not relieve the pain.[1,2] If the cremasteric reflex is normal on the affected side, torsion can be ruled out.[2] When the diagnosis is clinically uncertain, color Doppler ultrasound is the investigative procedure of choice.[3]

If surgical consultation is not available, an attempt may be made to detort the testis manually. The direction of rotation in torsion is usually toward the midline, so the physician corrects the rotation by sitting on the examining table at the patient's feet, grasping the affected testis, and rotating it from the inside toward the outside (right testis counterclockwise and left testis clockwise).[4]

Testicular and epididymal appendages

Remnants of the Müllerian duct called the testicular appendage are located on the superior pole of the testes, while remnants of the Wolffian duct may be found on the superior pole of the epididymis. Either of these structures may undergo torsion. Pain is present but is generally less sudden in onset and less severe than that of testicular torsion. If found early, a small tender mass can often be felt on the upper pole of the testis or epididymis, and sometimes a bluish discoloration ("blue dot sign") may be seen through the scrotum.[2] At a later stage there may be too much swelling to allow a precise clinical diagnosis. Management consists of scrotal support and NSAIDs. Resolution occurs in about 2 weeks.[1]

REFERENCES

1. Junnila J, Lassen P: Testicular masses, *Am Fam Physician* 57:685-692, 1998.
2. Kass EJ, Lundak B: The acute scrotum, *Pediatr Clin North Am* 44:1251-1266, 1997.
3. Galejs LE, Kass EJ: Diagnosis and treatment of the acute scrotum, *Am Fam Physician* 59:817-824, 1999.
4. Leduc C: La douleur scrotale aiguë: un cas de torsion testiculaire, *L'Omnipraticien* 3(2):9-16, 1999.

URINARY TRACT INFECTIONS

(See also catheters; circumcision; hormone replacement therapy; interstitial cystitis; prostatitis; urinalysis; urinary tract infections in children)

Classification

The following are the major categories of urinary tract infection (UTI)[1]:

1. Uncomplicated—cystitis in young women, recurrent cystitis in young women; pyelonephritis in young women
2. Complicated—persistent or recurrent infections
3. Infections in men
4. Catheter related
5. Asymptomatic bacteriuria

Dipsticks and Cultures

(See also urinalysis)

Leukocyte esterase dipsticks have sensitivities of 75% to 96%. Dipstick tests for nitrites in urine are positive in many UTIs. The reaction depends on the conversion of nitrates to nitrites by bacteria, but some fairly common organisms such as *Staphylococcus saprophyticus* do not have this capacity. As a result the sensitivity of the test is rather low, but its specificity is high.[1]

In the past, urine cultures producing fewer than 100,000 colony-forming units (CFUs) of bacteria per milliliter of urine were not considered diagnostic of UTI. New data suggest that the presence of as few as 100 CFUs/ml correlates well with uncomplicated cystitis in symptomatic women. Many laboratories do not report such low values, but in most instances this is academic because cultures are not required for the diagnosis or treatment of uncomplicated UTIs in young women. Patients with complicated UTIs and women with uncomplicated pyelonephritis generally have more than 100,000 CFUs/ml.[1]

Risk Factors for Urinary Tract Infections

Commonly stated risk factors for uncomplicated UTIs in young women include the following[1,2]:

1. Sexual intercourse
2. Diaphragm use
3. Spermicide use (including spermicide-coated condoms)
4. History of recurrent UTIs
5. Delayed postcoital micturition

A prospective study of sexually active young women failed to find any protective effect of postcoital voiding, but the frequency of UTIs increased with the frequency of coitus and the frequency of diaphragm use.[2] Both the diaphragm and spermicides are thought to foster colonization of the periurethral area with coliform bacteria.[1]

Treatment of Uncomplicated Cystitis in Women

Between 80% and 90% of uncomplicated UTIs are caused by *E. coli*, 10% to 20% by coagulase-negative *Staphylococcus saprophyticus,* and less than 5% by other organisms. Although many of the common organisms are resistant to ampicillin or sulfonamides, the vast majority are sensitive to trimethoprim-sulfamethoxazole and fluoroquinolones.[1] The treatment of choice for most uncomplicated UTIs in women is a 3-day course of oral trimethoprim-sulfamethoxazole (Bactrim, Septra). Alternatives are a 3-day course of one of the fluoroquinolones or a single dose of fosfomycin (Monurol). Cultures are not required. Cultures are indicated for recurrent infections, and in these cases the antibacterials of choice are usually fluoroquinolones, amoxicillin/clavulanic acid, or third-generation cephalosporins. Amoxicillin alone is usually not a drug of first choice because many organisms are resistant to it.[1,3] Single-dose treatments are effective for many women, but with the exception of fosfomycin, they are not generally recommended because of a relatively high risk of recurrence within 6 weeks.[1]

Some of the suggested treatment regimens for uncomplicated UTIs are listed in Table 73.

Phenazopyridine (Pyridium) is an azo dye that was first marketed in the United States in 1914 as a urinary antiseptic. It is not effective in this role but continues to be prescribed as a urinary analgesic. There are no good studies supporting this indication, and since antibiotics give rapid

Table 73   Pharmacotherapy for Uncomplicated Urinary Tract Infections

Drugs	Usual doses
Trimethoprim-sulfamethoxazole (Bactrim, Septra)	160-800 mg (1 DS tablet) bid × 3 days
Ciprofloxacin (Cipro)	100 mg bid × 3 days
Norfloxacin (Noroxin)	400 mg bid × 3 days
Ofloxacin (Floxin)	200 mg bid × 3 days
Fosfomycin (Monurol)	3 grams as a single dose
Amoxicillin	250 mg tid × 3 days
Nitrofurantoin (Macrobid)	100 mg bid × 7 days

relief of symptoms and phenazopyridine can cause methemoglobinemia, its use has little justification.[4]

Prophylaxis of Uncomplicated Urinary Tract Infections in Women

Recurrent UTIs are defined as more than three infections documented by urine cultures in 1 year. A variety of acceptable antibiotic prophylactic regimens can be used for this condition in women[1]:

1. Prescription of repeated 3-day treatment regimens so the patient can treat herself at the onset of symptoms
2. Continuous prophylaxis for a 6-month period using drugs such as a single daily dose of trimethoprim-sulfamethoxazole 40/200 mg (½ regular strength tablet), trimethoprim 100 mg, nitrofurantoin 50 to 100 mg, or norfloxacin 200 mg
3. If UTIs are related to intercourse, antibiotics such as trimethoprim-sulfamethoxazole 40/200 mg (½ regular strength tablet) taken immediately after intercourse

An Israeli study found that intravaginal estriol was effective in preventing recurrent UTIs in postmenopausal women. Estrogens facilitate the colonization of lactobacilli in the vagina, which lowers the vaginal pH and inhibits the growth of coliform bacteria.[5] Estriol is not absorbed systemically. It is not available in Canada or the United States.

A study of elderly women found that those who drank 300 ml of cranberry juice daily had a decreased incidence of bacteriuria with pyuria compared with control subjects given placebo.[6] However, whether drinking cranberry or blueberry juice will prevent UTIs in young women is unknown.[7]

Pyelonephritis in Young Women

E. coli is the cause of most cases of uncomplicated pyelonephritis in young women, and in about one third of cases the organism is resistant to ampicillin, amoxicillin, and first-generation cephalosporins. If a patient with pyelonephritis is not toxic and can tolerate oral medications, she may be treated as an outpatient for 10 to 14 days with trimethoprim-sulfamethoxazole or a fluoroquinolone.[1,8] Examples include trimethoprim-sulfamethoxazole 160 mg/800 mg (DS) q12h, ciprofloxacin 500 mg q12h, ofloxacin 200 to 300 mg q12h, and norfloxacin 400 mg q12h.[8]

Complicated Urinary Tract Infections

Complicated UTIs are due to anatomical, functional, or pharmacological factors that lead to persistent or recurrent infections. Obstruction is a common cause. *E. coli* is responsible for less than one third of complicated UTIs, and therapy is usually with a fluoroquinolone or a third-generation cephalosporin administered for at least 10 to 14 days.[1]

Urinary Tract Infections in Men

Initial (uncomplicated) UTIs in men are commonly due to obstruction, instrumentation, or prostatitis. Usual treatment is trimethoprim-sulfamethoxazole or a fluoroquinolone for at least 7 days; if prostatitis is present, treatment may have to be continued for 6 to 12 weeks (see discussion of prostatitis). Urological workup is indicated for elderly men and for men of any age with clinical evidence of pyelonephritis. In otherwise healthy young men with symptoms of cystitis only a culture is required.[1]

Catheter-Related Urinary Tract Infections

Long-term catheterization is always associated with bacteriuria, and no effective means of preventing this have been devised. Antibiotic treatment of asymptomatic bacteriuria in patients with long-term catheters is rarely indicated. If patients are symptomatic, they are usually treated with fluoroquinolones for 10 to 14 days.[1]

Bacteriuria and Pyuria in the Elderly

Asymptomatic bacteriuria and asymptomatic pyuria are common findings in elderly women. In a prospective observational study from Boston, 61 women from a long-care institution or community housing sites submitted monthly clean-catch urine specimens for a 6-month period; 28% of patients had at least one sample showing bacteriuria alone, while bacteriuria with pyuria was found in at least one sample from 26% of patients. Bacteriuria with symptoms occurred in only 10% of patients. Spontaneous clearance of both bacteriuria and pyuria was common. For patients with symptoms the sensitivity of urine dipstick (leukocyte esterase) and microscopic examination for bacteria and white cells was 80% or better, and the negative predictive value of these tests approached 100%.[9]

The Canadian Task Force on Preventive Health Care has concluded that no evidence has shown that the treatment of asymptomatic bacteriuria in the elderly is beneficial. It gives "E" ratings for screening elderly institutionalized men and women and persons of either sex with indwelling catheters; a "D" rating to screening of ambulatory elderly men; and a "C" rating to screening of ambulatory elderly women.[10] The U.S. Preventive Services Task Force also gives an "E" rating to screening for bacteriuria in institutionalized elderly

patients and a "C" rating to such screening in ambulatory elderly women.[11]

❧ REFERENCES ❧

1. Orenstein R, Wong ES: Urinary tract infections in adults, *Am Fam Physician* 59:1225-1234, 1999.
2. Hooton TM, Scholes D, Hughes JP, et al: A prospective study of risk factors for symptomatic urinary tract infection in young women, *N Engl J Med* 335:468-474, 1996.
3. The choice of antibacterial drugs, *Med Lett* 40:33-42, 1998.
4. Zelenitsky SA, Zhanel GG: Phenazopyridine in urinary tract infections, *Ann Pharmacother* 30:866-868, 1996.
5. Raz R, Stamm WE: A controlled trial of intravaginal estriol in postmenopausal women with recurrent urinary tract infections, *N Engl J Med* 329:753-756, 1993.
6. Avorn J, Monane M, Gurwitz JH, et al: Reduction of bacteriuria and pyuria after ingestion of cranberry juice, *JAMA* 271:751-754, 1994.
7. Ronald A: Sex and urinary tract infections (editorial), *N Engl J Med* 335:511-512, 1996.
8. Stamm WE, Hooton TM: Management of urinary tract infections in adults, *N Engl J Med* 329:1328-1334, 1993.
9. Monane M, Gurwitz JH, Lipsitz LA, et al: Epidemiologic and diagnostic aspects of bacteriuria: a longitudinal study in older women, *J Am Geriatr Soc* 43:618-622, 1995.
10. Canadian Task Force on the Periodic Health Examination: *Canadian guide to clinical preventive health care,* Ottawa, 1994, Canada Communication Group—Publishing, pp 966-967.
11. US Preventive Services Task Force: *Guide to clinical preventive services,* ed 2, Baltimore, 1996, Williams & Wilkins, pp 347-359.

VASECTOMY

(See also infertility, male; tubal sterilization)

Vasectomy and Prostate Cancer

A number of publications have reported a positive association between vasectomy and prostate cancer. A systematic review of the literature concluded that such reports are rife with methodological problems and that there is no evidence that vasectomy increases the risk of prostate cancer.[1]

VASOVASOTOMY

A review of close to 1500 microsurgical procedures to reverse vasectomies found that if the procedure was performed within 3 years of vasectomy, the patency rate was 97% and the pregnancy rate 76%. If the procedure was performed 15 years after the vasectomy, the patency rate was 71% and the pregnancy rate 30%.[2]

❧ REFERENCES ❧

1. Bernal-Delgado E, Latour-Pérez J, Pradas-Arnal F, et al: The association between vasectomy and prostate cancer: a systematic review of the literature, *Fertil Steril* 70:191-200, 1998.
2. Belker AM, Thomas AJ Jr, Fuchs EF, et al: Results of 1,469 microsurgical vasectomy reversals by the Vasovasostomy Study Group, *J Urol* 145:505-511, 1991.

Index